# MUIR'S
# TEXTBOOK
# OF PATHOLOGY

# MUIR'S
# TEXTBOOK
# OF PATHOLOGY

## Fifteenth Edition

Edited by

C Simon Herrington MA DPhil FRCP(Lond) FRCP(Ed) FRCPath

Professor of Pathology, University of Dundee and Consultant Pathologist, Ninewells Hospital and Medical School, Dundee, UK

**CRC Press**
Taylor & Francis Group
Boca Raton London New York

CRC Press is an imprint of the
Taylor & Francis Group, an **informa** business

CRC Press
Taylor & Francis Group
6000 Broken Sound Parkway NW, Suite 300
Boca Raton, FL 33487-2742

© 2014 by Taylor & Francis Group, LLC
CRC Press is an imprint of Taylor & Francis Group, an Informa business

No claim to original U.S. Government works

Printed on acid-free paper
Version Date: 20140121

Printed and bound in India by Replika Press Pvt. Ltd.

International Standard Book Number-13: 978-1-4441-8497-6 (Paperback)

International Standard Book Number-13: 978-1-4441-8499-0 (International Students' Edition, restricted territorial availability)

This book contains information obtained from authentic and highly regarded sources. While all reasonable efforts have been made to publish reliable data and information, neither the author[s] nor the publisher can accept any legal responsibility or liability for any errors or omissions that may be made. The publishers wish to make clear that any views or opinions expressed in this book by individual editors, authors or contributors are personal to them and do not necessarily reflect the views/opinions of the publishers. The information or guidance contained in this book is intended for use by medical, scientific or health-care professionals and is provided strictly as a supplement to the medical or other professional's own judgement, their knowledge of the patient's medical history, relevant manufacturer's instructions and the appropriate best practice guidelines. Because of the rapid advances in medical science, any information or advice on dosages, procedures or diagnoses should be independently verified. The reader is strongly urged to consult the drug companies' printed instructions, and their websites, before administering any of the drugs recommended in this book. This book does not indicate whether a particular treatment is appropriate or suitable for a particular individual. Ultimately it is the sole responsibility of the medical professional to make his or her own professional judgements, so as to advise and treat patients appropriately. The authors and publishers have also attempted to trace the copyright holders of all material reproduced in this publication and apologize to copyright holders if permission to publish in this form has not been obtained. If any copyright material has not been acknowledged please write and let us know so we may rectify in any future reprint.

---

**Library of Congress Cataloging-in-Publication Data**

---

Muir's textbook of pathology / editor, Charles Simon Herrington. -- Fifteenth edition.
   p. ; cm.
   Textbook of pathology
   Includes bibliographical references and index.
   Summary: "Muir's Textbook of Pathology sets a standard in this subject by outlining the scientific aspects that underlie pathological processes, relating these to specific organ systems and placing all in a context that the student of medicine or pathology can appreciate and understand. The clearly defined and easy-to-follow structure, enhanced by numerous photographs and explanatory line diagrams, focus on core material without neglecting novel concepts and up-to-the-minute detail. This one-stop-shop in pathology that will take the student right through medical school and beyond to postgraduate training."--Provided by publisher.
   ISBN 978-1-4441-8497-6 (pbk. : alk. paper)
   I. Herrington, C. S., editor of compilation. II. Title: Textbook of pathology.
   [DNLM: 1. Pathology. 2. Pathologic Processes. QZ 4]

RB111
616.07--dc23
                             2014001358

**Visit the Taylor & Francis Web site at**
**http://www.taylorandfrancis.com**

**and the CRC Press Web site at**
**http://www.crcpress.com**

# CONTENTS

## SECTION 1 CELLULAR AND MOLECULAR MECHANISMS OF DISEASE

## SECTION 2 SYSTEMIC PATHOLOGY

# CONTRIBUTORS TO 15TH EDITION

**Jonathan N Berg** MSc MD FRCP(Ed)
Senior Lecturer in Clinical Genetics, University of Dundee and Consultant in Clinical Genetics, Ninewells Hospital and Medical School, Dundee, UK

**Daniel M Berney** MB B Chir MA FRCPath
Professor of Genito-Urinary Pathology and Consultant Histopathologist, Department of Cellular Pathology, Bartshealth NHS Trust, London, UK.

**Alastair D Burt** BSc MD FRCPath FSB FRCP
Dean of Medicine and Head of School of Medicine, University of Adelaide, Australia

**Francis A Carey** BSc MD FRCPath
Consultant Pathologist and Professor of Pathology, Department of Pathology, Ninewells Hospital and Medical School, Dundee, UK

**Runjan Chetty** DPhil FRCPA FRCPC FCAP FRCPath
Professor of Pathology and Consultant Pathologist, University Health Network and University of Toronto, Canada

**Cathy Corbishley** FRCPath
Consultant Urological Histopathologist, St George's Hospital, London, UK

**Ian O Ellis** BMedSci FRCPath
Professor of Cancer Pathology and Consultant Pathologist, Faculty of Medicine and Health Sciences, Department of Histopathology, City Hospital Campus, Nottingham, University Hospitals NHS Trust, Nottingham, UK

**Alan T Evans** BMedBiol MD FRCPath
Consultant Dermatopathologist, Department of Pathology, Ninewells Hospital and Medical School, Dundee, UK

**Stewart Fleming** BSc MD FRCPath
Professor of Cellular and Molecular Pathology, University of Dundee, Ninewells Hospital, Dundee, UK

**Alan K Foulis** BSc MD FRCP(Ed) FRCPath
Consultant Pathologist and Professor of Pathology, Department of Pathology, Southern General Hospital, Glasgow, UK

**C Simon Herrington** MA DPhil FRCP(Lond) FRCP(Ed) FRCPath
Professor of Pathology, University of Dundee and Consultant Pathologist, Ninewells Hospital and Medical School, Dundee, UK

**Andrew HS Lee** MA MD MRCP FRCPath
Consultant Histopathologist, Nottingham University Hospitals, City Hospital Campus, Nottingham, UK

**Sebastian Lucas** FRCP FRCPath
Professor of Pathology, Department of Histopathology, King's College London School of Medicine, St Thomas' Hospital, London, UK

**Elaine MacDuff** BSc MBChB FRCPath
Consultant Pathologist, Department of Pathology, Southern General Hospital, Glasgow, UK

**Anne Marie McNicol** BSc MD FRCP(Glas) FRCPath
Molecular and Cellular Pathology, University of Queensland Centre for Clinical Research, The University of Queensland, Australia

**Sarju Mehta** BSc FRCP
Consultant in Clinical Genetics, Department of Clinical Genetics, Addenbrooke's Hospital, Cambridge, UK

**Wolter J Mooi** MD PhD
Professor of Pathology, Department of Pathology, Vrije Universiteit Medical Centre, Amsterdam, The Netherlands

**James AR Nicoll** BSc MD FRCPath
Professor of Neuropathology, Clinical Neurosciences, University of Southampton and Consultant Neuropathologist, University Hospital Southampton NHS Foundation Trust, Southampton, UK

**Sarah E Pinder** FRCPath
Professor of Breast Pathology, Research Oncology, Division of Cancer Studies, King's College London, Guy's Hospital, London, UK

**Alexandra Rice** FRCPath
Consultant Histopathologist and Senior Lecturer in Pathology, Imperial College, Department of Histopathology, Royal Brompton Hospital, London, UK

**Fiona Roberts** BSc MD FRCPath
Consultant Ophthalmic Pathologist, Department of Pathology, Southern General Hospital, Glasgow, UK

**Mary N. Sheppard** BSc MD FRCPath
Professor of Cardiovascular Pathology, Cardiovascular Sciences, St George's Medical School, London, UK

**Dina Tiniakos** MD PhD
Clinical Senior Lecturer in Cellular Pathology Institute of Cellular Medicine, Faculty of Medical Sciences, Newcastle University and Consultant Histopathologist, Department of Cellular Pathology, Royal Victoria Infirmary, Newcastle upon Tyne, UK

**Paul Van der Valk** MD PhD
Professor of Pathology, Department of Pathology, Vrije Universiteit Medical Centre, Amsterdam, The Netherlands.

**Sharon White** BMSc BDS MFDS RCPSGlasg PhD FRCPath
Clinical Senior Lecturer and Consultant in Oral Pathology, Department of Pathology, Ninewells Hospital and Medical School, Dundee, UK

# PREFACE

It is a great privilege to edit this, the Fifteenth Edition of Muir's Textbook of Pathology. Muir's Textbook (or just 'Muir's') was first published in 1924 and has been the stalwart of pathology education for several generations. This Edition is in many ways an update of the Fourteenth Edition, which, as recorded by the Editors in their Preface, differed in a number of ways from previous editions. The structure of the book remains the same and the highly successful case studies and special study topics have been retained, and updated where appropriate. The move to a more integrated approach has been highly successful and the presentation of core knowledge, with development of a more in-depth discussion of specific areas that illustrate recent advances, allows both breadth and depth of coverage. The last Edition saw the involvement of more Editors and authors from outside Glasgow. This trend has continued in this Edition, but many, if not most, of us who did not train or have not worked in Glasgow have been influenced by Glasgow Pathology through use of 'Muir's' during our own training, or our training of others. I hope that this has allowed us to preserve the unique feel of the book.

I am extremely grateful to the other contributors for their efficient and timely engagement with the publishing process. I would also like to thank those who contributed images and other figures: they are acknowledged specifically at the appropriate point in the book. Thanks go also to the publishers, particularly Jo Koster who galvanized the project in the beginning and Julie Bennett who managed the publishing process. Finally, I am particularly indebted to the Editors of the 14th Edition, Professors Levison, Reid, Burt, Harrison and Fleming, for their transformation of 'Muir's' into what it is today; and for allowing the use of their material in this Edition.

C Simon Herrington

2014

# PREFACE TO 14TH EDITION

This is the Fourteenth Edition of Muir's Textbook of Pathology, building upon the work of previous editions. It is different in a number of ways from previous editions, but we think it is similar enough to retain the traditional values of its predecessors. We trust we have produced a text that will be useful both to undergraduate medical students and to postgraduates who are interested in having a better understanding of disease upon which to base either their clinical practice or their research, or both.

This edition differs in the balance between general and systematic pathology from most earlier editions, with the general section being relatively shorter. This is deliberate; it is not meant to suggest that we think an understanding of the basic sciences is any less important to clinical practice than it used to be – quite the contrary. What we have tried to do is to focus on the most clinically relevant basic science and we have included some of that in the systematic chapters where its relevance is hopefully easier to appreciate.

We have also introduced into almost every chapter one or two special study topics where the information provided is rather more than most medical educators would include in the core curriculum of a medical undergraduate course. This is intended to interest and stimulate the best students to appreciate that undergraduate education is just the beginning – a window on the exciting and challenging world of disease. We have also included in most chapters, several case histories which illustrate and add to the information provided in the main text, in an attempt to emphasize the fundamental relevance of pathology to clinical medicine. By adopting this format of special study topics and case studies integrated into, but clearly distinguished from, the core text, we are adopting the approach taken to medical education in many medical schools. We strongly support the move in the UK to more integrated teaching of the disciplines in medicine. We, not unexpectedly, believe that the best doctors are knowledgeable about disease processes, and we hope that this belief is reflected in the level at which we have pitched the text.

It will be noted for this edition of the book that for the first time ever the majority of the editors are not based in Glasgow. However, three of us are Glasgow graduates, and we all acknowledge our debt to, and the inspiration we have drawn from, our predecessors in Glasgow Pathology. We are honoured to have had the opportunity to edit this latest edition of 'Muir' and hope that we have done justice to the task.

David A Levison
Robin Reid
Alastair D Burt
David J Harrison
Stewart Fleming

2008

# SECTION 1

# CELLULAR AND MOLECULAR MECHANISMS OF DISEASE

# 1

# APPLICATIONS OF PATHOLOGY

C Simon Herrington

## WHAT IS PATHOLOGY?

Pathology is the study of disease. It is central to the whole practice of evidence-based medicine. Arguably, anyone who studies the mechanisms of a disease can be described as a pathologist, but traditionally the term is restricted to those who have a day-to-day involvement in providing a diagnostic service to a hospital or undertake research in a pathology department. Within the discipline there are numerous subspecialities:

- Cellular pathology, including histopathology (the study of tissues) and cytopathology (the branch in which diagnoses are made from the study of separated cells).
- Morbid anatomy is an old term that refers to post-mortem dissection, and forensic pathology is the related branch concerned with medicolegal postmortem examinations. These are carried out under the aegis of a legal officer, for example the Coroner in England and Wales, the Procurator Fiscal in Scotland, and the Medical Examiner in the USA.
- Microbiology is the study of infectious diseases and their causes. This can be subdivided into bacteriology, virology, mycology (the study of fungi), and protozoology (the study of infections by protozoa).
- Haematology is the laboratory study of diseases of the blood. This is also a clinical discipline, its practitioners dealing with patients with these disorders. Most haematologists work in both clinical and laboratory arenas.
- Chemical pathology or clinical biochemistry is the study of body chemistry, usually by assaying the levels of substances – electrolytes, enzymes, lipids, trace elements – in the blood or urine. Increasing sophistication of analytical requirements often means that this discipline is at the cutting edge of new technology.
- Immunology is the study of host defences against external threats. Many of these are microbiological, but some are chemical, e.g. foodstuffs. In addition, this is also the study of autoimmunity, when the body's defence systems are turned on themselves (see Chapter 2, pp. 25–26).
- Genetics is the study of inheritance of characteristics and diseases, or a predisposition to diseases. Clinical geneticists, similar to haematologists, are directly involved with patients, whereas laboratory-based geneticists apply the traditional techniques of karyotyping, the microscopic examination of chromosomes in cells in mitosis, and the whole spectrum of modern molecular techniques, such as polymerase chain reaction (PCR), fluorescence in situ hybridization (FISH), gene-expression profiling, and DNA sequencing.

Historically, these subjects emerged from the single discipline of 'pathology' which exploded in the mid-nineteenth century, especially in Germany where Rudolf Virchow introduced the term 'cellular pathology'. The divergence of specialities was largely on the basis of the different techniques used in each area. Today, the boundaries between these subspecialities are increasingly becoming blurred as modern techniques, especially those resulting from molecular biology, are applied to all. Cellular pathology remains a critical part of the clinical evaluation of a patient before definitive treatment is offered. Increasingly, some of the roles are also delivered by scientists who are not medically qualified, bringing new opportunities and challenges to building effective multidisciplinary teams.

The editor and almost all of the contributors to this book are primarily histopathologists and it is on this area that the book focuses.

# DIAGNOSTIC HISTOPATHOLOGY AND CYTOPATHOLOGY: IMAGES OF DISEASES

## Key Points

- Pathology is the study of disease.
- Naked eye examination and the light microscope are the traditional tools of the pathologist.
- Increasingly, molecular biological techniques are applied across the whole spectrum of study of diseases to explore underlying mechanisms.

Cellular pathology, i.e. both histopathology and cytopathology, are essentially imaging disciplines. Its practitioners interpret an image, usually obtained by microscopy, and from it deduce information about diagnosis and possible cause of disease, recommend treatment and predict likely outcome.

## Preparing the Image

Tissues or cells are removed from a patient. The fairly simple technique of light microscopy is the bedrock of preparing images. A very thin slice of a tissue, usually about 3 µm thick, is prepared and stained so that the characteristics of the tissue, i.e. the types of cells and their relationships to each other, can be examined. To prevent the tissue digesting itself through the release of proteolytic enzymes, the tissue is immersed in a fixative, usually formaldehyde, which cross-links the proteins and inactivates any enzymatic activity. It is impossible to cut very thin sections of even thickness without supporting the tissue in some medium. Usually the tissue is embedded in paraffin wax, which has the appropriate melting and solidifying characteristics, but freezing the tissue (the principle of the frozen section) and embedding hard tissue in synthetic epoxy resins, such as Araldite, are also done. To stain the tissue section, the vegetable dyes haematoxylin and eosin are traditionally used to distinguish between the nucleus and cytoplasm, and to identify some of the intracellular organelles. It is from examination of sections stained by these simple tinctorial techniques that normal histology and the basic disease processes of inflammation, repair, degeneration, and neoplasia were defined (Figs. 1.1 and 1.2). In the past century numerous chemical stains have been developed to demonstrate, for example, carbohydrates, mucins, lipids, and pigments such as melanin and the iron-containing pigment haemosiderin.

## Refining the Image

### Electron Microscopy

Pathological applications of this technique emerged in the 1960s as the technology of 'viewing' tissues by beams of electrons rather than visible light became available. This greatly

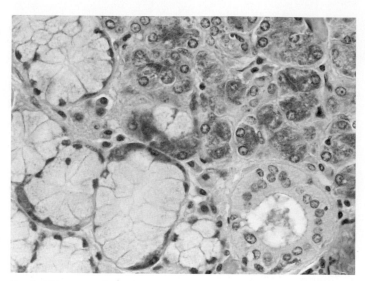

**Fig. 1.1** Haematoxylin and eosin (H&E)-stained section of the parotid gland allowing the serous cells (top right), mucinous cells (left), and salivary duct (lower right) to be readily distinguished.

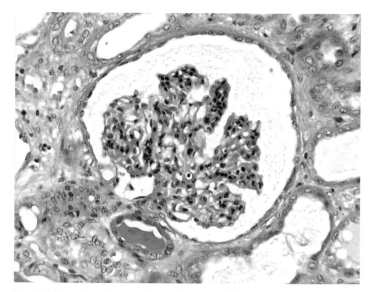

**Fig. 1.2** A section of renal glomerulus stained by haematoxylin and eosin. The nuclei have affinity for the basic dye haematoxylin and are blue. The cytoplasm has more affinity for the acidic dye eosin and is pink. This technique has not changed significantly in well over a century.

increased the limits of resolution so that cellular organelles could be identified, and indeed their substructure defined. This allowed more precise diagnosis of tumour types and allowed the structure of proteins such as amyloid to be determined. Ultrastructural pathology now has only a limited place in tumour diagnosis, but still has a central role in the diagnosis of renal disease, especially glomerular diseases (Fig. 1.3) (see Chapter 13).

### Immunohistochemistry

This technique evolved in the 1980s and gained a major boost from the development of monoclonal antibodies by the

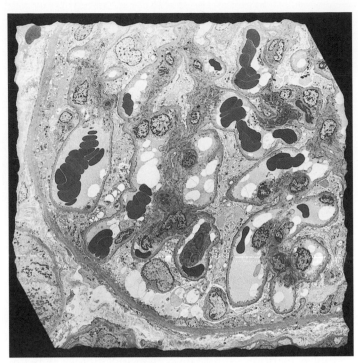

**FIG. 1.3** Electron micrograph showing the ultrastructure of a glomerulus. The increased detail is apparent even at this low power.

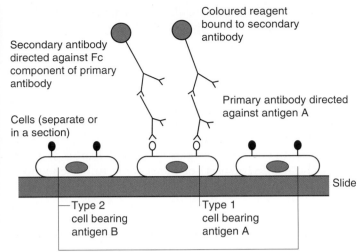

**FIG. 1.4** The principles of immunohistochemistry: the aim of the technique is to identify any cell bearing a specific antigen. The cell in the centre has antigens on its surface which are recognized by antibodies, often raised in mice, directed against that antigen. These are the primary antibodies. To demonstrate where these antibodies have bound, a secondary antibody is applied to the section. This antibody is raised in another species, e.g. rabbit. It is directed against the Fc component of the primary antibody and therefore binds to it. An enzyme or fluorescent label is bound to the secondary antibody so that a coloured signal is produced. The cells on the left and right bear different surface antigens, which are not recognized by the primary antibody, and so no signal is produced in relation to them.

late Professor Cesar Milstein. It depends on the property of antibodies to bind specifically to cell-associated antigens. Of course one must beware cross-reactive binding to other unrelated proteins. Tagging such an antibody with a fluorescent, radioactive, or enzymatic label allows specific substances to be identified and localized in tissue sections or cytological preparations. This has proved particularly useful in the diagnosis of tumours, in which it is important to classify the tumour on the basis of the differentiation that it shows to allow the most appropriate treatment to be given. The technique is outlined in Fig. 1.4.

### Molecular Pathology

Molecular techniques were the logical next step: rather than attempt to identify proteins within a cell, expression of the genes responsible could be identified if appropriate mRNA could be extracted from the cells or localized to them by *in situ* hybridization techniques. In addition, expression of abnormal genes could be detected, e.g. in several forms of non-Hodgkin lymphoma, specific genetic rearrangements appear to be responsible for the proliferation of the tumour (see Chapter 8, pp. 206–212); their identification allows precise subtyping (Fig. 1.5).

### Future Imaging in Pathology

Histopathology sets great store on making the correct diagnosis and gleaning information that is going to be useful in determining treatment options and the probable clinical outcome. In parallel, oncologists are now increasingly aware of how a patient's disease is unique to that patient

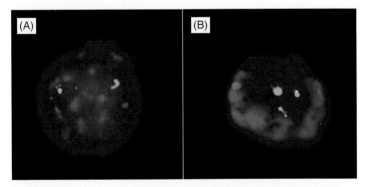

**FIG. 1.5** Interphase fluorescence *in situ* hybridization (FISH) on a lymphoma using the *IGH/CCND1* dual fusion probe (Vysis). (A) Normal pattern showing two green signals representing IGH on chromosome 14 and two red signals representing *CCND1* on chromosome 11. (B) Abnormal pattern in a mantle cell lymphoma showing a single green *IGH* signal, a single red *CCND1* signal, and two fused signals representing the two derived chromosomes involved in the t(11;14) translocation. (For more information on the probe used see www. abbottmolecular.com/products/oncology/fish/vysis-ighccnd1-df-fish-probe-kit.html.)

and treatment must be 'individualized'. The image that a pathologist sees down a microscope reflects the underlying differentiation of the cells and the processes that are taking place. The use of antibodies or RNA detection to identify different cell types and processes adds to this basic knowledge. In recent years the techniques of genomics, transcriptomics, proteomics, and metabolomics have been developed.

In these, the entire DNA profile, gene-expression profile, or protein or metabolic composition of a diseased tissue can be established in comparison to the corresponding normal tissue (Fig. 1.6). Many of these approaches employ high-throughput array-based methods that can generate large amounts of information about normal and diseased tissues: analysis of this information presents a challenge that requires close collaboration with bioinformaticians. The recent development of massively parallel sequencing techniques (next generation sequencing) (see Chapter 3, p. 35) allows the whole (or part) of the genome to be sequenced quantitatively, rapidly, and cheaply, and has the potential to transform the way in which tissue can be interrogated on an individual basis. However, these high-throughput technologies can provide meaningful information only if the tissues being analysed are carefully selected and characterized.

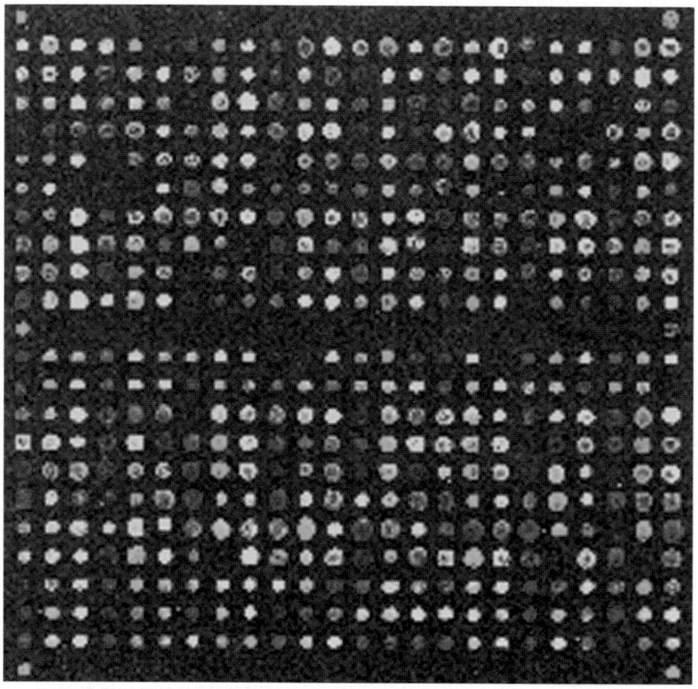

Pathology thus has a key role in translational research and should remain at the forefront of medical advances.

## HOW RELEVANT IS PATHOLOGY?

### Is Histopathology Necessary?

It might be argued that with advances in radiological imaging and other laboratory techniques the role of the histopathologist has decreased. This misses the key point that pathology directly addresses the question of what disease process is occurring and is complemented by many other diagnostic modalities. This role is especially important in the management of patients suspected of having a tumour (see Case History 1.1), but almost all tissues removed from a patient should be submitted for histopathological analysis.

### What Can Cytopathology Achieve?

Unlike histopathology, where assessment of the tissue architecture is of prime importance, in cytopathology it is the characteristics of the individual cells that are of most value. Essentially, in diagnostic practice the cytopathologist looks for the cytological features of malignancy (see Fig. 5.3D, p. 80). Admittedly, the relationships between adjacent cells can be appreciated to some extent: e.g. in an aspirate from a breast lump, loss of cohesion between cells is suggestive of malignancy, as is a high nucleus:cytoplasm ratio of the cells (Fig. 1.7). In screening practice, e.g. in cervical cancer programmes, the cytopathologist seeks to identify the same changes but at an earlier stage and thus give a warning of incipient cancerous changes. The biological basis and efficacy of screening programmes continue to be hotly debated.

FIG. 1.6 Gene expression microarrays were developed in the mid-1990s and have become a powerful tool to study global gene expression. Real-time polymerase chain reaction (RT-PCR) is used to generate complementary DNA (cDNA) from mRNA extracted from test and control samples. The test and reference cDNAs are labelled with different fluorochromes, in this case represented by the red and green circles. These samples are then competitively hybridized to an array platform that comprises representations of known genes or expressed sequence tags (ESTs), which have been spotted on to a solid support, usually glass or nylon. The presence of specific cDNA sequences in each sample can then be determined by scanning the array at the excitation wavelength for each fluorochrome, with the ratio of the two signals providing an indication of the relative abundance of the mRNA species in the two original samples. Although spotted microarrays are still in use today, the market is now dominated by one-colour platforms such as the Affymetrix GeneChip, in which a single sample is hybridized to each array. Gene expression microarrays have been used in numerous applications including identifying novel pathways of genes associated with certain cancers, classifying tumours, and predicting patient outcome.

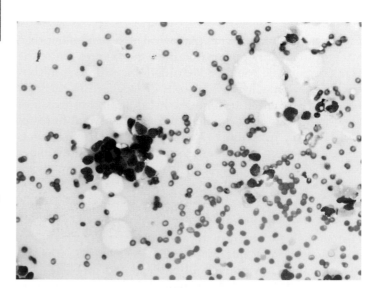

FIG. 1.7 This breast aspirate shows cells with a high nucleus:cytoplasm ratio and loss of cohesion indicating malignancy.

## Is the Postmortem Examination a Useful Investigation?

The popular image of a pathologist, perhaps fostered by television programmes, is of an individual who determines the cause of death, especially when foul play is suspected. From the early days of pathology, the postmortem examination has been of importance in understanding disease mechanisms, and in explaining the nature of the individual's final illness. However, advances in imaging and a cultural move not to accept postmortem examinations in many countries have significantly reduced the number performed, other than those carried out for legal reasons. Enormous advances in imaging techniques, especially computed tomography (CT) and magnetic resonance imaging (MRI), when coupled with targeted needle biopsies have to some extent diminished the need for postmortem examinations, but publications continue to show that they uncover hitherto unsuspected conditions.

Establishment of a robust, updated, scientific evidence base for postmortem pathology remains a challenge. Recent events, including the disclosure of widespread practices of retention of tissue and organs for research purposes, have provoked a sea change in public attitudes to postmortem examinations. In some countries specific new legislation is attempting to find the balance of investigation versus prohibition and to provide a platform for education of the public and support of families. Nevertheless, the postmortem examination remains the final arbiter of the cause of death in many cases, the key investigation in the forensic investigation of unexplained deaths, and potentially an essential part of medical audit. This can be so

---

The patient, a man of 55, presents with altered bowel habit. Both barium enema and colonoscopy show a stricture at the rectosigmoid junction. A biopsy is taken from this site.

### What does the clinician (and of course the patient) want to know?

Is this a benign stricture, perhaps due to diverticular disease or even Crohn's disease? Or is this a tumour and, if so, is it benign or malignant? Fig. 1.8 shows infiltration of the normal tissues by malignant cells arranged in glandular structures, indicating an adenocarcinoma (see Chapter 5, p. 82).

In the light of this diagnosis, the patient proceeds to have a resection of the rectum and sigmoid colon with anastomosis of the cut ends to restore bowel continuity. The specimen is submitted for pathology.

### Once again, what information do the clinician and patient require?

- First, confirmation of the diagnosis.
- Second, any information that would predict the likely prognosis of the patient and indicate whether any additional therapy should be given.

This information would include an indication of the type of tumour and an estimate of its biological potential – how malignant it is (its grade), how far it has spread (its stage), e.g. how far through the bowel wall the tumour has spread, and whether the tumour has been completely excised or is present in lymph nodes (Fig. 1.9). To improve the collection of such information in a standard form, the concept of a 'minimum data set' has evolved. The data set recommended by the Royal College of Pathologists is shown in Fig. 1.10.

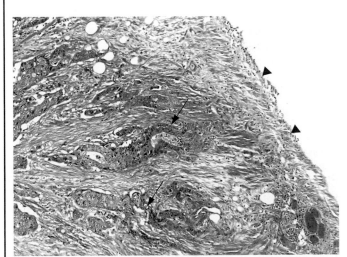

**Fig. 1.8** Adenocarcinoma of the colon. Malignant glandular structures (arrows) have invaded the wall of the bowel and have almost reached the peritoneal surface (arrowheads).

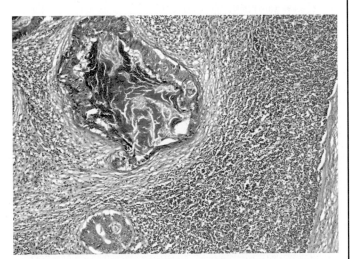

**Fig. 1.9** Secondary (metastatic) adenocarcinoma of the colon in a lymph node. Two malignant glands can be seen, with the surviving node to the right. A tumour that has reached the lymph nodes by the time of diagnosis has a worse prognosis.

**APPENDIX C     PROFORMA FOR COLORECTAL CANCER RESECTIONS**

Surname: ................................. Forenames: ................................. Date of birth: .................................

Hospital.......................................... Hospital no: ................................. NHS no: .................................

Date of receipt: ............................. Date of reporting: ............................. Report no: .................................

Pathologist: ............................. Surgeon: ................................. Sex: .................................

**Specimen type:** Total colectomy / Right hemicolectomy / Left hemicolectomy / Sigmoid colectomy / Anterior resection / Abdominoperineal excision / Other (state) .................................

## Gross description

Site of tumour ......................................................

Maximum tumour diameter: ...........................mm

Distance of tumour to nearer cut end ...............mm

Tumour perforation (pT4)     Yes ☐     No ☐

If yes, perforation is serosal ☐ retro/infra peritoneal ☐

For rectal tumours:

  Relation of tumour to peritoneal reflection (tick one):

  Above ☐     Astride ☐     Below ☐

  Plane of surgical excision (tick one):

    Mesorectal fascia     ☐

    Intramesorectal     ☐

    Muscularis propria     ☐

For abdominoperineal resection specimens:

    Distance of tumour from dentate line ...............mm

## Histology

**Type**

Adenocarcinoma     Yes ☐     No ☐

If No, other type .................................................

**Differentiation by predominant area**

Well / moderate     ☐     Poor ☐

**Local invasion**

No carcinoma identified (pT0)     ☐
Submucosa (pT1)     ☐
Muscularis propria (pT2)     ☐
Beyond muscularis propria (pT3)     ☐
Tumour invades adjacent organs (pT4a)     ☐
AND/OR
Tumour cells have breached the serosa (pT4b)     ☐
Maximum distance of spread
  beyond muscularis propria     ...........................mm

**Response to neoadjuvant therapy**

Neoadjuvant therapy given     Yes ☐     No ☐     NK ☐

If yes:

No residual tumour cells / mucus lakes only     ☐
Minimal residual tumour     ☐
No marked regression     ☐

## Tumour involvement of margins

|  | N/A | Yes | No |
|---|---|---|---|
| Doughnuts | ☐ | ☐ | ☐ |
| Margin (cut end) | ☐ | ☐ | ☐ |
| Non-peritonealised 'circumferential' margin | ☐ | ☐ | ☐ |

Histological measurement from
tumour to non-peritonealised margin     ...............mm

## Metastatic spread

No of lymph nodes present ...............................................

No of involved lymph nodes ...............................................

(pN1 1–3 nodes, pN2 4+ nodes involved)

Highest node involved (Dukes C2)     Yes ☐     No ☐

Extramural venous invasion     Yes ☐     No ☐

Histologically confirmed distant metastases (pM1):

Yes ☐     No ☐     If yes, site: ...............................

## Background abnormalities: Yes ☐     No ☐

If yes, type: (delete as appropriate)

Adenoma(s)  (state number .......................)

Familial adenomatous polyposis / Ulcerative colitis / Crohn's disease / Diverticulosis / Synchronous carcinoma(s) (complete a separate form for each cancer)

Other ...............................................................

## Pathological staging

Complete resection at all surgical margins

Yes (R0) ☐     No (R1 or R2)     ☐

**TNM (5th edition)**

(y) pT ........     (y) pN ........(y) pM ........

**Dukes**

Dukes A     ☐     (Tumour limited to wall, nodes negative)
Dukes B     ☐     (Tumour beyond M. propria, nodes negative)
Dukes C1     ☐     (Nodes positive and apical node negative)
Dukes C2     ☐     (Apical node involved)

Signature: ...............................     Date ...../...../..........     SNOMED Codes  T........ / M......

Fig. 1.10 National Minimum Data Set for Colorectal Cancer. (Reproduced with permission from the Royal College of Pathologists.)

only if it is carried out thoroughly and appropriately, realizing that no single investigation is the gold standard and that the postmortem examination is a much less effective way to examine death caused by metabolic 'failure' than that due to a structural abnormality. The examples of new variant Creutzfeldt–Jakob disease (see Chapter 11, p. 323), acquired immune deficiency syndrome (AIDS) (see Chapter 19, p. 540), and severe acute respiratory syndrome (SARS) (see Chapter 7, p. 176) emphasize that new diseases are still emerging. Meticulous postmortem examinations can help clarify the disease mechanisms.

### The Postmortem Examination Itself

The aim of a full postmortem examination is the examination first of the external aspects of the body, to look for injuries, haemorrhage, jaundice, or other stigmata of disease. The body is then opened and the body cavities inspected, and the organs are removed so that each in turn can be weighed and examined both externally and on the cut surface. Ideally, if appropriate permission has been granted, small pieces of the major organs and any diseased tissues are taken for fixation and histological assessment, so that the impression gained on naked eye inspection may be confirmed (or refuted). For a detailed analysis of some organs, especially the brain, it is essential that the organ is retained intact, preserved in formaldehyde, and then cut into thin slices followed by histology, a process that usually takes at least 3–4 weeks.

### Where is Pathology Going?

The past 20 years have seen major advances in our understanding of the underlying molecular mechanisms of disease. The completion of the human genome project, molecular genetics, and cell biology, and more importantly the use of this information to allow construction of a functional framework of tissues in health and disease, will inevitably lead to new approaches to basic research, and also to the day-to-day investigation of disease. Proteomic and functional genomic analysis of a few cells aspirated from a mass may give far more information on the nature of a tumour than conventional histopathological assessment of the entire specimen, which at present remains the gold standard, although the issue of tumour heterogeneity (i.e. variation in tumour characteristics from one place to another) is likely to limit this. Virchow might be familiar with the workings of a twentieth-century pathology department. It is doubtful if he would be as familiar with the evolving pathology department of the twenty-first century.

## SUMMARY

- Pathology is the study of disease. Subspecialities include histopathology, cytopathology, postmortem pathology, forensic pathology, haematology, microbiology, chemical pathology, immunology, and genetics.
- Techniques in pathology include light microscopy, electron microscopy, immunohistochemistry, and molecular pathology.
- Genomics, proteomics, and tests of metabolic function are entering practice.

## ACKNOWLEDGEMENTS

The contributions of Robin Reid and David J Harrison to this chapter in the 14th edition are gratefully acknowledged.

## FURTHER READING

Dabbs D. *Diagnostic Immunohistochemistry*, 2nd edn. Philadelphia, PA: Churchill Livingstone, 2006.

Killeen AA. *Principles of Molecular Pathology*. Totowa, NJ: Humana Press, 2004.

Rosai J. *Rosai and Ackerman's Surgical Pathology*, 10th edn. London: Mosby, 2011: Chapters 1–3.

# 2

# NORMAL CELLULAR FUNCTIONS, DISEASE, AND IMMUNOLOGY

C Simon Herrington

## INTRODUCTION

Disease may result from an abnormality in structure or function within cells of a particular type, e.g. in cancer, but more often than not it manifests itself because of the way in which other cells and tissues are affected and take part in the response to the original cause.

Understanding the normal function of cells and tissues gives insight into both the cause and the effect of disease, as well as beginning to allow rational design of therapy. Normal cellular function is encapsulated in the reproductive cycle. The body originates from a single fertilized ovum, which generates all body tissues including germ cells in the gonads; these in turn contribute to a fertilized ovum ensuring continued propagation of the species. This involves many processes: cell proliferation, cell deletion, intercellular communication, basic energy supply and use, oxygen delivery and combustion, protective mechanisms that may be active or passive, and complex gene programming that can be overridden in certain circumstances by the environment in which a cell finds itself. For this complex organization to function there must be many checks and balances, and ways in which different cells and tissues can communicate with each other. At the heart of understanding the pathogenesis of disease is recognizing how different injuries and insults can subvert or overwhelm these normal physiological processes and lead to an imbalance in homeostasis. This principle is well illustrated by the normal and abnormal function of the immune system, which comprises the latter half of this chapter.

## COMPONENTS OF THE CELL: STRUCTURE

With the exception of the red blood cells, all living cells in the human body contain a nucleus in which resides most of the genetic information; in addition the mitochondria harbour 37 genes, 13 of which code for proteins. The nucleus is not an inert structure cut off from the rest of the cell (Fig. 2.1).

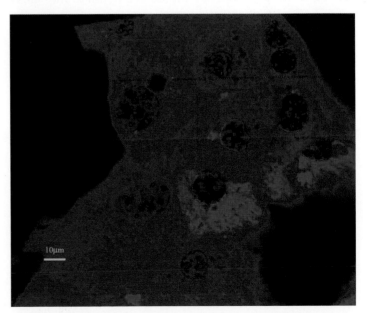

**FIG. 2.1** Liver cells in which the nuclei have been stained blue and the cytoplasm red. The nuclei communicate with the cytoplasm, and the cells connect intimately with each other through a variety of cell junctions (confocal fluorescence microscopy).

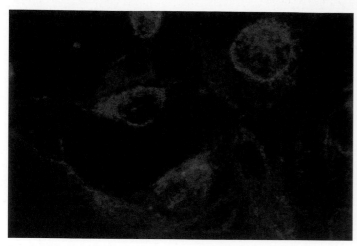

**FIG. 2.2** Mitochondria, visible as rod-like structures lying mostly around the nucleus, are demonstrated by a fluorescence technique. (Courtesy of Dr Rehab Al-Jemal.)

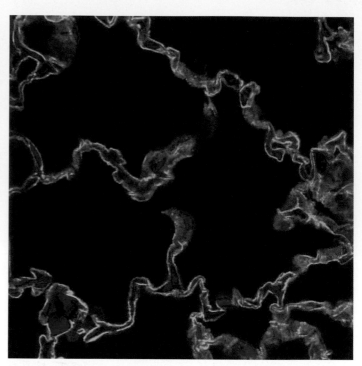

**FIG. 2.3** Lung alveolar epithelium. Nuclei are blue, flattened type 1 alveolar epithelial cells are green, and type 2 cells are pink. The green and pink fluorescence depends on the expression of proteins specific to the different cell types identified by particular antibodies labelled with fluorescent dyes. (Courtesy of Dr Gareth Clegg.)

The nuclear membrane is constantly crossed by factors which regulate the expression of genes and may repair DNA damage as soon as it occurs. The chromatin material that is the scaffold for the double-stranded DNA is packaged very tightly. It is critically important that this wrapped DNA is protected from damage, and yet can be unravelled when needed for gene transcription and for replication.

In the cytoplasm, a variety of organelles are responsible for the remainder of the cellular function. In some cases these are permanent features, e.g. mitochondria (Fig. 2.2), but in other cases a particular macromolecular complex may be assembled only when needed, e.g. the proteosome, which is involved in protein degradation, or the 'apoptosome', which catalyses cell death by apoptosis. Ribosomes translate messenger RNA (mRNA) into peptide sequences and further processing, including splicing, glycosylation, and possible packaging for secretion, occurs in the endoplasmic reticulum. The mitochondria are the primary site of oxidative phosphorylation. As part of this function they generate free radicals, which, in addition to potentially causing damage to membranes, enzymes, and DNA, are also part of the redox signalling system that indirectly regulates the expression of a number of genes involved in protection. The mitochondria are also key players in executing apoptosis in some situations.

## CELLULAR BIOCHEMISTRY: FUNCTION

Perhaps as many as 10,000 genes are actively expressed in a cell simply to maintain cell viability and function. These genes code for a variety of protein products involved directly and indirectly in energy production, protection against unwanted side effects of carbohydrate combustion in the presence of oxygen, maintenance of cell structure, and waste disposal. It is clear that these many gene products interact with each other so that cell homeostasis is a complex interactive network (Fig. 2.3). The regulation of gene expression is therefore complex, with many genes being expressed only when needed through the assembly of regulatory protein complexes which include transcription factors. This gives the cell the ability to express certain genes selectively at appropriate levels in response to particular stimuli. In addition to controlling gene (and hence protein) expression, the cell controls protein function through a network of competing enzymes that regulate the activity, structure, and function of other proteins. Thus phosphorylases and kinases act at suitable amino acid residues to dephosphorylate or phosphorylate their targets. These cause pH-dependent conformational shifts that alter both structure and function. Thus enzymes can modify proteins after they have been translated (post-translational modification) to flick protein switches, providing a rapid response to the changing intracellular environment.

Central to understanding many diseases is the appreciation that an oxygen-rich environment is potentially toxic and that protection against oxidant-induced stress is key to cell survival. The balance between oxidation and reduction is central to many processes including the reduction of ribose acids to generate deoxyribose, which is a critical component of DNA. Antioxidant enzymes are positioned throughout the cell to maximize protection. Thus superoxide dismutase 2 (SOD2) is located in mitochondria where it quickly takes reactive superoxide anions and converts them to the less potent hydrogen peroxide. This diffuses from mitochondria and can be destroyed by catalase. Within the soluble component of the cytoplasm (the cytosol) many peroxidases and transferases protect against oxidative species or make use of them in other cell reactions. Lipid peroxidation can occur as a chain reaction, as is seen in alcoholic liver disease (see Chapter 10, p. 280), and there are many antioxidant enzymes associated with microsomes that can abort these reactions. In addition to enzymatic protection, which can also use hydrogen for reducing reactions, there are other molecules associated with reduced nicotinamide adenine dinucleotide (NADH) and reduced nicotinamide adenine dinucleotide phosphate (NADPH), which offer protection, notably the reduced tripeptide glutathione, uric acid, and vitamins E and C.

## Protein Degradation and Removal

The half-life of cellular proteins varies from just a few moments to many months and perhaps even years. The haemoglobin protein in red blood cells lasts for more than 100 days before the effete cell is removed from the circulation. The regulation of cell proteins is a complex and important process for cell viability and function. If damaged protein accumulates it may inhibit normal protein function and even injure the cell directly. Genetic abnormalities resulting in abnormal proteins are implicated in many diseases. In cystic fibrosis (see Chapter 7, p. 171) a transmembrane chloride channel is dysfunctional and this results in abnormal mucus secretion, leading to the phenotype seen clinically. In storage diseases, such as $\alpha_1$-antitrypsin disease, an abnormal protein is produced that cannot be efficiently secreted from the cell. The protein accumulates and can cause damage to the liver cells resulting in hepatitis, which may progress to cirrhosis (see Chapter 10, p. 279). In addition the absence of functional anti-protease in plasma leads to an increased risk of emphysema developing in the lungs (see Chapter 7, p. 174). Mutation of tumour-suppressor genes can result in the formation of proteins with abnormal folding characteristics. Sometimes these inhibit the function of the corresponding normal protein (a dominant negative effect) and so contribute to the pathogenesis of cancer. Normally, damaged protein is marked for degradation by being bound to a carrier protein called ubiquitin, a process known as ubiquitination. This ubiquinated protein is then removed from the cellular pool and degraded in the proteosome.

## INTERCELLULAR COMMUNICATION

For any multicellular organism it is essential that cells communicate with each other to allow proper functioning. This communication must occur at several different levels, starting with immediate direct cell-to-cell contact, extending through local communication networks to information passing around the whole body. There are many distinct mechanisms to allow this to happen.

Cells are joined by cell junctions that are physical connections. These are of several types. Desmosomes and tight junctions join cell membranes, and gap junctions allow passage of chemical messages between cells. In addition, adhesion molecules are expressed on the cell surfaces, which not only join cells together but also transduce signals important for growth, migration, and differentiation. The surface-bound major histocompatibility complex (MHC) molecules and immunoglobulin are specialized forms of recognition mechanism present in lymphocytes, without which an immune response would be impossible (see later in this chapter).

Another form of communication is the production and release of peptides and other mediators that act in a *paracrine* fashion, i.e. they pass messages to nearby cells. Examples of this include mediators of injury and inflammation, and changes in extracellular matrix that occur during wound repair. Although cytokines are primarily locally acting paracrine factors, they may also have systemic functions. Thus interleukin 1 (IL-1) and IL-6 are important mediators of the systemic response to injury. Hormones are of course *endocrine* mediators and act in a tissue-specific manner dependent on the presence of receptors on the target cells and tissues. Feedback loops that ensure coordination throughout the organism are a key feature of intercellular communication. Any dysregulation or interruption of these feedback loops can lead to disease, as discussed in Chapter 17.

Perhaps the most complex intercellular communication is found within the nervous system. It is a prerequisite of a nervous system that it will respond immediately to changes in the external environment. Communication must therefore be rapid, specific, and geared to allow a direct pathway between sensory input, on the one hand, and effector output, on the other. Neurons do not actually join to each other but instead have a close association through the synapse, across which chemical neurotransmitters can pass causing depolarization of the adjacent cell and hence passage of a message. Many chemicals are neurotransmitters, including some more commonly thought of as hormones in the gastrointestinal tract (such as bombesin and gastrin).

## STEM CELLS AND DIFFERENTIATION

Inevitably, during life cells are damaged, die, and must be replaced. For some tissues this is a continuous process and in these *labile* tissues cell loss occurs at a high rate, e.g. mucosal cells in the colon and keratinocytes from the skin are constantly shed from the surface; neutrophils are constantly being phagocytosed and removed from the circulation; and there is even a slow turnover of hepatocytes. To survive, an organism must therefore be able to produce cells to take the place of those that have been lost. Usually cell division is restricted to a small subpopulation of the total cell mass, a group of cells known as stem cells. A stem cell has a high capacity for self-renewal and to give rise to daughter cells, which differentiate to replace those that have died.

In many tissues stem cells can give rise only to a single differentiated cell type, e.g. a keratinocyte, and are thus regarded as unipotential. Haematopoietic cells can give rise to cells of several lineages including monocytes and myeloid cells. These are called pluripotential. Stem cells necessary for passing on genetic information through the germline must be able to give rise to every cell type, and are thus known as totipotential.

The importance of stem cells is their persistence as a pool of proliferating or potentially proliferating cells throughout life. They are exposed to many kinds of damage, some of which cause mutations leading eventually to cancer. Indeed most cancers are thought to arise from mutations accumulating in stem cell compartments rather than in morphologically recognizable differentiated cells. Stem cells are also important because they may be used to replenish cells that have been ablated. This may occur in the treatment of myeloid leukaemia, or in fulminant liver failure, in which the liver's prodigious ability to reconstitute itself may reduce the need for liver transplantation.

## Stem Cells and Cloning

Until relatively recently it was assumed that pluripotent stem cells resided for the most part within specific organs. Thus bone marrow contains haematopoietic stem cells, the liver contains hepatocyte stem cells, and so on. Recent data indicate that the pool of stem cells is larger, more diverse, and more potent than previously supposed. Thus stem cells have been found in bone marrow and umbilical blood which can generate, for example, hepatocytes, neurons, or cardiomyocytes; these may be useful in treating specific diseases or used as part of gene replacement therapy.

An extension of this work, with important ethical implications, is the use of near-totipotent stem cells derived from human embryos fertilized *in vitro*. Basic genetics research is addressing how stem cells are controlled and, in particular, how many classes of genes can be switched on or off depending on differentiation status. This has led to the development of cloning, whereby a single nucleus from a differentiated cell can be conditioned to behave like a totipotent fertilized germ cell and give rise to a genetically identical offspring. This requires the pseudo-fertilization stimulation of a nucleus inserted into the empty cytoplasm of an ovum. To date cloned progeny have included sheep (e.g. Dolly), cats, and mice. There is a high loss of embryos due to malformation, and the effects on ageing and disease susceptibility are being studied to determine whether the cloned animals retain memory of their originating cell's 'age', or whether their replicative clock is reset to zero.

## MORPHOGENESIS AND DIFFERENTIATION

There is often a trade-off between a cell retaining the ability to proliferate and being able to exhibit differentiated functions necessary for the organism's wellbeing. In fetal development differentiation occurs during morphogenesis to allow formation of vital structures and organs. This involves cell migration, carefully regulated proliferation, cell differentiation to acquire new functional and structural characteristics, and, as mentioned below, selective and highly regulated deletion of some cells by a form of cell death described morphologically as apoptosis (Fig. 2.4). How this complex process is achieved in mammalian cells is only now beginning to be understood, having previously been extensively worked on in nematodes and fruit flies. It is clear that the whole process is under very tight genetic control. The master genes that are identified are very similar

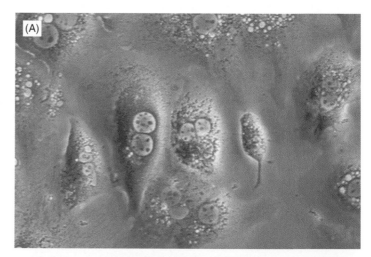

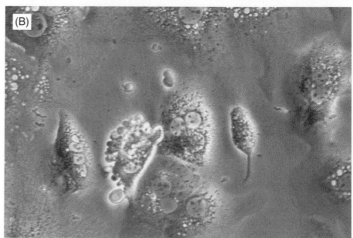

**Fig. 2.4** (A) Liver cells in culture. (B) After apoptosis-inducing injury, one cell has become shrunken and blebbed before completely disintegrating into apoptotic bodies. *In vivo* these apoptotic bodies are rapidly phagocytosed.

in higher-order animals to those first identified in worms and flies; this indicates how conserved morphogenesis is in evolution. These genes are called homeobox genes and their primary purpose is to regulate the expression of groups of other genes, and thus impose a discipline on the growing mass of cells. Mutations of these genes have been found, and these inevitably lead to developmental abnormalities. They have been implicated in some rare forms of childhood neoplasia. The main tumours of infancy are listed in *Table 2.1*.

More commonly morphogenesis and embryological development are adversely affected by damage caused by infection, metabolic, dietary, or chemical action. In this situation, as would be predicted from the description of how whole groups of cells are herded to differentiate in unison, the resulting malformations are often severe, e.g. the absence of a limb or failure of an eye to develop. This process is known as teratogenesis.

## Dysmorphogenesis: Congenital Malformations

About 1 in 50 babies is born with malformations that may present with immediate problems or not declare themselves until later life (*Table 2.2*). Such congenital malformations are a heterogeneous group consisting of genetic disorders, effects of intrauterine infection or trauma, and a variety of other conditions. The developing fetus is particularly susceptible to malformations because of the extremely rapid growth and the constraints of intrauterine existence, e.g. an insufficiency of amniotic fluid caused by leakage from a damaged placenta compresses the developing fetus.

The resulting appearance is characteristic: deformed, bent limbs; flattened face; and often poorly expanded chest with failure of normal lung development. Another mechanical cause of dysmorphogenesis is the presence of amniotic bands, strips of amniotic membrane that arise from tears in the amnion. These can constrict a limb or impede blood flow, thus causing incomplete or absent development.

Infection and drugs taken during pregnancy are also important causes of fetal malformation. Rubella in the early stages of pregnancy can result in many abnormalities, including physical deformity, deafness, and blindness. For this reason immunization against rubella is essential before pregnancy is likely to occur and teenage girls should be screened for evidence of immunity. Alcohol excess can lead to characteristic malformations and retarded growth, a constellation of features known as fetal alcohol syndrome.

Genetic disease, both chromosomal abnormalities and single gene defects, can cause physical and mental impairments. The most common genetic malformation is associated with trisomy 21 and results in Down's syndrome (see Chapter 3, p. 36). This occurs in 1 in 1,000 births and is more common if the mother is over 35 years of age. Many cases of malformation are of unknown cause; these most probably represent a combination of genetic and environmental factors, i.e. they are multifactorial. Even when detailed genetic analysis is performed many cases fail to show a recognizable genetic defect.

**TABLE 2.1** Congenital and neonatal malignant neoplasms

| Tumour type | Total (for four series) | Percentage of total |
|---|---|---|
| Classic neuroblastomas | 139 | 33 |
| Sarcoma (not otherwise specified) | 138 | 33 |
| Renal tumours (mostly Wilms') | 24 | 6 |
| Retinoblastomas | 20 | 5 |
| Brain tumours | 15 | 3 |
| Germ-cell tumours | 8 | 2 |
| Carcinomas | 3 | 1 |
| Liver tumours (mostly hepatoblastomas) | 6 | 1 |
| Leukaemia/lymphomas | 24 | 5 |
| Other | 48 | 11 |
| **Total** | **425** | **100** |

Adapted from Stocker JT, Dehner LP, eds. *Stocker & Dehner's Pediatric Pathology.* Philadelphia, PA: JP Lippincott, 1992: Chapter 20, p. 325.

**TABLE 2.2** Types of morphological abnormality

| Defect | Descriptive term | Example |
|---|---|---|
| Failure of organ formation or development | Agenesis or hypoplasia | Drugs e.g. thalidomide |
| Failure of differentiation | Dysplasia | Renal dysplasia in Potter's syndrome |
| Failure of fusion of embryological structures | Dysraphism | Neural tube defects e.g. meningocele |
| Failure of programmed cell death, involution, or luminization | Atresia | Syndactyly (webbed fingers), biliary atresia |
| Failure of migration, incomplete migration | Ectopia | Undescended testis |
| Chromosomal abnormalities, single gene defects | (Multiple abnormalities) (Very varied effects) | Down's syndrome, some forms of dwarfism, familial adenomatous polyposis (FAP) |

# CELL PROLIFERATION AND GROWTH

Mitosis results in daughter cells being produced, each containing the full complement of DNA (46 chromosomes, diploid) (Fig. 2.5), whereas in meiosis the DNA content of a cell is halved and cells become haploid (Fig. 2.6). Diploidy is achieved when two haploid cells combine, usually an egg and a sperm. Although disturbance in the cell cycle is widely recognized to be important in the pathogenesis of cancer, an understanding of how cell proliferation is controlled is also needed to fully appreciate processes such as wound healing and atherosclerosis. Classically the cycle is divided into four states: gap 1 (G1), synthesis (S), gap 2 (G2), and mitosis (M), with an additional fifth state, gap 0 (G0), which is in effect 'time out' for the cell (Fig. 2.7). Despite the explosion of knowledge about cell cycle control, these five states remain

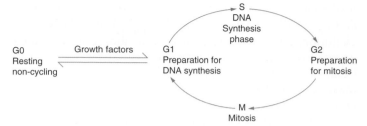

**Fig. 2.7** The cell cycle: cells start at rest in G0 and cycle through to mitosis or meiosis. At a number of steps there are checkpoints where the cycle can be stopped. Failing to activate cycle checkpoints may contribute to mutagenesis, ultimately leading to cancer.

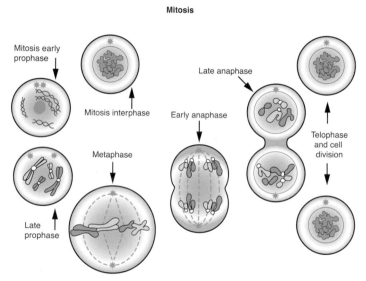

**Fig. 2.5** Summary of mitosis.

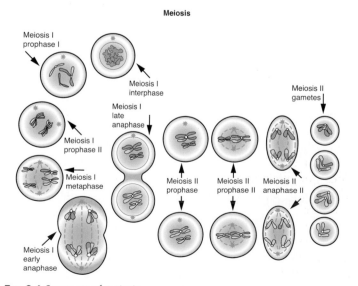

**Fig. 2.6** Summary of meiosis.

fundamental to understanding how cells proliferate and, just as importantly, why they do not.

Not all cells retain the ability to enter the cell cycle because they are terminally differentiated and permanently confined to G0, e.g. neurons in the central nervous system (CNS) in adults. However, some cells in stable populations, such as hepatocytes, which normally have a very low rate of proliferation, may be encouraged to proliferate under certain conditions in the presence of growth factors. Labile populations are constantly cycling, even though a relatively small proportion of their cells is actively cycling at any given time. As cell proliferation is such a key event in the life of an organism, and as inappropriate cycling activity could have such devastating effects, there are many tight controls over proliferation.

Cells normally reside in quiescent G0 unless stimulated by an exogenous growth stimulus to enter the cycle and therefore be available for proliferation. The cell cycle is controlled by a complex network of competing proteins, the activities of which are frequently modulated by kinases and phosphorylases. Thus cyclin-dependent kinases promote cell cycle activity, but cyclins modulate their activity and cyclin-dependent kinase inhibitors inhibit them. There are several stages during the cell cycle when a checkpoint has to be passed. This provides an opportunity for the cell cycle to be arrested, e.g. to allow repair of DNA damage. These checkpoints are in G1, at the G1/S boundary, and in G2 and M, and are critically important in the prevention of tumorigenesis. Some genes are particularly important in regulating these stages, notably *TP53* and *RB1*, both well-known tumour-suppressor genes (see Chapter 5, p. 98).

The expression of multiple genes must be coordinated to allow the cycle to proceed. Without this temporal cooperation the correct players are not present and cell cycle activity is aborted. Disruption of the cell cycle may not simply arrest the growth of cells. Some genes involved in cell cycle activation, including *c-myc* and *H-ras*, if expressed aberrantly, will cause the cell to engage apoptotic effector mechanisms and die. Thus genes involved in allowing cycle activity to proceed will directly lead to death if they are not expressed in the correct cellular context. This concept will be developed further in the discussion of cancer (see Chapter 5). It is

**TABLE 2.3** Growth factors and disease

| Growth factor | Disease involvement |
|---|---|
| Platelet-derived growth factor (PDGF) | Atherosclerosis |
| Insulin-like growth factors (IGF-1, IGF-2) | ? Anti-apoptotic effects in some tumours |
| Transforming growth factor α | Synergy with *c-myc* oncogene in transgenic models of liver cancer |
| Epidermal growth factor | Receptor overexpression in breast cancer |
| Interleukins | Autoimmune diseases |
| Fibroblast growth factors | Systemic response to injury? Therapeutic use in vascular disease to promote new vessel formation |

apparent, however, that cells go to quite extreme lengths to prevent inappropriate cell proliferation. Cancer is very much the end-stage of a series of extremely unlikely events and the evasion of a number of protective pathways.

## Initiating Cell Cycle Activity

As discussed above cells communicate with each other directly, in the local neighbourhood by paracrine pathways and throughout the organism hormonally. It is unsurprising therefore that one of the major functions of these communication routes is to initiate cell proliferation. Selectivity is achieved by cell-specific receptor expression coupled to an intracellular signalling pathway that will result in a permissive environment for proliferation to occur. Many growth factors are known and some, when overexpressed aberrantly, can act as oncogenes and promote excessive growth (*Table 2.3*).

# CELL DEATH BY ACCIDENT AND DESIGN

In general one assumes that a cell is a functional unit that should be kept alive as long as possible to maintain orderly functioning of the organism, and to conserve energy and resources. Although this is often the case there are circumstances where this is neither possible nor even advisable. Under these circumstances cells die, either because they are overwhelmed by an injurious stimulus or because they are deliberately deleted as part of a master plan. At times the severity of an insult may be so great or the cell and tissue so vulnerable that normal homeostasis may be impossible to maintain. Under these circumstances a cell may lose metabolic control, rapidly decompensate, and undergo catastrophic loss of viability leading to necrosis. *Necrosis* is thus defined as a collapse of membrane integrity and death of a cell or tissue. This results in the release of intracellular components. Many of these are reactive and

can lead to the activation of the clotting cascade and the generation of mediators of inflammation. Necrosis is therefore always pathological (with the exception of menstrual shedding of the endometrium) and brings the risk of inflammation and scarring, and may even be implicated in initiating autoreactive immune responses. Tissues rather than individual cells tend to be affected because the trigger for necrosis is usually a catastrophic exogenous event. A region of dead material is formed and the effect depends to some extent on the tissue involved. In most tissues, a coagulum of protein, referred to as coagulative necrosis, is produced by denaturation and aggregation of intracellular proteins. An example of this form of necrosis is myocardial infarction, where heart muscle undergoes necrosis as a result of an interruption in the blood supply. Heart muscle cells are rich in protein (largely derived from the contractile apparatus), which produces a coagulative end-result. In the brain, where there are many lipid-containing cells and little supporting tissue architecture, there is liquefaction, sometimes referred to as colliquative (or liquefactive) necrosis. Coagulative necrosis tends to be followed by healing by fibrosis, i.e. scarring, whereas colliquative necrosis typically results in tissue removal and formation of tissue spaces (cysts).

In a multicellular organism cell death is an essential part of development and, clearly, it is advantageous to have a mechanism that is not likely to lead to inflammation and scarring, but that is conservative. Studies referred to earlier in worms and insects have revealed a process of selective and specific deletion of cells during embryogenesis known as programmed cell death. Through further studies of the effects of hormone withdrawal on the adrenal gland it became clear that this pattern of death also occurred in pathological situations not truly programmed in the sense of being morphogenetically determined. By analogy with leaves falling from a tree in autumn, the process was named apoptosis (*apo-* away from, *piptein* to fall). It is important to realize that, although the morphology of apoptosis tends to be similar irrespective of the cause, there are many different routes to apoptosis involving several different genetically regulated pathways. Thus the finding of apoptosis in a tissue is indicative of neither the cause nor the particular biological significance in that situation.

One striking feature of apoptosis is the rapidity of removal of apoptotic cell fragments before their membrane integrity is lost. This is because of a number of changes in glycosylation and receptor expression on the surface of apoptotic cells that facilitate recognition and engulfment by macrophages. Intriguingly, phagocytosis of apoptotic debris does not elicit an inflammatory response; indeed macrophages may be prevented from producing proinflammatory cytokines by this process. Apoptosis is increasingly implicated in many diseases – from viral hepatitis, where it has long been suspected, to lymphocyte depletion in human immunodeficiency virus (HIV) infection to type 2 diabetes and neurodegenerative disease. The inability to engage apoptosis after injury may result in the selection of cells in

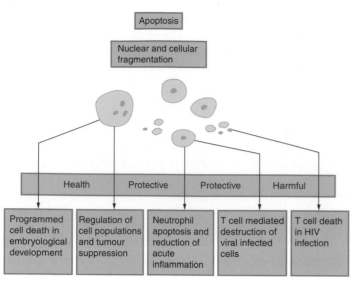

**FIG. 2.8** Apoptosis refers to the morphological form of individual cell death. It can occur as part of normal homeostasis in a variety of settings or as part of a disease. Programmed cell death, for example, when cells die during embryological development, usually occurs by apoptosis. HIV = human immunodeficiency virus.

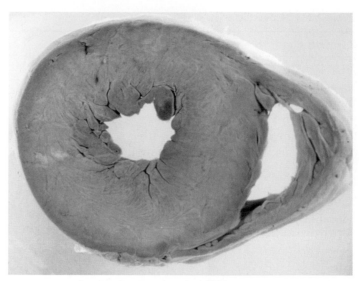

**FIG. 2.9** A slice of heart with the left ventricle to the left and right ventricle to the right. There is massive left ventricular hypertrophy. This occurs when an increased load is placed on the ventricle, as in systemic hypertension or aortic valve stenosis.

a developing tumour and in conferring resistance of cancer cells to chemotherapeutic drugs (Fig. 2.8).

# DISORDERS OF GROWTH

## Hypertrophy

Increased workload on a muscle may result in enlargement of individual cells by a process known as hypertrophy. In this situation increased cell numbers are not an option because the differentiated cells have lost the ability to proliferate. An important clinical example is the hypertrophy of the ventricular myocardium that occurs in hypertension (Fig. 2.9), in which increased fibre size leads to increased oxygen requirements (see Chapter 6, p. 130). In the presence of atheromatous coronary artery disease it may be impossible to deliver sufficient oxygen, so ischaemia (insufficient blood supply) and ultimately necrosis may occur. Hypertrophy is an active response, because the cell must synthesize extra proteins to allow increased cell size and activity. Hypertrophy itself cannot lead to neoplasia because no cell proliferation occurs.

## Hyperplasia

In the presence of excessive growth factor or hormonal stimulation of growth, a tissue that retains the ability to proliferate may be forced to undergo several rounds of the cell cycle, leading to an increase in cell numbers. This is called hyperplasia, and may be associated with an increase in size of the tissue that must be distinguished from hypertrophy. The cause may be apparent, such as overproduction of adrenocorticotrophic hormone (ACTH) from a pituitary

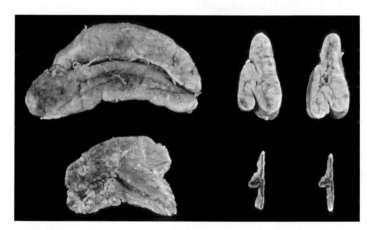

**FIG. 2.10** Normal (lower) and hyperplastic (upper) adrenal glands from different patients. The increased size of the upper glands is due to the presence of increased numbers of glucocorticoid-producing cells in response to sustained stimulation by adrenocorticotrophic hormone from a pituitary adenoma.

tumour causing adrenal hyperplasia (Fig. 2.10). Hyperplasia caused by abnormal growth factor stimulation should be distinguished from so-called reactive hyperplasia, which may occur in response to tissue loss, e.g. in the liver after paracetamol-induced injury or in the gastric mucosa after acute gastritis. In the latter case the proliferation is a healing response that is temporary and self-limiting.

## Atrophy

This term refers to decrease in the size of a tissue or organ which may be caused by a combination of cell shrinkage (the opposite of hypertrophy) and fall in cell number (the opposite of hyperplasia). In some situations atrophy is physiological. Each month the breast and endometrium

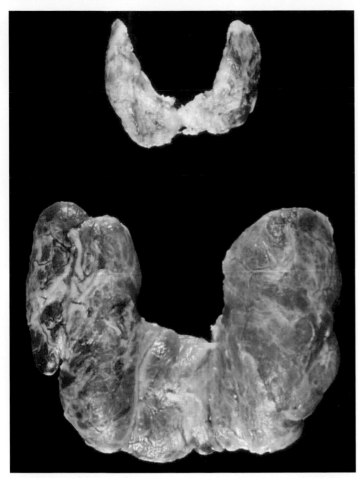

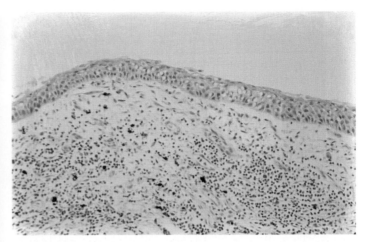

FIG. 2.12 Squamous metaplasia. The normal pseudostratified columnar lining of the bronchus has been replaced by stratified squamous epithelium as a consequence of chronic exposure to cigarette smoke. The black flecks among the submucosal inflammatory cells are particles of carbon from the inhaled smoke.

FIG. 2.11 Atrophic (upper) and normal (lower) thyroid glands. The atrophy is the result of loss of normal thyroid tissue due to longstanding autoimmune disease.

undergo hormonally induced proliferation followed by cell death and atrophy. Denervation of muscle (see Chapter 12, p. 388) or immobility results in disuse atrophy. Atrophy can be the result of destruction of cells as in the autoimmune damage resulting in primary myxoedema of the thyroid (Fig. 2.11; see Chapter 17, p. 483).

Atrophy is thus a non-specific change that may occur when:

- blood flow is reduced
- nerve supply is interrupted
- there are changes in hormone concentrations
- the tissue experiences disuse or excessive pressure.

## Metaplasia

Although it is usual for the precise differentiated state of a cell to be constant, under certain conditions one mature cell type may change into another. This process is known as metaplasia and is reversible. It is an adaptive response and may confer protection from local injury. It often affects glandular epithelia, which may change to squamous epithelia when exposed to trauma or environmental insult, e.g.

in smokers the columnar epithelium of the bronchus may change to a more robust squamous epithelium (Fig. 2.12). Conversely, exposure of the lower oesophagus to acid reflux is a factor resulting in the normal squamous epithelium of the oesophagus becoming glandular, similar to the stomach or intestine, because these epithelial types are more adapted to an acid environment.

Although the process of metaplasia is not in itself premalignant, metaplasia is sometimes associated with progression to malignancy. This can be explained by supposing that the new cell type, although not in any way cancerous, is more susceptible to injurious stimuli in the vicinity, which may lead to the development of cancer. Thus, in the case of Barrett's oesophagus, in which glandular epithelium replaces squamous epithelium, continued follow-up is advised to ensure that malignant change does not superimpose itself on the banal metaplastic change. Metaplasia can also occur in mesenchymal tissues. In chronic scarring, fibrous tissue may exhibit focal metaplasia into bone, and this can be identified radiologically.

## AGEING

### Cellular Ageing

The lifespan of cells varies greatly according to cell type. Neutrophils may live for only a matter of hours, red blood cells for 100 days or more, and some mesenchymal cells for years. There has been much debate over whether ageing of cells is a pathological process or a programmed physiological process. Judging from the factors that affect ageing it is clear that both programmable and non-programmable components are present. In rapidly proliferating cell populations cells eventually lose the capacity to divide any further and undergo a process known as cellular senescence.

For a long time it has been known that the number of replicative events that a cell can undergo in tissue culture is fixed to around 50 divisions, the so-called Hayflick limit. This suggests a degree of inbuilt senescence although the equivalence of an *in vitro* phenomenon to the *in vivo* setting should not be assumed too readily. Every time a cell undergoes mitosis (with the exception of germ cells which express telomerase) DNA polymerization starts at the end of chromosomes at telomeres, which are tandem repeat sequences. This region is incompletely copied and so the telomere shortens each time. Eventually it becomes too short to allow replication and the cell ceases to undergo mitosis. This telomere-shortened cell is also more likely to permit translocations and be error prone, possibly increasing the risk of breakthrough proliferation leading to cancer. This seems plausible and indeed some cancers show re-expression of telomerase; this might explain why some cancer cells are immortalized and do not undergo senescence.

Further evidence that genetic control of ageing occurs comes from developmental genetic studies in the nematode *Caenorhabditis elegans* in which mutations of a gene called *clk-1* (the 'clock' gene) result in elongation of lifespan. Although homologues of these genes in primitive organisms may exist in humans, it is true that wear and tear is a major factor in ageing. Oxidative metabolism generates free radicals and over time these cause progressive damage to cell membranes, DNA, the cytoskeleton, and enzymes. Damaged lipids accumulate in cells in the form of lipofuscin, a giveaway sign of cellular ageing and damage. Although protective mechanisms exist to repair DNA and to remove damaged protein and oxidized lipid, there is a gradual attrition over time that eventually leads to the cell's demise.

## Ageing of the Individual

Old age and the attendant increase in dependency and expenditure of resources is a major factor affecting the economies of every industrialized country and is now becoming important in developing countries. The features of ageing are of multisystem deterioration (*Table 2.4*), the effects of each compounding the others and leading to gradual debility. In addition specific degenerative diseases may be superimposed on this 'normal' ageing, further adding to the incapacity of the individual and the requirement for assistance. Just as is the case with cellular ageing there are both environmental and genetic factors in play. The earlier idea that environment and oxidant-induced injury were major players has been dashed after the failure of massive antioxidant consumption reliably to increase lifespan. Features seen in ageing include atrophy, possibly as a result of disuse, reduced trophic supply, and reduced ability to mount a new immune response or repair wounds quickly.

**TABLE 2.4** Characteristics of ageing, showing a spectrum from genetically programmed to more overtly 'pathological' and environmentally linked

| At the level of the whole organism | Possible cause |
| --- | --- |
| Cardiovascular disease | Atherosclerosis, calcification |
| Loss of lung tissue resembling emphysema | Environmental pollution |
| Deafness | Repeated environmental trauma |
| Forgetfulness | Neuron loss due to ischaemia or other mechanisms |
| Elastotic, sagging skin | Solar damage |
| Frailty | Muscle wasting |
| Osteoporosis | Genetic, hormonal, ? previous diet |

| At the level of cells and tissues | Associations | |
| --- | --- | --- |
| Cerebral atrophy | Loss of neurons | i.e. loss of permanent cells |
| Myocardial atrophy | Loss of cardiomyocytes | |
| Anaemia | Replication limit reached | |
| Atrophy of liver | Many, e.g. toxins, diet, hypoxia | |

Growing old and ageing are often assumed to be synonymous, but different species, and different individuals within the same species, age at different rates. This indicates that, although ageing is associated with the passage of time, it is not solely a function of time. Indeed, premature ageing syndromes such as progeria and Werner's syndrome indicate a strong genetic component, at least in disordered ageing. Recent genetic studies have identified regions of the genome where variation alters the propensity to age. Whereas yeasts and other single-cell organisms that replicate by asexual means do not age, multicellular organisms and their constituent cells and tissues decline in function and eventually die. It is apparent that the clinical and cellular features of ageing are the result of a complex interaction between genes and the environment, e.g. osteoporosis is strongly associated with ageing; however, it is very heavily influenced by genetic predisposition, menopausal status and previous dietary habits, and calcium load. Perhaps half of ageing is genetically regulated (programmed or clonal senescence), with the other half influenced by environment, when cells simply lose the ability to respond to damage and the attrition of nature's ravages (replicative senescence).

There are many theories and putative remedies for ageing, many of which may have some validity, but none of which is sufficient to explain the phenomenon. There is still uncertainty about how far ageing should be regarded as pathological and resisted or normal and accepted gracefully.

Houseflies have a short lifespan, giant tortoises a long one. Humans, domestic animals, and birds are intermediate in lifespan and in size. The generation of hydrogen peroxide as a function of body mass is inversely proportional to life expectancy, suggesting that oxygen free radical generation may be a major determinant in acquiring wear-and-tear injury. For some cells loss is irreplaceable, e.g. permanent cells such as neurons and cardiomyocytes, whereas other stable or labile cell populations may be regenerated, at least for a time. Oxygen free radicals damage proteins, membranes, RNA, DNA, and perhaps mitochondrial DNA in particular, which is repaired less efficiently than nuclear DNA and codes for proteins involved in oxidative phosphorylation. Thus ageing may be a curse imposed by living in an oxygen-rich environment and reliance on combustion of food for survival. Severe calorie restriction of laboratory rodents increases their lifespan by up to 50%. A sedentary lifestyle, such as that enjoyed by the giant tortoise, may also be important but sloth has its own disadvantages, as exemplified by its association with an increased risk of ischaemic heart disease (see Chapter 6, p. 133).

# IMMUNOLOGY

## Key Points

- The immune system is an adaptive defence mechanism.
- Immunoglobulins of five classes circulate in body fluids as a specific recognition and effector system.
- T lymphocytes provide the main cell-mediated defence.
- On occasion the immune system may cause disease such as hypersensitivity and autoimmunity.

The immune system is a defence mechanism that protects the body against a wide range of environmental insults, particularly microbial pathogens. It is also involved in the recognition of self and non-self in transplantation. There is another aspect to the immune system, however, namely the capacity to cause disease and injury in certain circumstances; indeed some of our most common ailments such as asthma and hayfever are mediated by the immune system gone awry.

There are many defence mechanisms that are general and non-specific: these are often referred to as innate immunity. However, one of the most important properties of the immune system is its specificity, which gives it the capacity to recognize and respond appropriately to each pathogen separately and distinctly. This adaptive immune system has conventionally been divided into two components, termed humoral and cell mediated. The humoral component consists of a series of plasma proteins in the blood and tissue fluids and the cell-mediated component comprises specific populations of cells that circulate throughout the body.

## Innate Immunity

Innate immunity is an immediate and important defence against many different microbial pathogens and toxins; it lacks specificity, i.e. the response is similar irrespective of the triggering agent.

### Epithelial Surfaces

The interfaces between the body and external environment across which microbial pathogens may enter are lined by the epithelia of the skin, gastrointestinal tract, respiratory system, and genitourinary tract. These epithelia consist of a continuous and tightly cohesive layer of cells; the cohesion of cells with each other and with the underlying connective tissue is achieved by the action of cell adhesion molecules. The epithelial cells form a physical barrier, but through secretions complement this with antimicrobial chemicals. Fatty acids secreted by sebaceous glands in the skin maintain a low pH on this surface; in the gastrointestinal tract there is secretion of acid in the stomach, digestive enzymes from the pancreas, and mucins produced by specialized cells throughout the tract. The respiratory epithelium secretes mucus to entrap bacteria, which are then expelled by the action of cilia on the cell surface. Urine produced in the kidney continually flows across the surface of the lower urinary tract, impairing the adhesion of bacteria to the surface.

The importance of these features in defence against infection is illustrated by examining the consequences of their disruption in predisposing to disease. Thus stasis of urinary flow increases the risk of urinary tract infection. Likewise loss of gastric acid secretion allows pathogens to reside in the stomach.

### Phagocytes

Once the epithelial layer has been breached potential pathogens encounter a further defence, a population of cells capable of engulfing and destroying bacteria, the phagocytes named after the process that they use for such engulfment – phagocytosis. Phagocytes reside in tissues and can circulate in the bloodstream from where they are recruited to sites of tissue injury. During phagocytosis bacteria are engulfed, and the cell membrane fuses around them to form a phagosome. This in turn fuses with a lysosome, an organelle containing bactericidal and digestive enzymes, to form a phagolysosome within which the bacteria are killed and degraded. The process of recognition of bacteria by phagocytes is a key step in this process. The phagocytes have on their surface recognition receptors that bind to microbial surface chemicals such as lipopolysaccharide and peptidoglycan. The phagocyte receptors include members of the toll-like receptor family. On binding of the toll-like receptor there is activation of a signalling cascade inside the phagocyte leading to the production of cytokines such as IL-1, IL-6, and tumour necrosis factor $\alpha$ (TNF-$\alpha$). The toll-like pathway activation also results in the expression of so-called co-stimulatory signals on the surface of the phagocyte; these signals are important in driving the adaptive and specific immune response.

### Plasma Proteins

The cytokines produced by phagocytes have systemic as well as local effects. Prominent among the systemic effects is the release from the liver of proteins known collectively as acute phase reactants or proteins. C-reactive protein (CRP) is elevated in the plasma in a whole range of acute and subacute inflammatory diseases. It enhances phagocytosis by binding to the phosphorylcholine component of lipopolysaccharide, enabling recognition by the CRP receptor on the phagocyte surface. The plasma also contains immunoglobulins, which are an important component of the humoral component of the adaptive immune system.

### Complement

Complement is a complex plasma protease cascade, the components of which are among the acute phase proteins released by the liver. It not only has an important role in mediating the protective effects of innate immunity, contributing in a major way to the effector arm of adaptive immunity, but it is also a significant factor in the tissue injury that occurs when the immune system goes awry (see Chapter 4). It can lead to direct cell (bacterial) killing, enhanced phagocytosis, and amplification of the response by cell recruitment.

The complement components circulate in the plasma in an inactive form; activation occurs on proteolytic cleavage by the relevant convertase. The important step in the complement cascade is the activation of C3 by cleavage to C3a and C3b. C3b then acts as the convertase for the activation of C5, which unleashes a cascade to complete the formation of a cell lytic complex C5–9. The key C3 activation may occur by the classic pathway, which is activated by an immunoglobulin (Ig) binding to antigen, or by an alternative pathway, which can be activated by a number of less specific triggers, including bacterial cell surface and aggregated Ig. The complement cascade is also regulated by complement inhibitory or regulatory proteins. Genetic deficiencies in these lead to serious disorders of exaggerated complement activation and acute tissue injury. In addition to generating a cell lytic complex, various complement components have other properties. C3a and C5a are important chemotaxins, and C3b bound on a bacterial cell surface (a process known as opsonization) enhances recognition and phagocytosis.

## Adaptive Immunity

The adaptive immune response is divided into humoral- and cell-mediated components by the activity of B lymphocytes and T lymphocytes, respectively. Although in practice the immune response is a continuous process, for the sake of discussion and analysis it may conveniently be considered to have an afferent arm of initiation and stimulation of immunocompetent cells, and an efferent or effector arm leading to the immune-directed elimination of pathogens.

### B Lymphocytes

B lymphocytes, originally so called because in birds they develop in the bursa of Fabricius, develop in the bone marrow in mammals including humans. They comprise 10–20% of peripheral blood lymphocytes and provide for the humoral immune response. They are present in defined microanatomical compartments of the lymph nodes, spleen and gut-associated lymphoid tissue. In these sites, on stimulation they proliferate within roughly spherical germinal centres.

B lymphocytes are specifically activated by antigen, which binds to and cross-links the B-cell receptor molecules on the surface. The B-cell receptor is composed of monomeric IgM (see below) existing in a transmembrane form with the antigen-binding fragment (Fab) at the external surface and the Fc fragment at the cytoplasmic face. The cross-linking of the B-cell receptor provides one signal for B-cell activation but, for complete activation, and particularly a shift between immunoglobulin isoforms, a second signal is needed. This may be provided by B-cell CD40 stimulated by a CD40 ligand (CD154) on a helper T cell or by complement components associated with the antigen and acting via B-cell CD21.

On activation B cells proliferate to amplify the immune response and differentiate into plasma cells. Plasma cells are highly synthetic cells that synthesize and secrete immunoglobulin, of the same specificity as its receptor, into the plasma. The different Ig isoforms are regulated in major part by signalling from T cells, resulting in the differing balance achieved in different immune responses.

### Immunoglobulin

The main component of the humoral immune response is antibody, also termed 'immunoglobulin'. Broadly, immunoglobulins are tetrameric proteins composed of two identical heavy chains and two light chains. Each heavy chain binds to one light chain to create the antigen-binding site that gives the antibody its specificity. The pairs of heavy and light chains mean that the typical Ig molecule is at least divalent (Fig. 2.13). In addition to antibody binding, immunoglobulins have secondary properties including the activation of complement and enhancement of phagocytosis. Immunoglobulins are classified by their heavy chain type into one of five classes (Table 2.5).

IgG is the most abundant immunoglobulin. It is present in plasma and tissue fluids, and can cross the placenta. It exists as a monomer and in humans there are four subclasses of IgG, each with slightly different secondary properties. IgA is the second most abundant but exists in two slightly different forms in different body fluid compartments. In serum, IgA exists as an immunoglobulin monomer but in secretions such as saliva and tears, and gastrointestinal secretions,

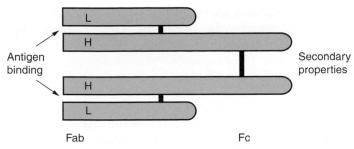

**FIG. 2.13** The typical immunoglobulin unit consists of two heavy (H) and two light (L) chains linked by disulphide bonds. The H and L chains both contribute to the antigen-binding site but the secondary properties reside in the H chain.

TABLE 2.5 Immunoglobulin classes

|  | Heavy chain | Common form | Complement fixation | Location |
|---|---|---|---|---|
| IgG | γ | Monomer | Classic | Plasma and tissue fluid |
| IgA | α | Monomer or dimer | Alternative | Secretions |
| IgM | μ | Pentamer | Classic | Plasma |
| IgE | ε | Monomer | No | Mast cells |
| IgD | δ | Monomer | No | B lymphocytes |

it exists as a dimer, with an additional protective secretory piece that resists its digestion in these secretions. IgM is the largest of the immunoglobulins, found almost entirely in plasma. It exists as a pentameric form which confers multivalency on each separate IgM molecule. It is also the first immunoglobulin to appear in immature B cells, and the first to appear in the initial immune response to any new antigen. IgE is a monomeric form which circulates in serum but importantly is found bound to the surface of tissue mast cells and circulating basophils. It is involved in protection against parasites but is clinically most important as the mediator of allergic responses. IgD is a minor component of circulating immunoglobulin but is found on the cell surface of B lymphocytes where it acts as a cell surface receptor.

During the maturation of B cells, and particularly during an immune response, there is a phenomenon of heavy chain class switching. This involves the cessation of IgM production and a switch to IgG, IgA, or IgE production but of antibodies with the same specificity. Heavy chain switching is dependent on a T-cell helper signal: responses that are T-cell independent, such as the response to pneumococcal polysaccharide, remain predominantly of an IgM type.

## T Lymphocytes

T lymphocytes are responsible for cell-mediated immunity and are so called because they undergo a maturation process in the thymus. T lymphocytes start their development in the bone marrow but recirculate to the thymus. Here they become subdivided into CD4 helper T cells and CD8 cytotoxic T cells. These have different activities and a different pattern of cell-surface markers, and respond to antigen in association with different MHC molecules. It is during thymic development that T-cell receptor gene rearrangement (see below) occurs.

T cells recognize antigen presented to them on a cell surface and in association with molecules of the MHC class. There are two families of MHC molecules: MHC I and MHC II. MHC class I is expressed on the surface of most tissue cells as a heterodimer of an α chain and a common $\beta_2$-microglobulin. MHC class I is recognized by T lymphocytes of the CD8 class. In contrast MHC class II is expressed only on a limited range of immune accessory cells and endothelium. It exists as an αβ heterodimer and is recognized by CD4 subclass T lymphocytes. Antigen is presented to T lymphocytes by these molecules in the form of small, partially degraded peptides held in molecular grooves on the MHC molecules (Fig. 2.14).

MHC genes show extreme polymorphism within the population and are the major component of the transplantation reaction. Hence, in preparation for solid organ transplantation, patients are tissue typed for their MHC alleles and a match between donor and recipient is sought. Even with modern transplant immunosuppression the outcome remains best for optimally matched individuals.

On encounter with an antigen, T cells proliferate to expand the reactive population. CD4 T lymphocytes after stimulation can be divided into Th1 and Th2, depending on the cytokine types that they produce. Th1 lymphocytes produce interferon, a potent stimulator of macrophages in their capacity to aid antigen presentation and phagocytosis. Th2 lymphocytes produce a menu of cytokines including IL-4 and IL-5, which contribute to type I hypersensitivity. CD8 lymphocytes respond to cell-surface antigen by the production of a cell lytic molecule, leading to cell killing. T-cell-mediated immune responses are particularly important in our defence against the first encounter with viruses and fungi.

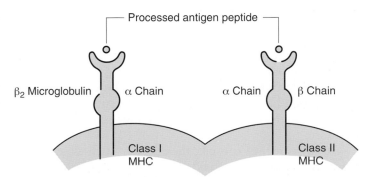

**FIG. 2.14** Major histocompatibility complex (MHC) class I and II molecules present antigen on the cell surface as processed peptide. Class I MHC consists of an α chain and $\beta_2$-microglobulin, whereas class II consists of αβ heterodimers.

## Specificity and Diversity of the Immune Response

The immune response demonstrates specificity and yet has the capacity to react to a whole range of pathogens (viruses, bacteria, fungi, parasites) and transplantation antigens. How is this achieved? T and B cells must become committed to a specific antigen before activation, that specificity must be retained during expansion of the reactive population by cell division, and the effector molecules such as Ig must share the same specificity. To achieve this, immature B and T cells exhibit changes in the genetic material of the Ig and T-cell receptor genes, respectively. There is gene rearrangement with excision of large parts of the genomic material of these receptors, restricting the range of specificity but ensuring that rearrangement is inherited by daughter cells. During further maturation there is extreme hypermutation within the genomic components encoding the antigen-binding regions of the immunoglobulin molecules and T-cell receptor. This ceases on maturation so diversity is expanded but remains inherited by daughter cells.

## Hypersensitivity

### Type I or Immediate Hypersensitivity

Type I hypersensitivity is a common clinical problem with up to 20% of the population having one or more allergies. It is the principal mechanism of disorders such as hayfever, asthma, and anaphylactic shock. Typically there is a rapid onset of symptoms within less than 1 minute but if allergen exposure ceases the clinical effects wane.

The disease is mediated through binding of allergen to preformed IgE on the surface of mast cells, usually within the submucosa of the respiratory tract or on the surface of basophils within the circulation. On first exposure to the specific allergen, the atopic patient mounts a predominantly IgE response, whereas non-atopic individuals may mount an IgG or IgA response to the same allergen. The factors regulating the balance of Ig subclass production in any immune response are incompletely understood. However, it appears that predisposed individuals mount a response driven by Th2-type helper T cells, with the IL-4 and IL-13 produced by these cells influencing the isotype switch to IgE production. The Th2 response involving IL-4, IL-6, and IL-9 also activates mast cells, priming them for their effector role in type I hypersensitivity. The circulating IgE thus formed binds to the surface of the submucosal mast cells via an IgE receptor, priming the mucosa for an allergic response.

On subsequent exposure, the allergen, such as grass pollen or house-dust mite, binds to the IgE cross-linking it on the cell surface. The clustering of IgE receptors causes calcium influx and degranulation of the mast cell. The granules release several inflammatory mediators including histamine, chemokines, and kallikrein-generating factor. These substances act on microvascular smooth muscle and endothelium, and on bronchial smooth muscle and mucous glands to trigger the characteristic symptoms. There is congestion, hyperaemia, and leakage of a protein-rich exudate from the mucosal vessels. The mucosa becomes swollen and oedematous, and glandular production of watery mucus increases. Bronchial smooth muscle contraction causes the airway narrowing and bronchospasm of acute asthma. Once this acute phase has been established the airway mucosa in particular becomes hyper-responsive to other inflammatory stimuli such as cigarette smoke or diesel fuel particulates which further accentuate and prolong the symptoms.

When a type I hypersensitivity reaction occurs in the general circulation the resulting anaphylactic shock is a serious life-threatening condition. This is the mechanism of acute collapse following peanut ingestion or bee stings in susceptible individuals. These two conditions alone may kill up to 100 people a year in the UK. There is generalized degranulation of mast cells and basophils with release of vasoactive mediators into the circulation. Generalized vasodilatation and plasma leakage occur with circulatory collapse. There is acute mucosal oedema of the larynx and respiratory tract, with acute distressing dyspnoea. Unless reversed by immediate resuscitation measures, sudden death may supervene.

### Type II or Cytolytic Hypersensitivity

Type II hypersensitivity reactions are triggered by antibody binding to an antigen on the cell surface or the extracellular matrix. As a consequence, effector mechanisms lead to lysis of the cell and/or an inflammatory reaction at the site of antibody deposition. This type of reaction is seen in some autoimmune disorders, in Goodpasture's syndrome (see Chapter 13, p. 405), and in blood transfusion reactions. It is also the mechanism of certain forms of tissue damage in drug reactions. In these reactions the drug binds to the cell surface, most commonly the red blood cell, and acts as a hapten, with the cellular proteins in effect being carriers of the small drug molecule. Most commonly the antibody involved is either IgG or IgM.

Preformed antibody binds to the antigen at the cell surface, locally activating complement. Completion of the complement cascade leads to insertion of the $C_{56789}$ membrane attack complex in the cell wall and subsequent cell lysis. In haemolytic anaemia or in transfusion reactions the red blood cell lyses within the circulation, releasing its contents into the plasma. In circumstances where complement is not activated cell injury may still occur. In Graves' disease antibody binding to the thyroid-stimulating hormone (TSH) receptor mimics TSH binding, leading to metabolic activation of the cell and hyperthyroidism (see Chapter 17, p. 481). This mechanism has been termed type V hypersensitivity.

### Type III or Immune-complex-mediated Hypersensitivity

Type III reactions result from either the deposition or the formation *in situ* of immune complexes with subsequent activation of complement and recruitment of proinflammatory effector cells. They may exist as either local or generalized disease processes. The location of the disease is influenced by the route of exposure to the antigen, its size and charge, and genetic factors. The clinical features are also determined by whether the exposure is a single event or chronic repeated exposure, the former being typical of a reaction to an injectable drug or of diseases such as farmer's lung. The latter is typical of many autoimmune disorders including systemic lupus erythematosus (SLE) and rheumatoid arthritis. Briefly, immune complexes are deposited in tissue, usually within the walls of small blood vessels. At this site they activate complement by the classic pathway, resulting in the liberation of chemotactic peptides. These in turn influence the accumulation of inflammatory cells, neutrophils, and macrophages, which attempt to phagocytose and clear the immune complexes. As a bystander effect, tissue components are damaged by the proteolytic enzymes released by the inflammatory cells. The whole process takes 6–8 hours to develop in the acute setting but in many diseases there is persistence of the antigen and chronicity to the hypersensitivity reaction.

### Type IV or Delayed Hypersensitivity

In type IV, or delayed, hypersensitivity tissue damage is mediated by T lymphocytes. Activated T lymphocytes directly kill cells or secrete cytokines, leading to macrophage accumulation and activation. The aggregated macrophages may assemble into a granuloma. This form of hypersensitivity is independent of antibody and complement. It requires 24–48 hours to develop fully. If antigen persists there will be progressive tissue damage and eventually fibrosis. This form of hypersensitivity is the basis for the skin tests used to identify prior exposure to tuberculosis, e.g. the Mantoux test.

## Autoimmunity

A number of diseases are characterized by the immune system targeting self-antigens expressed in body tissues. The resulting tissue damage may be mediated by any of the various forms of hypersensitivity but most usually by type II, III, or IV. This self-autoreactivity occurs when the phenomenon of immunological tolerance breaks down.

### Immunological Tolerance

Immunological tolerance is an active process that allows the immune system to maintain its protective role but avoid self-reactivating – during the generation of diversity of the immune repertoire T-cell and B-cell clones that detect self-antigens are actively eliminated. Tolerance occurs during the maturation of T cells in the thymus and B cells in the bone marrow. Self-reactive cells are eliminated by Fas-induced apoptosis, active T-cell-mediated suppression of self-directed immune responses, or T-cell anergy, whereby antigen-stimulated T cells are inactive unless co-stimulation occurs simultaneously.

Tolerance may be bypassed by several mechanisms. Activation-induced cell death may be bypassed if Fas-induced apoptosis fails. This seems to increase with age as the efficiency of intrathymic elimination decreases. T-cell anergy is circumvented if cells that normally do not express co-stimulatory molecules such as MHC class II are induced to do so. Thus, in the pancreas, induction of MHC class II molecules on the β cells of the islets triggers an immune response against self-antigens on these cells and the induction of both cell-mediated and antibody-mediated β-cell elimination, with consequent type 1 diabetes mellitus (Fig. 2.15). Molecular mimicry occurs when a microbial antigen encountered by the patient is sufficiently similar to a self-antigen that cross-reactivity with the self-antigen occurs. In rheumatic heart disease after a throat infection with certain streptococcal strains the antibody formed to the bacterium cross-reacts with an antigen present in the heart wall. The resulting antibody-mediated attack damages

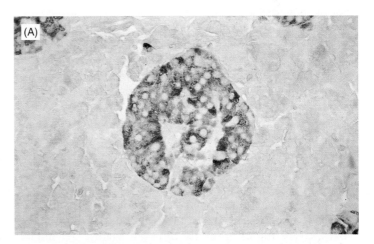

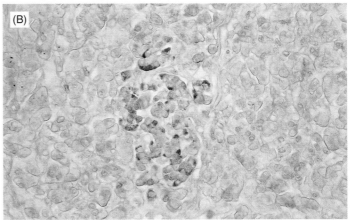

**Fig. 2.15** Double immunohistochemical staining of the islets of Langerhans – insulin-producing cells brown, glucagon-producing cells blue. (A) A normal islet and (B) an islet from the pancreas of a patient with type 1 diabetes mellitus. There are virtually no surviving insulin-producing cells in (B).

the myocardium and endocardium, leading to chronic valvular disease and potentially life-threatening long-term sequelae (see Chapter 6, p. 145). In some circumstances, particularly exposure to Gram-negative endotoxin, there is a polyclonal and relatively non-specific activation of B cells. These B cells may be reactive against a number of different antigens including some self-antigens.

In the majority of clinically important autoimmune diseases it remains unclear how immune tolerance is bypassed.

### Autoimmune Disease

Autoimmune diseases are common and may be either organ specific or systemic (*Box 2.1*). They result from the breakdown of tolerance, generation of an autoimmune response, and subsequent tissue damage. The autoimmune response may be humoral, cell mediated, or more commonly both. Autoantibodies are mediators of injury but are also useful in diagnostic assays. The tissue injury consequent on the autoimmune response may be mediated by any of the hypersensitivity reactions.

Tissue damage mediated by type II hypersensitivity in autoimmune disease is exemplified by autoimmune haemolytic anaemia. In this disease autoantibodies are formed against self-antigens on the surface of red blood cells. Autoantibody binds to these antigens, leading to the local activation of complement. The red blood cells may then be either lysed by the lytic activity of complement or phagocytosed by mononuclear phagocytes in the spleen and liver, phagocytosis being enhanced by the presence of antibody and the C3b component of complement on the red cell surface. The red cells are destroyed and the patient presents with the signs and symptoms of anaemia, and usually with a spleen enlarged secondary to the increased phagocytic activity of its mononuclear cells.

In SLE the main mechanism of tissue injury is through a type III hypersensitivity reaction. Soluble immune complexes, consisting of antibody directed against self nucleic acid and related antigen, and double-stranded DNA

> **Box 2.1** AUTOIMMUNE DISEASE
>
> **Organ specific**
> Type 1 diabetes mellitus
> Pernicious anaemia
> Graves' disease
> Hypothyroidism
> Addison's disease
> Autoimmune hepatitis
>
> **Multisystem disease**
> Rheumatoid disease
> Systemic lupus erythematosus
> Polyarteritis nodosa
> Wegener's granulomatosis

(dsDNA), circulate in the blood and become deposited in the microcirculation of key tissues such as the skin, joints, and especially the kidney. In these locations complement activation occurs. Neutrophils and, in a chronic setting, macrophages infiltrate the tissues and elicit damage (see Case History 2.1 below).

Primary biliary cirrhosis is a chronic progressive disease of the liver with good evidence of an autoimmune aetiology. Although autoantibodies to mitochondria are present, the pattern of destruction of intrahepatic bile ducts is typical of type IV hypersensitivity. Autoreactive T lymphocytes directed against antigens on the epithelium of the bile duct trigger the activation of macrophages and formation of a granulomatous response. This leads to progressive destruction of bile ducts, obstruction to biliary secretion, and fibrosis leading to cirrhosis and liver failure.

Attempts to suppress the autoimmune response and the inflammatory destruction of tissue form the basis of the medical management of these disorders. Understanding the type of autoimmune reaction and the type of hypersensitivity underlying the tissue injury is important in directing the rational treatment of autoimmune disease.

---

**CASE HISTORY 2.1**

A 26-year-old woman presents with a short history of joint pain, a skin rash on her face, and tiredness. On investigation, blood and an abnormal level of protein are found in her urine. Serological tests show that she has circulating antibodies to nuclear antigens, including dsDNA and a nucleic acid-associated protein Rho. These features, especially the autoantibody profile, are diagnostic of SLE.

One of the most important prognostic features of SLE is the type, extent, and activity of the renal involvement so a renal biopsy was done. Biopsy specimens from affected tissues may show a range of severity and acuteness, the assessment of which is an important part of histopathological analysis of SLE. The biopsy specimen showed deposition of immune complexes in the wall of the glomerular capillaries (Fig. 2.16A). The immune complexes contained IgG, IgM, IgA, and complement components. On light microscopy, 80%

of the glomeruli were affected by an inflammatory process with infiltration by neutrophils and macrophages (Fig. 2.16B). Of the glomeruli 30% had crescents, which represent extracapillary cellular proliferation and are one measure of severity. These features indicate that this woman has lupus nephritis with significant activity (World Health Organization classification).

The patient was started on treatment with cyclophosphamide and steroids. Our understanding of the pathogenesis of SLE informs this therapy. Cyclophosphamide specifically targets the B lymphocytes that produce the autoantibody, and the steroids suppress the activity of the effector neutrophils and macrophages. After 6 months of therapy the young woman is well with no blood and protein in her urine, her joint symptoms have improved, and she does not have a skin rash.

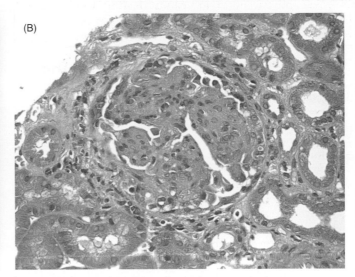

FIG. 2.16 In the glomerulonephritis associated with systemic lupus erythematosus there is deposition of complement-activating immune complexes – the presence of IgG in a glomerulus is demonstrated by immunofluorescence (A), with consequent infiltration by inflammatory cells (B).

## Immunodeficiency and Immunosuppression

Immunodeficiency may be primary or secondary, the primary immunodeficiencies being inherited abnormalities associated with a failure of development of components of the immune system, whereas secondary immunodeficiency occurs as a result of disease or its treatment.

### Primary Immunodeficiency

These are rare, often life-threatening diseases that nevertheless have contributed greatly to our understanding of the immune system. X-linked agammaglobulinaemia is the most common of these disorders and is caused by a failure of cell signalling and maturation of B cells, with failure of the light chain gene rearrangement which normally allows the formation of Ig molecules. Circulating B cells are markedly reduced or absent and there is a failure to make antibody. Once maternal antibody has declined the children become susceptible to recurrent episodes of bacterial infection.

DiGeorge syndrome occurs when there is failure of development of the thymus from the branchial arches, usually as a consequence of a deletion affecting chromosome 22q11, so there is no suitable microenvironment for the maturation of T cells. The patients are vulnerable to infection by viruses, fungi, and parasites. There is also a marked propensity to infection by mycobacteria. Severe combined immune deficiency is the situation where both the T- and B-cell components of the immune system are defective. The affected individuals are susceptible to a whole range of microorganisms and frequently succumb to infection as infants. Several different genetic abnormalities have been demonstrated in these patients and there are different patterns of inheritance.

### Secondary Immunodeficiency

Human immunodeficiency virus (HIV) infection and acquired immune deficiency syndrome (AIDS) are a common worldwide cause of secondary immunodeficiency. The pathogenesis of this infection is dealt with in detail in Chapter 19 (pp. 540–549). Briefly, HIV transmitted by blood or during sexual intercourse is capable of infecting the helper T cells of the CD4 class. There is progressive and eventually profound loss of these helper T cells. This has detrimental effects on the capacity of the affected patients to mount an effective immune response. Helper T cells drive both cell-mediated and humoral responses. People with AIDS acquire a progressive susceptibility to a range of infections with various clinical consequences. They may develop intractable viral infections such as cytomegalovirus infections, but they are also often infected with tumour-promoting viruses – papillomavirus causing squamous carcinomas, Epstein–Barr virus (EBV) causing lymphomas, and human herpesvirus 8 causing Kaposi's sarcoma. They may develop overwhelming tuberculosis, which often lacks the formation of typical granulomas. They acquire protozoal infestation by organisms such as *Pneumocystis jirovecii* (*carinii*) or *Toxoplasma* species. Infective complications, including virus-induced malignancy, are the most common causes of death in the HIV/AIDS population.

Immunosuppression may result from specific therapy or may occur as a complication of therapy. To maintain the survival of transplanted organs, drugs and other therapies are administered to suppress the immune response. The main immunosuppressive drugs are designed to suppress specifically the afferent arm of the immune response, blocking the activation of immune cells reactive to the allogeneic (foreign) MHC and other antigens present on the cells

## 2.1 Special Study Topic

### PATHOGENESIS AND RATIONALE FOR THE MANAGEMENT OF POST-TRANSPLANTATION LYMPHOPROLIFERATIVE DISORDER

A 32-year-old man received a renal transplant for end-stage renal failure due to glomerulonephritis. He was immunosuppressed with tacrolimus and oral steroids. His clinical course was complicated by two acute rejection episodes. For these he was treated with high-dose steroids which on both occasions successfully suppressed the rejection. However, because of these episodes mycophenolate mofetil was added to his immunosuppression treatment in an attempt to prevent further rejection. Mycophenolate mofetil suppresses the proliferation of both B and T lymphocytes by the reversible inhibition of inosine monophosphate dehydrogenase, a key enzyme in the pathway of new synthesis of guanine (Sievens et al. 1997).

Several months later the patient presented with enlarged lymph nodes in his groin. One of these was removed and examined microscopically. It showed a florid lymphoproliferative disorder, which was demonstrated to be of B-lymphocyte origin, monoclonal, and the cells expressed EBV antigen. A diagnosis of post-transplantation lymphoproliferative disorder (PTLD) in the monoclonal phase was made. This is an EBV-driven proliferation of B cells, which progresses to a type of lymphoma (see Chapter 8, p. 202). EBV survived in the infected B cells because the T cells that clear the virus in a healthy individual were being suppressed by his transplant immunosuppression drugs.

Although PTLD is regarded as a neoplasm, chemotherapy is not usually the first choice of treatment because this would further immunosuppress the patient; instead the patient's transplant immunosuppression drug doses should be reduced. This was done with close monitoring of the lymph nodes, peripheral blood cells, and transplant function. After 6 months he had had no rejection episodes, his lymphadenopathy had regressed, and his peripheral blood was free of EBV-positive B cells. This is an instance of a virus-induced tumour in the context of immunosuppression being treated by allowing the host defence to clear the relevant virus.

Sievens TM, Rossie SJ, Ghobrial RM, *et al.* Mycophenolate mofetil. *Pharmacotherapy* 1997;**17**:1178–1197.

of the transplanted organ. Such drugs include tacrolimus, mycophenolate mofetil, and azathioprine. However, if this suppression is overcome and the patient experiences an episode of transplant rejection, the strategy shifts to one targeted at suppressing the effector arm of the response. In these clinical circumstances high-dose corticosteroids are used and, if these are not wholly effective, humanized monoclonal antibody may be used to deplete immuno-competent cells.

Comparable but undesirable immunosuppression may occur in patients receiving chemotherapy for malignancy or anti-inflammatory therapy for autoimmune or other chronic inflammatory disease. In these circumstances the immunosuppression is less specific and may affect the afferent or effector arms of the immune response, and the outcomes are much less predictable.

Both groups of patients are susceptible to infection. The specific suppression of the afferent T-cell response in transplantation renders these patients particularly susceptible to viral disease. Cytomegalovirus infection, by reactivation or new infection, is a well-recognized and difficult problem in patients who have received transplants. Such patients are also at risk for two types of virus-induced malignancy. Those who have experienced several rounds of anti-rejection therapy have an especially high risk of developing EBV-induced B-cell proliferation and lymphoma called PTLD (see Special Study Topic 2.1 above). Patients who receive transplants also commonly develop multiple papillomavirus-induced squamous cell carcinomas of the skin and genital tract. Chemotherapy patients have a tendency to be more susceptible to bacterial infection, although they may also experience viral infection. The risk of bacterial infection is particularly associated with bone marrow suppression and a fall in white blood cell count.

## SUMMARY

- Understanding normal cellular structure and function is key to understanding disease.
- Stem cells form a small but fundamental subpopulation of the total cell mass.
- Morphogenesis occurs under tight genetic control, which may be disrupted.
- The balance between cell proliferation (regulated through the cell cycle) and cell death (through apoptosis) is crucial for normal development and survival, and is perturbed in many diseases.
- The main non-neoplastic disorders of growth are hypertrophy, hyperplasia, atrophy, and metaplasia.
- Ageing is a complex process, aspects of which are still incompletely understood.
- The immune system has innate and adaptive components, the latter having humoral- and cell-mediated components.
- There are four classes of hypersensitivity reaction.
- Autoimmune disease occurs when immunological tolerance breaks down and is either tissue specific or systemic.

- Immunodeficiency may be primary (inherited) or secondary to disease (e.g. HIV infection) or its treatment (e.g. immunosuppression for organ transplantation).

## ACKNOWLEDGEMENTS

The contributions of David J Harrison and Stewart Fleming to this chapter in the 14th edition are gratefully acknowledged.

## FURTHER READING

Delves PJ, Martin SJ, Burton DR, Roitt IM. *Roitt's Essential Immunology*, 12th edn. Oxford: Wiley Blackwell, 2011.

Kumar V, Abbas AK, Aster JC, Fausto N. *Robbins and Cotran's Pathologic Basis of Disease*, 8th edn. Philadelphia, PA: Elsevier Saunders, 2009.

Martin J, Sheaff M. The pathology of ageing. *J Pathol* 2007;**211**:111–113.

Nairn R, Helbert M. *Immunology for Medical Students*, 2nd edn. Edinburgh: Mosby, 2007.

# 3

# CLINICAL GENETICS

Jonathan N Berg and Sarju Mehta

## INTRODUCTION

Clinical genetics is a branch of medicine concerned with the diagnosis, testing, and management of diseases caused by changes in the human genome. Clinical geneticists must understand the molecular basis of genetic disease and identify clinical situations in which genetic testing is appropriate. A clinical geneticist should be able to communicate genetic information to family members so that they can understand the implications of having a genetic test, and make informed decisions for their clinical management. Increasingly, clinical geneticists are also involved in identifying the best treatment for patients with rare genetic disorders, and in testing for genetic predisposition to common disease.

Research in clinical genetics has led to the identification of the causative genes for many conditions. This is leading to an improved understanding of how specific genes, and the proteins that they encode, are involved in disease processes. Understanding the mechanisms of disease is an initial step in trying to identify new and specific treatments for disease. The practice of diagnostic pathology is intricately linked to the practice of clinical genetics. For example:

- A pathologist may be the first clinician to make a finding that suggests a genetic disorder running in a family, e.g. discovering *post mortem* that a bowel cancer in a young man was caused by familial adenomatous polyposis (see Chapter 9, p. 270). In such a case it would be important to arrange referral of the affected individual or his or her family to genetic services for further management. If this were a postmortem examination finding it would be important to store a DNA sample, with appropriate consent.
- Pathology findings may be important in confirming a genetic diagnosis in an individual or a relative, such as Alport's syndrome on a renal biopsy (see Chapter 13, p. 394).
- Pathology may be important in helping to establish a diagnosis, e.g. describing abnormal findings in a fetal postmortem examination that indicate a specific syndromic diagnosis.
- Molecular pathology uses DNA analysis techniques to characterise genetic aberrations, particularly in tumours, allowing this information to direct treatment. An example would be the use of fluorescence *in situ* hybridisation (FISH) to detect *HER2* gene amplification in breast cancer, described later in this chapter.

## BASIC STRUCTURE OF DNA

The DNA molecule consists of a sugar (deoxyribose) and phosphate backbone, with bases covalently bonded to each deoxyribose molecule. The base can be adenine (A), cytosine (C), guanine (G), or thymine (T). The DNA double helix is formed by two strands running in opposite directions, held together by hydrogen bonds between the bases. Adenine always pairs with thymine, and guanine always

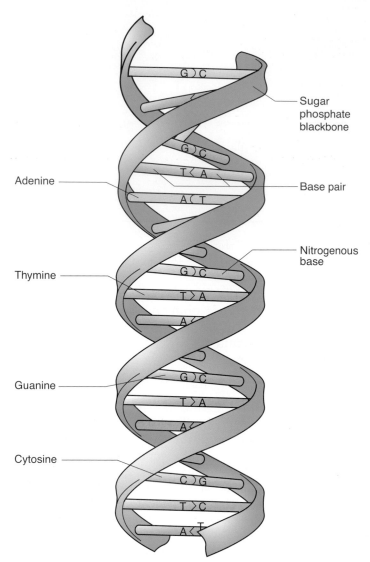

Adenine

Thymine

Guanine

Cytosine

Sugar phosphate blackbone

Base pair

Nitrogenous base

**FIG. 3.1** Deoxyribonucleic acid (DNA). (Redrawn with permission from the National Human Genome Research Institute, Division of Intramural Research.)

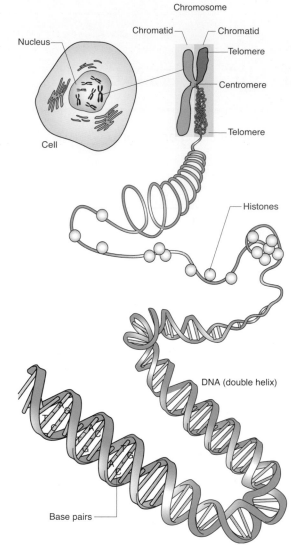

Chromosome

Nucleus

Chromatid

Chromatid

Telomere

Centromere

Telomere

Cell

Histones

DNA (double helix)

Base pairs

**FIG. 3.2** Structure of the chromosome. (Redrawn with permission from the National Human Genome Research Institute, Division of Intramural Research.)

pairs with cytosine. The basic structure of DNA is shown in Fig. 3.1.

## CHROMOSOMES

Chromosomes are the basic packages of DNA in the nucleus of a cell. In humans who have a diploid set (denoted 2*n*) of chromosomes, there are 22 pairs of chromosomes in every cell, called the autosomes, and two sex chromosomes, giving a total of 46. Females have two homologous sex chromosomes, the X chromosomes, and males have one X and one Y chromosome. Each chromosome has a long arm, designated the *q* arm, and a short arm, designated the *p* arm. At the ends of each chromosome are the telomeres. Chromosomes consist of a DNA strand that is wound around histones and packaged with other proteins into a compact structure (Fig. 3.2). Figure 3.3 shows the chromosomes of a normal male, as seen during metaphase in mitosis.

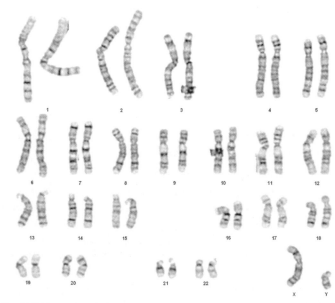

**FIG. 3.3** Normal male karyotype.

33

# CELL DIVISION

The cell cycle is discussed in Chapter 2 (p. 16). Although cell division takes place in the M phase (mitosis), DNA replication occurs during the S phase. A number of checkpoints exist during the cell cycle to allow for repair of DNA damage and replication errors that have occurred in the S phase, and, if repair of the DNA is not possible, to enable the cell to enter apoptosis. During DNA replication, a small number of mutations are incorporated randomly into the genome of the cell, and different repair mechanisms exist to counteract this. Mechanisms exist to repair base mismatches, strand breaks, and chemical cross-links.

## Mitosis

In mitosis, the cell divides to produce two almost identical daughter cells. Both parent and daughter cells are diploid. The phases of mitosis are named interphase, prophase, prometaphase, metaphase, anaphase, and telophase (Fig. 3.4).

## Meiosis

During meiosis, one diploid parent cell gives rise to four haploid daughter cells. In humans, it occurs only during gamete formation. It takes place in two stages: meiosis I and

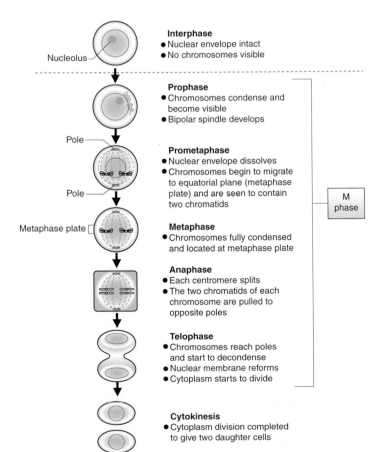

**FIG. 3.4** Mitosis. (Redrawn with permission. This information was provided, and is copyrighted, by Clinical Tools, Inc.)

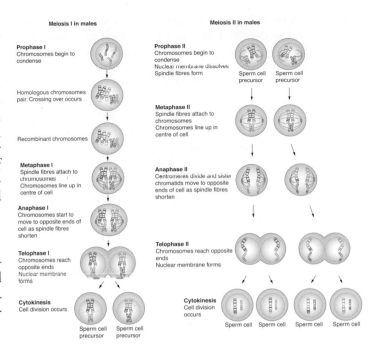

**FIG. 3.5** Meiosis. (Redrawn with permission. This information was provided, and is copyrighted, by Clinical Tools, Inc.)

meiosis II (Fig. 3.5). One of the key features of meiosis is the formation of chiasmata between homologous chromosomes during meiosis I. This allows the exchange of material or recombination between homologous chromosomes. Such recombination ensures that, although one of each chromosome is passed into the gamete, the chromosome is a mixture of parts of both parental chromosomes. Some additional variation also occurs because of new mutations incorporated at DNA replication. A child will have around 70 new mutations not present in either parent. These mutations are usually harmless, although the occurrence of a new mutation in a developmentally important gene is now recognized as a major cause of learning disability or malformation in a child.

# TECHNIQUES FOR GENETIC ANALYSIS

## Chromosome Analysis

### Karyotyping

Until recently, chromosome analysis depended on karyotyping, with visualization of chromosomes in metaphase at mitosis. Modern culture and staining techniques can detect rearrangements of approximately 5 million base pairs or larger. More recently array comparative genomic hybridization (aCGH) is being used as a first-line test for chromosome analysis because it offers better resolution with more rapid analysis.

### Array Comparative Genomic Hybridization

Array comparative genomic hybridization (aCGH) is a technique used to detect any chromosomal imbalance in a patient sample, by comparing patient DNA with a control sample. This is depicted in Fig. 3.6. As well as unbalanced translocations, this technique will identify deletions and duplications of chromosomal segments. The use of oligo-nucleotide arrays has the potential to detect any imbalance, down to fewer than 100 base pairs. However, analysis at such high resolution identifies a large number of polymorphisms and, in clinical use, only larger imbalances, or those falling within clinically important genes, are reported.

### Fluorescence in situ Hybridization (FISH)

The technique used to look rapidly for specific microdel-etions, and also for gross alterations in chromosomal num-ber, is called FISH. In this technique a fluorescent dye is attached to a probe DNA that attaches to the chromosomal region of interest. The probe DNA can be designed to be specific to any particular genetic sequence. If that region is present, the dye fluoresces, which can be visualized micro-scopically, and if the region is absent, then no light is emit-ted. This technique is illustrated in Fig. 3.7. An example of the use of this technique is shown in Fig. 3.8.

As FISH detects just loss or gain of a specific small chromosomal region, it can be used only where clinical parameters have defined which chromosomal region should be analysed.

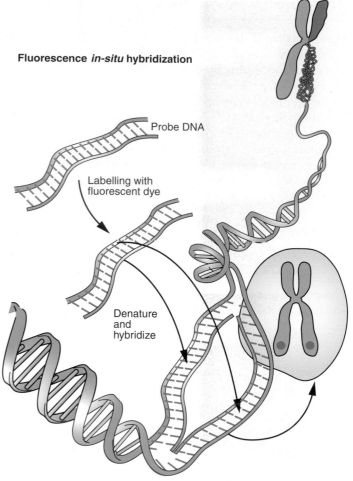

**Fluorescence *in-situ* hybridization**

Probe DNA

Labelling with fluorescent dye

Denature and hybridize

**Fɪɢ. 3.7** FISH allows detection of the presence of specific genes. The principle of the technique is illustrated.

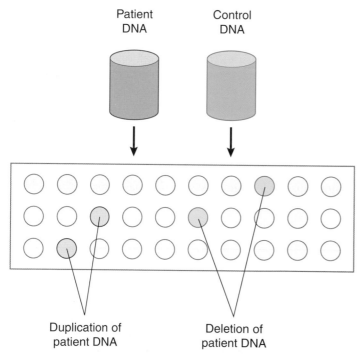

Patient DNA

Control DNA

Duplication of patient DNA

Deletion of patient DNA

**Fɪɢ. 3.6** Array comparative genomic hybridization allows identification of regions of the genome that are deleted or duplicated in a patient by comparison with a control DNA sample. Each dot on a microarray represents a specific genetic region. If more patient DNA than control DNA hybridizes to the dot, it suggests that the region is duplicated in a patient. If less patient DNA hybridizes than control DNA, then the region is deleted in the patient. (Adapted from www.ncbi.nlm.nih.gov/dbvar/content/overview.)

## Analysis of DNA Sequences

### PCR Amplification and Sequencing

Until recently, the majority of diagnostic DNA analysis was carried out using PCR (polymerase chain reaction) amplifi-cation and Sanger sequencing, also known as the 'dideoxy' or 'chain termination' method. This technique was developed by Frederick Sanger in 1977, and allows sequencing of short stretches of DNA, up to approximately 700 base pairs (bp) in length. Analysis of a gene using this technology requires amplification of each part of the gene in suitable frag-ments, with sequencing of each. The high overall cost of this restricts the amount of analysis that can be performed. To use this effectively in the diagnostic setting, it is necessary to identify which gene requires analysis from the clinical phenotype. Sanger sequencing is still the method of choice for analysis of very specific genetic regions, e.g. to test a family member to see if he or she carries a mutation found in other relatives.

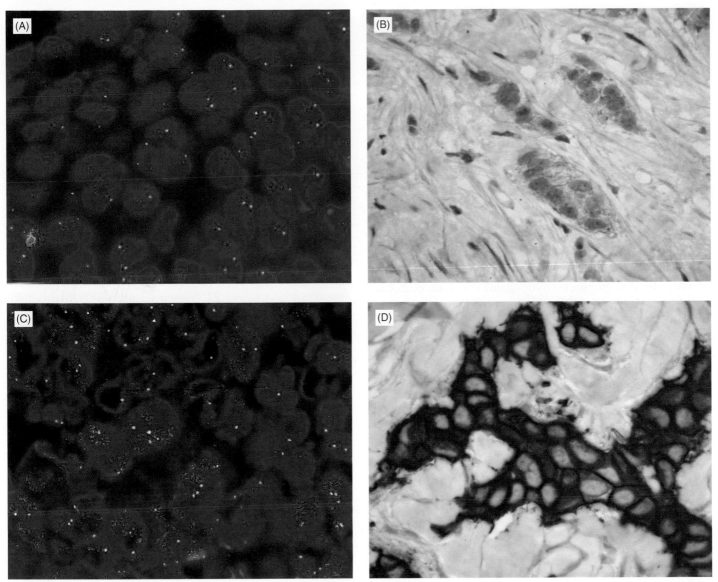

**Fig. 3.8** (A) FISH with a probe to the *HER2* gene shows the usual two copies of the *HER2* gene (red signals) and two copies of the control probe (green signal) in each cell. (B) Immunohistochemistry on this tumour with a normal *HER2* gene complement shows little expression of the epidermal growth factor receptor, which is encoded by the *HER2* gene. (C) FISH shows many copies of the *HER2* gene in each cell. (D) Immunohistochemistry on this tumour shows over-expression of the HER2 (epidermal growth factor receptor 2) protein, localized to the cell surface. Patients whose tumours show over-expression of HER2 have an improved prognosis after treatment with trastuzumab (Herceptin). (Images provided by Dr Lee Jordan, Department of Pathology, Ninewells Hospital and Medical School.)

### Next-generation Sequencing

Next-generation sequencing (NGS) describes a number of different competing technologies that have allowed DNA (or RNA) to be sequenced much more economically. All NGS techniques sequence massive amounts of DNA in parallel, so it can also be referred to as massively parallel sequencing. NGS sequences a large number of short DNA fragments in a single experiment. The main advantages over Sanger sequencing are speed, cost, sample size, and accuracy. In NGS, because of the millions of reactions being undertaken at the same time, 300 Gbp of DNA can be read on a single run.

There are a number of different technologies, and the field is evolving rapidly. Currently, in all cases, template preparation is required to prepare a representative sample of genomic material. The whole genome can be sequenced or the DNA sample from a patient can be enriched for genes of interest. This may be a panel of genes involved in a specific disease process, e.g. all genes involved in cancer predisposition. It is also possible to enrich the samples for coding regions (exons) of most of all known genes (the exome). The enriched DNA sample goes through further preparation steps that may involve clonal amplification. The NGS process then sequences multiple repeats of the same or overlapping segments of nucleic acid. The multiple, short, overlapping reads are aligned to the known reference sequence of the human genome, and variations present in the sample are noted (Fig. 3.9).

One of the biggest challenges of NGS is the requirement for analysis of very large amounts of data. Approximately 3 million single nucleotide variants (SNVs) are identified in a whole genome analysis and bioinformatics analysis is needed to sift through these variants and highlight those that may be disease causing. There are different approaches to filtering the variants, which include the exclusion of variants known to be polymorphisms, identifying variants that are new (i.e. not present in a healthy parent) and predicting the effect of the variant on gene function.

NGS has also led to applications in new areas, including microbiology and public health, by sequencing microorganisms responsible for outbreaks of new epidemics, sequencing of tumours to understand the biology behind cancer processes, and identifying new genes that cause human disease.

There are significant hurdles to be resolved with NGS, particularly the bioinformatics challenge in interpreting vast swathes of data. However, whole-exome (and eventually whole-genome) sequencing is likely to revolutionise medicine.

# GENETIC CHANGES THAT CAUSE DISEASE

The genetic changes that cause human disease can vary in size from a whole additional or missing chromosome to a change of a single base in a gene sequence. The techniques required to detect such changes depend on the size of change being sought (Fig. 3.10).

## Chromosomal Aneuploidy

Chromosomal aneuploidy refers to the presence of an entire extra chromosome (trisomy) or absence of a whole chromosome (monosomy), usually arising as a consequence of non-disjunction during meiosis. The majority of conceptions with aneuploidy will miscarry, and only some chromosomal aneuploidies are viable. The most common viable autosomal aneuploidy is trisomy 21 (Down's syndrome). Infants with trisomy 18 (Edwards' syndrome) and trisomy 13 (Patau's syndrome) can also survive to term, but usually die within the first few days or weeks of life. Aneuploidies involving the sex chromosomes are better tolerated by the fetus, and usually show a milder phenotype because of X-chromosome inactivation. The most commonly detected sex chromosomal aneuploidies are Turner's syndrome – in which a female has one X chromosome (45,X) – and Klinefelter's syndrome – in which a male has two X chromosomes and one Y chromosome (47,XXY). The 47,XXX and 47,XYY karyotypes are commonly detected as incidental findings on chromosome analysis because affected individuals usually show no obvious phenotypic features.

## Chromosome Translocations

Translocations are exchanges of chromosomal material between two or more chromosomes. If there is no significant loss or gain of chromosomal material it is described as

**Conceptual overview of whole genome resequencing**

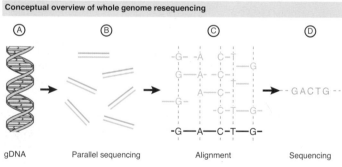

gDNA | Parallel sequencing | Alignment | Sequencing

**Detecting mutations using next generation sequencing**

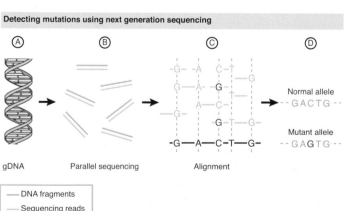

gDNA | Parallel sequencing | Alignment

DNA fragments
Sequencing reads
Reference genome

**Fig. 3.9** Next-generation sequencing: (A) extracted genomic DNA (gDNA); (B) gDNA is fragmented into a library of small segments that are each sequenced in parallel; (C) individual sequence reads are reassembled by aligning to a reference genome; and (D) the whole genome sequence is derived from the consensus of aligned reads.

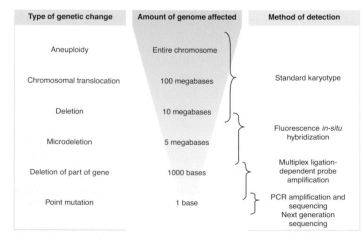

| Type of genetic change | Amount of genome affected | Method of detection |
|---|---|---|
| Aneuploidy | Entire chromosome | Standard karyotype |
| Chromosomal translocation | 100 megabases | Standard karyotype |
| Deletion | 10 megabases | Fluorescence *in-situ* hybridization |
| Microdeletion | 5 megabases | Fluorescence *in-situ* hybridization |
| Deletion of part of gene | 1000 bases | Multiplex ligation-dependent probe amplification |
| Point mutation | 1 base | PCR amplification and sequencing / Next generation sequencing |

**Fig. 3.10** Types of gene change and methods for their detection. PCR = polymerase chain reaction.

a *balanced* translocation. If there is a significant gain or loss of chromosomal material, the translocation is described as *unbalanced*. It is important to note that aCGH will detect only unbalanced chromosomal rearrangements.

A fetus with an unbalanced chromosome complement will often miscarry, sometimes before a pregnancy is recognized. If the pregnancy continues to term, the phenotypic effects of the imbalance involving the autosomes vary widely, but will usually include developmental delay, which may be severe, and may also include renal, gastrointestinal, and cardiac malformations with facial dysmorphism.

The likelihood of chromosomal imbalance leading to miscarriage is determined by the size of the imbalance. A small imbalance is more likely to proceed to term, but the liveborn child would still be expected to have significant phenotypic abnormalities and developmental delay.

## Robertsonian Translocations

In a robertsonian translocation, the long arms of two acrocentric chromosomes become joined together, with loss of the short arms. The short arms of acrocentric chromosomes contain highly repetitive DNA sequences and ribosomal RNA genes, so the loss of this material does not cause any clinical phenotype. A t(14;21) translocation and its inheritance are illustrated in Fig. 3.11. An individual with a balanced robertsonian translocation will usually be asymptomatic, but may have infertility (especially males), recurrent miscarriages (whether the translocation is carried by the mother or father), or a child affected with a chromosomal aneuploidy. If a parent carries a robertsonian translocation involving chromosome 21, such as the t(14;21) translocation shown in Fig. 3.11, the risk of a child being affected with Down's syndrome is increased (10–15% if the mother carries the balanced translocation, <1% if it is carried by the father).

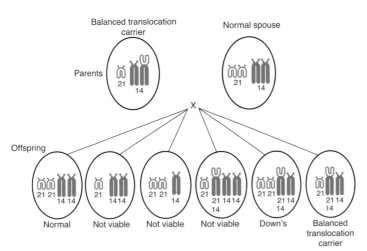

**FIG. 3.11** Possibilities for offspring in families with translocation Down's syndrome. (Reproduced with permission from Harper PS. *Practical Genetic Counselling*, 6th edn. London: Hodder Arnold, 2005.)

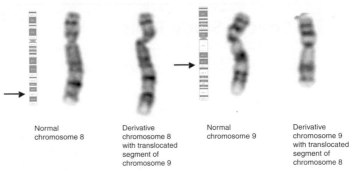

**FIG. 3.12** Chromosomes 8 and 9 from an individual with a reciprocal t(8;9) translocation: 46,XX,t(8;9)(q24.1;q22.1).

## Reciprocal Translocations

In a reciprocal translocation, there is exchange of material between two, usually non-homologous, chromosomes. Again, in the balanced form, there is usually no phenotypic effect, although, rarely, the translocation may disrupt an important gene and cause a genetic disease. A person with a balanced reciprocal translocation may present with infertility or multiple miscarriages, or have a child with multiple malformations and an unbalanced translocation. Figure 3.12 shows an example of a t(8;9) reciprocal translocation.

## MOSAICISM

In theory, the usual state is that every somatic cell in an individual has the same genetic constitution. Mosaicism is the situation in which there are two or more populations of cells with different genetic constitutions within the same individual. This occurs during somatic cell division, at mitosis, when a mutation arises in one cell lineage during DNA replication. This mutation can be of any size from the change of a single base in a gene to a chromosomal aneuploidy in one cell lineage. The clinical effects of mosaicism are determined not only by the genetic alteration but also by the tissue involved and the proportion of cells affected.

In germline mosaicism, a proportion of the gametes in an individual has the same mutation, even though other cells in the individual may not. A gamete that has the mutation will produce a child with an inherited disease. In this scenario, even if neither parent has the mutation in their blood or other tissues, there is a risk of having another child with the same mutation and therefore disease.

The main clinical importance of somatic mosaicism is in the development of cancer. As discussed in Chapter 5, cancer cells gain a number of characteristics or 'hallmarks', and this often happens through acquisition of somatic mutations at mitosis. Such somatic mutations can be chromosomal abnormalities, inactivating mutations of tumour-suppressor genes, or activation of oncogenes. A classic example of this is the Philadelphia chromosome (see Special Study Topic 3.1 below).

## 3.1 Special Study Topic

### THE PHILADELPHIA CHROMOSOME

The Philadelphia chromosome results from a translocation between chromosomes 9 and 22. This was the first chromosome abnormality to be found in a tumour, after identification of an abnormally small chromosome, named the Philadelphia chromosome (Fig. 3.13). The translocation occurs in a bone marrow cell and then, through clonal expansion, leads to the uncontrolled production of mainly the granulocytic cell lineage, leading to leukaemia. This in turn leads to the chronic phase of the disease, and additional genetic and epigenetic factors are required to transform chronic myeloid leukaemia (CML) from the chronic to the blast phase. The translocation leads to a fusion of the *ABL* gene, a proto-oncogene on chromosome 9 that encodes a tyrosine kinase enzyme, with the *BCR* gene on chromosome 22, denoted as t(9;22)(q34;q11). This fused gene encodes a protein with unregulated tyrosine kinase activity that ultimately leads to the leukaemia.

This discovery led to the development of imatinib mesylate (Gleevec), a specific tyrosine kinase inhibitor. In 80% of newly diagnosed cases of CML, imatinib induces the bone marrow to be totally free of the Philadelphia chromosome.

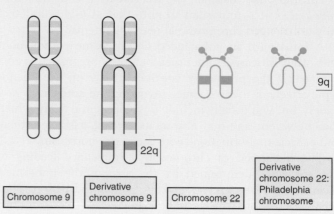

FIG. 3.13 The Philadelphia chromosome results from a reciprocal translocation between chromosome 22 and chromosome 9, leading to fusion of the *ABL* oncogene with the *BCR* gene, activating *ABL* and contributing to malignant transformation. The other derivative chromosome is not important in the disease pathogenesis. (With permission from Haematological Malignancy Diagnostic Service, 'Molecular Diagnostics in Haematological Malignancies: Polymerase Chain Reaction (PCR)', www.hmds.org.uk.)

Therefore the Philadelphia chromosome is a diagnostic marker and prognostic indicator for CML. It is also found in acute lymphoblastic leukaemia.

## SINGLE-GENE (MENDELIAN) INHERITANCE

Single-gene disorders are caused by mutations in a single gene. The inheritance of single-gene disorders is determined by Mendel's laws of segregation and independent assortment. An autosomal gene is one that is carried on one of the autosomes (chromosomes 1–22, found in pairs in each cell), and an X-linked gene is one that is found on the X chromosome.

Alleles are the specific versions of a gene in an individual. For an autosomal gene, an individual will have two copies of that gene or two alleles. If one copy has a mutation, it is described as the mutant allele. The genotype is the genetic makeup of an individual. The phenotype is the effect of the genetic constitution. To visualize the inheritance of single-gene disorders in a family, it is often necessary to draw a family tree or pedigree (Fig. 3.14).

### Autosomal Dominant Inheritance

Autosomal dominant inheritance (Fig. 3.15A) is a pattern of inheritance in which one copy of a mutant allele is sufficient to cause disease: an affected individual possesses one

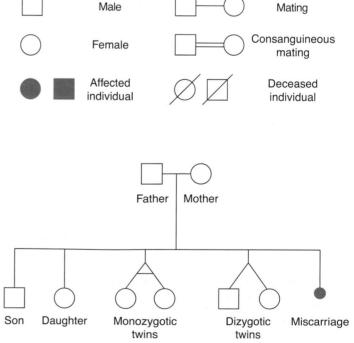

FIG. 3.14 Drawing a family tree. A pedigree is drawn using standard symbols.

(A)

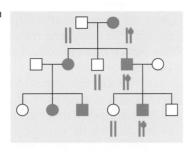

Autosomal dominant inheritance

- One faulty copy of gene is sufficient to cause disease
- Disease phenotype is seen in all generations
- Disease severity may be variable
- Males and females are equally likely to be affected
- If neither parent is affected, there may be a new mutation

(B)

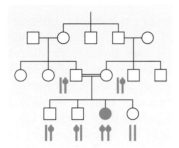

Autosomal recessive inheritance

- Both copies of the gene are mutated to cause the disease
- Often only individuals in one generation are affected
- 1-in-4 risk of an affected child if both parents are carriers
- Higher incidence of recessive disorders in consanguineous families

(C)

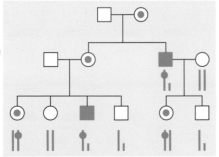

X-linked recessive inheritance

- The mutated gene lies on the X chromosome
- A female carrier:
  is unlikely to show significant features of disease
  half her male children will be affected
  half her female children will be carriers
- An affected male:
  all his male children will be unaffected
  all his daughters will be carriers of the condition

FIG. 3.15 The three most common patterns of single gene inheritance for human disease. (A) Autosomal dominant inheritance; (B) autosomal recessive inheritance; and (C) X-linked recessive inheritance.

copy of the mutant allele and one copy of a normal allele. Individuals who have an autosomal dominant disease have a one-in-two, or 50%, chance of passing the mutation to all their offspring.

Many conditions that are autosomal dominant start with a new mutation in the person him- or herself and so the parents may be unaffected. Many severe developmental disorders in children are caused by such new autosomal dominant-acting mutations. In these cases, a new mutation has arisen in a key developmental gene. If the genetic disorder is sufficiently severe to prevent the affected individual having children, the disorder appears as a sporadic condition in the family. In these cases, the risk of recurrence for the parents is related to the germline mosaicism risk discussed previously.

## Autosomal Recessive Inheritance

In autosomal recessive inheritance (Fig. 3.15B) both copies of the gene must harbour mutations for the disease to arise. This usually occurs when both parents are carriers, with one normal and one mutated copy of the gene, and they have each passed on their abnormal gene to a child. The risk of having a child with an autosomal recessive disease if both parents are carriers is one in four or 25%.

## X-linked Disorders

X-linked disorders (Fig. 3.15C) are caused by mutations in genes on the X chromosome. Females have two X chromosomes, and males have one X and one Y chromo¬some. In a female, to maintain chromosomal balance, one X chromosome becomes inactive in each cell. Usually, it is a random event as to which chromosome is inactivated (Fig. 3.16A).

The Y chromosome contains few genes and has very little homology to the X chromosome. A male, therefore, has only a single copy of most of the genes on the X chromosome. In an X-linked recessive condition, a female with a mutation in a gene on the X chromosome shows few or no phenotypic effects, because she has a second functioning copy. A male with the same mutation will be affected because he has no functioning copy. Haemophilia A is an example of such a condition. In an X-linked dominant condition, a female with a single faulty copy of the gene on the X chromosome will show features of the disease. The effect of the same mutation on a male depends on the gene: in some cases, such as incontinentia pigmenti, the effect may be to make the male fetus non-viable; in other cases, the phenotype in a male may be similar to that seen in a female, such as in X-linked rickets.

Females who carry an X-linked recessive disorder may display signs and symptoms of an X-linked disorder. This is most commonly because, due to X-chromosome inactivation, 50% of the nuclei in their cells contain the

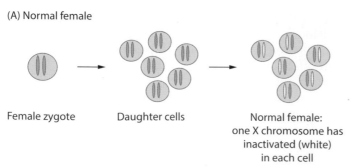

(A) Normal female

Female zygote → Daughter cells → Normal female: one X chromosome has inactivated (white) in each cell

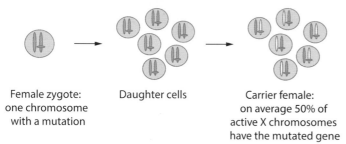

(B) Female carrier of mutation on X chromosome

Female zygote: one chromosome with a mutation → Daughter cells → Carrier female: on average 50% of active X chromosomes have the mutated gene

**FIG. 3.16** X-inactivation: (A) normal female; (B) female carrier of mutation on X chromosome.

active X chromosome with the mutated gene (Fig. 3.16B), e.g. female carriers of haemophilia A, with mutations in the factor VIII gene, may show mild coagulation disorders. Much less often, a female may show a phenotype of similar severity to an affected male. This arises because the mutated X chromosome is active in most or all of her cells. This may be either through non-random inactivation, called skewed X-inactivation, or if she only has a single copy of the X chromosome that carries the mutation, as in a patient with Turner's syndrome (45,XO).

## NON-MENDELIAN INHERITANCE

### Mitochondrial Inheritance

The mitochondria are exclusively maternally inherited. Therefore, although a disease inherited through the mitochondrial genome can affect either sex, it can be passed on only by affected mothers. Each mitochondrion has a genome of approximately 16.5 kbp in size. Mutations may be homoplasmic, affecting all mitochondria in a cell, or heteroplasmic, affecting only a proportion. Where there is heteroplasmy, the phenotypic effects can vary depending on what proportion of mitochondria has the mutation in each cell, and in which tissues.

## Imprinting

Imprinted genes are ones that are differentially expressed, depending on whether they are maternally or paternally inherited. Only certain genes in certain chromosomal regions are imprinted, e.g. only the maternally inherited copy of the *UBE3A* gene on chromosome 15 is active. If a child does not inherit a functioning copy from the mother then he or she will be affected with Angelman's syndrome. The gene could be inactivated by a point mutation or deletion, or an unusual transmission of chromosomes may occur, so that the child inherits two chromosomes 15 from its father but no chromosome 15 from its mother (paternal uniparental disomy).

## STRUCTURE OF A GENE AND HOW IT ENCODES A PROTEIN

Genes consist of a number of different components, shown in Fig. 3.17. Upstream of the gene there are regulatory elements, which may increase or decrease gene expression (enhancers and silencers). The promoter is the binding site for proteins that initiate transcription. Downstream from the promoter, a gene consists of many exons, which contain the DNA sequence that encodes the protein, and introns, which do not. The production of protein from a gene requires the processes of transcription, splicing, and translation (Fig. 3.17).

### Transcription

A transcription factor binds to the promoter and a single RNA strand is synthesized using the DNA sequence as a

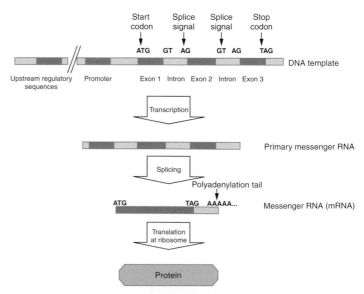

**FIG. 3.17** Gene structure and how a protein is encoded.

template. RNA has a similar structure to DNA, with the minor differences that the sugar phosphate backbone contains ribose rather than deoxyribose and the base uracil (U) is substituted for the base thymine (T). In RNA, therefore, adenine (A) pairs with uracil (U).

## Splicing

The primary messenger RNA (mRNA) that is synthesized undergoes splicing to remove the intronic sequences, creating a mature mRNA. There are specific splicing recognition sequences; each intron starts with a GT sequence and ends with an AG sequence.

## Translation

The mRNA is moved to the ribosome in the cytoplasm, where it is translated into a polypeptide. Every three bases (= one codon) of the mRNA molecule encode an amino acid or a stop. Transfer RNAs transport the amino acids to the assembling peptide. The translation starts at a start codon, which is always AUG encoding methionine, and stops when a UAA, UAG, or UGA is reached. The polypeptide then undergoes post-translational modification, e.g. glycosylation, and is transported to its place of function as a mature protein.

The amount of a polypeptide produced is determined by many factors, including the rate of transcription and splicing of the mRNA, stability of the mRNA, and stability of the protein produced.

## HOW MUTATIONS AFFECT GENE FUNCTION

Any change in DNA sequence that affects the processes of transcription, splicing, or translation will affect the production of protein. A disease-causing mutation may be a deletion of the entire gene, deletion of a part of the gene, or a change of a single base. When considering the effect of a mutation, it is important to work out how it will affect the processes of transcription, splicing, translation, and post-translational modification of a protein (*Table 3.1*).

## Loss of Function Mutations

The mutation abolishes production of protein. This can either be a deletion of the whole gene, or a smaller mutation in a gene that critically affects its ability to be transcribed or translated.

In autosomal dominant diseases, loss of function of one allele may reduce protein production, but will not abolish

**TABLE 3.1** Types of mutation and their effects on protein function

| Mutation | Possible effects on: | | |
| --- | --- | --- | --- |
| | mRNA | Protein production | Protein function |
| Deletion of whole gene | Loss of transcription | No protein produced | – |
| Deletion of promoter | Loss of transcription | No protein produced | – |
| Deletion of three base pairs from exon | Loss of one codon from mRNA | Loss of one amino acid from polypeptide sequence | May have no effect or severe effect depending on importance of amino acid deleted |
| Deletion of one or two base pairs | Loss of one or two base pairs of sequence. mRNA may be unstable and suffer nonsense-mediated decay | Frameshift at translation, leading to highly abnormal protein production after deletion | Likely to have severe effect or create unstable protein that is degraded |
| Single base change altering a splice signal | Abnormal splicing, creating highly abnormal mRNA. mRNA may be unstable and suffer nonsense-mediated decay | Production of an abnormal polypeptide | Likely to have severe effect. If mRNA is not subject to nonsense-mediated decay, unstable protein may be made that is degraded |
| Single base change in an exon, creating a premature stop codon | mRNA sequence includes a premature stop sequence. mRNA may be unstable | Production of polypeptide terminates early | Likely to have severe effect, or create unstable protein that is degraded |
| Single base change in an exon, altering amino acid sequence | mRNA produced incorporating mutant sequence | Production of a polypeptide containing an incorrect amino acid | May have no effect, cause protein to be inactive, or activate protein |

it because there is a second, functioning, allele. In this case there are two possible mechanisms by which mutation may cause disease:

1. Haploinsufficiency: the level of a protein is important, either in absolute terms or in relation to another protein. Loss of a single copy of the gene reduces the amount of protein produced sufficiently to cause a disease phenotype. This mechanism is more likely to be the case for signalling molecules where the exact level of a protein may be critical for normal cell function. Haploinsufficiency is also the mechanism whereby mutations in one of the collagen genes, *COL1A1* or *COL1A2*, cause the milder form of osteogenesis imperfecta, osteogenesis imperfecta type I. Loss of one copy of the collagen gene leads to reduced collagen levels in bone and a tendency to fractures in childhood (see Chapter 12, pp. 356–357).

2. Loss of function of the second copy of the gene during somatic cell division, leading to a cell that has no functioning copy of the gene: this is a common mechanism in inherited cancer syndromes, such as in Lynch syndrome, described in Case History 3.1 and Chapter 9, pp. 270–271.

## Dominant Negative Mutations

A dominant negative mutation is one in which a mutation leads to creation of an abnormal protein, which has an effect on the function of the normal version of the protein that is produced. An example of this is a point mutation in one of the collagen genes *COL1A1* or *COL1A2* which leads to production of an abnormal collagen protein. This abnormal protein is incorporated into the collagen fibril and disrupts formation of normal collagen in bone, leading to a severe deficiency of collagen. This severe collagen deficiency causes a severe form of osteogenesis imperfecta (osteogenesis imperfecta type II) which is usually lethal shortly after birth.

## Gain-of-function Mutations

Rarely, a point mutation may alter the sequence of a gene, and subsequently the protein made, in a way that activates the protein. This can occur in the germline, an example being mutations in the *FGFR3* gene causing achondroplasia. Gain-of-function mutations may also arise somatically, and are commonly observed in the progression of cells to neoplasia.

## Triplet Repeat Disorders

These disorders are caused by a stretch of DNA that has a repeated three-base-pair sequence. In some individuals this 'trinucleotide' repeat has increased in length to cause disease. In conditions such as fragile-X syndrome, there is a very large expansion of repeats outside the coding region of a gene, causing a loss of function by stopping transcription. In other conditions such as Huntington's disease, the expanded allele is translated into a polyglutamine tract in a protein. The expansion of this tract affects protein function and causes a toxic gain of function.

---

**CASE HISTORY 3.1**

### LYNCH SYNDROME (HEREDITARY NON-POLYPOSIS COLORECTAL CANCER)

A 35-year-old man presented with a 4-week history of rectal bleeding. Clinical examination was entirely normal, but a colonoscopy identified a cancer of the transverse colon, which was removed surgically (Fig. 3.18). Pathological examination of the resected colon showed a single 3-cm tumour with no polyps.

A family history was taken (Fig. 3.19). The patient has a brother and a sister who are both in good health. His father died of bowel cancer at the age of 55, and his father's sister was affected with bowel cancer at the age of 48, but is still alive. The young age of onset of bowel cancer in the patient, and the number of affected relatives in the family, are highly suggestive of a hereditary form of bowel cancer. The most common forms of hereditary bowel cancer are familial adenomatous polyposis (FAP) and Lynch syndrome (hereditary non-polyposis colorectal cancer [HNPCC]) (See Chapter 9, pp. 270–271). The absence of polyps elsewhere in the bowel makes FAP unlikely. With three affected individuals, all of whom are first-degree relatives of each other, and at least one of whom is under 50, this family fulfils the modified Amsterdam criteria, and may, therefore have Lynch syndrome.

Lynch syndrome is caused by mutations in genes that are responsible for repair of DNA mismatches. Mutations that cause Lynch syndrome are usually found in the *MLH1*, *MSH2*, and *MSH6* genes. These genes form a complex that scans DNA for mismatches (Fig. 3.20). Patients with Lynch syndrome

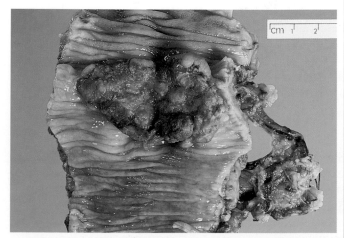

**FIG. 3.18** A plaque-like carcinoma in the transverse colon. (Image provided by Professor Jeremy Jass.)

**3.1 CASE HISTORY**

have one normal and one mutated copy of one of these genes. The disease is, therefore, transmitted through families as an autosomal dominant condition.

As epithelial cells in the colon divide, they are subject to somatic mutations at random in the genome. A cell that loses its remaining functioning copy of the mismatch repair gene will acquire mutations at other sites in the genome more easily (Fig. 3.21). Loss of mismatch repair by cells in a tumour can be seen as microsatellite instability (Fig. 3.22). Only 10–20%

of sporadic colorectal tumours show microsatellite instability, whereas 80–90% of colorectal tumours in individuals with Lynch syndrome show this. Tumours can also be immunostained for MLH1, MSH2, and MSH6 proteins. As loss of the remaining functioning copy of the gene is an early step in tumorigenesis, tumours from individuals with a mutation causing Lynch syndrome are expected to show absence of the protein in which the predisposing mutation lies.

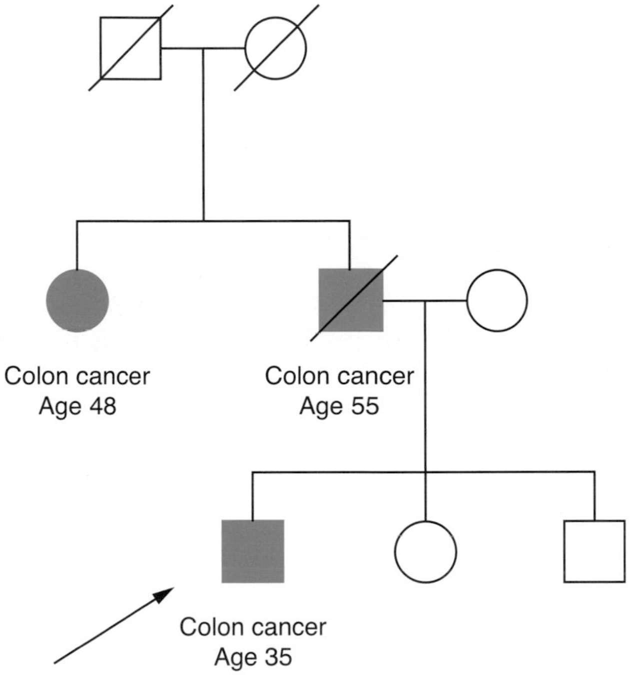

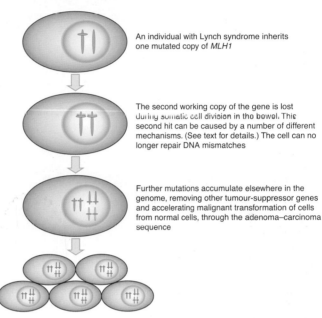

An individual with Lynch syndrome inherits one mutated copy of *MLH1*

The second working copy of the gene is lost during somatic cell division in the bowel. This second hit can be caused by a number of different mechanisms. (See text for details.) The cell can no longer repair DNA mismatches

Further mutations accumulate elsewhere in the genome, removing other tumour-suppressor genes and accelerating malignant transformation of cells from normal cells, through the adenoma–carcinoma sequence

**FIG. 3.21** Loss of the sole functioning copy of the *MLH1* gene during somatic cell division makes a colonic epithelial cell prone to developing further mutations.

Colon cancer
Age 48

Colon cancer
Age 55

Colon cancer
Age 35

**FIG. 3.19** Family tree of the patient.

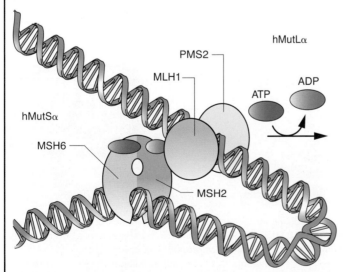

hMutLα

PMS2

MLH1

ATP

ADP

hMutSα

MSH6

MSH2

**FIG. 3.20** The proteins MSH6, MSH2, MLH1, and PMS2 form a complex that scans DNA for mismatched bases and repairs them. (Redrawn from www.uniklinikum-saarland.de.)

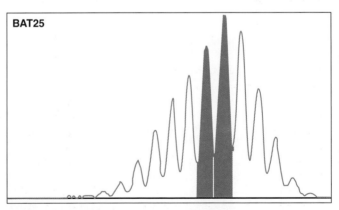

BAT25

**FIG. 3.22** Analysis of microsatellite 'BAT25' in DNA from the patient. Microsatellites are short stretches of repetitive DNA that vary in length between individual copies of the genome. Analysis of DNA extracted from the individual's blood showed two different microsatellite lengths (shaded in the figure), reflecting the two copies of the genome in a diploid individual. Analysis of DNA extracted from the tumour showed multiple different lengths of microsatellite. This occurs because loss of the sole functional copy of *MLH1* causes failure of mismatch repair, and the microsatellite length can change during cell division in multiple cell lineages in the tumour. The tumour is said to show 'microsatellite instability'.

Immunostaining for MLH1, MSH2, and PMS2 in the patient is shown in Fig. 3.23. This shows complete loss of MLH1 protein expression by the tumour cells. The patient was referred to the local genetics service, where a DNA sample was taken and the *MLH1* gene sequenced to look for a mutation. Such a mutation was identified. As a result of this referral, the patient's sister was shown to have the same mutation in the *MLH1* gene and was referred for 2-yearly screening for bowel cancer by colonoscopy. The brother was shown not to carry the mutation, and did not, therefore, require any further investigation.

**Key Points**

- Pathological findings can indicate a genetic predisposition to disease in a family.
- DNA analysis techniques can be used to investigate tumours.
- Where pathological findings or clinical information suggest a genetic predisposition, this should be investigated with, at least, a family history.
- Immunohistochemistry can be used to identify loss of protein expression that may be due to a mutation in the gene.
- Such loss of a protein may guide diagnostic laboratories about which gene to test.
- Identifying a genetic predisposition in a family may have important implications for other family members.

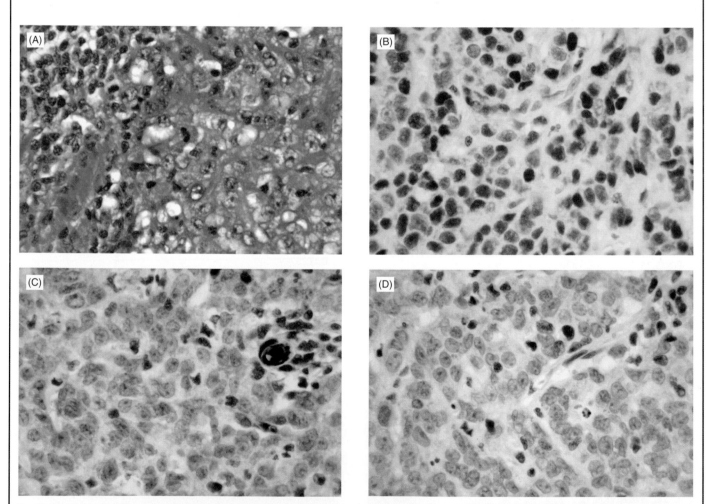

**Fig. 3.23** (A) Poorly differentiated adenocarcinoma of the colon with a chronic inflammatory reaction. (B) Staining for MSH2 shows the presence of protein in both tumour cells and inflammatory cells. (C) Staining for MLH1 shows loss of protein in the tumour cells but the chronic inflammatory cells remain positive, providing an internal control. (D) Staining for PMS2 shows loss of protein. This occurs because PMS2 is stabilized by forming a complex with MLH1, which cannot take place when MLH1 expression is lost. The chronic inflammatory cells remain positive, acting as a positive internal control.

## Molecular Pathology and Cancer Treatment

The majority of pathological analysis involves the microscopic identification of specific cellular morphologies. However, particularly in the case of cancer, the cellular appearance and behaviour are largely controlled by the somatic mutations that have caused altered cellular behaviour. Precise information about a tumour can therefore be obtained by analysing tumour DNA for mutations in genes that lie within specific pathways. Mutations that are important for allowing tumours to grow are commonly referred to as 'driver mutations'. Such driver mutations are increasingly being studied as targets for highly specific treatment. A mutation that identifies a specific therapeutic target is often known as an 'actionable mutation'.

The number of different specific therapeutic targets is increasing rapidly, and will lead to a large increase in molecular DNA analysis as a component of the pathological analysis of cancer. The examples of the Philadelphia chromosome, amenable to treatment with imatinib, or HER2-positive breast cancer treated with trastuzumab, are both excellent early examples of identifying actionable mutations using molecular techniques that subsequently led to specific targeted treatment. Many further examples are coming into clinical practice, such as identification of activating mutations in *BRAF* in melanomas and bowel cancers that can then be treated with specific inhibitors. Although these agents are clinically effective, tumours can evolve through a process of continued somatic mutation and develop resistance to one highly targeted treatment. Therefore, it is envisaged that, in the future, treatment of cancer may involve re-sampling of recurrent tumours and further molecular analysis to identify targets for further specific treatment.

# THE GENETIC BASIS OF COMMON DISEASE

Although mutations in genes causing mendelian inheritance of a disease are comparatively rare, most if not all human diseases are caused by a combination of environmental factors and genetic predisposition.

## Normal Variation in the Genome

Every copy of the human genome contains multiple variations in sequence. These variations are described as polymorphisms, and they do not usually themselves cause disease. They may, however, predispose an individual to disease. Polymorphisms may be a single change of base sequence, in which case they are described as single nucleotide polymorphisms (SNPs) or they may involve deletion or duplication of larger regions of the genome, in which case they are described as copy number variations (CNVs).

The total possible variation in the human genome is considerable. Studies have estimated that 12–18% of the genome is subject to copy number variation. Over 38 million SNPs have been identified in different populations and each has been assigned a unique identifier. Any single individual will have between 3 and 4 million SNPs.

An SNP in a gene may affect the amino acid sequence of a protein or its level of expression, but most SNPs probably have no effect. The frequency of each polymorphism often varies depending on the population studied. The most common method of identifying SNPs that may predispose to a human disease is an association study (see Special Study Topic 3.2). Even where a study shows that an SNP is associ-

## 3.2 Special Study Topic

### MUTATIONS IN THE FILAGGRIN GENE CAUSE ICHTHYOSIS VULGARIS AND PREDISPOSE TO ATOPIC ECZEMA

Using a classic gene-mapping approach it was shown that patients with severe dry and scaly skin (ichthyosis vulgaris) are homozygous for mutations in the filaggrin gene. The skin from a patient with ichthyosis vulgaris is shown in Fig. 3.24. The two most common causative mutations both cause premature termination of the filaggrin polypeptide, and lead to loss of production of the protein profilaggrin from that copy of the gene. There are a number of other mutations in the filaggrin gene, which are less common. Up to 10% of the white population in the UK are carriers of one working and one mutated copy of the filaggrin gene.

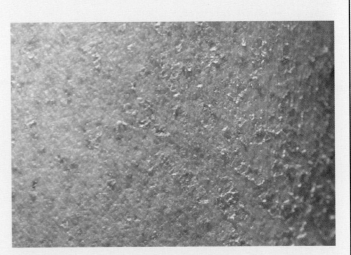

FIG. **3.24** Skin of a patient with ichthyosis vulgaris showing fine scaling and flaking. (Courtesy of Professor Colin Munro.)

# Special Study Topic continued . . .

The filaggrin gene encodes the profilaggrin protein that is expressed in skin epithelium during terminal differentiation. During formation of the cornified layer of the epithelium, it is cleaved into multiple peptides that cause the keratin filaments in the epithelium to aggregate. Loss of filaggrin, therefore, impairs this process (Figs. 3.25 and 3.26).

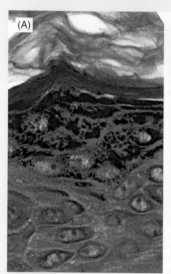 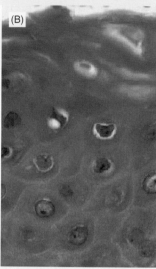

**FIG. 3.25** Histology of (A) normal skin and (B) skin from a patient with ichthyosis vulgaris showing loss of normal keratinization in the upper epidermis.

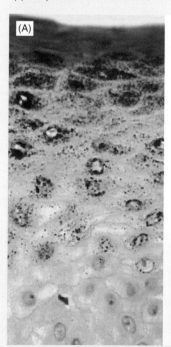 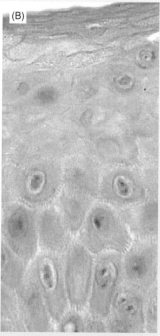

**FIG. 3.26** Immunohistochemical staining for filaggrin in (A) normal skin and (B) skin from a patient with ichthyosis vulgaris. There is no staining for the filaggrin protein in the upper epidermis from the patient, because the patient is homozygous for the *R501X* mutation in the *filaggrin* gene, which abolishes protein production. (Courtesy of Professor Irwin McLean.)

It was noted that members of families with ichthyosis vulgaris who are heterozygous for a filaggrin mutation can show mild ichthyosis. It was also suspected that they have a significantly increased risk of atopic dermatitis (eczema) and asthma. A formal study was therefore carried out to look at the frequency of the common filaggrin mutations in children with eczema or asthma when compared with the general population. An initial association study of 52 Irish children with atopic dermatitis compared with 186 population controls was carried out. The results of this are summarized in *Table 3.2*.

Using the $\chi^2$ test with two degrees of freedom, these data show a highly significant association between mutations in the filaggrin gene and atopic dermatitis ($p < 3 \times 10^{-17}$). This is strongly suggestive, but does not in itself confirm that the mutations in filaggrin themselves cause a high risk of eczema in patients who carry them. Importantly this finding has been confirmed in other populations, in both this study and others.

Proof of causation has required further studies demonstrating the mechanism by which filaggrin deficiency confers a predisposition to atopic disease. This mechanism is currently uncertain. Filaggrin deficiency may lead to a skin barrier that is more permeable to environmental antigens, leading to sensitization. This could explain why children who carry a filaggrin mutation also have a higher risk of asthma. The high prevalence of filaggrin mutations in the population suggests that it has conferred an evolutionary advantage in the past, possibly by improving immunity to severe infections.

**TABLE 3.2** Results of association study

| Filaggrin genotype | Atopic dermatitis patients No. (%) | Population controls No. (%) |
|---|---|---|
| Normal/normal | 23 (44) | 170 (91.5) |
| Normal/mutated | 23 (44) | 16 (8.5) |
| Mutated/mutated | 6 (12) | 0 |
| Total | 52 | 186 |

## Key Points

- All genes can contain polymorphisms, some of which affect protein function.
- This is the basis of genetic variation between humans, and genetic predisposition to common disease.
- A polymorphism in a gene can be tested for association with a common disease phenotype by comparing its frequency in affected and unaffected members of the same population.
- Where an association is found, this needs to be replicated and further studies carried out to demonstrate a biological effect of the polymorphism, before it can be said to be a predisposing factor for the disease process.

ated with a disease, further study is required to confirm this. Where multiple different SNPs are tested and the effect of the SNP is weak, it is not uncommon to have a false-positive result. Even if the result is correct, a different unknown SNP that is in linkage disequilibrium with the one that is being studied may be responsible for the disease association. It is therefore essential that an association study be duplicated in a separate population and further experiments carried out to identify the mechanism by which the SNP causes the predisposition to disease.

## Candidate Gene vs Genome-wide Association Studies

Initial association studies were carried out using a candidate gene approach, analysing individual genes that were felt to be good candidates for predisposition to the disease. In more recent studies, most of the significant genes for multifactorial disorders have been identified using a genome-wide approach, in which large numbers of SNPs, more than 500,000 from across the entire genome, are analysed. This identifies multiple SNPs that associate with a particular phenotype. There are many problems with this approach, including correction for multiple testing and the small size of effect of each SNP, which mean that, in any one study, only a small proportion of the genetic variation is identified. Study samples have to be large with over 1,000, and on occasion over 10,000, cases.

It is now thought that 12–18% of the human genome is copy number variable, with polymorphic duplications or deletions, often involving genes. The optimal methods for studying copy number variation as a contributor to predisposition to human disease have yet to be established.

## Use of Informatics

Given the diversity of human genetic diseases, electronic resources have become an essential tool for addressing clinical problems in genetics. Many websites provide information on genetic diseases, including PubMed, Online Mendelian Inheritance in Man or OMIM (www.ncbi.nlm. nih.gov/entrez/query.fcgi?db=OMIM), and GeneReviews (www.genereviews.org). Databases of laboratories performing mutation analysis of specific genes include the UK genetic testing network (www.ukgtn.org) and GeneTests (www.genetests.org). Information on DNA sequence, known polymorphisms, and chromosomal location of genes can be accessed through Ensembl (www.ensembl.org) or the National Centre for Biotechnology Information (www. ncbi.nlm.nih.gov). Patient self-help group websites can also provide useful resources, particularly for patients, and many can be accessed through the contact-a-family website (www.cafamily.org.uk).

A clinical geneticist will usually have access to other more specialized informatics resources, including the London Dysmorphology and Neurogenetics Genetics databases, which allow identification of syndromes by specific clinical features, the REAMS Database for skeletal dysplasias, and the European Skeletal Dysplasia Network.

## SUMMARY

This chapter has described the basic structure of genes and the processes by which they are translated into proteins. This provides the essential information required to understand how gene changes (mutations and polymorphisms) cause, or predispose to, human disease. The case studies demonstrate the relationship between diagnostic pathology services and clinical genetics, how genetic testing techniques can be used in pathology, and how pathological findings can be important in management of patients in clinical genetics.

## ACKNOWLEDGEMENTS

We thank the following people for assistance in preparation of this manuscript: Jacqueline Dunlop, Clinical Genetics, Ninewells Hospital and Medical School, for critical review of the manuscript. Chris Maliszewska and staff, Cytogenetics Laboratory, Ninewells Hospital and Medical School for review of the manuscript and cytogenetic images. Dr Alan Evans, Dr Shaun Walsh, Dr Lee Jordan, and Professor D Levison, Department of Pathology, Ninewells Hospital, Dundee, for images of gross pathology, histology, and immunohistochemistry. Professor Colin Munro, Department of Dermatology, Southern General Hospital, Glasgow, and Professor Irwin McLean, Dundee, for clinical images and tissue sections of ichthyosis vulgaris. Professor Jeremy Jass, St Marks Hospital Park, London for Fig. 3.18.

## FURTHER READING

Eeles RA, Easton DF, Ponder BAJ, Eng C. *Genetic Predisposition to Cancer*, 2nd edn. London: Hodder, 2004.

Firth HV, Hurst JA, Hall JG. *Oxford Desk Reference – Clinical Genetics*. Oxford: Oxford University Press, 2005.

Palmer CN, Irvine AD, Terron-Kwiatkowski A, *et al*. Common loss-of-function variants of the epidermal barrier protein filaggrin are a major predisposing factor for atopic dermatitis. *Nat Genet* 2006;**38**:441–446.

Ren R. Mechanisms of BCR-ABL in the pathogenesis of chronic myelogenous leukaemia. *Nat Rev Cancer* 2005;**5**:172–183.

Smith FJ, Irvine AD, Terron-Kwiatkowski A, *et al*. Loss-of-function mutations in the gene encoding filaggrin cause ichthyosis vulgaris. *Nat Genet* 2006;**38**:337–342.

Strachan T, Read A. *Human Molecular Genetics*, 4th edn. London: Garland Science, 2011.

Tobias E, Connor M, Fergusson-Smith M. *Essential Medical Genetics*, 6th edn. Oxford: Wiley-Blackwell, 2011.

# 4

# CELL INJURY, INFLAMMATION, AND REPAIR

C Simon Herrington

## INTRODUCTION

Cells are generally able to cope with a range of normal physiological demands, a state referred to as homeostasis. When fluctuations in the environment around the cell are more severe, leading to cellular stress, a number of adaptive responses may occur. These allow the cell to remain viable but may modify its structure and function. Some of these adaptive responses are characterized by changes in cell size or number. An increase in cell size in response to a stimulus is termed hypertrophy, whereas an increase in the number of cells is called hyperplasia. Atrophy is the process by which there is a decrease in the size or number of cells in response to a stimulus, or lack of stimulus. Cells may also adapt by changing their differentiation, so-called metaplasia. These phenomena have been considered in Chapter 2 (see pp. 18–19).

In some circumstances, particularly in the face of a pathological stimulus, the capacity for adaptation is exceeded, leading to cell injury. Initially the events that follow may be reversible and the cell may return to its previously normal state, particularly if the injurious agent is removed. However, if the pathological stimulus is severe enough, or if it is persistent, a point of no return is reached beyond which the cell loses its viability and cell death occurs. This has been discussed in Chapter 2 in the context of normal cellular functions (see p. 17), but here we consider the causes and mechanisms of cell injury and death and then look at the tissue responses to these.

## CELL INJURY AND DEATH

### Causes of Cell Injury

There are many diverse causes of cell injury, from subtle changes occurring because of a genetic mutation leading to a single amino acid change in a polypeptide chain, to massive burns:

- hypoxia (deficiency of oxygen)
- chemical agents and poisons
- infectious agents
- immune-mediated processes
- genetic abnormalities
- nutritional imbalances
- physical agents.

The most common cause in clinical practice is hypoxia where the cell is damaged because aerobic respiration is diminished. Hypoxia can occur when there is a reduction in the blood supply to a tissue, as occurs in myocardial infarction, for example (Fig. 4.1). Such an impairment in the blood supply, called ischaemia, clearly leads to a reduction in the availability of key substances other than oxygen (e.g. glucose). Hypoxia can also occur when there is a reduction in the overall oxygenation of the blood as occurs in cardio-respiratory failure and carbon monoxide poisoning.

Many chemical agents can cause cell injury; even some apparently innocuous substances (e.g. salt) in certain situations and concentrations may bring about cell death. Other agents that can be considered in this category include

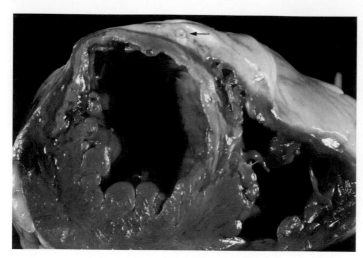

FIG. 4.1 Myocardial infarction. The posterior wall (top) is thinned and there is an area of yellow discoloration representing dead myocardium. A coronary artery (arrow) is seen; this is occluded by complicated atheroma.

adverse effects of prescribed medications, poisons such as arsenic, environmental pollutants, and recreational drugs such as alcohol. The range of infectious agents that cause cell and tissue injury, and some of the mechanisms by which this occurs, are discussed in Chapter 19. With some pathogenic organisms cell injury is a direct result of products of the infectious agent, whereas in others much of the injury is a 'bystander' phenomenon, where the cell gets in the way of the host's immune response to the pathogen. Immunological reactions are also a cause of cell injury when there is an exaggerated response to a foreign protein (anaphylaxis) or there is breakdown of the normal tolerance mechanisms to self-antigens (autoimmune disease).

Genetic diseases can lead to cell injury by a variety of mechanisms. At one extreme there are gross chromosomal abnormalities which lead to major congenital malformations (e.g. trisomy 18) and, at the other, single base mutations in a gene leading to a protein product that is abnormally folded and cannot be exported from the cell (e.g. $\alpha_1$-antitrypsin deficiency). Many inherited metabolic abnormalities are caused by a genetically determined enzyme defect or deficiency; these may have consequences for only one tissue or organ system but most commonly have systemic effects.

Nutritional imbalances can also be gross, such as that seen in protein–calorie malnutrition (kwashiorkor) which sadly remains a common condition in certain parts of the world, or more subtle, e.g. a vitamin deficiency. It is important to recognize, however, that nutritional imbalances are not always due to a lack of nutrients: the cell injury associated with excess nutrients is becoming increasingly common. Obesity and the associated metabolic syndrome are a major cause of serious disease, particularly in western countries. Physical agents that cause cell injury include extremes of temperature and atmospheric pressure, radiation, direct and indirect mechanical trauma, and electrical currents.

## Mechanisms of Cell Injury

### Key Points

- Subcellular targets of injury include mitochondria, membranes, DNA, and the cytoskeleton.
- Some changes of cell injury are potentially reversible.
- Examples of sublethal injury include vacuolar degeneration, fatty change, and accumulation of cytoskeletal proteins.

Cell injury results from disruption to the structure and function of one or more subcellular components; the precise mechanisms vary depending on the nature, duration, and severity of the injurious stimulus. The key targets for injury are: interference with aerobic respiration in mitochondria, cell membranes (both at the surface and those of intracellular organelles), DNA, protein synthetic pathways, and the cytoskeleton (Fig. 4.2).

Interference with the process of oxidative phosphorylation in mitochondria leads to a reduction in adenosine triphosphate (ATP), and therefore impairs many key biochemical processes in the cell. This is a central mechanism in hypoxic injury and is also a feature of some chemical injury. Reduction in ATP reduces the activity of the sodium pump at the cell membrane, leading to gross changes in intracellular sodium and potassium concentrations, the net result of which is an influx of water across the membranes, causing the cell to swell. Continued ATP depletion interferes with protein production. There is also failure of intracellular

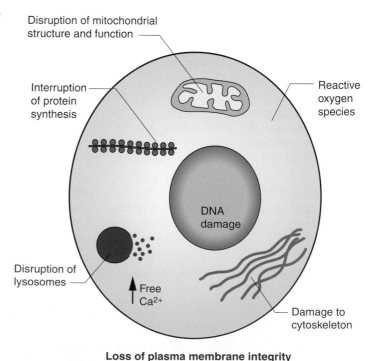

FIG. 4.2 Key targets of cellular injury. Individual agents may disrupt more than one subcellular compartment.

calcium homeostasis. Normally calcium concentrations in the cytosol are low. This is important because calcium can activate cytosolic enzymes that could destroy cellular components. The calcium levels are kept in check by ATP-dependent enzymes. With a reduction in ATP as occurs in hypoxia there is a dramatic increase in cellular calcium leading to activation of (1) phospholipases that break down membranes, (2) endonucleases that degrade DNA, and (3) proteases that also destroy membranes and other cytosolic components such as the cytoskeleton. Increased cytosolic calcium can also further damage mitochondria, leading to a vicious cycle; this can be a key event in progression to a point of no return for the cell – irreversible injury or cell death (Fig. 4.3).

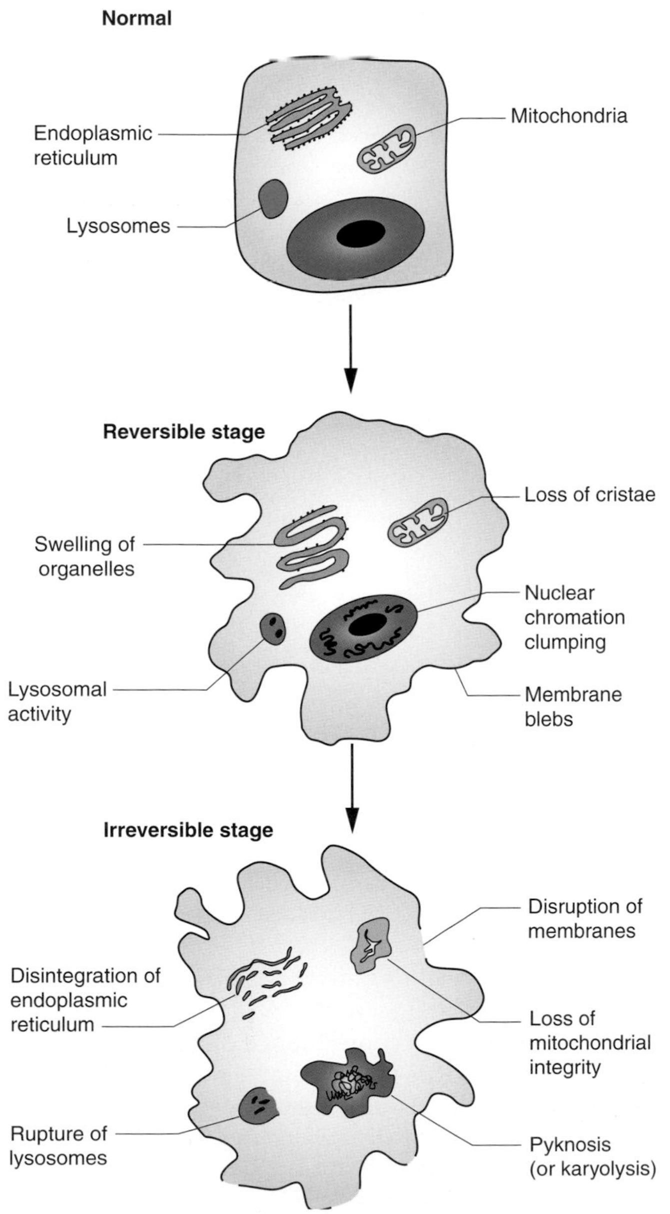

Another biochemical pathway that is now recognized to be important in cell injury involves so-called reactive oxygen species (Fig. 4.4). These are by-products of normal cellular respiration and are partially reduced oxygen molecules including $OH^-$, $O^-_2$, and $H_2O_2$. These are free radicals, i.e. they are chemical compounds with a single unpaired electron; they are highly reactive and interact with adjacent molecules, releasing energy but also potentially altering the molecules. Normally, there are efficient intracellular homeostatic mechanisms that prevent injury by such free radicals, but in some situations the normal defence mechanisms (which include antioxidants such as vitamin E and enzymes such as glutathione peroxidase and superoxide dismutase) are overwhelmed and free radicals interact with lipids in cell membranes (peroxidation), cellular proteins, and DNA, leading to breaks in its continuity. The imbalance between free radical generation and scavenging that occurs in injury is referred to as oxidative stress. Free radicals can be generated by a variety of processes and are thought to be important in so-called reperfusion injury (this occurs after restoration of blood flow in ischaemic tissues), chemical injury, and radiation damage.

It is important to recognize that, although the relative importance of these various mechanisms varies depending on the injurious agent, a common theme is the disruption of membranes. We have already seen that ATP depletion affects the plasma membrane, whereas the calcium-modulated

**Normal**

Endoplasmic reticulum

Lysosomes

Mitochondria

**Reversible stage**

Swelling of organelles

Lysosomal activity

Loss of cristae

Nuclear chromation clumping

Membrane blebs

**Irreversible stage**

Disintegration of endoplasmic reticulum

Rupture of lysosomes

Disruption of membranes

Loss of mitochondrial integrity

Pyknosis (or karyolysis)

FIG. 4.3 Overview of changes during the reversible and irreversible phases of cellular injury. Note that the precise point of no return is not fully established but loss of membrane integrity appears to be an important factor.

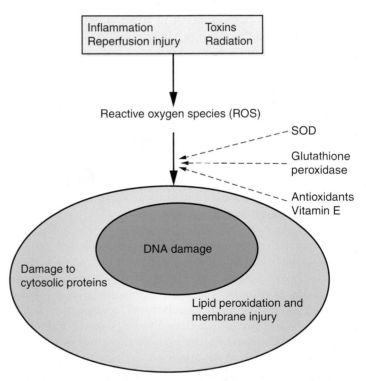

Inflammation    Toxins
Reperfusion injury    Radiation

Reactive oxygen species (ROS)

SOD

Glutathione peroxidase

Antioxidants Vitamin E

DNA damage

Damage to cytosolic proteins

Lipid peroxidation and membrane injury

FIG. 4.4 Role of reactive oxygen species in cellular injury. Several molecular structures are generated during cellular injury that can damage membranes, proteins, and nucleic acids. A number of inherent antioxidant compounds are present within the cell to limit the damage. Cellular injury due to reactive oxygen species occurs when these normal defence mechanisms are overwhelmed. SOD = superoxide dismutase.

activation of phospholipases interferes with all membranes. Free radical-induced lipid peroxidation further damages their structures. Activation of proteases can also disrupt the cytoskeleton and, as this is anchored to the plasma membrane, there is further damage to the overall structure of the cell. Disruption of lysosomal membranes leads to escalation of the cell injury. These organelles are packets of highly reactive enzymes including DNAases and proteases; release of these enzymes into the cytosol almost inevitably leads to the demise of the cell.

### Reversible and Sublethal Injury

As noted above some of the changes that occur in cell injury are thought to be potentially reversible. Several manifestations of this sublethal injury can be recognized histologically; some of these may in fact be adaptive responses of the cell. One of the earliest changes detected is swelling of the cytoplasm. The cells may become vacuolated (hence the term 'vacuolar degeneration'). This is a reflection of the inability of the cell to regulate the ionic and fluid balance across the plasma membrane as a result of ATP depletion. There is electron microscopic evidence of disruption of the membranes; blebs are seen and points of contact with adjacent cells become loosened. Mitochondria may also be swollen and there may be subtle changes in the nuclear structure. Another common manifestation of sublethal injury is the accumulation of triglycerides in the cell – fatty change or steatosis. This is most commonly seen in liver injury (Fig. 4.5) but can occur at other sites such as heart and skeletal muscle. The mechanisms for the accumulation are complex but include impairment of fatty acid oxidation, increased generation of free fatty acids. and reduction in apolipoprotein production.

Cytoskeletal abnormalities can also be seen microscopically. The most common forms are an accumulation of intermediate filaments. This is the basis for the so-called Mallory bodies seen in liver disease (see Chapter 10, p. 280) and the neurofibrillary tangles seen in neurodegenerative disorders such as Alzheimer's disease (Fig. 4.6). This is thought to be partly a consequence of misfolding of the intermediate filament proteins as a consequence of the injury and partly a failure of the normal mechanisms for getting rid of abnormal intracellular proteins – the so-called proteasomes. Other compounds can accumulate within cells: these include cholesterol and cholesterol esters (an important process in the development of atherosclerosis), glycogen (seen in some inborn errors of metabolism), and pigments. The last include lipofuscin, a yellow–brown pigment present in lysosomes, which accumulates where there has been previous lipid peroxidation. Iron may also accumulate in cells as a response to injury; it may be a localized phenomenon, e.g. surrounding an area of haemorrhage, or form part of a systemic disorder where iron is deposited in different tissues, as occurs in genetic haemochromatosis (see Chapter 10, pp. 281–283). In the latter the accumulation in cells is referred to as haemosiderosis or iron overload.

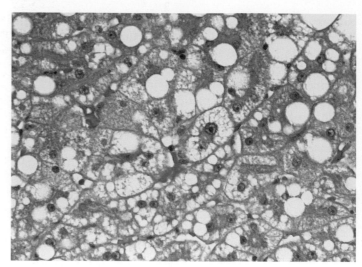

**FIG. 4.5** Simple fatty liver: most of the hepatocytes contain pale droplets; in some cells this is a large single droplet, in others there are smaller droplets. In this case lipid accumulation in hepatocytes has occurred as a consequence of excess alcohol.

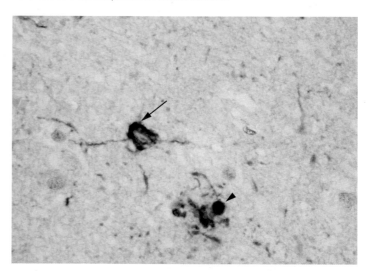

**FIG. 4.6** Neurofibrillary tangles in Alzheimer's disease. Tau protein is seen in an astrocyte (arrow) and in a plaque (arrowhead). (Courtesy of Professor David Ellison.)

## Cell Death

### Key Points

- There are two distinct pathways of irreversible cell death: necrosis and apoptosis.
- Necrosis is always a consequence of injury and is associated with loss of membrane integrity.
- Apoptosis is a more regulated process – programmed cell death – which may be physiological or pathological.

The precise point beyond which reversible injury becomes irreversible is not yet fully defined. As noted above a pathway common to most forms of injury is disruption to membranes and there may be a level beyond which cell viability is no longer possible. Another may be irreversible mitochondrial dysfunction. Loss of cell viability – cell death – is thought to occur through two major and distinct pathways: necrosis and apoptosis. These are different biological processes, occur in different disease states, and are morphologically distinguishable. Necrosis is the form of cell death that generally follows the sequence of events described above, culminating ultimately in loss of membrane integrity, whereas apoptosis is a more tightly regulated pathway, often described as programmed cell death if it occurs as part of a predetermined, genetically regulated process (see Chapter 2, p. 14). Necrosis often involves a group of cells within a tissue whereas apoptosis involves single cells; necrosis is generally accompanied by a host inflammatory response whereas this does not happen with apoptosis. Apoptosis may be a physiological phenomenon. It is thought to play a key role in the programmed remodelling of tissues during embryogenesis and in the shaping of the immune system with the programmed deletion of autoreactive T cells.

## Necrosis

Necrosis is the death of cells with loss of membrane integrity and enzymatic destruction of the cellular constituents.

This leads to leakage of cell constituents into the surrounding tissue and the circulation. There is an inflammatory response to these cellular constituents and the initiation of a repair process.

The microscopic changes that occur in necrosis reflect these key processes. Necrotic cells stain pink with routine (haematoxylin and eosin) stains: this identifies denatured proteins produced by the action of lysosomal enzymes. The cells lose definition under the microscope; this reflects loss of organelles, again because of the effects of phospholipases and proteases. Nuclear changes are an important feature: there may be loss of staining of the nucleus (karyolysis), shrinkage of the nucleus (pyknosis: more characteristically seen in apoptosis), and fragmentation of the nucleus (karyorrhexis). Eventually the nucleus disappears completely. Calcium may be deposited in the dead cells, a process referred to as dystrophic calcification. It is important to recognize that the histological changes are identifiable microscopically only after several hours. There are several different types of necrosis defined by morphological features (Figs 4.7 and 4.8).

The most frequently encountered is coagulative necrosis in which cell outlines are initially maintained but the protein constituents coagulate. To the naked eye, the area of

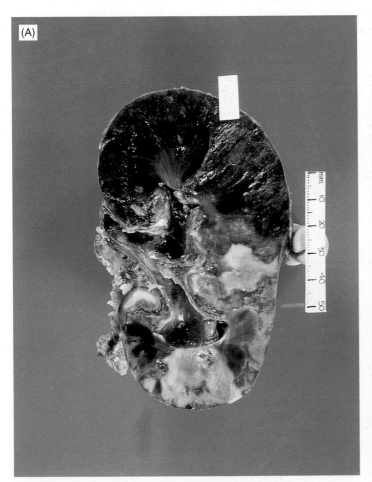 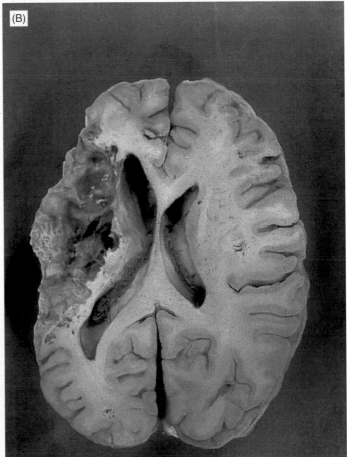

**FIG. 4.7** Common forms of necrosis. (A) Renal infarction: well-defined areas of renal parenchyma have undergone coagulative necrosis due to an embolus in a renal artery. (Courtesy of Dr Katrina Wood.) (B) Cerebral infarction resulting in colliquative necrosis. (Courtesy of Professor David Ellison.)

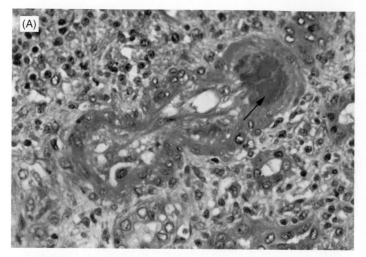

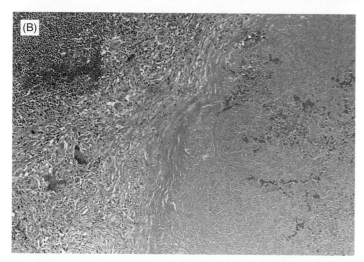

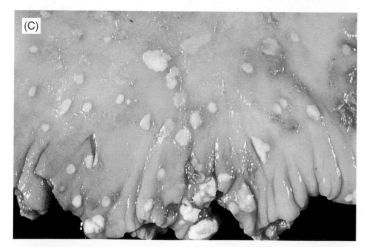

necrosis appears pale yellow/white but initially of normal consistency. Histological examination shows loss of nuclear staining with increased eosinophilia of the cytoplasm, but retention of the cellular outlines. These are gradually lost and eventually the extracellular tissue architecture breaks down. At this stage the tissue is soft and autolysed. Inflammatory cells infiltrate the necrotic tissue to phagocytose and digest the dead cellular debris.

Colliquative or liquefactive necrosis is seen in the lipid-rich tissues of the central nervous system. The lack of extracellular architecture and the high lipid content lead to liquefaction of the necrotic nervous tissue. Caseous necrosis is seen in tuberculosis (TB). There is an amorphous white centre to the granulomas in TB as a consequence of the tissue digestion by activated macrophages. Fibrinoid necrosis is seen in the special circumstances of vascular damage. It is characterized by platelet activation, fibrin deposition, and usually cell death of the vascular smooth muscle. The terms 'fat necrosis' and 'gangrenous necrosis' (which refers to necrosis with putrefaction) are commonly used in clinical practice.

## Apoptosis

Apoptosis is programmed cell death in which the cell initiates a genetic cell death programme via extrinsic and intrinsic pathways in response to a range of stimuli. It leads to the deletion of individual cells, the membrane remaining intact, with engulfment and destruction of the cellular remains by adjacent cells or macrophages (Fig. 4.9). An inflammatory response is not generally seen in apoptosis. The cells undergo shrinkage with condensation and fragmentation of the nuclear chromatin. Individual cells are affected

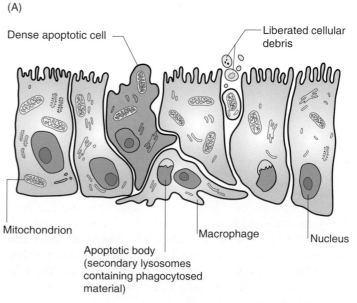

(A)

Dense apoptotic cell

Liberated cellular debris

Mitochondrion

Apoptotic body (secondary lysosomes containing phagocytosed material)

Macrophage

Nucleus

**FIG. 4.9** (A) Scheme of events in apoptosis.

**FIG. 4.8** Other forms of necrosis. (A) Fibrinoid necrosis: in this artery there is accumulation of a fibrin-like substance (arrow) in the media. In this case it is part of a generalized systemic vasculitis. (Courtesy of Dr Katrina Wood.) (B) Caseous necrosis: this is granulomatous inflammation with degeneration at the centre of the lesion, a characteristic feature of tuberculosis. (Courtesy of Dr Fiona Black.) (C) Fat necrosis: in this case destruction of the peritoneal fatty tissue has resulted from the release of lipases after pancreatitis.

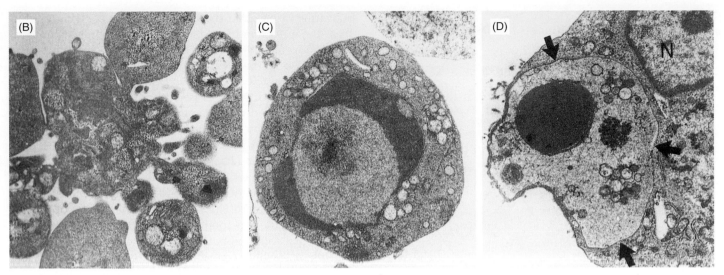

FIG. 4.9 (Continued) The accompanying electron micrographs in B–D demonstrate the changes at an ultrastructural level. (B) Cellular shrinkage and blebbing; (C) nuclear condensation; (D) phagocytosis within a neighbouring cell in which its own nucleus (N) is normal. The boundaries of the phagosome are arrowed. (Courtesy of Professor Andrew Wyllie.)

rather than numerous adjacent cells, as seen in necrosis. As noted above, apoptosis may occur under physiological circumstances. In some situations it could be thought of as a defence mechanism, providing a means of eliminating cells that are no longer required or that have acquired potentially dangerous properties, e.g. significant DNA damage. It is, however, also the mechanism for cell loss in a number of pathological conditions:

- some forms of radiation injury
- elimination of tumour cells (including action of anti-cancer agents)
- elimination of cells infected with virus (e.g. hepatitis)
- neurodegenerative conditions.

Apoptotic cells may be difficult to detect by conventional light microscopy. A number of cellular markers such as the binding of dyes (annexin V) and the demonstration of fragmented DNA using the TUNEL (terminal deoxynucleotidyl transferase dUTP nick end labelling) method can help (Fig. 4.10), and DNA fragmentation can also be shown in cellular extracts by the technique of DNA laddering although it is probably best identified by electron microscopy. The cells are smaller than their normal counterparts and have a dense cytoplasm with tightly packed organelles. The most dramatic features are seen in the nucleus where there is condensation of the chromatin; the nucleus may become fragmented. Small fragments of the cell bud off: these are called apoptotic bodies. The apoptotic cells and apoptotic bodies are then engulfed by macrophages or other adjacent cells. By contrast, with necrosis there is not thought to be appreciable loss of membrane integrity until the very last stages of the process.

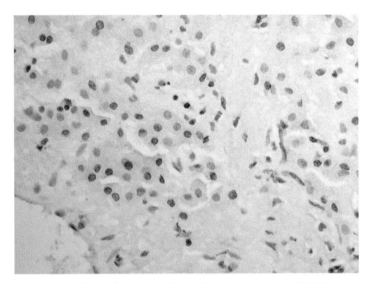

FIG. 4.10 Labelling of nuclei in cells undergoing apoptosis (TUNEL method). In this case the injury has been induced in the liver during radiofrequency ablation of a tumour. (Courtesy of Dr Helen Robertson.)

In common with necrosis, apoptosis involves the activation of cellular enzymes. Apoptosis does not, however, involve the 'blunderbuss' approach seen in necrosis, but rather employs a group of proteases that are particularly active in destroying the proteins of the nuclear membranes and skeleton and can in turn activate DNAases that degrade nuclear DNA. These so-called caspases are found in normal cells but apoptosis is only initiated when these become catalytically active. There are three major phases of apoptosis: (1) initiation or induction, (2) execution, and (3) phagocytosis.

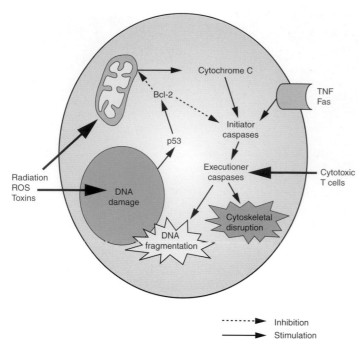

- - - - - - - - ▶ Inhibition
―――――――▶ Stimulation

**FIG. 4.11** Role of caspases in apoptosis. Note: the caspase system can be activated via a variety of routes. The common result is DNA fragmentation and disruption of the cytoskeleton. TNF = tumour necrosis factor; ROS = reactive oxygen species.

The first phase principally involves two distinct but overlapping pathways, which both lead to activation of caspases that go on to stimulate the execution phase (Fig. 4.11). One pathway involves cell surface 'death receptors' that span the membranes of many cells. These are members of the tumour necrosis factor (TNF) receptor family of proteins, of which the best characterized are type I TNF receptors and a related protein, Fas. When these are linked to their ligands, several molecules come together to form a binding site for another protein, which also has a cytoplasmic 'death domain' (so-called Fas-associated death domain or FADD). This in turn activates one of the caspases (caspase 8), and there is then a cascade reaction whereby other procaspases are sequentially and rapidly activated.

The other pathway involves mitochondria. In normal cells, there are anti-apoptotic molecules present in the membranes of mitochondria. These belong to the Bcl-2 family of proteins, most notably Bcl-2 itself and Bcl-x. Their presence is stimulated by growth factors and other normal survival signals. In circumstances of cellular stress or where the cell is deprived of its normal survival signals, there is loss of the anti-apoptotic proteins and these are replaced by pro-apoptotic members of the same family such as Bax. With the reduction in Bcl-2 and Bcl-x, the mitochondrial membranes become leaky (so-called mitochondrial permeability transition). One of the proteins that then escapes from the mitochondria is cytochrome C, an enzyme involved in respiration. In the cytosol, this protein binds to another protein Apaf-1 (apoptosis-activating factor 1), which is capable of

activating caspases. At the same time other proteins leak out from the mitochondria, which further encourage apoptosis.

It is now recognized that there are other ways to stimulate the initiation pathway. We know, for example, that cytotoxic T lymphocytes release compounds such as granzyme B, which lead to the executioner phase without the involvement of a transmembrane death receptor complex or mitochondrial changes. Radiation and free radicals can also set the pathways in motion by inducing DNA damage and activating the tumour-suppressor *TP53* gene, which codes for the p53 protein. p53 has been termed the guardian of the genome, arresting the cell cycle under these circumstances to allow time for DNA repair. If there is no repair, p53 induces apoptosis by upregulating the pro-apoptotic signals Bax and Apaf-1.

The final common pathway, which comprises the execution phase, involves more members of the caspase family. These are all proteases that have a cysteine amino acid at their active site. The members of the family involved in the executioner phase are caspases 3 and 6; on catalytic activation these enzymes degrade nuclear proteins, including those involved in regulating gene transcription and DNA repair, and activate DNAases leading to cleavage of nuclear DNA. Other effects include alteration of cytoskeletal proteins, contributing to cell shrinkage.

Cells undergoing apoptosis secrete factors and express molecules on their surface that facilitate uptake either by macrophages or by adjacent cells; it is this efficient uptake of apoptotic cells that explains the lack of a significant inflammatory response compared with necrosis.

# INFLAMMATION

Inflammation and repair are the local responses initiated to limit the damage caused by tissue injury, infection, toxins, and ischaemia, and to aid recovery from tissue damage. Despite their primary role as defence mechanisms, the inflammatory response and repair processes may contribute to the tissue damage seen in many diseases.

The term 'inflammatory response' encompasses a whole range of processes designed to limit tissue injury. For convenience and to aid understanding, the inflammatory response is divided into acute inflammation and chronic inflammation, based largely on temporal features but also on the different cells involved in the process.

## Acute Inflammation

### Initial Response to Tissue Injury

- Vascular phase of increased flow
- Exudate formation
- Neutrophil polymorph infiltration of tissue
- Bacterial phagocytosis and killing
- Resolution, suppuration, organization, or chronicity.

Acute inflammation is the initial response to tissue injury in most circumstances and the main causes are:

- bacterial infection
- hypersensitivity reactions
- physical agents such as radiation
- chemical reagents including toxins
- tissue necrosis following infarction.

It is of short duration, initiated within minutes and lasting for several hours or a few days. Its main function is the delivery of cells and mediators to the site of injury by the bloodstream; therefore, the vasculature has a central role in coordinating the inflammatory response. Acute inflammation can be considered to comprise two phases: the vascular phase and the cellular phase. These usually coexist in any one inflammatory response, with the vascular phase occurring earlier and merging with the later cellular phase of acute inflammation. Inflamed tissue has characteristic morphological features as a consequence of the vascular and cellular changes described classically as the cardinal signs of inflammation (Fig. 4.12):

- redness
- heat
- swelling
- pain
- loss of function.

### Vascular Phase of Acute Inflammation

#### Key Points

- At sites of injury there are marked changes in blood flow.
- An initial phase of vasoconstriction is followed by prolonged vasodilatation.
- Increased vascular permeability accompanies the vasodilatation and this leads to the formation of a protein-rich exudate and tissue oedema.

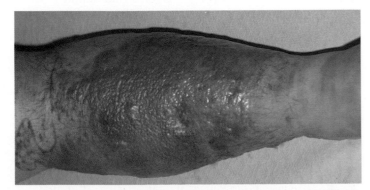

**FIG. 4.12** Cellulitis. Note: swelling and reddening of the skin. (Courtesy of Dr Clifford Lawrence.)

### Changes in Blood Flow

One of the earliest features of the acute inflammatory response is an alteration in the flow of blood to the injured site. It starts with early transient vasoconstriction, mediated by contraction of smooth muscle within arterioles, which leads to a short-lived reduction in blood flow to the injured site. This is followed by vasodilatation, achieved by relaxation of arteriolar smooth muscle and distension of capillaries within the injured site. This vasodilatation is more sustained and can last for many hours. The increased blood flow to inflamed tissue gives it the characteristic red and warm appearance. This series of events allows the increased delivery of molecules and cells involved in acute inflammation (Fig. 4.13).

Following on from increased blood flow there is a gradual slowing of the circulation through inflamed tissue. This is achieved partly by the dilatation of capillaries and partly

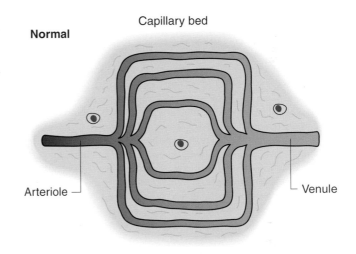

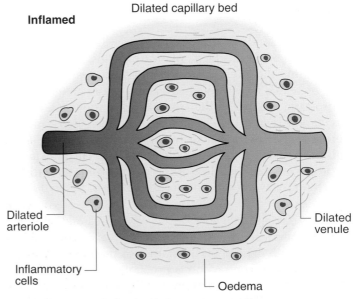

**FIG. 4.13** Overview of the vascular changes in acute inflammation.

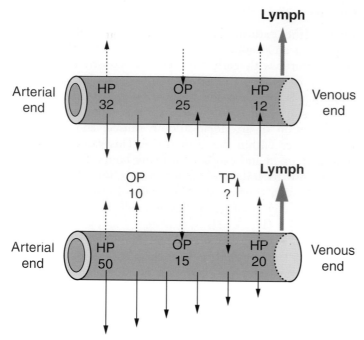

**FIG. 4.14** Exchange of fluid by ultrafiltration across the wall of small blood vessels. Hydrostatic pressure (HP) and osmotic pressure (OP) represent the difference between the hydrostatic and colloid osmotic pressures (in millimetres of mercury or mmHg) of plasma and extravascular space. The solid arrows indicate the net movement of fluid in and out of vessels along their length. The interrupted arrows indicate the direction of forces exerted by HP, OP, and tissue pressure (TP). Upper figure, normal tissue: fluid movement across the vessel wall approximates to equilibrium. Lower figure, acute inflammation: much more fluid leaves the vessels than is returned to them. The values of HP and OP are approximations. In inflammation, HP may be less than indicated because of the rise in TP and the reduction in OP: the latter is due to the escape of plasma protein via endothelial gaps into the extravascular space, which increases OP in the extravascular fluid (shown as 10 mmHg). The level of TP varies depending on the nature of the tissue involved. In loose tissue, TP will show no increase, whereas, in tissues that are tightly tethered or have fibrous capsules, TP can rise considerably (hence the question mark in this figure).

by altered vascular permeability as capillary endothelium becomes more permeable to plasma proteins. The leakage of protein into the interstitium contributes to oedema formation. Increased flow through arterioles causes an increase in hydrostatic pressure at the arterial end of the tissue microcirculation (Fig. 4.14). Combined with increased capillary permeability this causes an increase in fluid moving from within the blood vessels to the tissue spaces. The fluid is rich in protein so there is a loss of the normal osmotic gradient, which normally opposes the accumulation of tissue fluid.

### Increased Vascular Permeability

Vascular permeability is increased by several different mechanisms, which depend on the nature of the injurious agent. Endothelial cell contraction is probably the most common mechanism. It occurs predominantly in venules and is a response to inflammatory mediators including histamine, bradykinin, and leukotrienes. It is a rapidly occurring event

and is short-lived (up to 30 minutes). Typically this alteration affects venules between 20 μm and 60 μm in diameter, but does not appear to affect capillaries or arterioles.

Direct endothelial injury may occur in diseases in which vascular damage is part of the tissue injury. This type of alteration in vascular permeability is seen after burns and in some bacterial infections. There may be some delay between the time of injury and the leakage of protein-rich exudate, to allow the development of the full process of cell death and detachment from the vessel wall. These changes can affect all of the microvessels, arterioles, capillaries, and venules. The leakage of a protein-rich exudate is sustained until the vessels either become occluded with thrombus or are repaired.

Leukocyte-mediated injury to vessels occurs when the white blood cell release of cytotoxic agents causes endothelial damage. This is characteristically seen in vasculitis. The leakage of an exudate occurs from the time of endothelial loss and is sustained throughout the duration of disease activity as new endothelial cells become targets for leukocyte-mediated damage. In the neoangiogenesis associated with the repair process (see below) there is loss of a protein-rich exudate from these healthy but immature capillaries. There are many mediators of these different mechanisms of the vascular phase of the inflammatory response. The biochemical nature of these agents is discussed in detail below.

These properties of the vascular phase of the acute inflammatory response lead to the formation of a protein-rich exudate, consequent tissue oedema, and increased blood viscosity, coupled with reduced flow which leads to stasis. The proteins within the exudates include immunoglobulins, complement components, coagulation factors, and kinins, all of which contribute to the inflammatory response. These events allow the next stage, the cellular phase of acute inflammation, to occur. This cellular phase involves the migration of white blood cells, particularly neutrophils, from the circulation into the site of tissue injury.

### Cellular Phase of the Acute Inflammatory Response

The cellular phase of acute inflammation involves the movement of white blood cells, particularly neutrophils, from the circulation into the site of tissue damage where they act to limit the extent of injury. This involves several different stages and again the endothelial cells play a key role (Fig. 4.15).

#### Margination and Adhesion

During the slowing of blood flow, which occurs as part of the vascular phase of the acute inflammatory response, the larger white blood cells move from a central axial position in flowing blood to a peripheral position. In the microcirculation these white blood cells can be seen adjacent to the endothelium. As the blood flows slowly along the microcirculation, the white blood cells roll on the endothelial surface. This process is known as margination. During rolling the white blood cells become increasingly adherent to the

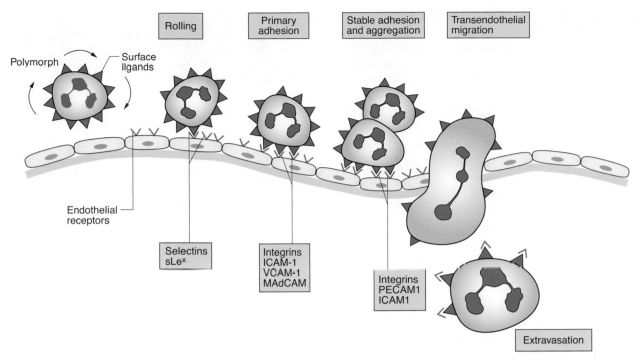

FIG. 4.15 Margination of leukocytes, endothelial adhesion, and leukocyte emigration. PECAM = platelet/endothelial cell adhesion molecule; ICAM = intercellular adhesion molecule; VCAM = vascular cell adhesion molecule; MAdCAM = mucosal addressin cell adhesion molecule.

endothelial cell surface. This leukocyte endothelial adhesion is achieved by the expression on the surface of activated endothelial cells of a family of molecules known as selectins. Selectins recognize specific carbohydrate groups found on the surface of neutrophils and macrophages, the most important of which is the sialyl-Lewis X (sLex) molecule. The interactions between sialyl-Lewis X and selectins increase the stickiness between leukocytes and endothelial cells. The adhesion between leukocytes and endothelial cells becomes firmer by interactions between other adhesion molecules, especially members of the immunoglobulin supergene family on the endothelial surface and integrins on the leukocytes. The immunoglobulin gene superfamily adhesion molecules include intercellular adhesion molecule-1 (ICAM-1) and vascular cell adhesion molecule-1 (VCAM-1), whereas the main integrins are members of the $\beta_1$ family expressed on the surface of leukocytes. These molecules allow much tighter adhesion and stabilize the interactions between leukocytes and endothelial cells.

Obviously the response of endothelial cells on activation adjacent to tissue injury is critical in signalling to leukocytes in the circulation. Expression of cell adhesion molecules is controlled in several different ways in these cell types. Molecules such as P-selectin are stored preformed in endothelial cells in Weibel–Palade bodies. On stimulation of the endothelial cells by histamine or platelet-activating factor, the P-selectin within these cytoplasmic storage granules is rapidly redistributed to the cell surface within minutes. Thus the expression of P-selectin on the endothelium is an important early mechanism for attracting leukocytes to a

site of inflammation. Other adhesion molecules, including E-selectin, ICAM-1, and VCAM-1, are expressed by new protein synthesis. On stimulation of the endothelial cells by proinflammatory cytokines such as TNF or interleukin 1 (IL-1) there is transcriptional activation of the genes encoding these proteins. This level of control of adhesion molecules requires between 4 and 6 hours of stimulation but can be sustained for hours or days.

Finally, in the regulation of leukocyte endothelial interactions, there may be alteration in the relative avidity of the two groups of molecules for each other. This is particularly seen during the activation of leukocytes when integrins of the $\beta_1$ family undergo conformational changes that increase their avidity for adhesion molecules on the endothelial surface such as ICAM-1.

The importance of leukocyte endothelial interactions is emphasized in a group of diseases collectively known as leukocyte adhesion deficiencies. Of these the best described is deficiency of the leukocyte expression of $\beta_1$-integrin. Patients with this inherited disorder are susceptible to recurrent bacterial infections, which they clear rather poorly, suffering more extensive tissue damage than would be seen in unaffected individuals.

Leukocyte Migration (Fig. 4.15)

After attachment, leukocytes pass between adjacent endothelial cells and exit from the circulation. The endothelial cells retract and the leukocytes migrate on the endothelial surface, using the above adhesion molecules and possibly others, including platelet/endothelial cell adhesion molecule-1 (PECAM-1 or CD31). Leukocytes pass through the endothelial basement membrane, probably by enzymatic degradation of the extracellular matrix, and then migrate towards the site of injury by a process known as chemotaxis. This is directional migration in which the leukocytes sense and respond to a concentration gradient of chemotaxins. A variety of important molecules in the inflammatory process behave as chemotaxins, in particular the C3a and C5a components of complement, leukotriene B$_4$ (LTB$_4$) and IL-8. Leukocyte migration further into the inflamed site occurs on the extracellular matrix. The cells move by the extension of an anterior pseudopod, with attachment to extracellular matrix molecules such as fibronectin mediated via adhesion molecules at the anterior end of the pseudopod. The cell body is then pulled forward by the action of actin and myosin filaments which insert into the adhesion complex.

## Phagocytosis

Once neutrophils accumulate within the inflammatory focus they are involved in clearing the injurious agent, e.g. bacteria, by the process known as phagocytosis (Figs 4.16 and 4.17). This involves the cellular events of attachment, engulfment, and killing of bacteria by inflammatory cells.

The first event is recognition and attachment. Most microorganisms and particles to be phagocytosed by neutrophils and macrophages must be coated by opsonins, of which there are three main families: immunoglobulin, complement, and carbohydrate molecules. Immunoglobulins may bind specifically to antigens on the bacterial surface, leaving exposed their Fc fragments, which are recognized by Fc receptors on the neutrophil surface. Activation of complement (directly by bacterial surfaces by the alternative pathway or by the classic pathway after antibody binding to bacterial surfaces) generates the C3b fragment of complement. This, the opsonic fragment, can be recognized by C3b receptors on the neutrophil surface. Finally carbohydrate-binding proteins or lectins circulating in plasma may bind to sugar residues on bacterial cell walls, particularly via mannose sugars. These receptors in turn can be recognized by neutrophils. For all three of these recognition phenomena, binding and cross-linking of receptors allow progression to engulfment.

During engulfment, cytoplasmic extensions or pseudopods flow around the bacterium, and fusion of the membranes of the pseudopods leads to complete enclosure of the bacterium within a membrane-bound phagosome. This is internalized and fusion of the membrane of the phagosome with the limiting membrane of lysosomal granules results in secretion of the granule contents into what is now known as the phagolysosome. This leads to the final stage of phagocytosis, namely bacterial killing.

## Bacterial Killing

The microorganism-killing mechanisms of neutrophils and macrophages may be either oxygen dependent or oxygen independent (Fig. 4.18). Although both probably coexist

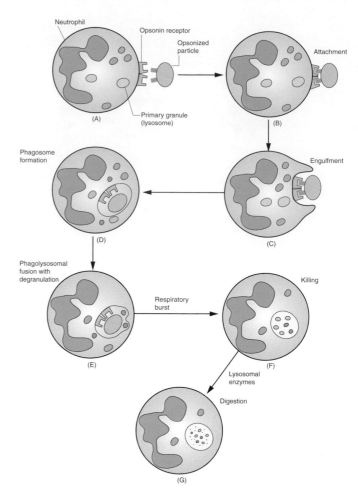

**FIG. 4.16** (A) Phagocytosis and killing of microorganisms. The microorganism is opsonized with antibody or complement. (B) The opsonized particle becomes attached to neutrophil membrane receptors for the opsonin. (C) Engulfment. (D) The opsonized microorganism is internalized into a phagocytic vacuole (phagosome). (E) Fusion of the lysosomes (primary granules) with the phagosome allows the discharge of lysosomal enzymes into the phagolysosome and triggers the respiratory burst, which results in bacterial killing. (F) Lysosomal enzymes degrade the dead microorganism (G).

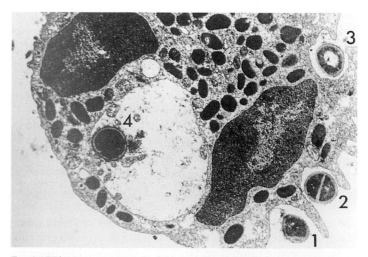

**FIG. 4.17** Electron micrograph of phagocytosis and killing of *Staphylococcus aureus* by a neutrophil: (1, 2 and 3) the different stages of engulfment of the microorganisms, leading to their presence in a phagolysosome (4).

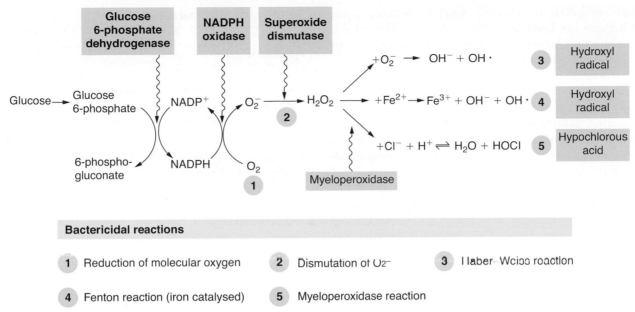

**Bactericidal reactions**

1. Reduction of molecular oxygen
2. Dismutation of O2⁻
3. Haber–Weiss reaction
4. Fenton reaction (iron catalysed)
5. Myeloperoxidase reaction

FIG. 4.18 Pathways of intracellular killing of microorganisms.

during the phagocytosis of most organisms, the oxygen-dependent mechanism is the more important. In oxygen-dependent killing, reactive oxygen metabolites are generated during phagocytosis because of the rapid action of nicotinamide adenosine dinucleotide phosphate (reduced form) (NADPH) oxidase on NADPH. This enzyme activity reduces oxygen molecules to the superoxide anion ($O^{2-}$). These superoxide anions are then converted into hydrogen peroxide, mostly by spontaneous dismutation. Hydrogen peroxide is produced within the lysosome during the phagocytic metabolic burst. Although the concentration of hydrogen peroxide rises considerably within the phagolysosome, this may be insufficient to kill many bacteria. However, the granules of neutrophils also contain the enzyme myeloperoxidase, which in the presence of chloride ions converts hydrogen peroxide to HOCl⁻, a potent antimicrobial agent. This hydrogen peroxide myeloperoxidase halide system is the major bactericidal system in neutrophils, but it is also effective against fungi, viruses, and parasites. Hydrogen peroxide is eventually detoxified into water and oxygen by the action of catalase and the dead microorganisms are degraded by lysosomal enzymes. Oxygen-independent killing also occurs through the action of substances within the phagolysosome. Lysozyme, an enzyme that degrades the glycopeptide coat of bacteria, lactoferrin, an iron-binding protein, and the major basic protein particularly found in eosinophils all have bactericidal and bacteriostatic activity.

Diseases in which these defence mechanisms are deficient again illustrate their importance in infection. There is deficient phagocytosis in the Chédiak–Higashi syndrome, an autosomal recessive condition in which there is increased risk of bacterial infection. In chronic granulomatous disease, an X-linked recessive disorder, there are defects in the capacity of neutrophils to generate the superoxide anion, leading to deficient bacterial killing and chronic bacterial infections. During these processes a number of reactive, potentially toxic, substances are released into the environment of the inflammatory focus. Although their primary role is as a defence mechanism they may contribute to tissue injury by lipid peroxidation, extracellular matrix degradation, and cytocidal properties. In some disease situations, e.g. immune complex-mediated disorders such as Goodpasture's syndrome (see Chapter 13, pp. 404–405), neutrophil infiltration of the affected organs is the major pathological event. Their action leads to cell death and degradation of the extracellular matrix of critical structures such as the glomerulus.

## Outcomes of the Inflammatory Response

Acute inflammation has both beneficial and harmful consequences. As a protective mechanism, inflammation allows ingress of phagocytes to the inflammatory focus, the oedema formation dilutes toxic substances, antibodies are delivered to sites of infection, and fibrin forms a substratum for cell migration. The harmful effects of inflammation include the digestion of adjacent viable tissue, and local tissue swelling of hollow viscera can be detrimental, e.g. acute epiglottitis may be life threatening. There may be loss of function of affected organs and, when generalized, the increased vascular permeability can cause shock as seen in some hypersensitivity reactions (e.g. anaphylaxis).

### Sequelae of Acute Inflammation

There are four main possible sequelae of acute inflammation:

- resolution
- abscess formation
- healing by fibrosis and scar formation
- chronic inflammation.

Complete resolution occurs after short-lived tissue injury in which there has been little tissue damage. The offending bacterium may be neutralized, killed, and cleared by the acute inflammatory response, and the affected tissues return entirely to normal. This occurs in some acute bacterial infections and is the ideal outcome. Abscess formation occurs when a localized collection of pus forms, often surrounded by granulation tissue and fibrosis. This is characteristically seen with certain pyogenic organisms such as staphylococci. An abscess may discharge spontaneously or require drainage by surgical intervention (Fig. 4.19).

Healing by fibrosis and scar formation occurs when substantial tissue destruction is seen during the acute phase. The damaged tissues are unable to regenerate and are replaced by fibrous tissue. This process is dealt with in more detail below. Progression to a chronic inflammatory response occurs in several circumstances, which are also discussed below.

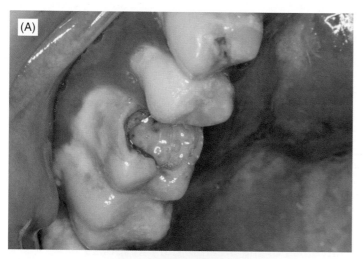

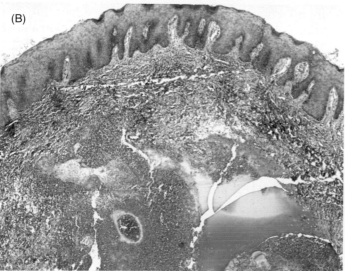

FIG. 4.19 (A) A dental abscess. (B) Photomicrograph of abscess cavity with accumulation of neutrophils and fibrin. (Courtesy of Dr Max Robinson.)

## Chronic Inflammation

### Key Points

- Chronic inflammation is characterized by an infiltration of lymphocytes and macrophages.
- Granulomatous inflammation is a specific form of chronic inflammation seen in diseases such as tuberculosis and sarcoidosis.
- Chronic inflammation may follow acute inflammation or may arise anew.

Chronic inflammation occurs over a more prolonged and sustained course than the acute inflammatory response and, although it shares many features in its vascular and leukocyte biology, the major leukocytes involved are the peripheral blood monocytes or macrophages. Chronic inflammation may supervene on an acute inflammatory response in two main instances or may arise anew.

First, persistence of the microorganism or toxic agent may lead to the development of chronic inflammation after an acute phase. This is particularly seen with microorganisms that are not cleared by neutrophils, e.g. *Mycobacterium tuberculosis*, the causative agent of TB. Second, recurrent episodes of acute inflammation may lead to tissue destruction and the inflammatory response then enters a chronic phase. This is seen, for example, in repeated episodes of acute cholecystitis associated with gallstones (see Chapter 10, p. 288). Eventually this leads to chronic cholecystitis, thickening of the gallbladder wall, infiltration by macrophages, and persistence of symptoms. Finally, chronic inflammation may be seen, and often arises anew, in certain diseases in which the immune system reacts against the individual's own tissues. Autoimmune diseases are relatively common and in these the chronic inflammatory response is the major cause of tissue damage.

### Features of Chronic Inflammation

The chronic inflammatory response is characterized by less oedema formation and fewer changes in blood flow than acute inflammation. But the major difference is infiltration of the tissues by peripheral blood monocytes and lymphocytes (Fig. 4.20). Chronic inflammation is almost uniformly accompanied by tissue destruction followed by attempts at healing by fibrosis.

### Macrophages in Chronic Inflammation

The macrophage is a key cell in the chronic inflammatory response. Monocytes undergo extravasation from the circulation and chemotaxis in the same way as neutrophils, although some of the mediators differ. Compared with neutrophils, the time course of exit of monocytes into the inflammatory focus is delayed and more prolonged. When monocytes reach tissues, they are termed 'macrophages'. This sustained monocyte/macrophage infiltration may be

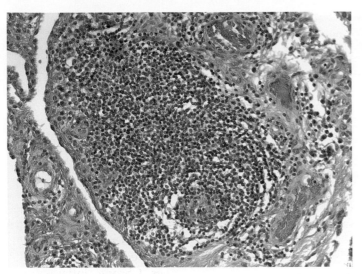

FIG. 4.20 Chronic inflammation in a joint from a patient with rheumatoid arthritis. The inflammatory infiltrate includes lymphocytes and plasma cells with few neutrophils. (Courtesy of Dr Petra Dildey.)

achieved by continued recruitment, prolonged survival, and immobilization of macrophages, or by local proliferation of macrophages within the inflammatory focus.

Macrophages are large cells that can react to chemotactic stimuli by migration. They are capable of phagocytosis and intracellular killing of bacteria by mechanisms similar to those seen in neutrophils. However, they may be activated by interactions with T lymphocytes during inflammatory responses, enhancing their intracellular killing and degradation capacity. In the response to particularly resistant organisms, such as *M. tuberculosis*, macrophages have the capacity to fuse together to form multinucleated giant cells during granulomatous inflammation. Macrophages are capable of releasing a variety of potent proteolytic enzymes, important both in defence against bacterial infection and in causing tissue injury during chronic inflammation. These products include proteases, elastase, collagenase, plasminogen activators, and lipases. The secretion of these substances by macrophages leads to extensive degradation of the extracellular matrix, resulting in the tissue damage that is such a prominent feature of chronic inflammation.

Macrophages can influence the repair process by the production of a variety of growth factors including platelet-derived growth factor (PDGF), epidermal growth factor (EGF), fibroblast growth factor (FGF), and transforming growth factor β (TGF-β). They can also secrete a number of proinflammatory cytokines and plasma proteins, which contribute to the development of the inflammatory response. Macrophages are also important in directing the early induction of the specific immune response. After intracellular killing and degradation of bacteria, certain macrophages can then express antigenic peptides on their cell surface in association with major histocompatibility complex (MHC) molecules. This combination of antigenic peptide and MHC is required for the activation of T lymphocytes. Macrophages thus have an important role in both the recognition and effector arms of inflammatory and immunological responses.

## CASE HISTORY 4.1

Ulricka is a 56-year-old married woman who spent the first 30 years of her life in Sweden. She then came to the UK as a student and is now a chemical engineer. She has always been fit and well and has no previous ailments of any significance. She had all relevant immunizations as a child including the BCG.

Ulricka presented to her general practitioner with increasing breathlessness, which had developed over a period of approximately 3 months. She complained of some tightness in her chest and had occasional bouts of a dry cough, but there was no haemoptysis. She had also developed some stiffness of her knee and ankle joints and noticed that she had dry eyes and on occasions sensitivity to light (photophobia). On examination there were no abnormal chest signs, and no finger clubbing or cyanosis. She did, however, have palpable lymph nodes in her neck and evidence of hepatosplenomegaly.

A chest radiograph was taken which showed some shadowing in both lungs, particularly around the midzones, and there was marked bilateral hilar lymphadenopathy. She underwent a series of lung function tests, which demonstrated a restrictive lung disease with decreased compliance and mild impairment of diffusion capacity. All routine blood tests, including full blood count and urea and electrolytes, were in the normal range but there was mild derangement of liver function tests including elevation of alkaline phosphatase (see Chapter 10, p. 275). There was elevation of inflammatory markers, in particular C-reactive protein and a markedly elevated serum angiotensin-converting enzyme (ACE). Mantoux's test for active TB was negative.

She underwent biopsy of one of the lymph nodes identified in her neck. It showed replacement of the node by granulomas characterized by the presence of large multinucleated giant cells, epithelioid macrophages, and lymphocytes (Fig. 4.21). Some of the granulomas showed

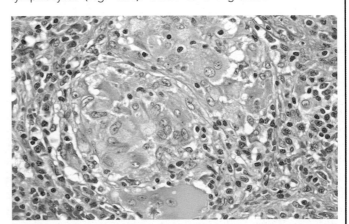

FIG. 4.21 A well-formed sarcoid granuloma. It is composed of epithelioid and giant cells with surrounding lymphocytes. The giant cell at the lower border contains an asteroid body (most often seen in sarcoidosis).

accompanying scarring but there was no necrosis. Staining for mycobacteria was negative.

The appearances on biopsy and the constellation of clinical signs and symptoms, together with the finding of high serum angiotensin converting enzyme levels, led to a diagnosis of sarcoidosis (see Chapter 7, p. 179). Ulricka was treated with corticosteroids and within 2 months the lung symptoms had disappeared and the lymph node swelling in the neck had also reduced. Over time the joint stiffness improved and she was able to lead a normal life again.

Sarcoidosis is a multisystem disorder characterized by granulomatous infiltration in various tissues. The precise aetiology remains uncertain but it has long been considered to probably be due to an abnormal response to some external agent such as bacteria or chemicals. It occurs worldwide but there are some areas with a much higher prevalence, in particular Scandinavia. Lymph nodes and the liver are the most commonly affected sites

but, as with Ulricka, there can be ocular and joint involvement. In addition some patients develop cardiac sarcoidosis, and involvement of the nervous system and brain may lead to cranial nerve palsies, including facial palsy.

A number of conditions need to be distinguished from sarcoidosis in patients such as Ulricka. In particular it was important to consider whether she may have had another condition characterized by granulomatous inflammation – TB – and the other concern was that she may have developed a lymphoma. It was clearly therefore extremely important to obtain a histological diagnosis by sampling the enlarged node in her neck. Although Ulricka showed an impressive response to the corticosteroid therapy, in the longer term there is a high chance of relapse, particularly when steroids are stopped, and interestingly little difference is demonstrable in the long-term outcome, comparing patients who have been treated with steroids with those who have not.

## Granulomatous Inflammation

Granulomatous inflammation is a specific pattern of chronic inflammatory response defined by the localized aggregation of activated macrophages around an inflammatory focus. It is encountered in a small number of highly characteristic diseases including TB, leprosy, brucellosis, and Crohn's disease. In clinical practice the recognition of granuloma formation is therefore a major diagnostic criterion for these diseases.

A granuloma is a localized aggregate of macrophages that are activated and transformed into so-called epithelioid cells, usually surrounded by a cuff of lymphocytes and occasionally plasma cells (see Fig. 4.21). In haematoxylin and eosin-stained histological sections, epithelioid cells have abundant pale-pink granular cytoplasm with indistinct cell boundaries. In some instances multiple macrophages may fuse together to form a multinucleated giant cell. As granulomatous inflammation progresses, it may eventually be surrounded by fibroblasts and scar tissue. Granulomas form in response to two quite different mechanisms: immune-mediated granulomas, of which the main clinical diseases discussed above are examples, and foreign body granulomas, elicited by inert foreign particles that have proved difficult for macrophages to clear.

Granulomas form after macrophages have initially digested the pathogenic organism. During the killing and partial degradation of the organism antigenic peptides are expressed on the macrophage surface. They pass through the draining lymphatics to the adjacent lymph nodes where the antigenic peptides stimulate specific antigen-recognizing T lymphocytes. These are activated and migrate to the inflammatory focus, where they secrete proinflammatory cytokines. These cytokines in turn activate macrophages, which accumulate, immobilized within the inflammatory focus. Macrophage activation causes increased production of a variety of proteases and lysosomal enzymes, increasing the

cytoplasmic volume and resulting in the pale granular eosinophilic staining seen in histological preparations. In some granulomas, tissue associated with the release of digestive enzymes leaves the centre of the granuloma necrotic. In TB this is the characteristic caseous (cheese-like) necrosis.

Granulomas form relatively slowly over a period of days and are dependent on the integrity of the immune system as well as the chronic inflammatory response. They are an important defence mechanism against several major infections and patients with defective cell-mediated immunity (e.g. in acquired immune deficiency syndrome [AIDS]) may develop overwhelming TB or leprosy (see Chapter 19). Nevertheless, in immunocompetent individuals, the process of granuloma formation, with central necrosis and tissue destruction, consequent on macrophage degranulation, leads to significant tissue damage and scar formation and therefore contributes to the pathogenesis of the disease.

## Systemic Effects of Inflammation

There are many systemic effects of inflammation, some of which may be symptomatic and some of which are a response to injury demonstrated only by laboratory testing. Fever (pyrexia) is one of the most commonly encountered consequences of an acute inflammatory illness (Fig. 4.22). It is a consequence of the effect of the cytokines IL-1 and TNF directly acting on the hypothalamus to reset the thermoregulatory mechanisms in the body, leading to a rise in body temperature through increased sympathetic nerve stimulation of cutaneous arterioles, vasoconstriction, and reduced heat loss. The liver produces a number of acute phase proteins including C-reactive protein, serum amyloid A protein, serum amyloid P protein, and the important complement and coagulation proteins. There is increased production of the stress-related glucocorticoids and there

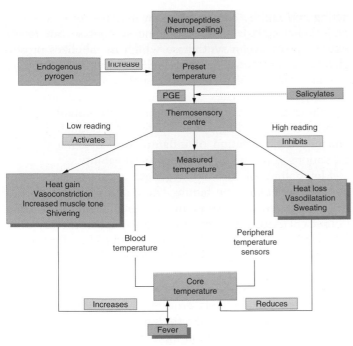

**FIG. 4.22** Mechanisms of pyrexia. PGE = prostaglandin E.

may be a diuresis as a consequence of reduced vasopressin production. One of the consequences of these effects is a catabolic state with increased breakdown of fat and protein stores in the body. Leukocytosis, an increase in the number of white blood cells within the circulation, is an important part of the defence mechanism in inflammatory illness. The release of increased numbers of white cells, initially from bone marrow stores, and in a more prolonged inflammatory illness because of increased bone marrow turnover and differentiation towards leukocytes, can lead to white cell counts two to three times the normal level. This leukocytosis may be regulated by IL-1 and TNF acting on the bone marrow stores, but a more prolonged leukocytosis requiring increased bone marrow turnover is dependent on the production of colony-stimulating factors.

## Mediators of the Inflammatory Response

### Key Points

- The processes of acute and chronic inflammation are mediated by a variety of small molecules.
- Some of these are found circulating in plasma whereas others are produced by inflammatory cells.
- Activation of many of these mediators involves a cascade of kinase reactions.
- The activation pathways are tightly regulated.

Various chemical mediators of acute and chronic inflammation have been described. These may circulate in plasma or be synthesized and secreted by inflammatory cells. In general plasma-derived mediators must be activated, usually

by proteolytic cleavage, to an active form. Cell-derived mediators tend to be stored in the active form within intracellular granules or are synthesized anew in the active form in response to an external stimulus. Most of these mediators exert their biological properties by binding to specific receptors on target cells, leading to a characteristic biological response. Some mediators can act on several target cells within the inflammatory focus. Most mediators are rather short-lived and are degraded to inactive forms within minutes. The importance of many of these mediators is that they provide an important point for therapeutic intervention, e.g. the use of antihistamines in the treatment of hay fever.

### Histamine

This is widely distributed in tissues, mostly stored within the granules of mast cells present in connective tissue. It is also found in circulating basophils and platelets. The preformed histamine is released by mast cell degranulation in response to a variety of signals, including trauma, cold, IgE binding by antigen, anaphylatoxic elements of complement (C3a and C5a), and cytokines such as IL-1 and IL-8. In the acute inflammatory response histamine causes dilatation of arterioles by relaxation of vascular smooth muscle and increases the endothelial permeability in venules. It is thought to be one of the major mediators of the early stages of the acute inflammatory response, particularly the increased vascular permeability.

### Serotonin

This is another preformed vasoactive mediator similar to histamine but present in platelets. Serotonin is released from platelets during platelet activation and aggregation after platelet contact with collagen, thrombus, or antigen–antibody complexes. Serotonin has target organ properties similar to histamine, causing dilatation of arterioles and increased vascular permeability of venules.

### Platelet-activating Factor

PAF is a bioactive phospholipid synthesized anew in leukocytes and endothelial cells in response to inflammatory stimuli. It is an extremely powerful activator of platelets and of venular endothelial permeability, with a potency at least 1,000 times greater than that of histamine. PAF can also increase leukocyte adhesion to endothelium, is probably chemotactic, and can influence the degranulation of neutrophils. It is one of the important elements of inflammation and, in certain experimental models, the inflammatory response may be considerably subdued by the use of PAF antagonists.

### Metabolites of Arachidonic Acid (Prostaglandins, Leukotrienes, and Lipoxins)

During the activation of cells as part of the inflammatory response, membrane lipids are metabolized to produce inflammatory mediators. The major category of these is

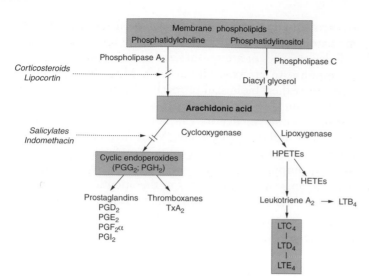

**Fig. 4.23** Formation of arachidonic metabolites. HPETE = cyclic hydroperoxides; HETE = hydroxy-eicosatetraenoic acids.

derivatives of arachidonic acid (Fig. 4.23), derived from phospholipids by the action of phospholipases. Arachidonic acid is an unsaturated fatty acid that is a constituent of many cell membrane phospholipids. There are two main pathways of metabolism of arachidonic acid, namely the cyclooxygenase (COX) pathway and the lipoxygenase pathway. The two main enzymes in the cyclooxygenase pathway are COX-1 and COX-2, the enzyme activity of which leads to the generation of prostaglandins. Prostaglandins may be further metabolized into three main groups of molecules: prostacyclin, thromboxane, and other members of the prostaglandin family. The metabolism of prostaglandins towards these substances is dependent on the action of other enzymes, many of which have a tissue-specific distribution. Platelets contain thromboxane synthetase and metabolize prostaglandins to thromboxane $A_2$, which causes vasoconstriction and promotes platelet aggregation. It is short

acting and rapidly converted to an inactive form. Vascular endothelial cells lack thromboxane synthetase but rather express prostacyclin synthetase which metabolizes prostaglandins to prostacyclin. Prostacyclin is a potent vasodilator and an inhibitor of platelet aggregation and therefore has the opposite properties to thromboxane. Some molecules remain as part of the prostaglandin family, notably prostaglandin $D_2$, $E_2$ and $F_{2\alpha}$, which promote vasodilatation and enhance the formation of inflammatory oedema through alterations in vascular endothelial permeability.

Metabolites of the lipoxygenase pathway are members of the leukotriene family. These again fall into groups depending on their subsequent metabolism. $LTB_4$ is a potent chemotactic agent produced by inflammatory cells. The other leukotrienes $LTC_4$, $LTD_4$, and $LTE_4$, all promote smooth muscle contraction and endothelial cell contraction, therefore enhancing vasoconstriction and causing increased vascular permeability.

Many anti-inflammatory drugs used in clinical practice act on this group of molecules. Steroids inhibit the phospholipases required for the generation of arachidonic acid. Aspirin, indometacin, and other non-steroidal anti-inflammatory drugs inhibit COX, thereby reducing the generation of prostacyclin, thromboxane, and prostaglandins. The anti-inflammatory properties of dietary fish oils are dependent on the metabolism of the phospholipids derived from these oils to leukotrienes, which are less potent as proinflammatory agents.

## Plasma Protease Pathways

### Complement

The complement system consists of more than 20 components circulating within the plasma (Fig. 4.24). It is a major defence mechanism, which contributes to the inflammatory response and the damage of bacteria after an immunologically mediated attack. There are two main pathways for the activation of complement: the classic pathway

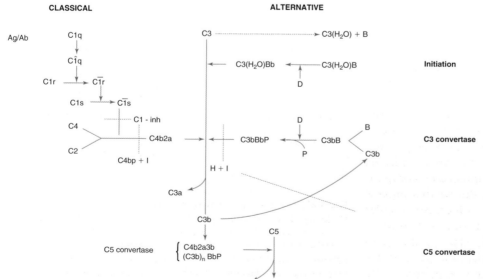

**Fig. 4.24** Outline of complement activation pathways. The cascade involves complement components (C) and a number of ancillary factors (B, D, H, I, P). Ag/Ab = antigen–antibody complex.

involving activation of C1, the first complement component, by antigen–antibody complexes, and the alternative pathway, in which C3 activation occurs on microbial surfaces, polysaccharides, or other microbial products. The cleavage of C3 to C3a and C3b is the most important step in the complement cascade, and is the essential element common to both the alternative and classic pathways. Complement activation influences three different biological functions within the inflammatory response.

C3a and C5a, the cleavage products of C3 and C5 respectively, may increase vascular permeability and cause vasodilatation by acting via release of histamine from mast cells. C5a can also activate the metabolism of arachidonic acid, causing the release of further inflammatory mediators. C3a and C5a are both powerful chemotactic agents for neutrophils and monocytes, and enhance the adhesion of leukocytes to endothelium, thereby influencing the cellular phase of the acute inflammatory response. C3b is an important opsonin enhancing the phagocytosis of bacteria by fixation to the bacterial cell wall; it is recognized by receptors on the macrophage surface. Finally the membrane attack complex C5b–9 may insert into bacterial cell walls, leading to cell lysis. The cascade of complement activation allows amplification at each stage, further enhancing its proinflammatory properties. This, however, requires regulatory mechanisms to prevent overactivity. Protein inhibitors, including the inhibitors of C3 and C5 convertases, closely regulate the activity of the complement system. There are also circulating proteins in the plasma that combine with complement components, thus inactivating them. Among the most important of these is the C1 complement inhibitor.

### Clotting and Fibrinolytic Systems

Although the major function of the clotting system is haemostatic control there are intimate links with the inflammatory response and many clotting factors are involved with either the complement or the kinin cascades. Particularly important in inflammation is the activation of the Hageman factor, a protein synthesized in its inactive form by the liver as part of the acute phase response (Fig. 4.25). When the Hageman factor is exposed to collagen in basement membranes or activated by platelets it undergoes a conformational change to become factor XIIa, exposing an enzymatically active site that can act on downstream components of both the clotting and the kinin cascades. Two further components of the coagulation system provide links between blood clotting and inflammation. Thrombin, which is the cleavage product of the inactive precursor prothrombin, cleaves the plasma protein fibrinogen to form fibrin, an important component of blood clot formation. However, during this process small fibrin peptides are formed that can increase vascular permeability and are chemotactic for leukocytes. Thrombin itself may activate leukocytes, directly causing increased leukocyte adhesion to endothelial cells, and may cause fibroblast proliferation during the healing response. Factor X, when activated to factor Xa, may also increase vascular permeability and enhance leukocyte exudation. During the activation of the coagulation cascade the fibrinolytic regulatory mechanism is activated. This second cascade generates the proteolytic enzyme plasmin to degrade fibrin, but it is also capable of activating the complement cascade.

### The Kinin System

The kinin system generates vasoactive peptides from a group of plasma protein kininogens. These kininogens are cleaved by enzymes called kallikreins, which are formed from the cleavage of prekallikrein by factor XIIa (activated Hageman factor) of the coagulation system. The resulting activation of the kinin cascade releases bradykinin, a potent vascular permeability agent. Bradykinin also causes vasodilatation and excites nerve endings, causing pain. The properties of bradykinin are therefore similar to those of histamine, but the rate of production of bradykinin is slower because of the multiple steps involved in activating the kinin proteolytic cascade. Other elements of the kinin cascade, in particular kallikrein, not only have chemotactic activity, but also activate the complement component C5 to C5a.

There are therefore four intimately linked plasma protease cascades that regulate both the inflammatory response and the haemostatic properties of blood.

## Cytokines

Cytokines are a variety of soluble mediators produced by inflammatory cells and by endothelium, epithelium, and connective tissue during the inflammatory response. They are locally acting with rapid degradation, although a few also have systemic effects. They usually act by binding to cell membrane receptors on the target cells promoting proliferation, activation, and differentiation. A large number of cytokines have been described and more continue to be identified but their general properties and functional classes are of more importance than the recognition of individual molecules. Some cytokines regulate the function of lymphocytes: lymphocyte activation,

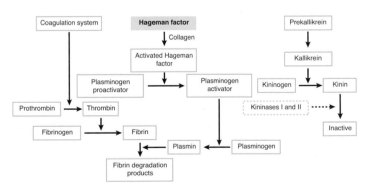

**Fig. 4.25** Hageman factor-dependent pathways. Activation of the Hageman factor (coagulation factor XII) by contact with collagen results in the acquisition of protease activity, which is able enzymatically to activate the coagulation system, the fibrinolytic system, and the kallikrein–kinin system. Kallikrein, an enzyme that converts kininogen to kinin, also amplifies the system by activating the Hageman factor. Kininases I and II inactivate kinins rapidly.

proliferation, and terminal differentiation. Among the most important of this category are IL-2 and IL-4, both of which stimulate lymphocyte proliferation, whereas IL-10 and TGF-β suppress lymphocyte proliferation. There are also cytokines that activate effector cells within the inflammatory response, particularly macrophages. Many of these cytokines are released by T lymphocytes or by target cells damaged during inflammation. Macrophage-activating cytokines include interferon-γ and TNF-α. Some cytokines stimulate inflammatory responses and immune responses in a non-specific manner, including TNF-α and IL-1β, both of which are responsible for many of the systemic effects of the inflammatory response. Other cytokines stimulate the generation of white blood cells required for the leukocytosis seen in inflammation.

Chemokines are a family of small proteins acting as activators and chemotactic agents for specific leukocytes. They are divided into several groups depending on their amino acid sequence, in particular the grouping of cystine residues. These different groups have different biological properties. CXC chemokines such as IL-8 act primarily on neutrophils, having been secreted by macrophages or endothelial cells attracting neutrophils to the inflammatory focus. These chemokines may be induced by other cytokines, in particular general proinflammatory cytokines such as IL-1 and TGF. C-C chemokines act mostly on macrophages and comprise the main monocyte chemoattractant proteins MCP-1 (macrophage chemotactic protein 1) and RANTES (regulated on activation, normal T-cell expressed and secreted). Both of these are responsible for attracting and immobilizing monocytes within the inflammatory focus, and they also act on eosinophils and lymphocytes. They do not possess chemotactic properties for neutrophils. C chemokines possess only one of the conserved cystine residues of the chemokine family and are specific for lymphocytes. CX3C is a more recently described family and appears to exist mostly as cell surface-bound chemokines promoting the adhesion between monocytes and T cells, which is an important part of the inflammatory and immune responses.

Most chemokine activity is highly localized and these are therefore paracrine regulators of the inflammatory response.

### Nitric Oxide

Nitric oxide (NO) is an important mediator of inflammation. It was first identified as a substance released from endothelial cells that caused smooth muscle cell relaxation, and was known as endothelium-derived relaxing factor. It is produced not only by endothelial cells but also by macrophages and certain neurons in the brain. Nitric oxide is synthesized from L-arginine, oxygen, and other cofactors by the enzyme nitric oxide synthase (NOS). There are three different types of NOS: endothelial, neuronal, and inducible. Both endothelial and neuronal NOS are constitutively expressed but their level may be enhanced after stimulation of the appropriate cells. Inducible NOS by contrast is upregulated only when macrophages are activated by cytokines

or other agents. In the inflammatory response, endothelial and macrophage generation of NO appears to be important. NO may influence the vascular phase of the inflammatory response by causing vascular smooth muscle relaxation and hence vasodilatation. NO is also an important part of the pathway of the generation of free oxygen radicals, which are important in macrophage killing of bacteria.

## Repair

When cellular injury has resulted in necrosis of cells a repair process occurs, the aim of which is to attempt to replace the dead cells by healthy tissue. This response is referred to as healing. It involves two distinct processes:

1. Regeneration – in which there is replacement of injured cells by proliferation of surviving cells of the same type
2. A connective tissue response characterized initially by the formation of granulation tissue (see below) and its subsequent maturation, which may lead to scar formation (fibrosis).

The mechanisms that control the regenerative and connective tissue responses are similar and involve cell proliferation, differentiation, interactions between cells and the surrounding matrix, and cell migration. The relative roles of regeneration and the connective tissue response vary in different tissues. In some tissues, e.g. skin, there may be complete restoration of the epithelial architecture after healing, particularly if the injury is very superficial. Elsewhere (e.g. in the central nervous system) the specialized cells cannot regenerate and the healing process is dominated by a connective tissue response. This is clearly a less satisfactory outcome because, although healing may have restored structural defects, there will be residual functional abnormalities as the specialized cells will have been replaced by scar tissue.

The outcome of a healing process is also affected by the nature, severity, and duration of the injury (Fig. 4.26), e.g. the liver shows a remarkable capacity for regeneration.

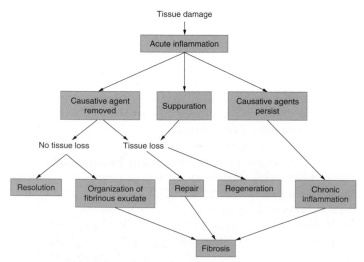

FIG. 4.26 Sequelae of acute inflammation.

Two-thirds of the liver can be removed surgically and the remaining parenchyma will in time regenerate to the original mass and will show a normal structure. A similar remarkable degree of regeneration can occur when there is acute necrosis such as occurs after paracetamol (acetaminophen) overdose. This is a serious condition and many patients either die or require a liver transplantation. However, those patients who survive without the need for liver transplantation have an essentially normal liver within a few weeks with no fibrosis. In contrast, in chronic liver injury such as occurs with hepatitis C virus, although there is ongoing regeneration, it is the connective tissue response that predominates and leads to severe scarring. A combination of liver cell regeneration and fibrosis results in the formation of liver nodules, a condition called cirrhosis (see Chapter 10). In this section we consider the mechanisms of regeneration and the connective tissue response and see how these relate to important and common forms of healing – skin wounds and bone fractures. Before considering basic mechanisms, however, we review the composition of the extracellular matrix.

## Extracellular Matrix

### Composition of the Matrix

The extracellular matrix is a complex structure of interacting molecules that provides structural support for tissues. It also modulates the function of surrounding cells and has an effect on proliferation, differentiation, movement, and structure. The proteins that comprise the matrix are well hydrated, providing turgor for soft tissues, and act as a sink for growth factors, which control the proliferation of surrounding cells. It also provides a base to which cells adhere and on which they can migrate.

Four main groups of compounds form the extracellular matrix: (1) collagens, (2) elastin and related proteins, (3) structural glycoproteins, and (4) proteoglycans/hyaluronic acid. There are two major forms of connective tissue: the interstitial extracellular matrix and the basement membranes. The most common matrix protein is collagen. Collagens are a family of closely related proteins with common structural properties unique to this group of molecules. To date some

**TABLE 4.1** Types of collagen

| Collagen type | Localization |
| --- | --- |
| I | Skin, bone, tendons (accounts for 90% of all collagen) |
| II | Cartilage |
| III | Internal organs, skin, blood vessels |
| IV | Basement membranes |
| V | Blood vessels, internal organs |
| VI | Widespread distribution |
| VII | Dermal, epidermal junction in skin |
| VIII | Descemet's membrane in eye |
| IX | Cartilage |

18 collagens have been described. The common property is that they all contain (at least in part), a triple helical structure formed from three protein chains ($\alpha$ chains). Along a substantial length of the amino acid sequence of these chains there is the repeating sequence gly-x-y. They are rich in hydroxyproline and hydroxylysine; these amino acids are formed by hydroxylation of proline and lysine, a process that requires vitamin C. In this context it is of interest that scurvy (vitamin C deficiency) results in abnormal healing.

In the case of some collagens the individual chains are identical. In others, such as type I collagen, which is the most abundant form, the molecule is composed of two identical chains and one non-identical chain. Collagens are produced on the endoplasmic reticulum of mesenchymal cells such as fibroblasts and osteoblasts. The sequence of events in collagen biosynthesis is outlined in Fig. 4.27. Individual collagen molecules line up to form fibrils and these have a banded appearance ultrastructurally. There is cross-linking of the different molecules and this stabilizes the fibrils. The sites of the major forms of collagen are summarized in *Table 4.1*.

Some tissues require elasticity for their function and this is facilitated by another matrix protein, elastin. This forms the core of elastic fibres found in blood vessels, skin, and the lungs. The elastin molecules are surrounded by a microfibrillar network containing the protein fibrillin. Elastic fibres can recoil after transient stretching and this is important in tissues such as large blood vessels and the skin.

The extracellular matrix contains several large glycoproteins, which act as adhesion molecules that link matrix components to each other and to surrounding cells. The most abundant of these is fibronectin. This protein binds to other matrix components such as collagens via specific peptide domains on its molecule and to cells via a three amino acid sequence (arginine–glycine–aspartic acid; RGD). Laminin is the principal structural glycoprotein of basement membranes. This also has cell- and matrix-binding domains. It has the capacity to alter the morphology and differentiation of a wide range of cell types. A new group of related proteins – so-called matricellular proteins – have been described which do not function as structural proteins, but rather appear to disrupt cell matrix interactions. These may be important during tissue remodelling and include osteonectin and tenascin.

Another important component of the extracellular matrix is a heterogeneous group of negatively charged polysaccharide chains, known as glycosaminoglycans. The most abundant of these are hyaluronic acid, chondroitin sulphate, dermatan sulphate, and heparin sulphate. With the exception of hyaluronic acid, all of the compounds are linked to a core protein to form proteoglycans. These are long unbranched structures, which form a water-replete gel. Proteoglycans may also be found within cell membranes (e.g. syndecan).

### Turnover of the Extracellular Matrix

The extracellular matrix is not a static structure. During development, for example, there needs to be substantial

(A)

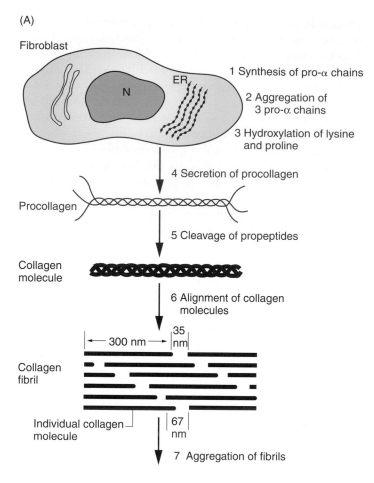

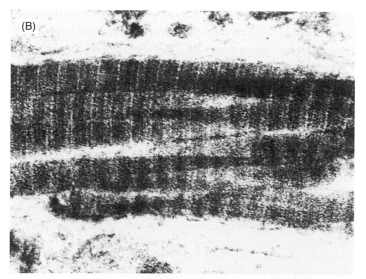

**FIG. 4.27** Principal steps in biosynthesis of interstitial collagens: (A) 1, synthesis of pro-α chains in rough endoplasmic reticulum; 2, aggregation of three pro-α chains; 3, hydroxylation of lysine and proline residues; 4, secretion of procollagen molecule; 5, cleavage of propeptides; 6, alignment of collagen molecules to form fibrils; 7, aggregation of fibrils to form collagen fibre, seen here in longitudinal section and showing regular cross-banding (B). N = nucleus; ER = endoplasmic reticulum.

remodelling and even in adult tissues there is constant (albeit low-level) turnover of all matrix proteins. The so-called degradation of matrix proteins is achieved by a family of metalloproteases. Various forms exist that degrade either interstitial collagen, basement membrane collagen (type IV), or other matrix components such as the structural glycoproteins. All of the matrix metalloproteases are produced as inactive precursors. Once activated, metalloproteases are controlled by a family of tissue inhibitors of metalloprotease (TIMPs).

### Cell Receptors for Matrix Proteins

Integrins are the principal form of cell surface receptor by which cells can attach to the matrix. This family of proteins is also important in cell–cell interactions such as those occurring in leukocyte adhesion (see pp. 58–59). Integrins are transmembrane proteins comprising an α and a β chain. There are over 20 different forms of integrin molecules and these have different matrix-binding properties. The extracellular part of the integrin molecule binds to several of the matrix components by recognizing the RGD sequence referred to above. The integrins not only act by anchoring cells to the matrix but also transmit the effect of surrounding matrix to the structure and shape of the cells by their interaction with cytoskeletal proteins. There is also recent evidence to suggest that the binding of matrix to the integrins leads to the activation of intracellular pathways similar to those activated by cytokines and growth factors (see below), thereby influencing cell behaviour such as gene expression.

## Regeneration

Proliferation of parenchymal cells forms an important part of the healing of any injured organ. The capacity for such regeneration varies between tissues, in general reflecting the degree of proliferative activity of the normal tissue (see Chapter 2).

The control of cell division and regulation of the cell cycle are discussed elsewhere. In broad terms, cell proliferation is controlled by binding of extracellular growth factors to specific receptors on the surface of the cells. Ligand–receptor binding in turn sets in motion a series of cascade processes or signal transduction pathways by which signals are transferred to the nucleus, leading to activation of transcription factors, ultimately influencing gene expression. Of particular importance are the changes in the expression of genes that control entry into the cell cycle. This includes a number of proto-oncogenes such as c-*myc* and tumour-suppressor genes such as *TP53*. The cell surface receptors are of three types: (1) those that act through intrinsic tyrosine kinase activity; (2) transmembrane receptors without intrinsic enzyme activity; and (3) receptors linked to G proteins. There are several different forms of signal transduction pathway, which link these receptors to nuclear events. The principal pathways are the MAP kinase pathway, inositol phosphate pathway, cAMP pathway, the Janus kinase/signal transducers and activators of transcription (JAK/STAT) pathway and integrin-mediated pathways. This is almost certainly an oversimplification and there is evidence of cross-talk between the different pathways.

At least three types of extracellular signal can initiate these events. First, there are substances that are secreted by the cells themselves, i.e. a cell produces a growth factor together with the relevant receptor and can therefore control its own proliferation. This is referred to as autocrine signalling and occurs in epithelial proliferation in skin wounds and in liver regeneration; it is also a feature of some tumours. The second form is where the molecules stimulating proliferation are produced by cells in the vicinity of the target cell. As we shall see, this occurs in the connective tissue response of repair where, for example, growth factors produced by inflammatory cells can stimulate the proliferation of endothelial and mesenchymal cells. This is referred to as paracrine signalling. Finally, substances produced at a distant site, such as a completely separate organ, can also control cell proliferation. This is referred to as endocrine signalling (Fig. 4.28).

There is now a wealth of information on a large number of growth factors that may be involved in regeneration. Some of these act on a wide range of cell types, but others are more specific. Many influence not only proliferation but also cell motility and differentiation. The most important factors in regeneration (particularly that of epithelial tissues) are EGF and the related TGF-α, insulin-like growth factors (IGFs), so-called hepatocyte growth factor (HGF), and some of the FGF family. In some tissues, e.g. in the gastrointestinal tract, there are other peptides that may play an important role. These have a unique structure – the so-called trefoil peptides.

EGF and TGF-α share a common receptor – the EGF receptor. This has inherent tyrosine kinase activity, and ligand–receptor binding leads to the series of signal transduction events referred to above. EGF is found in abundance in tissue secretions such as sweat, saliva, and urine, whereas TGF-α is probably more important in the regeneration of solid organs such as the liver and kidney. Another growth factor that signals through a similar pathway is HGF. This is a misnomer in that it has a wide-ranging proliferative effect on a variety of cells in different tissues. Its receptor *c*-met is expressed by many epithelial cells, including those of the breast and kidney. This growth factor not only controls cell proliferation, but also acts as a morphogen (controlling cell differentiation during development), controlling cell motility, particularly during regeneration. Because of the latter property HGF has also been referred to as 'scatter factor'.

It is important to recognize that there are also signals that inhibit cell proliferation. This is an important form of regulation when healing has occurred, e.g. in compensatory liver hyperplasia after hepatectomy, it is important that proliferation does not get out of control and is kept in check by inhibitory signals. There is less known about growth inhibition than proliferation, although it appears to be regulated through autocrine and paracrine means by growth factors such as TGF-β.

## Connective Tissue Response

When tissues are injured there is damage not only to the epithelial cells but also to the surrounding matrix. Therefore there needs to be restoration, not only of the epithelial mass, but also of the normal structural framework. It follows that, in all forms of repair, there is at least some connective tissue response, although as noted above

**Autocrine signalling**

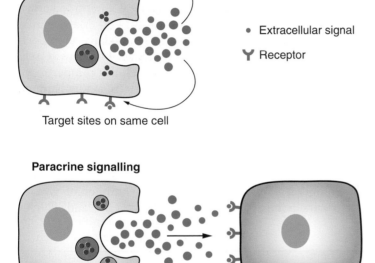

Target sites on same cell

- Extracellular signal

Y Receptor

**Paracrine signalling**

Secretory cell          Adjacent target cell

**Endocrine signalling**

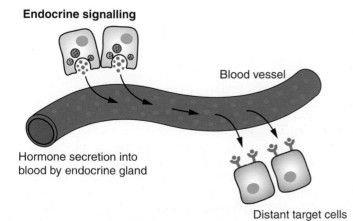

Blood vessel

Hormone secretion into blood by endocrine gland

Distant target cells

Fig. 4.28 Comparison of autocrine, paracrine, and endocrine signalling.

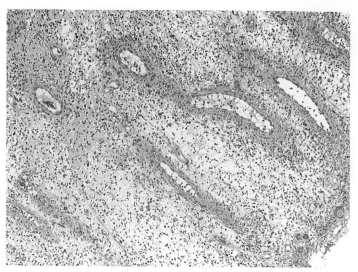

**FIG. 4.29** Granulation tissue. Note the parallel rows of capillaries surrounded by oedema and inflammatory cells, many of which are neutrophils.

the balance between regeneration and connective tissue response is influenced by a number of factors, including the severity and duration of the injury. The connective tissue response consists of four main processes. The first is the formation of new blood vessels, a process referred to as angiogenesis. The second is the activation and proliferation of fibroblasts and related mesenchymal cells (myofibroblasts). The third (and a consequence of the second) is the deposition of extracellular matrix proteins, in particular collagens. Finally, there is remodelling of the matrix, and this includes gradual changes in the relative abundance of different matrix proteins. The processes of angiogenesis and fibroblast proliferation lead to the development of

so-called granulation tissue (Fig. 4.29). This name derives from the red granular appearance seen on the surface of skin wounds, but it is a process that occurs in the healing of most tissues.

### Angiogenesis

The process of angiogenesis involves the formation of new capillary buds (sprouts) from pre-existing vessels. It follows a sequence of events that includes: (1) breakdown of the basement membrane of the pre-existing vessel; (2) migration of endothelial cells; (3) proliferation of endothelial cells behind the migrating cells; (4) maturation of endothelial cells with the formation of capillary tubes; and (5) recruitment of supporting cells (pericytes) to surround the endothelial cells. New vessel formation is thought to be critical in healing because it supplies oxygen and nutrients to the injured tissue, and ensures the delivery of both humoral and cell-mediated arms of the immune system to help prevent infection. Several growth factors have been found to stimulate angiogenesis but the principal factor involved in the formation of new vessels in granulation tissue is a peptide known as vascular endothelial growth factor (VEGF). Matricellular proteins such as tenascin are also thought to have an important role in the formation and maintenance of new vessels, and there are also factors in the extracellular compartment (e.g. endostatin) that regulate angiogenesis, acting through inhibition of endothelial proliferation.

### Fibrosis

One of the key elements in the development of granulation tissue is the migration, activation, and proliferation of fibroblasts. This is controlled by a number of growth factors including PDGF, TGF-β, IL-1, FGFs, and TNF-α.

---

## 4.1 Special Study Topic

### CELL AND MOLECULAR BIOLOGY OF LIVER FIBROSIS

Fibrosis of the liver is an end-result of most forms of chronic liver disease, including that associated with alcohol misuse, chronic viral hepatitis, and inherited metabolic diseases such as haemochromatosis. In the fibrotic liver, there is a substantial increase in most matrix proteins but in particular the interstitial collagens type I and III. These not only are present in greater amounts but also are deposited in abnormal sites within the liver microanatomy. This leads to replacement of functional parenchymal tissue by scarring and to disruption of the intrahepatic blood flow as a space-occupying effect.

It is now clear that the principal cell involved in liver fibrosis is a special form of mesenchymal cell that acts as a facultative (myo)fibroblast and is now referred to as

the hepatic stellate cell (Fig. 4.30). This was previously called the Ito cell or fat-storing cell and is found within the perisinusoidal space of Disse (the area between the hepatocytes and the endothelium of the liver sinusoids). These cells resemble pericytes in other tissues, but have some unique properties, including the expression (at least in some species) of intermediate filament proteins normally seen in either muscle cells or cells of the central nervous system. In the normal liver, their principal functions are storage of vitamin A (they are the main site of storage for retinoids in the body) and the regulation of intersinusoidal blood flow through contraction and relaxation in response to vasoactive mediators.

Hepatic stellate cells are thought to be responsible for producing extracellular matrix proteins in the normal liver and contribute to the low-level turnover required for maintaining the structural integrity of the liver microcirculation. However, in response to most forms of liver injury, these cells become activated and undergo

## Special Study Topic continued . . .

phenotypic transformation to become myofibroblast-like cells. They are then much more active in producing matrix proteins, in particular the interstitial collagens, become more contractile, and are more responsive to vasoactive mediators. They are thus the principal driving force behind the progressive scarring that occurs in chronic liver disease, but, as the result of their increased contractility, they also lead to reduction of blood flow through the liver sinusoids and this contributes to the development of portal hypertension (see Chapter 10, p. 283). Not only do they produce increased amounts of collagens, but on activation they produce TIMPs, which inhibit the breakdown of collagens and other matrix proteins.

There has been recent interest in unravelling the molecular events associated with activation of these cells. They can be readily isolated from liver tissues and grown in primary culture. Studies using such an approach have shown that they proliferate in response to PDGF and TGF-α and undergo phenotypic changes including increased collagen production in response to TGF-β and TNF-α. Numerous other growth factors may also have a role but, on an equimolar basis, these four are considered to be the most important. Hepatic stellate cells can, however, also be activated by ROS and other low-molecular-weight compounds including metabolites of alcohol metabolism.

The intracellular signalling cascades involved in bringing about the biological changes in activated hepatic stellate cells include the mitogen-activated protein kinase (MAPK) pathway, inositol lipid pathway, JAK/STAT pathway, and integrin-mediated pathway. Some of the growth factors stimulate more than one cascade pathway and this may explain why they are more active than others: e.g. PDGF is more mitogenic than TGF-α and recent evidence suggests that this is because whereas TGF-α signals through the extracellular signal-regulated protein kinase (ERK) and stress-activated protein kinase forms of the MAPK pathway, PDGF signals through these and inositol lipid pathways.

The interest in identifying the cell and molecular biological events in fibrosis is driven largely as a consequence of the current lack of specific therapies for treating liver fibrosis. Strategies are now being designed that target inhibitors of the signalling pathways to hepatic stellate cells, in an attempt to prevent activation of the cells. Strategies not only to reduce collagen production, but also to enhance its resorption by stimulating matrix metalloproteases, are also being developed. Core aspects of liver damage and cirrhosis are discussed in Chapter 10.

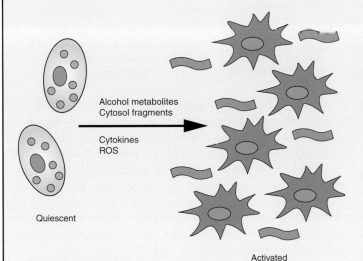

FIG. 4.30 Role of hepatic stellate cells in liver injury. Quiescent stellate cells contain abundant cytoplasmic lipid (vitamin A). In response to a number of cytokines, reactive oxygen species (ROS), proteins from dead hepatocytes, and acetaldehyde, the cells proliferate, lose cytoplasmic fat, and begin to resemble myofibroblasts. There is increased production of matrix proteins together with a reduction in activity of metalloproteases, which degrade the matrix. The net result is accumulation of collagen and other matrix proteins.

These are released by platelets, inflammatory cells, injured epithelial cells, and endothelial cells. Other cells may also contribute, such as mast cells and eosinophils. It is thought that TGF-β is the most important profibrogenic peptide. As noted above, it acts principally as an inhibitor of cell proliferation, but in granulation tissue its main action is to switch on fibroblasts to produce extracellular matrix proteins. Some of the fibroblasts that are involved in granulation tissue formation contain myofibrils and express the cytoskeletal protein α-smooth muscle actin. These are so-called myofibroblasts, which may have contractile properties and are thought to play a role in the contraction of wounds (see below).

## HEALING OF SKIN WOUNDS

The simplest form of wound healing occurs when uninfected skin incisions are closed promptly by suturing. This is referred to as healing by first intention (or primary union). It is characterized by the formation of only minimal amounts of granulation tissue. It is a rapid process and contrasts with healing by second intention, which occurs in an open wound, the edges of which are not brought together and where there is loss of epithelium.

When an incision is made in the skin and subcutaneous tissue, blood escaping from cut vessels clots on the wound surface and fills the gap between the wound edges

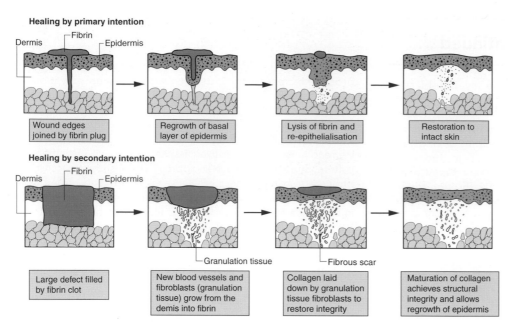

**Healing by primary intention**

Dermis — Fibrin — Epidermis

| Wound edges joined by fibrin plug | Regrowth of basal layer of epidermis | Lysis of fibrin and re-epithelialisation | Restoration to intact skin |

**Healing by secondary intention**

Dermis — Fibrin — Epidermis

Granulation tissue — Fibrous scar

| Large defect filled by fibrin clot | New blood vessels and fibroblasts (granulation tissue) grow from the demis into fibrin | Collagen laid down by granulation tissue fibroblasts to restore integrity | Maturation of collagen achieves structural integrity and allows regrowth of epidermis |

**FIG. 4.31** Outline of stages involved in healing of skin wounds, and comparison of primary and secondary intention.

(Fig. 4.31). In sutured wounds, this gap is narrow. Fibrin in the clot acts as a glue, which holds the cut surfaces together. The dehydrated blood clot on the surface forms a scab, which seals the wound. After 24 hours there is a mild inflammatory reaction at the wound edges with exudation of fluid and migration of polymorphs. The blood clot is digested by lysosomal enzymes released from polymorphs and this is contributed to from day 3 by macrophages. These cells phagocytose cellular debris, fibrin, and red cells. Within 24–48 hours there is enlargement of the basal cells of the epidermis, with some loss of their normally close adherence to the underlying tissue and flattening of rête ridges. Close to the cut edge, cells from the deeper part of the epithelium begin to proliferate and slide over each other; they migrate out along the exposed surface of the dermis and become flattened to form a continuous advancing sheet. Whereas the advancing edge of the sheet of new epidermis consists of a single layer of flat cells, the older part at the periphery of the wound becomes stratified so that there is a gradient of thickness. The cells will migrate only over viable tissue. There may be some growth of cells down the cut edges of the dermis. This is later resorbed, although occasionally a small implantation cyst, which contains epithelium, may form.

The dermis and subcutaneous tissues are repaired by the formation of small amounts of granulation tissue. From about day 3 angiogenesis occurs at the wound margins. The newly formed capillaries are delicate and lack a basement membrane. They leak protein-rich fluid and neutrophils emigrate from them. Within a few days, however, these structures differentiate into arterioles and venules. Fibroblasts stream from the perivascular connective tissue and begin to proliferate and move into the wound. Collagen and other matrix proteins are produced and these help to unite the cut edges from about day 7. By 3 weeks the total amount of collagen in the wound has reached a maximum. At this stage the tensile strength is still low, but this increases over a period of months by further modification to the matrix proteins, including

cross-linking between collagen fibrils. From the second week onwards there is devascularization, a process by which the newly formed blood vessels and proliferated fibroblasts gradually disappear. Some sensory nerves may gradually grow into the scar from about 4 weeks, but specialized nerve endings such as pacinian corpuscles do not re-form. The end-result of healing by first intention is usually a fine pale linear scar that is level with the adjacent surface. Occasionally, the connective tissue component of the healing process is excessive leading to a hypertrophic scar or keloid (Fig. 4.32).

Healing of an open gaping wound where there has been loss of tissue occurs by the formation of more substantial amounts of granulation tissue, which grows from the base of the wound to fill the defect. Angiogenesis and fibroblast proliferation are more abundant and healing takes longer than that following healing by first intention. Initially, there is haemorrhage and exudation of fibrin from the cut surfaces. This is followed by a massive emigration of neutrophils and subsequently macrophages. These cells soften and remove the fibrin and other debris. As in the incised wound,

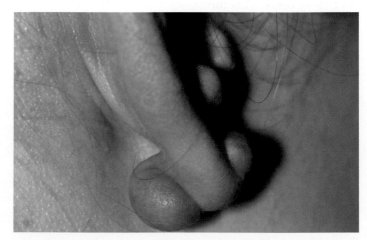

**FIG. 4.32** Keloid scar after ear piercing. (Courtesy of Dr Clifford Lawrence.)

**TABLE 4.2** Factors that slow down healing

| Local | Systemic |
|---|---|
| Poor local blood supply and infection | Diabetes mellitus; renal failure |
| Excessive movement | Malnutrition |
| Ionizing radiation | Vitamin C deficiency |

epithelial cells at the margins enlarge and begin to migrate down the walls of the wound after 24–48 hours. Migration and proliferation together produce a sheet of cells, which advances in a series of tongue-like projections beneath any residual blood clot on the wound surface. As the single layer of cells moves inward towards the wound centre, there is stratification of the cells near to the wound margin. As the denuded area is large, the advancing epithelial sheet does not completely cover the wound until the granulation tissue from the base has started to fill the wound space. Within a few days pre-existing vessels in the wound bed produce vascular sprouts, which grow upward, forming loops and coils near the wound surface. From these new more permeable vessels, small haemorrhages occur and neutrophils migrate, reinforcing those already present in the exudate on the wound surface, and help to keep down bacterial growth. This fibrovascular granulation tissue continues to proliferate and fill the wound space until the epithelium grows over its surface, at which time the exudative inflammatory changes subside. As soon as the wound surface has been covered, epithelial cell migration ceases and proliferation, stratification, and keratinization are then rapidly completed although rête ridges are not re-formed.

The fibroblasts become orientated parallel to the wound surface and, by the end of week 1, collagen is being actively produced and rapidly increases in amount. There is subsequently devascularization and remodelling of the collagen as described above and the dermis over a period of months becomes progressively less cellular. Healing of an open, excised wound is aided by contraction of the surface area at sites where the skin is mobile and loosely attached to underlying tissue. This movement of the edges towards the centre of the wound is brought about by so-called myofibroblasts, which develop from mesenchymal cells within the connective tissue of the wound. The term 'contracture' is used when the repair process ultimately leads to distortion or limitation of movement of the tissues. This may result either from contraction of the wound itself or from scarring of the deeper muscle and soft tissues.

Several factors can alter the rate and efficiency of wound healing – local and systemic factors that can interfere with healing are outlined in *Table 4.2*.

## HEALING OF FRACTURES

The basic processes involved in the healing of bone fractures bear a resemblance to many of those seen in skin wounds

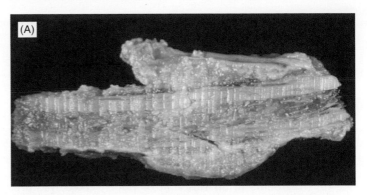

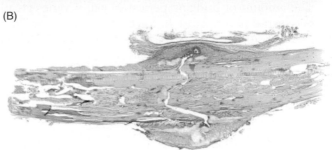

**FIG. 4.33** Fracture healing: this segment of rib was excised from a woman aged 22 years, who complained of a painful swelling in the chest wall, of a few weeks' duration. The preoperative diagnosis was of a tumour of the bone. (A) The gross specimen shows an irregular fracture line involving both cortices and the medullary canal. The fracture is bridged by periosteal callus, which is particularly marked on the superior surface. (B) Histological examination shows that the periosteal callus consists of arcades of reactive bone and a mass of cartilage overlaying the fracture line. There is also callus within the medullary canal. At this relatively early stage of fracture healing, the fracture gap remains unrepaired.

(Fig. 4.33). Primary union is rarely found, however, and there is usually a marked connective tissue response involving osteogenic cells. Continuity between bone fragments is first established by a mass of new bony trabeculae and cartilaginous tissue (provisional callus). This undergoes slow remodelling with resorption, so that under favourable conditions firm bony union is achieved. Sometimes this is so efficient that the original fracture site can hardly be identified.

A good deal of force is required to break a bone. The fragments are usually displaced and there may be haemorrhage between the bone ends. There may also be substantial haemorrhage into the adjacent tissues. Inflammatory changes take place with exudation of protein-rich fluid from which fibrin is deposited. Neutrophils are scanty unless there is infection, and this is common only in compound fractures when a bone fragment has torn the overlying skin. Macrophages invade and phagocytose the clot and tissue debris. Bone necrosis occurs chiefly as a result of tearing of blood vessels in the medullary cavity, cortex, and periosteum. Damage to the bone marrow may have serious results when globules of fat enter torn local vessels, producing fat emboli (see Chapter 6, p. 113). When there is splintering of bone (comminuted fracture) some of the fragments may lose their blood supply. These become necrotic and if small enough are eventually resorbed by osteoclasts. Bone death is recognizable histologically by the loss of osteocytes from bone lacunae.

There are three components to the formation of provisional callus:

1. Periosteal reaction: the cells of the inner layer of the periosteum proliferate in a wide zone, overlying the cortex of each fractured bone end. A cuff of bone trabeculae is formed around each bone at right angles to the cortex and anchored to it. Mixed with this, nodules of cartilage may form. The two enlarging cuffs of callus advance towards each other and finally unite to bridge the fracture line. This bandage of external callus helps to immobilize the fragments in an unstable or poorly fixed fracture. The amount of bridging periosteal callus varies greatly between different sites. In fractures occurring within a joint capsule (e.g. some fractures of the neck of femur) there is no periosteum, and union occurs almost entirely due to internal callus formed by osteoblasts lying in the medullary cavity (see below). In contrast, fractures of the long bones such as humerus form large amounts of external callus with relatively little internal callus.

2. Medullary reaction: the first evidence of healing in the medullary cavity is the advance of capillaries from viable marrow into necrotic marrow. This is followed by emigration of macrophages and proliferation of fibroblasts and osteoblasts. The osteoblasts produce new woven bone in the marrow spaces. The new bone is deposited partly on the surface of dead trabeculae which when surrounded by new bone may remain unabsorbed for months or even years.

3. Cortical reaction: in viable cortex adjacent to the fracture there is an increase in osteoclastic resorption with widening of the haversian canals. This may be followed later by some osteoblastic activity. Similar changes are seen in the dead cortex of the bone ends once there has been revascularization of the haversian canals from adjacent vessels in viable bone, or from periosteal and medullary vessels.

The periosteal callus unites the fragments externally, but there remains a gap within the fracture itself. This is initially filled with blood clot. This becomes replaced by granulation tissue in which there are varying numbers of osteoblasts and fibroblasts. Bony union of the fracture gap may occur through two processes. Direct ossification is brought about by osteogenic cells from the medullary and periosteal callus, and is rapid and effective. By contrast a process of fibrous union may occur in which collagen is laid down initially and this is only later ossified to become bony tissue. This slower form of union occurs when there is instability or separation of the bone ends. It also occurs more often when there is a poor blood supply or infection. Occasionally ossification fails to occur, leading to an unstable healed fracture (non-union).

Once bony union has occurred and function has been regained, the bone begins to be remodelled in response to mechanical stresses. Excess callus is resorbed, slowly formed lamellar bone begins to replace the hastily laid down woven bone, and any remaining necrotic bone is removed and replaced. The cortex is re-formed across the fracture gap, and gradually medullary callus is removed and the marrow cavity restored. The whole process may take about a year and is more rapid and complete in children.

## SUMMARY

- Cellular and tissue stress may lead to adaptation responses, which include hypertrophy, hyperplasia, atrophy and metaplasia.
- When the capacity for adaptation is exceeded, there is cellular injury, which may be reversible or irreversible.
- Cell death (irreversible injury) occurs through two distinct mechanisms: necrosis and apoptosis.
- Inflammatory and repair processes are designed to limit the adverse effects of cellular injury and death but may themselves contribute to tissue damage.
- Acute inflammation is the initial response to most forms of tissue injury and comprises a vascular phase and a cellular phase in which neutrophil polymorphs have an important role.
- Acute inflammatory processes may be followed by resolution, abscess formation, development of chronic inflammation, and/or healing with fibrosis.
- Chronic inflammation lacks the vascular component of acute inflammation and is characterized by an infiltrate of lymphocytes and macrophages.
- Repair processes are designed to restore tissue integrity and consist of both regenerative and connective tissue responses.
- The balance between regeneration and fibrosis varies depending on the tissue and nature of injury, as does the outcome.
- Some repair processes lead to complete restitution of tissue integrity whereas in others there is replacement of functional tissue by dense scar tissue.

## ACKNOWLEDGEMENTS

The contributions of Alastair D Burt and Stewart Fleming to this chapter in the 14th edition are gratefully acknowledged.

## FURTHER READING

Kumar V, Abbas AK, Aster JC, Fausto N. *Robbins and Cotran's Pathologic Basis of Disease*, 8th edn. Philadelphia, PA: Elsevier Saunders, 2009.

Majno G, Joris I. *Cells, Tissues and Disease. Principles of General Pathology*, 2nd edn. Oxford: Oxford University Press, 2004.

Solomon L, Warwick DJ, Nayagam S. *Apley's Concise System of Orthopaedics and Fractures*, 3rd edn. London: Hodder Arnold, 2005.

# 5

# CANCER AND BENIGN TUMOURS

C Simon Herrington

**5.1 CASE HISTORY**

## NEOPLASIA (CANCER AND BENIGN TUMOURS)

### History

A 63-year-old male presented to his general practitioner with a 3-month history of increasing breathlessness and a non-productive cough. He was an electrician, and had worked in a shipbuilding yard for over 40 years. He admitted to having smoked 25 cigarettes a day since the age of 16 years.

On clinical examination he was noted to have finger clubbing and his fingers were heavily stained with nicotine. On examining the chest, there was evidence of diminished air entry at the left base.

### Investigations

A left-sided hilar mass was seen in the chest radiograph. Bronchial biopsy showed a moderately differentiated squamous cell carcinoma (Fig. 5.1).

The recommended treatment was surgical, and a left pneumonectomy was performed (Fig. 5.2). Histological examination confirmed the biopsy diagnosis and showed that the surgical resection margins were free of tumour. Tumour had, however, involved the parietal pleura and the lymph node metastases suspected on gross examination were confirmed histologically. The tumour was staged as T3 N1 M0.

The patient made a good recovery from surgery but, at a routine outpatient clinic appointment 18 months later, he complained of fatigue and recent onset of backache.

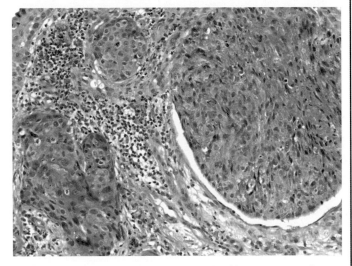

**FIG. 5.1** This bronchial biopsy shows islands of large tumour cells, which are cohesive and have long cell-to-cell borders. Keratin production is not, however, prominent.

On examination, his liver was found to be enlarged, and a radiograph of his spine showed multiple areas of bone destruction with collapse of the body of the T8 vertebra. Palliative radiotherapy was given to the spine with good pain relief, but the patient died 3 months later. At postmortem examination, multiple bony metastases (secondaries) were found in his liver and spine.

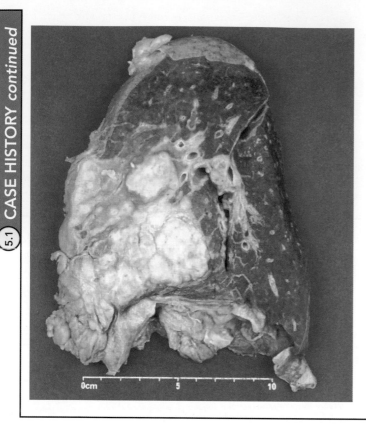

This patient died of lung cancer, the most common malignant tumour in the western world. The case raises a number of points including:

- What is cancer?
- How do tumours develop?
- Why did this patient develop this tumour? Were his cigarette smoking and his occupation in any way responsible? If so, why did he develop the tumour when many equally heavy smokers do not?
- How do metastases develop, and why do they occur in the sites that they do?

**Fig. 5.2** This section of left lung shows a large white tumour that extends to the pleural surface, to which parietal pleura is attached. Two peribronchial lymph nodes contain what appears to be white tumour.

## CANCER EPIDEMIOLOGY

### Key Points

- Cancer is predominantly a disease of middle-aged and elderly people.
- The varying incidence of cancers of different types in different populations may indicate the underlying causes of these tumours.
- Environment and genetics are important in determining cancer risk.
- Smoking and diet are major predisposing causes.

Epidemiology is the branch of medicine that describes the distribution of diseases in different populations over time: this includes the incidence (number of new cases) and prevalence (number of existing cases) of a disease as well as its geographical distribution. Through studying the geographical distribution of a type of cancer, its racial prevalence, and the occupations of those who have developed it, much can be understood about both the risk factors and the underlying pathogenic mechanisms. To draw meaningful epidemiological conclusions about cancer, precise diagnoses must be made, then accurately registered with cancer registration organizations and, ideally, there should be good follow-up information to determine patient outcome, including mortality.

### The Global Cancer Burden

The World Health Organization publishes annual cancer mortality statistics for most countries, and its subsidiary, the International Agency for Research on Cancer, issues a regular statistical analysis known as Cancer Incidence in Five Continents. It is estimated that about 10 million new cases of cancer are diagnosed each year and cancer accounts for around 12% of all deaths worldwide. The annual total is predicted to rise to 15 million per year in 2020 as the population increases and ages; cancer is predominantly a disease of middle-aged and elderly people.

Taking all forms together, cancer is the second most common cause of death in developed countries and has recently overtaken heart disease to become the major killer in some western societies, killing around 25% of the population. The major human cancers are carcinomas (malignant epithelial tumours); lymphomas (malignant lymphoid tumours) rank about tenth and sarcomas (malignant connective tissue tumours) are rarer still. The most common cancer in men is bronchial (lung) carcinoma, followed by stomach, colorectal, and prostate carcinomas. Worldwide, carcinoma of the breast is the most common cancer in women, but, in some areas, e.g. west Scotland, the incidence of lung cancer in women exceeds breast cancer because the smoking habits of women have changed. Cervical, colorectal, and endometrial carcinomas are also relatively common.

The risk of developing a cancer depends on many different factors, among them age, sex, geographical location, race, occupational history, social habits, and socioeconomic class. Some of the factors that influence the risk of cancer are discussed below.

## Age

Overall, cancer particularly affects middle-aged and elderly people, but different tumour types have different age profiles. Some particularly affect infants (e.g. neuroblastoma, nephroblastoma), children (e.g. acute lymphoblastic leukaemia), and adolescents (e.g. osteosarcoma). Hodgkin disease, a form of lymphoma, has a bimodal peak affecting young adults and then middle-aged to elderly people. Carcinomas, the most common cancers, tend to affect middle-aged and elderly people, the incidence generally increasing with age.

## Geographical Variations

There are striking regional variations in cancer incidence throughout the world. Many of these variations appear to be due to environmental factors such as carcinogens rather than genetic factors. In south-east Asia and Africa, hepatocellular carcinoma is common due to the high prevalence of hepatitis B infection and environmental exposure to carcinogens, e.g. aflatoxins present in mouldy groundnuts. Chewing betel-quid and areca-nut, a practice common in Asia, is recognized to be carcinogenic. Malignant melanoma is mainly a disease of white-skinned people and is especially common in sunny climates such as Queensland, Australia, where many of the population are fair-skinned individuals of northern European extraction. Exposure to high levels of ultraviolet light can cause cancer. Gastric carcinoma is common in the former Soviet Union, Japan, and China, whereas its incidence in western countries has progressively fallen, perhaps due to altered dietary habits and the decline of infection with *Helicobacter pylori*. Breast and colorectal carcinoma are far more common in western countries than in Asia.

### Changing Patterns of Disease and the Effects of Migration

Careful epidemiological studies of large populations who have migrated around the world have demonstrated that the incidence of cancers in migrant populations rapidly moves towards that of the recipient country, e.g. the incidence of gastric carcinoma in Japanese migrants to the west coast of America falls from the high level seen in Japan to the lower incidence in the USA by the second generation of immigrant families. These data strongly suggest that environment is more important than heredity in determining geographical variation in cancer risk. It is thought that environmental factors account for over 80% of human tumours.

### Diet

In general, diets rich in fruit and vegetables are associated with lower risks of many major forms of cancer, including tumours of the lung, stomach, breast, and colon. In contrast, a diet rich in animal fat is statistically linked to increased incidence of cancers of the breast, colon, prostate, pancreas, and endometrium. The risk of colon cancer in a population is directly proportional to the extent of meat consumption. A diet rich in salted fish is associated with a high incidence of gastric and nasopharyngeal carcinoma. Alcohol consumption is linked to tumours of the breast, colon, and liver, and acts in a synergistic manner with smoking in tumours of the aerodigestive tract.

### Cigarette Smoking

It is now generally acknowledged that cigarette smoking is responsible for at least a quarter of cancer deaths, especially from cancers of the lung, larynx, oral cavity, and to a lesser extent urinary tract. Most of the effects are due to direct contact with carcinogens in smoke, but these are also absorbed and excreted through the kidneys. Many carcinogens are present in smoke, including benzopyrene and dimethylnitrosamine. There is a direct relationship between the number of cigarettes smoked and the risk of lung cancer and, although stopping smoking reduces this risk, its effects are not totally reversible.

## GENERAL FEATURES OF TUMOURS

A neoplasm, literally a new growth, is classically defined as an abnormal mass of tissue, the growth of which is uncoordinated with, and exceeds that of, the normal tissues. It results from aberration of the normal mechanisms that control cell number: cell production by cell division, and cell loss by the process of apoptosis. Most tumours are monoclonal, i.e. all the cells in a tumour appear to have arisen from one parent cell which has undergone a genetic change; this is then passed on to all its progeny. As tumour cells lack the normal control mechanisms, the clone expands due to uncontrolled proliferation. Although the tumour is derived from one clone, further genetic changes develop in some of the progeny, so that the tumour may become heterogeneous, a property described as clonal evolution.

## Classification of Tumours

Tumours are divided into two major groups according to their behaviour: benign and malignant. Benign tumours remain localized at their site of origin. They grow by expansion, pushing the normal tissues away, often with the formation of a capsule of compressed fibrous tissue. Benign tumours usually grow slowly but, despite their name, are not always benign in clinical terms. Their effects are described on p. 80.

Malignant tumours, also known as cancers, grow by infiltrating into the surrounding normal tissues and have the ability to spread to distant sites, i.e. to metastasize, where secondary deposits, metastases, form. The histological appearance of metastases resembles that of the primary tumour. Although malignant tumours usually grow rapidly, it should be recognized that not all malignant tumours are equally malignant. Some are highly aggressive and metastasize early, e.g. small-cell carcinoma of the bronchus. Others are slow growing and, although they are locally infiltrative, they rarely metastasize. Basal cell carcinoma and chondrosarcoma are good examples of this. The degree of malignancy, described as tumour grade, usually correlates well with survival. The features of benign and malignant tumours are shown in Fig. 5.3 and summarized in *Table 5.1*.

### Histogenesis of Tumours

Tumours are further classified according to the cell type that they resemble, i.e. their differentiation. This property is usually determined by the tumour's appearance on light microscopy, i.e. its phenotype. The term 'histogenesis' – meaning tissue of origin – is used because most tumours resemble to some extent the tissue from which they arise, although tumours of course arise from primitive stem cells so the concept of histogenesis is not very helpful scientifically. It is now clear that the phenotype and histogenesis of a tumour are not necessarily synonymous: thus rhabdomyosarcoma, a malignant tumour showing skeletal muscle differentiation, may arise at sites in which no skeletal muscle

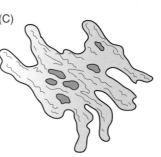

(C)

Infiltrating crab-like processes invading surrounding normal tissue

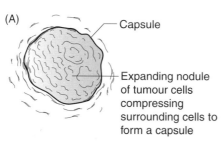

(A)

Capsule

Expanding nodule of tumour cells compressing surrounding cells to form a capsule

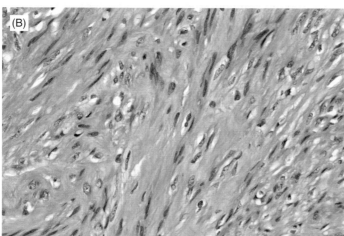

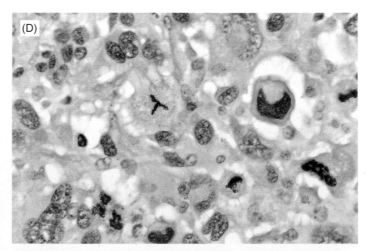

**Fig. 5.3** (A) Benign tumours are well circumscribed and the surrounding tissue often forms a capsule of fibrous tissue. (B) The cells of benign tumours closely resemble those of the normal tissue in which they arise. The nuclei are normal. As growth is slow, mitoses are uncommon, and as division is normal mitotic figures are of normal appearance. (C) Malignant tumours have infiltrative margins both on naked eye and on microscopic examination. (D) The nuclei are usually enlarged and the nucleoli active, indicating that the cell is active. The nuclei are often darkly staining – hyperchromatic – and variable in size and shape – pleomorphic – as the DNA content of the nucleus is frequently increased. Mitoses are often numerous and they are frequently abnormal in form, indicating that the process of cell division may be abnormal. A tripolar mitosis (as seen in this figure) is one in which the chromosomes are attempting to segregate towards three daughter cells.

**TABLE 5.1** Differences between benign and malignant tumours

|  | **Benign** | **Malignant** |
| --- | --- | --- |
| Growth pattern | Expand, remain localized | Infiltrate locally, spread to distant sites (metastasize) |
| Growth rate | Slower | Faster |
| Clinical effects | Local pressure effects; hormone secretion | Local pressure and destruction; inappropriate hormone secretion; distant metastases |
| Histology | Resembles tissue of origin | Many differ from tissue of origin (less well differentiated) |
| Nuclei | Small, regular, uniform | Larger, pleomorphic |
| Mitoses | Few, normal | Numerous, including atypical forms |
| Treatment | Local excision | Local excision and systemic therapy if metastases present |

is normally found. Increasingly, traditional histological ways of defining the phenotype of a tumour are being complemented by molecular biology techniques, such as the polymerase chain reaction and gene chip array technology, to determine the genes expressed by tumour cells.

It is important to understand that some highly malignant tumours do not show any definite form of differentiation. These tumours are described as undifferentiated or anaplastic.

## Epithelial Tumours

### Benign Epithelial Tumours

Benign tumours may arise from both covering epithelium, e.g. of squamous type, forming papillomas, and from glandular epithelium, e.g. of colon or thyroid, forming adenomas.

### Papillomas

Papillomas are warty growths in which the proliferating epithelium is thrown upwards into folds, and does not invade the underlying connective tissue. Between these folds of epithelium are cores of fibrous tissue and blood vessels, which bring nutrition to the epithelium. In general, the epithelium is well differentiated and closely resembles the normal epithelium from which it arises. Typical examples are squamous papillomas of skin or larynx (Fig. 5.4), which are usually viral in origin. Papillomas may arise within duct structures, e.g. intraduct papillomas of the breast, which often cause a blood-stained nipple discharge.

### Adenomas

Adenomas are benign tumours of glandular epithelium. The tumour cells in such a tumour form glandular structures mimicking the arrangement of the normal tissue (Fig. 5.5). The cells are well differentiated and often continue to secrete the normal product of the gland; thus the cells of a colonic adenoma may produce mucin or a thyroid adenoma thyroxine. If the glands become distended by secretion they may form cysts – resulting in a multiloculated lesion described as a cystadenoma, which may be found in the ovary or pancreas. Sometimes, especially in the ovary, there is proliferation of epithelium within the cyst, often in the form of papillary structures – papilloma-like growths with central fibrovascular cores – and the term 'papillary cystadenoma' is used.

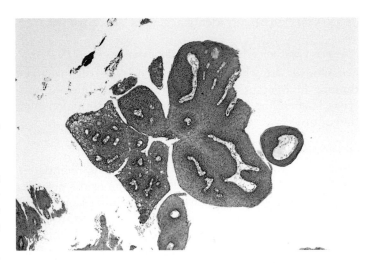

**Fig. 5.4** Squamous papilloma of the larynx: this lesion consists of finger-like projections of squamous epithelium with central connective tissue cores.

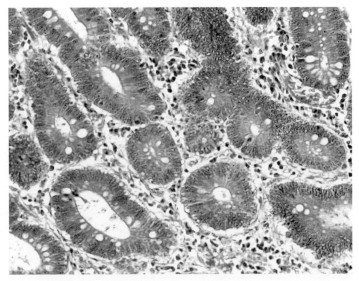

**Fig. 5.5** Adenoma of the colon: several gland-like structures are present, mimicking the structure of normal colonic mucosa.

Adenomas of viscera such as the colon tend to grow into the lumen, and often adopt a papillary architecture. Some are sessile and are thrown into greatly thickened papillary folds – so-called villous adenomas – whereas others become pedunculated with a stalk of normal mucosa – known as tubular adenomas (Fig. 5.6).

In most benign tumours, the cytological features closely resemble those of the normal tissue from which they arise. Colonic adenomas are an exception; they usually show a varying degree of cytological atypia with a high nuclear:cytoplasmic ratio and increased mitotic activity – features known as dysplasia. The importance of this lies in the risk of malignant change to carcinoma. This is described as the adenoma–carcinoma sequence; the underlying molecular biology of this process is now well understood (see Chapter 9, p. 268). It is important to realize that this paradigm does not mean that every single tumour follows the same route or necessarily harbours identical genetic abnormalities.

### Malignant Epithelial Tumours (Carcinomas)

Carcinomas are the most common type of malignant tumour in humans. They fall into several different sub-types, depending on the form of differentiation that they show.

#### Squamous cell carcinoma

These are tumours showing squamous differentiation (Fig. 5.7) in the form of keratin production or the presence of intercellular bridges, which on electron microscopy can be seen to be desmosomes. Squamous carcinomas can arise from pre-existing squamous epithelium, e.g. of skin or larynx, but some, e.g. of bronchus and the cervical transformation zone, arise at sites where there is normally glandular epithelium, but squamous metaplasia has been followed by malignant change. Squamous carcinomas resemble normal squamous epithelium to a varying extent. Well-differentiated tumours show maturation from proliferating basal cells, through acanthotic cells resembling the stratum spinosum, to heavily keratinized cells. Poorly differentiated tumours show much less maturation, often with no keratin production, but consist of sheets of cells joined by intercellular bridges.

#### Adenocarcinoma

These are tumours showing glandular differentiation. They usually arise from glandular epithelium, e.g. within the stomach, endometrium, or colon, and may arise from metaplastic glandular tissue, e.g. at the lower end of the oesophagus in Barrett's oesophagus when chronic acid reflux has resulted in metaplasia. Adenocarcinomas may be well differentiated – forming well-defined glandular structures known as acini (Fig. 5.8) – but in poorly differentiated forms there may be only occasional glandular structures or only patchy evidence of mucin production. In some tumours, typically of the stomach, individual cells contain intracytoplasmic globules of mucin; these push the nucleus to one side and the tumour cells are known as signet-ring cells (Fig. 5.9). In other mucin-producing tumours there is extensive extracellular accumulation of mucin; this forms large lakes in which scattered epithelial cells are seen. These are known as mucoid carcinomas and are seen in the stomach, colon, and breast. Some adenocarcinomas, similar to cystadenomas, form large cystic spaces (cystadenocarcinomas) and may have papillary ingrowths (papillary cystadenocarcinomas); these are typically found in the ovaries.

#### Transitional cell carcinoma

Transitional cell carcinoma arises from the transitional epithelium of the urogenital tract. It too may show considerable variation in appearance: well-differentiated papillary transitional cell carcinomas resemble papillomas, and may not show any invasion of the underlying stroma, but they are regarded as malignant for practical purposes because they have a high risk of recurrence, often in a more aggressive form. Poorly differentiated transitional cell carcinomas have a more solid architecture and frequently invade deeply within the wall of the bladder or ureter.

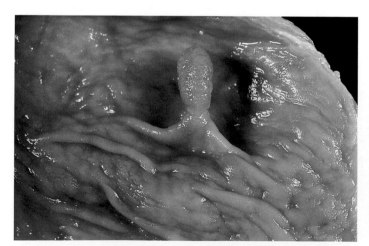

**FIG. 5.6** Tubular adenoma of the colon: this is a small pedunculated polyp on a slender stalk.

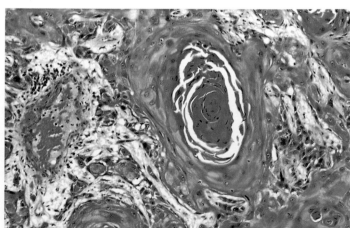

**FIG. 5.7** Squamous cell carcinoma. This is an example of a well-differentiated tumour with irregular islands of squamous epithelium, one of which shows central keratinization.

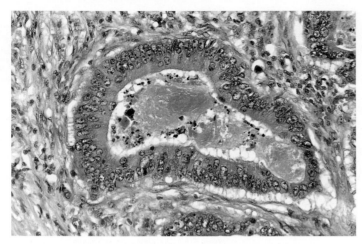

**FIG. 5.8** Adenocarcinoma: the tumour cells form an acinar structure. The nuclei contain prominent nucleoli.

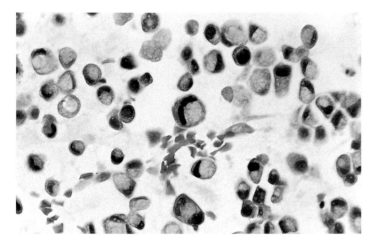

**FIG. 5.9** Signet-ring cell carcinoma of stomach: the tumour cells have eccentric nuclei, pushed to the side by a central globule of mucus.

### Small cell carcinoma

Small cell carcinoma is a tumour that shows neuroendocrine differentiation in the form of neurosecretory granules which may be found on electron microscopy or immunostaining for vesicle membrane proteins such as synaptophysin. Typically, it arises in the bronchus, where it is the most aggressive form of lung cancer, but occasionally in other sites such as the cervix and oesophagus.

Other forms of carcinoma include hepatocellular carcinoma, the malignant tumour of hepatocytes, and basal cell carcinoma, a variety of skin cancer that is often locally destructive, but seldom metastasizes.

## Connective Tissue Tumours

The connective tissues are fibrous tissue, fat, nerve, muscle, blood vessels, bone, and cartilage. Both benign and malignant tumours which show differentiation towards one of these forms can occur. It is likely that all arise from primitive mesenchymal stem cells, which retain the ability to differentiate in many directions.

### Benign Connective Tissue Tumours

The nomenclature of these tumours is straightforward – the name consists of a prefix indicating the type of differentiation, e.g. lipo- (fat), chondro- (cartilage), haemangio- (blood vessel), with the suffix -oma denoting a benign tumour. Most are slowly growing encapsulated tumours composed of the appropriate differentiated tissue. The most common form is a leiomyoma, a benign tumour showing smooth muscle differentiation, often occurring in uterine muscle (see Chapter 14, p. 430). Lipomas are also common tumours, usually occurring in the subcutaneous tissues of adults, typically on the back and shoulders. They consist of an encapsulated mass of mature fat. These, and other benign tumours, are discussed in appropriate chapters in this volume.

### Malignant Connective Tissue Tumours

These are known as sarcomas (Greek *sark* = flesh). They are far less common than carcinomas. Most occur within the deep soft tissue of the limbs and trunk, although some arise within viscera. There are numerous different types. Similar to benign tumours, the nomenclature indicates the form of differentiation shown: e.g. a leiomyosarcoma is a malignant tumour showing smooth muscle differentiation (Fig. 5.10). Rhabdomyosarcomas show skeletal muscle differentiation and are among the most common tumours of childhood. Well-differentiated examples contain myosin and actin myofilaments so well orientated that cross-striations similar to those found in normal skeletal muscle can be seen. In poorly differentiated tumours, the diagnosis is made on the basis that proteins found in skeletal muscle (e.g. desmin, myoglobin) or involved in skeletal muscle differentiation (e.g. MyoD1) can be demonstrated by immunochemistry.

Some sarcomas tend to occur in soft tissue, e.g. liposarcoma, leiomyosarcoma, and malignant peripheral nerve sheath tumours. Some, such as osteosarcoma and chondrosarcoma, occur preferentially within bone. Bone and soft tissue sarcomas are discussed in Chapter 12.

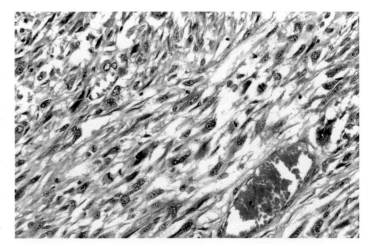

**FIG. 5.10** Leiomyosarcoma: this tumour consists of elongated cells with cigar-shaped, but pleomorphic and hyperchromatic, nuclei and eosinophilic cytoplasm. There are several mitoses in this field.

## Tumours of Haematopoietic and Lymphoid Tissues

### Leukaemias

These are malignant tumours of haematopoietic cells, derived from stem cells within the bone marrow. From the marrow, the malignant cells, similar to their normal white cell counterparts, tend to migrate into the peripheral blood so that there is usually an elevated white cell count (leukaemia – *leukos* [white], *haima* – blood). There is often widespread infiltration of other organs such as liver and spleen. Leukaemia is therefore a diffuse form of tumour, and the usual concepts of tumour spread do not apply. Leukaemias fall into two broad categories: tumours of lymphoid and myeloid cells; within each group the cells may be primitive or fairly mature and associated with a rapidly progressing or indolent natural history, respectively. The four main types – acute lymphoblastic leukaemia, chronic lymphocytic leukaemia, acute myeloblastic leukaemia, and chronic myeloid leukaemia – together with less common variants are discussed in Chapter 8 (pp. 222–228).

### Lymphomas

These are malignant solid tumours of lymphocytic origin, most of which arise in the lymph nodes, spleen, thymus, or bone marrow. A smaller proportion, around 30%, arise in other organs such as the gastrointestinal tract, thyroid, and brain, usually within lymphoid tissue resulting from chronic inflammatory conditions, such as helicobacter gastritis and Hashimoto's thyroiditis. Lymphomas may remain localized to the site of origin for some time or they may be widely disseminated. They are broadly divided into two groups: Hodgkin lymphoma and non-Hodgkin lymphoma, on the basis of the distinctive large cells known as Reed–Sternberg cells (Fig. 5.11) present in Hodgkin lymphoma. Non-Hodgkin lymphoma falls into two main groups: those derived from B cells or from T cells. In recent years immunocytochemical and molecular biological techniques have been applied to these tumours to determine the form of differentiation of the cells in different types, compared with normal lymphoid cells, e.g. it is now apparent that the Reed–Sternberg cells of Hodgkin lymphoma are of B-cell lineage. Lymphomas are discussed in detail in Chapter 8 (pp. 199–212).

Leukaemias and lymphomas are related tumours, and there is some overlap: e.g. chronic lymphocytic leukaemia and well-differentiated lymphocytic lymphoma are essentially the same disease, but one label is applied when the disease predominantly affects marrow and peripheral blood, and the other when enlarged lymph nodes are the presenting complaint. No true benign tumours have been described in either group.

## Germ Cell Tumours

Tumours may arise from the germ cells, and these are therefore usually found within the testis or ovary. Occasionally, however, they may arise from nests of germ cells, which have been left behind during embryonic migration of germ cells from the posterior dorsal ridges. Germ cell tumours can therefore be found, usually in the midline, from the pineal, base of skull, mediastinum, and retroperitoneum to the sacrococcygeal region.

Normal germ cells are totipotent – they give rise to all tissues found within the body and to the placenta and yolk sac, the latter tissues being described as extraembryonic. Unsurprisingly, therefore, germ cell tumours may contain differentiated tissue from any of the three layers of the embryo – ectoderm, mesoderm, and endoderm – and from the extraembryonic tissues. Tumours of this type are called teratomas. These are most common in the ovary (Fig. 5.12), where they are almost always benign, and, less commonly but with a rapidly rising incidence, within the testis, where they are almost always malignant. In benign tumours, such as those of the ovary, the tissues may be very well differentiated, resembling normal skin, thyroid, brain, or cartilage. Malignant tumours, as might be predicted,

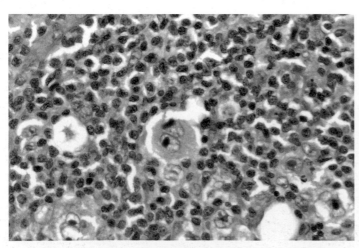

**FIG. 5.11** Hodgkin lymphoma: a typical Reed–Sternberg cell is present in the middle of the field. It is binucleate with an 'owl's eye' appearance due to the large eosinophilic nucleoli.

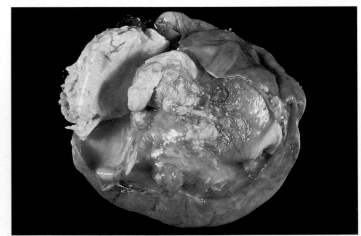

**FIG. 5.12** Benign cystic teratoma of ovary: this cyst is lined by squamous epithelium and is filled with sebaceous material and hair.

contain much less well-differentiated tissues, but curiously often form differentiated tissues under the influence of chemotherapeutic drugs.

Some germ cell tumours consist of undifferentiated cells that resemble primitive germ cells. These are known as seminomas when they arise in the testis and dysgerminomas when they arise in the ovary.

## Tumours of Neuroectoderm

Many tissues of the body are derived from neuroectoderm – the brain, neurons and supporting glia, peripheral nerves (including axons and their supporting Schwann cells), and melanocytes. Tumours derived from these cells are discussed in detail in the appropriate chapters.

The nomenclature of tumours is summarized in *Table 5.2*.

**TABLE 5.2** Tumour nomenclature

| Tissue of origin | Benign | Malignant |
|---|---|---|
| **Epithelial** | | |
| Covering epithelia | Papilloma | Carcinoma, typically squamous |
| Glandular epithelia | Adenoma (cystadenoma) | Adenocarcinoma (cystadenocarcinoma) |
| **Connective tissue** | Benign (*-oma*) | Malignant (*-sarcoma*) |
| Smooth muscle | Leiomyoma | Leiomyosarcoma |
| Skeletal muscle | Rhabdomyoma | Rhabdomyosarcoma |
| Bone forming | Osteoma | Osteosarcoma |
| Cartilage | Chondroma | Chondrosarcoma |
| Fibrous | Fibroma | Fibrosarcoma |
| Blood vessels | (Haem)angioma | Angiosarcoma |
| Adipose | Lipoma | Liposarcoma |
| **Other tissues** | | |
| Lymphoid | None | Lymphoma (Hodgkin or non-Hodgkin lymphoma) |
| Haematopoietic | None | Leukaemia |
| Primitive nerve cells | Ganglioneuroma | Neuroblastoma, retinoblastoma, and others |
| Glial cells | None | Glioma (e.g. astrocytoma) |
| Melanocytes | Pigmented naevi (moles) | Malignant melanoma |
| Mesothelium | None | Malignant mesothelioma |
| Germ cells | Teratoma | Teratoma, seminoma |

# SPREAD OF MALIGNANT TUMOURS

> **Key Points**
>
> Forms of tumour spread include:
> - local spread
> - lymphatic spread
> - haematogenous (blood) spread
> - transcoelomic spread
> - intraepithelial spread.

Malignant tumours spread in several ways. These are first described in general terms and then the complex underlying mechanisms are outlined.

## Local Spread

Malignant cells have the ability to insinuate themselves between adjacent normal cells and invade the surrounding tissues. For epithelial tumours, the first step is for the tumour cells to breach the basement membrane, i.e. to proceed from the stage of intraepithelial neoplasia to that of an invasive tumour (Fig. 5.13). It is at this point that the cells of the tumour can be said to have become malignant. Tumour cells follow the paths of least resistance and spread easily through loose fibrous and adipose tissue (Fig. 5.14). Dense fibrous tissue such as fascia and periosteum tend to form more of a barrier, but are eventually also penetrated.

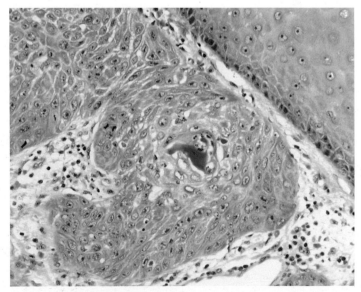

**FIG. 5.13** Early invasive squamous carcinoma: small groups of tumour cells (bottom left) have broken free from the overlying epithelium (top right) and have invaded the underlying connective tissue.

## Lymphatic Spread

This is the principal mode by which carcinomas spread. The very thin walls of the lymphatics are readily penetrated by tumour cells (Fig. 5.15), which are carried along in the lymph to the first lymph node in the lymph node chain, the sentinel node. Whether this node is involved by tumour is now recognized to be important in planning the extent of surgery, e.g. for melanoma or carcinoma of the breast. At first, the tumour cells are seen in small groups in the subcapsular sinus (Fig. 5.16), but they extend through the sinuses and gradually replace the node; they then spread proximally along the chain of lymph nodes (Fig. 5.17). Ultimately they may reach the thoracic duct and enter the superior vena cava, from which further dissemination through the bloodstream may occur.

## Haematogenous (Blood) Spread

Tumour cells are also able to invade thin-walled veins and grow along the venous system or embolize into the bloodstream. The site of initial metastasis (first-pass organ) depends on the venous drainage of the location of the tumour. Most tumour emboli pass through the right heart and impact in the pulmonary capillary bed, but many tumours of splanchnic origin, e.g. of bowel, metastasize by blood to the liver along the portal vein. Visceral tumours also invade blood vessels that communicate with the paravertebral venous plexus of Batson, a complex system of valveless veins. Retrograde flow occurring, for example, when intra-abdominal pressure is raised is responsible for the common metastases to the spine seen, for instance, in prostate carcinoma. Tumour emboli from the lungs enter the systemic circulation and may be widely disseminated to the brain or elsewhere. In contrast to the thin-walled veins, the thick walls of arteries are resistant to invasion by tumours.

It is not only the anatomical features of blood flow that explain the sites of metastases. The phrase 'seed and soil' was coined in the nineteenth century to describe the tendency of some cancers to spread to specific sites. This emphasizes the importance of the relationship between tumour cells (seed) and the site of metastasis (soil) in this process. This phenomenon is now explicable in terms of target tissues for metastasis bearing the appropriate extracellular matrix and cell adhesion molecules to allow tumour cells to stop in a given site and grow there.

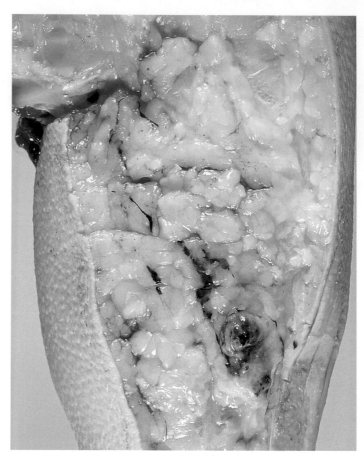

**FIG. 5.15** Lymphatic spread: this malignant melanoma has spread extensively through the lymphatics (outlined in black by melanin) in the leg.

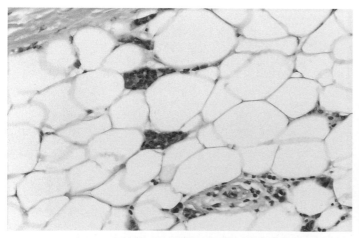

**FIG. 5.14** Local invasion by breast carcinoma: the tumour cells have spread along paths of least resistance, here through adipose tissue.

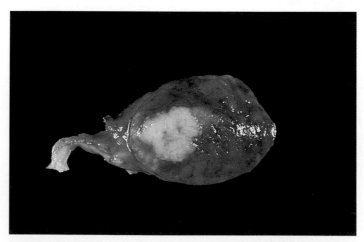

**FIG. 5.16** Early involvement of a lymph node by metastatic carcinoma. A nodule of white tumour is present under the subcapsular sinus.

Sarcomas usually spread through the bloodstream and carcinomas, which usually initially spread through the lymphatics, often spread by blood in the later stages. Renal carcinoma shows a particular tendency to invade the renal vein (Fig. 5.18).

### Transcoelomic Spread

Transcoelomic spread means spread across body cavities, namely the peritoneal, pleural, and pericardial spaces. These provide no planes of resistance so that, once tumour cells gain access to the open spaces, they readily spread widely. This is best seen in intra-abdominal tumours, especially ovarian carcinoma, which disseminates throughout the abdomen often resulting in a mass of tumour matting loops of bowel together. Gastric carcinoma can spread in a similar fashion, to involve the peritoneal cavity, often seeding to the ovaries. When these ovarian metastases are bilateral in premenopausal women they are known as Krukenberg's tumours.

### Intraepithelial Spread

This is the process by which tumour cells can infiltrate between the cells of a normal epithelium, without invading the underlying stroma. It is best seen in Paget's disease of the nipple (see Chapter 15, p. 453) in which the cells of ductal carcinoma *in situ* grow into the nipple skin (Fig. 5.19), giving an appearance resembling eczema. Extramammary Paget's disease is seen in the vulva and anorectal region and may complicate malignant skin adnexal tumours.

The mechanisms of tumour spread (*Table* 5.3) and the process of metastasis (Fig. 5.20) are complex and not simply due to the anatomy of blood flow.

(A)

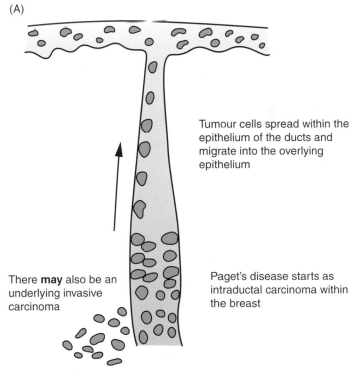

Tumour cells spread within the epithelium of the ducts and migrate into the overlying epithelium

There **may** also be an underlying invasive carcinoma

Paget's disease starts as intraductal carcinoma within the breast

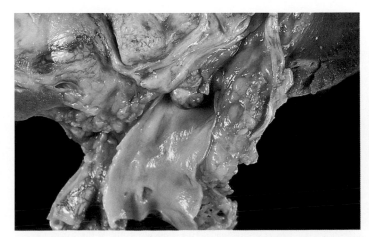

**FIG. 5.17** Breast carcinoma showing lymph node involvement. The tumour lies just lateral to the nipple. The largest arrow indicates the first node in the chain. This and the node marked by the next arrow are both involved by metastatic carcinoma. The third node is free from tumour.

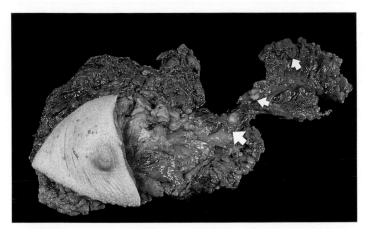

**FIG. 5.18** This large yellow renal carcinoma is seen invading the opened renal vein. Tumour can propagate via the inferior vena cava and reach the heart.

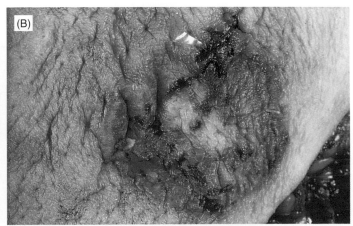

**FIG. 5.19** Paget's disease of the nipple: the mechanism of development is shown in (A) and the resulting eczema-like appearance of the overlying skin in (B).

**TABLE 5.3** Spread of tumours

| Tumour | Haematogenous | Lymphatic | Transcoelomic |
|--------|---------------|-----------|---------------|
| Carcinoma | Common, late | Common, early | Stomach, ovary |
| Melanoma | Common, late | Common, early | Rare |
| Sarcoma | Common, early | Rare | Rare |

## PREMALIGNANCY

### Key Points

There are three situations in which a premalignant process can be identified:
- intraepithelial neoplasia
- malignant change in benign tumours
- malignancy developing in association with chronic inflammatory conditions.

Familial syndromes in which there is an increased risk of malignancy are described on pp. 96–97.

## Intraepithelial Neoplasia

This is a key concept in understanding carcinomas. At numerous sites (*Table 5.4*) it is possible to identify a stage of preinvasive neoplasia, where the epithelial cells show the cytological features of malignancy but have not yet

**TABLE 5.4** Major sites of intraepithelial neoplasia

| Site | Terminology |
|------|-------------|
| Cervix | CIN (cervical intraepithelial neoplasia) |
| Vulva | VIN (vulval intraepithelial neoplasia) |
| Vagina | VaIN (vaginal intraepithelial neoplasia) |
| Prostate | PIN (prostatic intraepithelial neoplasia) |
| Skin | Carcinoma *in situ* |
| Breast | Ductal and lobular carcinoma *in situ* |

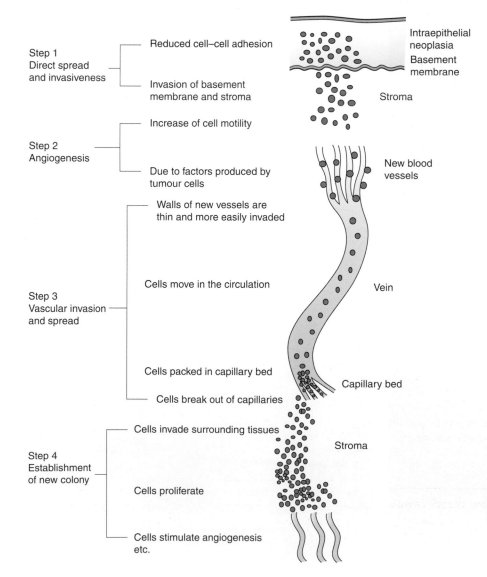

**Step 1**
**Direct spread and invasiveness**
— Reduced cell–cell adhesion
— Invasion of basement membrane and stroma

Intraepithelial neoplasia
Basement membrane
Stroma

**Step 2**
**Angiogenesis**
— Increase of cell motility
— Due to factors produced by tumour cells

New blood vessels

**Step 3**
**Vascular invasion and spread**
— Walls of new vessels are thin and more easily invaded
— Cells move in the circulation
— Cells packed in capillary bed
— Cells break out of capillaries

Vein

Capillary bed

**Step 4**
**Establishment of new colony**
— Cells invade surrounding tissues
— Cells proliferate
— Cells stimulate angiogenesis etc.

Stroma

**FIG. 5.20** The process of tumour spread (metastasis). This diagram outlines the basic process of blood-borne metastasis. More detail is provided in the accompanying Special Study Topic 5.1.

# 5.1 Special Study Topic

## MECHANISMS OF TUMOUR SPREAD

Invasion and metastasis are part of a complex multistep process involving cell–cell and cell–matrix interactions, in which various types of cell adhesion molecules are involved. Here the spread of carcinomas is described, but similar concepts apply to other tumours.

## Step 1 Direct Spread and Invasiveness

### Reduction in Cell–Cell Adhesion

Normal epithelial cells bind tightly to each other by molecules such as E-cadherin (epithelial cadherin), a member of a family of calcium-dependent cell–cell adhesion molecules. Malignant epithelial cells are less firmly attached to each other, due at least in part to reduced expression of E-cadherin, and this correlates with the invasiveness of the tumour, e.g. in breast carcinoma. In colonic carcinoma and gliomas loss of N-CAM (neural cell adhesion molecule) plays a similar part.

### Invasion of Basement Membrane and Stroma

Initially, the tumour cell must attach to the basement membrane by interaction between cell surface integrins and matrix proteins such as laminin and fibronectin. A wide variety of alterations in integrin expression is seen in cancer cells. Next, the tumour cells produce proteolytic enzymes such as collagenase and stromelysin (members of the group of zinc-containing matrix metalloproteases [MMPs]), which break up the matrix proteins laminin, fibronectin, and collagen. These proteolytic enzymes are under complex control mechanisms; they are produced in an inactive form (proenzyme) and require activation. MMP inhibitors are being developed for clinical use. In addition, there is a group of naturally occurring antagonists known as tissue inhibitors of metalloproteases (TIMPs). Other proteins including plasminogen activators and cathepsins are involved in matrix breakdown.

### Tumour Cell Motility

Invasion of the basement membrane and underlying stroma requires that the tumour cells are motile. The cells extrude pseudopodia at the front and attach to stromal proteins. Movement is generated by the cytoskeleton of cross-linked actin molecules, and is stimulated by a wide variety of growth factors, stromal components, and cytokines, e.g. autotaxin.

## Step 2 Angiogenesis

Angiogenesis is the process by which new blood vessels are formed. It is seen in embryogenesis, wound healing, and chronic inflammation. In recent years its importance in tumour development has been recognized. The development of a rich blood supply around the tumour is a critical step (described as the 'angiogenic switch') in the progression from a small localized tumour to a large one with the potential for metastasis. The mechanisms involved are complex and summarized here.

Initially, the tumour consists of a morula of cells, deriving nutrition from pre-existing blood vessels by diffusion. The distance over which nutrients can diffuse limits the tumour size. New blood vessels are formed by outgrowth of endothelial cells from post-capillary venules into the tumour mass. The stimulus for this is the increased production of angiogenic factors by the tumour cells, especially vascular endothelial growth factor (VEGF), fibroblast growth factors, and angiogenin. Normally, angiogenesis is controlled by a balance between these angiogenesis-promoting factors and inhibitors of angiogenesis such as angiostatin and endostatin. The steps involved in angiogenesis include:

- proteolytic digestion of basement membrane by plasminogen activators and MMPs
- migration of endothelial cells, initially as a solid cord
- proliferation of endothelial cells
- organization of the cords of endothelial cells into new blood vessels with lumina.

Although these mechanisms are not yet fully understood, inhibition of angiogenesis is being investigated as a potential new form of anticancer therapy.

## Step 3 Vascular Invasion

Tumour cells must breach the basement membrane and penetrate between endothelial cells; the thin walls and poorly formed basement membranes of newly formed blood vessels are easy to penetrate. Once tumour cells are free within the lumen of the blood vessel, they are carried into the circulation and lodge in a capillary bed.

At this site, further complex interactions are required. The tumour cells bind to endothelial cells, mediated by selectins and certain isoforms of CD44, a hyaluronic acid-binding protein. The cells then penetrate the capillary basement membrane by mechanisms similar to those described above. Angiogenesis is again necessary for the establishment of any metastasis ≥1 mm.

## Step 4 Establishment of a New Colony

This involves cell proliferation and the development of a tumour blood supply by stimulation of angiogenesis as previously described.

It will be apparent that the process of metastasis is not simply determined by simple mechanical factors. It has long been recognized that some sites are much more prone to metastasis than would be determined simply by their blood flow – the role of the tumour and the recipient tissue being developed the ability to invade adjacent normal tissues. This process has been known as dysplasia, carcinoma *in situ*, and more recently as 'intraepithelial neoplasia'. It can affect epithelia of all types – squamous, transitional (e.g. bladder), and glandular (e.g. stomach). In squamous epithelia the key feature is a loss of the normal maturation that occurs from the basal layer, where proliferation normally takes place, to the surface where fully mature cells are found. Detection at this early stage allows treatment to be given before local invasion occurs and metastasis is possible. This is the basis of the cervical screening programme (see Chapter 14, p. 426) in which the abnormal cells from cervical intraepithelial neoplasia (CIN) can be identified in cervical smears.

Similar changes can be seen in the vulva, vagina, bladder, and skin, but none of these is currently part of a screening programme. In other tissues, e.g. the endometrium and breast, a range of proliferative lesions can be seen, from simple hyperplasia through hyperplasia with cytological atypia to *in situ* malignancy (carcinoma *in situ*). Similar to CIN, if these are diagnosed and treated at a preinvasive stage, the prognosis is much improved.

Breast screening aims to detect carcinoma *in situ* and also small invasive carcinomas, with the hope of diagnosis before metastases have occurred. Dysplastic changes can also be seen in the metaplastic intestinal epithelium found in the oesophagus in Barrett's oesophagus, an important precursor of adenocarcinoma of the oesophagus (see Chapter 9, p. 243).

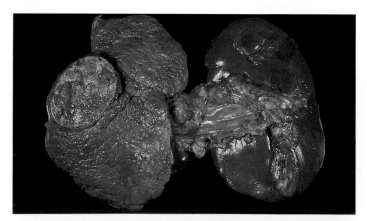

**FIG. 5.21** Cirrhotic liver on the left with a large spleen (due to portal hypertension) on the right. A large hepatocellular carcinoma has arisen in the cirrhotic liver.

## Malignant Change in Benign Tumours

Examples include colonic adenomas, which may become adenocarcinomas. This relationship is described as the adenoma–carcinoma sequence, the molecular basis of which is dealt with in Chapter 9 (p. 268). Polyps may be solitary (or few) in sporadic cases or more numerous in inherited susceptibility syndromes. Other benign tumours that may undergo malignant change are neurofibromas (see Chapter 11, p. 335).

## Malignancy Developing in Association with Chronic Inflammatory Conditions

The increased proliferation found in inflammatory and reparative conditions appears to predispose to the development of malignancy. Examples include longstanding ulcerative colitis, in which there is an increased risk of colonic cancer, and Hashimoto's thyroiditis, in which lymphoma may develop. Hepatocellular carcinomas typically arise in livers affected by cirrhosis (Fig. 5.21).

## CLINICAL EFFECTS OF TUMOURS

Not all tumours are symptomatic. Many are found incidentally on a radiograph or *post mortem*, and all tumours pass through a stage when they are too small to cause any effects.

### Benign Tumours

Despite their name these are not always harmless. As they remain localized at their site of origin, the effects fall into three broad categories:

1. The presence of a palpable lump, often painless, but occasionally causing discomfort.
2. The effects of substances produced by a tumour. The cells of a benign tumour are well differentiated and often retain the function of the tissue of origin, such as production of hormones. This is usually outwith the normal feedback mechanisms and overactivity may result, e.g. a thyroid adenoma may lead to hyperthyroidism.
3. The effects on adjacent tissues due to pressure from expansion of the tumour. This is seen particularly when the tumour arises in a confined area, e.g. within the cranial cavity. Thus, a pituitary adenoma may cause

hypopituitarism by compressing the surrounding normal glandular tissue. The distortion of the uterine cavity by a fibroid (leiomyoma) often results in heavy menstrual blood loss, whereas a benign tumour may block a hollow viscus, e.g. by causing intussusception (see Chapter 9, p. 265).

## Malignant Tumours

### Direct Effects of the Primary Tumour

Malignant tumours may cause a palpable mass, which often grows rapidly and compresses adjacent structures such as nerves with resultant pain. Despite the angiogenesis that they induce, malignant tumours often outgrow their blood supply so that there is central necrosis (Fig. 5.22). Blood loss due to haemorrhage from an ulcerated carcinoma may be acute or chronic, thus leading to iron deficiency anaemia. Carcinomas often cause narrowing (stenosis) or complete obstruction of a hollow viscus (Fig. 5.23).

### Metastatic Effects

Metastases can cause similar mass effects to primary tumours, but because they are usually multiple (Fig. 5.24) the consequences tend to be more severe. The common sites of metastases and their effects are summarized in *Table 5.5*.

### Non-metastatic Effects

This is a heterogeneous group of disorders, many due to release of cytokines such as interleukin 1 (IL-1) and tumour necrosis factor α (TNF-α) from tumour cells. Patients with advanced cancer are often wasted (cachectic) with weight loss, anorexia, and fever. Immunosuppression, abnormalities of coagulation, e.g. thrombophlebitis migrans, and neurological disorders, e.g. neuropathy, cerebellar degeneration, and the Eaton–Lambert syndrome, a syndrome resembling myasthenia gravis, may all be seen.

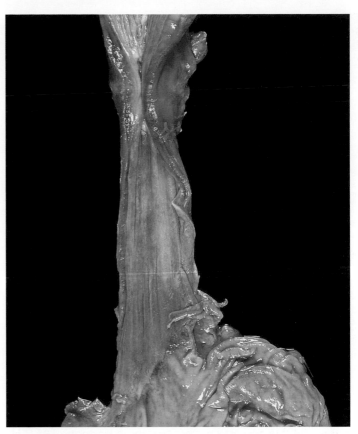

**FIG. 5.23** This carcinoma of the oesophagus had caused a tight stricture, resulting in dysphagia.

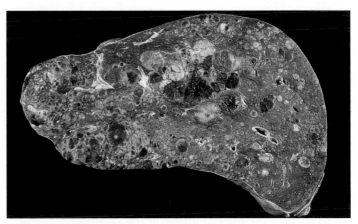

**FIG. 5.24** Metastatic melanoma in the liver. Note the numerous deposits of tumour, some deeply pigmented and others paler. The liver was greatly enlarged. The patient had had an eye removed for a malignant melanoma many years before.

**TABLE 5.5** Common sites of metastases and their effects

| Site | Effects |
| --- | --- |
| Lung | Haemoptysis, pneumonia, pleural effusion |
| Bone | Pain, fracture, spinal cord compression |
| Liver | Hepatomegaly, jaundice, hepatic failure |
| Brain | Seizures, stroke, raised intracranial pressure |
| Bone marrow | Anaemia, leukopenia, thrombocytopenia |

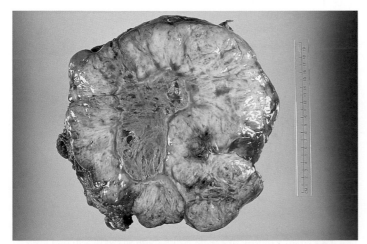

**FIG. 5.22** Central necrosis is a feature of many highly malignant tumours such as this large soft-tissue sarcoma.

TABLE 5.6 Common cancers and their effects

| Cancer | Effects |
|---|---|
| Lung | Cough, haemoptysis, chest pain, pneumonia, pleural effusion, obstruction of the superior vena cava, metastases to bone, liver, brain |
| Breast | Lump, early spread to nodes, bone, lung, liver |
| Colon | Altered bowel habit, obstruction, anaemia, metastases to liver |
| Prostate | Urinary symptoms, metastases to bone |
| Pancreas | Obstructive jaundice, back pain |
| Kidney | Mass, haematuria, metastases to lung, bone |
| Oesophagus | Dysphagia, anaemia, early local spread, and metastases |
| Lymphoma | Lymph node enlargement, infection, marrow replacement |
| Leukaemia | Anaemia, infection, bleeding (marrow replacement) |

### Inappropriate Hormone Production

Many tumours produce hormones not normally produced by their tissue of origin. These include antidiuretic hormone (ADH) and adrenocorticotrophic hormone (ACTH) typically secreted by small-cell carcinoma of the bronchus. Many tumours including squamous carcinomas produce parathyroid hormone-related peptide, which has a parathormone-like action and results in humoral hypercalcaemia of malignancy.

The typical effects of common cancers are summarized in *Table 5.6*.

## PATHOLOGICAL DIAGNOSIS OF TUMOURS

Although clinical, radiological, and biochemical findings all contribute towards the diagnosis of a tumour, the final diagnosis is made, in almost all cases, by microscopic examination: a so-called tissue diagnosis. Depending on the procedure used to obtain a sample for examination, the entire lesion, a large or small sample, or a few cells may be studied.

### Biopsies for Histopathological Assessment

These allow assessment both of the appearance of the tumour cells and of their relationship to normal tissues, i.e. the tissue architecture.

#### Excisional Biopsy

In this process, usually performed for relatively small tumours, the entire lesion is removed and submitted for examination.

#### Incisional Biopsy

In this process, the surgeon exposes the tumour and removes a wedge of tissue, giving a fairly large and hopefully representative specimen. On the basis of the biopsy result, either immediately by frozen section or after a day or so, the appropriate therapy can be instituted.

#### Needle Biopsy

Many tumours, including deep-seated ones under radiological control, can be sampled by needle biopsy, in which a thin core of tissue is removed (Figs 5.25 and 5.26). This technique provides small amounts of tissue, which may not be representative of the entire lesion, i.e. there is a potential for sampling error.

### Cytology

In recent years there has been an explosion in the use of cytology to obtain cells for study. This technique relies largely on interpretation of the appearance of the individual cells, although the degree of cohesion of the tumour cells (a feature of epithelial tumours) can also be assessed. Cells can be found easily in body fluids, e.g. extracted by syringe and needle from the pleural or peritoneal cavities, or in urine or sputum. Fine-needle aspiration of solid tumours is now routine; it has the benefit of being relatively atraumatic to the patient who usually does not require an anaesthetic. It is a simple procedure for superficial lesions, e.g. breast lumps, and deeply located lesions can be sampled under imaging control.

### Conventional Diagnosis and Additional Techniques

In most cases, e.g. carcinomas of the breast, colon, or lung, the diagnosis is made on haematoxylin and eosin (H&E)-stained sections, applying the conventional criteria of malignancy. Simple histochemical techniques, e.g. for the detection of glycogen, mucopolysaccharides, and pigments

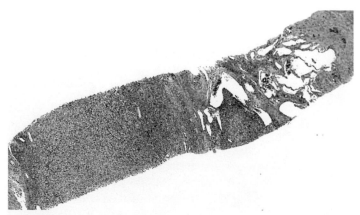

FIG. 5.25 Needle biopsy of a mass in the thigh shows a highly cellular tumour. There was enough tissue for immunohistochemistry to confirm the diagnosis of Ewing's sarcoma (see Chapter 12, p. 368).

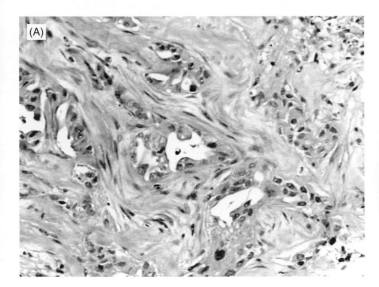

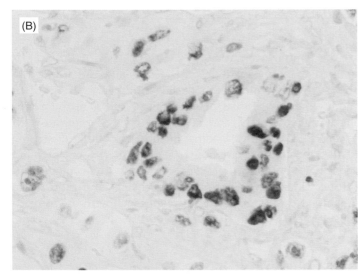

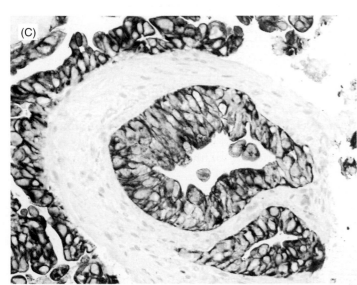

**FIG. 5.26** This needle biopsy is from the paraspinal tissue of a 40-year-old female. (A) The haematoxylin and eosin (H&E)-stained section shows an adenocarcinoma. Strongly positive immunostaining for (B) thyroid transcription factor 1 in the nuclei, and (C) cytokeratin 7 in the cytoplasm, indicates that the likely primary site is the lung.

such as melanin, help in some cases. Immunohistochemistry, using antibodies to cell constituents, contributes much to the diagnosis of poorly differentiated tumours (Fig. 5.27) and often allows a precise diagnosis to be made on small needle biopsies. Some of the more common markers are listed in *Table 5.7*. Immunostaining has largely superseded

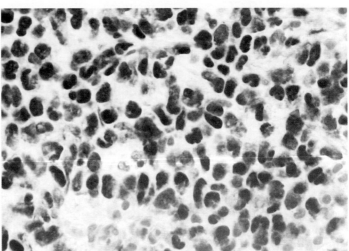

**FIG. 5.27** Immunohistochemistry is a powerful tool in determining the histogenesis of poorly differentiated tumours. Here, the nuclei stain strongly for MyoD1, a marker of skeletal muscle differentiation, allowing the diagnosis of rhabdomyosarcoma to be made with confidence.

**TABLE 5.7** Common immunocytochemical markers of value in cancer diagnosis

| Marker | Nature | Tumour |
|---|---|---|
| Cytokeratins | Intermediate filaments | Carcinoma[a], rare sarcomas |
| Desmin | Intermediate filament | Muscle tumours |
| Glial fibrillary acid protein | Intermediate filament | Gliomas |
| CD45 | Glycoprotein | Lymphomas |
| α-Fetoprotein | Oncofetal antigen | Teratoma; hepatocellular carcinoma |
| Human chorionic gonadotrophin (hCG) | Hormone | Choriocarcinoma; teratoma |
| Prostate-specific antigen (PSA) | Protein | Prostatic carcinoma |
| CA-125 | Glycoprotein | Ovarian carcinoma |
| Calcitonin | Hormone | Medullary carcinoma of thyroid |
| Thyroglobulin | Hormone | Follicular and papillary carcinomas of thyroid |

[a]In recent years it has become common practice to determine the cytokeratin profile of a metastatic carcinoma in an attempt to determine the site of origin, e.g. colonic carcinoma typically expresses CK20 and not CK7, whereas ovarian carcinoma is often CK7 positive and CK20 negative.

**TABLE 5.8** Commonly used tumour markers

| Marker | Tumour |
| --- | --- |
| α-Fetoprotein | Teratoma; hepatocellular carcinoma |
| Human chorionic gonadotrophin (hCG) | Choriocarcinoma; teratoma |
| Prostate-specific antigen (PSA) | Prostatic carcinoma |
| CA125 | Ovarian carcinoma |
| Carcinoembryonic antigen (CEA) | Carcinoma, e.g. gut, lung |
| Calcitonin | Medullary carcinoma of thyroid |
| Thyroglobulin | Follicular and papillary carcinomas of thyroid |

**TABLE 5.9** TNM staging of gastric carcinoma (7th edn)

| Stage | Explanation |
| --- | --- |
| T1 | Tumour invades lamina propria, muscularis mucosae, or submucosa |
| T2 | Tumour invades muscularis propria |
| T3 | Tumour penetrates subserosal connective tissue without invasion of visceral peritoneum or adjacent structures |
| T4 | Tumour invades serosa (visceral peritoneum) or adjacent organs |
| N0 | No nodal metastases |
| N1 | Metastases in one or two regional lymph nodes |
| N2 | Metastases in three to six regional lymph nodes |
| N3 | Metastases in seven or more regional lymph nodes |
| M0 | No distant metastases |
| M1 | Distant metastases |

electron microscopy in this regard. Recently, molecular biology techniques such as *in situ* hybridization have been used to detect gene expression as a way of determining tumour type, but this is of limited clinical usefulness so far. A number of tumour types, especially lymphomas, leukaemias, and sarcomas, have been shown to have characteristic chromosomal rearrangements that can be detected by karyotyping, i.e. examination of chromosomes, or by nucleic acid techniques (see Chapter 3).

## Tumour Markers

These substances are produced by tumour cells, detectable in the blood, and of value in diagnosis and in monitoring progress after treatment. Many are oncofetal antigens, proteins that are usually produced by fetal cells but not by normal mature adult cells. Examples are given in *Table 5.8*, and are discussed in more detail in the appropriate chapters.

## TUMOUR STAGING AND GRADING

Once the diagnosis of cancer has been made, it is important to predict the likely behaviour of a tumour, both to decide the appropriate therapy and to estimate the patient's survival. The two main factors are the biological nature of the tumour (the grade) and its extent (the stage).

Different grading systems have been developed for various tumour types. These assess to what degree the tumour resembles its putative tissue of origin (e.g. squamous epithelium) and the main parameters are:

- mitotic activity
- nuclear pleomorphism
- degree of differentiation
- extent of necrosis.

Tumour stage (the extent of tumour spread) can also be assessed in a number of ways. The TNM system, developed by the Union Internationale Contre le Cancer (UICC), is applied to many tumour types, especially carcinomas. In this scoring system an increasing number is ascribed to more extensive disease, at the primary site T, in the draining lymph nodes N, and at distant sites of metastasis M (*Table 5.9*). Other systems include the Dukes' staging system for colonic carcinoma (see Chapter 9, p. 267) and the FIGO (International Federation of Gynecology and Obstetrics) staging system for gynaecological tumours (see Chapter 14). Tumour stage correlates well with outcome in most tumour types.

## CARCINOGENESIS

### Aetiology of Cancer

Cancer is not a single disease, and different cancers have different causes. In some tumours a single major factor is implicated, but in most tumours multiple factors are involved. The clues to our understanding of the causes of cancer come from several sources, but it is clear that environment, genetic predisposition, and interindividual variability in coping with toxic injuries are all important.

#### *Environmental Factors*

##### Chemical Carcinogenesis

Many chemicals have been implicated in causing cancer in humans. Sometimes this is based on strong epidemiological evidence, e.g. lung cancer and cigarette smoking or bladder cancer in aniline dye workers, but it may also be assumed from animal experiments. A list of some chemicals associated with human cancer is given in *Table 5.10*.

From animal studies it became apparent that chemicals acted in different ways to cause cancer. Some acted

**TABLE 5.10** Some chemicals associated with human cancer

| Chemical | Occurrence | Tumour |
|---|---|---|
| Alkylating agents | Chemotherapy | Leukaemia |
| Asbestos | Insulation | Mesothelioma |
| Benzene | Solvents | Leukaemia |
| Nickel | Mining | Lung cancer |
| Nitrosamines | Dietary | Gastric carcinoma |
| Polycyclic hydrocarbons | Incomplete burning of organic material | Lung, bladder carcinoma |
| Radon | Mining | Lung cancer |
| Vinyl chloride | PVC monomer | Angiosarcoma of liver |

directly, whereas others required metabolic conversion to an active form. Many chemicals are weakly carcinogenic but that potency is much increased when chemicals are given in combination or sequentially. From these observations the multistep theory of carcinogenesis evolved. Initiation leads to DNA damage and mutation of cells, followed by promotion in which there is clonal expansion of the abnormal cell, eventually giving rise to cancer. Although useful conceptually it has become apparent that this model is too simple. Some chemicals appear to be initiators and promotors, so-called complete carcinogens, but not all of these cause DNA damage. A further complication is extrapolation from

animal experiments to the human state, for several reasons. First, humans and rodents have markedly different metabolic pathways in some respects and may therefore cope with a potential carcinogen in quite different ways. Second, the capacity of human cells to repair damage may differ. Third, animal experiments tend to rely on a constant, relatively high exposure to one or a few agents whereas in the human context exposure to potential carcinogens occurs intermittently, frequently at low dose, and as complex mixtures rather than single agents.

It is perhaps more useful therefore to think of carcinogens as being either genotoxic, i.e. causing DNA damage, or non-genotoxic. This concept is illustrated and explained in Fig. 5.28. Of critical importance is being able to recognize and identify carcinogens and use the information to plan accordingly. They may be present in the environment as pollutants, derived during preparation of food, produced as a byproduct of industry, or a therapeutic drug.

### Radiation

There is much evidence that ionizing radiation can induce cancers. Radiation-induced cancers were seen in early radiologists, who used their own hands to calibrate their equipment. Many of the survivors of the atomic bombs that fell on Hiroshima and Nagasaki in 1945 later succumbed to tumours, especially carcinomas and leukaemias. An increased incidence of cancer, especially of the thyroid, was seen in the aftermath of the nuclear explosion at Chernobyl in 1986.

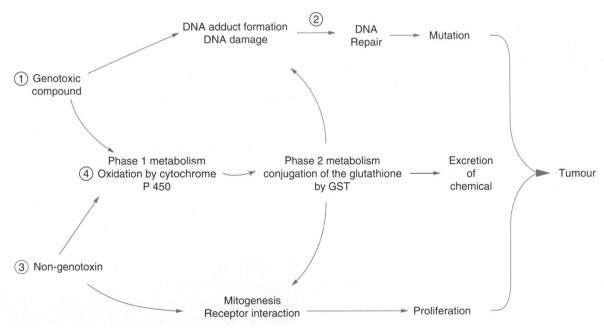

**FIG. 5.28** (1) A genotoxin may directly interact with DNA or do so after metabolic activation, e.g. by one of the cytochrome P450 enzymes. DNA adducts are formed or direct DNA strand breakage occurs. (2) Defective DNA repair may result in mutations that affect key genes such as those involved in regulating the cell cycle, apoptosis, or differentiation leading to tumour formation. (3) Non-genotoxins do not have direct effects on DNA but cause cell proliferation by deregulating normal cell cycle activity. (4) Many of the enzymes involved are polymorphic, i.e. there is a sequence variation in the gene that may reflect a change in expression, inducibility of the gene or function. At each stage of metabolism there is variability between individuals in terms of exposure levels and also the metabolic activity determined both by the genotype of the individual and by the level of expression and function of the enzymes. GST = glutathione S-transferase.

Therapeutic irradiation, principally in the treatment of cancer, may be followed several years later by the development of second tumours, both carcinomas and sarcomas.

Ionizing irradiation acts by damaging DNA. Both single- and double-strand cleavage is seen. Breaks in a single strand of DNA are repaired but, especially in rapidly growing cells, this may be inaccurate, leading to single base mutations. In contrast, double-strand damage leads to chromosomal breakage, and repair of multiple such breaks may lead to major chromosomal rearrangements such as translocations and deletions.

Ultraviolet irradiation is strongly implicated in the aetiology of skin tumours, especially malignant melanoma, of which 90% of cases can be attributed to exposure. As ultraviolet light is of low energy it does not penetrate deeply and the effects are confined to the skin. Ultraviolet rays induce the formation of pyrimidine dimers, which lead to base-pair substitutions during replication. Abnormalities of DNA-repair systems, e.g. xeroderma pigmentosum, lead to greatly increased risks of skin cancer.

## Viruses and Cancers

It has been recognized that viruses are responsible for some cancers for 90 years, since the pioneering work of Peyton Rous, who demonstrated that 'cell-free filtrates' could transmit leukaemia and sarcomas in experimental animals. Viruses contribute to the development of cancers in different ways. Some RNA tumour viruses (retroviruses) contain genes – viral oncogenes – that are directly responsible for transforming cells to malignancy. The viral RNA genome is copied into DNA by the enzyme reverse transcriptase and this is then inserted into the host genome. Viral genes can thus influence the expression of adjacent cellular genes. Other viruses, e.g. hepatitis C virus, act indirectly by causing tissue damage, leading to increased proliferation and an increased risk of mutations. The major viruses thought to be involved in human cancers are given in *Table 5.11*.

The final common pathway of many of these precipitating factors is mutation of DNA. Other factors such as chronic infection or hormonal stimulation cause increased cell turnover and may therefore make mutations more likely. Immunosuppression is associated with an increase particularly of lymphomas, a common complication of AIDS.

## Genetic Factors

Undoubtedly there are individuals with significant genetic predispositions to various tumours, including the common cancers of breast, lung, and colon. There are three broad categories of familial cancer.

### Familial Cancer Syndromes

In this group of disorders the increased risk of cancer is due to transmission of a single gene, which appears to act in an

**TABLE 5.11** Viruses implicated in human cancers

| Virus | Human tumour |
|---|---|
| Papillomaviruses, especially types 16 and 18 (see Special Study Topic, Chapter 14, pp. 439–441) | Cervical carcinoma<br>Anal and penile carcinomas |
| Epstein–Barr virus | Nasopharyngeal carcinoma, Burkitt's lymphoma, Hodgkin lymphoma |
| Hepatitis B and C viruses | Hepatocellular carcinoma |
| Human T-lymphotrophic virus 1 | T-cell leukaemia |
| Herpesvirus 8 | Kaposi's sarcoma |

autosomal dominant manner, although in fact both copies of the gene must be inactivated before a tumour develops.

Familial adenomatous polyposis coli is characterized by the growth of numerous adenomas in the colon (Fig. 5.29) and the almost inevitable development of colonic carcinoma by middle age. The responsible gene (*APC*) has been identified and its function as an inhibitor of growth-promoting signal transduction molecules established. The normal APC protein binds β-catenin and promotes its proteolytic destruction; mutations of *APC* tend therefore to increase the concentration of β-catenin, which is important in carcinogenesis.

In the Li–Fraumeni syndrome family members have an increased propensity to premature development of a

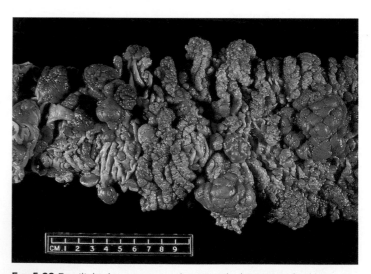

**FIG. 5.29** Familial adenomatous polyposis coli: this patient had a pancolectomy at the age of 25. Innumerable polyps are present throughout the colon. Fortunately no invasive carcinomas were identified. The patient's mother was less fortunate and died at the age of 43 from metastatic carcinoma of the colon.

variety of different tumour types, e.g. the early development of breast carcinoma and childhood sarcoma, typically in the mother and child. It is due to mutation of the *TP53* gene. Familial retinoblastoma is characterized by the almost inevitable development, usually bilaterally, of the rare retinal tumour retinoblastoma. This is due to inheritance of one abnormal copy of the retinoblastoma (*Rb*) gene (Fig. 5.30 and see also p. 98).

### Familial Cancers

In some families there is a striking increase in the incidence of a common cancer, e.g. of breast, colon, or ovary. In some cases the responsible gene can be discovered, e.g. the *BRCA-1* and *BRCA-2* genes associated with familial breast carcinoma.

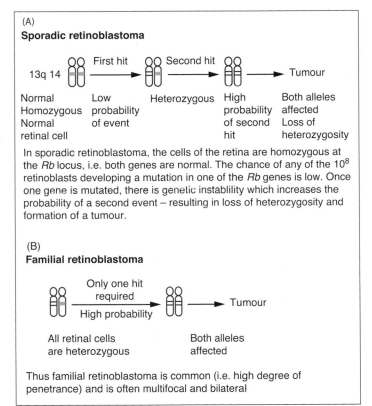

(A)
**Sporadic retinoblastoma**

In sporadic retinoblastoma, the cells of the retina are homozygous at the *Rb* locus, i.e. both genes are normal. The chance of any of the $10^8$ retinoblasts developing a mutation in one of the *Rb* genes is low. Once one gene is mutated, there is genetic instability which increases the probability of a second event – resulting in loss of heterozygosity and formation of a tumour.

(B)
**Familial retinoblastoma**

Thus familial retinoblastoma is common (i.e. high degree of penetrance) and is often multifocal and bilateral

**FIG. 5.30** Inheritance of retinoblastoma: the retinoblastoma gene lies on the long arm of chromosome 13. (A) The sporadic form of retinoblastoma occurs in individuals who have two normal *Rb* genes. Loss of both alleles is required before a tumour will develop, so the risk of this is very small and the tumour, which is unilateral, often occurs in older children. (B) In contrast, in patients with familial retinoblastoma, one *Rb* allele is mutated in the germline, and therefore in every cell in the body. Only one mutation in the remaining normal *Rb* gene is required for a tumour to develop. Accordingly, this almost invariably occurs, and most patients develop bilateral tumours at an early age. Unfortunately, they also develop a variety of other tumours in later life.

### Autosomal Recessive Disorders due to Defects in DNA Repair

In ataxia–telangiectasia, an autosomal recessive condition, there is an increased risk of developing lymphoma or leukaemia. This is related to excessive fragility of the chromosomes, either spontaneously or after radiation. The responsible gene (*AT*), which is thought to act as a sensor of DNA damage, activates the *TP53* gene, causing the cell to enter G0 until DNA repair is complete. In its absence, the mutated cell continues to proliferate, increasing the chance of malignancy.

Lynch syndrome, which is associated with colorectal carcinoma in both sexes (hereditary non-polyposis colorectal cancer) and endometrial carcinoma in women, is another disorder due to impaired DNA repair (see Chapters 3, pp. 42–44 and 9, pp. 270–271). The relevant genes are known as 'mismatch repair genes'; they detect point mutations where the nucleotides on complementary DNA strands do not match correctly (i.e. normally A:T, C:G) and excise the abnormal base. Failure of these mismatch repair genes can be detected by the accumulation of variable microsatellites, short sequences that are normally identical in any individual; microsatellite instability is an indication of mismatch repair. Xeroderma pigmentosum is due to loss of the genes involved in excision of so-called pyrimidine dimers caused by ultraviolet damage. It leads to a greatly increased risk of skin cancer.

## Oncogenes

The sections above indicate that mutations of DNA are fundamental to the causation of tumours. The topic of oncogenes and tumour-suppressor genes can be difficult and confusing. In simple terms: cancer is due to excessive and uncontrolled cellular proliferation or insufficient cell loss, i.e. it results from defects in the normal control mechanisms for cell populations (see Chapter 2). Normal genes that are switched on when cell division is needed, and promote cell division when expressed, are known as cellular proto-oncogenes. If these genes are inappropriately switched on, the cell will divide at the wrong time: the abnormal variant of the gene is called an oncogene, and produces an oncoprotein. Only one of the two cellular copies has to be affected because the oncogene acts in a dominant manner. The numerous proto-oncogenes fall into at least four main categories:

1. Genes that produce growth factors, e.g. the *sis* gene encoding platelet-derived growth factor (PDGF).
2. Genes that produce growth factor receptors, e.g. the *erbB1* gene, which encodes a receptor with tyrosine kinase activity for epidermal growth factor. There may be overexpression of the gene, or it may be mutated, with alteration of the conformation of the receptor, such that it does not require binding of its growth factor to be activated. The cell is therefore 'switched on' permanently.

3. Genes that encode 'signal transducers', i.e. proteins that transmit the growth signal to the nucleus. Mutations may cause the signal to be *on* permanently. The *ras* group of genes encode for GTP-binding proteins.

4. Genes that activate other genes to promote growth (transcription activators), e.g. the *fos* and *myc* genes.

### Oncogene Activation

Oncogenes can be activated in a variety of ways. Point mutations may change the structure of the oncoprotein so that it becomes permanently active. The *ras* gene encodes a cell membrane-associated signal transduction protein that exists in two forms: an inactive form bound to GDP and an active form bound to GTP. Normally, GTPase activity cleaves GTP to GDP so that activation of *ras* is short lasting. Mutations of *ras* result in a reduction of GTPase activity, so that the *ras* protein remains bound to GTP and is therefore locked into its active form.

Gene amplification is a process whereby multiple copies of an oncogene are formed by reduplication. Transcription of these extra copies of the gene results in increased production of the oncoprotein, e.g. the N-*myc* gene on chromosome 2 is greatly amplified in many cases of neuroblastoma, a rare childhood tumour of primitive neurons. The extra copies may be located on the correct chromosome, where they can be recognized as a 'homogeneously staining region', or as numerous extra chromosomal structures known as 'double minutes'. The consequence in either case is of increased synthesis of the *myc* protein, a transcription factor for genes involved in cell proliferation.

Translocations between chromosomes may also cause overexpression of oncoproteins. There are two main mechanisms. In some lymphomas, e.g. Burkitt's lymphoma and mantle cell lymphoma, an oncoprotein (c-*myc* and cyclin $D_1$, respectively) is moved so that it lies under the control of the promotor sequence of the immunoglobulin heavy chain gene, which is constitutively expressed in active B lymphocytes. Thus the oncoprotein is permanently switched on. The second mechanism, commonly seen in sarcomas (see Chapter 12) results in the fusion of two genes, thus producing a new hybrid molecule, which has increased transcription activity. Several well-recognized translocations and the resulting tumours are listed in *Table 5.12*.

### Tumour-suppressor Genes

Tumour-suppressor genes are genes with products that normally stop a cell growing, promote differentiation of a cell to a terminal end state, or trigger checkpoints that cause cell cycle arrest if DNA damage occurs. Thus, tumour-suppressor genes are cell cycle arrest genes (gatekeepers) or DNA-repair

**TABLE 5.12** Some tumours associated with specific chromosomal translocation

| Tumour | Translocation | Genes involved |
|---|---|---|
| Burkitt's lymphoma | t(8;14)(q24;q32) | c-*myc*; Ig heavy chain |
| Chronic myeloid leukaemia | t(9;22)(q34;q11) | *Abl*; *bcr* |
| Ewing's sarcoma | t(11;22)(q24;q12) | *Fli*-1; *EWS* |
| Follicular lymphoma | t(8;14)(q24;q32) | Ig heavy chain; *bcl*-2 |
| Mantle cell lymphoma | t(11;14)(q13;q32) | *cyclin D*$_1$; Ig heavy chain |
| Alveolar rhabdomyo-sarcoma | t(2;13)(q35;q14) | *PAX*-3; *FKHR* |
| Synovial sarcoma | t(X;18)(p11;q11) | *SSX*; *SYT* |

genes (caretakers). It also follows that tumour-suppressor genes cause problems when they are absent, i.e. when their normal protective function has been lost. This can occur by inactivating mutations, deletions, or even when they form a complex with viral proteins, resulting in their deactivation. It follows that to lose their tumour-suppressor function it may be necessary to lose both functional copies of a gene.

Inherited cancers, although not common, have given valuable insight into the role of tumour-suppressor genes and how they are implicated in disease. Alfred Knudson studied retinoblastoma, a rare cancer of the retina of the eye. Retinoblastoma may be familial (approximately 40% of cases) or sporadic (approximately 60% of cases). In familial cases the child affected is usually under 3 years of age and both eyes may be affected. In sporadic cases the child tends to be older and the disease is unilateral. Knudson reasoned that if there was an inherited element then there was perhaps a similar genetic mechanism in both familial and sporadic cases. He further argued that, as the familial cases occur at younger ages and the occurrence of disease was more frequent in members of families affected by the familial disease, it was possible that the inherited trait meant that these cases were already 'halfway' to cancer. Since then the gene *RB1* (retinoblastoma 1) has been identified. This is a tumour-suppressor gene, the normal function of which is to regulate entry of cells into the cell cycle. Disruption of the function of the *RB1* product results in inappropriate cell proliferation, eventually leading to cancer. In cases of familial retinoblastoma the sufferer inherits one normal copy of *RB1* and one copy that is non-functional. In retinoblasts (why in these cells in particular you may wish to enquire) a further mutation may occur, in which case there is loss of function of the normal gene resulting in dysregulated entry into the cell cycle. The same happens in sporadic cases: there must be loss of function. However, in sporadic cases cells must suffer two mutations or deletions in the same cell to knock out each copy of *RB1*. This may happen but is much less likely than a single hit. Therefore, in sporadic cases the disease occurs at a later age, indicating that many more chances of mutation must have occurred. This theory also explains why multiple tumours are generally not found in the sporadic form because the chance of more than one retinoblast acquiring mutations in both *RB1* genes is very unlikely, whereas in the hereditary form all the retinoblasts have one hit from the outset. This is Knudson's two-hit hypothesis (see Fig. 5.30).

It then becomes apparent that other cancers also have familial and sporadic forms, although the precise organ type, age at onset, penetrance of disease and pattern of heredity are more ill defined. However, in these diseases there is an indication that an inherited trait, a dysfunctional tumour-suppressor gene, has been acquired. A number of important tumour suppressor genes are listed in *Table 5.13*.

## Apoptosis and Cancer

Oncogenes and tumour-suppressor genes are important because they regulate cell numbers by controlling cell proliferation. Cell numbers also depend on the rate of cell loss. Apoptosis, or programmed cell death, is also governed by a number of genes, and aberrant function of these is important in the cause of some cancers. In follicular B-cell lymphomas, a translocation t(14;18)(q32;q31) causes the *bcl-2* gene to come under the control of the immunoglobulin heavy chain regulatory sequences and become overexpressed. This inhibits apoptosis so that the cells are immortalized. Even though the tumour cells are growing very slowly, the tumour increases in size due to the lower rate of cell loss. A number of other similar genes are thought to be important in other tumours.

**TABLE 5.13** Tumour-suppressor genes

| Gene | Tumour |
| --- | --- |
| *APC* | Familial adenomatous polyposis coli, colon cancer |
| *BRCA-1* | Breast, ovarian cancer |
| *BRCA-2* | Breast cancer |
| *NF-1* | Neurofibromatosis type 1 |
| *TP53* | Li–Fraumeni syndrome, sporadic cancers |
| *Rb* | Retinoblastoma, osteosarcoma, sporadic cancers |
| *WT-1* | Wilms' tumour |

## Telomerases and Cancer

Much experimental work is currently directed at clarifying the role of telomerases in cancer. Telomeres are repeating DNA sequences found at the ends of chromosomes which are important in regulating the number of cell divisions of which a cell is capable, the so-called Hayflick limit (see Chapter 2, p. 20). Each time a cell divides, the telomere is shortened until eventually the cell is incapable of further replication, a phenomenon thought to be important in cellular senescence. This does not apply to stem cells, because they contain a mechanism for lengthening telomeres, an enzyme called telomerase. Theoretically, overexpression of telomerase might immortalize tumour cells. Indeed, many tumours do appear to express increased telomerase activity. This may open novel therapeutic approaches to cancer, with the development of telomerase-inhibiting drugs.

## SUMMARY

Cancer epidemiology has demonstrated that cancer is a major health problem in all countries, although the ageing populations of western countries are particularly affected. This importance is reflected in the large share of healthcare budgets spent on the care of patients with cancer, and in attempts at cancer prevention and the widespread development of cancer screening programmes, which may detect both preinvasive and invasive tumours. Appropriate clinical management depends on an understanding of the classification of tumours (both benign and malignant) and an appreciation of their biological behaviours, including both local and distant effects. Knowledge of the modes and patterns of tumour spread allows a rational approach to the staging of tumours. It is important that all clinicians involved in cancer care have some understanding of the processes involved in laboratory diagnosis of tumours, including the strengths and limitations of existing techniques and newer immunological and molecular techniques, and the necessity of close clinico-pathological cooperation, not least in multidisciplinary team review of cancer management.

Our understanding of the molecular mechanisms underlying the development of tumours (carcinogenesis) and the spread of malignant cells has greatly increased in recent years. As well as being of scientific interest, this offers alternative strategies for cancer prevention, including genetic testing in families of cancer patients, and has led to the development of novel therapies, some already in clinical use and many others in development and assessment.

# 5.2 Special Study Topic

## DNA-REPAIR MECHANISMS

DNA damage is an obligatory risk of being alive and so it is important that repair mechanisms exist. In general they are extremely effective and it is only when they fail that we become aware of how stressful an environment we inhabit. DNA repair has similarities irrespective of whether we are looking at yeast or people. Repair machinery is always linked to replication and so it is no surprise that induction of repair is associated with cessation of replication (lest erroneous sequence replication takes place). At several points in the cell cycle (see Chapter 2, p. 16), known as checkpoints, damage sensing and repair induction have a particularly effective influence over cell cycle progression. Driving through cell cycle checkpoints is a bad idea!

## Basic Repair Principles

### Cells Die by Apoptosis

It is better to have no cell than a cell with potentially harmful damage and mutation. This is not simply a matter of dose of injury; it is also dependent on the importance or stage of differentiation of the cell type.

### Tolerance of Damage

Three examples will illustrate not so much that these mechanisms occur but rather that a lot of eukaryotic DNA repair is still speculative and based on the much more robust science of yeast:

1 Neurons in the brain are susceptible to damage. They cannot be repaired easily and cannot replicate. They adapt to live with damage.
2 An alternative mechanism may occur in hepatocytes. These cells are constantly under attack by free radicals generated by respiration and metabolism of xenobiotics. As the liver cells age and sustain damage they undergo polyploidy. This process, which is not fully understood, results in cells that instead of having a diploid content of DNA become polyploid: doubling, quadrupling, and more their cellular DNA content. Instead of having two copies of genes they have four, eight, sixteen, or more copies. The reasoning is that the polyploid cell has more copies of each gene and so can still produce protein even if numerous gene-inactivating mutations are sustained. This is a persuasive argument if the liver cell is regarded as a protein factory where the production line output is the major driving force, but there is little evidence base to support this.
3 DNA repair may be delayed because replication is not imminent, e.g. a pyrimidine dimer caused by UV light may persist and act as a brake on replication. If there is no involvement of a transcriptionally active gene, this may not

matter in a cell for some time. But there is a danger that, as DNA replication can have multiple start sites, a gap may be formed around the damaged area resulting in a frameshift-type mutation. In these circumstances recombination using undamaged DNA as a template may be useful. Many genes are involved in this fairly complex scenario including BRCA-1, which is implicated when defective in causing breast and ovarian cancer. In essence the repair refers back to the original sequence manual, and uses it to cut and paste – more correctly to fuse – back the correct sequence, thereby bypassing the replicative block posed by the intercalation or pyrimidine dimer.

### Removal of Damage

A single base or a stretch of damaged DNA is excised and repaired.

#### Base Excision Repair

If a damaged base is present the easiest repair method is simply to excise it and replace it with a correct base. This is the principle of base excision repair. It is conservative, i.e. minimal effort is required, and is not error prone.

#### Nucleotide Excision Repair

If the damage is more severe, e.g. a pyrimidine dimer, then the DNA configuration is altered, not just a single base. The same basic idea of base excision is relevant but the processes of recognition, excision, and replacement are more complex. Instead of a single base being excised. a strip of nucleotides on one strand is excised and DNA polymerase enzymes replicate the gap using the other strand as a template. Defects of nucleotide excision repair have serious effects. In the condition xeroderma pigmentosum skin cannot repair UV-induced damage and there is a high incidence of mutation and skin cancer.

#### Mismatch Repair

This is analogous to a computer spellchecker. It is generally useful but can be less helpful if dealing with specialist material because it tends to insert a suggestion that is perhaps erroneous. This is because the dictionary available to the software is limited. Similarly when DNA is replicated it is checked for spelling errors. The trouble is that the only comparator available is the original strand from which replication started. The repair mechanism checks for mismatches and corrects those it finds, or deletes the cell altogether. Some areas of DNA are more error prone than others, e.g. regions containing multiple repeat short sequences, and defects of mismatch repair are more likely to be found in these regions. Defects of mismatch repair are implicated in susceptibility to a number of cancers, in particular colon cancer.

## Special Study Topic continued . . .

### *Reversal of Damage*

This can be envisaged as a cosmetic exercise smoothing over the bumps or gaps in damaged DNA. If DNA suffers a single strand break the most simple option is to recognize damage and then simply to ligate it with a DNA ligase enzyme. It sounds simple but within that straightforward mechanism there must be recognition, specificity, distinguishing normal strand breakage (e.g. uncoiling DNA during replication) and catalytic activity to actually anneal the ends.

### Conclusion

It is worth emphasizing that prevention is better than correction – but most DNA damage is an obligatory part of being alive. Inherited or acquired defects in DNA repair are important in causing cancer, allowing progression and potentially inducing resistance of cancer cells to therapy.

## ACKNOWLEDGEMENTS

The contributions of Robin Reid and David J Harrison to this chapter in the 14th edition are gratefully acknowledged.

## FURTHER READING

Fletcher CDM. *Diagnostic Histopathology of Tumours*, 4th edn. New York: Saunders, 2013.

Hall PA, Lowe SW. Molecular and cellular themes in cancer research 2. *J Pathol* 2005;**205**:121–292.

Hong WK, Bast RC, Hait WN, *et al. Holland-Frei Cancer Medicine*, 8th edn. Hamilton: BC Decker, 2009.

Skarin AT. *Atlas of Diagnostic Oncology*, 4th edn. Edinburgh: Mosby, 2010.

# SECTION 2

# SYSTEMIC PATHOLOGY

# 6

# THE CARDIOVASCULAR SYSTEM

Mary N Sheppard and C Simon Herrington

## INTRODUCTION TO THE CARDIOVASCULAR SYSTEM

Diseases of the heart and blood vessels constitute a leading cause of morbidity and mortality throughout the world. Most cases arise from complications of atherosclerosis, hypertension, obesity, and diabetes mellitus.

The cardiovascular system's role is to pump around a constantly circulating fluid which provides the body with oxygen and other nutrients, and removes waste. Thus, the cardiovascular system maintains the circulation of blood, of which the average person has approximately 5 litres. Blood is mostly liquid but numerous cells and proteins are suspended in it, making blood thicker than pure water.

The heart is adapted as a pump although, in each part of the circulation, tubes are structurally adapted to the pressure and flow of blood within them. Conductance arteries such as the aorta absorb the impulse of cardiac systole and elastic recoil maintains blood flow in diastole. Hence the wall of the aorta contains multiple layers of elastic tissue (Fig. 6.1). On the arterial side of the circulation, the blood flow is at a high pressure of at least 100 mmHg, so the vessels have thick muscular walls. The more muscular, medium-sized arteries regulate distribution of blood to the various organs by vessel constriction and dilatation, so they have a thick medial wall with less elastic tissue (Fig. 6.2). The veins contain blood at a low or even a negative pressure. They act as capacitance vessels and a reservoir of the

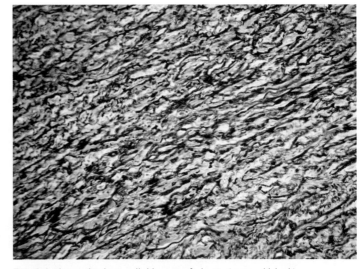

**Fig. 6.1** The multiple parallel layers of elastic (stained black) interspersed with collagen and smooth muscle cells in the aorta. Stain: elastin van Gieson.

circulation; thus, they have a large lumen and a thin wall (Fig. 6.3). Excessive hypercontraction of the vessels causes hypertension. Hyperaemia is increased blood flow and is due to dilatation of the arteries and arterioles. It occurs in skeletal and heart muscle during exercise. There may also be excessive blood flow with blushing noticeable in the skin on exercise. Excessive dilatation is also associated with septic shock.

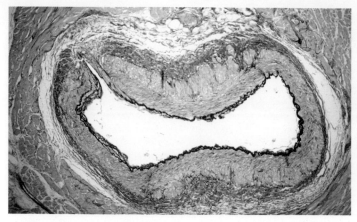

**FIG. 6.2** Muscular coronary artery showing the adventitial collagen in red, the smooth muscle of the media in yellow, and the internal elastic lamina in black. Stain: elastin van Gieson.

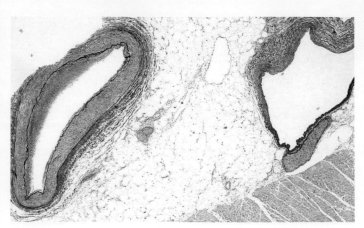

**FIG. 6.3** Epicardial coronary artery and vein in fat. Note the smooth muscle medial layer of the artery with adventitial collagen (left). There is intimal collagen thickening, which is eccentric. Contrast this appearance with the vein (right), which has a large lumen and a narrow wall, with less muscle and more adventitial collagen than the artery.

## ALTERED CONTENT, FLOW, AND PRESSURE

Haemorrhage is caused by rupture/breakdown of blood vessels, including arteries and veins, leading to excess loss of blood into the surrounding tissue, internal spaces (e.g. the peritoneal cavity), or externally. This can result in shock, with a drop in blood pressure and increase in heart rate to compensate for the loss in blood volume.

### Shock

Shock is a complex syndrome with a variety of aetiologies (*Table 6.1*). All causes culminate in acute circulatory failure with hypotension and inadequate tissue perfusion. A large component of the syndrome, whatever the aetiology, is failure of the microcirculation. If not quickly reversed, death occurs due to multiorgan failure. The major types of shock are:

- hypovolaemic shock – due to reduced blood volume
- septic shock – due to infection (see Chapter 19, pp. 571–574)
- cardiogenic shock – due to an acute severe fall in cardiac output (see also p. 108)
- anaphylactic shock – due to an acute (type 1) hypersensitivity reaction (see Chapter 2, p. 24) causing massive degranulation of mast cells and eosinophils.

Some causes of shock do not fall into these main categories: acute peritonitis due to escape of gastric juice into the peritoneal cavity from a perforated peptic ulcer, acute pancreatitis (see Chapter 10, pp. 290–291), and poisoning

**TABLE 6.1** Types of shock

| Types of shock | Clinical examples | Chief mechanisms |
| --- | --- | --- |
| Hypovolaemic | Haemorrhage – internal/external; burns/scalds; vomiting/diarrhoea | Insufficient circulating volume |
| Septic | Endotoxaemia; Gram-negative septicaemia; Gram-positive septicaemia; overwhelming infection with any microorganism | Fixed peripheral vasodilatation and pooling of blood in the microcirculation due to nitric oxide release; endothelial cell, and leukocyte activation by cytokines; activation of plasma enzyme cascades |
| Cardiogenic | Massive myocardial infarction; cardiac tamponade; ventricular arrhythmia massive pulmonary embolism | Pump failure |
| Anaphylactic | Acute hypersensitivity reaction | Massive mast cell degranulation causes release of vasodilators and permeability factors |

can all cause severe 'chemical' shock. So-called neurogenic shock may complicate anaesthesia or spinal cord injury. Severe shock develops when incompatible blood is transfused accidentally. Although the causes differ in aetiology, and in early aspects of their pathogenesis, the end-results, namely acute circulatory failure and its complications, are similar in all types of shock.

In the early stages of shock, compensatory mechanisms maintain the blood flow to the vital organs – the central nervous system, kidneys, and heart. However, the compensation is achieved at the expense of reduced perfusion of other tissues. Initially, the shocked patient is restless and confused, with a pale, cold, sweaty skin, often with peripheral cyanosis, a rapid weak pulse, a low blood pressure, and increased rate and depth of respiration; eventually the patient may become drowsy and finally comatose. Unless tissue perfusion is urgently restored, ischaemia causes multiorgan failure and death. The altered haemodynamics have been best studied in hypovolaemic shock, which is used here as an example.

## Hypovolaemic Shock

Trauma is one of the most common causes of death in young adults and many die of severe haemorrhage. In burns, plasma leakage from the damaged microcirculation causes hypovolaemia; hence the mortality of burns is related to their surface area. Severe vomiting and/or diarrhoea can also cause hypovolaemic shock. In a normal healthy adult a 500 mL blood loss, about 10% of the blood volume, is asymptomatic. The blood volume is restored within a few hours by absorption of fluid from the extravascular compartment. Plasma protein replacement takes a day or two and restoration of red cells takes weeks. Loss of a third of the blood volume (about 1,250 mL) results in significant hypovolaemia over the subsequent 36 hours, whereas a rapid loss of half the blood volume results in coma and death. Elderly and hypertensive patients tolerate blood loss much less well due to structural changes in their arterial tree.

### Early Compensatory Changes

Acute hypovolaemia lowers central (systemic) venous pressure and a diminished venous return decreases cardiac filling, with a fall in stroke volume, cardiac output, and arterial blood pressure. These changes trigger peripheral and central baroreceptors with intense sympathicoadrenal stimulation, and activation of the renin–angiotensin–aldosterone system and release of vasopressin. This stimulates the cardiovascular system and augments fluid retention. The heart rate increases to restore cardiac output and widespread arteriolar and venular constriction reduce tissue perfusion.

The beneficial effects are sodium retention and increased systemic venous tone, which increases central venous pressure, venous return to the heart, and cardiac output. Thus, even without treatment, the blood pressure may be partially or fully restored, although tissue perfusion is reduced. The central nervous system, heart and kidneys are protected because they autoregulate their own perfusion. In young people, cerebral and coronary blood flow are maintained close to normal levels at blood pressures down to about 50 mmHg. At this pressure, however, arteriolar relaxation is maximal and perfusion rapidly declines at lower pressures. In older patients with arteriosclerosis, or in those with hypertension, the lower limit of autoregulation may be 80–90 mmHg. These groups are susceptible to circulatory disturbances.

The compensatory mechanisms can cope with loss of up to 25% of the blood volume. Arterioles constrict more than the venules, thereby lowering the hydrostatic pressure in the capillaries. Also, circulating cytokines cause capillary leakage (see below) and extravascular fluid enters the intravascular compartment. Tissue perfusion is, nevertheless, precarious and it is important to restore the blood volume by prompt intravenous administration of fluid. Macromolecular solutions, such as plasma or dextrans, maintain plasma osmotic pressure and retain fluid in the circulation. Blood transfusion is required when the loss exceeds 25% of blood volume. Blood pressure, haemoglobin, and haematocrit levels are poor indicators of the degree of hypovolaemia during the first 36 hours. Central venous pressure gives a more accurate indication and should be monitored in all cases of severe shock.

### Established Hypovolaemic Shock

In advanced shock, hypovolaemia is complicated by cardiorespiratory failure and bacterial infection. If shock persists, the widespread arteriolar constriction gradually passes off, and peripheral vasodilatation causes hypotension. After around 2 hours, cytokine-mediated increased capillary permeability leads to loss of fluid into the extravascular space, and a further fall in blood volume. Capillary congestion with slowly flowing blood causes cyanosis and reduced tissue perfusion, which is aggravated by a number of factors. Loss of intravascular fluid leads to sludging of red cells and rouleaux formation. Viscosity is further increased by a rise in plasma fibrinogen. Release of thromboplastin from hypoxic endothelium and tissue cells generates thrombin, which promotes platelet aggregation and disseminated intravascular coagulation (DIC).

Leukocytes are important contributors to tissue damage. Neutrophil polymorphs adhere to the activated and injured endothelium of small vessels, especially in the lungs, and after 12 hours there may be significant neutropenia. Activated leukocytes and hypoxic cells release cytokines, especially tumour necrosis factor α (TNF-α) and interleukin 4 (IL-4) into the blood. This causes increased endothelial output of nitric oxide. They also release proteolytic enzymes, which activate the kinin and complement systems, and the circulation is further embarrassed by vasodilatation and increased permeability. Metabolic acidosis directly depresses cardiac myocytes, and a myocardial depressant factor is released from the ischaemic pancreas.

### Cardiogenic Shock

Cardiogenic shock is caused by severe acute reduction in cardiac output because of pump failure; most often this is due to cardiac catastrophes such as massive myocardial infarction, rupture of a valve cusp, or cardiac tamponade due to haemopericardium. The main metabolic and circulating effects are summarized in Fig. 6.4. Unlike other forms of shock, both the central venous pressure and the ventricular end-diastolic pressures are raised. The haemodynamic changes are otherwise similar to hypovolaemic shock; they are triggered by the fall in blood pressure and the reduced tissue perfusion. The mortality rate approaches 80%. Surgical intervention is sometimes appropriate and aortic pumps can support the circulation before surgery.

### Septic Shock

Septicaemia or localized infections may cause shock. This important type of shock is described in detail in Chapter 19 (pp. 571–574).

### Metabolic Consequences of Shock

Hypoxia has a profound effect on cell metabolism. It prevents the conversion of pyruvate into acetyl-CoA and blocks the tricarboxylate cycle; conversion of pyruvate to lactate causes accumulation of lactic acid and contributes to the metabolic acidosis. In this case, each molecule of glucose yields only two molecules of ATP, whereas in the presence of oxygen complete oxidation of one molecule of glucose via the citric acid cycle and the electron carrier chain yields about 38 ATP molecules for each glucose molecule. As a result of insufficient ATP, energy-dependent cell functions run down. Slowing of the membrane ATPase ion pumps causes potassium to leak from cells, and the entry of sodium and water causes cell swelling. Hypoxic cells also leak glucose leading to insulin-resistant hyperglycaemia and increased glycogenolysis. These metabolic disturbances, together with high levels of catecholamines, raise the blood levels of fatty acids and amino acids. These effects are sometimes termed the 'sick cell syndrome' (Fig. 6.5).

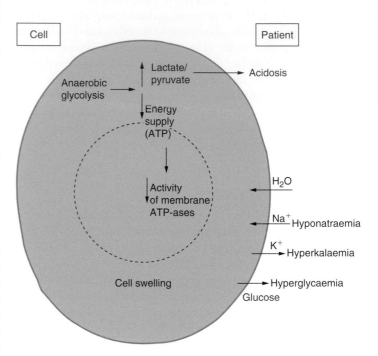

FIG. 6.5 Some effects of hypoxia.

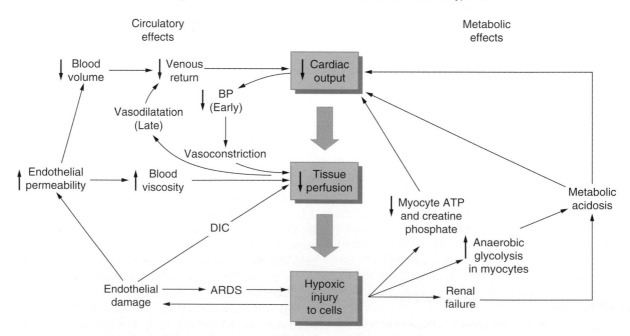

FIG. 6.4 Metabolic and circulatory effects of cardiogenic shock. ARDS = acute respiratory distress syndrome; BP = blood pressure; DIC = disseminated intravascular coagulation.

## Tissue Pathology in Shock

All organs are affected in severe shock. The typical histological findings are haemorrhage, microthrombi, and necrosis; however, morphological changes are often inconspicuous. Failure of autoregulation may cause acute tubular necrosis in the kidney, boundary zone infarction of the brain, selective neuronal necrosis, and subendocardial infarction of the heart.

Acute heart failure, first of the left and then of both ventricles, may develop in severe cardiogenic, hypovolaemic or septic shock, and is particularly common in older patients with hypertension or coronary artery disease. Inadequate myocardial perfusion produces focal necrosis or global infarction. Tachypnoea is produced by metabolic acidosis. In established shock, progressive reduction in gas exchange is due to a combination of causes – pulmonary oedema, alveolar collapse, intravascular and intra-alveolar fibrin formation, haemorrhage, and infection. These features, known collectively as shock lung or adult respiratory distress syndrome (ARDS) are discussed in detail in Chapter 7 (pp. 176–177).

Below the lower level of autoregulation, perfusion of the kidneys is directly proportional to the blood pressure. Production of urine ceases at about 50 mmHg and, if the pressure remains low for some hours, hypoxic injury leads to renal failure with acute tubular necrosis. The kidneys usually show cortical pallor and swelling; in more severe shock, often complicating obstetric catastrophes or septic shock, complete necrosis of the whole renal cortex may occur, giving rise to acute cortical necrosis, which is irrecoverable (see Chapter 13, p. 413).

There may be gastrointestinal haemorrhage and, in DIC, more widespread small haemorrhages affect mucosal and serosal surfaces (Fig. 6.6). Ischaemic necrosis of perivenular liver cells may be noted *post mortem* and are responsible for raised serum transaminase levels; cholestatic liver injury also occurs. Hypotension may precipitate acute pancreatitis, which will aggravate shock. The adrenals occasionally show a combination of haemorrhage and necrosis (Waterhouse–Friderichsen syndrome), particularly in septic shock associated with meningococcal septicaemia (see Chapter 17, p. 491).

The most severely affected organs are the heart, lungs, kidneys, and brain. Patients with this type of shock require intensive care in specialized units. In young patients with hypovolaemic shock the mortality rate may be as low as 20%. However, septic shock (mortality rate 60%) and cardiogenic shock (mortality rate 80%) are more difficult to treat. As renal failure and cardiac failure are both treatable, respiratory failure is the most common late organ failure; residual brain damage may also affect some patients who recover.

## Disorders of the Endothelium and Microcirculation

The microcirculation is the capillaries, the arterioles that supply them, and the venules that drain the blood from the capillary bed. A capillary consists of a single endothelial cell encircling a lumen that only just admits the passage of red blood cells. Intercellular junctions join adjacent endothelial cells. The microcirculation is adapted to each organ and tissue. Thus, the liver sinusoids and kidney have a highly permeable fenestrated endothelium, whereas the capillaries in the brain are watertight and contribute to the blood–brain barrier. Capillary endothelial cells are surrounded by pericytes, which support them, synthesize basement membrane, and can differentiate into a variety of cell types including vascular smooth muscle cells. Capillaries act as a semipermeable membrane. They retain most of the protein but permit free exchange of fluid.

The flow of interstitial fluid is governed by the balance between the hydrostatic and plasma oncotic pressures in the microcirculation and by the endothelial permeability (see Chapter 4, pp. 57–58). Interstitial fluid, rich in oxygen and nutrients, is formed by egress of fluid from the arterial end of capillaries, where blood pressure exceeds plasma oncotic pressure. At the venous end of the capillary, plasma oncotic pressure exceeds blood pressure, and interstitial fluid re-enters the circulation, carrying with it carbon dioxide, urea, and other metabolic waste products.

The endothelium controls the permeability of the circulation. Endothelial cells increase their permeability in response to mediators of inflammation, direct injury, and secretion of endothelial permeability factor (vascular endothelial growth factor [VEGF]). When injured, endothelial cells contract, opening gaps between them; this dramatic rise in permeability increases the volume and flow of interstitial fluid. Widespread endothelial injury by bacterial toxins, leukocyte enzymes, or hypoxia may cause DIC and contributes to the syndrome of shock.

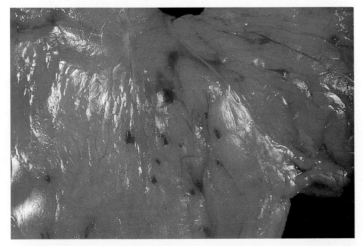

**FIG. 6.6** Spontaneous serosal haemorrhages in a case of meningococcal shock with disseminated intravascular coagulation.

## Oedema

### Key Points

- Oedema is an abnormal increase in the volume of interstitial fluid.
- There are three main pathogenic mechanisms: increased hydrostatic pressure in the microcirculation, decreased plasma oncotic pressure, and lymphatic obstruction.
- Oedema is either localized or generalized.

### Localized Oedema

Pulmonary oedema and cerebral oedema, both of which may be fatal, are the most important forms of localized oedema. Normally oedema fluid has a low protein content – a 'transudate'. However, because of the increased permeability of the microcirculation in inflammation, inflammatory oedema is protein rich and constitutes an 'exudate' (see Chapter 4, pp. 57–58).

The most important causes of localized oedema are:

- left heart failure (pulmonary oedema)
- inflammation
- venous hypertension
- lymphatic obstruction.

### Pulmonary oedema

The osmotic pressure of the plasma (25 mmHg, 3.32 kPa) is greater than the normal hydrostatic pressure in the pulmonary capillaries (8–10 mmHg, 1.06–1.33 kPa). This maintains the dryness of the alveoli and facilitates gas exchange. In left heart failure, increased pressure in the pulmonary veins (pulmonary venous hypertension) increases the capillary hydrostatic pressure and oedema ensues. Overloading the circulation by rapid transfusion of blood or fluids produces pulmonary oedema, especially in elderly people. Oedema occurs first in the interstitium – 'interstitial oedema' – which gives rise to characteristic streaky opacities on chest radiographs. The oedema fluid then escapes into the alveoli and fills the lung (see Chapter 7, p. 187).

Pulmonary oedema is seen in other circumstances. It is pronounced in influenza and lobar pneumonia. It may be part of generalized oedema, e.g. in renal disease. Pulmonary oedema also complicates raised intracranial pressure, probably due to neuroendocrine activation.

### Local venous hypertension

Prolonged sitting causes temporary oedema of the feet and ankles. Thrombosis of the deep leg veins is an important cause of local venous hypertension and oedema. Pitting oedema of the lower legs is a useful sign of right heart failure (Fig. 6.7).

### Chronic lymphatic obstruction (lymphoedema)

In this form of oedema the fluid is protein rich because normal lymph contains protein. In time, growth of connective tissue renders the tissues firm and they do not 'pit' on pressure. Lymphoedema may be due to lymphatic permeation by cancer cells, or following lymph node dissection, e.g. for breast cancer. Lymphatics can also be obstructed by chronic inflammation, e.g. in filariasis, which causes elephantiasis.

### Generalized Oedema

In generalized oedema, fluid also accumulates in serous cavities: ascites within the peritoneum, hydrothorax or pleural effusion, and pericardial effusion. Generalized oedema is detected clinically only when the accumulated fluid exceeds 5 L. The most important causes of generalized oedema are:

- total heart failure
- hypoproteinaemia
- nutritional oedema.

The principal mechanisms of development of generalized oedema are discussed below.

### Hydrostatic factors

In heart failure venous hypertension results in increased hydrostatic pressure in the microcirculation. Also, a fall in cardiac output and arterial blood flow stimulates arginine vasopressin and renin secretion, and secondary aldosteronism leads to sodium and water retention. However, secondary aldosteronism is present in only 50% of patients with cardiac failure, and renal sodium and water retention occur for other reasons.

### Hypoproteinaemia

Plasma oncotic pressure is governed largely by the concentration of albumin, and oedema occurs when the serum

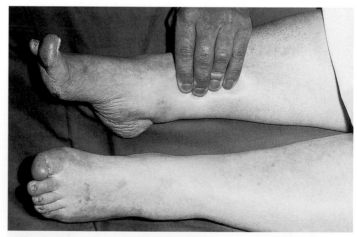

**FIG. 6.7** 'Pitting' oedema of the lower legs demonstrated clinically.

albumin level falls <25 g/L. Hypoalbuminaemia may be due to leakage into the urine in the nephrotic syndrome and other renal diseases or into the gut in protein-losing enteropathies, or insufficient synthesis in liver failure and malnutrition.

### Nutritional oedema

In severe malnutrition, notably kwashiorkor, a combination of low plasma protein, a poorly understood increased vascular permeability, and deficiencies in vitamins and other essential dietary components is responsible.

## Disseminated Intravascular Coagulation

In DIC there is thrombosis throughout the microcirculation, which lowers the platelet count and circulating levels of coagulation factors; thus the other term for DIC is 'consumptive coagulopathy'.

### Pathogenesis

In DIC excessive activation of coagulation is usually due to diffuse endothelial injury. Massive or prolonged release of soluble tissue factors and/or endothelial-derived thromboplastins into the circulation causes generalized activation of the coagulation system. Damaged endothelium also synthesizes less of the natural anticoagulants nitric oxide, prostacyclin, and protein S; severe damage exposes procoagulant subendothelial collagen, which activates the coagulation system. Widespread thrombosis throughout the microcirculation causes thrombocytopenia due to widespread platelet aggregation by thrombin. Consumption of coagulation factors reduces circulating levels of coagulation inhibitors (antithrombin, protein C), which are consumed by the activated clotting factors. Plasminogen activators released from damaged endothelial cells, platelets, or tissue cells convert plasminogen to plasmin, which degrades fibrin so that fibrin degradation products (FDPs) appear in the blood and urine. However, plasmin also digests fibrinogen, factor V, and factor VIII, further reducing the levels of coagulation factors in the blood. In the chronic form of DIC, some tumours release tissue factors as a result of necrosis or production of thromboplastins.

### Aetiology

DIC may be acute or chronic but is always secondary. Approximately 50% of acute cases are due to obstetric conditions such as placental abruption (retroplacental haemorrhage) or, rarely, to amniotic fluid embolism. In neonates, severe hypoxia also causes acute DIC due to endothelial injury. The other conditions most often associated with DIC are sepsis and shock in which there is widespread endothelial damage by hypoxia and other factors.

Chronic DIC accompanies some malignant tumours, particularly adenocarcinomas of the pancreas, lungs, or stomach, and acute myeloid leukaemia. Some of these tumours secrete thromboplastins.

### Causes of DIC

- Acute:
    o shock
    o sepsis
    o placental abruption
    o severe trauma and burns
    o severe hypoxia
    o acute pancreatitis
    o fat embolism
    o intravascular haemolysis.
- Chronic:
    o adenocarcinomas
    o acute myeloid leukaemia
    o malignant hypertension.

### Clinical Features

Widespread petechiae and ecchymoses are often accompanied by epistaxis and bleeding from the gums or venepuncture sites. Massive gastrointestinal or pulmonary bleeding (Fig. 6.8), or intracranial haemorrhage, both subdural and intracerebral, is a common cause of death. Thrombosis of small blood vessels may cause ischaemia of distal digits and a spreading, haemorrhagic, necrotic, gangrenous rash (purpura fulminans) may develop. Peritubular and glomerular capillaries and the renal arterioles may all be occluded, causing or aggravating acute renal failure.

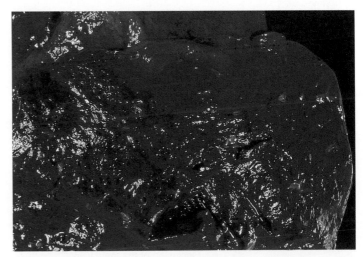

**FIG. 6.8** A sectioned lung showing spontaneous pulmonary haemorrhage in disseminated intravascular coagulation.

# INJURY TO BLOOD VESSELS

Blood vessel injury results in thrombosis, which is due to activation of the clotting cascade.

## Thrombosis

Thrombosis occurs most commonly in veins but can also occur in arteries. The risk of thrombosis is increased by (1) alterations in blood flow, (2) alterations in blood constituents that increase coagulability (e.g. thrombocytosis), and (3) injury to the vascular endothelium – known as Virchow's triad. In rapidly flowing blood, vascular injury results in the formation of platelet-rich thrombus, which grows by accretion of activated platelets and fibrin. Where the vessel is occluded, the blood flow slows and traps red blood cells to form red thrombus. This extends as far as the next branch, where flowing blood will deposit pale thrombus, which in turn will lead to further occlusion. This process is called propagation (Fig. 6.9). In veins the blood flow is so slow that the thrombus consists mostly of red thrombus.

### Fate of Thrombi

Thrombi can be lysed rapidly by anti-clotting factors. Larger thrombi adherent to the vessel wall are more likely to reorganize, with infiltration of macrophages and endothelial cells, recanalization of the clot opening up the lumen, and restoration of blood flow. Thrombi, especially those formed recently, may become detached from the vessel wall and carried by the blood flow to impact on a distal vessel (embolism).

## Embolism

The term 'embolus' refers to abnormal material carried in the blood, which may block downstream vessels, depending on the size and nature of the material. Large emboli result in infarction of the tissue in which the material impacts, such as the brain, causing stroke, the lung, leading to pulmonary infarction, and the kidney, leading to scarring (Fig. 6.10). The most common embolus is derived from thrombus – hence the term 'thromboembolism'. On the arterial side of the circulation most thrombi form in the heart and dislodge,

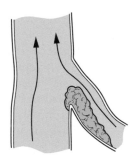

**Pale thrombus**

Platelets adhere to endothelium and undergo 'activation'. Coagulation cascade generates fibrin strands

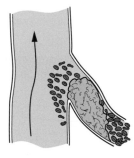

**Red thrombus**

Occlusion of the lumen by the thrombus causes slow or no flow which allows red blood cells to adhere to the surface

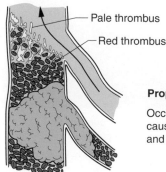

Pale thrombus

Red thrombus

**Propagation**

Occlusion of the main vein causes red thrombus in front and behind

**Fig. 6.9** Propagation of thrombus in a vein.

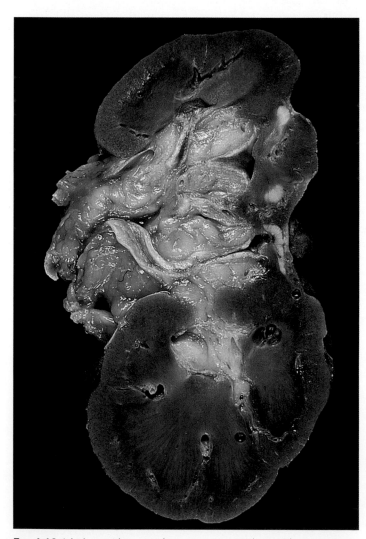

**Fig. 6.10** A kidney with two sunken areas in its midzone. These are scars due to old healed cortical infarcts.

particularly into the brain and kidney. On the venous side of the circulation, most thrombi impact in the pulmonary circulation.

The major types of embolism are:

- systemic arterial embolism
- atheroembolism
- fat embolism
- air embolism
- septic embolism
- amniotic fluid embolism
- paradoxical embolism (see p. 161)
- pulmonary thromboembolism (see p. 114).

### Systemic Arterial Embolism

Most systemic arterial emboli arise from the left side of the heart associated with myocardial infarction, dilated cardiomyopathy, cardiac failure, and cardiac arrhythmias, especially atrial fibrillation. Rarely, ulcerated atherosclerotic plaques, especially in the aorta and main vessels to the head and neck, may release thrombus but it is usually mixed with atherosclerotic material to cause atheroembolism.

### Atheroembolism

This can be identified histologically as cholesterol crystals associated with thrombus impacting in small blood vessels, usually within organs such as the gastrointestinal tract, brain, and kidney (Fig. 6.11). Most are asymptomatic but large showers of them can lead to transient ischaemic attacks ('mini-strokes'), abdominal pain, and renal hypertension, with eventual renal failure.

### Fat Embolism

This is usually associated with severe trauma, especially to the long bones. Fat is released from the bone marrow and impacts in the pulmonary, cerebral, and other circulations, including the kidney (Fig. 6.12) and skin. Multiple petechial haemorrhages occur due to capillary damage and DIC.

### Air Embolism

Air enters the circulation from neck wounds, cardiac surgery, and intravenous infusion. Large amounts (≥300 mL) become churned with blood in the right side of the heart and froth blocks the pulmonary circulation.

Decompression sickness occurs particularly in the context of deep sea diving, when divers breathe air at higher than atmospheric pressure. The inhaled gases are dissolved in blood and tissue in proportion to the pressure. Rapid ascent with an accompanying fall in pressure results in the gases coming out of solution, leading to blockage of small vessels, particularly in the legs, lung, and more severely the cerebral circulation. This can also occur in rapid aircraft decompression at high altitude. Recompression and slow decompression in a special decompression chamber are the only treatment. Chronic decompression sickness (caisson disease) results in necrosis of the intra-articular bone, especially of the hip and shoulder (see Chapter 12, p. 358).

### Septic Embolism

Infected thrombus from a heart valve with endocarditis (a vegetation, see pp. 151–153), or within veins draining areas of infection, may embolize and impact on organs such

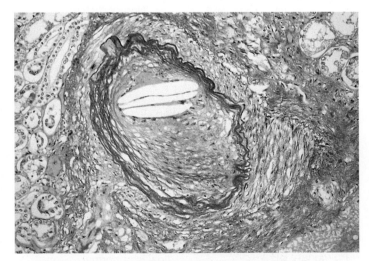

**FIG. 6.11** An artery occluded by loose fibrous tissue within which there are slits formed by crystals of cholesterol derived from an atherosclerotic plaque. This shows that the occlusion is due to organized atheroembolism.

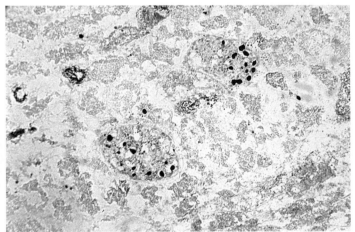

**FIG. 6.12** A section of kidney tissue from a patient who died after multiple long bone fractures. It shows two renal glomeruli stained to reveal fat (red). The glomerular capillaries are plugged with fat globules which, being fluid at body temperature, have passed through the pulmonary capillaries.

as the kidney, lung, or liver where they may form abscesses. On the aortic valve, fragments of vegetation lie close to the coronary orifices and can embolize into the coronary arteries, causing myocardial infarction. Any other cause of thrombus on native or prosthetic aortic valves has a similar risk.

### Amniotic Fluid Embolism

Amniotic fluid embolism is rare but may occur during pregnancy and delivery as a result of early placental detachment, forcing amniotic fluid into the uterine veins. Exfoliated fetal squames from the skin block the pulmonary circulation and cause DIC with a high mortality.

## DISEASES OF THE VEINS

### Venous Thrombosis

Venous thrombosis is common and due to slow blood flow, especially in the veins of the legs. Leg or pelvic vein thrombosis is the principal cause of pulmonary thromboembolism (PTE). Thrombosis starts at the valves of the deep calf veins, causing deep vein thrombosis (DVT). It may propagate into the posterior tibial, popliteal, femoral, or iliac veins and occasionally to the inferior vena cava. DVT starts during or shortly after surgical operations because the neurohumoral response to trauma activates the endothelium and increases the coagulability of the blood. There is also stasis due to immobilization. DVT occasionally causes oedema and calf tenderness but is often subclinical. The incidence is reduced by subcutaneous low-dose heparin and early mobilization.

Risk factors for deep venous thrombosis include:

- trauma, surgery
- immobilization, e.g. in bed or on long-haul flights
- heart failure
- old age
- obesity
- pregnancy and puerperium
- familial thrombophilia
- contraceptive pill.

The outcomes of venous thrombosis (Fig. 6.13) include: massive pulmonary embolism and sudden death; asymptomatic pulmonary embolism; pulmonary infarction; and showers of pulmonary emboli with consequent pulmonary hypertension.

### Pulmonary Thromboembolism

Pulmonary thromboembolism (see also Chapter 7, p. 187) is caused by recently formed thrombi that are poorly anchored to the vein wall in the deep veins of the calf, and break off and end up impacted in the right heart or pulmonary arteries. The size of the embolus and the state of the pulmonary

circulation determine the outcome. A large embolus may impact in the outflow tract of the right ventricle or the main pulmonary trunk, where coiling causes sudden death by circulatory arrest. Sudden death may also be seen with total occlusion of one or both left and right pulmonary arteries (Fig. 6.14). In healthy individuals, occlusion of smaller vessels is survivable with or without pulmonary infarction. Only occlusion of more than half the pulmonary arterial tree results in pulmonary hypertension and right ventricular failure. Occlusion of many vessels by showers of small emboli over months or years may result in chronic pulmonary hypertension. Such patients usually have thrombophilia, e.g. due to deficiencies of anticoagulants such as protein C or protein S. With smaller pulmonary thromboemboli, infarction is prevented by the bronchial circulation and rapid fibrinolysis. Pulmonary infarction occurs usually in the setting of cardiac failure in elderly patients.

### Thrombophlebitis

The term 'thrombophlebitis' refers to thrombosis of veins with associated inflammation. Migrating thrombophlebitis is thrombosis and inflammation of superficial veins in association with cancer, particularly of the pancreas and, in this context, is referred to as Trousseau's sign. Infected thrombi may cause pyaemia or embolism to form distant abscesses,

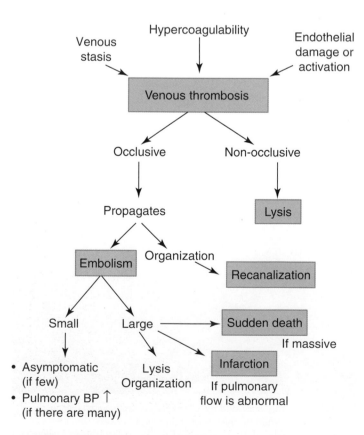

**FIG. 6.13** Outcomes of leg vein thrombosis.

e.g. an appendix abscess may give rise to liver abscess(es) through portal pyaemia. Phleboliths are calcified thrombi, which are common in pelvic veins.

## Varicose Veins

Varicosities are caused by venous hypertension, which leads to dilated tortuous veins with failure of the venous valves, usually in the lower limbs. Standing occupations, obesity, old age, cardiac failure, and pregnancy predispose to varicose leg veins, which affect almost 10% of adults. Although thrombosis occurs in varicose veins, the thrombi do not usually lead to embolization because they adhere to the vein wall. Varicose veins may lead to bleeding and infection, but the usual complication is poor wound healing with venous ulceration, a cause of widespread morbidity in elderly people. Haemorrhoids are caused by venous hypertension in the pelvic and abdominal veins due to constipation, obesity, and pregnancy. Oesophageal varices complicate portal hypertension in chronic liver disease, and bleeding from them is often the terminal event in such patients (see Chapter 9, p. 242). A varicocele is a mass formed by varicosity of the pampiniform venous plexus in the testicle.

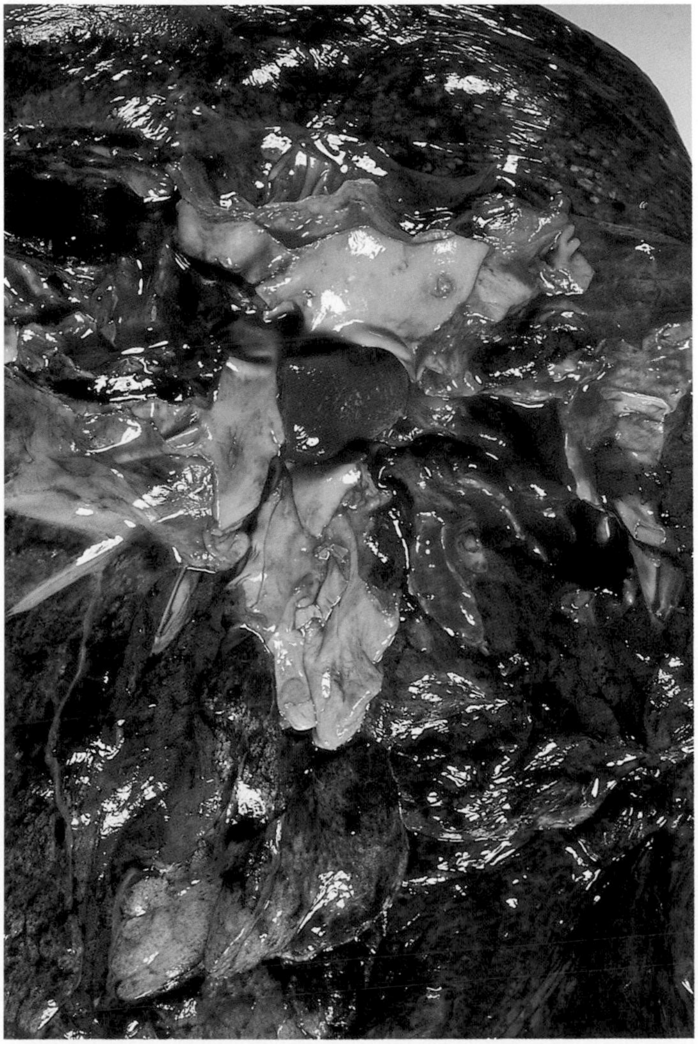

## DISEASES OF THE LYMPHATICS

Acute lymphangitis is usually caused by virulent bacteria, most commonly *Streptococcus pyogenes*, which invade and multiply in the lymphatics, causing subcutaneous red streaks draining an infected area. Lymphangitis leads to lymphadenitis and may herald septicaemia. Blockage of the lymphatics by cancer causes lymphoedema, especially in the upper limbs in breast carcinoma. Chronic filarial lymphangitis causes elephantiasis due to lymphoedema. Milroy's disease is a rare congenital form of idiopathic oedema, often affecting only one limb, which shows gross and diffuse dilatation of the lymphatics. Lymphangiectasia can also occur in the lungs and pericardium.

## DISEASES OF THE ARTERIES

### Arteriosclerosis

Arteriosclerosis is literally the hardening of an artery. The term 'arteriosclerosis' is often used non-specifically (and incorrectly) to refer to a range of abnormalities, including true arteriosclerosis, arteriolosclerosis, Mönckeberg medial calcific sclerosis, and atherosclerosis.

Arteriosclerosis affects both arteries and arterioles. It is due to gradual replacement of vascular smooth muscle cells by collagen and deposition of plasma proteins in the smooth muscle to produce hyaline change. This process is accelerated by age, hypertension, and diabetes mellitus. Arteriosclerosis lowers the compliance of the arterial tree, contributes to the age-related increase in systolic blood pressure, and alters circulatory stability and tissue autoregulation. Arteriosclerosis differs from atherosclerosis in that there is no intimal lipid deposition with resultant inflammation.

The term 'intimal hyperplasia' is used to describe the intimal thickening associated with arteriosclerosis, in which smooth muscle cells, collagen, and elastic deposition are present in the intima (see Fig. 6.3). This is also a feature of ageing and should not be confused with atherosclerosis. There are a variety of confusing terms used synonymously to describe this intimal thickening, such as neointima, fibromuscular hyperplasia, adaptive intimal thickening, hypertrophy, and fibroplasia. It is a ubiquitous response of the vessel wall to any injury and is responsible for angioplasty-related stenosis and experimental endothelial damage with instruments; it also occurs in hypertension. 'Arteriosclerosis obliterans' is a term applied to the occlusive arterial disease

FIG. 6.14 The hilum of a lung showing pulmonary arteries containing large red thromboemboli derived from the leg veins.

in the small- and medium-sized arteries of the lower extremities.

There are two histologically distinct subtypes of arteriosclerosis: the hyaline type and the hyperplastic type (Figs 6.15 and 6.16). Hyperplastic changes are seen, particularly in the temporal artery of elderly patients. Both hyaline and hyperplastic forms are prominent in the arterioles (arteriolosclerosis) of the kidney in hypertension and diabetes.

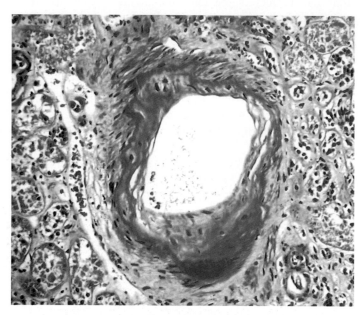

FIG. 6.15 Hyaline arteriosclerosis: pink hyaline change is present in the media of a small artery. Note the intimal thickening.

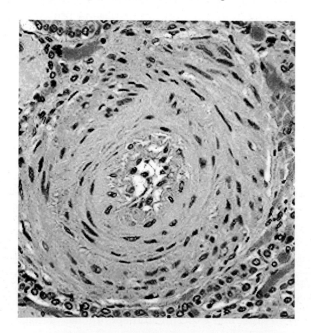

FIG. 6.16 Hyperplastic arteriosclerosis: proliferation of smooth muscle is present in the media of a muscular artery. Note the narrowing of the lumen.

The increased arterial rigidity of arteriosclerosis contributes to the age-related increase in systolic and pulse pressures. The overall decrease in compliance of the arterial tree affects autoregulation in the circulation by shifting the autoregulatory curve to the right (Fig. 6.17). The beneficial effect is decreased susceptibility of elderly and chronically hypertensive individuals to malignant hypertension (see pp. 131–132); however, the greatly increased susceptibility to hypotension accounts for the increased mortality of shock in elderly and hypertensive patients (see *Table 6.1*).

## Mönckeberg's Medial Calcification/Sclerosis

Mönckeberg's medial calcific sclerosis refers to medial calcification, usually at the internal elastic lamina (IEL). It is common and occurs independently of atherosclerosis. It is more frequent in people aged >50 years and in people with diabetes. In advanced cases, vessels may become rigid and lose their distensibility. It can be seen easily as an opaque vessel on normal radiographs and as purple material on histological slides. It is not usually associated with clinical sequelae because it does not cause narrowing of the lumen.

There are a number of other patterns of arterial calcification. Calcification limited to the IEL is observed in the coronary arteries of human immunodeficiency virus (HIV)-positive patients. In patients who have renal dysfunction, alterations in calcium metabolism cause widespread tissue calcification (metastatic calcification) around elastic laminae, which affects the arterial bed – so-called vascular tachyphylaxis. Extensive calcification occurs within atherosclerotic plaques. This calcification increases with advancing age and has been reported to

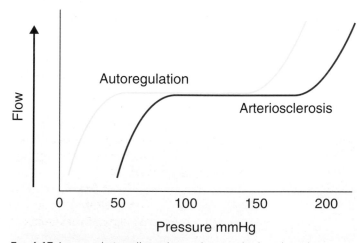

FIG. 6.17 Autoregulation allows the cardiac, cerebral, and renal circulations to maintain constant flow over a wide range of pressure. Arteriosclerosis due to age and hypertension shifts this curve to the right, and renders tissues susceptible to ischaemia if blood pressure falls. Conversely, malignant hypertension is rare in elderly people and those with longstanding hypertension.

develop in <5% annually for individuals aged <50 years but >12% for individuals aged >80 years. When present, vascular calcification indicates a worse clinical outcome for all cardiovascular events.

## Atherosclerosis (atheroma)

### Key Points

- Atherosclerosis is a focal accumulation of lipid in the intima of arteries with inflammation and fibrosis, forming atherosclerotic plaques.
- It causes luminal narrowing, with ischaemia in the brain, heart, and lower limbs.
- Plaque rupture with thrombosis causes acute ischaemia and infarction.
- Atherosclerosis causes ischaemic heart disease, stroke, and peripheral vascular disease, which are the main causes of death in developed countries.

Atherosclerosis is by far the most important arterial disease. It is the principal cause of death and disability in many western countries. Together, ischaemic heart disease (IHD) and stroke cause almost a third of all deaths. A discussion of the risk factors for atherosclerosis is included in the section on ischaemic heart disease (see pp. 133–137). Atherosclerosis arises and progresses as an inflammatory response of the vessel wall to chronic multifactorial injury produced by hyperlipidaemia, hypertension, smoking, and diabetes mellitus. It is a focal intimal disease of medium-to-large arteries, including the aorta, and the carotid, coronary, iliofemoral, and cerebral arteries. Some medium-sized arteries such as the internal mammary artery are spared, as are veins. In the absence of pulmonary hypertension the pulmonary arteries are also spared. Low-density lipoprotein (LDL) from the plasma moves freely in and out of the intima. Within the intima a small proportion of the LDL undergoes oxidative change. The oxidized LDL acts as an inflammatory stimulus, which invokes adhesion molecule expression by endothelial cells, monocyte migration, and cytokine production. Once oxidized, the LDL is taken up by the macrophage scavenger receptors, and lipid uptake continues until the cytoplasm is packed with lipid to form the foam cell. These foam cells eventually die and release the lipid.

At stage I, the monocytes adhere to the intact endothelial surface and subsequently move to enter the intima. The pathogenesis involves endothelial dysfunction, an influx of lipid macrophages and T lymphocytes, inflammation with smooth muscle proliferation, and deposition of collagen and elastic tissue. In the earliest visible lesions, 'fatty streaks', plasma lipid imbibed by intramural macrophages, accumulate in intimal 'foam cells' over which there is an intact endothelial surface (Fig. 6.18). This is termed a stage II lesion by the American Heart Association (AHA) Committee on plaque nomenclature. Stage III lesions look very similar to stage II lesions macroscopically, apart from being larger with more extracellular lipid and inflammatory cells. These three stages make up the 'fatty streak'.

As these intimal lesions develop, they acquire combinations of extracellular lipid, intracellular lipid within foam cells of macrophage origin, and collagen and other connective tissue matrix components produced by smooth muscle cells (Fig. 6.19). The resulting larger intimal lesions are termed 'atherosclerotic plaques', with a collagen cap, a core of variable lipid with calcium deposits, and vascularization from the vasa vasorum (see below).

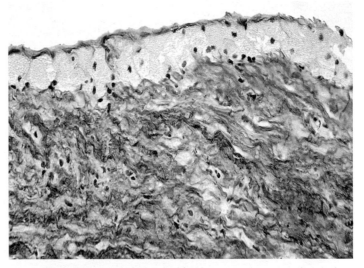

FIG. 6.18 Arterial wall with a layer of foamy macrophages just beneath the endothelial surface in a fatty streak. Stain: elastin van Gieson.

**Early atheromatous plaque**

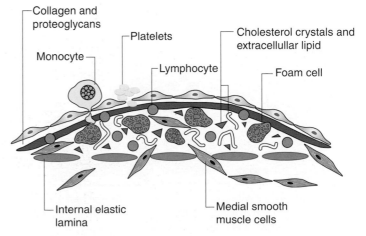

FIG. 6.19 Early events in the formation of an atherosclerotic plaque.

Progression of disease leads to luminal narrowing and changes in the plaques, including surface ulceration, intraplaque haemorrhage, rupture, and thrombosis (Fig. 6.20). Involvement of the coronary arteries results in major clinical complications due to ischaemic heart disease, which manifests as angina pectoris, myocardial infarction, or sudden cardiac death. Involvement of the cerebral circulation results in transient ischaemic attacks or cerebral infarcts (stroke). Atherosclerosis in the aorta results in aneurysm, rupture (particularly in the abdominal aorta), and narrowing of the iliofemoral vessels, which leads to gangrene of the lower extremities.

Atherosclerosis is a biphasic disease. Virtually all individuals in the developed world will have fatty streaks and raised plaques, but only a minority will at some point in their life enter the second phase and develop clinical symptoms.

## Pathology of Atherosclerosis

Examination of the intimal surface of the human aorta opened longitudinally *post mortem* shows plaques with considerable variation in their macroscopic appearances. The earliest lesion visible by naked eye examination is the fatty streak. This is a flat yellow dot or streak on the intima. Fatty streaks are the usual lesions found in children up to age 10 years. Although not all fatty streaks progress, they are considered the starting point in sequential plaque development. The next stage of plaque evolution is elevation above the intimal surface as smooth oval humps, the raised fibrolipid or advanced plaque (Fig. 6.21). Many plaques undergo calcification. In the AHA classification, type IV plaques have a thin cap whereas in type Va plaques the cap is much thicker. The external colour of the raised fibrolipid plaque is yellow due to the carotenoid pigment in the lipid core, but if the plaque cap is thick the external colour is white. Plaques occur in arteries down to 2 mm in diameter.

The later stages of plaque evolution include calcification (type Vb) and thrombosis (type VI). Thrombosis is the most important complication, being responsible for a range of acute manifestations of ischaemic heart disease including unstable angina, myocardial infarction, and sudden death. Thrombosis develops over plaques because of two different processes. The first is superficial intimal injury, in which there are large areas of endothelial loss and intimal erosion over a plaque. Thrombus forms which is entirely superimposed on to the luminal surface of the plaque. Although many of the coronary thrombi due to

Early plaque
confined to intima

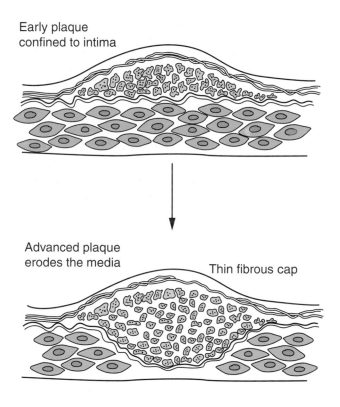

Advanced plaque
erodes the media

Thin fibrous cap

Red blood cells

Complicated plaque
with superimposed
thrombi

Ulceration of thin
cap causes
thrombosis

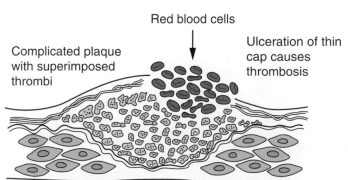

**FIG. 6.20** Stages in the development of an atherosclerotic plaque. It is believed that those with a thin overlying collagenous cap are more likely to crack and ulcerate, and trigger thrombosis.

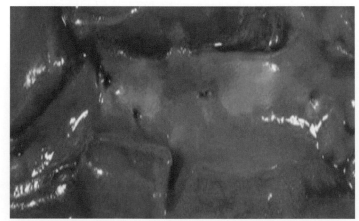

**FIG. 6.21** Coronary artery opened longitudinally to reveal two yellow-coloured atherosclerotic plaques. Note their position near branching points.

endothelial erosion over a plaque are small, a minority are larger and can lead to significant mural thrombi or even complete occlusion (Fig. 6.22). These lesions are more common in elderly females.

In established plaques with a large lipid core, acute inflammation predisposes to plaque rupture and resultant occlusive thrombosis. The fibrous cap tears and the interior of the lipid core, which contains tissue factor and is intensely thrombogenic, is exposed to blood. Thrombus forms within the core due to both activation of platelets and generation of thrombin. The thrombus within the plaque may then extend through the tear in the cap and into the lumen. Plaque disruption has a wide spectrum of severity. Small tears may have only an intraplaque component of thrombus. Large tears over several millimetres with extrusion of the lipid contents lead to occlusive thrombus (Fig. 6.23). In the aorta or carotid arteries, where both the plaques and the vascular lumen are much larger, chronic ulcers filled with thrombus develop as the result of disruption. These plaques may calcify and ulcerate, leading to surface thrombus, which may be asymptomatic or lead to cholesterol emboli. Thrombi and fatty debris from ulcerated plaques embolize into the cerebral circulation, legs, and abdominal organs. This atheroembolism is usually subclinical, but showers of microemboli, often released by an arteriography catheter, surgical manipulation, or anticoagulation, may cause transient ischaemic attacks, renal failure, or malignant hypertension, and may even mimic vasculitis.

Occlusive thrombosis will narrow or occlude a major branch of the involved artery and cause coronary, mesenteric, cerebral, or renal ischaemia. In medium-sized arteries, such as the coronary arteries, plaques tend to form at branching points and bifurcations. Rupture is common in the proximal epicardial vessels and occlusive or semi-occlusive thrombus on these disrupted or ulcerated plaques causes focal or transmural myocardial infarction.

Calcification is common in atherosclerotic plaques, increasing steadily in degree with both the extent of plaque formation and age. Two distinct patterns occur. In one, nodular masses of calcium form within the lipid core. In the other, plates of calcification develop in the connective tissue, deep in the intima close to the medial/intimal junction. Although formerly regarded as a passive precipitation of calcium phosphate crystals, plaque calcification is now recognized to be a regulated process. The current view is that the extent of calcification very roughly relates to the amount of atherosclerosis, but not to the degree of arterial narrowing. Calcification has no direct causal link to thrombosis with one exception. In old age (>75 years), diffuse intimal atherosclerosis and calcification are often associated with diffuse ectasia (dilatation) of the coronary arteries. Intimal tears at the margins of plates of calcium due to shear stress may then cause thrombosis. New methods including electron beam tomography and computed tomography angiography (CTA) are now being used non-invasively to screen for calcification, and by implication the atherosclerotic load within coronary arteries.

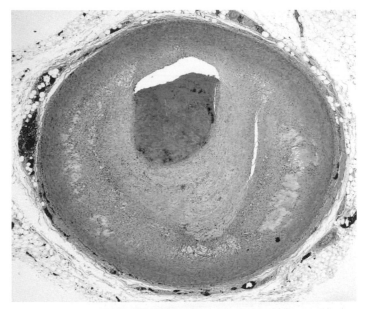

**FIG. 6.22** Cross-section of a coronary artery with a deep lipid core and thick fibrous cap. There is occlusive thrombus within the lumen of the vessel but no evidence of a rupture. This is an example of endothelial erosion causing thrombosis in a coronary artery.

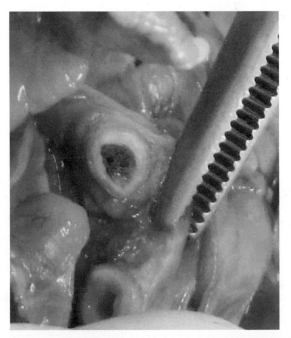

**FIG. 6.23** Cross-section of a coronary artery in which there is an occlusive thrombus blocking the vessel, leading to sudden death in this patient.

Coronary thrombi are dynamic and undergo repair and organization, leading to reversal to a stable lesion with or without some restoration of the lumen. Fibrinolysis, whether natural or therapeutically induced with streptokinase, is often effective at removing part or all of the intraluminal thrombus, which is a loose network of fibrin, and restoring flow. Thrombus within the plaque is more resistant or less accessible. Thrombotic material that is not lysed invokes a florid smooth muscle cell proliferation response, ultimately leading to fibrous replacement. The fibrous tissue contains many new capillary vessels and, if the thrombus has remained occlusive, ultimately there is the formation within the original lumen of a number of new vascular channels.

The circulations affected vary: atherosclerosis targets the aorta, leg, coronary, cerebral, gut, and renal arteries. In people with diabetes or who smoke, the aorta and leg arteries are often diffusely and severely affected, causing peripheral vascular disease. In others, the cerebral and/or coronary arteries are sites of predilection. In young adults coronary arteries are most often targeted whereas severe cerebral atherosclerosis mainly affects elderly people. Pulmonary arteries are affected only in longstanding pulmonary hypertension, as can occur with congenital heart disease, and veins only when pressurized, typically when used as coronary artery autografts.

## Consequences of Atherosclerosis (Box 6.1)

**Box 6.1** MAIN CLINICAL SYNDROMES CAUSED BY ATHEROSCLEROSIS

- ischaemic heart disease (see pp. 133–143):
  - sudden death
  - myocardial infarction
  - heart failure
- cerebrovascular disease (see Chapter 11, pp. 305–309):
  - transient cerebral ischaemic attacks
  - cerebral infarction
  - dementia (arteriopathic)
- peripheral vascular disease:
  - intermittent claudication
  - gangrene
- mesenteric vascular disease:
  - mesenteric claudication
  - intestinal infarction
- renovascular disease (see Chapter 13, pp. 410–412):
  - hypertension
  - renal failure
- aneurysms (see below):
  - aortic aneurysm with rupture.

## Aneurysm

An aneurysm is a localized increase in the luminal diameter of an artery by at least 50%. Aneurysms are symmetrical ('fusiform') or asymmetrical ('saccular'), and involve in particular the aorta and its main branches, and the cerebral vessels (*Table 6.2*). They occur most frequently in the abdominal aorta associated with atherosclerosis. In the ascending thoracic aorta they are linked to hypertension, connective tissue disorders, aortitis, and vasculitis. Weakness of the media is due to cystic medial degeneration, which causes aortic dilatation and dissection (Fig. 6.24), and occurs with hypertension and increasing age. High-risk patients (Marfan's syndrome, bicuspid aortic valve, type IV Ehlers–Danlos syndrome, history of dissection in family relatives) have to be

**TABLE 6.2** The characteristics of aneurysms

| Type | Main location | Comments |
|---|---|---|
| Atherosclerotic aneurysm | Abdominal aorta, iliac arteries, and popliteal and cerebral arteries | Usually infrarenal<br>Rupture and shock<br>May induce an inflammatory fibrotic response |
| Aortitis aneurysm | Thoracic aorta | Diffuse thickening of the aortic wall with involvement of coronary ostia |
| Dissecting aneurysm | Thoracic aorta | Tear in intima usually within 3 cm of aortic valve<br>Intramural haematoma<br>Exit tear in descending aorta or branches<br>Associated with hypertension or Marfan's syndrome |
| Traumatic/surgical aneurysm | Scalp, chest, or anywhere | Also causes false aneurysm |
| Berry aneurysm | Branching points of circle of Willis and cerebral arteries | Causes subarachnoid haemorrhage |
| Microaneurysm | Penetrating branches of cerebral arteries | Causes hypertensive cerebral haemorrhage |
| Mycotic aneurysm (infective) | Aorta and elsewhere, especially cerebral and mesenteric arteries | Embolism from bacterial endocarditis is the most common cause |

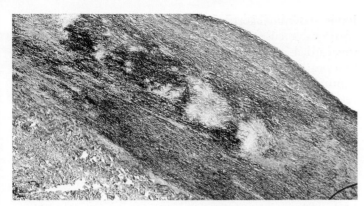

**FIG. 6.24** Wall of the aorta in which there is destruction of the elastic layer with formation of large cystic spaces in the media: this is termed 'cystic medial degeneration'. Stain: elastin van Gieson.

swelling, comprising tortuous and dilated arteries and veins with multiple intercommunications. It is most common in the scalp after birth injury or other trauma.

### Aortic Atherosclerotic Aneurysm

Atherosclerotic aneurysms typically affect hypertensive male smokers aged >60. They may be fusiform or saccular and occur in the lower abdominal aorta (typically distal to the origins of the renal arteries), and often extend into the iliac arteries (Fig. 6.25). Occasionally the whole aorta is ectatic. Large atherosclerotic aneurysms may rupture causing massive retroperitoneal haemorrhage. Unusual sites of rupture are into the oesophagus, mediastinum, lung, pleura, duodenum, pelvis, and vena cava. The larger the aneurysm, the greater the risk of rupture, and the risk is higher with fusiform than with saccular aneurysms. Aneurysms >5 cm in diameter rupture at a rate of 5% per year.

closely followed. Acute dissection and rupture lead to sudden death and in-hospital mortality remains high. Survivors are at lifelong risk for further aortic complications such as thoracoabdominal aneurysm, further dissection, or aortic rupture. Aortic cystic medial degeneration is associated with both hypertension and genetic diseases. It is histologically impossible to tell them apart. Conventional graft replacement surgery and endovascular therapy have significantly improved prognosis. Vasculitis can cause aortic aneurysms but infective syphilitic aortitis is now very rare. Giant cell aortitis, in which there is granulomatous inflammation of the media with giant cells, can lead to aortic aneurysm formation and may be associated with temporal arteritis or connective tissue disease, or be predominantly idiopathic.

Berry aneurysms typically affect the cerebral vasculature and are associated with subarachnoid haemorrhage (see Chapter 11, p. 309). Infective (mycotic) aneurysms are caused by infective arteritis due to embolism from distant infection or proximity to local inflammation. Miliary (Charcot–Bouchard) aneurysms are microaneurysms of the deep penetrating cerebral arteries, especially in the basal ganglia, pons, and cerebellum. They are caused by hypertension and lead to hypertensive intracerebral haemorrhage (see Chapter 11, p. 308). Capillary aneurysms occur in the fundi in diabetic retinopathy and in the glomerular capillaries.

The finding *post mortem* of an aneurysmal dilatation of a long segment of one or more coronary arteries needs careful consideration of a number of causes. Localized aneurysms are mainly atherosclerotic in elderly individuals, but may also be congenital, or occur as a result of Kawasaki's disease (see Special Study Topic 6.1, p. 127) or trauma. Traumatic penetration may cause a false aneurysm, which is the fibrous wall of an organized haematoma communicating with the arterial lumen. Trauma to adjacent arteries and veins may lead to an arteriovenous fistula. A carotid–cavernous sinus fistula may follow a skull fracture. Proptosis is due to venous engorgement and orbital oedema. A cirsoid or racemose aneurysm is an arteriovenous fistula that forms a pulsatile

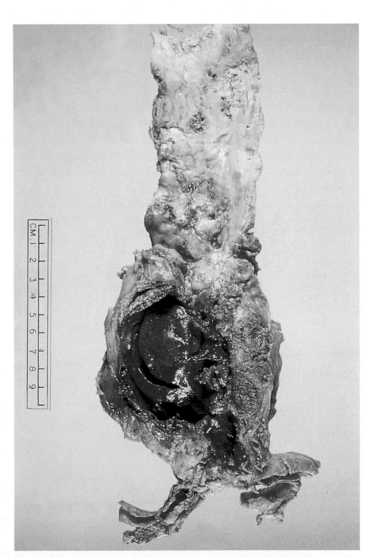

**FIG. 6.25** A saccular atherosclerotic aneurysm of the descending aorta in the typical position above the iliac, and below the renal, arteries. Its lumen contains abundant soft thrombus.

Occasionally, due to chronic inflammation and fibrosis, the wall of the aneurysm may attain 15 mm in thickness, forming an 'inflammatory aneurysm'. This is associated with periaortic and retroperitoneal fibrosis. Originally, chronic periaortitis was considered to be a localized inflammatory response to severe aortic atherosclerosis. However, subsequent studies have shown that chronic periaortitis may also involve other arteries and present with features of autoimmune disease. It affects not only the aortoiliac axis but also other vascular segments such as the thoracic aorta, proximal epiaortic arteries, and coronary, renal, and mesenteric arteries. Periaortitis can be a feature of IgG4-related systemic disease. Histopathological studies show medial and adventitial chronic inflammation with thickening and vasculitis of the vasa vasorum, and adventitial lymphoid follicles with germinal centres. A significant fraction of thoracic lymphoplasmacytic aortitis cases and inflammatory abdominal aortic aneurysms/abdominal periaortitis cases, and a proportion of retroperitoneal fibrosis cases are all caused by IgG4-related systemic disease. Rarely there may be an IgG-related vasculitis in response to atherosclerosis in the coronary arteries.

## Dissection

In arterial dissection, blood penetrates into the artery wall via an intimal tear. In the aorta, a transverse tear occurs in the ascending portion (Fig. 6.26), in the start of the descending aorta, and at other sites. Blood tracks proximally and distally between the inner two-thirds and the outer third of the media (Fig. 6.27). External rupture may occur after a short distance, but distal dissection may extend into the neck,

limbs, abdominal aorta, and beyond. At the aortic valve ring, aortic valve cusps may prolapse with regurgitation and/or myocardial ischaemia. More often, rupture into the pericardium causes fatal cardiac tamponade. Less common sites of rupture are the mediastinum, lung, pleura, peritoneum, and retroperitoneum. Occasionally, a second distal intimal tear decompresses the dissection and allows flow to re-enter the lumen; the second channel formed in the media may lead to a 'double-barrelled' aorta and long survival. Most dissections are due to hypertension but localized lesions such as coarctation may also be responsible (Fig. 6.27). Crack cocaine use predisposes to aortic dissection as well. Chronic dissection leads to depression and ridges in the aorta with dense fibrosis and reorganized thrombus.

Dissection with cystic medial degeneration is seen in Marfan's syndrome, an autosomal dominant mutation in the fibrillin gene (fibrillin is necessary for the deposition of elastic fibres). It is also seen in type 4 Ehler–Danlos syndrome due to a genetic defect in procollagen formation, in pseudoxanthoma elasticum, where there is fragmentation of the medial elastic fibres, and in osteogenesis imperfecta, where there is also defective collagen synthesis. Blunt chest injury, arterial catheterization, and surgery can all cause traumatic aortic dissection. Pregnancy also increases arterial glycosaminoglycans and predisposes to dissection in both the aorta and the coronary arteries. Aortic incompetence and myocardial ischaemia may follow aortitis and dilatation of the aortic root.

### Coronary Artery Dissection

In adults, isolated coronary artery dissection may precipitate acute infarction and sudden death. The process is distinct

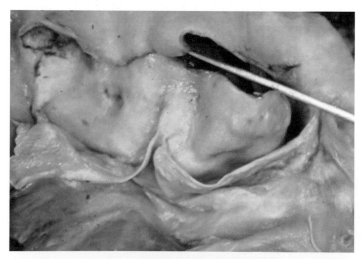

**FIG. 6.26** Aortic valve and ascending aorta in which there is a transverse tear highlighted by the probe. Note the intramural haematoma within the tear.

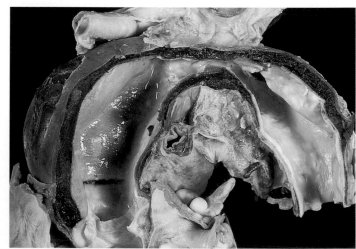

**FIG. 6.27** The ascending arch and descending aorta from a 26-year-old man, who died of a dissecting aneurysm. A transverse intimal tear is present just above the aortic valve and there is narrowing (coarctation) of the aorta (see p. 161), visible at the apex of the aortic arch.

from aortic dissection and starts as a subadventitial haematoma, which compresses the vessel lumen from outside. This haematoma may rupture into the lumen and create a dissection track. The pathogenesis is not clear but it is linked to pregnancy in many cases. There is an adventitial inflammatory process with eosinophils and basophils, which are reactive to the intramural haematoma (Fig. 6.28). In individuals who survive, the angiogram can return to close to normal as the haematoma is organized and becomes smaller. There is also a link to Marfan's syndrome or other connective tissue gene defects in some cases, as well as cocaine use.

## Other arterial diseases

### Fibromuscular Dysplasia

Fibromuscular dysplasia (FMD) is currently defined as an idiopathic, segmental, non-inflammatory, and non-atherosclerotic disease of the musculature of arterial walls, leading to stenosis of small and medium-sized arteries. It has been reported in almost every arterial bed and primarily affects females aged 15–50 years. It most commonly presents in the renal and extracranial cerebrovascular arteries,

manifesting as hypertension, transient ischaemic attack, or stroke, respectively. The true prevalence is unknown, partly because of the fact that it is underdiagnosed in many patients. Histological classification discriminates three main subtypes, in which there is intimal, medial, or adventitial fibrosis with smooth muscle proliferation in the absence of inflammation. This results in narrowing of the vessel. These subtypes may be associated in a single patient (Fig. 6.29). The angiographic classification includes the multifocal type, with multiple stenoses and the 'string-of-beads' appearance that is related to medial FMD, and tubular and focal types, which are not clearly related to specific histological lesions. The aetiology of FMD remains unknown. Several hypotheses have been postulated, such as hormonal effects, developmental abnormalities of the vessel wall, genetic factors, cocaine use, and even recurrent dissection with healing. It is the main cause of renal artery stenosis in middle-aged females who present with hypertension. The carotid, vertebral, and splanchnic arteries may also be involved. Other complications are thrombosis, aneurysms, and dissections. Similar arterial proliferative lesions occur in neurofibromatosis.

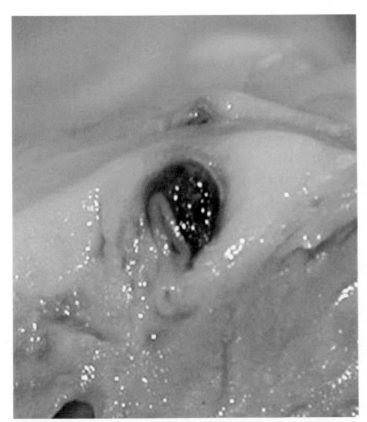

FIG. 6.28 The lumen of the coronary artery is blocked by an intramural haematoma. This is an example of spontaneous coronary artery dissection with intramural haematoma.

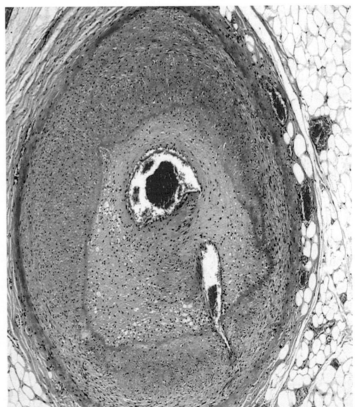

FIG. 6.29 Section of coronary artery demonstrating fibrointimal smooth muscle cell hyperplasia, which is typical of the intimal type of fibromuscular dysplasia.

### Transplant Arteriopathy

Transplant arteriopathy following organ transplantation is a non-atherosclerotic hyperplastic fibromuscular intimal proliferation, which occurs in virtually all types of solid organ transplant. Transplant arteriopathy affects large muscular arteries, small muscular arteries, and veins. Early on, there is inflammation in the vessel, which can be mild or marked and may involve one or more of the three layers. Usually, the intima is affected more than the media or adventitia, but sometimes even a transmural, necrotizing arteritis may occur. The typical intimal fibromuscular proliferation follows the inflammatory stage. With time, the lesions become less cellular and more fibrotic. Calcification, thrombosis, and atherosclerosis can also occur in the setting of transplant arteriopathy. In the heart, where this lesion is most damaging, transplant coronary artery disease affects large and small epicardial coronary arteries and intramyocardial arteries.

Another now common iatrogenic form of intimal hyperplasia occurs with restenosis after balloon angioplasty or after intravascular stent placement. The intimal proliferation in restenosis lesions is histologically the same as in transplant arteriopathy and the hyperplastic form of arteriolosclerosis.

### Coronary Artery Anomalies

Non-atherosclerotic coronary artery disease is rare as a cause of significant clinical problems. Congenital anomalies of the origins of the coronary arteries come in a myriad of forms, some of which are dangerous because they are associated with sudden death; others are simple anatomical variants without an effect on coronary blood flow. Dangerous anomalies include where one artery, usually the left coronary artery, takes origin from the pulmonary trunk. Another lethal anomaly is where both arteries take origin in one aortic sinus with one artery crossing between the aorta and pulmonary trunk. Both of these dangerous anomalies may present as myocardial infarction or angina in infancy or early adult life and there is always a risk of sudden death.

### Idiopathic Infantile Arterial Calcification

Idiopathic infantile arterial calcification (IIAC) is a rare cause of infantile sudden death. There is calcification at the internal elastic lamina and marked intimal fibroblastic proliferation of medium- and large-sized arteries. This results in narrowing of the vessels with distal ischaemia. The most frequent postmortem findings are myocardial hypertrophy, subendocardial fibrosis, and firm and tortuous coronary arteries. Histologically there is marked intimal proliferation and deposition of calcium hydroxyapatite around the internal elastic lamina and media of arteries. It usually presents early in life with death under 1 year. It is important to recognize because it is caused by mutations of the *ENPP1* gene (ecto-nucleotide pyrophosphatase/phosphodiesterase 1) on chromosome 6q. ENPP1 belongs to the phosphodiesterase nucleotide pyrophosphatase (PDNP) family that generates inorganic pyrophosphate ($PP_i$). $PP_i$ inhibits extracellular matrix calcification due to prevention of hydroxyapatite deposition. The reduction in the levels of $PP_i$ promotes calcification of the extracellular matrix in the arterial walls. It is an autosomal recessive disease and diagnosis is important for family counselling.

## VASCULITIS

The term 'vasculitis' refers to inflammation of blood vessels. Vasculitis can affect any of the blood vessels, including arteries, veins, and capillaries. Vessels of any type, in any organ, can be affected, resulting in a broad spectrum of symptoms and signs. The heterogeneous nature of vasculitides often presents a diagnostic challenge. The American College of Rheumatology classification criteria and the Chapel Hill Consensus Conference nomenclature are the most widely used to distinguish different forms of vasculitis. The latter defines 10 primary vasculitides based on vessel size (large, medium, and small). The diagnosis relies on the recognition of a compatible clinical presentation supported by specific laboratory or imaging investigations and confirmatory histology. Anti-neutrophil cytoplasmic antibody (ANCA) testing has been of particular benefit in defining a subgroup of small-vessel vasculitides. Arteritis affects arteries and arterioles, but, when veins and capillaries are affected, a broader term such as vasculitis or angiitis is preferred. Necrosis of the vessel wall may cause thrombosis and infarction, aneurysm formation, or rupture with haemorrhage. In the healing phase, luminal narrowing causes chronic ischaemia. There are four patterns of inflammation: granulomatous/giant cell, lymphoplasmacytic, acute neutrophilic, and eosinophilic. Mixed patterns, particularly acute/lymphoplasmacytic, also occur.

In most types the aetiology is unknown. However, immune complex deposition causes the vasculitis in serum sickness, systemic lupus erythematosus (SLE), and rheumatoid arthritis. In some cases of polyarteritis nodosa the immune complexes contain hepatitis B and C proteins in infected individuals. Immunogenic drugs can also induce vasculitis via immune complex deposition or hypersensitivity to drugs bound to the endothelium, and antibodies to the endothelial major histocompatibility complex (MHC) antigens contribute to the vasculitis of allograft rejection. In other diseases, ANCAs are pathogenic. Some infections cause vasculitis and some types of vasculitis currently considered idiopathic may ultimately prove to be infective in aetiology. As multiple organs or tissues are often affected, vasculitis may be confused with multisystem diseases or embolism. Vasculitis is discussed further in Special Study Topic 6.1.

# 6.1 Special Study Topic

## VASCULITIS

Vasculitis is diagnosed by a combination of clinical and histological features. The histological features vary, but always include inflammation of the vessel wall.

## Giant Cell Arteritis

Giant cell arteritis is the most common vasculitis. It affects patients aged >50 years and is associated with a high erythrocyte sedimentation rate (ESR). When widespread it affects the aorta and its major branches. The terms 'temporal' and 'cranial' arteritis should be avoided because the process is usually more diffuse. Headache, jaw claudication, and visual disturbances occur. Focal granulomatous inflammation with giant cells at the internal elastic lamina can be confirmed by temporal artery biopsy. Significant complications are blindness (from retinal artery involvement) and cerebral infarction. It is often associated with polymyalgia rheumatica. There is usually a good clinical response to steroids.

## Takayasu's Arteritis

Takayasu's arteritis is similar histologically to giant cell arteritis and affects the aorta and its branches. In contrast to giant cell arteritis, it mainly affects Asian women aged <40. The granulomatous inflammation progresses to fibrosis and narrowing, with thrombosis of the head and neck vessels, particularly the subclavian, carotid, and innominate arteries ('pulseless disease'). This causes limb ischaemia, and visual and neurological defects.

## Behçet's Disease

Behçet's disease is a multisystem disease of unknown aetiology characterized by chronic relapsing orogenital ulcers, uveitis, and systemic involvement, including articular, gastrointestinal, cardiopulmonary, neurological, and vascular pathology. Behçet's disease is more common in individuals of Mediterranean, Middle Eastern, or Far Eastern descent. There is mixed inflammation of vessels, with aneurysm formation and luminal thrombosis. Behçet's disease can affect any part of the body because it can involve vessels of any size or type. Venous manifestations are frequent and arterial lesions rarer. Arterial lesions include aneurysms, occlusions, stenosis, and aortitis. Lesions mainly involve the aorta, and femoral and pulmonary arteries. Patients with arterial lesions are more frequently male and have higher rates of venous involvement.

## Buerger's Disease

Buerger's disease (thromboangiitis obliterans) is vasculitis of the limb arteries and veins, predominantly in young males. As the whole neurovascular bundle is inflamed, it causes severe ischaemic pain, which progresses to gangrene. Confined to smokers, its progress is arrested only by cessation. The inflammation is mixed and mainly lymphoplasmacytic, with progression to intimal fibrosis and thrombosis.

## ANCA-associated Vasculitis

Microscopic polyangiitis, granulomatosis with polyangiitis (Wegener's granulomatosis), Churg–Strauss syndrome, 'renal limited' vasculitis, and a number of drug-induced vasculitides are all associated with circulating ANCAs. ANCAs with specificity for protease-3 (PR3) or myeloperoxidase (MPO) are hallmarks of ANCA-associated vasculitis and have a pivotal role in disease development. Clinically, PR3-ANCA is strongly associated with granulomatous vasculitis and MPO-ANCA with necrotizing small-vessel vasculitis, as in microscopic polyangiitis (see also Chapter 13, p. 403). ANCAs activate primed neutrophils to release lytic enzymes and reactive oxygen species, a process reinforced by the alternative pathway of complement. This process leads to endothelial detachment and lysis with inflammation. IgG ANCAs are causally associated with necrotizing vasculitides which are characterized immunopathologically by little or no deposition of immunoreactant. Disease onset usually occurs in elderly people, although it can occur at any age. Prevalence is generally higher in males, but females more often develop disease at a younger age. The overall prevalence of ANCA-associated vasculitis is highest in white people. The incidence of granulomatosis with polyangiitis is higher in northern Europe, whereas that of microscopic polyangiitis is higher in southern Europe and Japan.

## Granulomatosis with Polyangiitis

Previously known as Wegener's granulomatosis, this can occur anywhere in the body but most commonly affects the upper respiratory tract (nose, sinuses, and throat), lungs, and kidneys. There is necrotizing granulomatous vasculitis of the upper and lower respiratory tracts, segmental necrotizing glomerulonephritis, and systemic small-vessel vasculitis. The inflammation is usually mixed, with neutrophils admixed with plasma cells, lymphocytes, and giant cells.

## Special Study Topic continued . . .

### Churg–Strauss Syndrome

Churg–Strauss syndrome is a necrotizing systemic vasculitis with extravascular granulomas and eosinophilic infiltrates of small vessels (Fig. 6.30). It is a rare vasculitis of small- and medium-sized vessels, and is characterized by a constant association with asthma and eosinophilia, and the presence of MPO-ANCA in approximately 40% of patients. Vasculitis most frequently involves the peripheral nerves and skin. Other organs may be affected, such as the heart, kidney, and gastrointestinal tract, and their involvement is associated with a poorer prognosis. It can also cause aortitis and aortic valve incompetence. Overall, the survival of patients with Churg–Strauss syndrome is excellent, but relapses are not uncommon and require treatment with corticosteroids, often for prolonged periods, combined with immunosuppressants (e.g. induction [cyclophosphamide] and maintenance therapy [azathioprine]).

### Microscopic Polyangiitis

Microscopic polyangiitis affects small-sized vessels (i.e. capillaries, venules, and arterioles) without granulomas, and is a necrotizing small-vessel vasculitis with few or no immune deposits (pauci-immune vasculitis). Unlike polyarteritis nodosa, it does not usually involve larger vessels. In western countries microscopic polyangiitis has a lower prevalence than granulomatosis with polyangiitis, affects more men than women, and commences at the age of ≥50 years. The two organs most typically involved and often defining prognosis are the kidneys and lungs. Microscopic polyangiitis can also involve any other organ, especially nerves, the central nervous system, skin, musculoskeletal system, heart, eye, and intestines. Its typical clinical manifestations are rapidly progressive glomerulonephritis and alveolar haemorrhage. Capillaritis, with fibrinoid necrosis and a neutrophilic infiltrate, is the most common vascular lesion. Microscopic polyangiitis is a more appropriate name than microscopic polyarteritis because some patients have no evidence of arterial involvement. The absence or paucity of immunoglobulin localization in vessel walls distinguishes microscopic polyangiitis from immune complex-mediated small-vessel vasculitis, such as Henoch–Schönlein purpura and cryoglobulinaemic vasculitis. Clinical, epidemiological, and pathological differences warrant the separation of microscopic polyangiitis from polyarteritis nodosa on the basis of involvement of capillaries and venules by the former but not the latter. Pauci-immune necrotizing and crescentic glomerulonephritis, and haemorrhagic pulmonary capillaritis, are common in patients with microscopic polyangiitis and microscopic polyangiitis is the most common cause of the pulmonary–renal vasculitic syndrome. The vasculitis in patients with microscopic polyangiitis is pathologically indistinguishable from the vasculitis of granulomatosis with polyangiitis and Churg–Strauss syndrome: granulomatous inflammation distinguishes granulomatosis with polyangiitis from microscopic polyangiitis; asthma and eosinophilia distinguish Churg–Strauss syndrome from microscopic polyangiitis.

### Polyarteritis Nodosa

Polyarteritis nodosa (PAN) is a necrotizing angiitis that predominantly affects small- and medium-sized arteries. It is most common in people in their 30s and 40s. Males are twice as likely as females to develop PAN. It causes focal and segmental full-thickness necrosis of arteries up to 5 mm diameter in any part of the body. Lesions predominate in the skin, kidneys (Fig. 6.31), heart, muscle, gut, and nervous system. In the acute stage, thrombosis causes infarction and

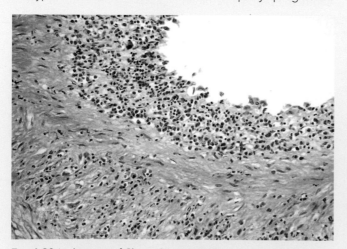

**FIG. 6.30** In this case of Churg–Strauss syndrome, there is an eosinophilic infiltrate involving the blood vessel wall, particularly the intima and media.

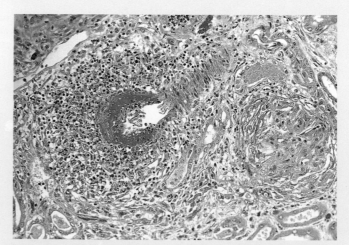

**FIG. 6.31** A section of kidney from a case of polyangiitis showing a damaged glomerulus (right) and an interlobular artery which, in its lower part, shows fibrinoid necrosis. There is intense surrounding inflammation.

## Special Study Topic continued . . .

arterial necrosis causes haemorrhage or aneurysms. Later, healing and fibrosis of arteries cause chronic ischaemia, leading typically to renovascular hypertension. Nerve infarction (mononeuritis multiplex) causes paraesthesiae and paralyses. Arteriography showing multiple aneurysms is diagnostic; otherwise, biopsy of symptomatic nerve or muscle may show diagnostic arteritis. Untreated, the relapsing clinical course extends over 2–5 years with death from lesions in the kidney, heart, or brain.

In some cases, PAN is associated with chronic hepatitis B infection or a very specific type of leukaemia known as hairy cell leukaemia (see Chapter 8, p. 200). In immunosuppressed and burns patients, PAN most commonly affects the kidneys, skin, and nerves. A variety of other vasculitides may exhibit similar arterial lesions, including aneurysm formation. These include: primary systemic vasculitides, secondary forms such as those associated with connective tissue diseases, and organ-limited forms. Infected emboli, e.g. in bacterial endocarditis, may cause acute necrotizing arteritis with rupture or the development of an infectious ('mycotic') aneurysm.

## Cryoglobulinaemia

The term 'cryoglobulinaemia' refers to the presence in the serum of one (monoclonal cryoglobulinaemia) or more (mixed cryoglobulinaemia) immunoglobulins, which precipitate at temperatures below 37°C and redissolve on rewarming. Common signs and symptoms of cryoglobulinaemia are a rash on the lower limbs, arthritis, and nerve damage. Cryoglobulinaemia is classified into three types (1, 2, and 3) on the basis of immunoglobulin composition. Predisposing conditions include lymphoproliferative disease, collagen disease, and hepatitis C virus (HCV) infection. The diagnosis of a cryoglobulinaemic syndrome is predominantly based on the laboratory demonstration of serum cryoglobulins. In type 1 cryoglobulinaemia, there is a monoclonal immunoglobulin paraprotein that is often associated with lymphoma. In types 2 and 3 cryoglobulinaemia, polyclonal immunoglobulins are present with (type 2) or without (type 3) a monoclonal component. Both of these types usually involve a mixture of IgG and IgM and are hence often referred to as mixed cryoglobulinaemia. Circulating mixed cryoglobulins are often detected in many infectious and systemic disorders, e.g. hepatitis C infection and rheumatoid arthritis: hepatitis C infection is particularly associated with type 2 disease. By contrast, 'essential' mixed cryoglobulinaemia is a distinct disorder, characterized by leukocytoclastic vasculitis of small- and medium-sized vessels, and frequent multiple-organ involvement. Cryoglobulinaemia generally leads to a systemic inflammatory syndrome characterized by fatigue, arthralgia, purpura, neuropathy, and glomerulonephritis. The disease mainly involves small- to medium-sized blood vessels and causes vasculitis due to cryoglobulin-containing immune complexes.

## Raynaud's Disease

Cold exposure causes excessive symmetrical vasoconstriction in the extremities. It mainly affects young females. The arteries are anatomically normal and the aetiology is unknown. In Raynaud's phenomenon the excessive vasoconstriction is secondary; causes include connective tissue diseases (scleroderma and SLE), Buerger's disease, use of vibratory power tools, drugs or toxins (ergot, α-adrenergic blockers and polyvinyl chloride monomer), and hyperviscosity syndromes such as cryoglobulinaemia, in which it is more severe and causes ulceration and gangrene.

## Henoch–Schönlein Purpura

IgA-associated vasculitis is commonly equated with the multiorgan systemic vasculitic syndrome. An infectious trigger, typically of mucosal origin, is frequently identified in patients with cutaneous IgA-associated vasculitis. Henoch–Schönlein purpura (HSP) occurs predominantly in children and most commonly affects the skin, kidneys, joints, and stomach. There is usually a neutrophilic leukocytoclastic vasculitis and full recovery is common.

## Coronary Artery Vasculitis

This is rare and can be subdivided into lymphoplasmacytic, eosinophilic, and giant cell types. It may occur as part of diseases such as polyarteritis nodosa, granulomatosis with polyangiitis, or giant cell aortitis, but in isolation is an indicator of Kawasaki's disease.

## Kawasaki's Disease

This condition follows a few weeks after a febrile disease in infants or young children in whom there is lymphadenopathy, mouth ulcers, and a rash that resembles that of rubella. Cases can present as sudden death. *Post mortem* the striking feature is massive aneurysmal dilatation of either a localized segment or long lengths of the proximal coronary arteries, with occluding thrombus leading to myocardial infarction. The arteries show an intense transmural arteritis, which is indistinguishable from that of PAN. In Kawasaki's disease, however, arteritis in other organs is absent. The disease is strikingly more common in Japan although sporadic cases occur worldwide. The pathogenesis is uncertain although all the hallmarks of an immune response to a viral infection are present. There is, however, as yet no definitive isolation of a particular virus. Patients who survive the acute phase are left with either local or diffuse aneurysmal dilatation of a coronary artery, which may undergo thrombosis some years later. It is being increasingly recognized that the acute phase disease may be misdiagnosed as rubella or be sufficiently mild not to be noticed. Coronary aneurysms come to light only when thrombosis occurs years later.

## Special Study Topic continued . . .

### Central Nervous System Vasculitis

Central nervous system (CNS) vasculitis affects the brain and sometimes the spinal cord. It is rare, with numerous causes. One such entity, non-infectious granulomatous angiitis of the nervous system (GANS), is an extremely rare disease with a predilection for leptomeningeal and parenchymal arteries and veins. Isolated involvement of the CNS is characteristic of GANS, which has also been referred to as primary angiitis of the CNS (PACNS). Characteristically, lesions are multiple, bilateral, and supratentorial. Both grey- and white-matter infarcts are identified in the deep white matter.

Congophilic (or amyloid) angiopathy is characterized by the deposition of amyloid fibrils within the walls of blood vessels of the brain and meninges. It may cause circulatory disturbances, including intracranial haemorrhage. It is the second most frequent cause of non-traumatic cerebral haemorrhage, accounting for as many as 15% of all cases. It is commonly associated with Alzheimer's disease and ageing, but is also seen in Down's syndrome and sometimes after head injuries (dementia pugilistica). Some degree of congophilic angiopathy is found in approximately a third of patients aged >60 years who undergo a postmortem examination and this percentage increases with advancing age. It occurs in both sporadic and hereditary forms. The sporadic form is usually most severe in the parietal and occipital lobes and within the meninges, and it is the most common cause of lobar intracerebral haemorrhage. It may also result in patchy loss of myelin within the white matter with progressive dementia. A variety of hereditary forms has been described in various parts of the world, with numerous genetic abnormalities and variation in clinical presentation and behaviour.

### Vasculitis and Infectious Disease

Many viruses can be responsible for systemic vasculitis, the most frequent being hepatitis B virus-related PAN. Such vasculitis probably results from immune complex-mediated mechanisms. Mixed cryoglobulinaemia has been shown to be associated with HCV infection in >80% of patients, but it remains asymptomatic in most of them, with only a minority developing vasculitis. HIV, erythrovirus B19, cytomegalovirus, varicella-zoster virus, and human T-cell lymphotrophic virus (HTLV)-1 have also been reported to be associated with, or implicated in the development of, vasculitides. On the other hand, some bacteria, fungi, or parasites can also cause vasculitis, mainly by direct invasion of blood vessels or septic embolization, leading, for example, to the well-known feature of 'mycotic aneurysm'. Syphilitic aortitis and/or cerebrovascular disease and rickettsial diseases are other, more specific, bacteria-induced vasculitides. Pseudomonas infections cause systemic infective vasculitis. In immunosuppressed patients and drug addicts, angioinvasive fungi such as *Aspergillus* and *Mucor* spp. cause tissue destruction with infarction.

Recognition of an infectious origin of vasculitides is of great importance because treatment strategies differ from those applied to non-infectious forms. Effective antimicrobial drugs are mandatory to treat bacterial, parasitic, or fungal infections, whereas the combination of antiviral agents and plasma exchange has been proven to be effective against hepatitis B virus-related PAN.

## VASCULAR TUMOURS

Vascular tumours are common. Many benign tumours are debatably true neoplasms; other endothelial proliferations are triggered by trauma or infective agents. Haemangiomas are masses of atypical blood vessels.

### Capillary Haemangiomas

Capillary haemangiomas occur in most internal organs, but are most common in the skin where they form 'birthmarks'. The 'port wine stain' is a diffuse cutaneous angioma. The juvenile capillary haemangioma, the so-called strawberry naevus of infancy, often grows rapidly for some months, then usually regresses completely by 5 years of age. Large placental angiomas (chorangiomas) may cause heart failure in the fetus. The pyogenic granuloma (lobular capillary haemangioma) is a polypoid cutaneous capillary angioma that often ulcerates and bleeds. Many follow trauma, especially in pregnancy. Bacillary angiomatosis is a proliferation of capillaries associated with inflammatory cells that occurs in immunocompromised patients, especially with acquired immune deficiency syndrome (AIDS). It is caused by infection by Gram-negative bacilli of the genus *Bartonella*.

### Cavernous Haemangiomas and Rarer Entities

Cavernous haemangiomas consist of large, dilated, thin-walled vascular channels. The most dangerous occur in the brain where they may rupture and cause a haemorrhage. Vascular hamartomas consist of cavernous channels admixed with fat, smooth muscle, and fibrous tissue. They often occur in muscles and cause pain from thrombosis. Multiple angiomas form part of several syndromes, including von Hippel–Lindau disease, Osler–Weber–Rendu disease, and Sturge–Weber syndrome. The lesions of epithelioid haemangioma consist of clusters of vessels lined by plump (epithelioid) endothelial cells, surrounded by chronically inflamed fibrous tissue containing eosinophils. Glomus tumour arises from the glomus bodies of the skin. It is therefore found mainly in the extremities, especially the digits. They form small nodules that are exquisitely tender because of the tumour's dense innervation. In other tumours, glomus cells are associated with larger channels, occur more on the proximal limbs and trunk, and are less often tender; these are called glomangiomas.

## Malignant Vascular Tumours

These tumours are rare. There is a spectrum of malignancy ranging from low-grade, slow-growing haemangioendotheliomas to highly malignant angiosarcomas. Epithelioid haemangioendotheliomas occur in large vessels, usually a vein, but may occur in soft tissues, liver, lung, and other organs. The tumour cells show primitive endothelial differentiation. These tumours are often multifocal so that many patients eventually die of their disease. Angiosarcomas occur most often in the skin, breast, soft tissues, and liver. Those in the skin arise at sites of chronic sun exposure; those in the liver have in the past been associated with industrial exposure to vinyl chloride monomer in the plastics industry. The most common aggressive endothelial tumour is Kaposi's sarcoma. This, and its relationship with HIV infection, are discussed in Chapter 19 (p. 546).

## Tumours of Lymphatic Endothelium

Lymphangiomas, similar to haemangiomas, are often congenital and may be composed of ramifying small channels of large cavernous spaces. They may form a large mass, a 'cystic hygroma', especially in the neck. Occasionally, a single large cyst lined by lymphatic endothelium forms a lymphatic cyst. Lymphangiomas are most common in the retroperitoneum and mediastinum.

# HYPERTENSION

### Key Points

- Hypertension is raised pressure in any vascular bed, e.g. systemic hypertension, pulmonary hypertension (see Chapter 7, p. 173), or portal hypertension (see Chapter 10, p. 283).
- Without qualification, hypertension is usually synonymous with systemic arterial hypertension.
- Its main clinical importance is as a major risk factor for the cardiovascular diseases associated with atherosclerosis.

## Variation in Blood Pressure and Definition of Hypertension

Within any population the distribution of blood pressure is a unimodal bell-shaped curve skewed to the right. The risk of cardiovascular disease increases with blood pressure, even within the normal range. The definition of hypertension is therefore arbitrary. Taking a cut-off point of 140/90 mmHg,

single measurements of blood pressure suggest a prevalence of 4% in the third decade of life and over 60% in the eighth decade. In the UK and many western countries, the overall prevalence of hypertension in adults reaches 20%.

In individuals, blood pressure shows a diurnal variation. The lowest levels occur during sleep. Blood pressure rises on standing up, during exercise, and on exposure to cold and emotion. Individuals with a larger than normal pressure rise in response to these stimuli have an increased risk of permanent hypertension and are said to have labile hypertension. A single blood pressure reading should therefore be interpreted with caution and additional information can be obtained from a 24-hour recording.

Normally, blood pressure rises through childhood and adolescence, and reaches adult levels in the third decade. Those children and adolescents with the highest blood pressure become adults with the highest pressure. This phenomenon of 'tracking' blood pressure has implications for early detection and treatment of hypertension.

## Classification and Causes of Hypertension

In 95% of cases of hypertension there is no detectable cause; such patients are said to have primary or essential hypertension. In the remaining cases, hypertension is secondary to an underlying condition, often renal disease, alcohol misuse, or, occasionally, an endocrine disorder (*Table 6.3*).

The prognosis of patients with hypertension is related to both the height and the rate of the pressure rise.

**TABLE 6.3** Classification of systemic hypertension

| Type | Benign/Malignant | Causes |
|---|---|---|
| Essential (95%) | 90% benign 10% malignant | Unknown |
| Secondary (5%) | 80% benign 20% malignant | Renal artery stenosis<br>Renal parenchymal disease, e.g.:<br>End-stage renal failure<br>Glomerulonephritis<br>Reflux nephropathy<br>Diabetic nephropathy<br>Adult polycystic disease<br>Coarctation of the aorta<br>Endocrine causes, e.g.:<br>Cushing's syndrome<br>Conn's syndrome<br>Phaeochromocytoma<br>Acromegaly<br>Others, e.g.:<br>Pre-eclampsia<br>Alcohol abuse |

Hypertension has been classified into a 'benign' form, in which the prognosis is measured in decades, and a 'malignant' or accelerated form, which, if untreated, is universally fatal within 2 years.

## Clinical Features

### Benign Hypertension

Benign hypertension causes:

- ischaemic heart disease
- heart failure
- stroke
- acceleration of renal disease
- malignant hypertension.

Benign hypertension is usually asymptomatic and most cases are discovered when the pressure is measured at a routine medical examination, often in middle age. Blood pressure rises slowly over many years, usually only to moderately high levels, e.g. 180/100 mmHg. Elderly people may develop a form with disproportionately high systolic pressure, systolic hypertension, which is probably due to arterial disease.

Benign hypertension affects the heart and arteries of all sizes (Fig. 6.32). The main target organs are the heart, brain, and kidneys. The most common complication is ischaemic heart disease, including heart failure, which accounts for about 60% of deaths, and another 30% die of stroke. Benign hypertension causes changes in the kidney, and hypertension is a major aggravating factor in patients with renal diseases. However, renal failure is uncommon and only affects those at the most severe end of the spectrum.

### Cardiovascular System

Increased pressure load causes hypertrophy of the arteries and heart. The muscle hypertrophy normalizes the work-load of individual cardiac myocytes and arterial smooth muscle cells, but also has adverse effects on both the heart and the arteries. The arterial geometry changes such that the resistance arteries have thicker walls and narrower lumina (Fig. 6.33).

The changes of arteriosclerosis that ensue are more severe and occur earlier than the age-related changes described on pp. 115–116. These permanent structural changes in the arterial tree perpetuate hypertension regardless of its aetiology. The longitudinal and circumferential stretching of arteries, if severe, may cause dilatation of the aortic root and, rarely, leakage (incompetence) of the aortic valve (see p. 146). Longstanding hypertension aggravates atherosclerosis and contributes to the development and rupture of aneurysms and dissections (see pp. 120–123).

### Heart

In the heart, left ventricular hypertrophy (Fig. 6.34) impairs diastolic function; the thickened ventricle is stiffer due to

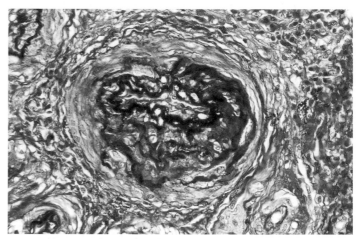

FIG. 6.33 Advanced arteriosclerosis in a renal radial artery in an elderly individual with longstanding benign hypertension. The intima is grossly thickened by excess matrix proteins, including collagen and elastic tissue. There has been almost complete loss of the medial smooth muscle, presumably due to atrophy.

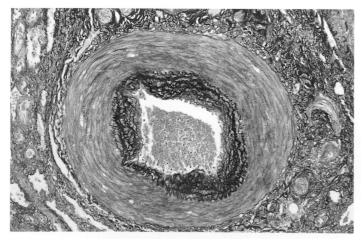

FIG. 6.32 A renal interlobar artery in early established hypertension. There is intimal thickening but the predominant feature is hypertrophy of the muscular media, leading to an increased wall:lumen ratio. This causes an increased response to prevailing pressor stimuli – the 'vascular amplifier'.

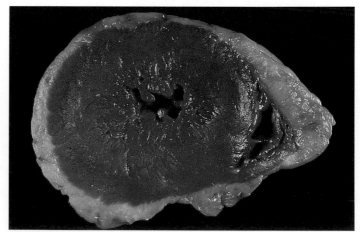

FIG. 6.34 This transverse slice of the left ventricle shows gross hypertrophy, which is present in some hypertensive patients.

both increased muscle mass and interstitial fibrosis. As the ventricle is perfused only during diastole, coronary artery perfusion is poor. In addition, people with hypertension are likely to have coronary atherosclerosis, and the increased oxygen demand of the hypertrophied left ventricle contributes to ischaemia, even at rest. Thus, left ventricular hypertrophy causes increased mortality, proportional to the degree of hypertrophy, from cardiac arrhythmias and myocardial infarction.

## Brain

In addition to arteriosclerosis and atherosclerosis of the cerebral arteries, hypertension causes multiple tiny aneurysms (microaneurysms) in the deep penetrating arteries supplying the basal ganglia, pons, and cerebellum. These aneurysms rupture and cause hypertensive cerebral haemorrhages (see Chapter 11, p. 308). Hypertension also predisposes to regional and watershed zone cerebral infarction. In addition, over-enthusiastic treatment of hypertension in elderly people can cause boundary zone infarction of the brain due to the rightward shift in the cerebral autoregulatory curve (Fig. 6.17 on p. 116).

## Kidney

Arteriosclerosis affects the afferent arterioles and to a lesser extent the glomeruli and efferent arterioles. This accelerates the normal age-related loss of nephrons and diminishes the functional reserve of the kidneys. Hypertension is an important aggravating factor for renal diseases (see Chapter 13, pp. 411–412), but only in the most severe cases does benign hypertension cause renal failure.

## *Malignant Hypertension*

Malignant hypertension is defined clinically as hypertension (diastolic blood pressure >130 mmHg) together with retinal changes of bilateral flame-shaped haemorrhages and/or papilloedema. In about 50% of cases malignant hypertension develops without a preceding history of hypertension; <5% of patients with benign essential hypertension develop the malignant phase. It is more common in black people and those with secondary hypertension, especially if caused by renovascular disease. Malignant hypertension usually affects younger people with hypertension; new cases usually present at 30–40 years.

Patients with malignant hypertension are ill. If they survive the usual complications of raised blood pressure – heart failure and cerebral haemorrhage – renal failure becomes universal and is the most common cause of death in untreated cases. Occasionally 'hypertensive encephalopathy' occurs, a syndrome characterized by altered consciousness, fits, and transient paralyses. The renal damage and encephalopathy are due to failure of autoregulation when the resistance vessels cease to protect the microcirculation from the increased pressure. This is rare in elderly people because the cerebral autoregulatory curve is shifted to the right (see Fig. 6.17), but is more common in young people and especially in

children whose arteries are unprotected by arteriosclerosis. Malignant hypertension causes:

- renal failure
- heart failure
- stroke
- hypertensive encephalopathy
- microangiopathic haemolytic anaemia.

### Pathology and Pathogenesis of the Arterial Lesions

Failure of autoregulation in the kidney transmits increased pressure to the glomeruli, causing fibrinoid necrosis and microaneurysms of glomerular capillaries. The pressure also causes fibrinoid necrosis of afferent glomerular arterioles (Fig. 6.35), which may rupture (Fig. 6.36) or be associated with luminal thrombosis, resulting in small infarcts. Thrombosis causes damage to red blood corpuscles –

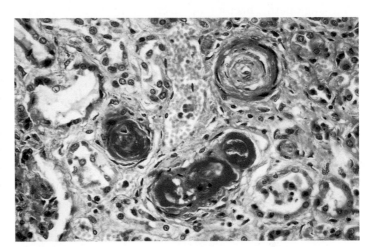

FIG. 6.35 A section of kidney showing fibrinoid necrosis and thrombosis of arterioles (stained red). A small radial artery (top right) shows intimal proliferation, probably due to a healing response, which causes extreme narrowing.

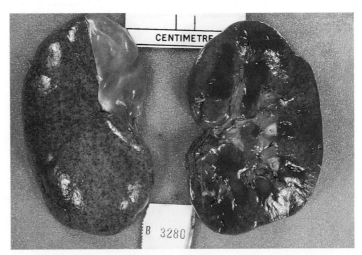

FIG. 6.36 The kidneys in acute malignant hypertension are swollen and their surfaces show small haemorrhages.

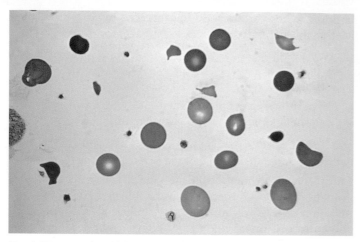

**FIG. 6.37** A peripheral blood smear showing red blood cells fragmented due to intravascular thrombosis in malignant hypertension.

microangiopathic haemolytic anaemia (Fig. 6.37). Ischaemia of the juxtaglomerular apparatus leads to increased secretion of renin, which further increases blood pressure, leading to a vicious circle. Together, these effects give rise to proteinuria and haematuria. Similar changes occur in the brain in hypertensive encephalopathy. The circulation in the heart is, however, protected from the brunt of the pressure by systolic contraction of the cardiac muscle, and other organs are usually spared.

Healing arterial damage results in intimal proliferation. This may cause chronic renal failure due to ischaemia and may require dialysis and renal transplantation a few years after successful treatment. With better detection and treatment of benign hypertension, the incidence of malignant hypertension has fallen steeply in countries with adequate medical care. By contrast, malignant hypertension is still the most common reason for acute renal failure in black people in some African countries.

## Aetiology of Essential Hypertension

### Key Points

- Hypertension is due to an interplay of genetic and environmental factors.
- Blood pressure has a polygenic inheritance.
- The most important environmental factors are stress, diet, and the intrauterine environment.

### Genetic and Racial Factors

A polygenic inheritance has been established. The candidate genes include those encoding angiotensinogen, which is estimated to account for 6% of blood pressure variation in humans, renin, and atrial natriuretic peptide receptor genes.

Black people are more susceptible to hypertension than white people; in the USA the black population has twice the incidence of hypertension and six times the mortality. Females have a higher incidence of hypertension, but mortality in males is 1.5–2 times the mortality of females with the same levels of blood pressure, probably because of increased atherosclerosis.

### Environmental Factors

City dwellers have higher blood pressures than rural populations and migration studies suggest environmental influences. Although difficult to quantify, stress seems to be the important factor and animal experiments support this notion. Epidemiological, clinical, and animal studies implicate sodium intake, which is excessive in most westernized countries. Diets high in salt are often also high in animal fats, and low in dietary potassium, which can lower blood pressure.

There is a linear relationship between alcohol intake and blood pressure. The oestrogen-containing contraceptive pill increases the blood pressure by a few millimetres of mercury in most females who take it. This will therefore tip some females into clinical hypertension. Regular exercise lowers blood pressure, probably because of induction of endothelial nitric oxide synthase (see Chapter 4, p. 68). Smoking only aggravates the complications of hypertension. The effects of the intrauterine environment are of current interest. Babies with low birthweight have an increased incidence of hypertension and other cardiovascular disorders in adult life. It is likely that the renin system is involved.

## Secondary Hypertension

In patients with secondary hypertension, renal disease is 10 times more common than all other causes added together. Hypertension is caused by disorders of the renal blood vessels (renovascular hypertension), many renal diseases (renal parenchymal hypertension), or simply loss of nephrons in renal failure.

### Renovascular Hypertension

In the community, 3% of the hypertensive population have renovascular hypertension. Any narrowing of renal arteries causes hypertension because of activation of the renin–angiotensin system. The most common condition is renal artery stenosis, which may be unilateral or bilateral. Over 50 years of age this is usually due to atherosclerosis whereas in younger patients fibromuscular dysplasia (see p. 123) is usually the cause. This may present in childhood but is more common in females aged about 40 years.

In renal artery stenosis the pathogenesis of hypertension has three phases. In the first phase, hypertension is maintained by high blood angiotensin II through a direct pressor effect, due to vasoconstriction combined with a 'slow pressor effect', probably due to vascular smooth muscle cell growth. In the second phase, renin and angiotensin levels fall, but the blood pressure is still dependent on renin. In the third phase, renin and angiotensin levels may be normal but, as in hypertension due to any cause, the blood pressure is sustained by permanent changes in the vascular tree. Surgical treatment of the stenosis at this stage is therefore disappointing. At any time during this sequence of events, malignant hypertension may be triggered.

Restoration of blood flow to the ischaemic kidney can cure the hypertension in selected cases, and can restore normal function to the atrophied kidney, which is protected from the effects of hypertension by the narrowed artery.

### Renal Parenchymal Hypertension

End-stage renal failure is always accompanied by hypertension due to sodium and water retention. Hypertension is also common in the early stages of glomerulonephritis. In children reflux nephropathy is the most common cause of secondary hypertension. The reason for increased renin secretion by the damaged kidney is unclear.

### Coarctation of the Aorta

Hypertension in the upper half of the body, mainly due to renal underperfusion and hyper-reninism, is a feature of this congenital disorder (see p. 161).

### Adrenal Hypertension

Hypertension occurs in several adrenal disorders:

- primary aldosteronism
- Cushing's syndrome
- phaeochromocytoma
- congenital adrenal hyperplasia.

These are discussed in Chapter 17.

### Other Endocrine Diseases

Hyperparathyroidism, acromegaly, and both hypo- and hyperthyroidism may be complicated by hypertension, but the mechanisms are poorly understood. Gestational hypertension is usually caused by pre-eclampsia, a disease characterized by hypertension, proteinuria, and oedema, which complicates 3–5% of pregnancies. In some cases essential hypertension may present in pregnancy.

## ISCHAEMIC HEART DISEASE

Ischaemic heart disease (IHD) occurs when there is insufficient blood supply to the myocardium to meet functional demand. This is a balance between myocardial blood supply and myocardial demand for oxygen and other nutrients. The former is reduced particularly by coronary artery atherosclerosis (see pp. 117–120) and the latter is increased by ventricular hypertrophy, which occurs most commonly in the context of systemic arterial hypertension and aortic valve disease (particularly aortic stenosis, see pp. 145–146).

## Aetiology and Risk Factors

The incidence of ischaemic heart disease is an indicator of the extent of atherosclerosis (see pp. 117–120) in a community. Epidemiological studies have identified many risk factors associated with an increased or decreased risk of developing ischaemic heart disease but only the major factors are discussed here. Age, sex, and heredity are all important, but hyperlipidaemia, hypertension, cigarette smoking, and diabetes are the most important because they are modifiable (*Table 6.4*).

### Age and Sex

Ischaemic heart disease begins in males in the fourth decade and increases in incidence thereafter. It is uncommon in females before the menopause, probably due to hormonal influences (particularly oestrogen).

### Hyperlipidaemia

Accumulation of lipid in arteries is central to the pathogenesis of atherosclerosis, and hyperlipidaemia often predisposes to ischaemic heart disease. Insoluble cholesterol and other lipids circulate within the centre of lipoprotein particles, the hydrophobic lipid core of which is surrounded by an outer hydrophilic layer of phospholipid and apolipoproteins. Apolipoproteins are protein ligands that bind to receptors on cells. They are divided into groups labelled alphabetically (apoA, -B, -C, and so on), within which subclasses are labelled numerically (apoA1, apoA2, and so on). Decreasing particle size is associated with increasing density. They range from large chylomicrons through very-low-density lipoprotein (VLDL) and low-density lipoprotein

TABLE **6.4** Risk factors for ischaemic heart disease

| Modifiable | Non-modifiable |
| --- | --- |
| Cigarette smoking | Age |
| Hyperlipidaemias | Male sex |
| Hypertension | Family history |
| Diabetes | Personality type |
| High-density lipoprotein levels | |
| Obesity | |
| Exercise level | |

(LDL) to high-density lipoprotein (HDL) (*Table* 6.5 and Fig. 6.38). Lipoproteins bound to membrane receptors are internalized by endocytosis and metabolized, or modified by lipase enzymes on the cell surface (Fig. 6.39). The endothel-ium is permeable to lipoprotein, some of which binds to the extracellular matrix and some of which is taken up by cells in the vessel wall.

**TABLE 6.5** Properties of the main lipoprotein particles

| Particle | Diameter (nm) | Apolipoprotein | Cholesterol content (%) |
|---|---|---|---|
| Chylomicron | 80–1200 | A1, A2, A4, B48 and C | <5 |
| Very-low-density lipoprotein (VLDL) | 30–80 | B48, C, E | 25 |
| Intermediate-density lipoprotein (IDL) | 25–35 | B100, E | 40 |
| Low-density lipoprotein (LDL) | 15–25 | B100 | 65 |
| High-density lipoprotein (HDL) | 5–15 | A1, A2, C | <20 |

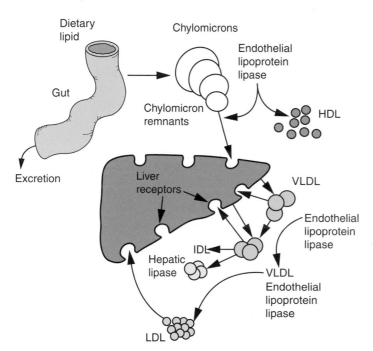

**FIG. 6.38** Schematic diagram of lipoprotein pathways. VLDL = very-low-density lipoprotein; IDL = intermediate-density lipoprotein; LDL = low-density lipoprotein; HDL = high-density lipoprotein.

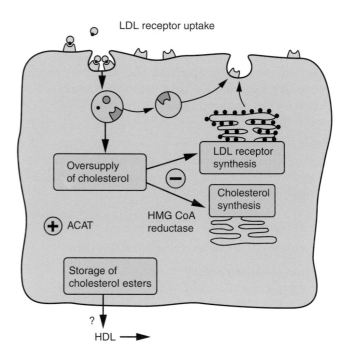

**FIG. 6.39** Intracellular cholesterol metabolism. ACAT = acyl-CoA:cholesterol acyltransferase; HMG CoA = 3-hydroxy-3-methylglutaryl-coenzyme A.

## 6.2 Special Study Topic

### CHOLESTEROL METABOLISM AND LIPID LEVELS AS RISK FACTORS FOR ISCHAEMIC HEART DISEASE

LDL carries 70% of blood cholesterol. All cells possess LDL receptors, but the liver possesses by far the most and 75% of plasma LDLs are removed by hepatocytes, which therefore control blood cholesterol levels. The number of LDL receptors on each hepatocyte is regulated by the intracellular cholesterol level. Increasing hepatocyte cholesterol content switches off LDL-receptor synthesis, and plasma LDL levels rise. Thus a low-cholesterol diet can lower blood cholesterol levels via hepatocyte LDL receptors. Lowering intestinal reabsorption of bile acids increases the conversion of cholesterol to bile acids in the hepatocyte; this fall in intracellular cholesterol lowers blood cholesterol. This knowledge is important in devising strategies to treat hyperlipidaemia.

HDL is synthesized mainly in the small intestine and hepatocytes. It is believed to take up cholesterol from

## Special Study Topic continued . . .

cells and other lipoproteins, and transport it to the liver. In different communities mean adult levels of total plasma cholesterol (TC) vary from about 3.9 mmol/L (150 mg/dL) to >7 mmol/L (275 mg/dL). In countries with a mean TC level below 4 mmol/L ischaemic heart disease is rare, whereas communities with mean TC levels of 5.2 or more invariably have high ischaemic heart disease rates. In prospective studies TC levels predict the risk of developing ischaemic heart disease, in communities with both high and low TC levels.

Blood levels of lipoprotein A, which contains a unique apoA, is an independent risk factor for ischaemic heart disease, in that raised levels confer a high risk of ischaemic heart disease, even when LDL and other lipids are normal. By contrast, plasma levels of HDL are related inversely to the risk of ischaemic heart disease; HDL levels may be of greater predictive value than TC or LDL levels within communities.

Hyperlipidaemias, which are grouped according to the class of lipid that is in excess, may be inherited or result from another disorder. Multiple unknown genes influence blood lipid levels, and the most common hyperlipidaemia is the polygenic form. The most common monogenic hyperlipidaemia is LDL-receptor deficiency. Low hepatocyte LDL receptors are due to mutation of one of the many genes that regulate the synthesis and transport of receptors; 1/500 live births are heterozygotes who possess 50% of normal LDL receptors. This results in plasma LDL levels that are two to four times normal. This increases the risk of ischaemic heart disease, which develops in early adulthood. Homozygotes constitute 1/1,000,000 live births and usually die of ischaemic heart disease in childhood. Sufferers are treated aggressively with lipid-lowering strategies.

### Cigarette Smoking

Smoking is one of the most powerful risk factors for ischaemic heart disease, is dose related, and is an especially potent risk factor in young males. On cessation, the risk falls over several years to that of matched non-smokers. Smoking affects the coagulation system: it decreases endothelial prostaglandin $I_2$ (prostacyclin or $PGI_2$) and nitric oxide synthesis, and increases platelet stickiness and blood fibrinogen levels.

### Hypertension

Increased blood pressure (both systolic and diastolic) is associated with increased risk of ischaemic heart disease. In some community studies the risk in the 20% of the population with the highest pressure was four times that for the 20% with the lowest pressure. Lowering blood pressure decreases the risk of ischaemic heart disease, especially in elderly people, but the effect is not as marked as the reduction in stroke.

### Diabetes Mellitus

Diabetes doubles the risk of ischaemic heart disease and 20% of people with type 2 diabetes have evidence of vascular disease at presentation. People with diabetes also tend to develop cerebrovascular and peripheral vascular disease. The complex mechanisms are linked to the 'endothelial dysfunction', hypertension, hyperlipidaemia, and obesity that occur in insulin resistance (see Chapter 17, pp. 495–496). Good metabolic control lowers the risk.

### Other Risk Factors

#### Diet

Diets rich in saturated fats and cholesterol are associated with high mean plasma levels of TC, LDLs, and VLDLs. Prospective studies have demonstrated that the risk of ischaemic heart disease is related directly to: (1) the percentage of calories derived from saturated fats; (2) high ratios of saturated/polyunsaturated dietary fats; and (3) dietary intake of cholesterol. The risk of ischaemic heart disease is inversely related to the amount of dietary fibre and polyunsaturated fats. Consumption of fish oils and fruit high in natural antioxidants may be protective, but dietary supplements of the antioxidant vitamin E and β-carotene are not.

#### Alcohol Consumption

Alcohol consumption of >5 units (50 mg) daily is an independent risk factor for ischaemic heart disease; heavy drinking is associated with hypertension, but the mechanisms are unclear. However, consumption of fewer than 2–3 units per day confers a lower risk of ischaemic heart disease than for abstainers.

#### Regular Exercise

This lowers the risk of ischaemic heart disease. Exercise lowers weight and blood pressure, raises blood HDL levels, and upregulates endothelial nitric oxide synthase. Obesity raises blood pressure, blood lipids, and insulin resistance, but, in addition, is an independent risk factor. Abdominal obesity, the predominant male pattern, is believed to be especially harmful.

#### Oral Contraceptives

These raise blood pressure and lipids and increase the risk of thrombosis. This slight risk is increased by age, smoking, and obesity.

#### Behavioural Patterns and Stress

Stress is an undoubted risk factor especially when associated with a poor diet and poverty. Epidemiological studies show that low birthweight is a risk factor for ischaemic heart disease as well as hypertension. This effect appears to be separate from social factors but the mechanisms are unknown.

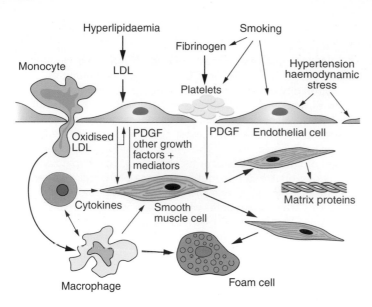

**Fig. 6.40** Interaction between risk factors and cells. LDL = low-density lipoprotein; PDGF = platelet-derived growth factor.

The above risk factors are synergistic (Fig. 6.40), each adding to the risk of developing ischaemic heart disease. They also contribute to the risk of the other major complications of atherosclerosis.

### Genetic Predisposition

Environmental risk factors probably account for most of the differences in the ischaemic heart disease rates between communities, but they do not predict accurately, within a community, who will develop ischaemic heart disease. Genetic influences clearly determine very important risk factors and protective mechanisms that at present remain unknown.

### Some Pathogenic Factors

#### Lipids in the Vessel Wall

The net influx of lipoproteins into the artery wall is proportional to plasma levels. Lipid influx is greater around the ostia of branches where the endothelium is more permeable. In the vessel wall LDL is immobilized by binding to proteoglycans, where it can be oxidized by endothelial cells, macrophages, and exposure to chemical factors and free radicals generated by platelets and leukocytes in the vessel wall. Receptor-mediated endocytosis of native LDL is regulated by negative feedback from the levels of intracellular cholesterol. However, foam cells gorge on oxidized LDL because it is absorbed via an unregulated pathway. Oxidized LDL is also antigenic and autoantibodies to oxidized LDL increase with the severity of atherosclerosis. LDL–antibody complexes are also taken up by macrophages via Fc receptors.

Oxidized LDL is toxic to endothelial cells and causes endothelial dysfunction. This leads to increased stiffness of large arteries and raises the blood pressure by deficient nitric oxide release. Endothelial function is improved by admin-

istration of antioxidants. Oxidized LDL is chemotactic for monocytes and their recruitment could contribute to plaque growth. There is therefore substantial evidence that, in the vessel wall, oxidized LDL mediates some of the atherogenicity of raised blood LDL.

HDL provides a theoretical clearance system for cellular cholesterol. It may also prevent the chemical and physical changes, such as oxidation, that promote the uptake of LDL. Although there is little *in vivo* evidence, these notions accord with the beneficial effect of raised plasma levels of HDL.

### Haemodynamic Factors

Atherosclerosis is increased by haemodynamic stress, e.g. the pulse pressure is greater in the lower aorta and legs than in the arms. In addition, hypertension and age aggravate atherosclerosis. Plaques occur on the outer aspects of branching points and at the ostia of branches. These are areas of low shear stress where the endothelial cells are more permeable to lipoproteins and have a more prothrombotic surface.

### Blood Coagulation

Platelets and fibrin form a fine layer on the surface of plaques and their products are detectable within the plaque itself. Incorporation of thrombus could therefore play a role in the growth of plaques. Endothelial dysfunction renders the endothelial surface prothrombotic. It is therefore likely that thrombosis, which has a crucial role in myocardial infarction and the other acute complications of atherosclerosis, also contributes to plaque growth.

### Inflammation

Most inflammatory cells probably enter the plaque via the small vessels derived from the vasa vasorum rather than from the lumen. Macrophages and activated T lymphocytes are universal. In some instances neutrophil polymorphs are plentiful. Acute inflammation has been implicated in plaque rupture, which precedes occlusive thrombosis and lytic enzymes released from leukocytes have been implicated in this. Infection by herpesvirus and *Chlamydia pneumoniae* has been implicated in coronary heart disease. This could explain the acute inflammation associated with plaque rupture. An infectious component in atherosclerosis is an important and intriguing possibility, but the evidence remains inconclusive.

The cellular and cytokine mechanisms in atherogenesis are similar to chronic inflammation and healing elsewhere (see Chapter 4, pp. 62–63). Cytokines released from inflammatory cells may also activate endothelial cells and alter endothelial function as well as influence the growth and differentiation of various cell types in the vessel wall (see Figs 6.19 and 6.40). In addition, continuing inflammation may result in fibrous thickening of the vessel wall and of the adjacent tissues – if severe, it is called periarteritis.

### Precursor Lesions

Fatty streaks are the earliest arterial lipid deposits (see Fig. 6.18 and p. 117). In societies with a high prevalence of ischaemic heart disease, intimal thickenings occur in the coronary and other arteries in some young children; they may even be present at birth. They are the putative precursors of 'premature' coronary atherosclerosis, which occurs in some young males. Intimal thickening (intimal cushion) is a normal feature of arterial branching points, and diffuse intimal thickening of age-related or hypertensive arteriosclerosis is the substrate for development of 'normal' late-onset atherosclerosis. Thus, all of the putative precursors of atherosclerosis have in common intimal thickening due to accumulation of cells and matrix.

### Cellular Interactions in Atherogenesis

It is likely that intimal thickening is orchestrated by the endothelial cell. However, the focal distribution of atherosclerosis is determined by haemodynamic factors, of which haemodynamic stress and shear stress are the most important. Haemodynamic stress modulates endothelial cell function. Endothelial cells modulate haemostasis and platelet and leukocyte adherence. The latter release growth factors and cytokines, which stimulate the migration and proliferation of subendothelial smooth muscle cells and then transform into myofibroblasts. As in wound healing, these myofibroblasts synthesize extracellular matrix proteins and proteoglycans which contribute to the bulk of the plaque, affect cell growth and differentiation, and bind lipoproteins.

### Future Trends

In developed countries conscious of risk factors, the epidemic of ischaemic heart disease that developed over the first half of the last century is on the wane; the incidence of ischaemic heart disease has fallen, in some countries, by 50%. Lifestyle changes are believed to be responsible. Lipid-lowering drugs such as hydroxymethylglutaryl (HMG)-CoA reductase inhibitors decrease mortality in both patients with complications of atherosclerosis and healthy adults. Recent studies using quantitative imaging have shown that lowering risk factors and aggressive therapeutic reduction of serum cholesterol levels can induce regression of individual lesions. Ischaemic heart disease has now become the fate of poor people who are stressed, smoke, and have a poor diet. It is increasing rapidly in eastern Europe, and an increase in affluence and adoption of a westernized lifestyle are producing new epidemics of the complications of atherosclerosis in developing nations. Prevention strategies are aimed at lifestyle modification for whole populations, to which are added lipid-lowering therapies for high-risk individuals with hyperlipidaemia, low blood HDL levels, hypertension, and diabetes.

## The Coronary Arteries and Ischaemic Heart Disease

Most ischaemic heart disease is associated with coronary artery atherosclerosis, which limits myocardial blood supply. For a given degree of coronary stenosis, the consequences for the myocardium are related to myocardial demand, which may be increased by factors such as ventricular hypertrophy. A global reduction in coronary artery perfusion, e.g. as a result of hypovolaemic shock, may also lead to myocardial ischaemia.

An understanding of how coronary artery atherosclerosis produces clinical disease must be based on knowledge of the anatomy, histological structure, and physiology of the coronary arteries themselves. There are two major coronary arteries, left and right, which form separate arterial systems, unless there is gradual narrowing, when collateral vessels develop between them. The epicardial surface coronary arteries have a well-developed medial coat containing very few elastic and numerous smooth muscle cells. Medial tone can therefore vary and significantly alter lumen calibre. The blood flow to the myocardium is unique in that it does not occur in systole when the left ventricle is contracting. The epicardial arteries fill in systole but flow into the myocardium occurs in diastole. As the ventricular myocardium relaxes, blood is sucked in from the epicardial arteries and aortic root above the closed aortic valve.

### Stable Angina

This is the pain that occurs on exertion when the blood supply to the myocardium is inadequate, usually due to severe significant narrowing of the coronary arteries. There is a reduction in cross-sectional area by ≥70% such that the luminal diameter is <1 mm in the epicardial vessels. This usually occurs in its proximal course over a distance of 30-40 mm, but it may be diffuse especially in people with diabetes (Fig. 6.41).

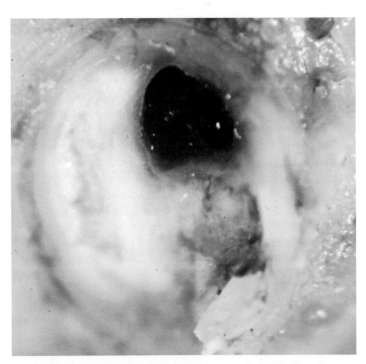

**FIG. 6.41** Cross-sectional area of a coronary artery in which there is a significant atherosclerotic plaque with a yellow lipid core. There is significant narrowing of the vessel lumen.

There is considerable diversity in the plaques causing high-grade stenosis. Some are relatively simple type Va plaques (see p. 118) with a lipid core and a cap, where the plaques have caused stenosis by primary atherogenesis, i.e. lipid and collagen formation. The size of the plaque core relative to overall size is very variable. Many plaques are eccentric, leaving an arc of normal media on the opposite side of the vessel wall. Plaques may form opposite each other and involve the whole circumference of the intima. Some plaques may be heavily calcified (type Vb) or totally solid and fibrous (type Vc). High-grade stenoses are often very complex, with multilayered plaques, some with more than one core (multilayered type Va). Replacement of the lumen by several smaller channels indicates recanalization of an occluding thrombus. Such arterial segments may or may not be related to healed infarcts.

### Unstable Angina

Unstable angina is clinically characterized by transient episodic myocardial ischaemia, manifesting as pain and ECG changes (ST-segment depression) at rest. Elevation in cardiac troponins is also important for diagnosis. Angiographic studies show that there is a culprit coronary artery lesion characterized by a stenosis with ragged outlines and overhanging edges, indicating a disrupted plaque. Microemboli of platelets into the distal vascular bed are responsible for episodic chest pain, and also cause small microscopic foci of necrosis. The thrombotic process in the artery ultimately resolves or progresses to occlude the artery completely.

## Acute Myocardial Infarction

Myocardial infarction is defined as death of myocardial tissue caused by ischaemia, which is a reduction or cessation of blood flow to myocytes, to a degree that oxygen delivery is not adequate to meet the metabolic demands of the cells. Ischaemia is initially reversible. Patients with stable angina on exercise have ischaemia that is reversed on rest when oxygen demand falls. Persistent ischaemia is usually due to more severe reduction or cessation of blood flow, and leads to structural changes and then death of the myocytes.

The blood supply of the human myocardium is regional in that each branch of the epicardial coronary arteries supplies a specific segment of myocardium from the endocardial to the epicardial surface. In the normal heart there is no functional overlap between adjacent arteries. In animal models, the only way to produce a regional infarct is to occlude a coronary artery for at least 6 hours. The same principles apply to human pathology and the presence of regional infarction means that flow had ceased for at least some hours in the subtending artery. The great majority (at least 99%) of infarcts are caused by thrombosis over an atherosclerotic plaque. Rare causes include spontaneous dissection and emboli. If there is no visible cause, coronary artery spasm should be considered but this is a diagnosis made by exclusion. Coronary spasm occurs particularly with drug

use such as cocaine, and this is the most frequent cause of myocardial infarction in young people. Provided that heavy calcification is absent, cross-sections of the coronary arteries made at 2- to 3-mm intervals will reveal thrombi often admixed with extruded lipid.

### Regional Myocardial Infarction

The term 'infarction' is used for a number of entities that have very different pathophysiology. The most common form of infarction recognized clinically and pathologically is an area of regional necrosis that is anterior, lateral, or posteroseptal in the left ventricle (Fig. 6.42), and clearly lies in the territory supplied by one major epicardial coron-

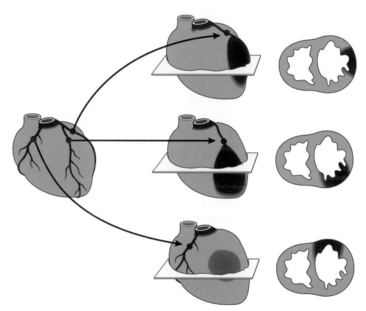

**FIG. 6.42** Diagram of the different types of myocardial infarct including lateral (top), anteroseptal (middle), and posteroseptal (bottom) infarcts.

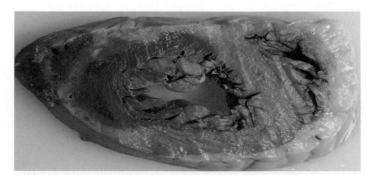

**FIG. 6.43** Transverse section of the left and right ventricles showing a haemorrhagic infarct in the anterolateral wall, with an overlying haemorrhagic pericardial reaction. The infarct is haemorrhagic because of reperfusion due to angioplasty, with stent insertion in the blocked left anterior descending coronary artery.

ary artery (Fig. 6.43). Regional infarction may be transmural or confined to the subendocardial zone. The non-transmural form of regional infarction is now common and characteristically formed by the coalescence of smaller areas of necrosis of different ages. Human myocardial infarction is complex in that the exact time of onset of the occlusion is not known, because occlusion often has a stuttering and intermittent onset, and collateral flow may or may not have been previously present. Even within the area of infarction, islands of surviving myocytes can be found. A very complex histological picture is produced in which different fields show different stages of necrosis. Survival of interstitial cells within the infarct zone allows very rapid fibroblastic responses with deposition of collagen.

More diffuse ischaemic myocardial necrosis unrelated to the area supplied by one coronary artery also occurs. The best-recognized form is circumferential subendocardial necrosis due to an overall failure of myocardial perfusion (Fig. 6.44). There are many causes including shock, prolonged hypotension, prolonged hypoxia, and use of high doses of inotropic drugs. The condition is always more likely to occur in ventricles with hypertrophy, and may be seen after prolonged cardiac bypass for aortic valve stenosis.

The process of replacing dead myocytes by a collagenous scar may take up to 8 weeks and fibrosis then continues for a further 3–6 months. The area of infarction has to be organized from the margins where there are viable interstitial cells. The process may never be completed and it is possible for so-called 'mummified' myocytes without nuclei to exist within a thick fibrous capsule for many months. The published data on dating of infarcts belong to an era when many human infarcts were single regional areas with a uniform age. There is development of myocyte necrosis with swollen eosinophilic myocytes (coagulative type necrosis) after 8–12 hours, infiltration by neutrophils (Fig. 6.45) after 24–48 hours, followed by granulation tissue formation (Fig. 6.46)

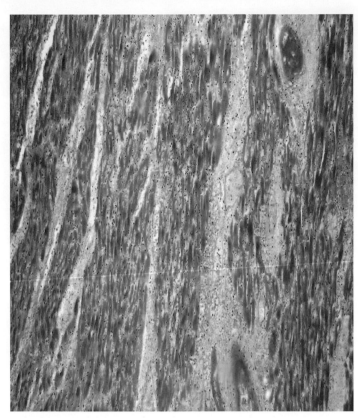

FIG. 6.45 An area of acute infarction that is 24–48 hours old. Note the swollen eosinophilic dead myocytes surrounded by acute inflammatory cells with oedema.

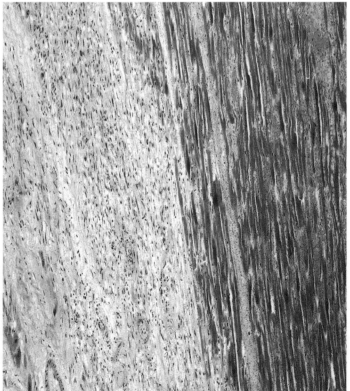

FIG. 6.46 There is an acute, 24- to 48-hour-old, infarct on the right, with healing granulation tissue on the left, indicating an adjacent area of infarction approximately 3–5 days old.

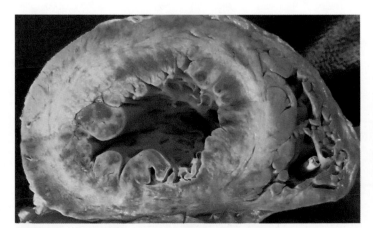

FIG. 6.44 Transverse section of the right and left ventricle showing dark discoloration of the subendocardium, due to subendocardial infarction resulting from poor perfusion of the heart postoperatively.

in 3–5 days, and finally fibrosis (Fig. 6.47). Today, most infarcts have been built up by the coalescence of foci of necrosis occurring over a period of time. All that can be done is to age the oldest foci, working on the basis that collagen deposition begins at 5–6 days. However, the foci of necrosis do not necessarily undergo histological changes at the same rate, e.g. in foci where the connective tissue stroma survives but the myocytes alone die, collagen deposition may begin within 2–3 days. Thrombi and fatty debris from ulcerated plaques can also embolize into the intramural vessels causing microinfarcts.

Myocytes that are irreversibly damaged but not yet totally dead develop a rather different pattern of histological change if the area of necrosis is reperfused: often due to interventions with angioplasty and insertion of metallic stents to open up the occluded vessel. This occurs very early after the onset of cell death, provided that reperfusion has occurred. The phenomenon is due to restoration of calcium ions to the interstitial tissues; calcium then enters the dying myocyte and invokes intense hypercontraction of the myofibrils. The myofibrils undergo intense hypercontraction and shunt together leading to the appearance of brightly eosinophilic cross-banding within the myocytes, so- called contraction band necrosis (Fig. 6.48), When present, the histological change is striking and appears by 30 minutes, long before other structural criteria of necrosis. There may also be extensive leakage of red blood cells from capillaries.

Some contraction bands will be found in any heart that has gone into ventricular fibrillation (VF) before death. If, however, they are present in large numbers, and in particular if they are found in one region only, they are a reliable means of identifying early infarction. Even when reperfusion had not occurred, some contraction band necrosis is usually found at the edge of an infarct that predominantly shows the colliquative pattern of necrosis. Contraction band necrosis has also been called coagulative myocytolysis.

### The Effect of Interventions on Myocardial Infarction

Hospital mortality for acute myocardial infarction has declined dramatically in the last 30 years, thanks to coronary care units and early revascularization with thrombolysis, angioplasty, and stent implantation. Long-term mortality after myocardial infarction is mostly due to sudden electrical death, which may be prevented by pharmacological (antiarrhythmic drugs) and non-pharmacological (implantable cardioverter defibrillator, pacemaker) therapy. Ventricular assist devices may support the left ventricle as a bridge to transplantation in end-stage ischaemic cardiomyopathy.

When the role of plaque rupture with thrombosis was firmly established as the cause of myocardial infarction, these studies led to the use of thrombolysis to break up the clot. Timely reperfusion of the myocardium by thrombolysis became the most effective means of restoring myocardial viability in the 1970s and 1980s. Percutaneous transluminal coronary angioplasty (PTCA), in which a balloon is used to expand the arterial wall, push the plaque aside, and remove blood clot, was shown in the 1990s to be

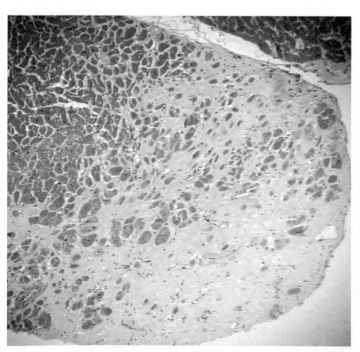

**FIG. 6.47** A healed infarct >6 months old, in which there are scattered myocytes that vary in size, mixed with pale areas of fibrosis.

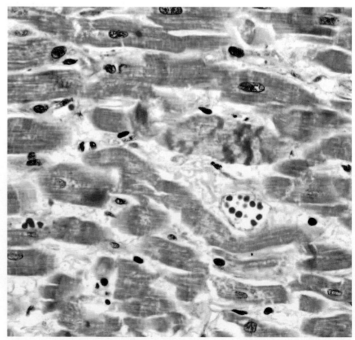

**FIG. 6.48** Myocyte with contraction band necrosis. Note the irregular eosinophilic bands within the myocyte in the centre.

superior treatment for acute infarction because the risk of reocclusion was almost two to four times higher for patients receiving thrombolysis alone than for patients receiving primary PTCA. It is also used for coronary artery bypass vein grafts, which are prone to narrowing due to intimal hyperplasia and lipid deposition. Dissection, bleeding, and thrombotic complications can, however, occur. Newer anticoagulants and antiplatelet agents reduce the bleeding risk.

If reperfusion occurs before the onset of irreversible injury of myocytes, then all myocytes survive. In contrast, if reperfusion occurs after irreversible injury, then myocytes that are already necrotic are lost but myocytes that are reversibly injured may be salvaged, particularly at the edge of established infarcts, thus reducing the size of the infarct. However, despite salvage, the process of reperfusion may damage some myocytes that were not already dead when reflow occurred. This is termed 'reperfusion injury', which is mediated by toxic oxygen species that are over-produced on restoration of the oxygen supply. Reperfused infarcts are haemorrhagic and, if large, may result in terminal arrhythmia, rupture, and sudden death. Although, most often, myocardium that is viable at the time of reflow ultimately recovers, critical abnormalities in biochemistry and function may persist for several days as prolonged post-ischaemic ventricular dysfunction, known as 'stunned' myocardium. Decreased intercellular calcium or decreased calcium sensitivity of the contractile process is the most likely explanation. Preservation of the myocyte fraction is an important determinant of functional recovery after revascularization. A higher myocyte fraction is required to maintain contractile function after a period of hibernation of the myocardium.

Unfortunately, the early use of balloon angioplasty led to thrombosis and rapid restenosis of the coronary artery due to intimal healing with smooth muscle cell hyperplasia. The application of a metallic stent to keep the coronary artery open improved the long-term patency of the vessels. The complication of stent thrombosis was overcome with the introduction of effective anti-platelet therapy. The introduction of drug-eluting stents, which slow smooth muscle growth, helped to reduce restenosis. Primary angioplasty with stent insertion is now the treatment of choice for patients with acute myocardial infarction. Late stent thrombosis can occur and histopathological data implicate a contributory allergic or hypersensitivity component.

## Complications of Regional Myocardial Infarction

### Arrhythmias

Ventricular tachycardia (VT) degenerating into ventricular fibrillation (VF) is the cause of sudden death in the first 24 hours of myocardial infarction, and is responsible for sudden deaths before the patient reaches hospital. The risk of VF is not directly related to infarct size and is present even with small infarcts.

### Cardiogenic Shock

Cardiogenic shock (see also p. 108) is responsible for most deaths in patients and is a complication directly related to infarct size. Infarcts that involve more than 40–50% of the total left ventricular mass usually lead to cardiac failure or shock. Most such large infarcts are due to proximal thrombotic occlusions of the left anterior descending coronary artery. Rupture of a mitral valve cusp or cardiac tamponade due to transmural rupture with haemopericardium can also lead to cardiogenic shock. There is a fall in blood pressure and reduced tissue perfusion. All organs are affected by shock. Acute tubular necrosis occurs in the kidney, and boundary zone infarction in the brain. Superimposed subendocardial circumferential necrosis often develops, leading to a downward spiral of more necrosis – further decline in left ventricle function – further myocardial hypoperfusion, and further necrosis.

### Infarct Expansion

Infarct expansion is a stretching and thinning of the necrotic region, producing an outward bulge. No further necrosis is involved and the process is distinct from infarct extension. Infarct expansion is a complication that develops during the first week in large transmural infarcts. As it is directly related to infarct size, it is most common in anteroseptal infarcts. Expansion is important because it is a prelude to cardiac rupture and may lead, in extreme form, to left ventricular aneurysms. Expansion is also important because, when fibrous repair occurs, the shape of the expanded acute infarct is retained. The left ventricle is left with a permanent enlargement of the cavity (cardiac aneurysm) with a detrimental effect on function.

### Cardiac Rupture

Cardiac rupture leading to tamponade falls into two groups. Rupture may occur within 24 hours of the onset of necrosis. Externally there is a slit-like tear in the left ventricle. On cross-sections it is often difficult to identify the infarcted area due to its early state of development. The tear appears to be at the junction of viable and non-viable tissue, and is presumably due to shear stresses between the non-contractile muscle and contracting viable muscle. Left ventricular rupture more rarely occurs later (5–7 days) and is a complication of expanding infarcts (Fig. 6.49). The hole in the left ventricle is at the apex of a distinct bulge and there is often overlying acute pericarditis. Cardiac rupture is more common in elderly females than males. It is also reported that rupture is more likely to result with reperfusion of infarcts after angioplasty and stent insertion.

### Ischaemic Left Ventricular Aneurysms

The most common form of ventricular aneurysm is the end-result of infarct expansion and produces an aneurysmal sac with a relatively wide neck. The wall is fibrous and contains no residual myocardium. The endocardium is white, and this white thickening often extends out from the sac itself over the rim into adjacent myocardium. The sac may or may not contain laminated thrombus (Fig. 6.50). Calcification of the deepest layers of thrombus is common. A much rarer type of aneurysm has a very narrow neck, leading to a large external sac. This type is thought to arise from a partial tear of the infarct in the acute stage, after which a subpericardial haematoma is contained by fibrosis developing in the pericardium. These aneurysms are sometimes called 'pseudoaneurysms' due to the wall being predominantly formed from the pericardium. In fact there is a complete spectrum and histology shows some residual myocardial tissue in the wall of virtually all left ventricular aneurysms. All these aneurysms carry a risk of rupture, and systemic emboli, and cause abnormal left ventricular function. A striking feature of left ventricular aneurysms is also a marked tendency to episodic ventricular tachycardia. These tachycardias arise in anastomosing strands and islands of surviving myocytes embedded in the endocardial thickening that occurs on the rim of the aneurysmal sac.

### Ventricular Septal Defect

This usually arises from expansion of either an anteroseptal or a posteroseptal infarct. In the acute stage the tear has a ragged edge and, in the rare patient who survives, this ultimately becomes a smooth-edged defect. The mortality rate in the acute stage is high and surgical repair is high risk. Percutaneous devices to close these defects have been applied but mortality is still high due to their association with large infarcts.

### Papillary Muscle Rupture

The majority of the complications listed so far are directly related to transmural large infarcts. Papillary muscle rupture (see Case History 6.1) is an exception in that the infarcts can be small and may not be transmural. Either papillary muscle can rupture. The anterolateral papillary muscle is supplied by the left marginal branch of the left circumflex artery, and there is a distinct entity of left marginal artery thrombosis producing papillary rupture without significant infarction of the rest of the left ventricle. The posteromedial muscle is supplied from the right coronary artery. Rupture may involve either one subhead or the whole papillary muscle across the base. The stump of the ruptured papillary muscle passes back and forward across the mitral valve in life and the chordae become twisted and tangled. The stump is found in the left atrium *post mortem*.

### Heart Failure

Ischaemic heart disease is the most common cause of heart failure (see pp. 133–143).

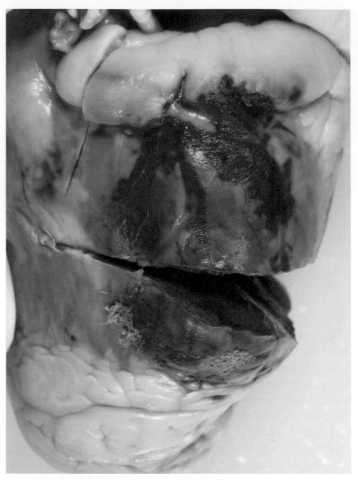

FIG. 6.49 The epicardial surface of the heart with an area of rupture resulting in haemorrhage and haemopericardium.

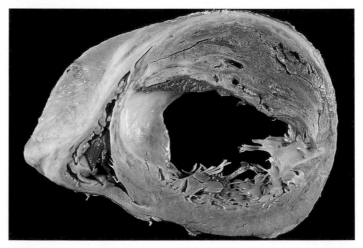

FIG. 6.50 A heart with a previous myocardial infarct that has stretched to form an aneurysm, which contains mural thrombus.

## MYOCARDITIS

Myocarditis is an inflammatory disease of the heart that frequently results from viral infections and/or post-viral

A 53-year-old woman developed crushing chest pain radiating into her neck. This was associated with shortness of breath. She was admitted to hospital and an ECG suggested acute myocardial infarction. She was given opioids for pain, aspirin, and a β blocker, then thrombolysis was achieved by intravenous streptokinase. Her condition stabilized, and over the next few days serial plasma enzyme studies confirmed that she had had a myocardial infarction. On day 5 she developed sudden breathlessness with associated tachypnoea. Auscultation revealed crepitations and a loud pansystolic murmur. The chest radiograph (Fig. 6.51) showed fine streaky mottling in the lung fields. This was diagnosed as acute pulmonary oedema due to left ventricular failure. In spite of prompt treatment with morphine, aminophylline, and diuretics, her condition deteriorated rapidly and she died just after emergency echocardiography was carried out. Fig. 6.52 shows the interior of her left ventricle *post mortem*, and demonstrates complete rupture and avulsion of the head of a papillary muscle.

In summary, this woman had a myocardial infarction. In spite of appropriate treatment she then developed rapidly fatal acute left ventricular failure due to sudden mitral valve incompetence. This was caused by papillary muscle rupture. There are three sites of cardiac rupture after a myocardial infarction: free wall rupture, which causes cardiac tamponade; septal rupture, which causes an acquired ventricular septal defect that can be surgically patched; and papillary muscle rupture. Avulsion of the head of a papillary muscle causes acute left ventricular failure due to sudden mitral incompetence from leakage via the unsupported part of the cusp. Rupture of the body of a papillary muscle causes cardiogenic shock because an unsupported whole mitral cusp abolishes mitral valve function.

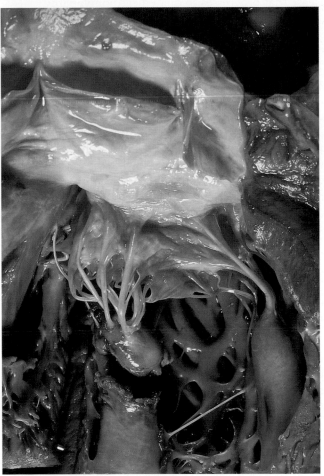

FIG. 6.52 The interior of the left ventricle showing the aortic valve at the top and the posterior surface of the anterior mitral valve leaflet. The head of the infarcted papillary muscle has been ruptured and avulsion of the attached chordae tendineae caused mitral incompetence.

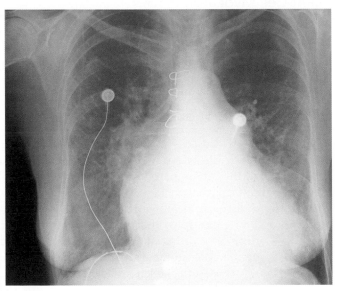

FIG. 6.51 A chest radiograph showing enlargement of the heart cause by heart failure. There are streaky opacities in both lung fields due to pulmonary oedema resulting from left ventricular failure. ECG leads are also visible.

immune-mediated responses. Myocarditis was defined by the World Health Organization (WHO)/International Society and Federation of Cardiology (ISFC) as an inflammatory disease of the heart muscle, diagnosed by established histological, immunological, and immunohistochemical criteria. Most often, myocarditis results from common viral infections. It is an underdiagnosed cause of acute heart failure, sudden death, and chronic dilated cardiomyopathy.

In developed countries, myocarditis is commonly caused by viral infections but, in the developing world, rheumatic carditis, *Trypanosoma cruzi* infection, and bacterial infections such as diphtheria still contribute to the global disease burden. The short-term prognosis of acute myocarditis is usually good, but varies widely by cause. Those patients who initially recover may develop recurrent dilated cardiomyopathy and heart failure, sometimes years later.

## Microscopic Findings

The gold standard in diagnosis of myocarditis is endo-myocardial biopsy. According to the Dallas criteria, acute myocarditis is defined by lymphocytic infiltrates in association with myocyte necrosis (Fig. 6.53). Lymphocytic myocarditis is presumed mainly to be caused by viral infection. The clinical course of patients with lymphocytic myocarditis varies; some patients have a subclinical disease, some present with fulminant disease, and others have indolent disease that progresses to dilated cardiomyopathy.

## Causative Agents

Coxsackievirus B was linked to myocarditis from the 1950s to the 1990s. The spectrum of viruses detected in endomyocardial biopsy samples shifted from Coxsackievirus B to adenovirus in the late 1990s and, in the past 5 years, to parvovirus B19 and hepatitis C. Cytomegalovirus (CMV) is considered to be an uncommon cause of myocarditis in previously healthy people. It is usually seen in transplant recipients, with multiorgan involvement. In addition to viruses, other infectious causes of myocarditis include *Borrelia burgdorferi* (Lyme disease). Lyme myocarditis should be suspected in patients with a history of travel to regions where the disease is endemic or of a tick bite, particularly if they also have atrioventricular conduction abnormalities. In areas of rural Central and South America, *Trypanosoma cruzi* infection can present as acute myocarditis or chronic cardiomyopathy with apical aneurysm formation. Toxoplasmosis may become reactivated in antibody-positive transplant recipients. After the introduction of pyrimethamine prophylaxis, this complication has decreased substantially. Acute toxoplasma myocarditis in immunocompetent individuals is very rare outside infancy. Myocarditis is quite frequent in AIDS patients: multiple opportunistic infections including

Coxsackieviruses and *Toxoplasma gondii* may occur. Fungal myocarditis frequently occurs in the setting of disseminated disease. The major fungal pathogen responsible for myocardial infection is *Aspergillus fumigatus*. The incidence of invasive fungal disease has dramatically increased over the past few decades, corresponding to the increasing number of immunocompromised patients.

Bacterial myocarditis is usually seen in the context of overwhelming sepsis and the potential pathogens are many: streptococci, staphylococci, pneumococci, gonococci, and mycobacteria, among others. It may also occur with salmonellosis and shigellosis.

## Eosinophilic Myocarditis

In this entity, there is a predominantly eosinophilic infiltrate of the myocardium with or without abscess formation. It may occur in association with systemic diseases, such as the hypereosinophilic syndrome, the Churg–Strauss syndrome, Löffler's endomyocardial fibrosis, cancer, drugs, and parasitic, helmintic, or protozoal infections.

## Giant Cell Myocarditis

This is a rapidly fatal disease confined to the heart, with giant cells infiltrating the myocardium. It is not linked to sarcoid or tuberculosis, but rather to autoimmune conditions and thymomas.

## Myocarditis and Sudden Death

Myocarditis is a rare disease in adults and an even rarer cause of sudden adult death. When there is no other cause of sudden death, and the inflammatory infiltrate is heavy and diffuse throughout the ventricular myocardium and associated with myocyte damage, it is justifiable to ascribe death to myocarditis. Most cases are due to lymphocytic myocarditis. Myocarditis is more common as a cause of sudden death in children. In one study of sudden death, myocarditis occurred in 5% of cases: this was mainly lymphocytic in type and occurred in young adults.

# VALVULAR HEART DISEASE

Valvular heart disease may be congenital or acquired. In developing countries, rheumatic valve disease remains the major cause of valve disease. In developed countries with an ageing population, degenerate calcification of the aortic valve and degenerate myxoid change in the mitral valve predominate.

Normal valve function depends not only on integrity of the structural components of the valve (the cusps and, where relevant, the chordae tendineae and papillary muscles) but also on the valve annulus and the function of the ventricles.

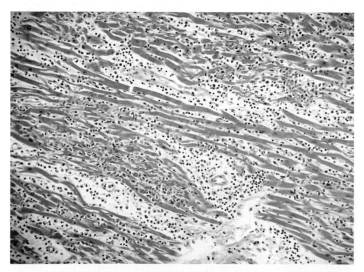

**Fig. 6.53** There is a dense lymphocytic infiltrate around myocytes with extensive myocyte necrosis – lymphocytic myocarditis.

# Rheumatic Valve Disease

### Key Points

- Chronic rheumatic valve disease is associated with valve cusp commissural fusion, cusp fibrosis, and cusp calcification.
- There is valve stenosis and/or incompetence.
- The mitral and aortic valves are most commonly involved.

Rheumatic fever is an acute multisystem disease in which there is an immune reaction 1–2 weeks after a streptococcal pharyngitis. It affects mainly the joints, subcutaneous tissue, and heart. In the heart there is a pancarditis with involvement of all layers, but it is the long-term consequences in the cardiac valves that are pathologically and functionally significant. In the myocardium, there is formation of small giant cell granulomas with fibrinoid necrosis in the interstitium, so-called Aschoff's bodies. The valvulitis of the acute phase is neither functionally important nor macroscopically striking. Microscopically, the cusp is inflamed with a mixture of acute and chronic inflammatory cells, and blood vessels begin to extend into the cusp from the base by 6–8 weeks after the acute phase. The cusps are also often retracted, i.e. reduced in area. The synthesis of collagen within the valve appears to continue over long periods and the characteristic pathology of chronic rheumatic valve disease is therefore to produce any combination of stenosis due to commissural fusion and/or incompetence due to cusp retraction in mainly the mitral and aortic valves.

The long latent period between acute rheumatic fever and chronic rheumatic valve disease implies that a low-grade stimulus to collagen production must be continuing. One view is that repeated subclinical attacks of streptococcal infection occur; another is that, once a valve has been damaged, abnormal mechanical force will operate to continue the fibrotic process. It is also recognized that some other diseases will produce a valvulitis that has very similar valve pathology, an example being SLE. Many patients with what is regarded as chronic rheumatic valve disease on morphological grounds do not give a history of acute rheumatic fever in childhood. This absence of a previous history is particularly a feature of rheumatic valve disease in older individuals in developed countries. These considerations have led to a view that chronic rheumatic type valves with no Aschoff's bodies in an atrial appendage, and no history of acute rheumatic fever, should be designated as post-inflammatory valvulitis. The incidence of rheumatic fever has fallen dramatically in developed countries, mainly due to improvement in living conditions, but it is still common in the Middle East, Africa, India, and South America.

# Aortic Valve Disease (Box 6.2)

## Aortic Stenosis

### Key Points

- The main causes of aortic stenosis are idiopathic calcific aortic stenosis and rheumatic valve disease.
- There is concentric left ventricular hypertrophy.
- Inadequate coronary perfusion causes syncope and angina.
- There is a significant risk of sudden cardiac death.
- Left ventricular failure eventually develops.

---

**Box 6.2** AORTIC VALVE DISEASE

**Causes of isolated aortic valve stenosis**

*Common*
Bicuspid calcific aortic stenosis
Degenerate aortic valve calcification
Chronic rheumatic disease

*Rare*
Congenital aortic valve stenosis
Collagen vascular disease, rheumatoid arthritis (RA), systemic lupus erythematosus (SLE)
Storage diseases

**Causes of isolated aortic incompetence**

*Common*
Idiopathic aortic root dilatation (non-inflammatory)
Chronic rheumatic valve disease
Aortitis (all types)
Post-bacterial endocarditis
Bicuspid aortic valves

*Rare*
Collagen/elastin disorders, Marfan's syndrome, Ehlers–Danlos syndrome, osteogenesis imperfecta, SLE, RA

**Mechanisms of aortic incompetence**

| *Cusp disease* | |
| --- | --- |
| Perforated | Bacterial endocarditis |
| Retracted | Chronic rheumatic, collagen vascular disease, RA, SLE |
| Notched | Bicuspid valve |
| *Root enlarged/distorted* | |
| Aortitis | Syphilis, ankylosing spondylitis, RA, SLE |
| Aortopathy | Idiopathic Marfan's syndrome |
| *Lack of cusp support* | |
| Above | Dissection of aorta |
| Below | Ventricular septal defect |

The main cause of aortic stenosis (narrowing), with reduction in blood flow, is degenerate nodular calcification of the aortic valve leaflets (Fig. 6.54). It is usually seen in elderly patients aged >70 and results from degenerate change in the fibrous layer of the leaflet causing dystrophic calcification and stiffening of each leaflet on its aortic side. In those aged <60, nodular calcification usually occurs on a bicuspid valve, which occurs in 1% of the population so it is the second most frequent cause of aortic stenosis. Chronic rheumatic valve disease is least common: this is associated with commissural (space between the leaflets) fusion and cusp thickening with calcification, with only a triangular slit-like opening remaining (Fig. 6.55). Rheumatic aortic valve stenosis is frequently accompanied by mitral stenosis.

## Aortic Incompetence

> ### Key Points
>
> - The main causes of aortic incompetence include: post-rheumatic, calcific aortic stenosis, dilatation of aortic sleeve, and infective endocarditis (see *Box 6.1*).
> - It leads to a collapsing pulse and left ventricular failure with dilatation.
> - There is angina due to inadequate coronary perfusion.
> - Left ventricular failure eventually develops.

Aortic incompetence/regurgitation with leakage has many more causes than aortic stenosis because of the involvement of the aortic root as well as the leaflets. Most cases are due to dilatation of the aortic root, which occurs in an older age group but can be due to aortitis (Fig. 6.56), bacterial endocarditis, rheumatic valve disease, or bicuspid valve. Rarer causes include collagen vascular disease.

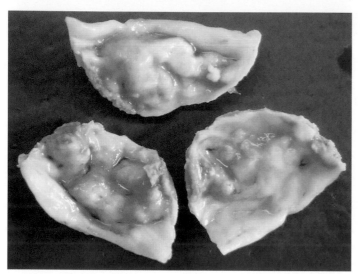

**FIG. 6.54** The three semilunar aortic leaflets in calcific aortic stenosis. Note the nodular calcification in the body of each leaflet.

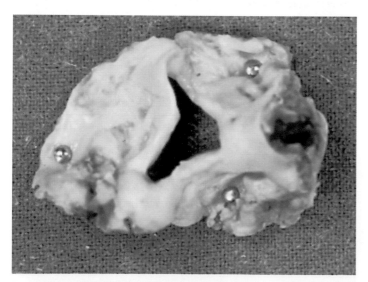

**FIG. 6.55** Aortic valve with commissural fusion and calcification particularly at the commissures, leaving a narrow triangular opening. This is typical of rheumatic aortic stenosis.

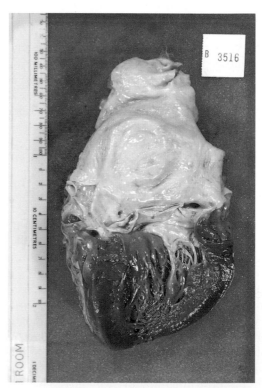

**FIG. 6.56** Syphilitic aortitis causing thickening and stretching of the aortic root and aortic incompetence.

# Mitral Valve Disease (*Box 6.3*)

**Box 6.3** MITRAL VALVE DISEASE

**Causes of mitral valve stenosis**
*Common*
Chronic rheumatic valve disease
*Rare*
Congenital
Ring calcification
*Very rare*
Carcinoid syndrome
Rheumatoid arthritis (RA), systemic lupus erythematosus (SLE)
Amyloid
Storage disease
Radiation

**Main causes of mitral valve incompetence**

| | |
|---|---|
| *Functional* | Normal valve structure |
| Structural abnormality of cusps/chordae | Floppy valve, Marfan's syndrome |
| Papillary muscle disease | Ischaemic heart disease |
| | Dilated cardiomyopathy |

**Mechanisms of pure mitral incompetence**

| | |
|---|---|
| *Cusps* | |
| Perforated | Bacterial endocarditis |
| Retracted | Chronic rheumatic disease, SLE, RA |
| Expanded | Floppy valve |
| *Chordae tendineae* | |
| Short | Chronic rheumatic disease |
| Long/broken | Floppy valve |
| *Papillary muscle* | |
| Ruptured | Ischaemic heart disease |
| Fibrosed | Ischaemic heart disease, cardiomyopathy |
| *Atrioventricular ring* | |
| Ring dilated | Marfan's syndrome |
| Ring rigid | Mitral ring calcification |
| *Left ventricle* | |
| Ventricle dilated | Functional mitral incompetence |

## Mitral Stenosis

### Key Points

- Mitral stenosis is almost always due to rheumatic fever.
- There is atrial dilatation, atrial fibrillation, and atrial thrombosis.
- It leads to pulmonary venous hypertension and oedema.
- Pulmonary arterial hypertension causes right ventricular hypertrophy and failure.

The aetiology of mitral stenosis is virtually limited to chronic rheumatic type disease. There are other causes of mitral stenosis but these are very rare (see *Box 6.3*)

### Rheumatic Mitral Valve Disease

In the simplest form of rheumatic mitral valve disease, there is a fibrous diaphragm with a central oval aperture due to fusion of both commissures. In these cases, a simple valvotomy with splitting of the commissures can be a highly successful treatment, without recourse to cardiac bypass and valve replacement. Such cases occur in younger individuals and are far more common in geographical areas where rheumatic fever is still endemic such as Egypt and India. In areas where rheumatic fever has declined, symptomatic patients with mitral stenosis are older and there is usually advanced cusp calcification. Diffuse thickening of each leaflet is seen with calcified deposits particularly at the edges of the leaflets and at both commissures (Fig. 6.57). In some cases, cusp calcification and fibrosis cause stenosis in the absence of commissural fusion. Calcific masses often ulcerate onto the atrial surface of the cusp. Below the level of the cusps, the chordae tendineae are also thickened, shortened, and fused, giving an element of subvalvar stenosis (Fig. 6.58). Such valves have to be replaced with a prosthesis to relieve obstruction and this requires cardiac bypass.

In countries such as the UK, most cases of mitral stenosis occur in patients aged >50 years. Often there is no history of rheumatic fever, which may indicate that the history is unreliable after such a time lapse, or the acute phase was subclinical, or that there are other causes of an acute valvulitis leading to chronic stenosis. Atrial appendages removed during mitral valve surgery, when examined histologically, may contain Aschoff's bodies in the absence of any sign of acute rheumatic activity, suggesting that Aschoff's bodies are long-lived granulomas that persist long after acute rheumatic fever has resolved.

There is often a dilated left atrium in association with mitral stenosis and thrombus may be present, but this can be variable. The dilatation may be related to the myocarditis found in the acute phase, be a result of the stenosis combined with incompetence, or follow the onset of atrial fibrillation. Thrombus usually starts in the left atrial appendage, and can extend over the surface of the whole chamber and undergo calcification.

## Mitral Incompetence

### Key Points

- The causes of mitral incompetence include: post-rheumatic, infective endocarditis, floppy mitral valve, papillary muscle pathology, valve ring dilatation.
- It results in compensatory left ventricular hypertrophy.
- There is impaired left ventricular function and failure.

In contrast to stenosis, there are many causes of mitral incompetence (see *Box 6.3*). These can be approached by whether the abnormality lies in the cusps, chordae tendineae, papillary muscle, or annulus.

### The Floppy Mitral Valve and Cusp Prolapse

The advent of echocardiography allowed clinicians to gain a far deeper insight into valve function than was previously possible. It was realized that prolapse of part of a mitral cusp into the left atrium during ventricular systole was a very common phenomenon. Prolapse is a strange word for what is an upward movement, but it is the one used. Large-scale surveys of fit young individuals show that minor degrees of cusp prolapse without regurgitation are commonplace,

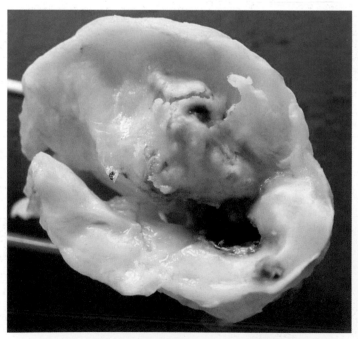

**FIG. 6.57** Classic rheumatic mitral stenosis: there is thickening and calcification at the edge of each leaflet, with commissural fusion of one leaflet. Note the slit-like opening.

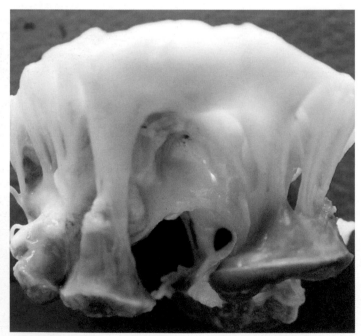

**FIG. 6.58** The mitral valve leaflets, chordae tendineae and papillary muscles in classic rheumatic mitral stenosis. There is diffuse thickening of the valve leaflets with chordal thickening and fusion extending onto fibrous papillary muscles. This results in a funnel-shaped narrow opening.

and can be regarded as minor physiological anomalies. Individuals who develop mild late-systolic mitral regurgitation, however, have anatomical abnormalities of the valve. Most of these abnormalities involve expansion of the cusp area and elongation of the chordae tendineae, to which the name floppy/degenerate mitral valve has been given. In a proportion of patients with mitral cusp prolapse, regurgitation develops at the end of systole. The name floppy valve was given to the condition by surgeons who were replacing mitral valves for what was initially diagnosed as a rheumatic valve. It was recognized at surgery that the cusps were large and voluminous and soft to feel, quite unlike the typical retracted hard cusps of rheumatic disease.

The striking macroscopic feature of the floppy mitral valve is expansion of the cusps, which adopt a dome shape. Viewed from the left atrium *post mortem* one or both cusps bulge up into the atria (Fig. 6.59). The cusp involvement may be very local and occur in one or more segments of the anterior or posterior cusp, or involve both cusps. Along with the cusp expansion the chordae tendineae elongate. The soft rather gelatinous feel of the cusps is characteristic. By the time patients with floppy valves come to surgical replacement or are seen *post mortem* many of the cases show advanced surface fibrosis over the cusps, making them thick and white. This is probably the reason why the condition was not clearly distinguished from chronic rheumatic disease in the past. The cusp area expansion and the soft feel, however, remain distinguishing features even in late cases. The surface fibrosis is a result of thickening of the superficial layer of the cusp, due to mechanical trauma as the hypermobile cusp hits the ventricular wall and the other cusp (Fig. 6.60).

Histologically, the floppy valve shows replacement of the solid fibrous layer of the leaflet with loosely arranged myxomatous tissue. These myxoid areas are cellular with many spindle-shaped fibroblastic cells. Collagen and elastin fibrils are fragmented with a high content of acid mucopolysaccharide. The surface of the cusp is often covered by a well-organized new layer of fibrous tissue containing elastic laminae. Floppy mitral valves are common. Their frequency appears to rise steadily with age. They are becoming the most common cause of isolated mitral incompetence in patients undergoing valve replacement/repair in populations in the developed world, where chronic rheumatic disease has declined. The pathogenesis of the floppy mitral valve is contentious. There is no doubt that floppy valves are a complication of all the genetic disorders of connective tissue synthesis including Marfan's syndrome, osteogenesis imperfecta, and Ehlers–Danlos syndrome. There is also increasing recognition that partial phenotypic expressions of these genetic diseases occur. A familial trend is well recognized in floppy valves without any other systemic abnormality. Floppy valves are, however, so common that genetic abnormalities can explain only a proportion of cases. Other theories include an age-related wear-and-tear phenomenon acting on a valve that was congenitally abnormal, perhaps lacking chordal support to certain parts of the cusp.

Chordal rupture in floppy mitral valves is due to excessive mechanical stress operating on the thinned and elongated chordae; a proportion of cases also develop mitral ring dilatation. This is particularly true of floppy valves associated with gene disorders of connective tissue such as Marfan's

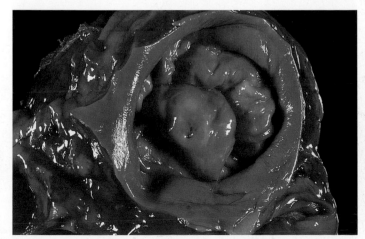

FIG. 6.59 A floppy mitral valve viewed through the atrium, showing soft, thickened, and stretched cusps bulging into the atrium.

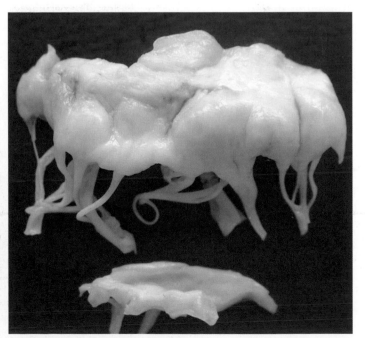

FIG. 6.60 Two mitral valve leaflets from a floppy mitral valve. Note the doming between the chordal attachment and the diffuse thickening of the leaflet with overlying fibrous thickening. Note also the elongation and thinning of the chordae.

syndrome. Bacterial endocarditis is a risk in any floppy valve that has even mild regurgitation. A rare complication is fusion of the chordae onto the posterior wall of the left ventricle. The hypermobile chordae hit the endocardium to produce vertical lines of endocardial fibrosis, which occasionally fuse with the chordae to produce a fibrous mass; this now restricts upward movement of the cusp and alters the mechanism of regurgitation. The most contentious and least understood risk is that of sudden death.

Surgical repair is the procedure of choice to preserve function of the valve apparatus, which is essential for ventricular function. The aim is to excise the most dome-shaped portion of the cusp and then stitch the rest of the cusp together, thus reducing its area and ability to prolapse.

## Tricuspid and Pulmonary Valve Disease

Rheumatic tricuspid valve disease occurs with concomitant aortic and mitral valve disease. Tricuspid stenosis is due to commissural fusion and calcification and marked fibrous thickening of the cusps but is very rare. The most common form of tricuspid incompetence is due to dilatation of the annulus after right ventricular dilatation in right ventricular failure. The valve orifice is too large to be closed by the cusps, and the valve consequently becomes incompetent, leading to regurgitation. A congenital downward displacement of the tricuspid valve is known as Ebstein's anomaly and may lead to right heart failure.

Pulmonary atresia or stenosis is seen in the context of congenital stenosis as in tetralogy of Fallot when the valve cusps are often thickened and dysplastic.

## Prosthetic Heart Valves

Replacing abnormal heart valves began in the 1950s and there is now a large variety of prosthetic valves.

Valve prostheses can be divided into mechanical prostheses, made of plastic, Teflon, or metal, and tissue valves.

### Mechanical Valves

All have a ring covered by Teflon, which is sewn into the native valve annulus after the cusps have been removed. The leaflets are carbonated steel and may have an old-fashioned disc-shaped poppet in a cage, a tilting metal disc controlled by a spring, or two hinged metal leaflets. Metal prostheses have a high risk of thromboembolism (Fig. 6.61), requiring lifetime anticoagulation, but the valves last for years.

### Tissue Valves

The tissue valves in current use include human aortic homografts and stented valves, within which semi-lunar cusps from pigs and cows are inserted. In adults, the aortic valve may be replaced by human aortic valves removed either from cadavers or from explanted hearts from patients with cardiomyopathy or ischaemic heart disease who are undergoing cardiac transplantation. Most have a pig aortic valve mounted inside a three-pronged stent covered by knitted polyester. Tissue valves have a high risk of failing within 10 years and will not last a lifetime, but they have a negligible risk of thromboembolism and anticoagulation is not required. The long-term survival of both aortic homografts and animal tissue valves is limited by primary failure of the cusp tissue, with tears and heavy calcification, which develops within the cusps (Fig. 6.62).

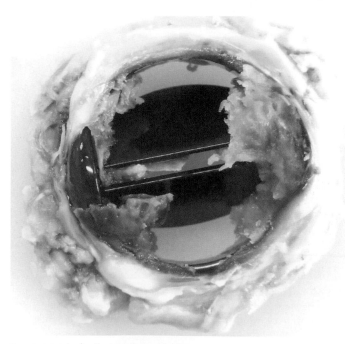

FIG. 6.61 A bi-leaflet mechanical valve over which there is thrombus.

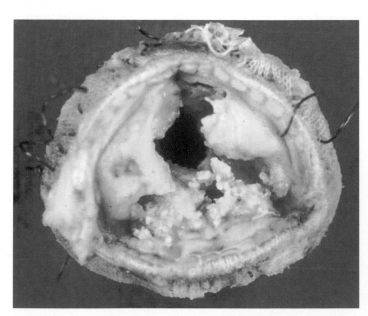

FIG. 6.62 A bioprosthetic valve with a synthetic ring. Note that the biological valve leaflets show yellow lipid deposition and tearing with extensive calcification, which has led to valve regurgitation.

# INFECTIVE ENDOCARDITIS

### Key Points

- In infective endocarditis, there is infection of the valve with formation of thrombotic vegetations.
- The virulence of the organisms dictates the severity of infection and degree of valve damage.
- Pre-existing valve disease, immunosuppression, and bacteraemia are all predisposing factors.
- Complications are valve damage, heart failure, septic embolism, toxaemia, and glomerulonephritis.

Infective endocarditis affects 15,000 patients each year in the USA and 600 per year in the UK. The mortality rate is still high, at almost 40%, so this disease remains a very serious health problem. The incidence has not declined over the last 30 years and now, with more healthcare interventions, such as pacer/defibrillators, and an increasingly elderly population with degenerative valvular heart disease, the number of people susceptible to endocarditis is actually increasing. Given the weak evidence for endocarditis prophylaxis, there therefore remains a large population at risk. Three-quarters of patients have pre-existing structural heart disease. Once infection is manifest, major cardiac complications include congestive heart failure, embolization, mycotic aneurysms, renal dysfunction, and abscess formation. The diagnosis of endocarditis has been enhanced by modifications in Dukes' criteria to include the use of transoesophageal echocardiography and microbial antibody titres. The major organisms involved in infective endocarditis include streptococci and staphylococci (representing 75% or so of all cases). Enterococcal infections account for many of the remaining cases, although small series and case reports suggest that almost all organisms that infect humans can be implicated at times. However, a sizable number of 'culture-negative' cases still occur despite all the improvements in diagnostic methodology.

A wide range of valve abnormalities, and all prosthetic valves, predispose to human infective endocarditis. The risk is greatest with valve lesions that involve high-pressure jets. Thus, mitral incompetence has a higher risk than mitral valve stenosis. The increased risk with regurgitant jets is due to direct damage to the endocardium by the local haemodynamic forces. It is, however, becoming more frequent for bacterial infection to become established on valves that were not clinically regarded as previously abnormal. In this context age-related changes in normal individuals predispose to small platelet thrombi on valve cusps at the lines and points of cusp apposition. Lambl's excrescences are probably the result of organization of such thrombi. Small thrombi that are not of a size to be either visible or of any haemodynamic consequence may act as a nidus on which

highly virulent organisms such as *Staphylococcus aureus* can establish infection. Mural endocarditis is rare.

The pattern of infective endocarditis has changed radically, especially in developed countries. Once a disease affecting young adults with previously well-identified (mostly rheumatic) valve disease (Fig. 6.63), it now affects older patients who more often develop it as the result of healthcare-associated procedures either without previously known valve disease or in the setting of prosthetic valves.

## Causative Agents

The relative proportions of cases of infective endocarditis due to different organisms have changed over the last few decades due to the decline in chronic rheumatic valve disease, the use of antibiotics, the advent of cardiac surgery making patients with prosthetic valves common in the community, better oral hygiene in the community, the increasing numbers of intravenous drug abusers, and the use of immunosuppressive treatment. Streptococci of the types found in the mouth (*viridans* group) have declined as a cause of native valve endocarditis, but are still responsible for about a third to a half of cases acquired in the community. The organisms enter the blood from the mouth, classically after dental work. Today, only about 15% of patients give a history of recent visits to the dentist. The majority of cases are, however, associated with poor oral hygiene and gingivitis. The range of β-haemolytic streptococci causing infective endocarditis is far wider than that found 30 years ago. *Streptococcus viridans* is an extremely broad group of organisms and common strains causing infective

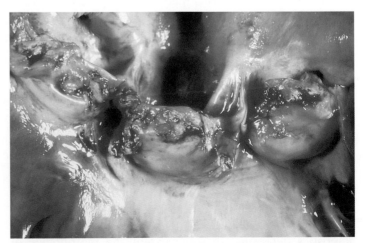

**FIG. 6.63** Vegetations on an infected aortic valve in subacute bacterial endocarditis. The valve is thickened, scarred, and fused at the commissures due to previous rheumatic damage.

endocarditis include *S. sanguis*, *S. mitis*, *S. milleri*, *S. mutans*, and *S. salivarius*. The disease produced is subacute in its clinical type.

Chronic haemodialysis, diabetes mellitus and intravascular devices are the three main factors associated with development of *Staphylococcus aureus* endocarditis. *Staphylococcus aureus* is the archetypal organism capable of settling on functionally normal valves and causes extensive tissue damage and septic emboli. Most series of native valve endocarditis now record it to be almost as common as, if not more frequent than, *Streptococcus viridans* endocarditis. Native valve staphylococcal infective endocarditis is due to *Staphylococcus aureus* while staphylococcal prosthetic valve infective endocarditis is more frequently due to coagulase-negative staphylococci such as *Staphylococcus epidermidis*. Native valve endocarditis affects men nearly three times as frequently as women. Microorganisms are identified histologically in most active endocarditis cases.

Enterococci are now responsible for many cases of infective endocarditis and are more frequent than the *viridans* group in infections that follow urogenital and gastrointestinal tract surgery, and in drug addicts. In general, the disease is subacute in type but it may on occasion be more acute with septic emboli.

Gram-negative bacteria account for up to 10% of cases of infective endocarditis in some series and are relatively more common in drug addicts and on prosthetic valves. A vast range of other organisms, many reported as single cases or small series, can cause infective endocarditis. More than 30 years ago, pneumococci and gonococci accounted for 10% of cases of infective endocarditis but their frequency has now been reduced to sporadic single cases. *Rickettsia* and *Chlamydia* spp. cause a very chronic and slowly progressive endocarditis with an insidious onset as does brucella endocarditis. Infection usually occurs on previously abnormal valves, and diagnosis is made in life by serology rather than isolation of the organism. A history of working with agricultural animals is present in more than 50% of cases of brucella and Q-fever endocarditis.

There has been an increasing frequency of deep mycotic infections complicating immunosuppression usually linked to haematological malignancy. *Candida* sp. dominates, followed by *Aspergillus* sp. *Histoplasma* sp. predominates in cases with large vegetations. The probable source of infection is often bronchopneumonia or an infected central venous catheter.

### Macroscopic Appearance

Infective endocarditis is caused by microorganisms with a wide range of capabilities for tissue destruction. These characteristics determine to some extent the morphology of vegetations and the adjacent heart valves. Marked destructive lesions are noted in *Staphyloccus aureus* infections, whereas less marked destruction plus a reparative fibrotic response are features of streptococcal infection The vegetations of infective endocarditis are most commonly found attached to the atrial aspect of atrioventricular (mitral and tricuspid) valves and to the ventricular aspect of semi-lunar (aortic and pulmonary) valves. Usually they are related to the line of cusp apposition but, if large, they may involve adjacent parts of a cusp, leaflet, or contiguous structures, e.g. chordae tendineae or the sinus of Valsalva. Vegetations may also arise at a site away from the cusps themselves, at the place where a regurgitant jet hits the endocardium. Vegetations vary in size, with those associated with fungal infections being the largest. Vegetations can vary in colour from red through pink to yellow and may be soft and friable or firm. They can have a smooth surface, but more often are irregular and granular on the surface of the leaflet and may be missed if small in size. Vegetations may be single or multiple. With organisms that cause extensive tissue necrosis, the edge of the cusp may ulcerate, chordae may rupture, or the body of the cusp may perforate, leading to incompetence of the valve. An infection may also weaken the fibrosa of a cusp, leading to aneurysm formation. Aortic valve aneurysms are usually small, 2–3 mm in size, and bulge towards the left ventricle. Mitral valve aneurysms usually affect the anterior leaflet. Occasionally a perforation can be found at the apex of such aneurysms.

Vegetations may spread from the aortic valve cusps to the endocardial surface of the interventricular septum or the ventricular face of the anterior cusp of the mitral valve. This spread often follows a regurgitant jet. Vegetations on the posterior mitral valve cusp may extend up onto the endocardium of the left atrium along the line of a regurgitant jet. It may be impossible to tell if infection has spread from the aortic to the mitral valve or vice versa if both valves are involved. 'Kissing' lesions on contiguous surfaces of cusps are another example of local spread.

Bacterial endocarditis on prosthetic valves usually begins on the valve ring and, in addition to spreading into the adjacent tissues, also causes vegetations, which protrude out into the valve orifice. Such vegetations may become large enough to cause obstruction or to hinder the mechanical movement of the valve resulting in regurgitation. Obstruction to flow by vegetations is far more common in prosthetic valves compared with native valves where the predominant haemodynamic abnormality is regurgitation. Annular abscesses are a very common feature of prosthetic valve endocarditis. Infection spreads in the tissue plane surrounding the sewing ring of the valve and rapidly forms an abscess, which extends around the whole annulus. The sutures often dehisce and the prosthetic valve tears away from the annulus over part or all of its circumference, leading to paraprosthetic leaks.

## Microscopic Appearance

Fresh vegetations consist of platelets and fibrin, with abundant polymorphonuclear leukocytes in some areas. Colonies of bacteria or fungal hyphae may be demonstrated both at the edge of and within the thrombus, and it is often striking that organisms are embedded in relatively acellular fibrin. If the infection is chronic, the vegetation often shows a varying degree of organization and vascularization from the underlying cusp and/or calcification. Chronic inflammatory cells and a few giant cells may occur. Numerous giant cells are a feature of vegetations in patients with endocarditis caused by *Coxiella burnetii* (Q-fever).

The result of the healing process after successful treatment of bacterial endocarditis depends on the amount of cusp damage that occurred in the acute phase. Vegetations are reduced in size and organize from the base leading to fibrous nodules, which often calcify. Considerable cusp fibrosis occurs leading to thickening and retraction of the cusps. Infections that destroyed cusp tissue in the acute phase leave irregular indentations along the free edge of the cusp or smooth-edged perforations through the body of the cusp; or are associated with chordal rupture. It is often impossible in the late stage of healed bacterial endocarditis to recognise if the valve was normal or abnormal before infection occurred.

## Complications

The mortality of bacterial endocarditis remains high largely because of a number of serious complications. *S. aureus* infection, severe heart failure, neurological manifestations, septic shock, perivalvular extension, and acute renal failure are all characteristics of a patient group at higher risk of mortality. As vegetations grow and disintegrate, they embolize into the brain, myocardium, spleen, and kidneys (Fig. 6.64).

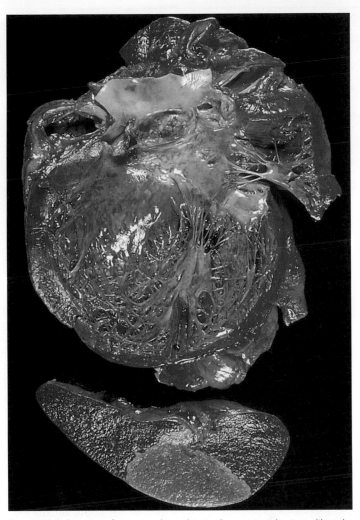

**FIG. 6.64** Subacute infective endocarditis in the aortic valve in a dilated heart. The spleen is also enlarged and shows an infarct due to embolism.

## Treatment

The cornerstone to the successful clinical treatment of infective endocarditis is isolation of the organism from blood cultures, with antibiotic therapy being specifically matched to the sensitivity of the organism. Surgery continues to play an important role, with large vegetations, ruptured leaflets, and large abscesses criteria for urgent surgery.

# Lesions Simulating Infective Endocarditis

## Non-bacterial Thrombotic Endocarditis

Non-bacterial thrombotic endocarditis (marantic or terminal endocarditis) consists of small thrombi on the heart valves, usually in a patchy fashion along the lines of cusp closure of the mitral and aortic valves. They are probably caused by a hypercoagulable state because identical lesions occur in any patient with acute DIC. They are usually asymptomatic but both systemic embolism and secondary infection of the thrombi are recognized complications. Characteristically, this condition occurs in patients with a debilitating illness such as cancer or tuberculosis.

## Libman–Sacks Endocarditis

This may develop in patients with SLE and can involve the mitral, aortic, or tricuspid valves. The vegetations are sterile, platelet rich, and rarely exceed 2 mm in size. Fibrinoid necrosis is a characteristic feature.

A 56-year-old woman complained of fatigue and diminished exercise tolerance. She developed a left hemiplegia, and on admission auscultation revealed a rumbling mid-diastolic murmur and a pansystolic murmur suggestive of mitral stenosis and incompetence. Chest radiographs showed some streaky shadowing in the lung fields that did not resolve despite diuretic therapy. A diagnosis of atrial fibrillation and cerebral embolism due to longstanding rheumatic heart disease with mitral stenosis and incompetence was made. This was confirmed by an echocardiogram (Fig. 6.65).

When recuperating, she became unwell with a pyrexial illness. There was no obvious site of infection until echocardiography revealed a vegetation on the mitral valve. Blood cultures grew no pathogens and she was treated with intravenous antibiotics for several weeks without response. As she was deteriorating clinically, a mitral valve replacement was undertaken. Fig. 6.66 shows the valve removed at operation. A year later she became more breathless and had a pansystolic murmur of mitral incompetence. The prosthetic valve was removed (Fig. 6.67) and replaced. This effected a symptomatic cure and she remains well.

In summary, this woman had chronic rheumatic heart disease due to recurrent subclinical rheumatic fever. Her mitral stenosis and incompetence were complicated by atrial fibrillation. This has a high risk of thrombus formation and she had a stroke due to cerebral infarction from thromboembolism. She developed subacute infective endocarditis that was resistant to treatment and cured only by mitral valve replacement. The flap valve prosthesis failed because it became blocked by the formation of adherent thrombus.

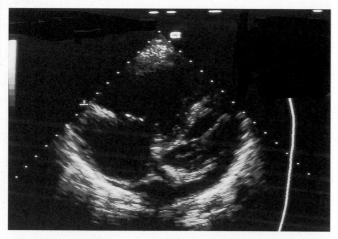

FIG. 6.65 Echocardiogram showing the heart in ventricular systole. The thickened and scarred cusps and chordae tendineae are visible. The mitral valve remains open during systole indicating regurgitation, which was confirmed by colour Doppler studies.

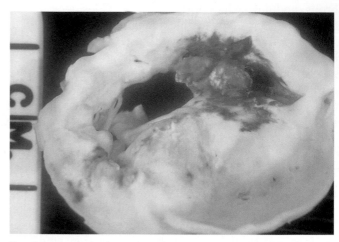

FIG. 6.66 A mitral valve removed at operation. It is thickened and calcified, and the orifice is reduced to a slit by fusion of the commissures due to rheumatic scarring. It is rigid and can neither open nor close. A large friable vegetation protrudes into the orifice.

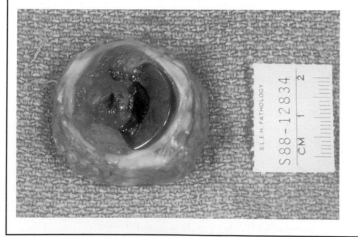

FIG. 6.67 The valve flap of the prosthetic mitral valve replacement is jammed with thrombus. It can neither open nor close fully.

# THE CARDIOMYOPATHIES

The term 'cardiomyopathy' has undergone radical changes in the last 25 years. The term is used specifically for myocardial dysfunction that is not the result of coronary artery disease, valve disease, hypertension, or congenital shunts. It implies that the functional abnormality lies within the myocardium itself. The primary cardiomyopathies (those unrelated to hypertension, ischaemic, valvular, or inflammatory disease) fall into those in which there is a thick-walled left ventricle (hypertrophic) or a dilated poorly contracting ventricle in systole (dilated), and those that are restrictive with the left ventricle failing to relax, impeding filling from the left atrium. The classification thus remains predominantly functional. This system of classification remains imperfect, and as more knowledge is gained is likely to be replaced by a system based on genetic and pathogenic mechanisms.

## Dilated Cardiomyopathy

### Key Points

- In dilated cardiomyopathy, there is four-chamber cardiac dilatation.
- There is poor systolic function.
- It is the end-stage of many insults to the myocardium.
- There is myocyte stretching and hypertrophy, myocyte damage and diffuse fibrosis.

Dilated cardiomyopathy has a prevalence of 1:2,500 and is characterized by ventricular chamber enlargement and systolic dysfunction in the absence of abnormal loading conditions (hypertension, valve disease) or coronary artery disease (*Table 6.6*). This disorder develops at any age, in either sex, and in people of any ethnic origin. In adults, dilated cardiomyopathy arises more commonly in males than in females. The disease is inherited in 20–48% of cases. Familial disease should be suspected when there is a family history of premature cardiac death, conduction system disease, or skeletal myopathy. Autosomal dominant forms of the disease are caused by mutations in cytoskeletal, sarcomeric protein/

**TABLE 6.6** Causes of dilated cardiomyopathy

**Idiopathic**

| | |
|---|---|
| Post-inflammatory (myocarditic) | Most commonly viral but includes protozoal and bacterial |
| Genetic | With or without skeletal muscle myopathy<br>Associated with inborn errors of metabolism, e.g. carnitine deficiency or haemochromatosis<br>Sex linked |
| Nutritional | Severe protein malnutrition |
| Metabolic | Endocrine disease, e.g. diabetes, hypoparathyroidism, phaeochromocytoma<br>Uraemia |
| Toxic | Alcohol, drugs, e.g. chemotherapeutic agents<br>Heavy metals, e.g. lead, cobalt, arsenic |

Z-band, nuclear membrane, and intercalated disc protein genes. X-linked diseases associated with dilated cardiomyopathy include muscular dystrophies (e.g. Becker and Duchenne) and X-linked dilated cardiomyopathy. Dilated cardiomyopathy may also occur in patients with mitochondrial cytopathies and inherited metabolic disorders (e.g. haemochromatosis). Examples of acquired causes of dilated cardiomyopathy include nutritional deficiencies, endocrine dysfunction, and the administration of cardiotoxic drugs. It can also occur during pregnancy and in the peripartum period. It is associated with an increased incidence of sudden death, thromboembolic risk, and heart failure.

All four chambers are dilated and the walls are thinned (Fig. 6.68). Microscopically there is myocyte loss with replacement fibrosis in the ventricle (Fig. 6.69). It is impossible to differentiate the causes of dilated cardiomyopathy, which are multiple, from the histological appearances.

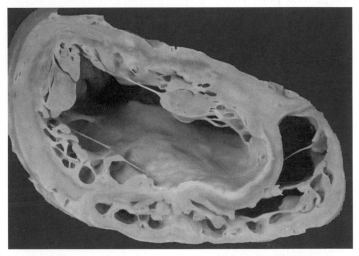

**FIG. 6.68** Dilated cardiomyopathy: transverse section of the left and right ventricles showing thinning, particularly of the interventricular septum with diffuse subendocardial fibrosis of the left ventricular wall.

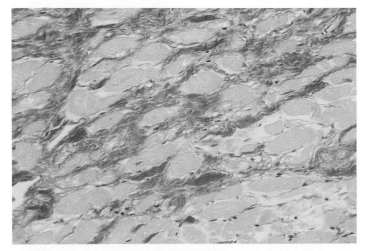

**FIG. 6.69** Dilated cardiomyopathy: myocytes, stained yellow, are surrounded by interstitial collagen, which isolates the myocytes. Stain: elastin van Gieson.

## Hypertrophic Cardiomyopathy

### Key Points

- Hypertrophic cardiomyopathy causes sudden death.
- There is left ventricular hypertrophy (usually asymmetrical), especially involving the interventricular septum.
- There is systolic and diastolic dysfunction.
- Many cases are due to myocyte contractile protein gene mutations, especially of the myosin heavy chain.
- There is myocyte hypertrophy and disarray with variable diffuse fibrosis.

Left ventricular hypertrophy in the absence of hypertension and valve disease occurs in approximately 1:500 of the general population. It can present with sudden death, especially in young people, but may also present with arrhythmias and cardiac failure. There may be symmetrical involvement of the whole of the left ventricle to produce an even, thick-walled chamber, with a small cavity similar to that seen in hypertension but focal involvement of the wall can be seen. It is now recognized that the segment of abnormal muscle can involve any region of the left ventricle, be in discontinuous segments, and also involve the right ventricle. Macroscopically there is hypertrophy with scarring in patients who die suddenly (Fig. 6.70). Where there is interventricular septal hypertrophy there is an impact lesion in which a thickened anterior leaflet of the mitral valve impacts on the left side of the septum, leaving a thickened mirror area (Fig. 6.71). Storage diseases such as Fabry's disease can mimic hypertrophic cardiomyopathy.

Microscopically, the left ventricular myocardial architecture is disorganized, composed of hypertrophied cardiac muscle cells (myocytes) with bizarre shapes and multiple intercellular connections, often arranged in chaotic alignment

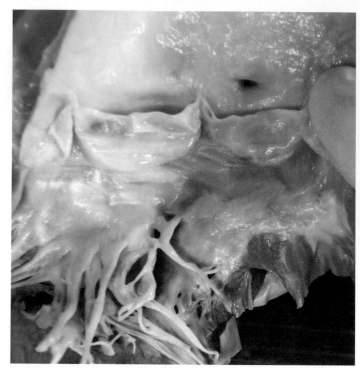

**FIG. 6.71** The aortic outflow tract in hypertrophic cardiomyopathy. Note the aortic valve, and below that the anterior leaflet of the mitral valve, which appears thickened. The chordae also appear thickened. Note the irregular area of fibrous thickening of the subendocardium (impact lesion) on the interventricular septum opposite the thickened leaflet.

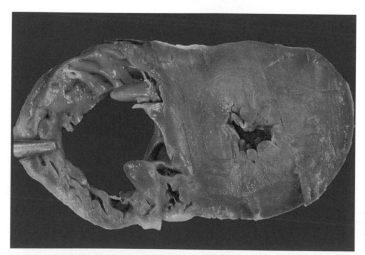

**FIG. 6.70** The right and left ventricles in hypertrophic cardiomyopathy. There is marked circumferential hypertrophy of the left ventricle with a very small chamber space.

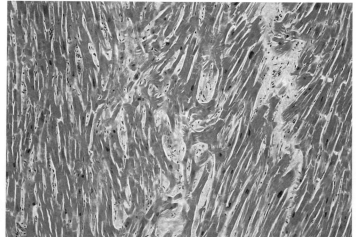

**FIG. 6.72** The central myocytes are disorganized, swirling in all different directions and curling around capillaries. This is classic myocyte disarray in hypertrophic cardiomyopathy.

at oblique and perpendicular angles (Fig. 6.72). This myocyte cellular disarray may be widely distributed, occupying substantial portions of the left ventricular wall, and is more extensive in young patients who die of their disease.

Many individuals have familial disease with an autosomal dominant pattern of inheritance, caused by mutations in genes that encode different proteins of the cardiac sarcomere, especially the myosin heavy chain.

## Arrhythmogenic Right Ventricular Cardiomyopathy

Arrhythmogenic right ventricular cardiomyopathy is a rare inherited heart-muscle disease that is a cause of sudden death in young people and athletes. It is characterized by progressive replacement of the right ventricle myocardium by either segmental or diffuse fibrofatty tissue, often with involvement of the left ventricular wall as well as the right ventricular wall. The left ventricle is so frequently involved that the broader term 'arrhythmogenic cardiomyopathy' may be more appropriate. The fibrofatty replacement leads to ventricular arrhythmias. These arrhythmias may range from asymptomatic ventricular premature complexes to monomorphic ventricular tachycardia or ventricular fibrillation.

Arrhythmogenic right ventricular cardiomyopathy is now regarded as a genetically determined myocardial degenerative disease. It is inherited in an autosomal dominant manner but autosomal recessive forms (e.g. Naxos and Carvajal syndromes caused by mutations in genes encoding plakoglobin and desmoplakin, respectively) are recognized. However, most cases are caused by autosomal, dominantly inherited mutations in genes encoding plakophilin 2 and other proteins of the desmosome of cardiomyocytes. Mutations in transforming growth factor (TGF)-β and ryanodine receptor genes may also be associated with an arrhythmogenic right ventricular cardiomyopathy phenotype.

### Macroscopic Appearance

Segments of the right ventricle show dilatation and thinning of the wall with fatty replacement of the muscle. There is also involvement of the left ventricle, particularly on the epicardial surface (Fig. 6.73). Fatty replacement is seen particularly in the right ventricular outflow tract. Usually the fat and scar tissue are in the epicardial aspect of the ventricle and extend in to replace the full thickness of the wall, which increases with age. However, fat is normally present in the right ventricle, especially in obese patients with coronary artery disease, so scarring must also be present, with histological confirmation.

### Microscopic Appearance

Arrhythmogenic right ventricular cardiomyopathy is defined histologically by the presence of progressive replacement of the right ventricular myocardium with adipose and fibrous tissue.

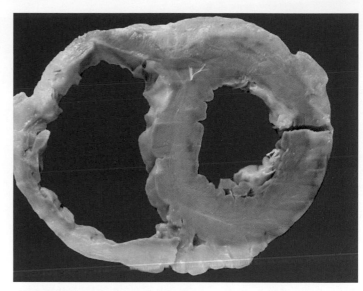

**FIG. 6.73** Transverse section of the right and left ventricles in arrhythmogenic right ventricular cardiomyopathy showing a dilated right ventricle with fatty replacement of the wall. There is also fatty infiltration of the anterior and lateral walls of the left ventricle.

## Restrictive Cardiomyopathy

Idiopathic restrictive cardiomyopathy is a poorly recognized entity characterized by non-dilated, non-hypertrophied ventricles with diastolic dysfunction resulting in dilated atria and variable systolic function. There are two main subtypes. In endomyocardial fibrosis, there is fibrosis in the subendocardium. In endocardial fibroelastosis, which affects children, a diffuse layer of dense white fibrous tissue, composed mainly of elastic fibres, lines the cardiac chambers. It can be associated with congenital heart disease, especially mitral and aortic stenosis with left ventricular hypoplasia. It seems likely that fibroelastosis simply represents a reaction to other heart diseases in early childhood and is not a separate entity.

The exact prevalence of restrictive cardiomyopathy is unknown but it is probably the least common type of cardiomyopathy. Restrictive cardiomyopathy may be idiopathic or familial, or result from various systemic disorders, in particular amyloidosis, sarcoidosis, carcinoid heart disease, scleroderma, and anthracycline toxicity. Cardiac amyloid may be senile in type: this occurs in elderly people, is confined to the atria and cardiac valves, and follows a benign course. When there is diffuse involvement of the ventricles it can be rapidly fatal. The amyloid fibrils may be derived from immunoglobulin (amyloid AL), from serum amyloid A protein, usually secondary to chronic infection (amyloid AA), or from transthyretin protein in familial disorders (amyloid AF).

Pericardial disorders that lead to diastolic heart failure usually do so as a result of restriction of diastolic cardiac function (constrictive pericarditis). These patients classically have clinical signs of heart failure in the presence of a non-dilated, non-hypertrophic left ventricle, with preserved contractility but abnormal diastolic function. However, the ventricular wall can vary in thickness, being thin in some cases but hypertrophied in others; this can also vary during the course of the disease.

Primary restrictive cardiomyopathy is a myocardial disease of unknown aetiology that affects predominantly elderly patients but can occur in any age group. Pericellular and interstitial fibrosis are present and vary from mild to moderate to severe. It affects both adults and children. In children the prognosis is particularly poor.

## DISORDERS OF THE CONDUCTING SYSTEM

The conducting system consists of specialized cardiac myocytes that initiate the heartbeat in the sinoatrial node and conduct the impulse through the atrioventricular (AV) node and then through the common AV bundles (bundles of His) and the left and right bundle branches to the apex of the ventricles, which is the first region to contract. Disturbances of rhythm complicate many types of heart disease: some are due to damage to the conducting system, its most vulnerable regions being the AV bundle and the left and right bundle branches; however, many arrhythmias, such as extrasystoles, paroxysmal tachycardia, and fibrillation, are due to spontaneous 'impulses' or irregularities arising in the myocardium itself.

Acquired conducting system defects include ischaemic damage, inflammatory conditions such as myocarditis, sarcoidosis or connective tissue diseases, infiltrative disorders such as amyloidosis or metastatic tumour, and finally surgical trauma.

## DISEASES OF THE PERICARDIUM

### Key Points

- Pericarditis has multiple aetiologies including infection, myocardial infarction, connective tissue diseases, and uraemia.
- Pericardial effusion and haemopericardium can both cause cardiac tamponade.
- Constrictive pericarditis is due to fibrous obliteration of the pericardial cavity with resulting impaired cardiac function.
- Pericardial involvement by metastatic tumour may produce effusion, inflammation, or restriction.

The pericardium is a fibrous sac, which surrounds the heart, comprises visceral and parietal layers, and may become inflamed (pericarditis). A pericardial effusion is an accumu-

lation of fluid in the pericardial sac, often due to metastatic carcinoma, but also seen in cardiac failure and other types of oedema. Blood can also accumulate (haemopericardium). The pericardial sac can dilate to contain over 1 L fluid without a significant rise in pressure if the fluid accumulates slowly. If accumulation is rapid, even a small rise in fluid volume increases the pericardial pressure, interferes with cardiac filling, and leads to cardiac tamponade. In its most severe form, cardiogenic shock with low cardiac output ensues. There is hypotension with a low pulse pressure, particularly during inspiration (pulsus paradoxus) and death results. Cardiac tamponade is usually due to haemopericardium caused by rupture of the heart or aortic root, but it may result from a tense effusion.

## Pericarditis

The causes of pericarditis are given in *Table 6.7*.

Pericarditis is inflammation of the pericardium, with consequent accumulation of an inflammatory exudate in the pericardial sac and fibrosis of the pericardial surface (Fig. 6.74). This usually reorganizes, but a thicker layer may become organized with consequent fibrous thickening and extensive adhesions between the two pericardial layers.

Viral and idiopathic pericarditis most commonly occur in young adults, often after an upper respiratory tract infection, and usually subside within 2 weeks. Coxsackieviruses A and B, echoviruses, and polioviruses are most commonly implicated. Fibrosis may eventually progress to chronic constrictive pericarditis.

**TABLE 6.7** The aetiology of pericarditis

| | |
|---|---|
| Infections | Viral – Coxsackievirus A and B, echoviruses, and polioviruses |
| | Bacterial – pyogenic organisms, tuberculosis |
| | Fungal and protozoal |
| Malignant disease | Direct spread from carcinoma of bronchus or oesophagus |
| | Metastatic tumour |
| Myocardial infarction | Uraemia |
| Metabolic | Hypothyroidism |
| Immunologically mediated | Rheumatic fever |
| | Connective tissue disease – rheumatoid arthritis, systemic lupus erythematosus, mixed connective tissue disease |
| | Post-cardiotomy or post-myocardial infarction (Dressler's syndrome) |
| Iatrogenic | Post-irradiation |
| | Drug hypersensitivity reaction |
| Idiopathic | |

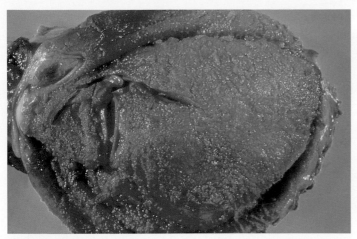

**FIG. 6.74** The anterior surface of the heart with the pericardium opened to reveal a fibrinous pericarditis.

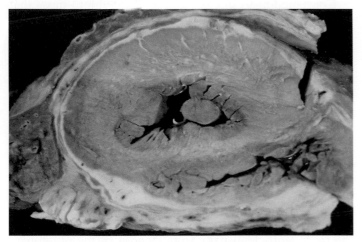

**FIG. 6.75** Transverse section of the left and right ventricles showing thickening of both the epicardial and the fibrous pericardium with fusion of both surfaces. Note that the fibrosis extends into the underlying myocardium, constricting the action of the muscle.

*Constrictive Pericarditis*

This is characterized by obliteration of the pericardial sac by a thick layer of dense fibrous tissue, which may become calcified, especially in tuberculosis. It can result from prolonged pyrogenic, tuberculous, or viral infection but in most cases the aetiology is unknown. The fibrotic pericardium adheres to the heart and interferes with filling, possibly aggravated by constriction of the great veins as they enter the atria (Fig. 6.75).

## TUMOURS OF THE HEART AND PERICARDIUM

### Key Points

- The most common malignant cardiac/pericardial tumour is metastatic carcinoma.
- Primary cardiac tumours are rare.
- Atrial myxoma is the most common primary tumour.
- Primary malignant cardiac/pericardial tumours are rare.

Primary cardiac and pericardial tumours are rare with a prevalence of between 0.001% and 0.3%. Modern advances in cardiac imaging have increased the number of patients identified with a primary cardiac tumour at an early stage, and have also improved prognosis. Most primary cardiac tumours are benign, with only 25% being malignant: these are usually sarcomas. The most common primary cardiac tumour is the cardiac myxoma, which usually occurs in adult life in the left atrium. It forms a gelatinous mass up to 6 cm in diameter (Fig. 6.76), which may create intermittent ball valve obstruction of the mitral valve. It may also present with embolic phenomena due to fragmentation, or with a variety of systemic symptoms due to production of

Bacterial pericarditis usually complicates septicaemia or pyaemia, or arises due to direct spread from pneumonia, empyema, or an ulcerating carcinoma of the bronchus or oesophagus. *S. aureus*, *Haemophilus* spp. and streptococci are the most common organisms. Tuberculous pericarditis is due to either haematogenous spread from the lung or direct extension from the trachea, bronchi, or mediastinal lymph nodes. Granulomatous inflammation progresses to fibrous obliteration of the pericardial sac, calcification, and constrictive pericarditis.

A more diffuse persistent pericarditis (Dressler's syndrome) may follow myocardial infarction or cardiac surgery, and is believed to be an immunologically mediated event. Pericarditis commonly complicates collagen vascular diseases, such as rheumatoid arthritis, SLE, and uraemia.

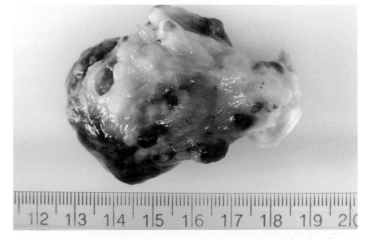

**FIG. 6.76** A classic atrial myxoma: a large gelatinous mass that has been excised from the left atrium.

inflammatory factors (Fig. 6.77). The bulk of the tumour comprises primitive polygonal or stellate cells embedded in a myxoid stroma. Why it occurs in the left atrium in particular is a mystery, with pluripotential cells in the atrial fossa being the presumed origin of the tumour cells. Adequate local surgical resection is usually curative.

In children, rhabdomyomas are the most common cardiac tumour and it is important to remember that half are associated with tuberous sclerosis, especially if they are multiple. These tumours tend to involve the left ventricle. Microscopically they consist of large branching vacuolated cells containing striped myofibrils. The other frequent childhood tumour is the fibroma, which is usually solitary in the ventricle and consists of smooth muscle cells that can be large and lethal, especially *in utero* or in the neonatal period. If not too large they usually regress with time and do not need surgery. Other benign tumours include lipomas, haemangiomas, and lymphangiomas, which also tend to occur in a younger age group and usually involve the ventricles.

In adults, metastatic malignant tumours are the most frequent tumours to involve the heart and pericardium. Such tumours are found in up to 12% of all fatal malignancies. Squamous cell carcinoma of the lung and adenocarcinoma of the kidney have the highest reported frequency of metastatic cardiac involvement, but metastatic melanoma, lymphoma, breast, and gastrointestinal carcinomas are also common. The very rare primary malignant cardiac tumours are sarcomas, including angiosarcomas. Most sarcomas are undifferentiated, originating possibly from pluripotential cells.

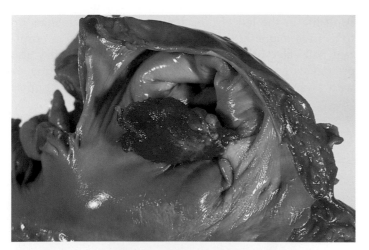

**FIG. 6.77** An opened atrium showing a myxoma as a soft ovoid gelatinous mass, which may obstruct the mitral valve or give rise to embolism.

## CONGENITAL HEART DISEASE

Congenital heart disease, which complicates up to 1% of live births, is becoming more important as advances in imaging, anaesthetics, and surgery permit many patients to survive into adulthood. The aetiology is obscure in many cases, but maternal rubella infection in the first trimester causes serious abnormalities in 10–20% of affected infants, of which heart disease constitutes about 50%.

At an early stage of development the heart consists of three compartments: atrial, ventricular, and the aortic bulb. Each is divided into two by a separate septum, defects in the formation of which result in most congenital abnormalities. Important abnormalities arise in relation to the growth of the ventricular septum and the division of the aortic bulb into the aorta and pulmonary artery. The ventricular septum grows upwards from the apex of the ventricle, whereas the aortic bulb is divided into two almost equal parts by the formation and fusion of two longitudinal folds in its wall. The two vessels formed must rotate spirally to establish their normal continuity with the ventricles. The septum of the bulb fuses with the upgrowing ventricular septum, the last portion to close being represented by the membranous part of the interventricular septum.

Congenital heart diseases can be divided into those that produce cyanosis and those that do not. The cyanosis results from admixture of venous blood with oxygenated blood leaving the heart. The lowered oxygen tension in arterial blood leads to a compensatory erythrocytosis, which makes cyanosis more prominent. The cyanosis may be further aggravated by impaired oxygenation of blood by the lungs in conditions in which there is pulmonary disease or when heart failure develops.

## Pathology of Cyanotic Congenital Heart Disease

The most common anomaly in this group is the tetralogy of Fallot. There is obstruction to the outflow tract of the right ventricle, usually from stenosis of the pulmonary valve, which results in right ventricular hypertrophy; high right ventricular pressures force unoxygenated blood into the aorta through a high interventricular septal defect. The aorta partially overrides the septal defect and receives both venous blood from the right ventricle and oxygenated blood from the left ventricle. The features of Eisenmenger's complex, which is a complication of chronic left-to-right shunts, resemble those of Fallot's tetralogy, but there is no obstruction to the outflow from the right ventricle. Initially little right-to-left shunting of blood occurs and there is little cyanosis, but later, with the onset of pulmonary hypertension, the shunt reverses and overt cyanosis appears partly from admixture cyanosis and partly from faulty oxygenation of the blood by the lungs.

Malformations of the aortic bulb can result in pulmonary or aortic stenosis. Most commonly pulmonary stenosis results from an unequal division of the bulb; the septum is pushed to the right, producing an abnormally large aorta that arises partly from the left and partly from the right ventricle; there is usually a defect in the interventricular septum. The site of stenosis varies: sometimes the pulmonary artery is small, occasionally completely obliterated, and in other cases the narrowing is at the valve where cusp fusion may form a thickened diaphragm with a reduced aperture. All these abnormalities interfere with flow of blood into the pulmonary artery and lead to varying degrees of right ventricular hypertrophy. Some of the blood from the right ventricle passes through the interventricular septal defect into the aorta. The ductus arteriosus usually remains patent after birth and the lungs receive part of their blood supply through it. The foramen ovale also remains open and may be large.

Transposition of the great vessels results from failure of the proximal aorta and pulmonary artery to undergo the spiral rotation necessary for the establishment of their correct relationship to the ventricles. Consequently, the aorta arises from the right ventricle and the pulmonary artery from the left ventricle. In isolation this abnormality is incompatible with extrauterine life; however, persistence of the ductus arteriosus, a patent foramen ovale, or a defect in the interatrial or interventricular septum may offer temporary compensation. Combinations of these defects are common. If shunting allows oxygenated blood to reach the systemic circulation, cyanosis is less marked.

In persistent truncus arteriosus the aorta and pulmonary artery arise from a common stem vessel, the truncus arising from both ventricles and overriding a ventricular septal defect. If the septum fails to develop, a single ventricular cavity results. Interatrial septal defects are also common.

## Pathology of Acyanotic Congenital Heart Disease

Interatrial septal defect, the most common congenital heart disease, usually has little effect on the circulation, although the most severe cases may cause pulmonary hypertension late in life. The important defects are of three main types: persistent ostium primum, persistent ostium secundum, and persistent AV canal. In the last condition there is often fusion of the tricuspid and mitral valves to form a common AV valve. Rarely, embolizing thrombus from the venous circulation may pass from the right atrium through the interatrial defect to reach the left atrium, and cause crossed or paradoxical embolism.

Interventricular septal defect may form part of another congenital anomaly such as Fallot's tetralogy where it is high in the septum. An isolated high interventricular septal defect (maladie de Roger) is not uncommon. The size and location of the defect vary. The left-to-right shunt causes pulmonary hypertension in young adults.

Aortic valve stenosis and subaortic stenosis may each occur as isolated abnormalities. So, too, may a bicuspid aortic valve, with an overall incidence of approximately 2%. Usually symptomless in early life, it predisposes to the development of calcific aortic stenosis (see pp. 145–146) and infective endocarditis (see pp. 151–154).

Patent ductus arteriosus, which can coexist with many other anomalies, may be the only abnormality present, in which case closure by surgery restores the circulation to normal. Failure to close leads eventually to heart failure, and there is a risk of infective 'endocarditis' involving the ductus. If there is pulmonary hypertension, blood flow in the ductus may be reversed so that unoxygenated blood passes from the pulmonary artery into the aorta via the ductus, beyond the origin of the left subclavian artery. Such a patient may thus have a cyanotic tinge in the nailbeds of the toes but not in those of the hands.

Coarctation (stenosis) of the aorta (Fig. 6.78) is a localized narrowing of the aorta between the left subclavian artery and the orifice of the ductus arteriosus. This abnormality is not uncommon and occurs predominantly in males and in females with Turner's syndrome (see Chapter 3, p. 36). All degrees of narrowing up to complete atresia occur. Severe narrowing causes an extensive collateral network from the carotid and subclavian arteries to link the aorta above and below the narrowed segment. Pulses in the legs are poor compared with those of the arms. Hypertension develops and death is likely to ensue from cardiac failure, cerebral haemorrhage, or, less commonly, local complications at the site of coarctation including aneurysm, dissection, or infection. Surgery is curative.

Anomalies of the aortic arch are commonly associated with Fallot's tetralogy; however, as isolated anomalies they rarely cause symptoms. When a vascular ring is formed around the trachea and oesophagus by a right aortic arch and the left descending aorta, together with a persistent ductus arteriosus, ligamentum arteriosum, or anomalous left subclavian artery, pressure effects may result, mainly on the trachea. A double aortic arch may give similar symptoms.

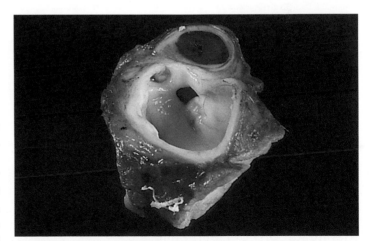

**FIG. 6.78** A surgically excised coarctation showing a tight stenosis of the aortic arch.

## HEART FAILURE

Assuming a resting stroke volume of 70 mL from the left ventricle beating at 70/min, the cardiac output is about 5 L/min, amounting to a daily output of 7,200 L (about 7.5 tons). The normal heart has great reserve power, which can be substantially increased by physical training. During exertion, there is a greater venous return with consequent increase in diastolic filling and stretching of the muscle fibres; the response is a more vigorous contraction (Starling's law) and a greatly increased stroke volume. The heart rate also increases during exertion. These two factors together can raise the cardiac output to about seven times that of the resting state. This physiological performance can be maintained only if the myocardium is healthy, the valves function efficiently, the conducting system of the heart coordinates contraction of the chambers, and peripheral resistance to blood flow is not raised. Disturbance of any of these components can cause heart failure.

In heart failure, impaired cardiac function fails to maintain a circulation adequate for the metabolic needs of the body despite an adequate blood volume. Inadequate tissue perfusion leads ultimately to a complex syndrome of clinical features (typically breathlessness, fatigue, and peripheral and pulmonary oedema) and multiorgan involvement (renal impairment, skeletal muscle dysfunction, impaired pulmonary and peripheral gas exchange, and hepatic dysfunction). Heart failure has a high morbidity and mortality (impaired effort capacity and quality of life, recurrent hospitalization, and death within 1–10 years depending on severity). As western populations age, the incidence of heart failure increases, and it is now a major public health problem.

The clinical spectrum ranges from asymptomatic cardiac dysfunction through reduced exercise tolerance, in which compensatory mechanisms (ventricular hypertrophy, peripheral vasoconstriction, salt and water retention) maintain tissue perfusion, to a stage in which these mechanisms are exhausted and symptoms and signs of heart failure occur at rest.

## Causes of Heart Failure

The main causes of heart failure are summarized in *Table 6.8*. They are due to excessive load on the myocardium (pressure or volume overload), poor myocardial function (contraction or relaxation), or a combination of both mechanisms. The major causes of heart failure vary geographically. In western countries, ischaemic heart disease and hypertension are by far the most common causes whereas, in developing countries, valve disease or myocardial infections are more important. Intrinsic heart muscle disease (cardiomyopathy) is an uncommon cause of heart failure.

## Manifestations of Heart Failure

Heart failure may be acute or chronic, and may affect the left ventricle, right ventricle, or both. Acute heart failure occurs most frequently in myocardial infarction and arrhythmias; less frequent causes are gross pulmonary embolism, myocarditis, or rupture of a valve cusp. In severe acute heart failure, the marked fall in cardiac output is accompanied by peripheral vasoconstriction and cardiogenic shock develops. Chronic heart failure occurs when the causal factors develop slowly. It is most commonly due to ischaemic heart disease, systemic arterial hypertension, chronic valvular dysfunction, or diseases of the lungs with pulmonary hypertension. Two-thirds of patients with chronic heart failure die from progressive pump failure; the other third die suddenly due to an arrhythmia.

### Left Ventricular Failure

Left ventricular failure is most commonly due to ischaemic heart disease, particularly myocardial infarction, but also to systemic hypertension and aortic and mitral valve disease. The failing ventricle dilates, which further impairs contraction. The main clinical features are dyspnoea and cough due to pulmonary venous hypertension and pulmonary oedema. Increased venous return in the recumbent position and increased blood reabsorption of fluid from the extravascular space cause acute exacerbations of left ventricular failure, commonly during the night (paroxysmal nocturnal dyspnoea). In acute left ventricular failure, death may occur rapidly from acute pulmonary oedema, which may be complicated by cardiogenic shock.

### Right Ventricular Failure

Right ventricular failure is usually secondary to left ventricular failure. When the left ventricle fails, increased pressure in the left atrium and pulmonary veins leads to pulmonary arteriolar vasoconstriction and resultant pulmonary artery hypertension. Persistent pulmonary hypertension causes right ventricular hypertrophy and eventually failure. Isolated

**TABLE 6.8** Causes of heart failure

| Left ventricle | Right ventricle |
| --- | --- |
| **Myocardial injury** | **Myocardial injury** |
| Ischaemia/infarction | Ischaemia/infarction |
| Myocarditis | Myocarditis |
| **Cardiomyopathy** | **Cardiomyopathy** |
| **Increased workload** | **Increased workload** |
| Systemic hypertension | Pulmonary hypertension due to: |
| Aortic and mitral valve disease |   left ventricle failure |
| Coarctation of the aorta |   chronic lung disease |
| Increased cardiac output: |   left-to-right shunting with increased blood flow |
|   anaemia |   pulmonary thromboembolism |
|   thyrotoxicosis |   pulmonary and tricuspid valve disease |

right ventricular failure is usually due to chronic obstructive pulmonary disease (COPD) (see Chapter 7, pp. 173–176) and less often pulmonary embolism. When the right ventricle fails, it dilates; stretching of the tricuspid ring results in valve incompetence and dilatation of the right atrium. Raised central venous pressure gives rise to systemic venous congestion and dependent peripheral oedema.

### High Output Failure

High output failure results from increased workload on both ventricles. Causes include thyrotoxicosis, anaemia, and arteriovenous fistulae. The onset of heart failure is associated with a fall in cardiac output but, because of the previously abnormally high output, even in failure, the absolute output may be normal or even increased.

## Pathology of Cardiac Transplantation

Heart transplantation is now an accepted treatment for end-stage heart failure with 5-year survival rates reaching 75%. In adults the most common indications are ischaemic heart disease and dilated cardiomyopathy. After the postoperative period, most deaths occur in the first year due to infection caused by immunosuppression and acute graft rejection. Acute rejection is detected and monitored using histological assessment of regular heart biopsies, with appropriate adjustment of immunosuppression. Thereafter, transplant-accelerated coronary artery disease is the main cause of death. The affected smaller epicardial coronary arteries show concentric thickening due to cellular proliferation and lipid accumulation, accompanied by intimal chronic inflammation. Ischaemic myocardial damage affects 50% of transplanted hearts at 5 years.

---

**CASE HISTORY 6.3**

A 50-year-old man, an ex-smoker with multiple previous myocardial infarcts, underwent heart transplantation because of intractable heart failure. The heart removed at surgery is shown in Fig. 6.79. The heart is dilated, typical of total heart failure. Sectioning revealed extensive, pale scarring in the wall of the left ventricle. One month after surgery, despite immunosuppressive therapy, the patient developed a fever, became lethargic, and the function of the transplanted heart deteriorated. Heart biopsy showed marked immunological rejection with widespread damage to the cardiac myocytes by infiltrating lymphocytes (Fig. 6.80). Urgent treatment with augmented immunosuppressive therapy controlled the rejection episode and heart function normalized. Soon thereafter the patient developed signs of a severe chest infection and *Aspergillus* sp. was isolated from the bronchoalveolar lavage fluid. The patient recovered with appropriate therapy. Four further significant rejection episodes occurred. Nine months after transplantation a mass developed adjacent to the heart and the patient died 2 months later. Fig. 6.81 shows white tumour tissue invading the left ventricular wall and the adjacent left lung. The tumour was an Epstein–Barr virus-positive post-transplantation lymphoma (or lymphoproliferative disorder) caused by immunosuppression (see Special Study Topic 8.1, pp. 202–204).

In summary, this heart transplant recipient developed two well-recognized, major complications of immunosuppressive therapy – infection and an Epstein–Barr virus-driven lymphoma.

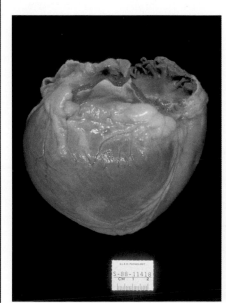

**FIG. 6.79** The ventricles of the heart removed at surgery during the transplantation procedure. The atria have been left to anastomose to the new organ.

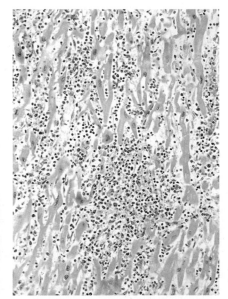

**FIG. 6.80** Diffuse chronic inflammation and myocyte damage indicate severe acute rejection of the allograft.

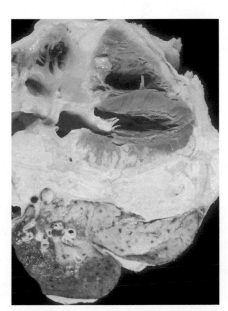

**FIG. 6.81** The heart is embedded in a white tumour mass consisting of diffuse large B-cell lymphoma, occupying most of the mediastinum.

## SUMMARY

- Ischaemia, infarction, thrombosis, and embolism are the key pathogenic mechanisms in the cardiovascular system.
- Disorders of the endothelium and the microcirculation result in oedema, disseminated intravascular coagulation, and shock.
- As arteries age they harden (arteriosclerosis).
- Atherosclerosis is the most important arterial disease in western populations. It narrows arteries, causing ischaemia, and weakens the aorta, causing aneurysms. Many factors predispose to its development.
- Hypertension (systemic arterial hypertension) damages the heart and arteries. It causes ischaemic heart disease, heart failure, stroke, and renal and retinal disease. It is caused by an interplay between genetic and environmental factors.
- Ischaemic heart disease is the largest cause of cardiac morbidity and mortality in the developed world. It presents with a variety of syndromes.
- Heart failure may be acute or chronic and may affect the left or right ventricle or both.

## FURTHER READING

Burke A, Tavora F. *Practical Cardiovascular Pathology*: *An atlas*. Philadelphia, PA: Lippincott, Williams & Wilkins, 2010.

Sheppard MN. *Practical Cardiovascular Pathology*, 2nd edn. London: Hodder Arnold, 2011.

# 7

# THE RESPIRATORY SYSTEM

Alexandra Rice

## THE NORMAL RESPIRATORY TRACT

### Key Points

- The upper airways conduct, warm, humidify, and filter air.
- The mucociliary transport mechanism traps organisms and particulate matter.
- The lower airways are responsible for gaseous exchange.

### The Nose

The nose warms, humidifies, and filters air. Filtration is by the nasal hairs and conchae (turbinates), causing alteration in airflow, so particles larger than 6 μm in diameter are trapped in nasal mucus. Sneezing, caused by nasal irritation, helps clear the nasal passages.

The inner nasal cavity sinuses, with their ostia in the lateral nasal walls, are lined by ciliated, pseudostratified, columnar epithelium. Goblet cells appear in the sinuses. The nasal sinuses consist of the frontal, sphenoidal, maxillary, and ethmoid sinuses, the last being a collection of air cells. Beneath the epithelium are seromucinous glands, which produce mucus, IgA, and other immunoglobulins as defence mechanisms. These extend to the bronchial tree. The epiglottis prevents aspiration of food and other materials into the respiratory tract. In the nasopharynx there are large masses of lymphoid tissue: the adenoids; the palatine, tubal and lingual tonsils; and aggregates of lymphoid tissue that circle the pharyngeal wall (Waldeyer's ring). They enlarge with antigenic stimulation, especially in childhood, and may be the site of pathological conditions, such as lymphomas.

### The Larynx, Trachea, and Bronchi

The larynx is divided into the supraglottis, glottis, and subglottis. The larynx acts as a vibrator via the vocal folds for speech. During normal breathing the folds are held wide open to allow air passage. With speech the folds close and airflow causes vibration. The intrinsic laryngeal muscles are innervated by the recurrent laryngeal branch of the vagus nerve. The epiglottis is lined by stratified squamous epithelium, but in the lower half it gives way to a ciliated, pseudostratified columnar type, characteristic of most of the larynx. The true folds are lined by stratified squamous epithelium.

The larynx is supported by a cartilaginous framework, connected by ligaments. The trachea comprises a series of 'C'-shaped cartilages, joined by fibroelastic membranes to form a hollow tube. Posteriorly lies the trachealis muscle. The midline cervical trachea lies anterior to the oesophagus. Subglottic tracheal lesions may cause oesophageal dysfunction and vice versa. The isthmus of the thyroid gland is anterior to the second to fourth rings.

The trachea divides into left and right main bronchi. The right continues in the general direction of the trachea, the left diverges at a greater angle. Thus aspiration is more common in the right lung, especially the middle and lower lobes. Bronchial cartilage progressively decreases with increasing distance from the trachea. At the terminal bronchiole (sixteenth division) it has disappeared. The airways continue dividing into respiratory bronchioles, alveolar ducts, and finally alveoli (Fig. 7.1). The terminal bronchiole is the smallest airway that is lined by bronchial epithelial cells. The terminal bronchiolar walls consist almost entirely of smooth muscle. The small bronchioles, i.e. terminal and those just proximal, play a larger role in determining airflow than the bronchi. This is because they have much more smooth muscle, which constricts easily. As they are small, they are easily occluded, as in bronchial asthma and chronic obstructive pulmonary disease. The respiratory bronchiole bears alveoli.

The cilia maintain the mucociliary escalator, causing upward passage of mucus and entrapped organisms or particulate matter to be expectorated. The ciliary shaft or cilium is a cytoplasmic extension from the cell surface. On transverse section the shaft shows an axial filament complex consisting of nine peripheral doublets of microtubules and two central microtubules. Radial spokes extend from central microtubules to the periphery of microtubular doublets. Each doublet has inner and outer dynein arms, essential for ciliary movement.

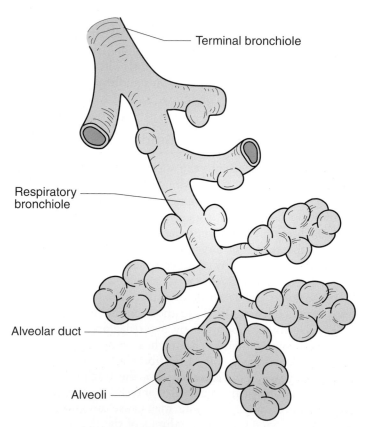

**FIG. 7.1** A model of the normal respiratory acinus: each acinus is formed by branching of a terminal bronchiole into a number of respiratory bronchioles, which eventually form alveolar ducts, the walls of which bear the alveoli.

Terminal bronchiole

Respiratory bronchiole

Alveolar duct

Alveoli

Just above the basement membrane are neuroendocrine cells, with an unknown role in the adult. They have clear cytoplasm and may occur as clusters, termed 'neuroepithelial bodies'. Neuroendocrine cells contain dense core secretory granules and can secrete hormones. In the first 3 months of life, when there is relative hypoxia, they may act as chemoreceptors. These cells increase in pulmonary fibrosis and hypoxia. Neuroendocrine cell hyperplasia is also seen in association with pulmonary carcinoid tumours.

There is a surface, non-ciliated, bronchiolar secretory cell termed a 'Clara cell'. These cells contain electron-dense, membrane-bound inclusions and myelin bodies, and produce surfactant proteins. Bronchial serous glands produce lysozyme and, if there is chronic cough, are converted to mucinous glands. The epithelium is regenerated by small pyramidal basal cells attached to the basement membrane.

## The Lung

The respiratory zone of the lung begins at the respiratory bronchiole and continues into alveolar ducts and alveoli. The alveolus is cup shaped and thin walled. Up to 96% of the alveolar wall is covered by type I pneumocytes, with thin cytoplasm to facilitate gas transfer between the alveolus and the pulmonary capillary. These cells are bound by tight junctions, which restrict the movement of ions and water. Approximately 7% of the alveolar surface is covered by type II pneumocytes, which lie in the corners of the alveolar walls. These cells form surfactant, phospholipids that lower the surface tension in the alveoli, thus preventing their collapse. These cells are also capable of cell division and are commonly hyperplastic following alveolar damage.

The interstitial space is the part of the septal wall that lies between the alveolar epithelial and capillary endothelial basement membranes. Normally inconspicuous, it is distended in any form of alveolar damage. It contains macrophages, myofibroblasts, mast cells, and occasional collagen and elastic fibres. Any thickening of this space hampers diffusion across the alveolar wall. The interstitial connective tissue forms a continuous sheet with that surrounding the blood vessels and bronchioles. This is important for removing fluid from alveoli to pulmonary lymphatics. Alveolar macrophages are common and may be intra-alveolar or interstitial. They are derived predominantly from bone marrow precursors and are increased in cigarette smokers.

Pulmonary lymphatics are present around pulmonary blood vessels at the alveolar level and in the septa and pleura. These drain directly into the mediastinal nodes, particularly in the upper lobes. The lymphatics can be traced to the respiratory bronchioles and continue around small bronchi and bronchioles, forming a plexus outside muscle. The lungs expand and contract by movement of either the diaphragm, supplied by the phrenic nerve (C3–5), or the ribs. The diaphragm lengthens or shortens the thoracic cavity. Elevation or depression of the ribs alters the anterior/posterior diameter of the chest wall. These muscles may be affected in neuromuscular disease. The lungs lie in the pleural cavities, the parietal and visceral layers of which are lined by mesothelial cells; these produce a thin film of fluid.

## Pulmonary Physiology

Lung physiology is most commonly investigated by means of pulmonary function and exercise tests. In the assessment of lung function the possibility of cardiac disease should be considered. The end-result of pulmonary ventilation is adequate tissue cell oxygenation and removal of excess carbon dioxide. To achieve this the partial pressure of oxygen in the alveoli must be above that of the blood flowing through the alveolar capillaries. Ventilation must also lower the partial pressure of carbon dioxide in the alveoli below that of the alveolar capillary blood to enable excess carbon dioxide to be removed. The partial pressure of oxygen ($PO_2$) and carbon dioxide ($PCO_2$) are important measures of the adequacy of oxygenation. In arterial and mixed venous blood the $PO_2$ is approximately 100 mmHg (13.33 kPa) and 40 mmHg (5.33 kPa), respectively. The corresponding figures for $PCO_2$ are approximately 40 mmHg (5.33 kPa) (arterial) and 46 mmHg (6.13 kPa) (mixed venous blood). Lung function depends on age, size, and sex, and normal values vary enormously.

The total amount of air that can be expired is the forced vital capacity (FVC), which depends on lung size, integrity of the respiratory muscles, and skeleton. Lung size is directly related to height. There is a decline in both these parameters with age. It may be affected by skeletal abnormality, weak respiratory muscles, diseases causing reduced lung volume, such as pulmonary fibrosis or large pleural effusions, or most commonly severe airway obstruction as in emphysema and bronchial asthma.

Forced expiratory volume in 1 second ($FEV_1$) is the volume of air expired during the first second of a forced maximal expiration. It is one of the most widely used lung function tests. It should be 70% or more of the FVC. If the ratio of $FEV_1$ to FVC falls below 70% this is strong evidence of obstructive airway disease, such as asthma (reversible) or chronic obstructive pulmonary disease (irreversible). If the ratio of $FEV_1$ to FVC remains the same in the presence of lung disease, the inference is that both FEV and FVC are diminished. This happens in restrictive lung disease, such as pulmonary fibrosis, where the compliance of the lung is reduced. $FEV_1$ and $FEV_1$:FVC ratio are important markers of severity of the disease, as well as progress during treatment.

At the start of forced expiration, air is rapidly accelerated to a maximum flow rate at a high lung volume. As expiration progresses, the speed of expulsion of air declines in a roughly linear fashion. The maximum speed is known as the peak expiratory flow rate (PEFR). This is dependent on both expiratory muscle effort and airway patency. With increasing age and airway obstruction, maximum flow rates become less dependent on effort. The more severe the airway obstruction, the less effort dependent they become.

Airway patency depends on size and the support of the surrounding elastic lung parenchyma. With expansion the pull of the stretched parenchyma holds airways open, especially the smaller ones. The elastic recoil also helps expel air from the alveoli during expiration. The PEFR is useful in assessment of the severity of asthma, chronic bronchitis, and emphysema.

Pulmonary arterial and left atrial pressures are measured by cardiac catheterization and the blood flow through the pulmonary vessels is calculated using the Fick principle. It is also possible to determine the pulmonary vascular resistance (arterial pressure wedge pressure). The normal pulmonary arterial pressure is 25/10 mmHg and pulmonary blood flow at rest is 4 L/min per m$^2$ of body surface area.

# DISEASES OF THE UPPER RESPIRATORY TRACT

## Disorders of the Nose

### The Common Cold

This is a highly infectious, common disease that is caused predominantly by rhinoviruses, of which there are more than 100 antigenic types, respiratory syncytial virus (RSV), parainfluenza viruses, Coxsackievirus A21, and coronaviruses. Children may act as a reservoir in the community. Because of the large number of strains, an individual is liable to contract two to three colds a year.

Clinically there is rhinorrhoea, nasal obstruction, sneezing, pyrexia, sore throat, and myalgia. Cough is due to postnasal discharge or more distal respiratory involvement by the virus. There is mucosal oedema and shedding of degenerate, columnar, epithelial cells, which contain viral inclusion bodies in the first 2–3 days. Sinusitis and chest disease may complicate the common cold in susceptible patients, e.g. those with chronic obstructive pulmonary disease (COPD). The exudate in the sinuses can become secondarily infected, typically by *Streptococcus pneumoniae* or *Haemophilus influenzae*. In chronic sinusitis the normal ciliated columnar epithelium is replaced by squamous epithelium, which hinders mucus clearance.

### Other Upper Respiratory Tract Infections

Other upper respiratory tract infections include influenza, herpes simplex and zoster, tuberculosis, and leprosy, the last (see Chapter 19, pp. 553–556) causing thickening of the nasal mucous membrane and perforation of the cartilage. Rhinoscleroma, caused by *Klebsiella rhinoscleromatis*, produces large deforming masses of nasal tissue. It is encountered in South America, parts of Africa, the Middle East, and India.

Fungal infections, e.g. aspergillosis, may form fungal balls, cause sinusitis, or rarely be invasive. Other fungi may affect this region, but they are more commonly seen in Asia and

Africa. Rhinosporidiosis, caused by *Rhinosporidium seeberi*, is transmitted by cattle and horses, and causes granulomatous nasal polyps.

### Allergic Rhinitis

Allergic rhinitis can be divided into seasonal (hayfever) and perennial allergic rhinitis. Hayfever mainly affects children and adolescents, at the peak of the pollen season. The important pollen allergens come from trees, grasses, and weeds, and are seen in spring, summer, and early autumn, respectively. House-dust mites, furry pets, moulds, or occupation (allergy to flour causing rhinitis in bakers), and rarely some foods, may be allergenic. These patients have a two- to threefold increased risk of developing perennial asthma. There is itching, watery rhinorrhoea, and congestion, causing serial sneezing and 'stuffy' head.

The nose is the target of allergic symptoms because of its effective filtering action for allergens. Pollen grains are 20–30 μm in size and cannot bypass the nose. There is inflammation, with infiltration by CD4 T lymphocytes of the Th2 (T-helper 2) type, mast cells, and eosinophils. Mast cells, stimulated by the allergen, release interleukin 3 (IL-3), IL-5, histamine, prostaglandins, bradykinin, and platelet-activating factor (PAF), which together cause many of the symptoms.

### Nasal and Paranasal Polyps

These complicate allergic and perennial rhinitis. Polyps (Fig. 7.2) consist of oedematous mucosa with variable numbers of eosinophils, chronic inflammation, and hyperplastic seromucinous glands. The surface respiratory epithelium shows goblet cell hyperplasia with a thickened basement membrane.

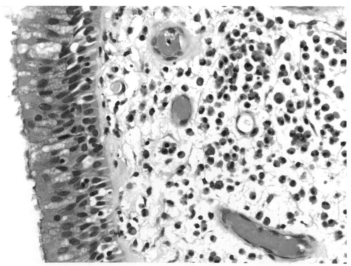

**FIG. 7.2** High-power view of a section of an allergic nasal polyp. It is lined by respiratory epithelium (left) and inflamed by a large number of eosinophils and some plasma cells.

### Wegener's Granulomatosis

This may be either a multisystem vasculitis or localized to one area of the respiratory tract. Over 80% of patients have nasal or paranasal involvement with 'nasal congestion'. The nasal mucosa is granular, crusted, and there may be septal perforation. This disorder is discussed in more detail in Chapters 6 (p. 125) and 13 (p. 412).

### Tumours of the Nose and Nasal Sinuses

Tumours of the nasal cavity and paranasal sinuses are rare but, because they grow into air-filled sinuses and soft tissues, they often present at an advanced stage. Sinonasal papilloma is the most common nasal tumour, occurring most frequently in men in their 60s. The aetiology is unknown. It resembles allergic nasal polyps with a corrugated surface, although is usually unilateral. It may be exophytic or inverted, the stroma being invaginated by stratified, non-keratinizing, squamous, or columnar epithelium. Mitoses are common and the greater the number the more likely the chance of recurrence. An inverted sinonasal papilloma may be accompanied or followed by carcinoma. Treatment is by total excision.

The nature of most of the remaining tumours can be deduced from knowledge of sinonasal histology. Thus there are salivary gland-like tumours, and tumours arising from bone, nerve, blood vessels, or ectopic cerebral tissue. The most common malignant nasal tumour is squamous carcinoma, whereas adenocarcinoma is more common in the upper nasal cavity and sinuses, especially the ethmoid, because of the presence of glands and lining respiratory epithelium. Adenocarcinoma is seen particularly in wood and nickel workers. Carcinomas spread locally and metastasize to cervical lymph nodes. Malignant variants of salivary gland tumours arising from minor salivary gland tissue, such as adenoid cystic carcinoma, and malignant melanoma may also be seen.

Lymphomas and sarcomas also occur at this site. T-cell and natural killer (NK) cell lymphomas are more common in Asia and South America, whereas, in the west, B-cell lymphomas predominate. These are usually high-grade, large cell type and cause soft-tissue or osseous destruction. The Epstein–Barr virus (EBV) genome is seen in many of these lymphomas.

## Diseases of the Larynx and Trachea

Congenital and acquired laryngeal conditions cause respiratory distress (stridor) in children and adults. These include congenital subglottic stenosis, laryngeal cysts arising from the mucous glands of the saccular appendage, laryngeal atresia and webs, viral laryngotracheobronchitis (croup), and acute epiglottitis often due to *H. influenzae* type b. Diphtheria, due to *Corynebacterium diphtheriae*, may be confined to the larynx. A 'false membrane', composed of fibrin and neutrophils, covers the epiglottis and false and true vocal folds, causing obstruction. Tuberculosis, sarcoidosis, leprosy, and fungal infections can also affect the larynx. The trachea is rarely affected by disease in adults, but in children acute laryngotracheobronchitis can be seen, as an extension of the laryngeal diseases mentioned above.

## Laryngeal Oedema

There is no lymphatic drainage from the true vocal fold area so any oedema persists. Excess fluid in the space between the epithelium and the vocal ligaments (Reinke's space) causes vocal fold swelling (Reinke's oedema). It is most common in smokers and there may be marked vocal fold mucosal swelling resembling a polyp.

## Benign Neoplasms

Recurrent laryngeal papillomatosis is most common in infants aged between 2 months and 5 years. It presents with hoarseness, weak cry, and stridor. The disease is caused by human papillomavirus (typically type 6 or 11), transmitted vaginally from women with genital condylomata. The papillomas occur anywhere in the respiratory tract but the larynx, usually the true folds, is always affected. The papillomas are glistening, fleshy, irregular, nodular tumours. They are covered with fronds of squamous epithelium with marked koilocytosis. Repeat chest radiographs are required to identify lung involvement. Regular follow-up is necessary. Benign connective tissue tumours, such as granular cell tumour, are occasionally seen.

## Malignant Tumours of the Larynx

Squamous cell carcinoma accounts for 95% of laryngeal malignancies and is classified by site as supraglottic (30%), glottic (60%), or subglottic (10%). Cigarette smoking and alcohol are the main aetiological factors; others include infection with EBV and human papillomaviruses, and coal tar products, sawdust, and paints. Cell carcinoma of the larynx is most common on the anterior part of the true fold. It is often seen as a white plaque with a raised, well-defined margin and a variable surface ranging from furrows to ulceration. Hoarseness occurs early and supraglottic lesions can be painful. Referred pain to the ipsilateral ear, mediated by the vagus nerve, indicates cartilaginous invasion. Stridor and dyspnoea, due to tumour bulk, occur late. Dysphagia occurs due to extension to the base of the tongue or hypopharynx. Tumour metastasizes to the cervical lymph nodes. Other rarer laryngeal tumours include adenoid cystic carcinoma, small cell carcinoma, and adenocarcinoma.

# CONGENITAL ABNORMALITIES AND PAEDIATRIC LUNG DISEASE

Many congenital abnormalities, such as tracheal agenesis, are rare. Tracheo-oesophageal fistula, which allows food to travel from the oesophagus into the main airways, causes choking. Lung cysts may be congenital and persist into adult life. These include bronchogenic cysts, pulmonary sequestration, congenital cystic adenomatoid malformation, and congenital lobar emphysema. Acquired cysts are due to previous infection, especially staphylococcal, and also include hydatid disease or obstruction of distal lung by a foreign body.

Pulmonary cilia dyskinesia or immotile cilia syndrome is part of Kartagener's syndrome (situs invertus, bronchiectasis, chronic rhinosinusitis, and absent frontal sinuses).

## Hyaline Membrane Disease (Respiratory Distress Syndrome)

This disorder affects preterm babies weighing <1,500 g who develop cyanosis, chest wall retraction, and grunting respiration within an hour of birth. Chest radiographs show a ground-glass appearance. Immature lungs lack surfactant, causing terminal airway collapse. The lungs are heavy at postmortem examination. The earliest change is necrosis of the epithelium in distal bronchi and bronchioles. Hyaline membranes (composed of protein-rich exudate) block terminal bronchioles and developing alveolar ducts, as well as lining immature alveoli.

If the patient survives ventilation, bronchopulmonary dysplasia (BPD) develops. There is bronchiolar and bronchial damage with obliterative bronchiolitis. Hyaline membranes continue to form and involve peripheral alveoli. Interstitial fibrosis develops and alveoli are lined by prominent type II cells. The lung is firm and nodular with focal emphysema. The vessels are thick walled with intimal fibrosis.

The underlying cause of BPD is epithelial/endothelial barrier damage. There is continued interstitial fluid and protein leakage, causing hyaline membranes and stimulating fibrosis. High ventilatory oxygen concentrations probably play an important part. The preterm infant is susceptible to relatively normal inspired oxygen concentrations.

# BRONCHIAL ASTHMA

**Key Points**

- Asthma presents with bronchospasm, which can be life threatening. Immune mechanisms are important.
- Asthma is associated with many environmental factors, including pollens, animal fur, chemicals, and diet.
- Asthma is increasing in prevalence.
- The important cells in asthma are mast cells, eosinophils, and lymphocytes.
- Histamine, leukotrienes, and other cytokines cause smooth muscle contraction, increased vascular permeability, and oedema of the bronchiolar wall.

Asthma is the main reversible cause of airflow limitation. Patients have wheezing, chest tightness, shortness of breath, often worse at night, and cough. Cough may be prominent, causing a misdiagnosis of chronic bronchitis. There is a decrease in $FEV_1$ and PEFR, the latter showing variability over time.

Asthma occurs in 12–15% of children, and the incidence increased by 50% between the mid-1970s and mid-1980s in industrialized countries. The prevalences of eczema and hayfever similarly rose, suggesting an increase in allergy.

## Aetiology

Atopy is an established risk factor and exposure to allergen in the first 2–3 years appears important, providing the stimulus for airway sensitization.

Environmental determinants include sensitizing chemicals, air pollution by allergens (e.g. soya bean), or indoor allergens (e.g. tobacco smoke, viral infections, and house-dust mite). Over 200 materials can cause occupational asthma. Diet may be important, either directly or perhaps as a surrogate for other markers. High salt diets and those containing much 'junk' food are linked to an increased prevalence of asthma whereas those high in oily fish appear protective. Breastfeeding protects babies against the disease. Infections such as measles are protective, especially if occurring in the first year. The keeping of pets may be important, because animal dander is an aeroallergen.

Asthma is exacerbated by atmospheric pollution, high concentrations of sulphur dioxide, nitrogen dioxide, ozone, cigarette smoke, and dust, cold air, and exercise. Similarly drugs, such as aspirin or other non-steroidal anti-inflammatory drugs, may provoke attacks.

Genes also play an important role, with one gene governing bronchial hyperresponsiveness and regulating serum IgE levels located near a major locus on chromosome 5q. Genes for cytokines IL-3, -4, -5, -9, and -13, and granulocyte–macrophage colony-stimulating factor (GM-CSF), which regulate IgE, mast cell, basophil, and eosinophil functions, also lie on chromosome 5. However. no single gene accounts for the major part of the expression of the disease. This phenotypic variability is probably in keeping with the aetiological heterogeneity and environmental influences.

## Pathology and Pathophysiology

In death from status asthmaticus, the lungs are hyperexpanded due to mucus plugging. Bronchial and bronchiolar walls are infiltrated by eosinophils, neutrophils, plasma cells, and lymphocytes. These inflammatory cells cause hyperaemia, and mucosal and submucosal oedema. Eosinophils are not seen in normal mucosa. The surface epithelium is focally sloughed in areas. In the surviving epithelium there is goblet cell hyperplasia, especially in the peripheral airways. The basement membrane may be thickened by deposition of collagen. There is prominent bronchiolar smooth muscle,

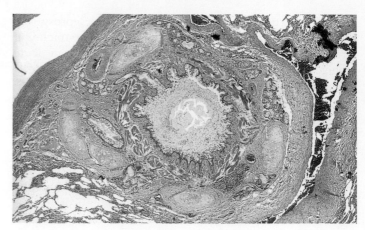

**Fig. 7.3** Asthma: microscopic view of a bronchiole with mucus in the lumen, submucosal oedema and inflammation, and prominent smooth muscle.

causing contraction and luminal narrowing (Fig. 7.3). Biopsies from non-fatal cases show a similar cellular infiltrate, with or without basement membrane thickening and goblet cell hyperplasia.

The physiological and clinical features in asthma are the result of interaction between the resident and infiltrating inflammatory cells and the airway epithelium. This results in a release of chemical mediators from the cells. The lymphocytes are of Th2 progeny and secrete cytokines including IL-4, -5, -6, tumour necrosis factor (TNF) $\alpha$, platelet-derived growth factor (PDGF), and GM-CSF. IL-4 and -6 are needed for the recruitment of mucosal mast cells and IL-5 and GM-CSF for maturation and priming of the eosinophils. Mast cell activation releases histamine (causing bronchoconstriction), leukotrienes, and prostaglandins. These factors increase microvascular permeability, resulting in oedema, and cause smooth muscle contraction, mucus section, and initiation of neutrophil and eosinophil recruitment. Mast cells also synthesize cytokines, including IL-3, -4, -5, and -6, and TNF-$\alpha$.

Eosinophils are attracted to endothelial cells, initially attaching to intercellular adhesion molecule-1 (ICAM-1) and vascular cell adhesion molecule-1 (VCAM-1), then migrating out of the vessel. They release toxic granule proteins, such as eosinophil cationic protein (ECP) and neutrophil basic protein (NBP), oxygen free radicals, leukotrienes, PAF, cytokines, and growth factors. Toxic granule proteins cause shedding of bronchial epithelium. Airway epithelial cells, fibroblasts, and endothelial cells also produce cytokines, including IL-6 and -8, GM-CSF, TNF-$\alpha$, and PDGF, promoting the inflammatory process.

## Complications

Pneumothorax is caused by overdistended lungs and rupture of pleural blebs. Mucus impaction may show contamination with *Aspergillus* species (Fig. 7.4). This fungus may itself provoke asthma. Bronchiectasis due to persistent mucus plugging is an occasional complication.

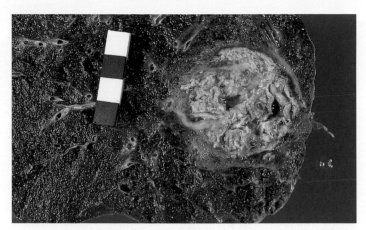

**FIG. 7.4** Aspergilloma: this slice of lung shows a large pale ball of fungus (*Aspergillus* sp.) mixed with mucus in a markedly dilated bronchus (see p. 186).

# OTHER DISEASES OF THE AIRWAYS

## Cystic Fibrosis

### Key Points

- Cystic fibrosis is the most common congenital lung disease, but other systems are involved
- It is inherited as an autosomal recessive trait
- It is caused by a defect in the cystic fibrosis membrane conductance receptor
- Increased viscosity of mucus leads to blockage of bronchi and ducts, with atrophy or infection.

Cystic fibrosis affects 1 in 2,500 infants in the UK. It is an autosomal recessive disease, due to a defect in the gene on the long arm of chromosome 7. This gene encodes the cystic fibrosis membrane conductance regulator (CFTR). CFTR is a cAMP-regulated membrane protein, acting as a low-conductance chloride channel across the epithelium. Mutations in this gene cause reduced chloride permeability across epithelial membranes, altering mucus composition, making it thicker and therefore more liable to cause obstruction. There are over 250 genetic mutations in cystic fibrosis, some giving different clinical presentations. The most common is δ F508, which removes a phenylalanine residue at position 508 of the CFTR protein.

Cystic fibrosis is a multisystem disease, but the lung is often affected most. It involves the bowel (meconium ileus or steatorrhoea) and liver (biliary cirrhosis), causes male infertility (blockage of the seminal vesicles although the patient produces normal sperm), recurrent pancreatitis (pancreatic duct obstruction), and nasal polyps (part of chronic sinusitis). There is excessive sweat containing chloride, sodium, and potassium, leading to the diagnostic abnormal sweat test.

Bronchial mucus is poorly hydrated and pulmonary mucociliary transport is impaired due to increased mucus viscosity and abnormal sulphated mucins. Mucostasis leads to infection and patients with cystic fibrosis experience recurrent pneumonia with organisms such as *Pseudomonas aeruginosa*, *Staphylococcus aureus* and *Aspergillus* sp. Inflammation associated with these infections weakens the bronchi and the negative intrathoracic pressure pulls them outwards, causing bronchiectasis (see Fig. 7.5) – permanently dilated bronchi filled with pus. Small airways also show acute or chronic inflammation with purulent bronchiolitis, progressing to obliteration. Pneumothorax is common, secondary to emphysematous blebs.

## Bronchiectasis

### Key Points

- In bronchiectasis, there is abnormal and irreversible dilatation of bronchi.
- It is a complication of cystic fibrosis, tuberculosis (TB), bronchiolitis, and pneumonia
- It becomes chronically infected and causes abscesses, e.g. in the brain.

Bronchiectasis is defined as abnormal and irreversible dilatation of bronchi (Fig. 7.5). It may affect one lung segment or be widely distributed. Bronchiectasis is the result of repeated episodes of infection, usually with some degree of lung collapse. The bronchial walls are weakened, lack support, and are expanded by the force of inspiration. Bronchiolitis and bronchopneumonia in childhood, cystic fibrosis, and chronic pulmonary TB are common precursors. An obstructing lung cancer can cause localized bronchiectasis in the distal segment.

The dilated bronchi become crowded together with loss of the intervening lung parenchyma. Although they are initially lined by respiratory epithelium, squamous metaplasia often follows, and eventually the cavities become chronically infected. The patient has a chronic cough with foul-smelling breath and sputum. Bacteraemia may lead to the formation of systemic abscesses, classically in the brain. Amyloidosis may supervene.

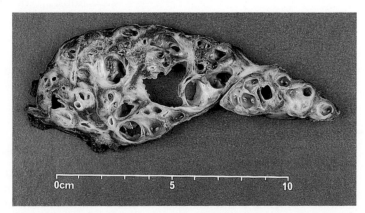

**FIG. 7.5** Bronchiectasis: a slice of left lung showing markedly dilated bronchi, scarring, and loss of lung parenchyma.

## Bronchiolitis

The term 'bronchiolitis' describes various inflammatory diseases of the distal bronchioles. Patients have dyspnoea, cough, variable amounts of sputum, râles, or rhonchi. The chest radiograph shows hyperinflation with interstitial or alveolar infiltrates. The main causes are:

- inhalation injury
- infection, e.g. respiratory syncytial virus (RSV), *Mycoplasma pneumoniae*
- drug- or chemical-induced reactions
- connective tissue diseases
- organ transplantation
- idiopathic.

Bronchiolitis may occur as part of other diseases, e.g. asthma and COPD. Acute bronchiolitis is common in children after viral infections, with acute inflammation filling the bronchiolar lumina and extending, with fibrosis, into the adjacent peribronchiolar tissue. Bronchiolitis is classified histologically into:

- acute bronchiolitis
- respiratory bronchiolitis
- mineral dust airway disease
- follicular bronchiolitis
- constrictive bronchiolitis (obliterative bronchiolitis).

These histological pictures have varying aetiologies. Acute bronchiolitis may be seen in infection, whereas follicular bronchiolitis and constrictive bronchiolitis occur most commonly with rheumatoid disease. In the early stages there is intraluminal, mucosal, submucosal, and peribronchiolar inflammation in membranous and respiratory bronchioles. The inflammatory infiltrate has variable numbers of polymorphs, lymphocytes, and plasma cells. With time there may be peribronchiolar fibrosis and obliterative fibrosis of the bronchiolar lumen.

# THE EFFECTS OF CIGARETTE SMOKE

### Key Points

- Cigarette smoke contains carcinogens and addictive agents, among many injurious factors.
- Smoking causes many diseases, including chronic obstructive pulmonary disease (COPD), coronary atheroma, and many cancers.
- Passive smoking can result in fetal damage, increased childhood infections, and disease in adults.
- COPD consists of chronic bronchitis, small airway disease, and pulmonary emphysema.
- COPD produces fixed airway obstruction, with decreased $FEV_1$ and PEFR.

## Constituents of Cigarette Smoke

Cigarette smoke contains more than 4,000 constituents. These include carbon monoxide, hydrogen cyanide, aldehydes, cadmium (linked to emphysema), ammonia, nicotine, and benz(a)anthracene and benzopyrene (both potent carcinogens). These are suspended in water droplets with resinous cores, which are absorbed onto bronchial walls and propelled on the mucociliary escalator back to the mouth; 98% of these particles are removed by cilia within 24 hours. Smaller particles enter alveoli and, if undissolved, are ingested by macrophages and removed to the lymphatics.

Passive smoking increases the risk of lung cancer and ischaemic heart disease and is linked to an increased incidence of asthma and chest infections in children. Some of the diseases caused or associated with cigarette smoking are given in *Table 7.1*.

**TABLE 7.1** Diseases associated with cigarette smoke (the effects of cigarette smoke are many and varied, with few organs unaffected)

| Target | Disease | Examples | Effects |
|---|---|---|---|
| Arteries | Atherosclerosis | Coronary artery occlusion | Myocardial ischaemia, infarction |
| | | Carotid arteries | Risk of cerebrovascular accident |
| | | Aorta and other arteries | Hypertension, peripheral ischaemia |
| Lung | Chronic obstructive pulmonary disease | Chronic bronchitis and emphysema | Breathlessness, irreversible airway obstruction, cyanosis |
| | Carcinoma | Squamous and other carcinomas | Local airway obstruction, haemoptysis, systemic spread, cachexia |
| | Asthma | | |
| | Lung infections | | |
| Bladder | Transitional cell carcinoma | | Haematuria |
| Pancreas | Adenocarcinoma | | Biliary obstruction |
| Cervix uteri | Squamous cell carcinoma | Cofactor synergizing with human papillomavirus infection | Bleeding per vaginam |
| Colon | Adenoma and adenocarcinoma | Cofactor with other factors such as diet, inherited genetic susceptibility | Bleeding per rectum, faecal occult blood |

# CHRONIC OBSTRUCTIVE PULMONARY DISEASE

> **Key Points**
>
> - Chronic obstructive pulmonary disease (COPD) consists of chronic bronchitis, small airway disease, and pulmonary emphysema.
> - It produces irreversible airway obstruction and can result in hypoxic pulmonary hypertension.
> - Death is from bronchopneumonia, respiratory or cardiac failure, or other cigarette-induced disease, such as myocardial infarction or lung cancer.

COPD encompasses three pathological entities, which are considered separately pathologically, but often coexist: chronic bronchitis, pulmonary emphysema, and small airway disease.

## Epidemiology

In the UK, 6% of male and 3% of female deaths are caused by COPD. The reason for the male predominance is unknown. The most important aetiological factor in COPD is tobacco smoking; others include occupation, especially those that are dust associated such as coal mining, and $\alpha_1$-antitrypsin (AAT) deficiency. The wide variation in susceptibility of smokers to the development of COPD is at least partly genetic. The symptoms have insidious onset, with a morning smoker's cough and gradually worsening exertional dyspnoea, especially in damp weather, and increasing numbers of chest infections with *H. influenzae* and *Streptococcus pneumoniae*. The chest radiograph shows hyperinflation with an enlarged heart and prominent hila if there is cor pulmonale, due to the prominent pulmonary arteries. There are upper, and sometimes lower, lobe emphysematous bullae. There is fixed airway obstruction with a decrease in $FEV_1$ and PEFR, reflecting loss of elastic recoil and/or narrowing of the airways.

## Chronic Bronchitis

Chronic bronchitis was defined functionally by the Medical Research Council as 'chronic or recurrent increase in the volume of bronchial secretions, sufficient to cause expectoration on most days for a minimum of three months of the year, for not less than two successive years, which cannot be attributed to other cardiac or pulmonary disease'. The presence of chronic bronchitis (very common in smokers) is not a good marker of functional impairment. In chronic bronchitis there is an increased mass of serous and mucous glands (Fig. 7.6), and goblet cells in smokers extend to the terminal bronchioles. Most mucus is produced by the submucosal glands, but hypersecretion does not probably contribute to the pathological basis of the fixed airway obstruction in COPD.

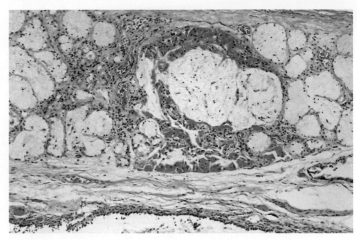

**FIG. 7.6** Microscopic view of the bronchial wall in chronic bronchitis. There are prominent mucous glands in the submucosa.

## Pulmonary Emphysema

This is defined as a condition of the lung characterized by permanent dilatation of the airways, distal to the terminal bronchiole. Emphysema is an 'apparent' dilatation of airspaces but is, in fact, due to destruction of alveolar walls (see Special Study Topic 7.1). The destruction has two major effects:

1. Loss of pulmonary surface area for gas exchange (leading to hypoxia)
2. Loss of elastic support for small airways; this is the means by which airways collapse and narrowing occurs (and thus obstruction).

Emphysema excludes pulmonary overinflation, as in bronchial asthma or post-pneumonectomy. *Post mortem* emphysematous lungs are overexpanded and fill the chest. Emphysema can be categorized as:

- centriacinar (centrilobular)
- panacinar (panlobular)
- bullous
- paraseptal
- scar.

The classification depends on an understanding of the functional unit of the lung (the respiratory acinus) (see Fig. 7.1). Thus centriacinar emphysema is characterized by an increase in size of the respiratory bronchioles, which are dilated and often have black pigment (carbon) in their walls (Fig. 7.7). The adjacent alveoli may also show dilatation. Panacinar emphysema (Fig. 7.8) usually shows an upper lobe distribution and is characterized by persistent enlargement and fusion of airspaces involving the entire acinus. If there is lower lobe panacinar emphysema, one should consider if the patient has AAT deficiency.

Bullous emphysema usually occurs either at anterior margins or at the apices of the upper lobes, and shows airspaces with few strands of alveolar tissue. A bulla is defined as an emphysematous space with a diameter >1 cm. Bullae and

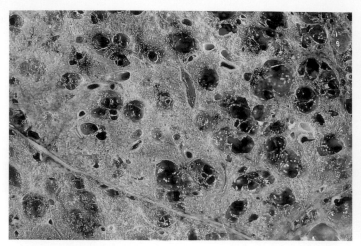

**FIG. 7.7** Centriacinar emphysema: this slice of lung shows expanded airspaces around respiratory bronchioles.

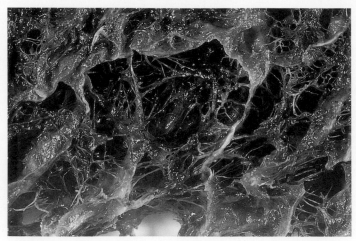

**FIG. 7.8** Panacinar emphysema: this slice of upper lobe shows more diffuse enlargement of airspaces than seen in Fig. 7.7.

blebs, which are <2 mm in diameter, may rupture causing a pneumothorax and lung collapse. Blebs are more common in young, tall men with some 'marfanoid' features, suggesting in this group that there is an underlying collagen disease. Centriacinar, panacinar, and bullous forms of emphysema often coexist. Surgeons excise apical bullous emphysema to remove useless tissue and allow the more preserved lower lobes to provide better respiratory function. Paraseptal and scar emphysema may be associated with other primary diseases, e.g. TB (scar emphysema), and are localized and seldom cause a clinical problem.

In the normal adult there is no muscle in pulmonary arteries <100 μm in diameter. In chronic hypoxia there is growth of muscle from more proximal arteries into arterioles, which are then termed 'muscularized'. Intimal longitudinal muscle grows in muscular pulmonary arteries and pulmonary arterioles, and in time is replaced by intimal fibrosis. The resultant increase in pulmonary vascular resistance causes pulmonary arterial hypertension causing cor pulmonale. This is defined by the World Health Organization as 'hypertrophy of the right ventricle resulting from diseases affecting the function and/or structure of the lungs, except when the pulmonary alterations are the result of diseases that primarily affect the left side of the heart, as in congenital disease'. Right ventricular hypertrophy is associated with both panacinar and centriacinar emphysema but a smaller percentage of lung tissue needs to be involved by centriacinar than panacinar

emphysema to produce right ventricular hypertrophy. Usually the type, rather than the severity, of emphysema is associated with the development of right ventricular failure. In centriacinar emphysema the percentage of lung tissue functionally destroyed is greater than in the panacinar variety.

## Small Airway Disease

This refers to abnormality of terminal and small bronchioles. There may be an asthmatic component to COPD with smooth muscle contraction, subepithelial fibrosis, and chronic inflammation, causing luminal narrowing and airflow obstruction. The lumen may be further occluded by mucus and necrotic cells. Goblet cell and sometimes squamous cell metaplasia impede the mucociliary escalator flow. Tissue remodelling in COPD may also result in loss of bronchioles.

## Cause of Death in COPD

Death in COPD is from bronchopneumonia, congestive cardiac failure, or respiratory failure. There is also an increased risk of lung cancer.

## $\alpha_1$-Antitrypsin Deficiency

$\alpha_1$-Antitrypsin is a major serum protease inhibitor. It is a glycoprotein, produced in hepatocytes and macrophages.

---

## 7.1 Special Study Topic

### EMPHYSEMA IN CHRONIC OBSTRUCTIVE PULMONARY DISEASE (COPD)

Emphysema, together with chronic bronchitis and small airway disease, makes up the clinical entity COPD, which tends to be progressive, is irreversible, and is characterized

by obstruction to air flow resulting in hypoxia, breathlessness, and eventually respiratory failure. Often overshadowed by lung cancer in public awareness, it is a major health problem and affects about 8/1,000 worldwide, being among the top 10 causes of mortality and causing even more morbidity. Cigarette smoking is strongly implicated; thus COPD is a growing problem in developing countries

## Special Study Topic continued . . .

where smoking is actively promoted and the market is increasing each year. Emphysema, defined as a loss of lung parenchyma without significant scarring, is perhaps the more significant component of COPD with serious clinical sequelae.

## Aetiology and Pathogenesis of Emphysema

The most important known cause of emphysema is cigarette smoking. However, not every smoker develops emphysema and not all patients with emphysema have smoked. The aetiology is therefore more complex; other modifying factors must be important.

Patients with genetically determined deficiency of AAT may develop both emphysema and cirrhosis of the liver. As AAT deficiency causes an imbalance of proteases favouring tissue destruction, the theory is that these patients are more susceptible to the effects of proteases released from inflammatory cells in the lung, causing tissue destruction. Although this seems likely to be true for this particular disease, it is less certain that this is generally applicable, e.g. the emphysema in cases of AAT deficiency tends to affect the whole acinus (panacinar), in keeping with an overall reduction in circulating antiprotease protection. By contrast, most cases of cigarette smoking-associated emphysema have predominantly focal damage at the entrance to the acinus (centriacinar), where reactive particulate components of smoke are deposited, in keeping with local damage. Thus, emphysema is heterogeneous, in both aetiology and pattern, and may be modulated by genetic susceptibility. As well as increased tissue enzyme activity, inflammation, apoptosis, and tissue remodelling have all been implicated.

## Genetic Susceptibility

In about 2% of cases of COPD, AAT deficiency may be important. AAT opposes the effects of neutrophil proteases. The normal M allele is the most common (>95%). The S allele (3%) is associated with mildly reduced plasma levels of AAT. However, the Z allele (1%) is associated with low levels: homozygosity for Z (protease inhibitor phenotype PiZZ) leads to <10% of normal levels of AAT in plasma. Not all PiZZ individuals develop emphysema and smoking certainly increases the likelihood, in keeping with the thesis that susceptibility to emphysema is multifactorial. Similarly, but less strikingly, other enzymes involved in metabolism of oxidant components of smoke have been shown to be polymorphic. The polymorphisms may affect the inducibility of the gene, the amount of protein product produced, or its activity. A large number of studies have provided inconclusive evidence on the roles of glutathione-S-transferases, microsomal epoxide hydrolases, and a host of other enzymes. Thus, although

there is some support for an oxidant/antioxidant balance, the attempts to exploit this therapeutically have also failed to impress. This does not mean that genetic susceptibility is irrelevant; rather it emphasizes the complex and multifactorial nature of the disease.

## Inflammation

Reactive components in cigarette smoke trigger a host inflammatory response with recruitment of inflammatory cells including neutrophils, resident and incoming macrophages, and CD81+ T lymphocytes. Recurrent, low-level inflammatory damage causes tissue remodelling and ultimately disruption of alveolar wall to airway attachments, which are crucial for maintaining airway patency. Loss of these attachments leads to collapse of airways on expiration, which obstructs airflow.

## Remodelling of Extracellular Matrix

It is increasingly apparent that there is a process of remodelling and maintenance of lung structure in adult life. Cigarette smoke, inflammatory cytokines, and even changes in mechanical force can influence tissue remodelling in a number of ways, including release of tissue enzymes and increased apoptosis of epithelial cells (both alveolar and bronchiolar) and capillary endothelial cells. In a number of human and animal settings emphysema is associated with activation of tissue metalloproteases (MMPs). MMP1 degrades perlecan and collagens, and can inactivate AAT. MMP9 and -12 expression is altered in emphysema. These MMPs can also liberate and activate latent transforming growth factor $\beta$ and other cytokines.

This cycle of inflammation and remodelling can continue unregulated, explaining why the disease can progress even after cessation of cigarette smoking.

## Lessons from Transgenic Studies

The use of transgenic mice alongside other animal models has led to a plethora of possible candidates for the tissue damage seen in emphysema. Surfactants, integrins, extracellular matrix, MMPs, and cytokines have all been implicated. The take-home message is that the aetiology and pathogenesis of emphysema are complex. There is no single cause but rather a matrix of susceptibility factors, both genetic and environmental, that conspire in some cases to cause disease.

## Conclusion

Emphysema as part of COPD excites less enthusiasm and concern than perhaps it should. This is in part because it is

## Special Study Topic continued . . .

difficult to study. Several very strongly held, and opposing, views on its cause have been tried, tested, and found wanting. Each has contributed to our understanding of the disease but has also highlighted how heterogeneous and complex it is. But from the extensive information now emerging new ideas for treatment are being suggested.

### Further Reading

Al-Jamal R, Wallace WAH, Harrison DJ. Gene therapy for chronic obstructive pulmonary disease: twilight or triumph? *Expert Opin Biol Ther* 2005;**5**:333–346.

Tuder RM, Petrache I. Pathogenesis of chronic obstructive pulmonary disease. *J Clin Invest* 2012;**122**:2749–2755.

Deficiency results from mutations in a gene located on chromosome 14q.31–32.3. Approximately 75 alleles have been identified at the AAT locus. The phenotype (Pi type) is determined by isoelectric examination of serum. The most common British phenotype is PiM, but low serum AAT levels are seen in PiZ and PiS. Deficiency is an autosomally recessive condition seen in 1/3,000 white people. As well as liver cirrhosis, patients develop panacinar emphysema that is more prominent in the lower lobes.

## ACUTE AND CHRONIC INTERSTITIAL LUNG DISEASE

This group includes a number of lung conditions of varying aetiology, all characterized functionally by a restrictive physiological abnormality. The term 'interstitial' is used but in practice there is evidence of both intra-alveolar and interstitial fibrosis at some stage of the disease. Fibrosis may also be seen secondary to other pulmonary diseases such as sarcoidosis.

### Adult Respiratory Distress Syndrome

Adult respiratory distress syndrome (ARDS) is an extreme form of acute lung injury associated with a variety of pulmonary and extrapulmonary insults (*Table 7.2*).

ARDS has multiple causes but the basic pathology is identical, irrespective of aetiology. The term has many synonyms, the best being diffuse alveolar damage (DAD). It may

**Key Points**

- Adult respiratory distress syndrome (ARDS) presents with severe dyspnoea, hypoxaemia, and diffuse pulmonary infiltrates.
- It is mediated by polymorphs and may be complicated by fibrosis.
- Pathology shows hyaline membranes, and fibrin thrombi, progressing to intra-alveolar and interstitial fibrosis.
- ARDS is characterized by uncontrolled activation of inflammatory mediators especially TNF, and IL-1, -6, and -8.

occur as part of multiorgan failure. Infection by the severe acute respiratory syndrome (SARS) virus gives a similar histological picture.

Clinically the patient develops severe dyspnoea, marked hypoxaemia with cyanosis, and tachypnoea that is refractory to oxygen therapy. There is decreased lung compliance with diffuse bilateral pulmonary infiltrates. There is a latent period varying from several hours to days after the insult, during which the clinical features are those of the underlying illness.

The early changes have been little studied in humans, for obvious reasons. These vary depending on which side of the basement membrane the insult occurs. The initial changes probably affect type I pneumocytes, which separate from the basement membrane. There is also type II pneumocyte damage, affecting surfactant production, and focal endothelial damage. There is interstitial oedema and fibroblast ingrowth to repair the gap left by the damaged type I cells. With loss of type I cells, fibrin leaks through epithelial cell junctions. The mixture of fibrin, dead cells, and plasma proteins makes up hyaline membranes (Fig. 7.9). Early alveolar wall congestion progresses to give rise to fibrin thrombi in arteries and capillaries (disseminated intravascular coagulation) and an increase in megakaryocytes in the pulmonary capillaries releasing platelets. As early as 48 hours, loose myxoid interstitial and sometimes intra-alveolar fibrosis begin. This is the characteristic pathology of ARDS of any cause. The pathogenesis of ARDS is summarized diagrammatically in Fig. 7.10.

**TABLE 7.2** Clinical scenarios associated with acute respiratory distress syndrome

| Respiratory | Non-respiratory |
| --- | --- |
| Infection (viral, bacterial) | Sepsis |
| Aspiration | Trauma (with hypotension) |
| Toxin inhalation | Burns |
| Oxygen therapy | Pancreatitis |
| | Ingested toxins (e.g. Paraquat) |

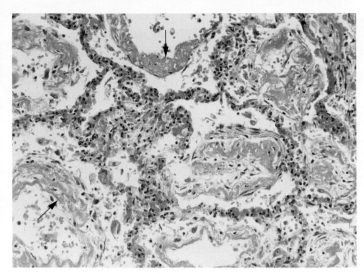

**Fig. 7.9** Lung section from postmortem examination on a patient who developed adult respiratory distress syndrome following peritonitis. Neutrophil polymorphs are packed in the alveolar capillaries and fibrin is present in alveoli, in places forming hyaline membranes (arrows).

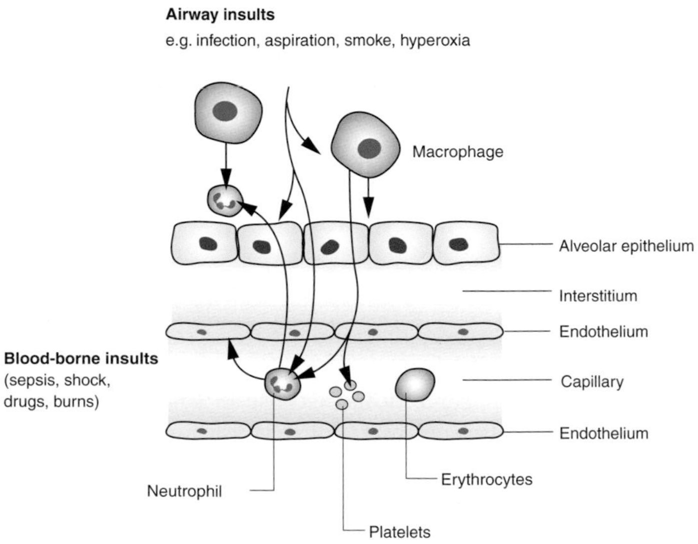

**Airway insults**
e.g. infection, aspiration, smoke, hyperoxia

Macrophage

Alveolar epithelium

Interstitium

Endothelium

**Blood-borne insults**
(sepsis, shock,
drugs, burns)

Capillary

Endothelium

Neutrophil

Erythrocytes

Platelets

**Fig. 7.10** Pathogenesis of adult respiratory distress syndrome. Initial injury is to the capillary endothelium or the alveolar epithelium. The endothelial damage is often initiated by endotoxin and is sustained by interactions of neutrophils, macrophages, cytokines, oxygen radicals, complement, and arachidonate metabolites. Fluid and proteins leak from the capillary into the interstitium and alveoli.

This condition is associated with a high mortality. *Post mortem* the lungs are blue, heavy, haemorrhagic, and oedematous, each weighing >1,000 g (normal weight 300–400 g each). After 10–14 days they become solid, fleshy, and reddish/grey, due to early fibrosis.

## Complications

The major complications in survivors are as follows. Pulmonary fibrosis is the most common residual problem,

because myofibroblasts, which are active in lung remodelling, migrate from the interstitium through gaps in the epithelial basement membrane. The damage may progress to diffuse fibrosis and cystic change, but fibrosis is not inevitable and the lung may sometimes recover. Pulmonary hypertension, due to hypoxia, and pneumonia are also significant complicating diseases.

### Acute Interstitial pneumonia

In up to 40% of cases of ARDS no predisposing cause is found and it represents an idiopathic acute interstitial lung disease, termed 'acute interstitial pneumonia' (AIP). There is a prodromal upper respiratory tract viral illness, followed by increasing dyspnoea and non-productive cough. The mortality rate is high (70%) and those who survive may develop fibrosis.

## Chronic Interstitial Lung Disease and Pulmonary Fibrosis

### Key Points

- There are many causes of chronic interstitial lung disease.
- Typically there is a restrictive defect in lung function.
- It may result in respiratory failure or cor pulmonale.

There are many causes of pulmonary fibrosis. These include sarcoidosis, Langerhans' cell histiocytosis, and collagen vascular diseases, such as rheumatoid disease, systemic lupus erythematosus, systemic sclerosis, and asbestosis. Drugs, such as methotrexate, used for cancer treatment or immunosuppression, or amiodarone, used to treat cardiac disease, are also implicated and there is an increased incidence among metal- or wood-dust workers. In many cases, however, no cause is found. Chronic interstitial lung disease is traditionally classified according to the histological pattern present, which corresponds to fairly well-characterized clinicopathological entities:

- Usual interstitial pneumonia
- Non-specific interstitial pneumonia
- Desquamative interstitial pneumonia and respiratory bronchiolitis
- Organizing pneumonia
- Lymphocytic interstitial pneumonia.

### Usual interstitial pneumonia (UIP)

UIP is the histological pattern seen in patients with cryptogenic fibrosing alveolitis (a clinical term not used by pathologists). It is most common in male smokers in their fifth decade. There is an insidious onset of exertional dyspnoea because of the large pulmonary functional reserve and possible relative inactivity in this age group. Clinically there is a dry, non-productive cough and lower lobe end-inspiratory crackles (Velcro crackles). With progression there is finger clubbing and central cyanosis, and death usually occurs within 5 years of diagnosis, from infection, respiratory failure, or cor pulmonale. A small number of patients develop acute exacerbations of disease characterised by development of DAD and there is also an increased incidence of lung cancer. Lung function tests are typically restrictive but may show a mixed restrictive and obstructive picture, due to associated emphysema. Computed tomography reveals a fine, ground-glass appearance, progressing to honeycomb lung (Fig. 7.11), which has a basal and subpleural predominance.

The disease is characterized by spatial and temporal heterogeneity. Fibrosis is unevenly distributed in the affected lobe(s), unlike NSIP, and predominantly affects the lower lobes with a subpleural and paraseptal distribution. Microscopically there are foci of active myxoid fibrosis (fibroblastic foci), which become incorporated into the alveolar wall, forming dense fibrotic scarring. The alveolar epithelium shows a number of reactive changes including type II pneumocyte hyperplasia and squamous, mucinous, or ciliated metaplasia. Smooth muscle proliferation is due to myofibroblast proliferation and differentiation. There is variable interstitial inflammation with lymphocytes, plasma cells, macrophages, and some neutrophils. Cases with large numbers of fibroblastic foci have the worst prognosis. In the late stages there is honeycomb lung with cystic change and metaplasia of the lining epithelium. The arteries show medial hypertrophy, pulmonary arterioles are muscularized, and the lumina of arteries and veins are obliterated by intimal fibrosis, as a reaction to the surrounding fibrosis and pulmonary hypertension.

### Non-specific Interstitial Pneumonia (NSIP)

In NSIP the distribution and pattern of inflammation and fibrosis is more uniform and less severe than that seen in UIP.

In the cellular form of NSIP an interstitial chronic inflammatory cell infiltrate predominates, whereas fibrotic NSIP is characterized by interstitial fibrosis. This pattern is often associated with an underlying connective tissue disease such as scleroderma. The importance of recognizing this pattern on biopsy is that it has a much better prognosis than UIP.

### Desquamative Interstitial Pneumonia (DIP) and Respiratory Bronchiolitis (RP)

DIP and RB are both disorders that are related to cigarette smoking and characterized by accumulation of brown pigmented alveolar macrophages in respiratory bronchioles and alveoli. The pigment represents products of cigarette smoke. In DIP the process is fairly diffuse whereas in RB it is milder and bronchocentric. Patients with DIP/RB may present with cough, dyspnoea, bi-basal end-inspiratory crepitations, interstitial radiological infiltrates, and a restrictive or mixed restrictive/obstructive pattern. There is generally little fibrosis and it is steroid reversible. A DIP picture can also be caused by asbestos and other inorganic particles.

### Organizing Pneumonia (OP)

OP is a pattern of lung injury characterized by intra-alveolar plugs of loose fibromyxoid granulation tissue (Masson's bodies), which represent organization of alveolar exudates (Fig. 7.12). The pattern is non-specific and has many causes, including infection, radiotherapy, drugs, and connective tissue disease, as well as being idiopathic.

## Granulomatous Lung Disease

There are many causes of granulomatous inflammation in the lung including infection (especially mycobacterial and fungal infection), sarcoidosis, exposure to heavy metals (e.g. beryllium), foreign material (e.g. aspiration and intravenous drug abuse), drugs, and immune reaction to tumour. In some cases the cause of the granuloma may be apparent

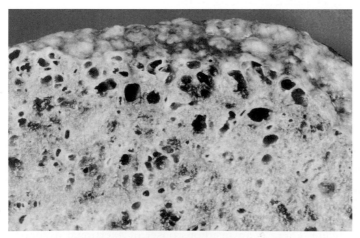

**FIG. 7.11** Honeycomb lung: this can be the end-result of a number of fibrosing lung diseases, including usual interstitial pneumonia.

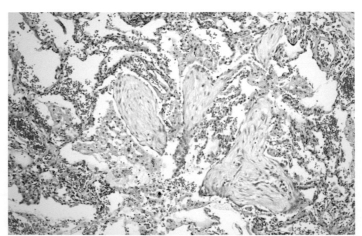

**FIG. 7.12** Organizing pneumonia with intra-alveolar buds of fibromyxoid granulation tissue.

histologically, but correlation with clinical history, radiology, and most importantly microbiology is frequently essential.

### Sarcoidosis

Sarcoidosis is a multisystem granulomatous disorder, affecting people in the 20- to 40-year age group. The aetiology is unknown. In Europe the incidence ranges from 3 cases per 100,000 population to 500 per 100,000 population. There are geographical and racial differences in that it is more common in the African–American population.

A quarter of patients have a dry cough, dyspnoea, and exercise intolerance, and another quarter present with eye, skin, or nasal complaints. Hilar lymphadenopathy is common. A third have fever, fatigue, malaise, and weight loss. Only in 15% of patients is the disease progressive and 40% have few symptoms. Depending on the degree of lung damage, there may be loss of lung volume and decreased diffusion capacity due to interstitial fibrosis (see also Case History 4.1, Chapter 4, pp. 63–64).

#### Pathogenesis

Bronchoalveolar lavage (BAL) shows increased T lymphocytes. The helper:suppressor T-cell ratio in active sarcoid is 4–10 times greater than normal whereas in inactive lesions suppressor T cells predominate. The elevated helper:suppressor T-cell ratio suggests an immunoregulatory imbalance, but BAL cell profiles cannot predict prognosis or steroid response. The granulomas produce angiotensin-converting enzyme (ACE), with elevated serum levels. This may be a marker of body granuloma burden and is sensitive in predicting relapse or remission.

T lymphocytes from active sarcoid release monocyte chemotactic and inhibition factors. The factor switching on the T cells is unknown. Although the disease resembles tuberculosis, mycobacteria do not seem to be the cause. Inhaled antigens, such as pine pollen, talc, and peanut dust, have been incriminated. Genetic factors may be involved, because there are familial clusters.

#### Pathology

The lymph nodes and lung are involved in 80% of cases. Other organs involved in decreasing order of frequency are the liver, spleen, heart, skin, central nervous system, kidney, eyes, parotid glands, thyroid, intestine, stomach, and pituitary. The earliest changes in the lung are a lymphocytic alveolitis with non-necrotizing granulomas (Fig. 7.13), which are interstitial and follow the lymphatics in the septa, pleura, and peribronchial regions. These may progress to pulmonary fibrosis and honeycombing, more marked in the upper lobes. There may be bronchiectasis and cavity formation, sometimes with aspergillus infection. The pleura and vessels may also be affected. The Kveim test, an intradermal injection of sarcoid tissue, is now rarely used, not least because of the risk of transmission of other infections.

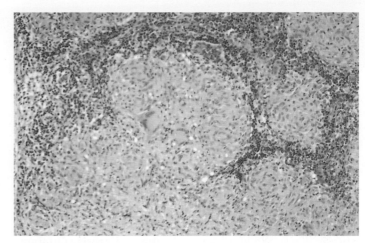

**FIG. 7.13** Sarcoidosis: microscopic view of non-caseating granulomatous inflammation, including giant cells.

## OCCUPATIONAL LUNG DISEASE

> ### Key Points
> - Occupational lung disease must be considered in any patient with respiratory problems.
> - Occupational lung disease follows exposure to fumes, or inorganic or organic dusts.
> - Coal dust pneumoconiosis, silicosis, and asbestosis are decreasing in the west due to legal controls. There is widespread use of asbestos in India and the Far East.
> - Organic dusts, such as fungi, can cause asthma in the workplace.

Occupational lung disease occurs in diverse forms and is due to fumes, vapours, gases, dusts, or immunological processes.

### Coalworkers' Pneumoconiosis

Coals, rich in carbon, are complex minerals, their composition varying from mine to mine. Inorganic material may be present in coals, including muscovite and kaolin, as well as trace elements such as arsenic, titanium, and beryllium. Miners constructing communicating shafts may work on hard siliceous rocks and develop silicosis rather than coalworkers' pneumoconiosis (CWP). The incidence and progression of CWP relates to the cumulative exposure of dust inspired, as well as the coal rank, i.e. the amount of volatile matter within the coal. The higher-ranked coals, containing the least amount of volatile matter, have a higher incidence and severity of CWP. The assessment of pneumoconiosis is on the prevalence and size of the radiological opacities in a system devised by the International Labour Organization. The condition is divided into several forms.

Simple CWP is a radiological or pathological diagnosis with no associated symptoms or signs. The earliest change is the collection of dust-laden macrophages around respiratory bronchioles and adjacent alveoli. In time, multiple bilateral, stellate black (macular) lesions not exceeding 1 cm are found, especially in the upper two-thirds of the lungs, with associated focal (centrilobular) emphysema. Macules are small foci of fibrosis. The peripheral lymph nodes contain whorled, pigmented nodules.

Complicated CWP gives no symptoms or signs at an early stage but, when extensive and associated with bullous emphysema, the affected person has breathlessness, cough, and exertional dyspnoea, progressing to cor pulmonale. It is characterized by the development of progressive massive fibrosis. These are large areas of rubbery fibrosis containing coal dust which measure >1 cm and are more common in the upper lobe. These may reach several centimetres, show varying cavitation due to ischaemic necrosis, and can destroy a lobe or lobes. On histological examination dust is seen, free and within macrophages, and admixed with collagen.

Kaplan's syndrome is an eponymous term denoting pneumoconiosis in coalminers with rheumatoid disease. Chest radiographs show large, round, peripheral shadows, not restricted to the upper lobes, as in progressive massive fibrosis. Pulmonary lesions can precede joint manifestations. The lesions are round to oval, firm nodules, may be discrete or confluent, and vary from several millimetres to several centimetres. These nodules can show cavitation and calcification. They represent a combination of rheumatoid nodules and dust-related fibrosis. The central zone contains necrotic collagen and coal dust, the latter often lying in rings. The periphery has palisading fibroblasts. Care should be taken to exclude tuberculosis, which is associated with histiocytes and giant cells and is a complication of progressive massive fibrosis.

## Asbestos Exposure and Asbestosis

### Key Points

- Asbestos is a group of fibrous silicates.
- Exposure is associated with shipbuilding, and the construction and demolition industries.
- Asbestos causes lung cancer and mesothelioma of the pleura, peritoneum, and pericardium.
- Asbestosis denotes pulmonary fibrosis due to asbestos.
- Pleural plaques indicate asbestos exposure, *not* necessarily asbestosis.

Asbestos refers to a group of naturally occurring fibrous silicate minerals that are still mined in Canada, Australia, South Africa, and the former Soviet Union. There are two major groups of fibres – serpentine and amphibole – which vary in their crystalline structure. The serpentine group consists of chrysotile (white asbestos), accounting for 90% of world production. The amphiboles, which include crocidolite (blue) and amosite (brown), are the more carcinogenic.

Asbestos bodies, in most cases amphiboles, have a central fibrous core coated with iron, which gives a typical golden brown, beaded, dumb-bell appearance (Fig. 7.14). Chrysotile fibres have a higher effective fibre diameter than amphiboles and impact on bifurcations of larger, proximal airways. Amphiboles are short, straight fibres, usually <0.5 μm in diameter, and can penetrate deep into the lung and through the visceral pleura. The longer, thinner fibres are most hazardous and show the greatest carcinogenic effects. Industrial exposure is seen in shipbuilding, construction, especially as asbestos is removed during demolition, increasingly with men who worked in the building and electrical trades, and in car mechanics who worked with brake linings. Patients may be exposed due to living close to an asbestos factory or because a close relative has carried the mineral home from work on clothing.

Asbestos is associated with many pleuropulmonary reactions: pleural plaques (denoting exposure) asbestosis, diffuse pleural fibrosis, and asbestos-induced pleural effusions. Asbestos causes lung cancer and malignant pleural and peritoneal mesothelioma.

### Asbestosis

Asbestosis is a form of interstitial pulmonary fibrosis that occurs after prolonged, substantial exposure (the latency from first exposure to development of symptoms is in excess of 20 years). Asbestosis prevalence is associated with age, fibre type, smoking, and cumulative exposure. Clinically asbestosis is associated with a non-productive cough, basal crackles, dyspnoea, and, in advanced stages, finger clubbing and cor pulmonale.

The earliest changes are fibrosis in and around respiratory bronchiolar walls. This extends distally, causing obliteration of the acinus. The traction of the fibrosis causes bronchial and bronchiolar dilatation, i.e. honeycomb lung, more

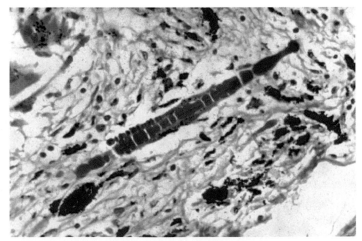

**FIG. 7.14** Asbestos body in a high-power view of a section of scarred lung tissue. It appears golden brown and beaded as it is coated with iron.

marked in the lower and subpleural zones. Asbestosis can resemble UIP pathologically, but asbestos bodies are readily identified in lung smears or sections. There is visceral and parietal pleural fibrosis and pleural plaques (Fig. 7.15).

Lung cancer and asbestos exposure are related. This was previously thought to be due to the fibrosis, but asbestos is carcinogenic and small pulmonary burdens can be associated with lung cancer. Cigarette smoking and asbestos exposure have a multiplicative effect in causing lung cancer. Mesothelioma is discussed on p. 194.

## Silicosis

Silicosis is defined as a fibrotic disease of the lungs caused by inhalation of dust containing crystalline silicon dioxide. Its development depends on particle size, mineral form, and individual susceptibility. Most rocks contain silica, either in its free form (silicon dioxide) or combined as various silicates. Silica exists in crystalline and amorphous forms, the latter including flint and opal. The most common form of crystalline silica is quartz, seen in many rock types. Sandstone contains almost 100% quartz, and slate and shale up to 40%. Silica exposure occurs in quarrying, stone cutting, mining, and tunnelling.

The clinical presentation depends on the length and intensity of exposure. Acute exposure to high levels of dust causes acute dyspnoea with accumulation of lipoproteinaceous material in alveolar spaces. Long-term exposure to dust with little quartz causes slowly progressive nodular changes. Higher concentrations cause progressive nodularity, often with massive upper zone fibrosis (progressive massive fibrosis).

Complications of silicosis include pulmonary tuberculosis, due to the toxic effect of silica on macrophages, and other opportunistic infections, such as aspergillosis, which complicate cavitating progressive massive fibrosis. Pneumothorax is related to bullous emphysema. Silicosis is associated with

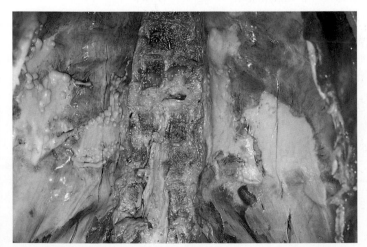

**FIG. 7.15** Pale yellowish-white fibrous plaques on the posterior parietal pleural surface at postmortem examination on a patient who had a history of occupational exposure to asbestos.

collagen diseases: the aetiological connection may be the development of antinuclear antibodies in silicosis.

### Pathology and Pathogenesis

In chronic silicosis there are firm, greyish/black, sometimes calcified, well-circumscribed nodules, most common in the upper zones. These vary from several millimetres to large massive lesions (progressive massive fibrosis), occupying a lobe or extending into several upper and middle lobes. The centres may cavitate, containing greyish/black fluid, due to ischaemic necrosis or tuberculosis. Hilar nodes are enlarged with calcified nodules.

Histologically, the silicotic nodule has concentric layers of hyaline fibrous tissue with a peripheral zone of dust-laden macrophages and chronic inflammation. There may be a necrotic centre. Interaction between silica and macrophages damages lysosomal membranes, releasing cytokines, and increasing macrophage production and release. Macrophage death causes release of the silica, which is then re-phagocytosed.

## Hypersensitivity Pneumonitis (Extrinsic Allergic Alveolitis)

This disease, the classic form of which is farmers' lung, shows a diffuse interstitial pulmonary infiltrate involving the small airways. It is caused by inhalation of different antigens (*Table 7.3*). Most of these are small enough to enter alveoli but some deposit on larger airways and become solubilized. The disease may be acute or chronic. Acute extrinsic allergic alveolitis (EAA) does not progress to chronic disease without continuous long-term, low-level exposure. In acute attacks, there is cough, dyspnoea, chest tightness, and fever 4–8 hours after exposure to the causative allergen. Symptoms subside in 12–16 hours, without repeated antigen exposure. Bilateral fine nodularity is seen radiologically.

In chronic disease there is dyspnoea, chronic cough, and weight loss, progressing to respiratory failure with clubbing. There are coarse reticular and nodular upper and midzone infiltrates, terminating in honeycomb lung.

### Immunopathogenesis

Bronchoalveolar lavage (BAL) shows a T-cell lymphocytosis of up to 70%. The CD4:CD8 ratio may be normal or low.

**TABLE 7.3** Some factors associated with extrinsic allergic alveolitis

| | |
|---|---|
| Humidifier | Bacterial antigens associated with humid conditions |
| Farmers' lung | Dust from hay, thermophilic *Actinomycetes* spp. |
| Pigeon fanciers' lung | Feather antigens, excreta |
| Woodworkers | |
| Mushroom pickers | |

The T lymphocytes are responsive to a specific antigen. A relative BAL lymphocytosis is seen in asymptomatic farmers and pigeon breeders. Thus the T-cell response does not fully explain the causation of this disease. Patients with active disease show a defect in antigen-specific, T-lymphocyte-suppressor function. This may allow inspired allergen to provoke T-lymphocyte-dependent inflammation. Mast cells are increased in EAA.

### Pathology

Acute and subacute disease show bronchocentric chronic inflammation with foci of organizing pneumonia, alveolar foamy macrophages, and multinucleate giant cells, and small, poorly formed, non-necrotizing granulomas are seen in 70% of cases. The nature and distribution of granulomas are different from those of sarcoidosis, which follow the lymphatics. In the chronic phase there is interstitial fibrosis in the upper lobes, with superimposed cystic change.

# LUNG INFECTIONS

### Key Points

- Infection is common in the lungs, because they are open to the air and receive organisms from the blood.
- Most pulmonary infection is spread by aerosols and thus incidence is increased in overcrowded conditions.
- Common predisposing causes for pneumonia are obstruction, aspiration, cigarette smoking, and immunosuppression.
- Complications of pneumonia are lung abscess, empyema, non-resolution, and pulmonary fibrosis.

Pneumonia is pulmonary infection, caused by viruses, bacteria, fungi, or parasites. A predisposing factor, such as occult lung cancer, with obstruction behind it, cystic fibrosis, immunosuppression, aspiration, and so on, should always be sought.

Lung infections are classified based on the anatomy or aetiology. Pneumonias may be localized, affecting a lobe (lobar pneumonia) or diffuse, affecting lung lobules, bronchi, and bronchioles (bronchopneumonia). A causative organism should be sought, although this may be difficult in viral infections. Molecular probes are becoming highly sensitive for the detection of DNA and RNA sequences unique to a particular organism. The method has the advantage of detecting small numbers of organisms, undetected by other means. However, the clinical significance of small numbers of organisms has still to be clarified.

## Bacterial Pneumonia

Bacterial infections cause lobar pneumonia, bronchopneumonia, or both.

### Lobar Pneumonia

Smoking, chronic bronchitis, alcoholism, and overcrowding predispose to classic lobar pneumonia (typically caused by *S. pneumoniae*). There is abrupt onset with high fever, tachypnoea, dry cough, and severe pleuritic chest pain, progressing to respiratory distress. Rusty, thick, tenacious sputum is produced and the typical signs of consolidation are present. Pneumonia due to organisms such as *H. influenzae* or *Legionella* spp. has a similar clinical picture. These classic signs and symptoms change with early antibiotic treatment. There are four distinct pathological phases:

1. Spreading inflammatory oedema: rarely seen and resembles pulmonary oedema.
2. So-called 'red hepatization': when the affected lobe is firm and brick-red, resembling liver (Fig. 7.16) and small bronchi are plugged with fibrin. Alveoli are filled with red blood corpuscles and fibrin, but there are few polymorphs. The alveolar capillaries are congested.
3. Grey hepatization: the lung is firm, grey/yellow, and there is overlying fibrinous pleurisy. Alveoli are filled with fibrin, many polymorphs, and a few red blood corpuscles. The pulmonary arterioles may become thrombosed.
4. Resolution: macrophages remove the exudate from the alveoli, the normal architecture is restored, and the lung is reinflated.

### Bronchopneumonia

Bronchopneumonia typically occurs in infancy, old age, and debilitated individuals in whom there is retention of pulmonary secretions, aspiration of gastric contents or a foreign body, and diminished coughing (Fig. 7.17). There is often a history of a pre-existing viral infection, chronic bronchitis, bronchiectasis, or cystic fibrosis. Bronchopneumonia typically involves the lower lobes. The infection is centred around bronchioles, and spreads into the adjacent alveolar spaces with a more patchy consolidation than in lobar pneumonia. *Post mortem*, the lungs are bulky and dark with blood-stained, purulent fluid filling bronchi and much of the parenchyma. Bronchial and bronchiolar walls are infiltrated by polymorphs and mononuclear cells, with shedding of the epithelium. Alveolar and bronchiolar lumina are filled with debris, pus cells, and oedema. If the pneumonia is treated, a subsequent radiograph may detect an underlying cause, such as a carcinoma, which may have caused bronchial obstruction. A recurrent pneumonia should *always* trigger a search for an underlying cause.

## Other Bacteria

*Haemophilus influenzae* is a commensal in the respiratory tract and is seen especially in the yellow/green sputum of patients with COPD. Pneumonia may be lobar or bronchial. Gram-negative pneumonia is an important cause of septicaemia and hospital-based death. It occurs in patients in intensive care units or in those on broad-spectrum antibiotics, immunosuppressants, or steroids. The causative organisms may be multiple and include *Pseudomonas aeruginosa*, *Proteus* spp., and *Escherichia coli*. Diagnosis may be difficult and the presenting feature may be septicaemic shock with fever, lymphocytosis, and mucopurulent sputum. Gram-negative bacilli in the sputum are present in any hospitalized patient and are insufficient for a diagnosis of this type of septicaemia.

Two specific Gram-negative organisms should be mentioned. *Klebsiella pneumoniae* usually occurs in the smoking, alcoholic male but may occur in malignancy and diabetes. It presents with rigors, fever, and purulent sputum. The patient is *in extremis* with frank haemoptysis. There is lobar or lobular consolidation, proceeding to abscess formation. The disease is usually seen in the right upper lobe or in an apical segment of the lower lobe, suggesting previous aspiration.

*Pseudomonas pneumoniae* is important in cystic fibrosis and patients with burns or tracheostomies, or on ventilators. There are multiple indurated haemorrhagic foci, which resemble infarcts, or yellow, irregular areas of consolidation, progressing to abscess formation.

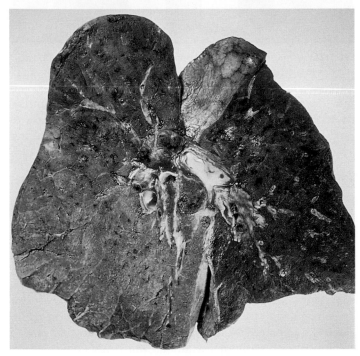

**FIG. 7.16** Lobar pneumonia affecting the whole of the lower lung on the left of the picture. This is solid and dull red (red hepatization) due to inflammatory exudates filling alveoli and small bronchi.

### Legionnaires' Disease

This is caused by *Legionella pneumophila*. There are three types of infection:

1. Outbreaks in previously fit individuals, exposed to contaminated shower or cooling systems
2. Sporadic cases, where the source of infection is unknown; occurs in middle-aged and elderly people, often smokers
3. Immunocompromised patients.

The organism grows in water and is spread by aerosols. Males are more commonly affected. Symptoms vary but characteristically there is headache, myalgia, and rigors, and half the patients have nausea, vomiting, diarrhoea, and abdominal pain. There may be mental confusion in severely ill patients. Respiratory symptoms include tachypnoea and cough, initially dry then purulent. Multilobular shadowing is seen on radiographs. There is confluent bronchopneumonia and less commonly a lobar pattern. Diagnosis is by demonstration of the organism by antibody staining.

## Complications of Pneumonia

Although in optimal circumstances pneumonia may resolve, frequently this is not the case. Lung abscess is a local cavity, usually with a fluid level. The most common cause is aspiration, inhalation of a foreign body, or obstruction by a bronchial carcinoma. Abscesses are more common with organisms such as *K. pneumoniae*, *Streptococcus pyogenes*, or septic infarcts. There is foul-smelling sputum, because of an overgrowth of the cavity by anaerobes.

Direct extension of the infection from the lung to the pleural cavity results in empyema, a collection of pus in an anatomical space. Non-resolution of pneumonia may

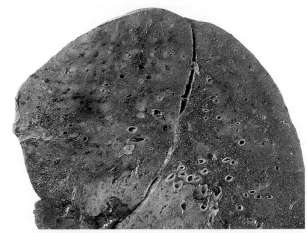

**FIG. 7.17** Bronchopneumonia: there is patchy consolidation (paler areas) of this lung. This case was due to aspiration of gastric contents (not shown).

follow incorrect treatment, commonly due to mycobacteria, actinomyces, or fungi, or in pneumonia complicating tumour, thromboembolism, or collagen diseases. Pulmonary fibrosis is usually intra-alveolar.

## Pulmonary Tuberculosis

**Key Points**

- The causative organism is *Mycobacterium tuberculosis*.
- The incidence is rising once again.
- There are two forms: primary and secondary.
- Spread is to draining lymph nodes and via the blood.

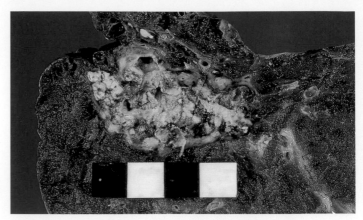

**Fig. 7.18** Secondary pulmonary tuberculosis: there is caseation, fibrosis, and developing cavitation toward the apex of the upper lobe.

The general features of tuberculosis are discussed in Chapter 19. This disease, apparently conquered in the west, is now increasing in incidence. The declining rate was largely due to better living standards with a smaller contribution from chemotherapy. The increase is due to human immunodeficiency virus (HIV) infection, immunosuppression, and multiple drug resistance, especially in the poorer developing countries. In the west, immigrants from the south-east Asian subcontinent and the West Indies are more susceptible to the disease.

### Primary Tuberculosis

Infection with *M. tuberculosis* causes a focal caseous granulomatous lesion, called a ghon focus, situated subpleurally. The organisms then travel to the regional hilar nodes, causing granulomatous caseation. The ghon focus (primary lung lesion) and the involved regional nodes are termed the 'primary complex'. This is usually clinically silent, apart from calcification on a chest radiograph. In children under 2 years there may be bronchial or vascular erosion, resulting in tuberculous bronchopneumonia or miliary tuberculosis respectively.

### Secondary Pulmonary Tuberculosis

This is probably due to re-infection, not reactivation of a dormant primary lesion. The second dose of *M. tuberculosis* causes a hypersensitivity reaction with tissue necrosis. Histologically, there are lymphocytes, histiocytes, plasma cells, and granulomas with Langhans' type giant cells and central caseation. This lesion, usually in the upper lobe, heals by fibrosis and calcification if there is a high degree of immunity. The predilection for upper lobe involvement is probably due to its better ventilation.

Cavitation occurs at the apex of the upper lobe (Fig. 7.18). There may be significant haemoptysis due to erosion of vessels. Some cases present as hilar or mediastinal lymphadenopathy, when an extrinsic tuberculoma impinges on the trachea or bronchus. This may erode a bronchus, with oxygen helping growth of the organism, causing dissemination and tuberculous bronchopneumonia. Alternatively miliary tuberculosis, due to rupture of a tubercle into a vein, may develop. The name miliary is because of the similarity with millet seeds. Miliary spread enables the disease to establish itself in organs such as bone, meninges, and kidney. There may be a pleural effusion.

### Clinical Features

Primary tuberculosis may be asymptomatic but there can be a vague illness with cough, wheeze, and erythema nodosum. Lymphadenopathy compresses bronchi, causing segmental or lobar collapse. If chronic this causes bronchiectasis, usually in the middle lobe (Brock's syndrome).

In adult secondary pulmonary tuberculosis there is tiredness, anorexia, weight loss, cough, pleural effusion, and fever but drenching night sweats are now uncommon. The chest radiograph shows patchy or nodular upper lobe shadowing as well as fibrosis with/without cavitation. Miliary tuberculosis presents in a non-specific manner with weight loss, fever, and few physical signs. The chest radiograph may show normal findings, because tubercles are only 1–2 mm in diameter. A Mantoux skin test is usually positive, but may be occasionally negative in severe disease. Bone marrow culture may be helpful.

### Atypical Mycobacterial Infection

This is difficult to distinguish from tuberculosis. Mycobacteria, other than those causing tuberculosis, are increasingly recognized as a cause of chronic lung disease. The causative organisms include *M. kansasii*, *M. avium-intracellulare* and *M. fortuitum*. These organisms are more common in patients with HIV and silicosis, and in immunocompromised individuals. There are four main pulmonary patterns:

1. Solitary nodules
2. Chronic bronchitis or bronchiectasis
3. Tuberculous-like and diffuse infiltrates, seen especially in HIV
4. Pleural involvement, but this is rare.

There are granulomas with varying degrees of necrosis. Bilateral diffuse interstitial infiltration is seen in the *M. avium-intracellulare* group.

# Viral Infections

The histological diagnosis of viral infection is possible only if there are specific intracytoplasmic or intranuclear inclusion bodies.

## Influenza

This is caused by an RNA virus that belongs to the orthomyxovirus family, with three main types A–C. The structural proteins are haemagglutinin, major protein, and neuraminidase. Influenza A virus can undergo antigenic drift, because of changes in both the haemagglutinin and neuraminidase antigens. Strains evolve that are different from the original pandemic virus. The virus is cytopathic to respiratory epithelium, leaving a bare basement membrane on which staphylococci and other organisms grow. The virus impairs chemotaxis in polymorphs and macrophages.

The disease is seen every year and, in the temperate climates, usually during the winter months. There is headache, non-productive cough, myalgia, and a high temperature. Viral spread is by droplets and spread is increased by close contact or crowding. The disease is usually fatal in its acute stage only if there is underlying cardiopulmonary disease. Death is usually due to staphylococcal pneumonia.

The acute changes vary from a patchy fibrinous intra-alveolar exudate and hyaline membranes with interstitial oedema to severe alveolar haemorrhage and necrosis of bronchiolar mucosa. Repair of the alveolar wall occurs with type II cell proliferation and there are mild chronic interstitial cell infiltrates.

## Respiratory Syncytial Virus Infection

This is more common in young children due to the close proximity of the upper and lower respiratory tracts. Epidemics in temperate climates are in winter and early spring. Transmission is by droplets, via the nose or eyes. There is fever, cough, and rhinorrhoea. It is more common in premature infants or those with pre-existing cardiopulmonary disease. The virus replicates in epithelial cytoplasm and

lymphoid tissue. The epithelial cells die and form mucus plugs, causing partial or complete airway obstruction. There is an associated lymphoplasmacytic and neutrophilic infiltrate in bronchiolar walls. Typical multinucleated giant cells suggest a giant cell pneumonia. These cells contain intra-cytoplasmic, acidophilic inclusions. RSV pneumonia complicates measles and influenza.

## Measles

This is a serious disease in malnourished children in developing countries. It is spread by aerosol. The virus replicates in respiratory lymphoid tissue, causing rhinorrhoea and cough. The respiratory epithelium sloughs, leaving a bare basement membrane. Multinucleated cells with intra-nuclear inclusions are present, especially in alveoli, with a peribronchiolar lymphoplasmacytic infiltrate. Secondary bacterial pneumonia often supervenes.

## Adenovirus

These are DNA viruses, causing severe bronchiolitis. Infection is a complication of immunosuppression. The lungs have small, dark, collapsed foci. There is bronchial ulceration. Shedding of bronchial and bronchiolar epithelium, containing some nuclei with eosinophilic inclusions and a clear halo, are seen. These coalesce and stain basophilically, causing smudge cells.

## Cytomegalovirus Infection

This is an important complication of solid organ transplantation and HIV infection. It can cross the placenta and cause perinatal disease. In adults there is fever, non-productive cough, dyspnoea, and hypoxia. The characteristic intra-nuclear, acidophilic inclusions surrounded by a clear zone are seen in bronchiolar and alveolar epithelium with an associated lymphoplasmacytic infiltrate (Fig. 7.19).

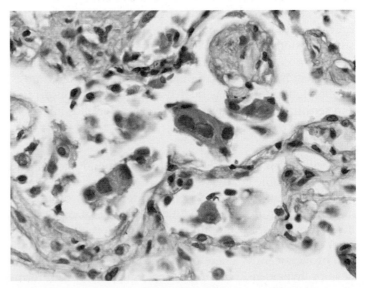

FIG. 7.19 Cytomegalovirus (CMV) infection in a patient after a lung transplantation. Note the prominent intranuclear inclusion.

Other viruses causing pulmonary damage include parainfluenza, chickenpox (varicella), herpes simplex, rubella, and hantavirus.

## Atypical Pneumonias

*Mycoplasma pneumoniae* is an important cause of community-acquired pneumonia transmitted by aerosol. A quarter of infections are asymptomatic, and the clinical illness varies from a mild upper respiratory tract infection to pneumonia with uni- or multilobular consolidation. The lungs are heavy and dark red with subpleural haemorrhages.

*Chlamydia* spp. are Gram-negative bacteria. *C. pneumoniae* is a common cause of pneumonia. The infection may present as pharyngitis, with pneumonia occurring several weeks later. The pneumonia is mild, except in elderly people, with fever, cough, and crackles. The pathology is ill described because there have been few deaths or biopsies. Diagnosis is made serologically or by specific monoclonal antibody. *C. psittaci* causes psittacosis/ornithosis, which is highly infectious, transmitted by aerosol or by direct handling of infected bird tissues. Budgerigars, pigeons, and many species of wild birds carry the organism. It causes cough, sputum, chest pain, dyspnoea, haemoptysis and fever, and lower lobe consolidation. The bronchial and bronchiolar epithelium show desquamation, necrosis, and lymphocytic inflammation. Alveolar cells show intracytoplasmic inclusions. Diagnosis is made by an ELISA(enzyme-linked immunofluoresence assay) test or by serology. *C. trachomatis* causes oculogenital infections and is a rare cause of neonatal pneumonia.

## Fungal Infections

Some of the fungi causing lung disease are purely saprophytic and grow along pre-existing cavities or necrotic lung tissue. Others, such as blastomycosis and coccidioidomycosis, are seen in well-defined geographical zones, where the fungal spores are found in the soil. They cause primary invasive infections in previously healthy people, in the absence of predisposing factors. Fungi cause a variety of effects from tissue necrosis, as in coccidioidomycosis and histoplasmosis, to allergic-type reactions, such as asthma due to absorption and sensitization to fungal products in aspergillus infection.

### Aspergillosis

*Aspergillus* spp. are widespread, being found in soil and decaying organic matter, such as manure and hay. Spores are disseminated by air currents. Infection is most likely in immunosuppressed individuals. Allergic manifestations include asthma, eosinophilic pneumonia, mucoid impaction of bronchi, allergic bronchopulmonary aspergillosis, and bronchocentric granulomatosis. Cystic fibrosis patients develop hypersensitivity to *Aspergillus* spp. The main forms of aspergillosis are as follows:

- An aspergilloma or fungal ball, which colonizes a pre-existing cavity, such as old sarcoid, tuberculosis, or bronchiectasis (see Fig. 7.4). Cavities are more common in the upper lobes. They cause haemoptysis and a radiograph shows a round opacity, surrounded by a radiolucent crescent of air. The ball is necrotic and brownish/yellow, and the surrounding lung is fibrotic.
- Invasive aspergillosis, which is confined to immunosuppressed patients. The affected lung resembles an infarct, is dark red and haemorrhagic, and shows coagulative necrosis with fungal hyphae. Fungal involvement of arteries produces infarction.
- Granulomatous pulmonary aspergillosis, which resembles tuberculosis.
- Tracheobronchial aspergillosis, which is seen in immunosuppressed patients. A necrotic membrane lines the trachea and main bronchi. If it separates, bronchial obstruction occurs.

### Cryptococcosis

This is caused by *Cryptococcus neoformans*, found in bird excreta contaminating soil worldwide. The disease is often asymptomatic, even with marked radiological changes, which include nodular infiltrates, pleural effusions, and lobar consolidation. Patients have fever, weight loss, dyspnoea, and night sweats. Sporadic cases with no predisposing condition occur, but it is seen more commonly in immuno-compromised individuals.

The disease may resemble tuberculosis and form a primary cryptococcal complex in any lobe. There are foci of caseation surrounded by fibrosis with hilar lymph node involvement. Localized granulomatous lesions (cryptococcomas or torulomas) are solitary, round, subpleural shadows, several centimetres in diameter, which may undergo central necrosis and cavitation. The disease may also disseminate to give diffuse pneumonia or a miliary picture. Silver stains show budding yeasts.

### Pneumocystis jirovecii *Pneumonia*

Reactivation of latent infection is probably the cause of the disease in immunosuppressed patients (see Chapter 19, p. 545). *Pneumocystis jirovecii (carinii)* causes diffuse consolidation. The lungs are bulky with firm yellow/pink foci. There is an interstitial lymphoplasmacytic infiltrate with characteristic foamy intra-alveolar eosinophilic material. Methenamine silver or monoclonal antibodies demonstrate the organism.

## PULMONARY VASCULAR DISEASE

The normal pulmonary vasculature is a low-pressure system. Pulmonary arteries are divided into three groups. Elastic arteries are >500 μm in diameter and have multiple elastic laminae and smooth muscle. Muscular arteries are between 80 μm and 500 μm in diameter, with internal and external elastic laminae, between which is a thin medium, reflecting the low-pressure system. Pulmonary arterioles, <80 μm in diameter, lose their media with decreasing calibre and have a single elastic lamina. Pulmonary veins contain muscle, collagen, and elastic fibres, the last forming an internal elastic lamina. The alveolar capillaries have a single layer of endothelium resting on a continuous basal lamina. They lie in the alveolar walls. Any prolonged rise in pulmonary arterial or venous pressure produces morphological vascular changes, which often include thickening of the media and intima.

## Pulmonary Oedema

Acute pulmonary oedema is a life-threatening emergency. The patient is acutely breathless, wheezing, anxious, and sweaty, produces frothy, blood-tinged sputum, and is tachypnoeic with peripheral shutdown. The $PaO_2$ falls. The chest radiograph shows diffuse haziness, secondary to intra-alveolar fluid, and Kerley B lines, due to interstitial oedema.

The lung is well suited to the development of oedema because it lacks solid tissue support. The organ consists predominantly of alveolar walls, suspended in air with only a thin tissue barrier separating capillaries from alveoli. Fluid is kept inside the pulmonary capillaries by a combination of factors including low haemodynamic pressure, plasma colloid osmotic pressure, active reabsorption of excessive alveolar fluid, and the efficiency of pulmonary lymphatics. Pulmonary oedema can be due to a variety of causes, principally haemodynamic (hydrostatic) and increased vascular permeability. Other types include neurogenic causes, due to a high altitude and uraemia.

### Haemodynamic Pulmonary Oedema

Haemodynamic pulmonary oedema is usually caused by increases in capillary transmural pressure. An increased plasma volume, usually due to intravenous fluid overload, has a similar effect. Initially there is interstitial oedema, the septa are widened, and the lymphatics dilated. Fluid leaks through the alveolar wall but lies in the corners of the alveoli. As the thin parts of the alveolar capillary wall are intact at this stage, there is little disturbance to gas exchange. If the fluid continues to increase, the oedema covers the entire alveolar surface, giving a low $PaO_2$. This causes diminished diffusion through the thickened alveolar wall.

The most common cause of haemodynamic pulmonary oedema is increased pulmonary venous pressure typically due to left ventricular failure (See Chapter 6, p. 110) secondary to systemic hypertension, or ischaemic or valvular heart disease. The pulmonary capillaries are distended and red blood corpuscles leak into the alveoli. They are ingested by macrophages, causing pulmonary haemosiderosis. The small pulmonary arteries show medial hypertrophy, and pulmonary veins form a medium between internal and external elastic laminae, i.e. arterialization.

### High-altitude, Neurogenic and Uraemic Pulmonary Oedema

High-altitude pulmonary oedema, the mechanism for which is unknown, develops on rapid ascent to altitudes >3,000 m. Pulmonary hypertension secondary to hypoxia occurs, increasing the hydrostatic pressure, and there may also be a component of permeability oedema, caused by mechanical damage to the alveoli. Neurogenic pulmonary oedema is associated with a rapid rise in intracranial pressure. Uraemic pulmonary oedema shows a bat's wing pattern on a chest radiograph, leaving the peripheral lung translucent, and flooding the perihilar alveoli. This is a type of permeability oedema because the oedema fluid contains high concentrations of plasma proteins. It is probably caused by toxic byproducts of renal failure.

## Pulmonary Embolism

### Key Points

- Thromboemboli are the most common form of emboli to the lung and are usually derived from deep venous thrombosis of calf and iliofemoral veins.
- Pulmonary emboli may cause sudden death or pulmonary infarction, or be asymptomatic.
- If recurrent, pulmonary emboli may cause pulmonary hypertension.

Pulmonary thromboemboli (see Chapter 6, p. 114) originate from thrombi in the deep calf veins, the iliofemoral and pelvic veins, and usually follow venous stasis, vessel injury, and coagulation changes. They are much more common in sedentary people and have recently been described in individuals spending many hours in front of computer screens (e-emboli). Less commonly thromboemboli derive from intravascular catheters, right atrial thrombosis due to atrial fibrillation, and right ventricular thrombus after a myocardial infarction. However, other substances can embolize to the lung and these include fat (after long bone fracture), amniotic fluid (during delivery), air (during surgery), and foreign material such as talc or silicone.

Pulmonary thromboembolism accounts for 10% of hospital deaths. Patients may be asymptomatic but they can present acutely with dyspnoea, substernal or central chest pain, and haemoptysis. Very large emboli may present with shock, due to an acute increase in right ventricular and pulmonary arterial pressure, and are often fatal; coiled thromboemboli lie in the pulmonary trunk and main pulmonary arteries. Unexplained dyspnoea should raise the clinical suspicion of pulmonary embolism. Ventilation/perfusion scans and ECGs are most useful diagnostically.

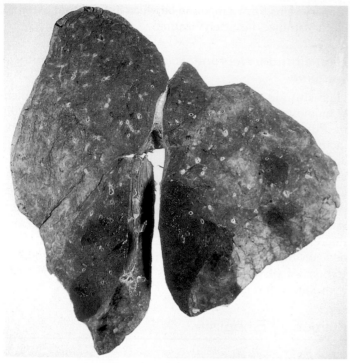

**FIG. 7.20** Pulmonary infarction: the dark haemorrhagic areas towards the periphery of the lung in the lower part of the field are infarcted.

Duplex ultrasound, using Doppler flow, is helpful in diagnosing deep venous thrombosis. Large emboli may result in lung infarcts: these are wedge-shaped haemorrhagic areas with a pleural base and apex pointing towards the embolus (Fig. 7.20). The lesion heals by fibrosis and rarely may become infected. A search of the pulmonary arteries histologically will often show many old or organizing emboli.

Recurrent pulmonary thromboembolism typically affects young females who present insidiously with dyspnoea, syncope, chest pain, and pulmonary hypertension. There are eccentric recanalization channels in the pulmonary arteries, the rest of the lumen being replaced by intimal fibrosis. The media shows hypertrophy.

## Pulmonary Haemorrhage

Pulmonary haemorrhage syndromes are a heterogeneous group of diseases characterized by haemoptysis, pulmonary infiltrates, and anaemia. Pathologically there is a haemorrhagic alveolitis. It may occur secondary to venous hypertension and vasculitides. Anti-basement membrane antibody formation on alveolar septa and immune complex deposition in systemic vasculitis are important causes.

Anti-basement membrane antibody disease (Goodpasture's syndrome, see Chapter 13, p. 405) consists of pulmonary haemorrhage and proliferative glomerulonephritis. There may be massive pulmonary haemorrhage and little renal disease, or vice versa. There is an alveolar capillaritis with fibrin thrombi and alveolar haemorrhage resembling ARDS. Diagnosis is by detection of antibody to anticollagen-$\alpha_3$ (IV).

Idiopathic pulmonary haemosiderosis is rare, affecting mainly males. There is progressive alveolar replacement by haemosiderin-laden macrophages, and interstitial and intra-alveolar fibrosis. The cause is unknown and the diagnosis is one of exclusion.

## Pulmonary vasculitis

Rarely the lung may be a major focus of damage in vasculitis. Wegener's granulomatosis is a necrotizing granulomatous vasculitis that also affects kidneys and the upper respiratory tract (see Chapter 6, p. 125). Churg–Strauss syndrome is usually characterized by a raised eosinophil count and asthma.

# LUNG TUMOURS

### Key Points

- Lung cancer is one of the major cancers.
- It is mainly smoking related.
- Small cell carcinoma, squamous cell carcinoma, and adenocarcinoma are the main forms.
- Secondary tumours commonly affect the lung.

The WHO produced a revised lung and pleural tumour classification in 2004 with a refined classification of adenocarcinoma, published by the IASLC/ATS/ERS (International

**TABLE 7.4** Histological classification of lung tumours

| Epithelial origin | |
|---|---|
| Benign primary | e.g. squamous papilloma |
| Malignant primary | A: Non-small cell carcinomas |
| | Squamous cell carcinoma |
| | Adenocarcinoma – papillary, acinar, solid, lepidic subtypes |
| | Large-cell carcinoma |
| | B: Small cell carcinoma |
| | C: Mixed types combining several of the above |
| | D: Neuroendocrine (carcinoid) with varying malignant potential |
| Metastatic | e.g. carcinoma from kidney or colon |

| Mesenchymal origin | |
|---|---|
| Benign primary | Chondroma |
| | Mesenchymoma |
| Malignant primary | Primary sarcomas from blood vessels, muscle, and so on (all are rare) |
| Metastatic | Osteosarcoma |

| Other | Lymphoma |
|---|---|

Association for the Study of Lung Cancer/American Thoracic Society/European Respiratory Society) in 2011. The main tumour variants are given in *Table 7.4*.

Tumours in the lung may be primary or secondary, benign, or malignant. As the lung receives the entire cardiac output, tumour metastases are common. Lung tumours are classified anatomically as central, i.e. arising from the main bronchi, or peripheral, i.e. arising from the lung parenchyma. This is important because the site determines the signs and symptoms. All central lung tumours present with similar symptoms, i.e. cough, recurrent chest infections, and haemoptysis, due to ulceration of the surface of the tumour. They often cause collapse of a lobe or lung, whereas recurrent infection may lead to bronchiectasis. Peripheral lung tumours are often detected as a chance radiological finding, known as 'a solitary pulmonary nodule'. If they involve the pleura it becomes fibrosed and puckered. As a rough guide 40% of solitary nodules are malignant and 60% are benign. The benign lesions may be inflammatory or nonneoplastic rather than benign tumours. However, for any individual patient these figures do not help with diagnosis. Radiologically benign lesions tend to have a smooth circumscribed periphery, whereas malignant lesions tend to be larger with irregular margins. Positron emission tomography (PET) scans are now increasingly used to try to differentiate benign from malignant disease, but they are not 100% accurate. The usual treatment for remaining solitary nodules of unknown aetiology is resection.

## Benign and Uncommon Lung Tumours

Memorization of every benign lung tumour is unnecessary. If one remembers the normal bronchial wall components, i.e. epithelium, connective tissue, muscle, cartilage, fat, nerves, neuroendocrine cells, and that the mucous and serous glands of the bronchial wall act as a minor salivary gland, the nature of most benign tumours can be predicted.

### Mesenchymomas

These lesions were originally called bronchial hamartomas but, because they grow in adulthood and have an abnormal karyotype, characteristically an exchange of material between 6p21 and 14q24, they are now regarded as neoplasms. They are usually peripheral and range from 1 cm to 4 cm in diameter. The cut surface is grey or yellow if fat is prominent. They consist of benign cartilage, bone, fat, loose myxoid tissue, and islands of ciliated or columnar epithelium.

### Carcinoid Tumours

Carcinoid tumours are low-grade malignant neuroendocrine tumours similar to those seen, for example, in the gut. They are divided into typical (TC) and atypical (AC) forms. The division is based on the mitotic rate, TC having fewer than two mitoses per 2 mm$^2$, but no necrosis, AC having two to

ten mitoses per 2 mm$^2$ and/or foci of necrosis. TCs have a good prognosis if surgically excised but 10–15% of cases show lymph node metastases at presentation.

## Carcinoma of the Lung

### Epidemiology and Aetiology

The lung is the most common site of cancer worldwide and is in first place in all areas of Europe and North America. In the UK, lung cancer accounts for 25% of all cancer deaths in males and the corresponding figure for females is 21%. This latter figure is increasing and worldwide lung cancer is the fourth most frequent cancer in females.

The major contribution of cigarette smoking to lung cancer has been known since four retrospective studies showing the relationship were published in the 1950s; each showed a consistent statistically significant association. The relative risk increases in a stepwise fashion with the increased number of cigarettes smoked. This association is strongest for squamous and small cell lung cancer. Other types of tobacco inhalation, ranging from pipes and cigars in the west, to bidis in Asia, also correlate with a significant risk of lung cancer. Passive smoking is also associated with an increased risk of lung cancer; it is now estimated that this causes about 600 deaths per year in the UK.

Only 10–15% of smokers who consume 20 or more cigarettes a day will develop lung cancer, implying that host factors may be important in altering the risk/predisposition to the development of this disease. There is mounting evidence that some of the genetic changes predisposing to lung cancer are inherited in a mendelian fashion. First-degree relatives of lung cancer relatives have a 2.4-fold increased risk of lung cancer or other non-smoking-related cancers. More tangible evidence of linkage between heredity and lung cancer has been shown in relatives of patients with retinoblastoma, with a 15-fold risk, and in some families with the Li–Fraumeni syndrome, who inherit one mutated copy of the *TP53* tumour-suppressor gene. Both the retinoblastoma and the *TP53* gene are mutated or inactivated in most lung cancers.

To determine the role of occupation is complex because employees may be exposed to more than one potentially carcinogenic substance, and tobacco smoke acts as a strong confounder in the association. A prime example of this is asbestos-related disease. Asbestos exposure alone is a risk factor for the development of lung cancer, but cigarette smoke and asbestos have a multiplicative effect in increasing its incidence. Arsenic and its compounds, chromates, nickel, beryllium, and cadmium, all cause an excess of lung cancer deaths. Hydrocarbons, derived from coal or petroleum, and polycyclic aromatic hydrocarbons, such as dibenzanthracene and benzo(a)pyrene, are known carcinogens and an increased lung cancer risk is seen in coke oven workers, gas house workers, and aluminium workers, exposed to pitch volatiles (tar). The increased risk of lung cancer in workers exposed to radiation was first shown in the Schneeberg mines due to radon gas, a decay product of naturally occurring uranium. The proportion of lung cancer attributable to occupational exposure has been estimated at 10–15%.

An increased incidence of lung cancer complicates cryptogenic fibrosing alveolitis and other significant causes of pulmonary fibrosis.

### Clinical Presentation

Central tumours cause obstructive symptoms, including cough, haemoptysis, wheezing, dyspnoea, and stridor. Pancoast's tumours (superior sulcus tumours) arise posteriorly at the apex of the upper lobe near the brachial plexus. They infiltrate the C8, T1, and T2 nerve roots, causing pain, temperature changes, and muscle atrophy in the shoulder and arm innervated by these nerve roots. Horner's syndrome, consisting of unilateral enophthalmos, ptosis, and miosis, is caused by involvement of the sympathetic chain and stellate ganglion. Superior vena caval obstruction causes oedema and plethora of the face, as well as dilated neck and upper torso veins. Hoarseness due to recurrent laryngeal nerve entrapment is seen particularly in left upper lobe tumours, because the left recurrent laryngeal nerve loops around the aortic arch. Tumour can involve the phrenic nerve, paralysing a hemi-diaphragm. The oesophagus may be infiltrated, causing dysphagia and, if the pleura is involved, an effusion occurs.

Metastases are common in small cell lung carcinoma (SCLC), with 20% metastatic at presentation. Squamous cell carcinoma tends to remain intrathoracic whereas adeno- and large-cell carcinoma metastasize to regional nodes, liver, adrenals, central nervous system, and bone. Small cell carcinoma, especially, because of its ability to produce hormones, can present with paraneoplastic or neuromuscular syndromes (see below). All lung tumours show histological heterogeneity and some tumours show mixtures of squamous and adenocarcinoma or SCLC. Major heterogeneity is found in only 5% of cases.

### Small Cell Lung Carcinoma

This is a rapidly growing and aggressive tumour, which may present with metastases without any visible primary tumour. It arises more commonly in the hilum with extension into lymph nodes (Fig. 7.21) and, in advanced cases, with bronchial obstruction by extrinsic compression. Some tumours, however, arise in the periphery of the lung. The tumour is soft and white, and shows extensive necrosis. In classic SCLC there are sheets of small, hyperchromatic nuclei with nuclear moulding and little cytoplasm (Fig. 7.22). There is a high mitotic rate, apoptosis, and necrosis. This tumour stains positively with neuroendocrine markers NCAM (neural cell adhesion molecule, CD56), synaptophysin, chromogranin, and thyroid transcription factor 1 (TTF-1). The term combined SCLC refers to a tumour with this

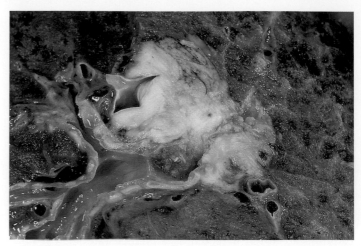

**FIG. 7.21** Slice of lung hilum showing an invasive carcinoma (white) originating in the wall of a bronchus.

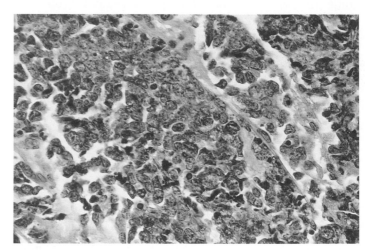

**FIG. 7.22** Small cell carcinoma of lung: microscopic view showing sheets of small, hyperchromatic nuclei with nuclear moulding.

pattern combined with an adenocarcinoma, or squamous or large-cell carcinoma component. Lymphovascular invasion occurs early and distant metastases are common. These are seen in bone marrow, liver, kidney, adrenals, cerebrum, cerebellum, meninges, and regional and cervical lymph nodes. This tumour is extremely responsive to chemotherapy, at least initially, and this is the main modality of treatment. However, recurrence is common and, interestingly after chemotherapy, recurrent tumour may be predominantly squamous or adenocarcinoma in type. The 5-year survival rate is about 5%.

### Squamous Cell Carcinoma

These are commonly central tumours, in main or segmental bronchi, and they often present earlier than other types of carcinoma because of obstructive symptoms. However, in recent years they have increasingly been seen in the periphery of the lung, which may reflect changing smoking behaviour. The tumour is solid and greyish/white, and

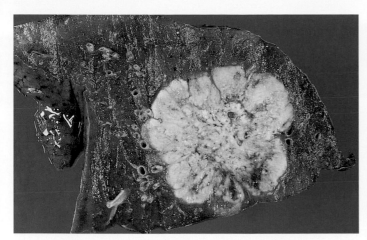

**FIG. 7.23** A large squamous cell carcinoma of lung: such tumours generally metastasize later than small cell carcinomas and are thus more often amenable to surgery.

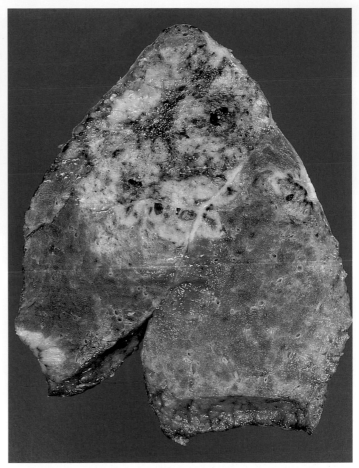

**FIG. 7.24** An adenocarcinoma with associated scarring and carbon pigmentation occupies most of the upper lobe of this lung and extends into the fissure and lower lobe.

may show cavitation (Fig. 7.23). These tumours arise from the bronchial epithelium through a process of squamous metaplasia through dysplasia to carcinoma *in situ*, and these changes may be seen adjacent to the invasive tumour. Secondary bronchiectasis and obstructive pneumonitis may be seen, and background smoking-related changes are common. The tumour is composed of large cells with squamous differentiation characterized by keratinization and/or intercellular bridges; tumour giant cells imply a poor prognosis.

## Adenocarcinoma

This type of lung cancer is increasing, especially in smoking females. However, it is also the most common tumour type in non-smokers, where it may be associated with mutations of the epidermal growth factor receptor (*EGFR*) gene. Mutations in this gene identify patients who may respond to anti-tyrosine kinase therapy. Most adenocarcinomas are peripheral, well-circumscribed masses; central adenocarcinomas arise from bronchial mucous glands and have a male predominance. There is no significant survival difference between the two variants. They may show marked scarring (Fig. 7.24), but the term 'scar carcinoma' is no longer used, because most authors regard the stroma as a desmoplastic response rather than indicating origin in a pulmonary scar. Adenocarcinomas may be multiple and this may create confusion with metastases. Pleural seeding is common and may mimic a mesothelioma.

Histologically there are different growth patterns with tubular, papillary, acinar, lepidic, mucinous, and signet-ring variants. The cells are large and polygonal and tend to be discohesive with a high nuclear:cytoplasmic ratio. Spindle cell and giant cell foci may be identified. The tumour may spread aerogenously within the lung. Adenocarcinoma invades lymphatics, blood vessels and the pleura, and spreads to distal sites.

The traditional difficulty in distinguishing a primary lung tumour from secondary adenocarcinoma, e.g. from the stomach or pancreas, is simplified by the frequent expression of thyroid transcription factor by primary adenocarcinoma of lung.

## Atypical Adenomatous Hyperplasia/ Adenocarcinoma in situ

The 2004, the WHO classification recognized a preinvasive lesion for lung adenocarcinoma called atypical adenomatous hyperplasia. The lesions are often peribronchiolar and characterized by a small localized proliferation of mild-to-moderately atypical type II pneumocytes and/or Clara cells, which line the alveolar walls. These lesions may progress, showing increased size and cytological atypia, but retaining a lepidic pattern of growth along alveolar walls. The term adenocarcinoma *in situ* has been introduced by the 2011 IASLC/ATS/ERS classification of lung adenocarcinoma to describe those lesions that formerly were called bronchioloalveolar carcinoma (a term that is no longer used).

## Large Cell Carcinoma

Large cell carcinoma is a diagnosis of exclusion, in a tumour in which no glandular or squamous differentiation is seen.

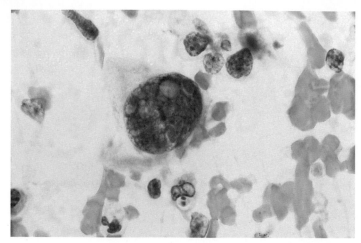

**FIG. 7.25** Cytological preparation from a large-cell carcinoma of lung showing an enormous malignant cell (compare its size with the adjacent red blood cells) with prominent vesicular nucleus and nucleoli. Papanicolaou stain.

It consists of sheets and nests of large epithelial cells with prominent vesicular nuclei and nucleoli (Fig. 7.25). The cell borders are easily visualized. Necrosis and haemorrhage are frequent and there may be acute and/or chronic inflammation. Many probably represent very poorly differentiated squamous or adenocarcinomas.

## Molecular Pathology

In recent years there have been several important advances in the molecular pathology of lung cancer, in particular adenocarcinoma, and some mutations are targets for new therapies. EGFR is a transmembrane tyrosine kinase that is mutated in between 10 and 50% of non-small cell carcinomas, depending on the population group studied. Patients with *EGFR* mutations are typically female non-smokers of Asian ethnicity who have adenocarcinoma. The majority of mutations are found in exons 18–21. Certain mutations (e.g. L858R) are associated with response to tyrosine kinase inhibitors (TKIs), whereas others are associated with either primary or acquired resistence to TKIs (e.g. T790M). Another genomic alteration seen in approximately 2–7% of lung cancers is an inversion in the short arm of chromosome 2, which results in fusion of the *EML4* gene with the *ALK* gene, resulting in an EML4–ALK fusion tyrosine kinase. Patients with the *EML4–ALK* fusion gene are more often young male non-smokers with adenocarcinoma of solid/signet-ring pattern, who respond to the TKI crizotinib. These mutations and translocations are readily detectable by genetic sequencing and fluorescence *in situ* hybridization (FISH) analysis, and are now part of the routine assessment of advanced lung cancer to determine responsiveness to these new targeted therapies

## Paraneoplastic Syndromes

This term identifies symptoms and signs secondary to cancer, occurring at a site distant from the tumour or its metastases. They are caused by the production of products such as polypeptide hormones, hormone-like peptides, antibodies, immune complexes, and so on, by the tumour. Cushing's syndrome, the most common, is due to ectopic adrenocorticotrophic hormone (ACTH) production, usually seen in SCLC. The syndrome of inappropriate antidiuretic hormone secretion (SIADH) is also mainly seen with SCLC. In half the cases there is ectopic antidiuretic hormone (ADH) (vasopressin) secretion from the tumour. In the remainder there is abnormal release of this peptide from the posterior pituitary because of altered or defective chemoreceptor control. Non-metastatic hypercalcaemia is most common in squamous cell carcinoma. The squamous carcinoma cells secrete parathyroid hormone-related peptide (PTH-rP), which shows limited sequence homology with parathyroid hormone. Gynaecomastia may develop in patients with lung cancer because of increased levels of βhCG (β human chorionic gonadotrophin). Neurological syndromes associated with carcinomas are discussed in Chapter 11 (pp. 336–337).

A 48-year-old steelworker presented with a history of weight loss, persistent cough, and occasional flecks of blood in his sputum. His elder brother died 3 years ago from lung cancer. On examination, his fingers were heavily nicotine stained, and there was loss of the nailbed angle and increased fluctuation at the nailbed, a feature known as finger clubbing. There was dullness to percussion at the right lung base. The liver was palpable three finger-breadths below the costal margin. A chest radiograph showed shadowing in the right base of the lung and ultrasound showed multiple echogenic areas within the liver.

Blood biochemistry revealed deranged liver function tests, particularly an elevated alkaline phosphatase, indicating obstruction of biliary drainage. Sputum was sent for cytological examination but this showed only inflammatory cells. Microbiological culture grew *Haemophilus influenzae*, sensitive to broad-spectrum antibiotics. However, bronchoscopy showed obstruction of the right lower lobe bronchus with bleeding. Brushings for cytology showed only inflammatory cells but a biopsy showed squamous cell carcinoma undermining the bronchial mucosa. Further imaging showed widespread metastases in hilar and mediastinal lymph nodes. The patient's condition deteriorated rapidly and he died within 3 weeks of presentation.

This case illustrates a number of key points about lung cancer:

- Smoking is its main cause.
- It has often metastasized by the time of clinical presentation (most common with small cell carcinoma, but sometimes, as here, also with non-small cell carcinoma), commonly to the lymph nodes and liver.
- Negative cytology (or biopsy) does not exclude carcinoma.

## Other Lung Tumours

Primary pulmonary lymphomas are rare and most commonly are marginal zone lymphomas of extranodal origin (mucosa-associated lymphoid tissue or MALT lymphomas). Other lymphomas found in the lung are similar to non-Hodgkin's lymphomas elsewhere, most being B cell in origin and most representing involvement by systemic lymphomas. Primary pulmonary sarcomas are also rare. The lung is frequently the site of secondary carcinomas and sarcomas, especially osteogenic and high-grade soft-tissue sarcoma. As a result of advances in chemotherapy it may be beneficial to treat these patients with localized resection.

# MISCELLANEOUS LUNG DISEASES

## The Lung in Systemic Disease

Systemic diseases may affect the lungs. The most common are the connective tissue disorders (CTDs), which can affect the lungs in diverse ways including airway disease (e.g. bronchiectasis), interstitial lung diseases (e.g. UIP, NSIP), vascular disease (e.g. alveolar haemorrhage and pulmonary hypertension), and granulomatous disease (e.g. rheumatoid nodules). The most common CTDs affecting the lung are rheumatoid arthritis (see Chapter 12, pp. 372–375), systemic lupus erythematosus (SLE), and scleroderma. In rheumatoid disease pulmonary involvement may precede the joint manifestations. There may be pleural effusions, interstitial fibrosis, and rheumatoid nodules, which may cavitate and cause haemorrhage.

SLE causes ARDS, pulmonary haemorrhage, and pleural effusions as the main manifestations. Scleroderma most commonly causes interstitial pulmonary fibrosis, but 30% of patients have pulmonary hypertension and the CREST syndrome (**c**alcinosis, **R**aynaud's phenomenon, **o**esophageal involvement, **s**clerodactyly, and **t**elangiectasia). Pulmonary hypertension is caused by medial hypertrophy of pulmonary arteries and concentric intimal thickening with myxoid connective tissue. Sjögren's syndrome is an autoimmune disorder characterized by keratoconjunctivitis sicca syndrome and xerostomia. It affects females in the fourth to sixth decades of life. There is xerotrachea (desiccation of the bronchial tree) and lymphocytic infiltration, which extends to the bronchial tree. It may progress to malignant lymphoma. The lung may be affected by amyloidosis including primary (myeloma associated) or secondary (inflammation or malignancy associated). Other systemic diseases that can affect the lung include inflammatory bowel disease and disorders of collagen and elastin such as Ehlers–Danlos syndrome.

## Drug-induced Lung Disease

Drugs can affect the lungs in a variety of dose-dependent and idiosyncratic ways. Toxicity can be enhanced by factors such as age, radiotherapy, and oxygen therapy. The main drugs causing pulmonary damage are cytotoxic agents, especially busulphan used in chronic myeloid leukaemia. This produces atypical epithelial cells with large hyperchromatic nuclei, suggesting malignancy, and progresses to interstitial fibrosis. Other drugs can produce pulmonary oedema, haemorrhage, pulmonary hypertension, and SLE.

## Langerhans' Cell Histiocytosis

The lung may be involved in this tumour-like disorder characterized by proliferation of Langerhans' cells; the cause is unknown but there is a strong association with cigarette smoking. In adults there is often interstitial lung disease. Most patients are between 10 and 40 years of age with an equal sex distribution. They present with dyspnoea, cough, chest pain, and wheezing, and radiologically there are reticulonodular infiltrates. Pulmonary function tests may be normal or have a restrictive or obstructive pattern.

Early in the disease there are nodules up to 1 cm in diameter, composed of a proliferation of Langerhans' cells; these show nuclear grooving and stain with CD1a and S100. Ultrastructurally the Langerhans' cell shows cytoplasmic, laminar, racket-shaped bodies (Birbeck's granules). Over time there may be progression to a fibrotic honeycomb and associated pulmonary emphysema.

# THE PLEURA

### Key Points

- Effusions and pleurisy are common and have many causes.
- Pneumothorax may follow rupture of bullae or penetrating injury.
- Mesothelioma is the most common tumour, and is due to asbestos exposure in most cases.

The pleural cavity is a potential space between the parietal and visceral pleura. The former covers the inner surface of the thoracic cage, mediastinum, and diaphragm, and the latter covers the lung surfaces. Both consist of a single layer of mesothelial cells, basement membrane, and layers of collagen and elastic tissue. Mesothelial cells vary in shape from flat to cuboidal or columnar, and ultrastructurally have long microvilli.

## Pleural Effusion

This is a common problem and is detected clinically when approximately 0.5 L is present. It appears first in the costophrenic angle. The effusion is categorized as a transudate or exudate. Normal pleural fluid has a protein concentration of 0.4 g/dL. A transudate has a protein concentration <30 g/L and is usually due to haemodynamic disorders, such as cardiac failure or severe hypoalbuminaemia. Exudates are due to inflammatory or neoplastic processes, where vascular permeability is increased, and have a protein content >30 g/L. The causes of pleural effusions are given in *Table 7.5*.

Empyema is a collection of pus in the pleural cavity, usually secondary to an underlying pneumonia, sometimes following penetrating chest trauma or rarely post-thoracic surgery. Haemothorax, a collection of blood, follows thoracic trauma or rupture of a thoracic aortic aneurysm. Chylothorax is a collection of opalescent lymph, usually due to obstruction of the thoracic duct, typically by a tumour.

## Pneumothorax

The accumulation of air in the pleural space is commonly caused by rupture of an emphysematous bulla, but may also follow penetrating chest wall injuries. Air leaks into the pleural space, causing collapse of the underlying lung. Occasionally a valve-like mechanism allows progressive accumulation of air and build-up of pressure with compression (and shift) of the mediastinal structures and contralateral lung. This is called a tension pneumothorax.

## Pleural Plaques

Pleural plaques are well-circumscribed discs of acellular hyaline collagen, seen mostly on parietal and diaphragmatic pleura and occasionally on the visceral pleura. Typically they are located in the posterolateral aspects of the lower thorax and the upper surface of the diaphragm. In the chest they lie parallel to the ribs (see Fig. 7.15). They may calcify and appear in the chest radiograph. Their importance is that they are evidence of asbestos exposure, but otherwise they have no intrinsic clinical importance.

## Pleural Tumours

### Malignant Mesothelioma

Malignant mesothelioma may arise in the pleura, peritoneum, or rarely the pericardium. It is due largely to exposure to asbestos, especially crocidolite (blue asbestos) and amosite. In the Cappadocia region of Turkey, where erionite, a non-asbestos zeolite fibre, is present in the soil, mesothelioma and asbestos-related disease are endemic. The incidence in the UK is rising and is expected to peak in the year 2020. The lag period from exposure to development of disease is long, in the order of 40+ years. The age-adjusted incidence in the USA is shown in Fig. 7.26. Pleural mesothelioma is rare before the age of 40 and shows a male predominance, most exposure being occupational. However, females may be exposed through factory work, and environmental and paraoccupational exposure (e.g. to asbestos dust on their partner's clothes). Patients present with dyspnoea, pleural effusion, chest pain, weight loss, cough, and fever, and most are dead within a year.

Malignant mesothelioma is usually unilateral, starting as small nodules over the visceral pleura and extending to cover the entire lung (Fig. 7.27). As the pleural cavity is obliterated, it is impossible to define the origin of the tumour. The tumour can also encase the pericardium, myocardium, mediastinum, aorta, oesophagus, and other great vessels, and grow into underlying lung, along the septa. These tumours

**TABLE 7.5** Causes of pleural effusion

| General cause | Specific cause | Effect |
|---|---|---|
| Trauma | Direct trauma | Haemothorax |
| | Fractured ribs | Haemothorax |
| | Bleeding dyscrasia, e.g. warfarin therapy | Haemothorax |
| Neoplasia | Extension of primary lung carcinoma | Exudative, may also be bloody |
| | Primary malignant mesothelioma | Exudative, may also be bloody |
| | Metastatic carcinoma, e.g. from breast or ovarian primary | Exudative |
| Inflammation and infection | Pneumonia | Exudative |
| | Pulmonary embolus | Exudative |
| | Pleurisy (infection) | Suppurative |
| | Systemic lupus erythematosus | Exudative, may also be bloody |
| Organ failure | Cardiac, renal, or liver failure | Hydrothorax, transudate |
| Lymphatic obstruction | Caused by tumour | Chylous (lymph) |

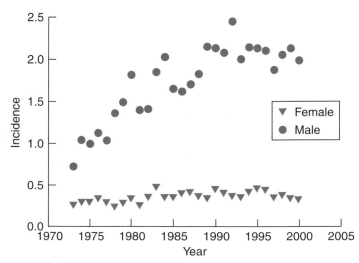

**FIG. 7.26** Age-adjusted mesothelioma incidents in USA (cases per 100,000) by gender. (Source: Weill H, Hughes JM, Churg AM. Changing trends in US mesothelioma incidence. *Occup Environ Med* 2004;**61**:438–441.)

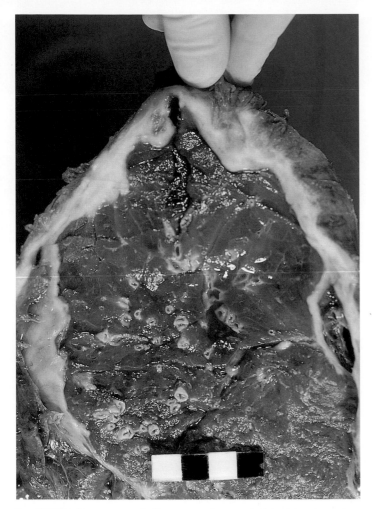

FIG. 7.27 Malignant mesothelioma encasing most of the lobe shown in this field.

are divided into epithelioid, sarcomatoid, and mixed subtypes. The epithelioid subtype is composed of cuboidal cells and often shows tubulopapillary, acinar, or microcystic architecture. Sarcomatoid mesothelioma consists of malignant spindle cells among collagen. Mixed mesothelioma shows both patterns. The diagnosis of mesothelioma and its differentiation from reactive mesothelium and metastatic adenocarcinoma can be difficult. Mucin stains are negative in mesothelioma and a panel of immunostains is helpful. Peritoneal mesothelioma is less common than pleural disease and is often associated with frank asbestosis. There is vague abdominal discomfort and distension with decreased appetite and constipation.

## Localized Fibrous Tumour

This is rare tumour of submesothelial fibroblasts. It is often asymptomatic but some patients have cough, dyspnoea, finger clubbing, and hypoglycaemia. The tumours are round or oblong and may be attached to the pleura by a pedicle. They are greyish/white, nodular, or lobulated tumours composed of spindle cells. They are usually benign but some tumours can behave in a more aggressive fashion, invading the underlying lung. However, both are generally cured by complete surgical excision.

## SUMMARY

As the organ of respiration and being open to the atmosphere, the lung is susceptible to infection, the causes of occupational lung disease, as well as inhaled allergens and cigarette smoke. It also forms a close interface with the heart, and thus diseases of one system impact on the other. Lung diseases are of great importance to all doctors, because asthma, COPD, lung infections, and lung cancer will form the bulk of many general practitioners' workload. In many developing countries, diseases such as tuberculosis are a major health problem. With the advent of readily available air travel, such infections are easily transported to this country, causing disease in susceptible individuals. The pleural cavity may give rise to a unique tumour, mesothelioma, an asbestos-related tumour that is due to peak in incidence in the UK by 2020.

## ACKNOWLEDGEMENTS

The contributions of Philip S Hasleton and David J Harrison to this chapter in the 14th edition are gratefully acknowledged.

## FURTHER READING

Cagle PT, Allen T, Barrios R, *et al. Color Atlas and Text of Pulmonary Pathology*, 2nd edn. Philadelphia, PA: Lippincott Williams & Wilkins, 2007.

Corrin B, Nicholson AG. *Pathology of the Lungs*. 3rd edn. Edinburgh: Churchill Livingstone, 2011.

Tomashetski JF, Cagle PT, Farver CF, Fraire AE, eds. *Dail and Hammars' Pulmonary Pathology*. Berlin: Springer Verlag, 2008.

Travis WD, Brambilla E, Muller-Hermelink HK, Harris CC. *World Health Organization Classification of Tumours. Pathology and Genetics of Tumours of the Lung, Pleura, Thymus and Heart*. Lyon: IARC Press, 2004.

Travis WD, Brambilla E, Riely GJ. New pathologic classification of lung cancer: relevance for clinical practice and clinical trials. *J Clin Oncol* 2013;**31**:992-1001.

# 8

# THE LYMPHORETICULAR SYSTEM AND BONE MARROW

Paul Van der Valk

## INTRODUCTION

The lymphoreticular system is involved in the defence of the body against microorganisms and foreign substances, i.e. the immune response. The system consists of two discrete organs, the thymus and spleen, together with an extensive network of lymph nodes, which are distributed throughout the body. In addition, there is diffuse lymphoid tissue, which is closely associated with mucosal surfaces, most prominently in the gut (see Chapter 9, pp. 253–254), and also in the upper respiratory tract in Waldeyer's ring, including the tonsils and adenoids. Lymphoid cells are also well represented within the bone marrow. This is, of course, the site of haematopoiesis – the process by which mature blood cells are produced.

In this chapter, diseases of the lymph nodes, spleen, and thymus are described. Although the pathology of the bone marrow is discussed and brief mention is made of haematological disease, no attempt has been made to provide any comprehensive account of all 'blood diseases', which properly fall into the subject of haematology. Hence, readers are referred to standard textbooks on this topic.

## DISEASES OF THE LYMPH NODES

Under normal conditions lymph nodes are small bean-shaped structures, which even in their major peripheral locations (e.g. cervical, axillary or inguinal) are seldom palpable. Their

### Key Points

- Lymph nodes are the frontier posts of the lymphatic system.
- Enlargement is usually due to an inflammatory process.
- Sometimes, the underlying cause (tuberculosis, toxoplasmosis, HIV) can be deduced from the nature of the cellular response.
- Lymph nodes are commonly involved in malignancy, both primary (lymphomas) and secondary (carcinoma, melanoma).

primary function is to entrap and, if need be, to mount an immune response to foreign agents or unwanted materials that have gained access to the tissue spaces. The structure of a lymph node and its basic functions are illustrated diagrammatically in Fig. 8.1.

Lymph node enlargement is an important clinical finding. The main causes are listed in *Box 8.1*, in which they are classified by the pattern of the histological appearances seen. In most cases, lymphadenopathy is a reaction to inflammatory disturbances taking place in the tissue spaces, even though in some cases the nature of the provoking agent cannot be identified. Nodal enlargement is caused by a neoplastic process in only a minority of cases, but this must always be borne in mind, especially if lymphadenopathy is persistent and unexplained.

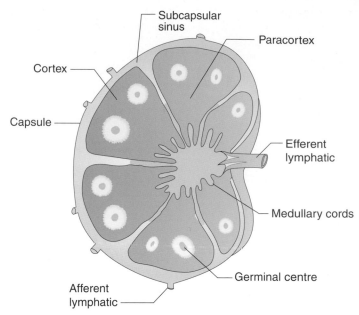

**FIG. 8.1** Diagrammatic structure of a lymph node. Material enters the sinus network of the lymph node via the afferent lymphatics. The phagocytic cells, which line the sinuses, entrap the antigenic material and deliver it to antigen-presenting cells within the B- and T-cell areas. A B-cell reaction results in germinal centre formation within the cortex, which leads to the production of plasma cells and memory cells; these recirculate. T-cell reactions occur mainly within the deep paracortical areas.

---

**Box 8.1** IMPORTANT CAUSES OF LYMPHADENOPATHY

**Reactive states**

Acute lymphadenitis:
 Pyogenic infections

Follicular hyperplasia:
 Non-specific reaction
 HIV infection
 Rheumatoid arthritis, systemic lupus erythematosus, and other connective tissue diseases

Paracortical reactions:
 Drug hypersensitivity, e.g. anticonvulsants
 Viruses, e.g. Epstein–Barr virus, cytomegalovirus

Histiocytic reaction:
 Foreign material, e.g. anthracosis, silicone
 Dermatopathic lymphadenopathy

Granulomatous reactions:
 Infection, e.g. tuberculosis, toxoplasmosis, fungi
 Unknown, e.g. sarcoidosis, Crohn's disease, reaction to tumours

**Neoplastic**

Metastatic tumours:
 Carcinoma, melanoma

Primary tumours:
 Hodgkin lymphoma
 Non-Hodgkin lymphoma

---

## Reactive Lymphadenopathy

Lymph nodes are commonly enlarged due to transient acute inflammation taking place during pyogenic infections involving the tissue spaces (acute lymphadenitis). Lymphadenopathy may also arise as a consequence of chronic inflammation. Although it is convenient to classify these reactions according to the predominant reactive element (see *Box 8.1*), mixed patterns are commonly seen.

### Acute Lymphadenitis

This is an acute inflammatory reaction to organisms or toxins that have gained entry to the lymphatics from tissue spaces. It may be preceded by inflammation of the lymphatics themselves (lymphangitis), and the initial reaction takes place within the sinuses. In some cases suppuration follows. This type of lesion is seen in cervical lymph nodes draining acute streptococcal tonsillitis. Historically, bubonic plague is more dramatic: a bubo is an acutely inflamed lymph node after entry of the plague bacillus through a flea bite in the lower limb.

### Follicular Hyperplasia

Germinal centre formation within the cortical B-cell population is an expression of antigenic exposure, and not surprisingly becomes exaggerated in reactive states (Fig. 8.2). It is not specific, and can be seen in relation to many inflammatory conditions. It is especially pronounced in some infections, most notably HIV, cytomegalovirus (CMV), and toxoplasmosis, and autoimmune disorders such as rheumatoid arthritis.

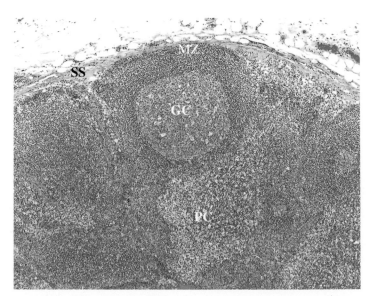

**FIG. 8.2** A lymph node displaying follicular hyperplasia. GC = germinal centre; MZ = mantle zone; PC = paracortex; SS = subcapsular sinus.

## Paracortical Hyperplasia

This reactive process takes place in the deeper parts of the lymph node cortex (T-cell zones) and is recognized by the presence of numerous large transformed lymphocytes (immunoblasts). This change is usually seen in viral infections, most notably infectious mononucleosis, and drug reactions, especially to anticonvulsants. The degree of lymphoid proliferation is so florid in these latter conditions that the unwary pathologist can mistake the histological features for malignant lymphoma.

## Histiocytic Reactions

Sinus histiocytosis – a proliferation of histiocytes in the sinuses – is a common reaction most often seen in nodes draining malignant tumours. Reactions with increased histiocytes within the nodal parenchyma are usually related to foreign material or cellular debris. Accumulation of anthracotic carbon pigment is prominent within the mediastinal and hilar nodes of older city dwellers due to soot inhalation. Other materials that produce these reactions include silicone used in artificial finger joints and breast implants. In dermatopathic lymphadenopathy, lymph nodes that are involved in draining skin disorders – especially lichenoid conditions and mycosis fungoides (see Chapter 18, p. 533) – may be considerably enlarged due to a paracortical proliferation of Langerhans' cells and histiocytes containing melanin pigment. This is an entirely benign reaction, but, in cases of T-cell lymphoma, small numbers of malignant cells can be present in such a pattern and should be looked for diligently.

## Granulomatous Reactions

Granulomas are seen in lymph nodes in many circumstances (*Box 8.2*), and infections, especially tuberculosis (TB), are one of the most important causes. The granulomas in TB, unlike those in sarcoidosis, commonly show central necrosis. Necrotizing granulomas are also a typical feature of cat-scratch disease and lymphogranuloma venereum. Sarcoid-like granulomas can occur in reactive nodes draining carcinomas and lymphomas (especially Hodgkin lymphoma) and in mesenteric nodes in Crohn's disease.

## Miscellaneous Lymph Node Lesions

Kikuchi's disease (histiocytic necrotizing lymphadenitis) is a self-limiting disease characterized by painful cervical lymphadenopathy, mainly in young females. Langerhans' cell histiocytosis (see Chapter 7, p. 193 and Chapter 12, p. 369) may affect lymph nodes. The hyaline vascular variant of Castleman's disease is another idiopathic condition that gives rise to a (often mediastinal) mass composed of abnormal lymphoid tissue with prominent follicular structures containing a central blood vessel. Another form exists in which there is massive infiltration by numerous plasma cells, often associated with fever, anaemia, weight loss, and other systemic symptoms.

---

**Box 8.2** CAUSES OF GRANULOMATOUS LYMPHADENOPATHY

**Infectious causes**
- Tuberculosis
- Cat-scratch disease
- Yersiniosis
- Spirochaetal disease
- Fungal infection, e.g. histoplasmosis
- Leishmaniasis
- Toxoplasmosis
- Schistosomiasis

**Idiopathic**
- Sarcoidosis
- Crohn's disease
- Primary biliary cirrhosis

**Reactive**
- Foreign material, e.g. silicone from prosthesis
- Draining tumour/carcinoma/Hodgkin lymphoma/ non-Hodgkin lymphoma
- Drug reactions

---

## Malignant Lymphomas

This term describes primary tumours of the lymphoreticular system (as opposed to the bone marrow), almost all of which arise from lymphocytes. They vary greatly in their behaviour and, although most prove fatal if untreated, considerable advances have been made in their management. Most lymphomas arise in lymph nodes, but 30–40% develop in extranodal sites such as the stomach, although almost any organ may be primarily involved. They usually produce lymph node enlargement, which may be localized or generalized, with widespread involvement of the lymphoreticular system at presentation. This latter tendency is a reflection of the normal recirculating behaviour of lymphocytes. Ironically, more aggressive lymphomas may remain localized, at least for a time, and tend to spread to adjacent nodes, rather like carcinomas.

## Classification of Lymphomas

It is customary to distinguish between Hodgkin lymphoma (HL) and non-Hodgkin lymphomas (NHL). Although this is to some extent a historical and rather arbitrary distinction, it remains of major importance in determining therapy and prognosis. In view of the complexity of lymphoma diagnosis, there have been many classifications over the years. With the advent of modern investigative techniques, the accuracy and reproducibility of classification is now high and the World Health Organization's (WHO's) classification published in 2001, and revised in 2008, is accepted throughout the world (*Box 8.3*). It combines haematoxylin and eosin (H&E) morphology, immunophenotyping, genetic information, and clinical features to define specific disease entities with a particular clinical course and prognosis. As the number of therapeutic options increases and specific treatments become linked to defined entities, accurate classification and a standardized nomenclature become increasingly important.

---

**Box 8.3** THE WORLD HEALTH ORGANIZATION'S (WHO)CLASSIFICATION OF LYMPHOMAS (2008) – SIMPLIFIED

**B-cell neoplasms**
*Precursor B-cell neoplasm*
Precursor B-lymphoblastic leukaemia/lymphoma

*Mature B-cell neoplasms*
Chronic lymphocytic leukaemia/small lymphocytic lymphoma
Lymphoplasmacytic lymphoma
Hairy cell leukaemia
Plasma cell myeloma
Extranodal marginal zone B-cell lymphoma
Follicular lymphoma
Mantle cell lymphoma
Diffuse large B-cell lymphoma (and variants)
Primary mediastinal large B-cell lymphoma
Plasmablastic lymphoma
Burkitt lymphoma
Post-transplantation lymphoproliferative disorder

**T-cell neoplasms**

*Precursor T-cell neoplasms*
T-lymphoblastic lymphoma/leukaemia

*Mature T-cell neoplasms*
T-cell prolymphocytic leukaemia
Adult T-cell leukaemia/lymphoma
Mycosis fungoides
Sézary's syndrome
Peripheral T-cell lymphoma
Enteropathy-type T-cell lymphoma
Angioimmunoblastic T-cell lymphoma
Subcutaneous panniculitis-like T-cell lymphoma
Anaplastic large-cell lymphoma
Primary cutaneous CD30-positive T-cell lymphoma
Extranodal natural killer (NK)/T-cell lymphoma, nasal type

**Hodgkin lymphoma**
Nodular lymphocyte predominant Hodgkin lymphoma
Classical Hodgkin lymphoma
   Nodular sclerosis
   Mixed cellularity
   Lymphocyte rich
   Lymphocyte depleted

---

## Hodgkin Lymphoma

**Key Points**

- These tumours are characterized by the presence of Reed–Sternberg cells, with an appropriate cellular background.
- Patients present with lymphadenopathy, which is often painless.
- Systemic symptoms are common.
- The extent of the tumour (clinical stage) correlates with the prognosis.
- Epstein–Barr virus (EBV) is aetiologically important in a little under half the cases.

First described in 1832, Hodgkin's disease was subsequently defined pathologically by the presence of distinctive large tumour cells known as Reed–Sternberg cells. Approximately 25% of cases of malignant lymphoma fall into this category. Although it was always suspected that Hodgkin disease was a lymphoma, proof that Hodgkin cells were in fact unusual germinal centre-derived B cells has come to light only in recent years – hence the use of the term 'Hodgkin's lymphoma' rather than 'Hodgkin's disease' in the 2001 and 2008 WHO classifications.

### Clinical Features

Hodgkin lymphoma has a bimodal incidence with peaks in early adult life and late middle age (4 in 100,000 of the population per annum). Cases in childhood are sometimes seen, especially in developing countries. Clinically, HL usually presents with enlargement of peripheral lymph nodes, the diagnosis then being made by lymph node biopsy. Extranodal involvement is extremely rare and usually due to direct extension from a nodal mass. Patients with large mediastinal masses may present with superior vena caval obstruction. There may be systemic symptoms, most notably an intermittent low-grade fever, sweating, weight loss, and pruritus. The disease may be complicated by concurrent infection due to immunological impairment. The extent of involvement by HL is defined by the Ann Arbor staging system (*Table 8.1*), and is highly relevant for planning treatment. The tumour spreads early from one nodal group to another, whereas liver and bone marrow involvement are late events.

### Macroscopic Pathology

The affected lymph nodes are usually discrete and rubbery, but may be matted together. They have a grey–pink cut surface, often with areas of necrosis. There may be dense bands of fibrous tissue around and within the node (see Fig. 8.8).

### Histological Appearance

The two main histological features of HL are, first, the presence of a small population of large neoplastic cells, the

TABLE 8.1 The Ann Arbor staging system for Hodgkin lymphoma

| Stage[a] | Description of lymphoma |
| --- | --- |
| I | Disease is confined to one lymph node group or involvement of a single extranodal site (I$_E$) |
| II | Disease confined to several lymph node groups on the same side of the diaphragm[b] |
| III | Disease is present in lymph node groups on both sides of the diaphragm with minimal involvement of an adjacent extranodal site (III$_E$) |
| IV | Diffuse involvement of one or more extranodal tissues, e.g. bone marrow or liver |

[a]Each stage is subdivided according to whether systemic symptoms are present (B) or not (A).

[b]The spleen is regarded as a lymph node for staging purposes.

Hodgkin/Reed–Sternberg cell, and, second, a large population of non-neoplastic inflammatory cells. Two distinct forms of HL are now recognized: classic HL and nodular lymphocyte-predominant HL. These appear to be separate tumours biologically, and their distinction is important clinically.

### Classical Hodgkin Lymphoma

Classical HL (CHL) accounts for 94% of all HLs, and is characterized by the presence of typical Reed–Sternberg cells and their mononuclear variants, collectively termed 'Hodgkin/Reed–Sternberg cells' (HRS cells). As cells similar to HRS cells can sometimes be seen in other conditions, it is important that there is also a mixed inflammatory background consisting of small lymphocytes, histiocytes, plasma cells, eosinophils, and neutrophils (Fig. 8.3). The Reed–Sternberg cells each have multiple nuclei (mostly two nuclei are seen), each with a large eosinophilic nucleolus (Fig. 8.4); the cytoplasm is abundant. Mononuclear and pleomorphic variants are common. The HRS cells have a particular phenotype that can easily be established by immunocytochemistry on paraffin sections. They are positive for CD30 and CD15, and negative for the standard B- and T-cell antigens (see Fig. 8.10). The expression of Pax5, a transcription factor initiating B-cell development, is proof of the B-cell origin of these cells and helps in difficult cases to make the distinction between HL and certain T-cell lymphomas. Surprisingly, HRS cells are also negative for CD45, the common leukocyte antigen that is expressed on all lymphocytes. Although the pathologist is usually fairly certain of the diagnosis based on the H&E morphology, it is good practice to perform immunophenotyping to support this impression. If the immunocytochemical profile does not fit, an alternative diagnosis should be considered, because there are many mimics of HL.

CHL can be divided into four major subtypes based on variations in their histological features:

1. Nodular sclerosis (NS): this is the most common subtype, and represents 70% of all CHLs. The tumour consists of mixed cellular nodules surrounded by thick bands of collagen. The Reed–Sternberg cells show cytoplasmic vacuolation (lacunar cells). Typically, nodular sclerosis HL occurs in young adult females, and mediastinal involvement is common (see Case History 8.1).

2. Mixed cellularity (MC): representing 20% of all CHLs, this variant is characterized by a mixed cell population often including granulomas, but lacks the fibrosis seen in nodular sclerosis. This subtype is more common in elderly people and HIV-positive patients, and is more frequently associated with EBV.

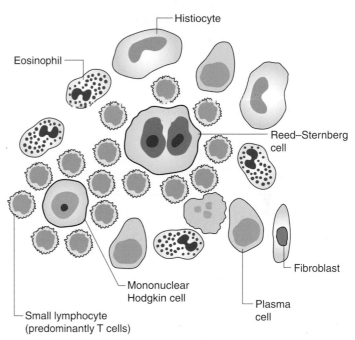

FIG. 8.3 Schematic diagram of the cellular composition of classic Hodgkin lymphoma. The Reed–Sternberg and mononuclear Hodgkin cells are the neoplastic component and may account for only 5% of the total cellularity. Hodgkin/Reed–Sternberg (HRS) cells secrete cytokines (e.g. interleukins, tumour necrosis factor), which invoke the inflammatory cellular reaction. Cytokine production is also likely to account for the fever and sweats experienced by some patients.

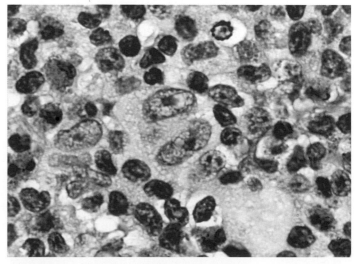

FIG. 8.4 A typical Reed–Sternberg cell surrounded by a mixed infiltrate of small lymphocytes, a single histiocyte, and eosinophils.

3. Lymphocyte-rich CHL (LRCHL): a variant in which the stromal response consists almost exclusively of small lymphocytes. It occurs predominantly in males and usually presents at a low stage. Immunocytochemistry is required to distinguish it accurately from nodular lymphocyte-predominant HL (NLPHL).

4. Lymphocyte-depleted CHL (LDCHL): the HRS cells predominate and are highly pleomorphic. Reactive lymphocytes are markedly reduced in number. Many tumours that were formerly included in this group have now been reclassified as high-grade non-Hodgkin lymphoma after detailed immunophenotyping. The LD subtype tends to occur in later life and presents at a high stage.

### Prognosis of Classical Hodgkin Lymphoma

In the past, the mixed cellularity and lymphocyte-depleted variants have been regarded as having a poorer prognosis. However, many of the prognostic differences formerly seen between the subcategories have been eradicated by modern chemotherapy. If CHL is untreated, death generally occurs in 6–24 months, but with treatment there is an 85% cure rate. Elderly people generally have a poorer outcome.

### Nodular Lymphocyte-predominant HL

In this form – which typically arises in young adult males and represents 6% of all HL cases – the tumour cells differ from classic Reed–Sternberg cells. They have folded, multilobated nuclei, less prominent nucleoli, and less abundant cytoplasm: they are known as 'popcorn cells'. These cells express B-cell markers (e.g. CD 20) and, unlike CHL, are capable of producing immunoglobulin and are usually negative for CD30 and CD15. In general, this variant has a very good prognosis. In 5% or so of cases, it evolves into a high-grade B-cell lymphoma.

### Aetiology of Hodgkin Lymphoma

There is now little doubt that EBV plays a major role in the causation of CHL (see Special Study Topic 8.1), but not of NLPHL.

## 8.1 Special Study Topic

### EPSTEIN–BARR VIRUS AND LYMPHOMA

In addition to being the causative agent of infectious mononucleosis (IM) and being linked to the development of nasopharyngeal carcinoma, EBV is also closely associated with a variety of lymphoid neoplasms (Box 8.4). Evidence of latent infection can be detected in 90% of normal adults. In the developed world, exposure tends to occur during adolescence, and this can give rise to the acute syndrome of IM, although in most patients the acute episode is asymptomatic. The virus resides in memory B cells, and low levels of infected cells can be detected in the blood and excised lymph nodes of normal individuals.

---

**Box 8.4** LYMPHOMAS ASSOCIATED WITH THE EPSTEIN–BARR VIRUS (EBV)

Burkitt lymphoma
Classical Hodgkin lymphoma
Immunosuppression-related lymphomas
Post-transplantation lymphoproliferative disorder
Primary immunodeficiency disorders
HIV related
Drug related (methotrexate, cytotoxics)
Lymphomatoid granulomatosis
Extranodal natural killer cell lymphoma/nasal type
Angioimmunoblastic T-cell lymphoma
EBV-positive diffuse large B-cell lymphomas (DLBCLs)

---

### Biology

EBV is a human herpes-type virus containing a genome of double-stranded DNA that is 172 kilobases in length and encodes approximately 100 genes. The virus is capable of infecting many different types of human cell, but it preferentially infects B lymphocytes via its capacity to bind to the B-cell surface protein CD21. Entry into cells other than lymphocytes is likely to be related to different types of receptors. There are two consequences of infection – lytic and latent. In lytic infection (as occurs in acute IM), the virus enters epithelial cells and replicates, with the release of many virions, which in turn infect neighbouring cells, including B lymphocytes. Many viral proteins are expressed on the cell surface and are recognized by host cytotoxic T cells; this brings about destruction of the infected cell. In latent infection, the normally linear DNA of the EBV genome forms a circular structure (an episome) by fusion of terminal repeat segments at either end of the viral genome. In contrast to lytic infection, only a small number of viral genes are expressed by the host cell, and this allows it to avoid recognition by cytotoxic T cells and so escape destruction. Each newly infected cell contains a viral episome of unique size due to variations in the length of terminal repetitive sequences. Viral replication occurs as the cell itself divides, each daughter cell containing an identical copy of the viral genome. Analysis of viral DNA by polymerase chain reaction (PCR) or Southern blotting can provide evidence as to the clonality of the viral genome. There are three different expression patterns of the latent genes in immortalized B cells, and these patterns can be seen in the various EBV-related lymphomas (Table 8.2).

## Special Study Topic continued . . .

TABLE 8.2 Gene expression profile in three different patterns of viral latency: EBERs (Epstein–Barr encoded small RNAs) are present within all patterns of latency

| Latency pattern | EBERs | EBNA1 | EBNA2 | EBNA3 A,B,C | EBNALP | LMP1 | LMP2 |
|---|---|---|---|---|---|---|---|
| Type 1 | + | + | – | – | – | – | – |
| Type 2 | + | + | – | – | – | + | + |
| Type 3 | + | + | + | + | + | + | + |

EBNA1, -2, -3A, -3B, -3C = Epstein–Barr nuclear antigen; LMP = latent membrane protein.
A type 1 pattern is seen in Burkitt lymphoma, type 2 in classical Hodgkin lymphoma, and type 3 in post-transplantation lymphoproliferative disorder.

In cell culture experiments, B lymphocytes infected by EBV continue to grow – they are immortalized. This is a reversible phenomenon, unlike true neoplastic transformation. All the latent gene products are important for cell immortalization, e.g. latent membrane protein 1 (LMP1) has been found to activate anti-apoptotic genes in cell lines, and also to induce permanent activation of various signal transduction pathways, resulting in up-regulation of nuclear factor κB (NFκB).

## Detection of EBV

EBV can be detected in paraffin-embedded tissue sections using either immunocytochemistry (ICC) or *in-situ* hybridization (ISH) (Figs. 8.5–8.7). Southern blotting and PCR methods performed on fresh tissue are also available and are useful in determining clonality of the viral genome.

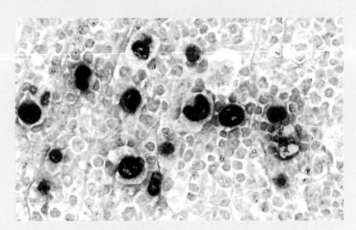

FIG. 8.6 *In situ* hybridization using an oligonucleotide probe to Epstein–Barr virus-encoded RNA (EBER) in a case of classical Hodgkin lymphoma. The nuclei of Reed–Sternberg and mononuclear Hodgkin cells contain large amounts of EBERs. The surrounding reactive T cells are negative.

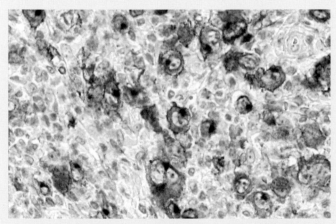

FIG. 8.5 Immunocytochemistry for Epstein–Barr virus (EBV) latent membrane protein 1 (LMP1) in classical Hodgkin lymphoma. Numerous Hodgkin/Reed–Sternberg cells are positive.

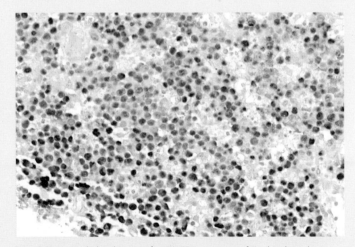

FIG. 8.7 *In situ* hybridization for EBER in a case of Burkitt lymphoma. The nucleus of every tumour cell is positive.

## Subtypes of Lymphoma Associated with EBV

### Burkitt Lymphoma

Virus-like particles were detected in cell cultures of endemic Burkitt lymphoma (BL) in 1964. EBV genomes of identical clonality are found in all tumour cells, in keeping with infection before the monoclonal expansion of the lymphoid population (see Fig. 8.7). The occurrence of BL in particular geographical areas is related to coexistent endemic falciparum malaria, which results in a decreased T-cell immunity; this allows growth of the infected cells. Although EBV is present in all tumour cells in endemic BL, it

## Special Study Topic continued . . .

is the occurrence of a chromosomal translocation involving the *c-myc* locus on chromosome 8 that is the most important event in malignant transformation. It is possible that the EBV-induced immortalization of B lymphocytes increases the likelihood of this genetic event occurring.

The incidence of EBV positivity in sporadic BL in western countries is much lower (30%). Cases related to immunosuppression as a consequence of HIV or immunosuppressive drugs are often positive.

### Classical Hodgkin Lymphoma

EBV can be detected in the Reed Sternberg and mononuclear Hodgkin cells in 30–40% of cases, especially in those with the mixed cellularity variant and in elderly people (see Figs. 8.5 and 8.6). There is a threefold increase in the incidence of EBV-positive HL in those with a history of IM. The median interval between IM and the development of HL is 4–5 years, although the increased risk remains for 20 years. There appears to be no increase in EBV-negative HL after IM. In absolute terms, only 1 patient in 1,000 with a history of IM will develop HL, which implies that there are likely to be other important factors required for lymphomagenesis.

### Post-transplantation Lymphoproliferative Disorder

Perhaps the best evidence for a role for EBV in lymphoma pathogenesis is the development of lymphoproliferative disorders in patients who are receiving immunosuppressive therapy after allogeneic organ transplantation. The vast majority of post-transplantation lymphoproliferative disorder (PTLD) cases are positive for EBV. The incidence varies depending on the organ transplanted (1% in renal and 8% in lung transplantation), presumably reflecting the different levels of therapeutic immunosuppression required for each system. In normal individuals, latently infected cells remain in the bone marrow and tonsillar area, and further proliferation of virally infected cells is prevented by a natural killer (NK) and cytotoxic T-cell response. When this immunosurveillance is decreased as a result of immunosuppressive therapy, EBV induces cell proliferation. Initially this may be a polyclonal reactive proliferation of plasma cells but, as further genetic events occur, evolution to a monoclonal proliferation takes place, e.g. diffuse large B-cell lymphoma. Most lymphomas are of B lineage, but 10–14% are derived from T cells. In some cases a reduction of immunosuppression can bring about a sustained remission, although this may not be possible in many cases because of the risk of rejection of the transplanted organ. In these cases chemotherapy will be required.

### EBV-driven Lymphomas (not transplant related)

Immunosuppression from other causes may be complicated by EBV-driven diffuse large B-cell, Burkitt or Hodgkin lymphoma.

These include primary immune disorders, such as Wiskott–Aldrich syndrome and common variable immunodeficiency. The incidence of NHL, often extranodal, is increased approximately 100-fold in HIV infection. Immunosuppressive drugs such as methotrexate (which is used to treat severe psoriasis and autoimmune diseases) may give rise to lymphomas, 50% of which are positive for EBV. Regression is seen in 60% of cases if methotrexate can be withdrawn. Some EBV-driven lymphomas occur in patients who are not apparently immunosuppressed. The best example of this category is the extranodal NK/T-cell lymphoma of nasal type, which causes massive destruction of the tissues of the face, maxilla, and skull. This is most prevalent in Asia, and Central and South America, and almost 100% of cases are associated with the presence of EBV. Up to 5% of all diffuse large B-cell lymphomas (DLBCLs) occurring in previously well patients are EBV positive. It is possible that these patients have some specific defect in immune surveillance that has not yet been identified.

## Conclusion

There is a clear association between the development of various types of lymphoma and EBV infection. EBV can cause immortalization of cells, but other factors are required to cause neoplastic transformation. The importance of detecting EBV in human lymphomas is that it may highlight a potentially reversible cause of immunosuppression. Immunosuppression reduction, where possible, can result in regression in a significant proportion of cases. New therapies directed at improving deficient T-cell immunity in EBV-driven lymphomas are being developed. Autologous *in vitro*-activated and, even allogeneic cytotoxic, T lymphocytes directed specifically towards EBV antigens expressed by the tumour cells have already been used in the management of PTLD. Immunization against EBV, although not available at the present time, may have a role in lymphoma prevention in the future.

## Further Reading

Hjalgrim H, Askling J, Rostgaard K, *et al*. Characteristics of Hodgkin's lymphoma after infectious mononucleosis. *N Engl J Med* 2003;**349**:1324–1332.

Niedobitek G, Meru N, Delecluse HJ. Epstein–Barr virus infection and human malignancies. *Int J Exp Pathol* 2001;**82**:149–170.

Papadopolous EB, Ladanyi M, Emanuel D, *et al*. Infusions of donor lymphocytes to treat Epstein–Barr virus associated lymphoproliferative disorders after allogeneic marrow transplantation. *N Engl J Med* 1994;**330**:1185–1191.

Swerdlow SH, Campo E, Harris NL, *et al*. *World Health Organization Classification of Tumours of the Haemopoeitic and Lymphoid Tissues*. Lyon: IARC Press, 2008.

## CLASSICAL HODGKIN LYMPHOMA

A 19-year-old man presented to his general practitioner with an enlarged lymph node in his neck. The GP initially suspected a reactive condition because the boy recently had a tooth abscess on the same side. He decided to watch and wait. A month later, the patient returned and it was clear that the node had increased in size. The young man was now also suffering from night sweats and had experienced some weight loss. An urgent appointment was made for the neck lump clinic in the local hospital. An excision biopsy was performed (Fig. 8.8).

Histological examination revealed a nodular infiltrate divided by thick collagenous bands (Fig. 8.9). The nodules were composed of large numbers of small lymphocytes, histiocytes, neutrophil polymorphs, eosinophils, and plasma cells. There was also a moderate number of mononuclear HRS cells present. On immunocytochemical analysis, the large cells were positive for CD30 (Fig. 8.10) and CD15, but negative for CD45, and B- and T-cell lineage markers. The pathological features were characteristic of CHL – nodular sclerosis subtype.

The patient was referred to the haematologist who arranged for staging to be carried out. Computed tomography (CT) revealed a large mediastinal mass (Fig. 8.11), in addition to abdominal and para-aortic lymphadenopathy. A bone marrow trephine biopsy was negative. The Ann Arbor stage was IIIB. The man was informed that Hodgkin lymphoma is a malignant condition, which will progress if left untreated, but that with chemotherapy and radiotherapy a cure can be achieved in 85% of patients. The patient underwent six cycles of chemotherapy over a 6-month period, during which the patient experienced hair loss and mild nausea. He also required intravenous antibiotics for an episode of sepsis related to a transient neutropenia. A repeat CT scan at the end of therapy showed complete resolution of the mediastinal mass (Fig. 8.12). The patient remains in complete remission at 5 years after therapy, and is now regarded as cured.

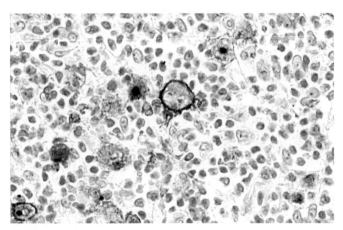

FIG. 8.10 Immunohistochemistry for CD30. Several Hodgkin/Reed–Sternberg (HRS) cells display membrane and perinuclear dot positivity for CD30.

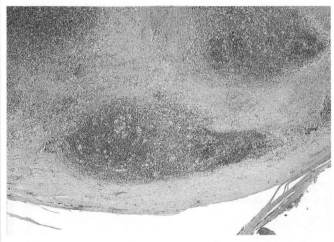

FIG. 8.8 Photograph of the cut surface of the excised lymph node (3 cm maximum) which has a nodular architecture with fibrotic bands between the nodules.

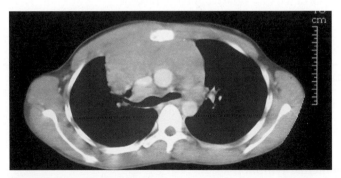

FIG. 8.11 Computed tomography scan of the thorax, showing a large mediastinal mass.

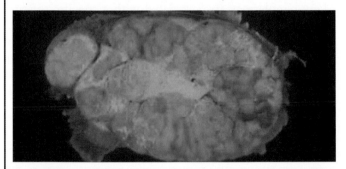

FIG. 8.9 Low-power view of the nodal histology. Thick bands of collagen divided the node into cellular nodules. There is also a thickened capsule.

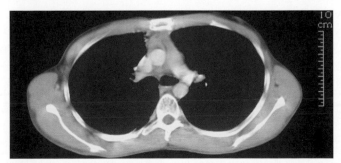

FIG. 8.12 Computed tomography scan of the thorax after treatment; the mass is no longer apparent.

# Non-Hodgkin Lymphoma

> **Key Points**
> - This is a heterogeneous group of tumours, with a complex classification.
> - There is a wide range of clinical behaviours between subtypes.
> - Low-grade tumours are often widely disseminated at presentation and grow slowly, but are seldom cured.
> - High-grade tumours are often localized and grow rapidly, but may be cured by chemotherapy.
> - In western countries B-cell lymphomas predominate.

These tumours show great diversity in their behaviour and morphology. The accurate diagnosis and WHO classification of NHL is essential in planning rational treatment and requires a combination of histological, immunocytochemical, and molecular genetic techniques. The incidence in Britain is approximately 16/100,000 per annum.

## Diagnosis of NHL

### H&E Morphology

Distinguishing between a reactive lymphoid infiltrate and a lymphoma can sometimes be difficult, because individual neoplastic lymphocytes – unlike the situation in carcinoma – often look identical to their normal counterparts. However, the distribution of the neoplastic lymphocytes and the low-power architecture of the excised lymph node give important clues to the diagnosis – hence the importance of a relatively large biopsy.

### Immunophenotyping

Different categories of normal lymphocytes express various surface antigens, which can be detected either by flow cytometry in liquid cell suspensions or by immunocytochemistry on paraffin blocks of formalin-fixed tissue. Many lymphomas have a characteristic pattern of antigen expression, and therefore a panel of antibodies is applied to lymph node biopsies in routine diagnostic practice (*Table 8.3*).

### Detection of Clonality

Reactive lymphoid infiltrates are derived from many different clones, all directed against different antigens. The cells in a lymphoma are genetically identical and represent the progeny of a single cell (monoclonal). In a B-lymphocytic proliferation, the demonstration that the cells produce only one of the two types of immunoglobulin light chain ($\kappa$ or $\lambda$), by either immunocytochemistry or *in situ* hybridization, effectively establishes the presence of monoclonality and thus of neoplasia. Monoclonality can also be determined by detecting clonal rearrangements of immunoglobulin and T-cell receptor genes in B- and T-cell lymphomas, respectively.

### Cytogenetics

Many lymphomas are associated with a specific reciprocal chromosomal translocation, and detection of these by either classic cytogenetics or molecular techniques (fluorescence *in situ* hybridization [FISH] and PCR) may be very helpful in establishing a diagnosis (see *Table 8.3*). In some instances the protein product of the translocation may be detected by immunocytochemistry.

**TABLE 8.3** Immunocytochemical profile and cytogenetic abnormalities of the most common B-cell lymphomas

| Tumour | CD20 | CD5 | CD10 | CD23 | CyclinD1 | Cytogenetics |
|---|---|---|---|---|---|---|
| Small lymphocytic lymphoma (SLL)/ Chronic lymphocytic leukaemia (CLL) | + | + | – | + | – | 13q14 del, trisomy 12, 17p13 del, 11q22–23 del, 6q– |
| Follicular lymphoma | + | – | + | ± | – | t(14;18)(q32;q21) |
| Mantle cell lymphoma (MCL) | + | + | – | – | + | t(11;14)(q13;q32) |
| Marginal zone lymphoma | + | – | – | – | – | Trisomy 3, t(11;18)(q21;q21) |
| Diffuse large B-cell lymphoma | + | – | ± | ± | – | t(14;18) in 15%, 3q27 abnormalities, complex |
| Burkitt lymphoma | + | – | + | – | – | t(8;14),t(8;22),t(2;8) |

Antibody numbers are preceded by 'CD', which stands for 'cluster of differentiation'.
CD20 is expressed by most B cells.
CD5 is a T-cell marker, but is expressed by B cells in SLL and MCL.
CD10 is a marker of germinal centre cells.
CD23 is expressed by follicular dendritic cells and a population of normal mantle zone lymphocytes.
CyclinD1 is a cell cycle regulatory protein, which is not detectable in normal lymphocytes. Its expression by lymphoma cells is almost always diagnostic of MCL;
+ = positive in most cases, ± = usually negative but positive in a minority of cases

A combination of these techniques demonstrates that, in western Europe and North America, most NHLs are of B-cell derivation. T-cell tumours are uncommon, except in specific locations such as the skin and small bowel. In Far Eastern countries, T-cell tumours are much more prevalent. The relative frequencies of lymphoma types in the UK are shown diagrammatically in Fig. 8.13.

Within each NHL subtype, the degree of aggressiveness varies and the outcome depends upon factors such as age at diagnosis, the presence of systemic symptoms, the stage of the disease, the origin of the disease (nodal versus extranodal), and the general condition of the patient (performance status). NHL can be staged in much the same way as HL. As a generalization, low-grade lymphomas are slowly progressive but incurable, whereas high-grade tumours advance rapidly but are susceptible to aggressive chemotherapy.

The aetiology of NHL is largely unknown, although a number of viruses are closely associated with some categories, e.g. EBV and Burkitt lymphoma (see Special Study Topic 8.1), human herpes virus 8 (HHV8) and primary body cavity lymphoma in HIV patients, hepatitis virus C and primary splenic lymphomas, and human lymphotrophic virus 1(HTLV1) and T-cell lymphoma/leukaemia in adults. *Helicobacter pylori* has an aetiological role in primary gastric B-cell lymphomas. The incidence of lymphoma in patients with autoimmune conditions is higher than normal.

### B-cell Lymphomas

These are tumours of B cells at various stages of differentiation, which largely correspond to the stages of normal B-cell maturation. The major forms of B-cell lymphoma include the following.

#### Follicular Lymphoma

Follicular lymphomas (FLs) are tumours derived from germinal centre (follicle centre) cells, and they at least partially retain a follicular architecture. FLs usually arise within lymph nodes, and are often found to be disseminated at presentation, with involvement of multiple nodes, spleen, and bone marrow. The cells are a mixture of small cleaved centrocytes and larger centroblasts, with the number of the latter determining the grade. Lower-grade tumours are indolent but seldom curable and will transform into a more aggressive form, diffuse large-cell lymphoma, in 25% of cases (see Case History 8.2). A proportion of grade 3 tumours is potentially curable by chemotherapy. The follicle centre cells in FL express the anti-apoptotic protein bcl2 as a result of the t(14;18) translocation, and this promotes cell proliferation (Fig. 8.14).

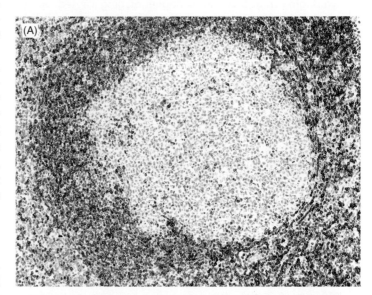

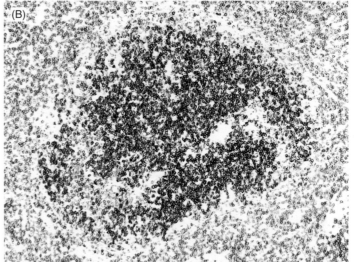

FIG. 8.14 Immunostaining for bcl2: (A) reactive follicle: the germinal centre (GC) cells are negative. A small number of intrafollicular T cells are positive. (B) In contrast, the GC cells in the neoplastic follicle in follicular lymphoma are strongly positive. Overexpression is a consequence of the t(14;18) translocation where the promotors on the IgH gene of chromosome 14 cause transcription of the *bcl2* gene on chromosome 18; this is a useful way to distinguish between reactive and malignant follicular lesions.

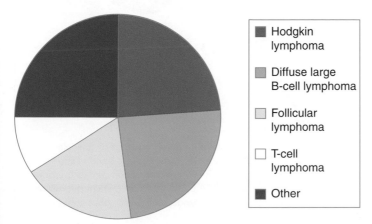

■ Hodgkin lymphoma

■ Diffuse large B-cell lymphoma

□ Follicular lymphoma

□ T-cell lymphoma

■ Other

FIG. 8.13 Relative frequency of lymphoma types in the UK.

## FOLLICULAR LYMPHOMA

A 61-year-old woman presented to the ear, nose, and throat (ENT) department with a 3-month history of a swelling on the left side of her neck. She also complained of a weight loss of 4 kg. A clinical examination revealed multiple enlarged lymph nodes on the left side of her neck. A fine-needle aspirate of the node was performed at the clinic by the consultant cytopathologist, and this showed a pattern highly suspicious of a low-grade NHL. A formal excision biopsy of the lymph node was performed under general anaesthesia 4 days later. This revealed the typical features of a grade 1 follicular lymphoma (Fig. 8.15). Immunophenotyping carried out by immunocytochemistry on the paraffin-embedded material supported this diagnosis (*Table 8.4*).

**TABLE 8.4** Immunocytochemistry results

| Antibody | CD3 | CD5 | CD10 | CD20 | CD23 | bcl2 | CyclinD1 |
|----------|-----|-----|------|------|------|------|----------|
| Case 8.2 | −   | −   | +    | +    | −    | +    | −        |

The patient was referred to the local haematologist who specialized in haemato-oncology. A staging CT scan revealed bilateral cervical and axillary lymphadenopathy in addition to a 12-cm para-aortic nodal mass near the pancreas. Extensive paratrabecular lymphomatous infiltration was noted on bone marrow trephine biopsy (Fig. 8.16). The patient was informed of her diagnosis and that the disease involved multiple sites including the bone marrow (Ann Arbor stage IVB). It was explained that, although it was unlikely that this

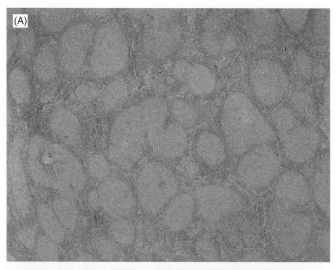

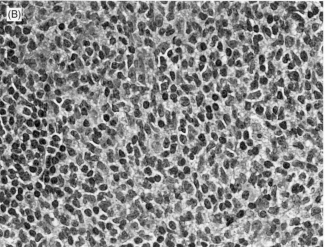

**FIG. 8.15** (A) Low-power view of the lymph node biopsy: the node is replaced by numerous follicular structures. (B) At high power, there is a mixture of germinal centre-type cells comprising large cells (centroblasts) and smaller cells with a cleaved nucleus (centrocytes). Tingible body macrophages are absent. This pattern is characteristic of follicular lymphoma. The number of large cells is fewer than 5 per high-power field and therefore the lesion is regarded as grade 1.

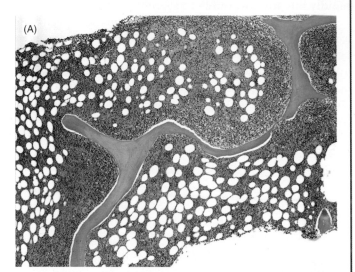

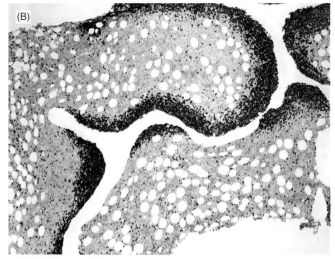

**FIG. 8.16** The bone marrow is extensively involved by follicular lymphoma. (A) This low-power H&E view shows a band of small lymphoid cells involving the area immediately adjacent to the bony trabecula (paratrabecular). (B) A parallel section is stained for CD20 (a B-lymphocyte marker) by immunocytochemistry, thus confirming the B-cell nature of the infiltrate.

low-grade lymphoma could be cured, much could be done to alleviate the symptoms and bring about a temporary remission.

The patient was treated with a chemotherapeutic regimen, and this resulted in the disappearance of the cervical and axillary nodes. Cervical lymphadenopathy recurred after a further 3 years, and a further course of chemotherapy was required. Two years later, the patient developed a rapidly growing para-aortic abdominal mass, which involved the porta hepatis and caused obstructive jaundice which was complicated by ascending cholangitis and septicaemia. It was suspected that a high-grade transformation had occurred. The patient died as a consequence of the septicaemia at 66 months after the initial presentation.

## Small Lymphocytic Lymphoma/Chronic Lymphocytic Leukaemia

This disorder of elderly people frequently arises in the bone marrow, and most commonly presents with a raised peripheral small lymphocyte count, i.e. chronic lymphocytic leukaemia (CLL). The spleen, liver, and lymph nodes are usually enlarged, and bone marrow failure eventually occurs late in the disease. In 5% of cases the patient presents with lymphadenopathy only, with no leukaemic component. This is a low-grade tumour, but it may be accompanied by immunological impairment and autoimmune disease, and occasionally is complicated by high-grade transformation (Richter's syndrome). Cytogenetic abnormalities provide useful prognostic information, e.g. 17p13 deletion is associated with a more aggressive disease. The median survival is 7 years.

## Mantle Cell Lymphoma

As the name suggests, this tumour is thought to arise from cells of the mantle zone of the follicle. Often a nodal tumour, it may also arise in the gastrointestinal tract, but quickly becomes disseminated so that most patients present with stage III or IV disease (see Case History 8.3). Hepatosplenomegaly and marrow involvement are common. The tumour is characterized by a translocation t(11;14) (q13;q32) which leads to overexpression of the *cyclinD1* gene, which in turn leads to cell progression from the G1 to the S phase in the cell cycle. Despite an apparent 'low-grade' appearance this lymphoma has, despite therapy, a poor median survival of only 3 years.

## MANTLE CELL LYMPHOMA

A 69-year-old man presented to the accident and emergency department with a 2-day history of bleeding per rectum. He also admitted to a 2-month history of general malaise and some weight loss. On examination, he was found to have cervical lymphadenopathy. A full blood count revealed iron-deficiency anaemia (Hb 9.6 g/dL) in addition to a mild lymphocytosis. The initial clinical impression was of colonic carcinoma with metastatic spread. A flexible sigmoidoscopy revealed multiple focally ulcerating polyps in the colon. An endoscopic biopsy was performed. The histology, immunophenotype, and FISH result were diagnostic of mantle cell lymphoma (Figs. 8.17 and 8.18, and *Table 8.5*).

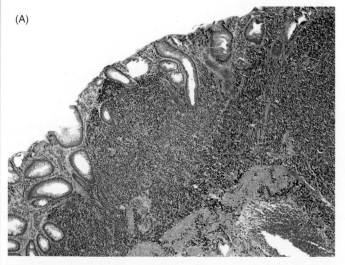

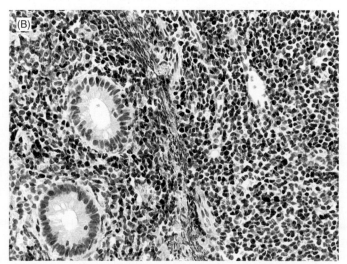

FIG. 8.17 (A) H&E staining of the colonic biopsy. Within the mucosa and submucosa, there is a lymphomatous infiltrate composed of a diffuse infiltrate of lymphoid cells resembling centrocytes. (B) Immunocytochemistry for *cyclinD1*. There is nuclear expression of *cyclinD1* in the neoplastic lymphoid population (not normally seen in other types of lymphoma).

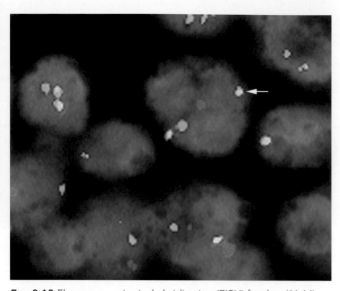

FIG. 8.18 Fluorescence *in situ* hybridization (FISH) for the t(11;14) translocation is performed on a 1-μm paraffin section from the biopsy. Red and green signals indicate chromosomes 11 and 14, respectively. In a cell containing a t(11;14) reciprocal translocation (arrowed), one red and one green signal (corresponding to the normal chromosomes) and two fusion signals (where the red and green probes are brought together by the translocation, giving rise to emission of yellow light) are seen.

TABLE 8.5 Immunocytochemical profile of the lymphoma: the coexpression of CD5 by the CD20-positive B cells and nuclear positivity for cyclinD1 are characteristic of mantle cell lymphoma

| Antibody | CD3 | CD5 | CD10 | CD20 | CD23 | bcl2 | CyclinD1 |
|----------|-----|-----|------|------|------|------|----------|
| Case 8.3 | −   | +   | −    | +    | −    | +    | +        |

A staging CT scan revealed lymphadenopathy in the cervical, axillary, intrathoracic, abdominal para-aortic, and iliac regions. There was also bilateral tonsillar enlargement. A bone marrow trephine biopsy showed diffuse infiltration by lymphoma.

This patient had therefore presented with stage IVB mantle cell lymphoma. Extranodal involvement is not unusual in this lymphoma and the pattern of colonic involvement with multiple polyps is well described – so-called 'lymphomatous polyposis'. Despite the small cell size, this is an aggressive lymphoma. As expected, the patient responded only transiently to chemotherapy and died from the disease 9 months after the first presentation.

## Extranodal Marginal Zone Lymphoma

Most extranodal lymphomas (e.g. in the stomach and thyroid) are in this category. They usually develop against a background of reactive lymphoid proliferations due either to infections (e.g. *Helicobacter pylori* – see Chapter 9, p.247) or to autoimmune disease (e.g. Hashimoto's thyroiditis). Most patients present with localized disease, and experience an indolent course and prolonged disease-free intervals. Interestingly, regression of early gastric lymphomas occurs in a significant number of cases after the eradication of *H. pylori* by antibiotics. Transformation to high-grade tumours may occur. Similar tumours can arise within lymph nodes.

## Diffuse Large B-cell Lymphoma

This is the most common type of NHL in western countries. These tumours arise in nodal and extranodal sites, usually anew, but sometimes they evolve from low-grade lymphomas. They tend to present with expansive and invasive lesions, which initially remain localized, but rapidly spread to adjacent lymph nodes and become widely disseminated (Fig. 8.19). Approximately 50% are curable with appropriate chemotherapy. Much work is being directed at identifying at presentation those tumours that will not be cured by standard chemotherapy. Expression of bcl2 is regarded as a poor prognostic factor. Recently, the expression pattern of approximately 12,000 genes was examined using gene array technology. As a result, two patterns – a germinal centre and an activated B-cell pattern – were identified, the former being more often associated with a good outcome. In the future, it

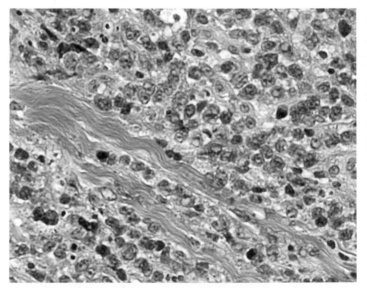

FIG. 8.19 Diffuse large B-cell lymphoma: the lymph node is completely replaced by a diffuse infiltrate of large lymphoid blast cells.

is likely that further molecular research will identify factors that will determine choice of therapy in individual cases.

## Burkitt Lymphoma

This highly aggressive B-cell tumour is found mainly – but not exclusively – in tropical parts of the globe. This endemic form mainly affects young children and has a distinctive extranodal pattern of growth involving, in particular, the jaws in males and the ovaries in females. Patients are at risk of developing central nervous system involvement. The characteristically rapid growth of the tumour is reflected in the high mitotic rate and the 100% labelling of the tumour cells with the proliferation marker Ki-67 (which labels those cells in the cell cycle, but not those in G0). There is a high apoptotic rate, and the numerous macrophages ingesting apoptotic debris account for the typical 'starry sky' histological appearance (Fig. 8.20).

The EBV has an important role in the development of Burkitt lymphoma, and its genome is found in the cells in most endemic cases. Both endemic and sporadic variants are characterized by a translocation involving chromosomes 8 and 14, which causes deregulation of the *c-myc* gene, resulting in cell proliferation. Intensive chemotherapeutic regimens have led to a cure rate of 60–90% depending on the stage in this highly aggressive lymphoma.

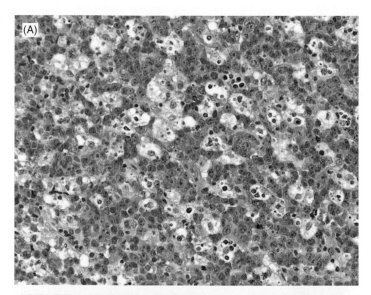

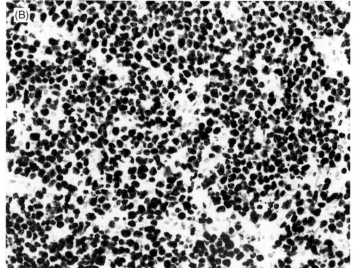

FIG. 8.20 Burkitt lymphoma: (A) diffuse infiltrate of small blast cells in addition to numerous macrophages with abundant pale cytoplasm phagocytosing cellular debris. (B) Almost 100% of tumour cells display nuclear positivity for the proliferation marker Ki67.

These tumours and their characteristic immunoprofile and chromosomal rearrangements are summarized in *Box 8.4.*

## T-cell Lymphomas

These account for 10–14% of all lymphomas in western countries. In general, they are difficult to treat and carry a poor prognosis. Some present with lymphadenopathy, but they may be leukaemic at the early stage and not infrequently arise in extranodal sites such as skin and bowel. Adults are most often affected.

In the past, T-cell lymphomas have been difficult to classify, and many are now included under the general category of peripheral T-cell lymphoma, not otherwise specified (NOS). Most of these are nodal tumours showing, as a rule, a pleomorphic cellular picture due to varying admixtures of small lymphoid elements and transformed cells (immunoblasts) with a correspondingly unpredictable, but usually poor, prognosis.

Some T-cell tumours, however, present as distinctive clinicopathological entities.

### T-cell Prolymphocytic Lymphoma

This usually presents with a high peripheral T-lymphocyte count, hepatosplenomegaly, and skin infiltration. It is much more aggressive than B-CLL; the median survival is less than 1 year.

### Mycosis Fungoides

This tumour presents as a skin rash (see Chapter 18, p. 533), initially with patches and plaques and later with nodules. Histologically, there is infiltration of the dermis and epidermis by CD4+ T cells. It can be difficult to make this diagnosis in its early stages because it can resemble dermatitis. Mycosis fungoides tends to be indolent in its behaviour, at least initially. A minority of patients develop high-grade transformation and die as a consequence.

### Sézary Syndrome

Possibly a variant of mycosis fungoides, this is characterized by erythroderma, lymphadenopathy, and circulating neoplastic lymphocytes with an atypical 'cerebriform' nucleus. It is aggressive and has a poor survival rate.

### Angioimmunoblastic T-cell Lymphoma

This tumour usually affects adults in later life. It causes widespread lymphadenopathy, hepatosplenomegaly, and striking systemic symptoms such as fever, weight loss, haemolytic anaemia, and skin rashes. Hypergammaglobulinaemia may be a feature. The outlook is poor despite treatment.

### Adult T-cell Leukaemia/Lymphoma

This is found mainly in the Far East, and is associated with human T-cell leukaemia virus 1 (HTLV1) infection. It varies in behaviour, but is generally aggressive. Usually it presents with lymphadenopathy, hepatosplenomegaly, leukaemic changes, and skin rashes. There may be lytic bone lesions and associated hypercalcaemia.

### Enteropathy-associated T-cell Lymphoma

This is a tumour of the small bowel arising from intraepithelial T lymphocytes, which, as a rule, is associated with coeliac disease. It is often highly aggressive, and usually presents with bowel obstruction or perforation (Fig. 8.21). Most patients presenting with this tumour have no antecedent history of coeliac disease, but are found to have evidence of subclinical disease during investigations for their lymphoma.

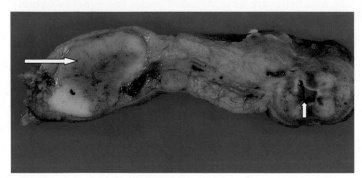

**FIG. 8.21** Cross-section of small bowel (right) and mesentery (left) in enteropathy-associated T-cell lymphoma complicating coeliac disease. The patient presented with small bowel obstruction and malabsorption. Note the markedly narrowed bowel lumen (short arrow) and the involved lymph node within the mesentery (long arrow).

### Anaplastic Large-cell Lymphoma

This lymphoma is composed of large pleomorphic cells that express the lymphocyte activation marker CD30. These tumours may show the translocation t(2;5)(p23;35) with expression of the chimaeric protein derived from the *ALK* gene (a tyrosine kinase receptor). The 5-year survival rate of treated ALK-positive tumours is 80%, in contrast to only 40% in ALK-negative cases. A primary cutaneous variant, negative for t(2;5), occurs and has a very good prognosis.

## Metastatic Tumours

It cannot be overemphasized that tumours found in lymph nodes are more often metastatic than primary (Fig. 8.22). Almost all carcinomas tend to spread initially via the lymphatic system, and some non-epithelial tumours such as melanomas and, much less commonly, sarcomas can behave in a similar way. Lymph node enlargement is therefore a feature commonly associated with these tumours, and may indeed be the first indication of their presence, e.g. a carcinoma of the stomach may be diagnosed after the appearance of an enlarged supraclavicular lymph node (Troissier's sign). It needs to be stressed that lymphadenopathy does not equate with metastatic disease and may be reactive in nature. It is therefore important to examine these nodes histologically or cytologically for confirmation. If the nearest regional node, the sentinel node, is clear of tumour, this is a good sign.

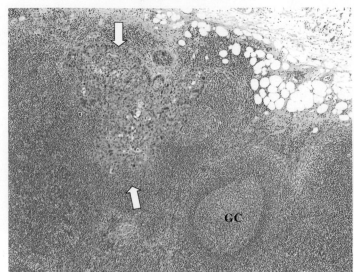

**FIG. 8.22** A deposit of metastatic adenocarcinoma is present in the subcapsular sinus of this lymph node (between the arrows). GC = germinal centre.

## DISEASES OF THE THYMUS

### Key Points

- The thymus is responsible for T-lymphocyte development.
- Enlargement is often asymptomatic, but can cause superior vena caval obstruction.
- Thymic hyperplasia is often associated with autoimmune diseases, especially myasthenia gravis.
- Thymoma is an epithelial tumour, which may be locally aggressive.
- Lymphoma and germ cell tumours may involve the thymus.

The thymus lies in the superior anterior mediastinum, overlying the pericardium. It is basically an epithelial structure, the cortical part being derived from ectoderm and the medulla from the endoderm of the third and fourth branchial pouches. Within the microenvironment of the cortex, T-lymphocyte precursors of bone marrow origin undergo antigen-independent proliferation and development. This process is maximal in childhood, the thymus enlarging from infancy until puberty, and then gradually decreasing throughout adult life. Failure of development of the epithelial component results in severe immunodeficiency (DiGeorge's syndrome).

### Thymic Enlargement

Thymic enlargement is an uncommon clinical finding and may be found only on a routine chest radiograph. Occasionally, a rapidly enlarging thymus may compress the superior vena cava and threaten life. The main causes of thymic enlargement are listed in *Box 8.5*.

**Follicular hyperplasia, associated with:**
Myasthenia gravis
Systemic lupus erythematosus
Rheumatoid arthritis

**Tumours:**
Thymoma
Thymic carcinoma
Lymphoma (Hodgkin lymphoma, T lymphoblastic, mediastinal large B cell)
Germ cell tumours (seminoma, teratoma)

Non-neoplastic thymic enlargement is usually due to the presence of lymphoid follicles with germinal centres within the medulla – a phenomenon related in most instances to autoimmune diseases and especially to myasthenia gravis (see Chapter 12, p. 388). Removal of the thymus often results in remission of the disease.

## Thymic Tumours

Thymoma is a primary epithelial tumour of the thymus that behaves like a low-grade carcinoma, invading surrounding structures but seldom metastasizing (<10% of cases). The lesion consists of epithelial cells, often interspersed with so many thymic lymphocytes that it can be misdiagnosed as a lymphoma. Although often found incidentally, thymoma may be associated with myasthenia gravis, pure red cell aplasia, hypogammaglobulinaemia, and autoimmune diseases such as polymyositis. Several forms of lymphoma may affect the thymus, most notably classical Hodgkin lymphoma and mediastinal large B-cell lymphoma, both typically in young females. T-lymphoblastic leukaemia, which usually occurs in childhood, may present with a large anterior mediastinal mass. Germ cell tumours, similar to those found in the gonads, can arise at this site.

## DISEASES OF THE SPLEEN

### Key Points

- The spleen removes effete blood cells and foreign material from the blood.
- Moderate splenomegaly in the western world is often due to portal hypertension or blood diseases.
- Massive splenomegaly in the western world is usually due to haematopoietic neoplasia, and in the tropics to infections (e.g. malaria, leishmaniasis).
- Hypersplenism results in pancytopenia.
- Removal of the spleen results in susceptibility to disseminated pneumococcal infection.

In normal adult life the spleen weighs 120–160 g, and is the only lymphatic tissue specialized to filter the blood. This function is intimately related to its structure, and particularly to its vascular arrangements (Fig. 8.23). The spleen removes foreign materials, microorganisms, and time-expired and otherwise abnormal red blood cells. It can also remove inclusion bodies (e.g. residual DNA, denatured haemoglobin) from red cells. The spleen has important immunological functions, and has a major role in counteracting blood infection, largely by producing IgM. Enlargement of the spleen and a reduction in its size or its surgical removal may have important clinical effects.

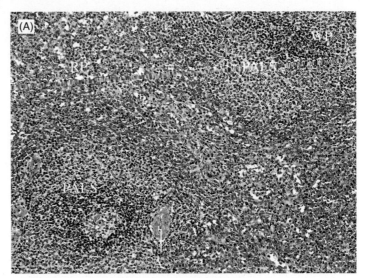

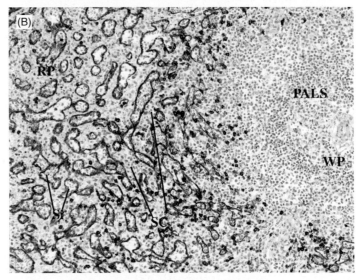

**FIG. 8.23** Microanatomy and function of the spleen: (A) high-power view of the spleen (this field is 2 mm in diameter). (B) Immunocytochemical staining of spleen for CD8, highlighting the CD8+ splenic sinusoid-lining cells. The spleen contains white pulp (WP), which consists of periarteriolar lymphoid sheaths (PALS) comprising both T and B lymphocytes, and red pulp (RP), which acts as a filter for the blood. Blood leaves the arterioles, enters sinusoids (Si), flows through fenestrae in the sinusoid-lining cells, percolates through the cellular splenic cords (SC) containing macrophages and fibroblasts, and eventually reaches the efferent capillaries. Effete and damaged red cells are removed from the circulation within the splenic cords.

## Splenic Enlargement

Splenic enlargement has many causes, the most important of which are summarized in *Table 8.6*. Worldwide, protozoal

**TABLE 8.6** Causes of splenomegaly

### Hereditary causes

| | |
|---|---|
| Storage disease | Gaucher's disease |
| | Niemann–Pick disease |
| Haemolytic anaemia | Sickle cell disease |
| | Congenital spherocytosis |
| | Thalassaemia |

### Infective causes

| | |
|---|---|
| Protozoal | Malaria |
| | Leishmaniasis |
| | Schistosomiasis |
| Bacterial | Tuberculosis |
| | Secondary syphilis |
| | Bacterial endocarditis |
| | Brucellosis |
| Viral | Infectious mononucleosis |
| Fungal | Histoplasmosis |

### Tumours

| | |
|---|---|
| Lymphoma | Chronic lymphocytic leukaemia |
| | Lymphoplasmacytic lymphoma |
| | Splenic marginal zone lymphoma |
| | Classical Hodgkin lymphoma |
| Myeloproliferative disorders | Chronic myeloid leukaemia |
| | Idiopathic myelofibrosis |
| | Polycythaemia vera |
| Metastatic tumours | Carcinoma (rarely metastasizes to spleen) |

### Non-neoplastic haematological conditions

| | |
|---|---|
| | Haemolytic anaemia |
| | Autoimmune idiopathic thrombocytopenia |

### Vascular disorders

| | |
|---|---|
| Portal hypertension | Cirrhosis |
| | Portal vein thrombosis |
| | Budd–Chiari syndrome |

### Autoimmune disease

| | |
|---|---|
| | Systemic lupus erythematosus |
| | Felty's syndrome |

### Miscellaneous

| | |
|---|---|
| | Sarcoidosis |
| | Amyloidosis |
| | Idiopathic splenomegaly |

infections (e.g. malaria) represent the most important cause of massive splenomegaly (see Chapter 19. In the western world, this is usually due to myeloproliferative disorders (Fig. 8.24) and CLL, although other rarer causes such as Gaucher's disease may also be responsible. Moderate enlargement occurs in chronic bacterial and viral infections, portal hypertension, the haemolytic anaemias and some lymphomas. Most lymphomatous involvement of the spleen is secondary, though true primary lymphomas do occur, for example splenic marginal zone lymphoma (Fig. 8.25). Metastatic carcinoma or melanoma rarely involve the spleen.

### Clinical Effects

Usually, the first indication of splenomegaly is that the spleen becomes palpable on examination. When enlargement is substantial there may be abdominal discomfort and

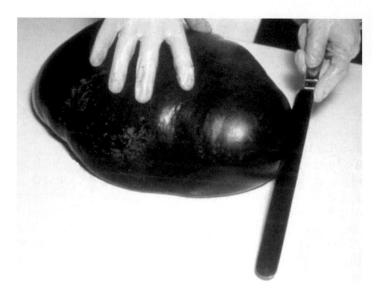

**FIG. 8.24** Massively enlarged spleen surgically removed from a patient with chronic idiopathic myelofibrosis.

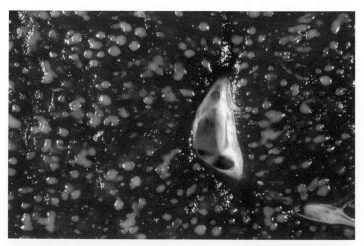

**FIG. 8.25** Cut surface of spleen showing expansion of periarteriolar lymphoid sheaths by splenic marginal zone lymphoma.

even pain, although this is usually due to infarction which often occurs in a spleen enlarged for any cause. More importantly, when a spleen exceeds approximately 1 kg, there is increased sequestration and premature destruction of the formed elements of the blood (hypersplenism), resulting in pancytopenia and compensatory marrow hyperplasia. Splenic rupture – either spontaneous or with minimal trauma – is a serious complication occurring particularly in infectious mononucleosis.

## Hyposplenism

Hyposplenism occurs most often as a result of splenectomy. Congenital absence may be associated with cardiac anomalies such as dextrocardia. Atrophy of the spleen is seen in coeliac disease as part of a generalized immunodeficiency, and in sickle cell disease due to progressive microvascular occlusion. Splenic hypofunction is usually evident from examination of the peripheral blood in which there is an accumulation of abnormal red cells and inclusions (e.g. Howell–Jolly bodies); these are usually removed by the spleen. Splenectomy – in both childhood and adult life – predisposes to severe infections, especially with pneumococci.

## DISEASES OF THE BONE MARROW

From approximately 7 months of fetal life, the bone marrow is entirely responsible for haematopoiesis. Diseases involving the marrow result in two basic effects for the patient:

1. A deficiency of one or more of the cell lines producing anaemia, agranulocytosis, or thrombocytopenia, causing fatigue, increased susceptibility to infection, and a bleeding tendency, respectively
2. An overproduction of cells as a result of neoplastic transformation of a stem cell causing an increase in circulating cells (i.e. leukaemia).

Frequently both effects coexist. Much can be learned about marrow function by close examination of a peripheral blood film. However, a full assessment requires aspiration and trephine biopsy of bone marrow, often from the iliac crest.

## Normal Haematopoiesis

Normal haematopoiesis (Fig. 8.26) is the process by which pluripotent stem cells develop into all the different lineages while at the same time maintaining their numbers by self-renewal, so that production can go on throughout the individual's life. In normal individuals, the marrow is composed of a mixture of fatty and haematopoietic components, the ratio of which varies with age. An infant's marrow is almost 100% haematopoietic, whereas in elderly people the value is closer to 30% (Fig. 8.27).

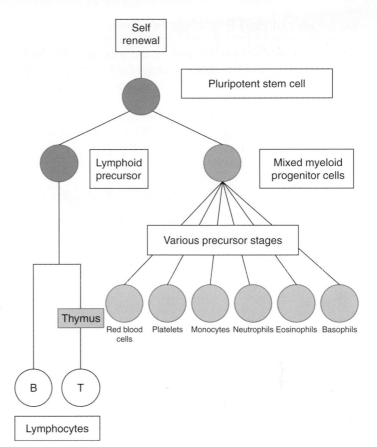

**FIG. 8.26** Simplified diagram of normal haematopoiesis. The pluripotent stem cell in the marrow gives rise to a number of progenitor cells which in turn proliferate and differentiate to produce all the cellular constituents of blood, including lymphoid cells. This process is controlled by various growth factors, produced by a range of cells including lymphocytes and endothelial cells, the secretion of which is partially dependent on environmental factors, e.g. hypoxia induces erythropoietin secretion, resulting in increased red cell production. The marrow stroma provides the appropriate environment for stem cells to grow and proliferate. The stem cell, which is capable of producing approximately $10^6$ mature blood cells, is also capable of self-renewal.

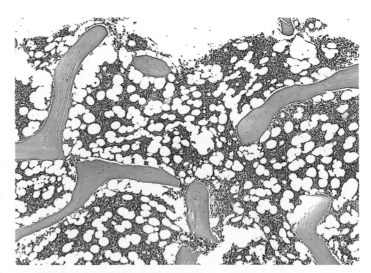

**FIG. 8.27** Trephine biopsy of ileum from a normal adult. The cellular haematopoietic red marrow accounts for 40–50% of the marrow space. The remainder consists of fat cells.

## Disorders of Red Blood Cells

This group of disorders comprises the anaemias (reduced haemoglobin), polycythaemia (increased haemoglobin), and a group of miscellaneous conditions resulting in the occurrence of red cell inclusions. The normal blood smear contains biconcave erythrocytes of uniform size and shape, measuring 7 μm in diameter (Fig. 8.28). The normal haemoglobin (Hb) concentration is 13.5–17.5 g/dL for males and 11.5–15.5 g/dL for females.

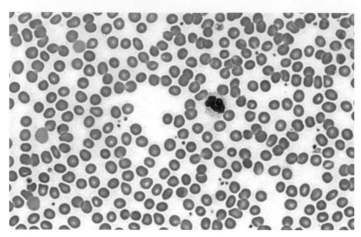

**FIG. 8.28** A normal blood film. Contrast this with the abnormal smears.

### The Anaemias

**Key Points**

- Anaemia is defined by a haemoglobin concentration below the normal range.
- Anaemia may be caused by insufficient production of red cells or excess loss or destruction.
- The causes of anaemia correlate with the appearances of peripheral blood and bone marrow.

A shortage of red blood cells (RBCs) may occur due to insufficient production, or to excessive destruction or loss. The clinical symptoms and signs will depend on the severity of the anaemia and the speed at which it has developed. Low oxygen tension in the tissues will usually manifest itself by fatigue, dizziness, palpitations, and, when severe, angina or cardiac failure. In long-standing anaemia, compensatory erythropoiesis – driven by erythropoietin produced in response to hypoxia – will cause replacement of fatty marrow by haematopoietic marrow, and may even cause thinning of the bone cortex. The major forms of anaemia are listed in *Table 8.7*. Investigation requires estimation of total Hb concentration and microscopic examination of a blood film, which may reveal a reduction in staining intensity (hypochromasia), a change in size (anisocytosis), and

**TABLE 8.7** An aetiological classification of anaemia

| | | |
|---|---|---|
| **Blood loss** | *Acute or chronic* | |
| **Increased erythrocyte destruction (haemolytic)** | *Intrinsic red blood cell (RBC) defect* | *Congenital*<br>Thalassaemia, RBC enzyme deficiencies<br>Abnormal haemoglobins, e.g. sickle cell disease<br>RBC membrane defects, e.g. hereditary spherocytosis<br>*Acquired*<br>Paroxysmal nocturnal haemoglobinaemia |
| | *Factors extrinsic to RBCs* | Autoimmune haemolytic anaemia<br>Haemolytic disease of the newborn<br>Drugs/chemicals<br>Microangiopathic haemolytic anaemia<br>Hypersplenism<br>Mechanical factors |
| | *Combined* | Glucose-6-phosphate dehydrogenase deficiency<br>Red cell instability caused by exposure to oxidizing agents |
| **Inadequate RBC production** | *Deficiency states* | Iron, vitamin $B_{12}$, folate, protein |
| | *Anaemia of chronic disease* | Connective tissue disorders<br>Renal failure<br>Liver failure |
| | *Primary bone marrow failure* | Aplastic anaemia<br>Selective red cell aplasia |
| | *Bone marrow infiltration* | Carcinoma, lymphoma, myeloma<br>Leukaemias |
| | *Myelodysplastic conditions* | For example, sideroblastic anaemia |
| | *Storage diseases* | Gaucher's disease |

**TABLE 8.8** Red blood cell indices in the common anaemias

| | Iron deficiency | Vitamin B$_{12}$/folate deficiency | Anaemia of chronic disease | Hereditary spherocytosis | Thalassaemia |
|---|---|---|---|---|---|
| Cell size | ↓ | ↑ | N or ↓ | ↓ | ↓ |
| Hypochromasia | ++ | 0 | 0 or + | 0 | +++ |
| Poikilocytosis | ++ | +++ | + | 0 | +++ |
| Hb (g/dL) | ↓ | ↓ | ↓ | ↓ | ↓ |
| MCV | ↓ | ↑ | N or ↓ | ↓ | ↓ |
| MCH | ↓ | N or ↑ | N | N | ↓ |
| MCHC | ↓ | N | N | ↑ | ↓ |

Hb = haemoglobin concentration; MCV = mean corpuscular volume; MCH = mean corpuscular haemoglobin; MCHC = mean corpuscular haemoglobin concentration.
↑ = increase; ↓ = decrease; N = normal; + = present; ++ = prominent; +++ = very prominent.

changes in shape (poikilocytosis) of the RBCs. Red cell parameters can be determined accurately by modern automated equipment, providing essential information in determining the aetiology of anaemia (*Table 8.8*). Subtle variations in these indices can occur before a drop in the blood Hb concentration, facilitating early diagnosis.

### Iron-deficiency Anaemia

**Key Points**

Iron-deficiency anaemia:
- is a hypochromic/microcytic anaemia
- is most often caused by prolonged blood loss
- is common in females of reproductive age
- may be the first sign of an occult gastrointestinal carcinoma
- is commonly caused by hookworm infestation in much of the world.

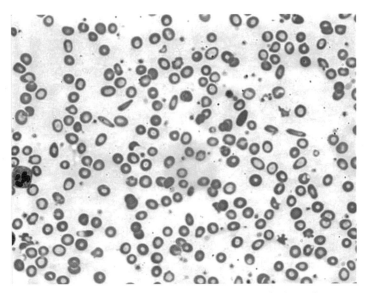

**FIG. 8.29** Blood film in iron-deficiency anaemia. Note the hypochromic and microcytic red blood cells and pencil-shaped poikilocytes.

This condition is one of the most common forms of anaemia, and results from chronic blood loss or insufficient iron uptake. In females of reproductive age, menstrual blood loss is the usual explanation. It may also result from chronic gastrointestinal tract bleeding, e.g. from a chronic peptic ulcer or an occult caecal or gastric carcinoma. In some parts of the world helmintic infections (e.g. hookworm infestation) are important. Iron deficiency may result from a diet that is low in iron, or from malabsorption, e.g. in coeliac disease. Achlorhydria also aggravates poor iron uptake.

In iron-deficiency anaemia, the bone marrow shows erythroid hyperplasia and there is a loss of stainable iron stores. Haemoglobin synthesis is impaired and red cell precursors are incompletely haemoglobinized. As a consequence, the erythrocytes in the peripheral blood are small and pale (Fig. 8.29). Iron deficiency is the prototype of a hypochromic/microcytic anaemia (low mean corpuscular volume [MCV], low mean corpuscular haemoglobin

[MCH]). In addition, blood chemistry data will reveal low serum iron, low ferritin level, and undersaturation of transferrin, i.e. an increased iron-binding capacity.

### Anaemia of Chronic Disease

This condition is related to iron deficiency because it is caused by the inability of the body to mobilize iron from the macrophages, where most of it is stored. It occurs as a complication of chronic infection, rheumatoid arthritis, or malignancy. The anaemia persists as long as the underlying condition is present. Unlike iron deficiency, the bone marrow shows no or only mild erythroid hyperplasia and there is sufficient stainable iron. There is a low serum iron level, but reduced iron-binding capacity and normal or raised ferritin.

### Vitamin B₁₂ and Folic Acid Deficiency

**Key Points**

- Deficiency of vitamin $B_{12}$ and folic acid causes megaloblastic anaemia with macrocytosis.
- Folate deficiency is frequently dietary or secondary to malabsorption.
- Vitamin $B_{12}$ deficiency is mainly due to pernicious anaemia.
- Vitamin $B_{12}$ deficiency may cause severe neurological complications.

Deficiency of these two vitamins leads to megaloblastic anaemia. Each has an important role in the synthesis of RNA and DNA, and in the metabolism of some amino acids (synthesis of methionine and breakdown of homocystine). This explains why deficiency of either or both has effects on tissues other than the bone marrow, most notably the central nervous system (see Chapter 11, p. 319).

Vitamin $B_{12}$ can be absorbed from the terminal ileum only if it is complexed with intrinsic factor, a protein produced by the gastric parietal cells. Accordingly, vitamin $B_{12}$ deficiency may result from previous gastrectomy or pathology of the terminal ileum, as in Crohn's disease. More frequently, it is secondary to chronic atrophic gastritis – an autoimmune condition (pernicious anaemia) in which autoantibodies are produced against parietal cells and/or intrinsic factor (see Chapter 9, p. 246). Insufficient intake is uncommon, but may occur in strict vegans and those on bizarre diets.

Folic acid deficiency often results from dietary abnormalities, e.g. in people with alcohol problems. Folic acid is absorbed in the jejunum, and malabsorption syndromes such as coeliac disease, tropical sprue, or extensive Crohn's disease may result in deficiency.

A prolonged high demand for vitamin $B_{12}$ or folic acid, as in pregnancy, may lead to deficiency in the face of normal intake. In vitamin $B_{12}$ deficiency a severe neurological condition – subacute combined degeneration of the cord (see Chapter 11, p. 319) – can precede the haematological abnormalities. Early treatment will stop the progression of the disease, although it may not reverse all the neurological damage. An examination of the peripheral blood often reveals pancytopenia with macrocytosis, poikilocytosis, a low reticulocyte count reflecting the inefficient erythropoiesis, and neutrophils with hypersegmented nuclei (Fig. 8.30).

The marrow is hypercellular, and the erythroblasts are large and show failure of nuclear maturation (megaloblastic change). The combination of increased cellularity and shift to more primitive forms may lead to leukaemia being falsely suspected. It is best to treat megaloblastic anaemia with both vitamin $B_{12}$ and folate, because supplying one may unmask a deficiency of the other. The anaemia is fully reversible, though in pernicious anaemia maintenance vitamin $B_{12}$ treatment is required for the rest of the patient's life.

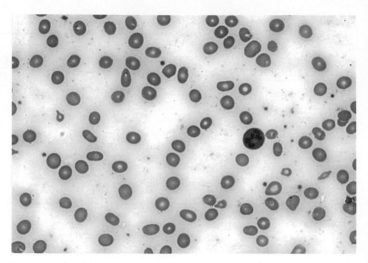

**Fig. 8.30** Blood film in megaloblastic anaemia due to vitamin $B_{12}$ deficiency. Poikilocytosis and oval macrocytes are prominent. A single hypersegmented neutrophil polymorph is also present.

### Aplastic Anaemia

In this condition there is severe hypofunction of the bone marrow. It is most often acquired and may follow exposure to drugs (e.g. chloramphenicol, gold, indometacin) or chemicals (e.g. benzene, insecticides) and viral infections such as hepatitis, CMV, and parvoviruses. In almost half the cases no cause is found (idiopathic), although an autoimmune attack at the level of the stem cell is considered likely because patients often respond to immunomodulatory drugs. Congenital aplastic anaemia occurs as part of Fanconi's anaemia. Rarely, aplasia may be confined to the red cell series – this is termed 'pure red cell aplasia'. It may be congenital or acquired, especially secondary to thymoma (see p. 213).

The bone marrow is severely hypocellular, whereas the peripheral blood shows pancytopenia, the cells present being mostly normal in appearance.

Treatment is supportive in the early part of the disease, with transfusion of red cells and platelets. Good results may be seen with androgens and anti-lymphocyte globulin. In younger patients, bone marrow transplantation has a fairly high success rate.

### The Haemolytic Anaemias

**Key Points**

- These conditions are caused by excessive destruction of red blood cells.
- Inherited disorders are usually due to abnormalities of the red cells.
- Acquired disorders are often extrinsic, e.g. autoimmune or mechanical in origin.
- Red cells may be destroyed in the spleen or the bloodstream.
- Increased haemoglobin breakdown may lead to jaundice.

The various conditions in which haemolysis occurs are listed under 'Inadequate RBC production' in *Table 8.7*. Globally, this group of diseases is a considerable burden on health-care resources. There is a wide range of mechanisms from defects of the red cell itself, to disorders of the red cell environment.

## Red Cell Membrane Defects

The most important of these is hereditary spherocytosis, caused by a defect in the molecule spectrin, which anchors the cytoskeleton to the cell membrane. This causes membrane loss, and the erythrocytes cannot maintain their usual biconcave shape, so that the cell becomes spheroidal. This reduces the plasticity of the cells, which are consequently trapped in the red pulp of the spleen and destroyed. Splenomegaly is therefore usual in spherocytosis. The anaemia is often mild, but can be aggravated by intercurrent infections, pregnancy, or folic acid deficiency. The constant haemolysis may lead to bile pigment gallstones. The diagnosis is made by finding spherocytes in the peripheral blood (Fig. 8.31), and showing that the red cells are excessively fragile when placed in a hypotonic salt solution. Splenectomy restores erythrocyte survival to normal, but of course does not correct the abnormal shape or osmotic fragility of the cells.

## Red Cell Enzyme Defects

By far the most common of these is glucose-6-phosphate dehydrogenase (G6PD) deficiency, which is endemic in parts of the Mediterranean basin and south-east Asia. G6PD plays an important role in maintaining stores of glutathione, which helps prevent oxidation of haemoglobin. Therefore, any process that places an oxidative stress on red cells can cause a haemolytic episode. This can be an infection, exposure to drugs such as aspirin, sulphonamides, or anti-malarials, and even ingestion of fava beans (favism).

## Autoimmune Haemolytic Anaemia

Haemolytic anaemia can be due to antibodies, most often autoantibodies directed against molecules in the red cell membrane. These antibodies are of different classes and may lyse the cells to which they bind, or sensitize the cells to complement-mediated lysis. Those that sensitize are often of IgM class and 'cold' antibodies, whereas those that lyse are IgG and 'warm' in type. Such autoantibodies are found in patients with systemic lupus erythematosus (SLE) or rheumatoid arthritis, or in patients with leukaemia or lymphoma. More often than not, however, no cause is identified. Drugs are also known to cause haemolytic anaemia, through autoantibody formation. Haemolysis may be due to antibodies from another individual – this situation occurs almost exclusively in pregnancy, when the mother produces antibodies against antigens on the red cells of her fetus (e.g. rhesus D antigen), leading to haemolytic disease of the newborn. An episode of sensitization from an earlier pregnancy usually precedes this event. If sufficient antibodies are produced, a severe haemolytic anaemia develops, usually with fetal death (hydrops fetalis). Desensitization procedures with rhesus immunoglobulin containing anti-D antibodies have largely suppressed this complication.

## Microangiopathic Haemolytic Anaemia

This is a consequence of physical damage to RBCs producing fragmented cells in the circulation (Fig. 8.32). It complicates such conditions as thrombotic thrombocytopenic purpura, haemolytic uraemic syndrome, and disseminated intravascular coagulation (DIC).

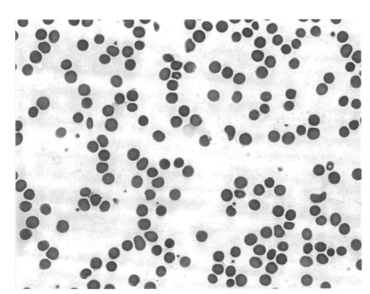

**FIG. 8.31** Blood film in hereditary spherocytosis. The spherocytes are small and round with a reduction in the degree of central pallor. The larger cells are reticulocytes, which reflect the reactive hyperplasia within the marrow.

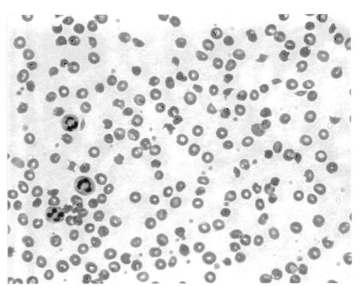

**FIG. 8.32** Microangiopathic haemolytic leukaemia: fragmented red blood cells are prominent.

# Disorders of Haemoglobin Synthesis

## Key Points

- These are inherited defects in production of haemoglobin α and β chains.
- Thalassaemia is characterized by haemolysis and ineffective erythropoiesis.
- The condition is common in the Mediterranean, the Middle East and Asia.

### Thalassaemia

This group of diseases is caused by mutations in the structure of the globin genes. Most of the body's haemoglobin (haemoglobin A [HbA]) is a tetramer of two α and two β chains. Small amounts of fetal haemoglobin, consisting of two α and two γ chains ($\alpha_2\gamma_2$), and $HbA_2$, which consists of two α and two δ chains, are found in adults. In mutations affecting the α chain (α-thalassaemia) the severity of the disease depends on the precise nature of the genetic events. The α chain is encoded by two duplicated genes on chromosome 16, and to abolish α-chain synthesis completely all four alleles must be silenced. This is incompatible with extrauterine life, and the fetus dies (hydrops fetalis). With one remaining allele, most of the haemoglobin is made of an unstable tetramer of four β chains and severe anaemia results (HbH disease). With two or one silent alleles a mild or silent disease will result (α-thalassaemia trait).

β-Thalassaemias result from mutations of the β chain that lead to reduced or absent synthesis. If both alleles are involved, β-thalassaemia major occurs (Fig. 8.33). Patients with this severe disease are transfusion dependent and many die in infancy. Mutation in one allele leads to β-thalassaemia minor with a mild-to-moderate anaemia. If both parents bear this trait, then one in four of their children will have β-thalassaemia major.

In thalassaemia, the failure of haemoglobin synthesis is aggravated by haemolysis of the abnormal red cells. The diagnosis is established by haemoglobin electrophoresis; antenatal screening is performed using molecular genetic techniques. Patients with β-thalassaemia major have severe anaemia from 3–6 months of age, hepatosplenomegaly due to extramedullary haematopoiesis, expansion of facial bones due to marrow hyperplasia, and iron overload due to repeated transfusions.

### Sickle Cell Disease

## Key Points

- Caused by an abnormality of the Hb β gene.
- Primarily affects those of African origin.
- Homozygotes show severe disease.
- Heterozygotes have the sickle cell trait.
- Red cells sickle under low oxygen tensions.
- Red cells lyse, and also aggregate to obstruct microcirculation.

This important disorder results from a single point mutation in the haemoglobin β chain, where substitution of a valine for a glutamic acid causes a dramatic change in the properties of haemoglobin, especially under conditions of low oxygen tension. Homozygotes in whom both β genes are abnormal are severely affected. Deoxygenated HbS precipitates into linear configurations that cause the erythrocyte to assume a sickle shape. These sickle cells tend to block blood vessels, causing ischaemia or infarction of the tissues supplied. This can occur anywhere in the body – from the skin of the feet to the brain – and these occlusive crises can be very painful. Repeated episodes can cause splenic atrophy, predisposing to infections, which by themselves provoke crises. Sepsis, meningitis, osteomyelitis (often caused by *Salmonella* spp.) and pulmonary infections are frequent. These may precipitate an aplastic crisis in the bone marrow. This grim picture, leading to early death, is seen in homozygous individuals. In heterozygotes, the term 'sickle cell trait' is applied; these individuals are usually asymptomatic, but sickling can occur under conditions of severe hypoxia. The trait protects against malaria – the reason why this genetic abnormality is widespread in areas where malaria is endemic. Sickle cell disease is diagnosed clinically and by electrophoresis. Sickle cell disease and thalassaemia may coexist.

## Conditions due to Increased Red Cell Numbers

Increased red cell mass, polycythaemia or erythrocytosis can be either reactive or neoplastic in origin. Reactive polycythaemia is seen under conditions of chronic hypoxia, such as chronic respiratory diseases, congenital heart disease and in those living at altitude. This is a response to increased

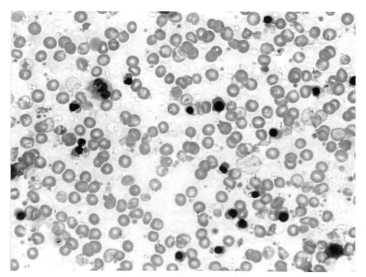

**FIG. 8.33** Blood film in β-thalassaemia. Numerous hypochromic/microcytic red blood cells and circulating normoblasts (red cell precursors) are prominent. Transfused normal erythrocytes are also present.

erythropoietin. Occasionally, a tumour – most often a renal cell carcinoma – can produce excess erythropoietin as a paraneoplastic phenomenon (see Chapter 13, p. 418). A true neoplastic erythrocytosis is seen in polycythaemia vera (see pp. 226–227).

## Disorders of the Myeloid Series

### Decreased Granulocyte Numbers

A decreased neutrophil count (neutropenia) or complete lack of neutrophils (agranulocytosis) may be due to decreased myelopoiesis or excessive destruction of white cells. Both conditions are associated with a risk of infection. Often, there is concomitant reduction in other blood cells (pancytopenia), but isolated neutropenia can occur. Neutropenia through insufficient production is most commonly drug induced (cytotoxic drugs, chloramphenicol, chlorpromazine, sulphonamides, and phenylbutazone). Neutropenia complicates aplastic anaemia and marrow replacement by malignant and non-malignant processes. Megaloblastic anaemias and myelodysplastic syndromes lead to inefficient granulopoiesis. Some infections (e.g. HIV) appear to suppress normal myelopoiesis.

Most cases of neutropenia related to excessive destruction are immunologically mediated, because they may occur in systemic autoimmune diseases. Drugs, through haptenization, can also provoke autoimmune neutropenia. Other causes include overwhelming sepsis, where the formation of new granulocytes cannot keep pace with their consumption, and hypersplenism (pp. 214–215).

### Disorders of Dysfunctional Granulocytes

In this rare heterogeneous group of disorders, the neutrophils display abnormalities of various functions. These include (1) migration and chemotaxis, (2) phagocytosis, (3) degranulation, and (4) the ability to generate oxygen free radicals and hydrogen peroxide. An example of the last category is chronic granulomatous disease, an X-linked recessive trait, in which there is an inability to create highly active oxygen radicals, primarily hydrogen peroxide. Patients are especially susceptible to infection by organisms such as staphylococci, which produce catalase, because this enzyme scavenges what little $H_2O_2$ the neutrophils can make. The clinical picture is dominated by repeated infections of the skin, lymph node, and respiratory tract. Granulomas, the only line of defence, can be found in many organs.

### Increased Myelopoiesis

An increase in numbers of white cells is called leukocytosis. An increase in neutrophils alone – neutrophil leukocytosis – is most frequently due to bacterial infection. This is mediated through increased release of bone marrow granulocytes by the actions of proinflammatory cytokines such as interleukin 1 (IL-1) and tumour necrosis factor (TNF). In more chronic states, these two cytokines promote the production of factors that stimulate an increase in neutrophil production itself. As IL-1 and TNF are produced in conditions other than infection, leukocytosis can be seen in patients with burns, myocardial infarction, pulmonary embolism, and other inflammatory conditions. Leukocytosis commonly occurs in leukaemia. Leukopenia, a decrease in the number of circulating leukocytes, may occur in many conditions including aplastic anaemia, drug reactions, viral infection, immunosuppression, myelodysplasia, and marrow replacement syndromes.

Eosinophilia – an increase in eosinophils in the peripheral blood – is almost always reactive in nature and tends to occur most commonly in parasitic infestations, asthma and allergic conditions, skin diseases such as dermatitis herpetiformis (see Chapter 18, p. 515), and vasculitis (Churg–Strauss syndrome). Eosinophilia may be drug induced and can accompany Hodgkin lymphoma. Very rarely, eosinophilic leukaemia occurs.

## Disorders of Platelets

### Thrombocytopenia

In this condition, a decreased number of platelets can result from their excess peripheral destruction or insufficient production. Excess destruction is the more important cause: it is frequently immunologically mediated or results from excessive consumption in thrombotic disease. Idiopathic thrombocytopenic purpura (ITP) results from the production of autoantibodies directed against surface molecules such as glycoproteins IIb/IIIa. ITP is usually idiopathic but may be secondary (e.g. to SLE). The autoantibodies opsonize the platelets, which are then phagocytosed by macrophages in the spleen and liver. Bone marrow examination usually shows a compensatory increase in megakaryocytes. Petechiae are common and gastrointestinal haemorrhage occurs, but intracranial haemorrhage is fortunately rare. Treatment is by steroids and, if these fail, by splenectomy. In adults, ITP runs a chronic course, but in children an acute form may follow a viral illness; this self-limiting disease requires treatment only when platelet counts are very low. Some drugs can precipitate immunological reactions against platelets.

Excessive consumption occurs in microangiopathic diseases, where diffuse activation of the clotting system causes thrombosis in many small vessels, resulting in platelet consumption and mechanical destruction of platelets and red cells (see Fig. 8.32).

Decreased formation of platelets is seen in aplastic and megaloblastic anaemia, marrow infiltration, and some infections (e.g. HIV), and as a reaction to some drugs, particularly cytotoxic drugs.

### Thrombocytosis

Thrombocytosis (increased platelet numbers) may be reactive – as seen after large haemorrhages – or neoplastic – as in essential thrombocythaemia and other myeloproliferative disorders such as polycythaemia vera (see pp. 226–227). Thrombocytosis carries a risk of thrombotic events, and treatment to lower the platelet count is warranted.

## Disorders of Lymphocytes

### Lymphopenia

Lymphopenia, a reduction in peripheral lymphocyte numbers, is normal in elderly people. It may occur in immunodeficiency disease such as HIV infection, in which the number of CD4+ cells is low. Lymphopenia can also occur in autoimmune diseases such as SLE and some acute infections, and after treatment with steroids and cytotoxic drugs.

### Lymphocytosis

A lymphocytosis, increased peripheral lymphocytes, is normal in the first year of life. In older children and adults, reactive lymphocytosis is usually caused by viral infections. Infectious mononucleosis causes a striking lymphocytosis with numerous very atypical forms, which can raise the possibility of malignancy. The other main cause of lymphocytosis in adults is lymphomatous disorders such as CLL and MCL (see Case History 8.3).

## Neoplastic Conditions of the Bone Marrow

### Key Points

Primary:
- leukaemia
- myeloproliferative disorders
- myelodysplasia
- some lymphomas
- plasma cell myeloma.

Secondary:
- metastatic malignancy
- lymphomas.

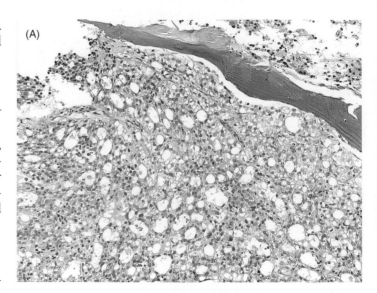

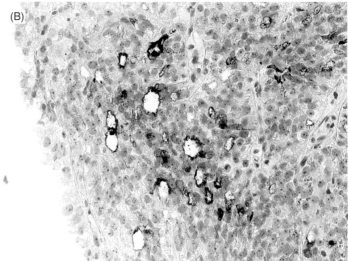

**FIG. 8.34** Bone marrow trephine biopsy in metastatic prostatic carcinoma. (A) Haematoxylin and eosin staining; (B) immunocytochemistry for prostate-specific antigen is positive, confirming its origin in the prostate.

Metastatic malignancy involving the bone marrow most commonly complicates carcinomas arising in the lung, breast, thyroid, kidney, and prostate (Fig. 8.34). Malignant melanoma is another well-recognized cause. Marrow replacement gives rise to a leukoerythroblastic blood film (Fig. 8.35), which may also be seen in storage diseases (Fig. 8.36) and myelofibrosis. Low-grade lymphomas commonly involve the marrow (see Case Histories 8.2 and 8.3) and some primarily arise there.

Primary malignancies of the bone marrow are clonal stem cell disorders producing varying degrees of proliferation and differentiation. The acute leukaemias are tumours showing proliferation, but little if any differentiation. These tumours consist of primitive blast cells with a high proliferative rate because no cells leave the pool of dividing cells to differentiate. They are thus fast growing and clinically aggressive. Those processes, characterized by proliferation and differentiation, are known as 'myeloproliferative disorders'. Both the bone marrow and the peripheral blood are highly cellular, but all stages of differentiation are seen. Differentiation draws cells out of the dividing pool – hence the apparent proliferation rate is lower and the clinical course is more protracted. In the myelodysplastic syndromes there is

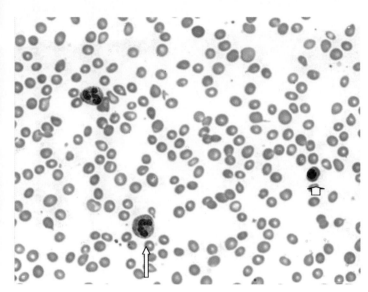

FIG. 8.35 Leukoerythroblastic blood film: a nucleated red blood cell precursor (short arrow) and an immature granulocyte (long arrow) are present. Immature precursors are not normally seen in the peripheral blood but, when present, indicate replacement of the normal marrow and consequent extramedullary haematopoiesis. Tear-drop poikilocytes are also a feature.

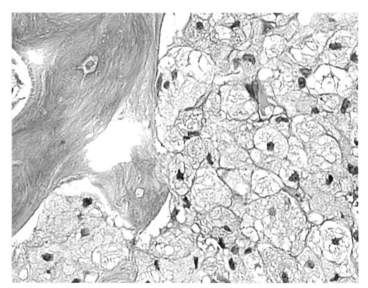

FIG. 8.36 Bone marrow trephine biopsy in Gaucher's disease. The marrow is replaced by macrophages filled with glucocerebroside.

proliferation and differentiation, but the latter is abnormal. The high rate of proliferation causes increased marrow cellularity, but the abnormal differentiation results in destruction of defective cells, so peripheral blood counts are low.

Multiple myeloma – a tumour composed of mature plasma cells – typically arises in the bone marrow.

## The Leukaemias

### Key Points

- The bone marrow is replaced by blast cells, which spill into peripheral blood.
- The clinical effects are due largely to marrow replacement and marrow failure.
- The tumours are aggressive, but often susceptible to chemotherapy.
- Cytogenetic abnormalities have prognostic importance.

Leukaemia is defined as a tumour with an increased number of neoplastic white cells in the peripheral blood. In a small proportion of cases the white cell count may not be raised, and this is the so-called 'aleukaemic leukaemia'. The acute leukaemias comprise acute myeloid leukaemia (AML) and acute lymphoblastic leukaemia (ALL), the latter now being classified with the lymphoproliferative disorders because it is derived from primitive precursor B or T lymphocytes (see Box 8.3). The chronic leukaemias include chronic myeloid leukaemia (CML), which is classified with the myeloproliferative disorders, and CLL, which is classified with the lymphoproliferative disorders (p. 209).

### The Acute Leukaemias

Clinically, all acute leukaemias are similar in that their effects are due to bone marrow failure. The proliferating malignant cells crowd out the normal haematopoietic elements, leading to anaemia, infections, and bleeding. The onset is often abrupt with fever, malaise, and sometimes bone pain. Rarely, acute leukaemia involves tissues other than the bone marrow such as the skin and gingiva. Occasionally, infiltrating myeloid leukaemia cells produce a tumour mass (myeloid sarcoma) in soft tissue or beneath the periosteum. This usually occurs when leukaemia is manifest, but it may precede the onset of overt disease by months.

Diagnosis and classification involve an assessment of cell morphology by microscopy, cytochemistry, immunophenotyping performed by flow cytometry, and increasingly genotyping. Without treatment, patients with acute leukaemia would die within weeks or months. Chemotherapy has greatly improved the outlook, especially in the lymphoblastic leukaemias of childhood. The AMLs have a much poorer prognosis and, although most patients achieve complete remission, a significant proportion relapse and eventually die of the disease.

## Acute Myeloid Leukaemia

AML is defined as a clonal expansion of myeloid blasts in bone marrow, blood, or other tissue (Fig. 8.37). The incidence among the UK population is 3/100,000 and the median age of onset is 60 years. Risk factors for AML include ionizing radiation, viruses, chemicals (e.g. benzene), and cytotoxic chemotherapy. Traditionally, AML has been classified morphologically by a system devised by French, American, and British haematologists (FAB classification). The discovery of a number of genetic abnormalities that predict clinical behaviour better than morphology alone led to the modified classification produced by the WHO in 2001 and revised in 2008 (*Box 8.6*). The presence of a translocation t(8;21)(q22;q22) or an inversion 16 is associated with an improved outcome. The t(15;17) defines a variety of AML (acute promyelocytic leukaemia) that has a high risk of association with DIC. Although the latter may be fatal, early recognition and treatment with the differentiating agent *trans*-retinoic acid can control this complication. Those cases arising on a background of a myelodysplastic or myeloproliferative disorder tend to occur in older patients, and have a poorer prognosis. A significant proportion of long-term cancer survivors develop AML as a consequence of cytotoxic chemotherapy. The remaining cases are subdivided according to their morphology based on the FAB classification.

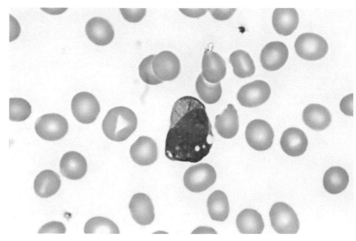

**FIG. 8.37** Blood film in acute myeloid leukaemia. A single blast cell containing an Auer rod (cytoplasmic crystalline structure specific for myeloid differentiation) is depicted.

---

**Box 8.6** WHO CLASSIFICATION OF ACUTE MYELOID LEUKAEMIA (AML) (SIMPLIFIED)

**AML with recurrent cytogenetic abnormalities**
Translocation t(8;21)(q22;q22); RUNX1-RUNX1T1
Inversion inv(16)(p13.1q22) or 7(16;16)(p13.1;q22); CBFB-MYH11
Translocation t(15;17)(q22;q12), PML-RARA; acute promyelocytic leukaemia
Translocation t(9;11)(p22;q23); MLLT3-MLL
Translocation t(6;9)(p23;q34); DEK-NUP214
Inversion inv(3)(q21q26.2) or t(3;3)(q21;q26.2); RPN1-EVI1
Mutated *NPM1*[a]
Mutated *CEBPA*[a]
**AML with myelodysplasia-related changes**
**Therapy-related myeloid neoplasms**
**AML, not otherwise specified**[b]
AML with minimal differentiation
AML without maturation
AML with maturation
Acute myelomonocytic leukaemia
Acute monoblastic and monocytic leukaemia
Acute erythroid leukaemia
Acute megakaryoblastic leukaemia
Acute basophilic leukaemia
Acute panmyelosis with myelofibrosis
**Myeloid sarcoma**
**Myeloid proliferations related to Down's syndrome**
Transient abnormal myelopoiesis
Myeloid leukaemia associated with Down's syndrome
**Blastic plamacytoid dendritic cell neoplasm**

[a]Provisional entities in the WHO (2008) classification.
[b]This category is based on the FAB morphological classification and includes those cases not fitting into the first three categories.

The diagnosis of AML requires the demonstration of...

The diagnosis of AML requires the demonstration of more than 20% myeloid blasts in the blood or marrow. Differentiation from ALL can be difficult on morphology alone, and immunophenotyping by flow cytometry is often required. The detailed laboratory techniques used in subclassifying these tumours is beyond the scope of this textbook.

### Acute Lymphoblastic Leukaemia

ALL is a clonal proliferation of lymphoid precursor B or T cells, which usually results in an acute leukaemia, although sometimes it can produce lymph node or mediastinal enlargement in the absence of circulating blasts. The latter presentation is termed 'lymphoblastic lymphoma', although for management purposes this is regarded as being equivalent to ALL. In the UK the incidence is 4/100,000 and each year this results in approximately 450 new cases. ALL usually affects children, the median age of onset being between 4 and 7 years. The aetiology of the condition is largely unknown, although both genetic and environmental factors are believed to play a role.

ALL broadly falls into two main groups: those of B-cell and those of T-cell type. Diagnosis requires detailed immunophenotyping to establish whether the neoplastic cells are of B or T lineage, and to differentiate them from myeloid leukaemia. Immunoreactivity for the enzyme terminal deoxynucleotidyl transferase (TdT) distinguishes lymphoblasts from mature lymphocytes (Fig. 8.38).

B-cell ALL (B-ALL), representing 85% of cases, is predominantly a disorder of childhood but also affects adults. Patients present with symptoms and signs of marrow replacement (anaemia, infection, haemorrhage), bone pain, lymphadenopathy, and splenomegaly. There is a tendency to involve other tissues, especially the central nervous system, with signs of raised intracranial pressure and cranial nerve palsies (especially nerves VI and VII). Central nervous system involvement is a poor prognostic sign because treatment is difficult. The testes are also frequently involved. A cure can be achieved in 80% of children, and this represents one of the greatest achievements in cancer therapy over the past 30 years. Good prognostic factors for children are: age between 4 and 10 years, a low leukocyte count at presentation, and hyperdiploid chromosomes or a translocation t(12;21)(p13;q22). Adverse factors include age <1 year, and the t(9;22) and t(4;11) translocations. The survival rate for adults is less good.

Some 15% of ALL in children is due to T-lymphoblastic leukaemia/lymphoma, which tends to affect adolescent males and may present with a mass in the anterior mediastinum. Here, the tumour cells mimic the normal development of T lymphoblasts by migrating from the bone marrow to the thymus. Although initially associated with a poorer prognosis than B-ALL, modern therapies are producing a substantial cure rate in children.

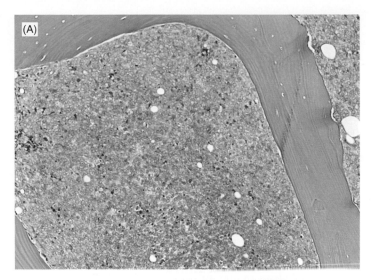
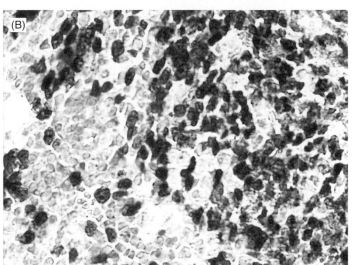

**FIG. 8.38** Trephine biopsy of bone marrow in acute lymphoblastic leukaemia. (A) The marrow cellularity is almost 100% and is replaced by an infiltrate of small blast cells. (B) Nuclear positivity for terminal deoxynucleotidyl transferase (TdT) is identified in the majority of cells by immunocytochemistry.

## Chronic Myeloproliferative Disorders

### Key Points

- These are clonal haematopoietic stem cell disorders with effective haematopoiesis.
- There is excess production of mature cells, usually producing high peripheral counts.
- The clinical presentation varies depending on the predominant differentiated component.
- There can be an overlap in clinical and laboratory features between the different subtypes.
- They may be complicated by gout.
- There is a risk of progression to acute leukaemia or myelofibrosis.

The chronic myeloproliferative disorders are clonal haematopoietic stem cell disorders characterized by the proliferation of one or more of the myeloid lineages (granulocytic, erythroid, or megakaryocytic) associated with relatively normal and effective maturation. This results in a raised peripheral white cell, red cell, and/or platelet count. Although only one lineage may appear to be primarily involved (e.g. red cells in polycythaemia vera), all lineages are found to be abnormal on further investigation. This derangement at stem cell level is proven by the demonstration of chromosomal abnormalities in all lineages in one given disorder.

The aetiology is largely unknown, although association with exposure to benzene, ionizing radiation, and genetic factors is recorded. The overall incidence is 6–9/100,000 population.

There are four main categories.

## Chronic Myeloid Leukaemia

CML results from a genetic abnormality at the level of the pluripotent stem cell. Its typical chromosomal abnormality – the Philadelphia chromosome (Ph), the result of a t(9;22) translocation – can be found in all haematopoietic cells including the lymphoid series.

The disease occurs at any age, but usually in patients during the fifth and sixth decades of life. It has an incidence of 1.5/100,000 population.

The symptoms are mostly non-specific, with fatigue, anorexia, weight loss, and hepatomegaly. On occasion, abdominal swelling due to splenomegaly, often massive, is the presenting feature. Splenic infarction may lead to sudden abdominal pain. In approximately 30% of cases, the patient is asymptomatic and the diagnosis is made from a routine full blood count. This reveals anaemia and a markedly raised white cell count (often >10 × 10⁹/dL), composed mainly of myeloid cells of varying maturation (Fig. 8.39). The bone marrow is hypercellular with a predominance of the granulocytic series, although there is often also an increase in megakaryocytes and erythroid precursors. Genetic studies reveal the translocation t(9;22) (q34;q11) in 95% of cases (Fig. 8.40). The course of the disease is indolent for some years (chronic phase), but almost inevitably it evolves into an 'accelerated' phase, which becomes refractory to therapy. Blast crisis and evolution to acute leukaemia, either myeloid or lymphoblastic, may follow. The median survival is 3–4 years, with death occurring from acute transformation or from infection or haemorrhage. Chemotherapy is useful for controlling symptoms in the chronic phase, but does not affect overall survival. Bone marrow transplantation also has a role. Recently, a signal transduction inhibitor, specifically targeting the pathways activated by bcr-abl (the product of the translocation), has been developed (imatinib), and this is proving beneficial in clinical trials (Fig. 8.40), notably because it also seems to be effective for gastrointestinal stromal tumours (see Chapter 9, p. 254).

## Polycythaemia Vera

This condition is characterized by increased red cell production and a lesser degree of proliferation of the myeloid and megakaryocytic lineages. It is more common among

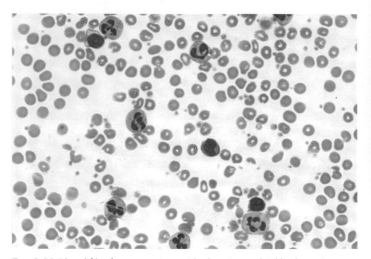

**FIG. 8.39** Blood film from a patient with chronic myeloid leukaemia (CML). There is a marked increase in the number of granulocytes compared with the normal blood film (see Fig. 8.28).

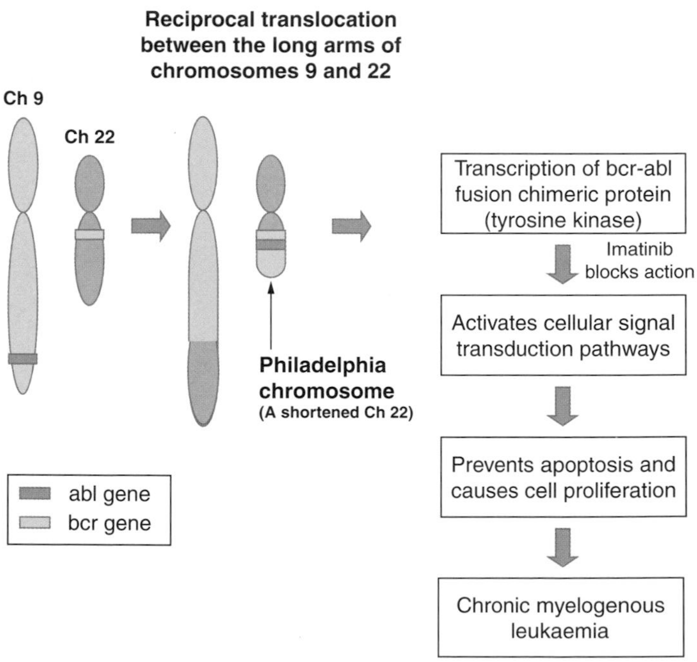

**Reciprocal translocation between the long arms of chromosomes 9 and 22**

Ch 9

Ch 22

Philadelphia chromosome (A shortened Ch 22)

abl gene
bcr gene

Transcription of bcr-abl fusion chimeric protein (tyrosine kinase)

Imatinib blocks action

Activates cellular signal transduction pathways

Prevents apoptosis and causes cell proliferation

Chronic myelogenous leukaemia

**FIG. 8.40** Cytogenetic abnormality in chronic myeloid leukaemia. This diagram depicts the classic t(9;22)(q34;q11) translocation associated with CML. This was the first cytogenetic abnormality detected in a human malignancy. There is a reciprocal translocation between the long arms of chromosomes 9 and 22, bringing together the *abl* and *bcr* genes in the derivative chromosome 22 (the Philadelphia chromosome).

males, and the mean age of diagnosis is 60 years. The incidence is 0.8/100,000 population. The clinical symptoms are caused by the increase in red cell mass, resulting in headache, tiredness, a plethoric complexion, and itching, especially after hot baths. There is increased blood viscosity and a tendency to thrombosis, leading to strokes, myocardial infarction, and deep vein thrombosis. Sometimes, as the platelets produced are dysfunctional, there may be haemorrhage, especially from the gastrointestinal tract. The increased cell turnover may lead to gout. Splenomegaly is common.

The diagnosis is established by identifying both a raised haemoglobin concentration (>18.5 g/dL in males, >16.5 g/dL in females) and an increased red cell mass. Oxygen saturation is usually normal, and erythropoietin levels low, allowing distinction from secondary polycythaemia. Both the white cell and platelet counts are usually raised. The bone marrow is hypercellular due to proliferation of mainly the erythroid and megakaryocyte series. The clinical course is usually prolonged, although regular venesection is required. Death may result from vascular complications. In 15% of cases, myelofibrosis supervenes; another 5% evolve into AML, particularly in those who have received chemotherapy.

### Chronic Idiopathic Myelofibrosis

This is a clonal proliferation of mainly megakaryocytes and granulocytes associated with extensive fibrosis of the marrow, which often prevents acquisition of an aspirate sample (a dry tap). This fibrosis is probably caused by the release of growth factors (e.g. platelet-derived growth factor) from the neoplastic megakaryocytes. The bones eventually become sclerotic. Haematopoiesis is displaced and there is extramedullary haematopoiesis primarily in the spleen, liver, lymph nodes, and sometimes other organs. The peripheral blood shows a leukoerythroblastic reaction (see Fig. 8.35). Splenomegaly may be massive, resulting in hypersplenism (see Fig. 8.24). The incidence is <1/100,000 population per annum. Patients may present with vague symptoms of fatigue, night sweats, and weight loss. Many are asymptomatic at diagnosis and come to light due to the detection of splenomegaly or abnormalities found on a routine blood film. The prognosis is poor (median survival 3–5 years), with many patients dying from infection, haemorrhage, or bone marrow failure; AML may supervene in 10%.

### Essential Thrombocythaemia

This condition predominantly involves the megakaryocytic lineage, resulting in sustained elevation of platelet counts, usually in excess of $600 \times 10^9$/L. Between 20% and 50% of patients present with either a thrombotic event or haemorrhage, the remainder being detected by a routine blood test. Otherwise, the disease is indolent, but may progress to myelofibrosis, and rarely to acute leukaemia.

## The Myelodysplastic Syndromes

This group of conditions is characterized by a clonal stem cell disorder causing bone marrow proliferation with abnormal differentiation resulting in ineffectual haematopoiesis in the face of a hypercellular marrow. Myelodysplasias present mainly in elderly people, with symptoms attributable to pancytopenia. As these conditions have a tendency to evolve into AML, they were formerly known as 'preleukaemias'. Myelodysplasia may be primary or occur secondary to previous chemotherapy or HIV infection. There are a number of subtypes with varying risks of leukaemic transformation.

## Plasma Cell Myeloma

### Key Points

Plasma cell myeloma is typified by:
- monoclonal proliferation of plasma cells within the bone marrow
- multifocal osteolytic bony lesions
- hypercalcaemia
- signs and symptoms of marrow replacement
- excess production of monoclonal immunoglobulin (M-protein in serum, Bence Jones protein in urine)
- presentation with acute renal failure in many cases
- the development of AL amyloidosis in some cases.

Plasma cell myeloma is a malignant tumour arising in the bone marrow, and is composed entirely of monoclonal plasma cells. It is one of the most common haematological malignancies, and affects adults with an incidence of 10/100,000 of the population per annum. The median age of diagnosis is 68 years. Chemicals, viruses, and ionizing radiation have been reported as aetiological factors, although none has been identified in most cases. Myeloma affects the patient by several mechanisms: first, by the direct effects of the tumour eroding bones – especially those of the vertebral column, ribs, and skull; this results in pain, pathological fractures, and vertebral collapse; second, by causing replacement of the marrow, resulting in pancytopenia with consequent immunosuppression, thrombocytopenia, and anaemia. The third mechanism is related to the secretory product of the neoplastic plasma cells, which – similar to their normal counterparts – are capable of producing immunoglobulin, and almost all cases are associated with a serum or urine monoclonal γ-globulin, the M-component. A monoclonal immunoglobulin light chain (Bence Jones protein) is detected in the urine in 75% of cases. When the level of this protein is high, precipitation may occur in the renal tubules, resulting in acute renal failure. In some situations the protein may be deposited in the tissues as AL amyloid. Hyperviscosity syndromes may also occur.

The diagnosis is usually suspected from the clinical and radiological features, and is confirmed by bone marrow biopsy and serum electrophoresis. The diagnostic criteria are listed in *Box 8.7*. The bone marrow may show an interstitial infiltrate or confluent sheets of plasma cells, which display varying degrees of atypia. The monoclonal plasma cells are capable of producing only one light chain – a feature that can be exploited in determining monoclonality (Fig. 8.41). Monosomy 13 occurs in 15–40% of cases. Despite treatment the prognosis of plasma cell myeloma is poor, with a median survival of 3 years. A small proportion of patients may survive for 10 years.

Some patients presenting with a low level of serum paraprotein are found to have <10% monoclonal plasma cells in the bone marrow. These patients display none of the clinical features of myeloma and lack bony lesions. This condition is called *monoclonal gammopathy of undetermined significance* (MGUS) and has a high prevalence (3%) after the age of 70 years. Most patients require no treatment, although plasma cell myeloma or amyloidosis will develop in 25% of cases.

*Solitary plasmacytoma* is a tumour occurring in bone or the upper respiratory tract, and is composed of monoclonal plasma cells identical to those of plasma cell myeloma. As these lesions are localized, radiotherapy can induce a cure in a significant proportion of cases. Plasma cell myeloma will occur in 50% of patients within 10 years of initial presentation.

---

**Box 8.7** WHO DIAGNOSTIC CRITERIA FOR PLASMA CELL MYELOMA[a]

**Major criteria:**
 Marrow plasmacytosis <30%
 Plasmacytoma on biopsy
 M-component
  Serum – IgG >3.5 g/dL; IgA>2 g/dL
  Urine – 1 g/24 h of Bence Jones protein
**Minor criteria:**
 Marrow plasmacytosis (10–30%)
 M-component present but less than above
 Lytic bone lesions
 Reduced normal immunoglobulins (<50% normal):
  IgG <600 mg/dL; IgA <100 mg/dL; IgM <50 mg/dL

[a]Diagnosis requires a minimum of one major criterion and one minor criterion or three minor criteria in a patient with progressive symptomatic disease.

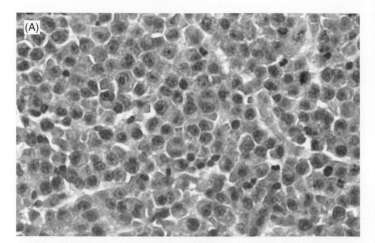
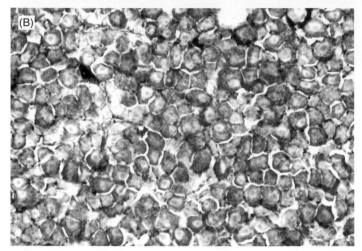
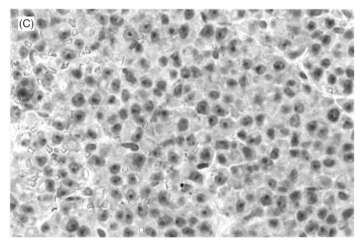

**FIG. 8.41** Bone marrow trephine biopsy in multiple myeloma. (A) Haematoxylin and eosin staining shows confluent sheets of atypical plasma cells. (B) The neoplastic plasma cells stain only for the κ light chain using immunocytochemistry and are therefore monoclonal. (C) The same population of cells is negative for the λ light chain.

## SUMMARY

- Conditions involving the lymphoreticular system and bone marrow are common and present in a wide variety of ways.

- Diseases involving the lymph nodes usually present with lymphadenopathy and include reactive conditions such as tuberculosis and sarcoidosis, in addition to neoplastic disorders such as lymphoma and metastatic carcinoma.

- Lymphoma is a malignant tumour derived from lymphocytes; it may affect lymph nodes or extranodal sites.
- The bone marrow may be affected by congenital, infective, autoimmune, and neoplastic disorders resulting in varying degrees of bone marrow failure. Anaemia, thrombocytopenia, and decreased white cell count are the consequences of bone marrow failure and lead to fatigue, haemorrhage, and increased susceptibility to infection.
- Leukaemia is a malignant condition characterized by an increase in white cells in the peripheral circulation as a result of a clonal proliferation of bone marrow stem cells.
- There are many different types of leukaemia and lymphoma with different clinical presentations and prognoses. Their accurate diagnosis is complex and requires correlation of morphological, immunophenotypic, cytogenetic, and clinical data.
- Many lymphomas and leukaemias are curable with modern therapy.

## ACKNOWLEDGEMENTS

We wish to acknowledge the contribution of Professor CJLM Meijer, VU University Medical Centre, Amsterdam, for input to the previous edition of this chapter. We thank Drs Mike Leach, Noelle O'Rourke, Grant McQuaker, and Andy Clarke for assistance with the figures and case histories.

## FURTHER READING

Bain BJ, Clark DM, Lampert IA, Wilkins BS. *Bone Marrow Pathology*, 4th edn. Oxford: Blackwell Science, 2009.

Hoffbrand AV, Moss PAH. *Essential Haematology*, 6th edn. Oxford: Blackwell Science, 2011.

Orazi A, Weiss LM, Foucar K, Knowles DM. *Neoplastic Haematopathology*. 3rd edn. Philadelphia, PA: Lippincott Williams & Wilkins, 2013.

Stansfeld AG, d'Ardenne AJ. *Lymph Node Biopsy Interpretation*, 2nd edn. Edinburgh: Churchill Livingstone, 1992.

Swerdlow SH, Campo E, Harris NL, *et al. WHO Classification of Tumours of the Haematopoietic and Lymphoid tissues*. Lyon: IARC Press, 2008.

Weiss LM, ed. Pathology of lymph nodes. In: *Contemporary Issues in Surgical Pathology*, Vol. 21. Edinburgh: Churchill Livingstone, 1996.

Wilkins BS, Wright DH. *Illustrated Pathology of the Spleen*. Cambridge: Cambridge University Press, 2000.

# 9

# THE GASTROINTESTINAL SYSTEM

Sharon J White, David A Levison, and Francis A Carey

## THE ORAL CAVITY, SALIVARY GLANDS, AND OROPHARYNX

### The Oral Cavity

#### Normal Structure and Function

The oral cavity extends from the lips anteriorly to the oropharynx posteriorly and contains the buccal mucosae, floor of mouth, anterior two-thirds of the tongue, hard palate, teeth, and gingivae (gums). Stratified squamous epithelium lines the oral mucosa and has a high rate of cell turnover. It is keratinized in areas such as the hard palate and attached gingivae, which are subject to functional trauma. Specialized structures such as taste buds and papillae are present in the mucosa of the tongue, and numerous minor salivary glands are located throughout the oral mucosa. The functions of the mouth include mastication, speech, taste, and swallowing.

Developmental, infective, inflammatory, and neoplastic lesions may affect the oral mucosa and many of these are the same as at other sites in the body. However, distinct features peculiar to the mouth are often seen. Furthermore, there are a number of specific lesions related to the teeth and their supporting tissues.

### The Teeth

The teeth consist of three specialized mineralized tissues with underlying soft-tissue pulp (Fig. 9.1). Dentine is a thick layer of tubular, calcified, collagenous tissue that surrounds the pulp. On the crown of the tooth, the dentine is covered by enamel, an acellular tissue consisting largely of calcium apatite crystals in a delicate organic matrix. Cementum overlies the root dentine. At the apex of each root is one or more foramina through which vessels and nerves enter the

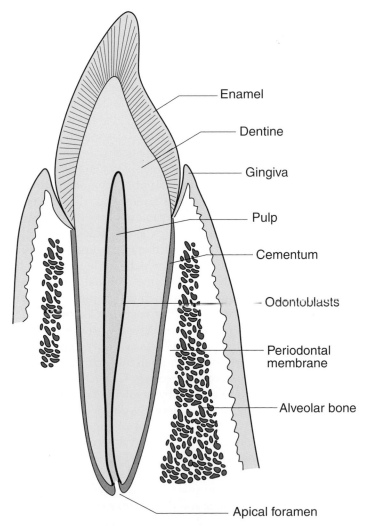

**FIG. 9.1** The tooth and its supporting tissues.

Enamel
Dentine
Gingiva
Pulp
Cementum
Odontoblasts
Periodontal membrane
Alveolar bone
Apical foramen

pulp. The teeth are attached to the jaws by the periodontium, a specialized supportive complex comprising cementum, the periodontal ligament, alveolar bone, and gingiva. The deciduous or 'baby' teeth erupt within the first few years of life and total 20 in number. From 6 years of age, additional permanent teeth erupt and the deciduous teeth are gradually replaced by permanent successors to give a full adult complement of 32 teeth by the late teens.

Dental caries and periodontal disease (non-specific chronic inflammation of the soft tissues related to the teeth), probably the most common diseases of humankind, are caused principally by oral bacteria. A highly complex bacterial flora is found in saliva, adherent to epithelium, and in deposits on tooth surfaces. The dental plaque on teeth consists of many types of bacteria in an organic matrix of salivary and bacterial origin. This may calcify to form dental calculus.

## Dental Caries

### Key Points

- Dental caries is a bacterial disease, related to adherent dental plaque.
- Plaque forms predominantly in stagnation areas.
- Bacteria invade dentine and cause pulpitis (toothache).

Dental caries (tooth decay) is the progressive destruction of the calcified tissues of the teeth exposed to the oral environment by bacteria and their products. Caries itself, and the consequent inflammation of the tooth pulp, are the most common causes of tooth loss up to middle age. Caries can involve any tooth surface, but usually starts in two principal areas of the tooth: the fissures on the occlusal or biting surfaces of posterior teeth, and the areas between teeth (proximal caries). Both of these are areas of relative stagnation in which dental plaque is likely to accumulate. The bacteria within plaque produce various organic acids, with the resultant pH depending on factors such as the thickness of the plaque and the concentration of dietary sugars. The initial attack on enamel is by the acid, which produces decalcification. Bacteria initially penetrate the dentinal tubules, but then cause softening and distortion of the dentine by a combination of decalcification and proteolytic breakdown of the collagen matrix. The process then extends through the dentine towards the dental pulp. At first caries is a painless process, but, as the lesion extends through the enamel to involve the dentine and pulp, toothache ensues. Caries may also start at the neck of the tooth, often by involving the cementum and then the dentine, or, if cementum is deficient, by directly attacking the root dentine. This form of caries is typically seen in older patients in whom gingival recession is more common. In the early stages of enamel caries, the damage is reversible, but thereafter caries of enamel and dentine is progressive, except in unusual circumstances in which the area becomes self-cleaning and the lesions may be arrested.

## Pulpitis

The dental pulp is a vascular connective tissue confined within the pulp chamber and root canals. Pulpitis is the most common and clinically significant lesion of the pulp. It occurs most often due to the extension of caries into dentine and then into the pulp. Physical injury, such as heat and chemical irritation from filling materials, may also give rise to pulpitis, which may be acute or chronic. As the changes occur within the rigid confines of the pulp chamber, there is an increase in pressure due to inflammatory exudate. Consequently acute pulpitis is very painful. The pain of pulpitis is poorly localized and patients frequently cannot indicate the tooth involved. If the inflammation spreads to the apical periodontal ligament the patient can localize the tooth involved and it becomes tender to percussion. If the insult to the pulp is less severe, chronic pulpitis may result. The pulp may undergo necrosis after acute or chronic pulpitis. Clinically, a non-vital tooth lacks lustre and may be discoloured by the leaching of products of the necrotic pulp into the dentine. In children, a large carious cavity penetrating quickly to the pulp may result in a large opening into the pulp chamber, leading to open pulpitis from which exudate can drain. Granulation tissue may extend as a pulp polyp into the carious cavity.

## Periapical Pathology

### Key Points

- Periapical pathology usually results from pulpitis.
- Some periapical granulomas undergo cystic change to form a radicular cyst.
- Periapical granuloma and radicular cyst appear as a periapical radiolucency on a radiograph.

The periapical tissues are the site of a variety of lesions related to the root apices of teeth. The most frequent of these arise from the spread of infection from pulpitis, through the apical foramina of the tooth, to reach the periodontal ligament. This can result in an acute periapical abscess, a very painful condition that may be accompanied by cervical lymphadenopathy and generalized fever and malaise. Pus can track through the adjacent bone and, after the periosteum is breached, a soft-tissue abscess develops and later discharges. More frequently, after low-grade pulpitis, a periapical granuloma develops. This consists of a mass of granulation tissue heavily infiltrated with chronic inflammatory cells. There is resorption of surrounding bone, seen radiologically as a periapical radiolucent lesion (Fig. 9.2). Acute exacerbation may result in a secondary acute periapical abscess and, conversely, a periapical granuloma can develop after an acute periapical abscess has pointed and drained. Remnants of odontogenic epithelium that persist in the periradicular tissue after tooth development proliferate within a periapical

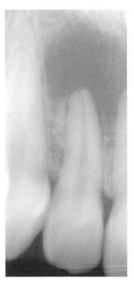

FIG. 9.2 Periapical radiolucency indicating resorption of bone and replacement by inflammatory soft tissue in the form of a periapical granuloma or radicular cyst (Image courtesy of Dr Donald J Thomson.)

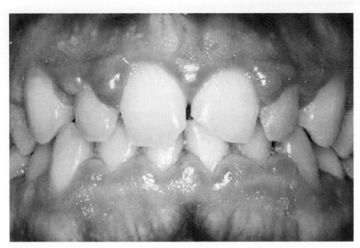

FIG. 9.3 Chronic periodontitis, with redness and swelling of the attached gingiva.

granuloma, and these give rise to the most common cyst of the jaws, the inflammatory radicular cyst.

## Periodontal Disease

### Key Points

- Most periodontal disease is caused by bacterial plaque.
- Periodontal disease may involve only the gingivae (gingivitis) or all of the periodontal tissues (periodontitis).
- Periodontitis may result in tooth loss.

Periodontal disease may occur as inflammation of the gingival tissues (gingivitis) or involve the gingivae, the periodontal ligament, and the related alveolar bone (periodontitis). The current classification of periodontal disease incorporates eight disease categories, including gingival diseases, various forms of periodontitis including necrotizing periodontal diseases, and those that are manifestations of systemic disease. Gingivitis, which does not result in loss of attachment of periodontal tissues, is often related to dental plaque but may also be due to various traumatic, genetic, and infective causes. Chronic periodontitis (Fig. 9.3) is very common and typically increases in frequency and severity with age, although some forms may affect children. A number of local and systemic factors are involved, but of these the most important is the presence of bacterial plaque around the neck of the tooth. The inflammation in periodontitis results in progressive loss of attachment of the periodontal ligament, with osteoclastic resorption of the alveolar bone supporting the teeth in later stages. Deepening of the gingival sulcus occurs with the formation of periodontal pockets.

Infrequently there is an acute exacerbation of infection in such pockets and a periodontal abscess can arise.

Necrotizing periodontal diseases include acute necrotizing ulcerative gingivitis (ANUG) and necrotizing ulcerative periodontitis. In developed countries, ANUG typically occurs in young adults and presents as painful, foul-smelling ulceration and necrosis of the interdental papillae, with variable spread to other parts of the gum. The condition involves the formation of an anaerobic fusospirochaetal complex including *Fusobacterium nucleatum* and *Treponema vincentii* organisms among others, and responds to appropriate antimicrobial therapy. In contrast, the disease in developing countries tends to occur most often in malnourished children and, if untreated, can lead to extensive necrosis of orofacial tissue – 'cancrum oris' – and may be fatal. Two of the three forms of periodontal disease associated with HIV infection also present as necrotizing conditions. Periodontal disease may arise as a manifestation of systemic disease such as haematological disorders or genetic disorders, e.g. Down's and Ehlers–Danlos syndromes. Despite various claims in recent years, there is currently no definitive evidence to support a link between periodontal disease and cardiovascular disease.

## Cysts of the Jaws

### Key Points

- Most jaw cysts are derived from odontogenic epithelium.
- Odontogenic cysts may be inflammatory or developmental.
- The odontogenic keratocyst (keratocystic odontogenic tumour) is potentially aggressive and prone to recurrence.

Several types of epithelium-lined cyst occur in the jaws and most are derived from the rests of odontogenic epithelium that remain after tooth development. These odontogenic cysts are subdivided into inflammatory and developmental cysts. The most common is the radicular cyst (described above), an inflammatory cyst that develops in some periapical granulomas associated with a non-vital tooth. If the affected tooth is extracted, the cyst may remain as a residual cyst. The most frequent developmental odontogenic cyst is the dentigerous cyst, which develops around the crown of an unerupted tooth. Closely related is the eruption cyst, which presents as a bluish fluctuant swelling in the gum overlying the crown of an erupting tooth.

The odontogenic cysts described above are lined by non-keratinized, stratified, squamous epithelium, which may include a few mucus-secreting cells. These cysts are usually symptomless unless infected and can grow to several centimetres with considerable bone destruction. They must be differentiated from the odontogenic keratocyst (keratocystic odontogenic tumour), which has a distinctive parakeratinized, stratified, squamous epithelial lining (Fig. 9.4). Its relationship to the teeth is variable and it occurs anywhere in the jaws, the most common site being the posterior mandible, often extending up into the ramus of the mandible. This cystic lesion is now recognized as a benign, potentially aggressive odontogenic tumour, which possesses a high recurrence partly due to the friable nature of the lining and the presence of small daughter cysts within the cyst wall. Multiple, recurrent, keratocystic odontogenic tumours are seen as part of the basal cell naevus syndrome (Gorlin–Goltz syndrome).

Cysts derived from non-odontogenic epithelium are less frequent in the jaws. The most common of these rare cysts is the nasopalatine duct cyst, which arises in the midline of the anterior hard palate in the region of the incisive canal.

## Other Tooth-related Pathology

Tooth development begins at about 3 months of intrauterine life and extends over about 20 years until the completion of root formation of the third molars. During this period many developmental abnormalities can occur in the number of teeth, in the form and colour, in the structure of individual tooth elements, and the times of eruption and shedding of teeth. These abnormalities result from various factors, both genetic and environmental. An example of iatrogenic disease is the permanent staining of the mineralized dental tissues caused by administration of some tetracyclines during tooth development. Non-carious loss of tooth substance may result from erosion (e.g. in individuals with a highly acidic diet), abrasion, and attrition.

Odontogenic tumours are uncommon lesions derived from various tissue components involved in tooth development. Most are benign although malignant types do very rarely occur. The most important benign odontogenic tumours are the keratocystic odontogenic tumour (see above) and the ameloblastoma. Ameloblastoma is an epithelial neoplasm of distinct appearance (Fig. 9.5) that most frequently arises in the molar region of the mandible. It is locally aggressive, often producing extensive bone destruction. The most frequently occurring odontogenic tumours are odontomes, typically arising in childhood, when they often impede the eruption of a permanent tooth, and early adulthood. These tumours are hamartomatous lesions containing enamel and dentine and sometimes cementum. A complex odontome consists of a disorganized mass of dental tissues, whereas a compound odontome consists of numerous small tooth-like structures.

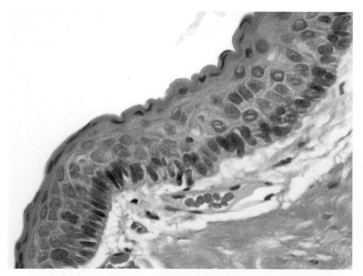

**FIG. 9.4** Odontogenic keratocyst (keratocystic odontogenic tumour) lining: a layer of corrugated parakeratin on the surface of benign stratified squamous epithelium with prominent palisading of the basal cell layer.

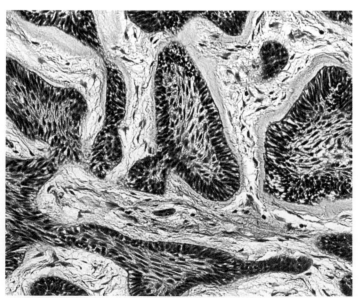

**FIG. 9.5** Ameloblastoma: characteristic islands of odontogenic epithelium within a mature fibrous stroma.

## The Oral Mucosa

The oral mucosa is subjected to numerous physical insults and is exposed to vast numbers of microorganisms, and to food and other material introduced into the mouth. In many lesions of the oral mucosa, physical trauma and infection have a role to play, and this may be superimposed on a previously normal or abnormal mucosa. It is not surprising that these circumstances produce complex changes, some of which are not fully understood.

### Developmental Abnormalities of the Oral Epithelium

Apart from the presence of Fordyce's granules (ectopic sebaceous glands), most frequently in the buccal mucosa, developmental abnormalities of the oral mucosa are rare.

### Oral Candidiasis

*Candida* spp. form part of the normal oral flora in about half the population. *Candida albicans* is the most frequent of these and causes opportunistic infection in a variety of situations, typically where the normal balance of the oral flora has changed and/or in individuals with altered immunity. Acute pseudomembranous candidiasis (thrush) is characterized by white fungal plaques, which rub off, exposing underlying red mucosa. Thrush is often found in healthy infants in addition to debilitated adults. Chronic candidiasis may be seen in a number of circumstances and is frequently present as denture stomatitis under upper dentures as an inflammatory reaction to fungi, which persist mainly on the fitting surface of the denture. Candidal hyphae may also be seen in adherent hyperkeratotic lesions found on the anterior buccal mucosa as chronic hyperplastic candidiasis. Persistent acute and chronic oral candidal infections are a common problem in patients with HIV infection. Angular cheilitis presents at the corners of the mouth as red, cracked lesions. It is described as a *Candida*-associated lesion; however, co-infection with *Staphylococcus aureus* is common and often there are other associated contributory causes.

---

### ORAL FUNGAL INFECTION

A 70-year-old woman complained of discomfort at the angles of her mouth and a sore tongue. Clinically, angular cheilitis was present (Fig. 9.6). The tongue was atrophic with loss of the normal pattern of papillae (Fig. 9.7). The patient had full dentures that she had worn for several years. The wear on the teeth had resulted in the lower jaw closing beyond the normal position, and there was a tendency for saliva to leak out on to the skin at the angles of the mouth. Examination of the palate revealed a red, inflamed area corresponding to the outline of the upper denture (Fig. 9.8).

Microbiological examination revealed heavy growth of *C. albicans* in cultures of swabs from the angle of the mouth and from the fitting surface of the upper denture. In addition,

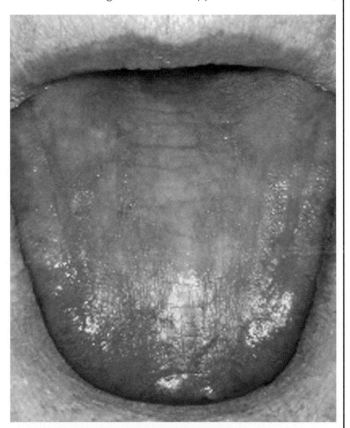

FIG. 9.7 Atrophic tongue: the rough filiform papillae of the dorsum of the tongue are replaced by flat mucosa; causes include chronic candidal infection, acute candidal infection after antibiotic treatment, and various vitamin/mineral deficiencies.

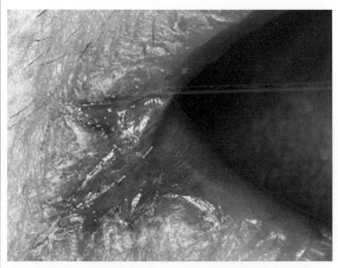

FIG. 9.6 Angular cheilitis: inflammation and fissuring at the labial commissure are often a marker of chronic candidal infection.

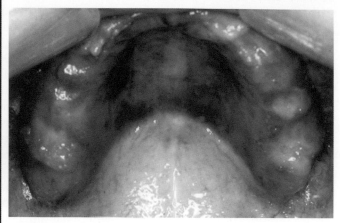

**FIG. 9.8** Chronic erythematous candidiasis: the pattern of inflammation on the hard palate mirroring the outline of the upper denture strongly suggests candidal infection.

haematological investigation revealed microcytic anaemia with a haemoglobin level of 95 g/L.

Investigations were conducted for iron-deficiency anaemia. No obvious source of blood loss was found. In particular, possible blood loss from neoplasms was excluded. It was felt that the cause of the iron deficiency was related to poor diet in an elderly person living alone and with limited finances. The iron deficiency responded to oral administration of iron. The fungal infestation was treated with appropriate antifungal drugs. New dentures were designed to increase the vertical dimension, in other words to open the mouth slightly and prevent the leakage of saliva. The patient was also counselled about denture hygiene to keep the denture free from fungal colonization. The clinical situation resolved satisfactorily.

Lessons to be learned from this case are:

- Oral lesions often have a multifactorial aetiology.
- Both local and systemic factors need to be considered.
- Treatment of only some of the involved factors is unlikely to resolve the whole clinical situation.

## Viral Infections

The most frequent viral infection of oral epithelium is caused by herpes simplex virus types I and II. Acute herpetic gingivostomatitis is characterized by extensive painful ulceration and occasionally generalized upset. Secondary or recurrent herpetic lesions are more common, especially at mucocutaneous junctions round the lips (herpes labialis or 'cold sores') and nose, where the initially vesicular phase is followed by ulceration and crusting. Herpes zoster can also affect the mouth and oral lesions caused by Coxsackievirus infection are seen in herpangina, and hand, foot, and mouth disease. Oral hairy leukoplakia, most cases of which occur in immunocompromised individuals, is due to Epstein–Barr virus infection.

## Recurrent Oral Ulceration (Recurrent Aphthous Stomatitis)

Recurrent painful fibrin-covered ulcers, either singly or in crops, are a very common and troublesome problem said to occur in about 20% of the population. The aetiology is not fully determined; however, immunological factors appear to play a role. Some cases may be associated with haematinic deficiencies, gastrointestinal disorders such as Crohn's disease, stress, stopping tobacco smoking, or food allergies.

## Dermatoses

A number of diseases can involve the mucosae in addition to the skin. The skin manifestations of these are discussed in Chapter 18. The oral mucosal features are similar, but frequently not so clear cut, making diagnosis more difficult. Lichen planus (Fig. 9.9) is the most frequent of the dermatoses that affect the mouth and typically presents as white striated lesions. Similar clinical and histological appearances are seen in lichenoid reactions to certain drugs or dental restorative material. Other examples of dermatoses with intraoral manifestations include pemphigus, mucous membrane pemphigoid, erythema multiforme, and lupus erythematosus.

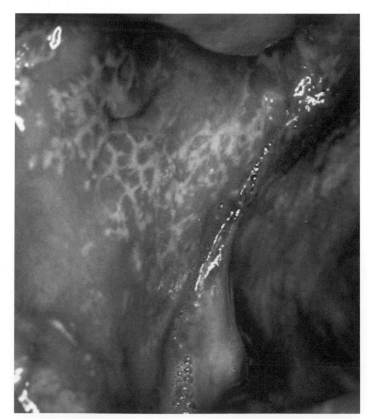

**FIG. 9.9** Lichen planus: a lacy network of white striae on the buccal mucosa is usually symmetrical. Other lesions of lichen planus include atrophy, erosions, and white plaques (the last often on the tongue).

## Pigmented Lesions

Pigmentation of the oral mucosa may be exogenous or endogenous in origin. The most common cause of exogenous pigmentation is the incorporation of dental amalgam into the oral soft tissues. Endogenous pigmentation is usually due to melanin. Melanocytes are present in similar numbers in the oral epithelium as in the skin, but less often produce melanin. Melanin pigmentation, especially of the gingiva, roughly parallels skin pigmentation, being more pronounced in dark- skinned races. Reactive or secondary melanosis is seen in smokers, after chronic dermatoses, and in Addison's disease. Oral and perioral pigmentation along with intestinal polyposis is characteristic of Peutz–Jeghers syndrome. Melanotic macules and intraoral melanotic naevi also occur. Primary oral mucosal melanoma is much less common than its counterpart in skin and its aetiology is unclear. It typically arises on the palate or gingiva and, as the presentation is frequently late, the prognosis is poor.

## Soft-tissue Swellings

Fibrous overgrowth of the oral mucosa is very common and frequently presents as a fibroepithelial polyp secondary to chronic trauma. An epulis is a localized swelling on the gingiva. A fibrous epulis typically occurs as a reaction to chronic irritation, e.g. from dental calculus (calcified plaque) or the rough margin of a carious cavity or filling. It consists of a mass of cellular fibrous tissue often with metaplastic bone formation. Pyogenic granulomas comprise a mass of granulation tissue, often ulcerated, and are found at any intraoral site, but most often form on the gingiva as a vascular epulis or, in pregnancy, as a pregnancy epulis. Giant cell epulis (peripheral giant cell granuloma) is a distinct lesion consisting of numerous multinucleated giant cells in a vascular stroma. It is a superficial lesion with minimal bone involvement. However, intraosseous lesions, such as central giant cell granuloma or lesions of hyperparathyroidism, may mimic a giant cell epulis clinically and histologically if they extend to involve the gingival soft tissues; thus, radiological and biochemical investigations are warranted in such cases.

## Potentially Malignant Lesions and Conditions

### Key Points

- A potentially malignant lesion is one in which cancer is more likely to develop.
- A potentially malignant condition is a pre-existing condition that possesses an increased risk of developing cancer.
- Leukoplakia and erythroplakia are important, clinically recognized, premalignant lesions.
- Leukoplakia has a relatively low risk of malignancy.
- Erythroplakia has a high risk of malignancy.
- The more severe the dysplasia microscopically, the greater the risk of malignancy.
- High-risk oral sites for malignant change are the floor of mouth, and ventral and lateral aspects of the tongue.

A potentially malignant lesion is one in which cancer is more likely to develop whereas a potentially malignant condition is a pre-existing condition, such as lichen planus or chronic hyperplastic candidiasis, with an increased risk of developing cancer. Leukoplakia and erythroplakia are potentially malignant lesions. Leukoplakia (Fig. 9.10) is a clinically descriptive term for a white patch that cannot be scraped off or attributed to any specific disease clinically or histologically. Erythroplakia is the analogous term for a red patch and speckled leukoplakia refers to similar lesions with white and red areas. These are not pathological entities and cover a variety of histological changes. On biopsy, a small proportion of leukoplakias, and many erythroplakias and speckled leukoplakias, show dysplastic changes. Generally the more severe the dysplasia the greater is the likelihood of progression to carcinoma. Erythroplakias and speckled leukoplakias have a much greater incidence of severe dysplasia and are frequently early invasive malignancies at first biopsy.

## Tumours of the Oral Mucosa

### Key Points

- Oral squamous cell papillomas are common benign epithelial tumours.
- Most oral cancers are squamous cell carcinomas.
- The incidence of oral cancer is increasing.
- Oral cancer has a poor prognosis if not treated early.
- The floor of the mouth, and ventral and lateral aspects of the tongue, are high-risk sites for oral cancer.

Squamous cell papillomas are benign epithelial tumours, caused by the human papillomavirus (HPV), which can occur at any intraoral site; they are considered to have no risk of malignant transformation. Most oral malignancies (approximately 90%) are squamous cell carcinoma. The incidence of disease is increasing particularly in younger

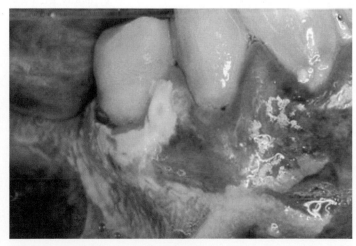

**FIG. 9.10** Leukoplakia: irregular white patch on the gum.

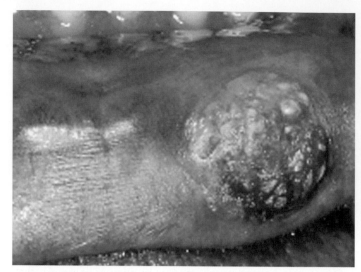

FIG. 9.11 Lip cancer: squamous cell carcinoma presenting as a raised tumour on the mucosal aspect of the lower lip.

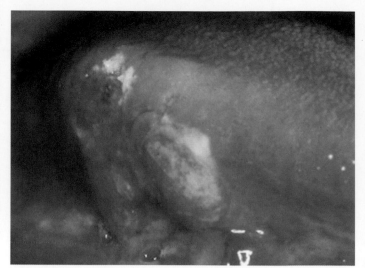

FIG. 9.13 Advanced cancer of the tongue: squamous cell carcinoma often presents as an indurated plaque-like mass in the ventral and lateral aspects of the tongue.

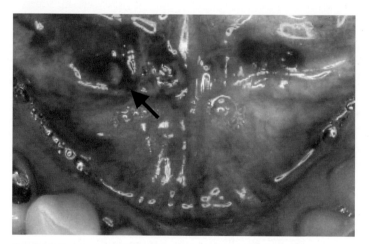

FIG. 9.12 Early cancer of floor of mouth: squamous cell carcinoma presenting as a small non-healing ulcer in the floor of the mouth; this is a 'high-risk area' for the development of oral cancer.

individuals, although it is still most common in older age groups. Distinction should be made between lip cancer and intraoral cancer. Cancer of the lower lip typically presents as a non-healing ulcer or a small lump (Fig. 9.11). Sunlight is the most frequent aetiological agent. The precise aetiology of intraoral cancer is undetermined but is considered to include genetic and environmental factors. Known risk factors include the use of tobacco, alcohol, and areca nuts. As in other cancers, nutritional status may also be important. Current evidence regarding HPV infection as a causative factor in cancer of the oral cavity is inconclusive.

Although oral cancers appear to develop from recognized premalignant lesions, many develop in clinically normal mucosa. Tumours typically present as a non-healing ulcer or a persistent white, red, or speckled patch, which may or may not be symptomatic. Tumours may occur at any intraoral site, although they almost never arise on the hard palate

or dorsum of tongue. High-risk sites are the floor of the mouth (Fig. 9.12), ventral and lateral aspects of the tongue (Fig. 9.13), and the retromolar trigone (the area behind the mandibular third molar tooth). Oral cancer generally has a poorer prognosis the further posteriorly in the mouth it occurs. Histological factors that suggest an adverse prognosis include poor differentiation of tumour cells, increased tumour diameter and depth of invasion, and the presence of neural or lymphovascular invasion. Tumours spread initially to adjacent tissues. This is followed by spread to local then regional lymph nodes. Haematogenous spread is a late complication. The survival rate for intraoral cancer (approximately 50% at 5 years) has shown very little change in the past few decades despite advances in treatment. This is at least in part due to late presentation and detection of the disease.

Successful treatment of squamous cell carcinoma of the mouth is dependent on early diagnosis. It is important that lesions of the oral mucosa that do not relate to obvious causes, or that fail to respond to the removal of presumed obvious causes, undergo biopsy.

## The Salivary Glands

### Key Points

- Mucoceles arise from trauma or blockage of a salivary duct.
- Mumps is a viral infection of major salivary glands, the incidence of which has been modified by immunization programmes.
- Chronic sialadenitis involves endogenous infection and is frequently secondary to duct obstruction.
- Sjögren's syndrome is an autoimmune exocrinopathy.

There are three pairs of major salivary glands – parotid, submandibular, and sublingual – and numerous intraoral minor salivary glands. The most common lesion of minor salivary glands is the mucocele. The lesion is most often seen on the lower lip and is frequently due to leakage of mucus from a damaged duct (mucus extravasation cyst – Fig. 9.14). A cyst-like cavity forms and consists of the escaped mucus and macrophages surrounded by granulation tissue. A ranula is a larger variant that occurs in the floor of the mouth and usually involves the sublingual glands. Alternatively, a mucus retention cyst results from accumulation of mucus within a blocked salivary duct.

## Inflammatory Lesions

Mumps, an acute inflammatory lesion of the salivary glands caused by paramyxovirus infection, has an incubation period of 3 weeks. Infected individuals secrete the virus in their saliva for about a week before the main symptom of painful salivary gland swelling is evident, and for just over a week thereafter. Both parotid glands are usually involved and sometimes also the submandibular glands. The salivary enlargement usually subsides without permanent damage to the glands. Rare complications of mumps infection include orchitis, oophoritis, pancreatitis, and viral meningitis. The incidence of mumps varies worldwide and has been altered by the use of the mumps vaccine (largely as part of the MMR vaccine).

Chronic sialadenitis arises as an endogenous infection related to obstruction. It is often associated with salivary calculi and the submandibular glands are the most frequently involved. Sialadenitis leads to glandular atrophy with marked acinar loss and interstitial fibrosis. Suppurative parotitis is an uncommon infection caused by pyogenic cocci and can occur as a postoperative complication in dehydrated patients. In addition to dehydration, a dry mouth may be due to various causes such as certain medications, previous radiotherapy, poorly controlled diabetes, and Sjögren's syndrome (see below).

## Sjögren's Syndrome

Sjögren's syndrome is an autoimmune condition in which there is a generalized exocrinopathy. The salivary glands and lacrimal glands are the most obviously involved, thus the main symptoms are of oral and ocular dryness (xerostomia and xerophthalmia, respectively). The dry eyes and mouth may occur in isolation (primary Sjögren's syndrome) or as secondary Sjögren's syndrome associated with another non-organ-specific autoimmune condition, most frequently rheumatoid arthritis. Biopsy of the lower labial minor salivary glands, which show focal lymphocytic infiltration, is used as one of a range of diagnostic tools. In major glands, particularly the parotids, there is acinar loss and extensive infiltration of lymphocytes. This may give obvious parotid swelling. In longstanding cases there is a risk of lymphoma, particularly in primary Sjögren's syndrome.

## Tumours of Salivary Gland Epithelium

### Key Points

- Epithelial salivary gland neoplasms are a complex group of benign and malignant tumours.
- Of salivary gland tumours 80% involve the parotid gland.
- Pleomorphic adenomas account for 60% of tumours.
- There is a higher relative incidence of malignant tumours in minor glands.

The current World Health Organisation (WHO) classification of salivary gland tumours includes 13 benign and 24 malignant epithelial tumour types, although additional entities not yet included in the classification have also been reported. Most tumours are benign and the frequency of malignant types alters by site and is relatively much higher in minor salivary glands. Most tumours (approximately 80%) occur in the parotid gland, with 10% each in the submandibular and minor salivary glands. Tumours very rarely arise in the sublingual gland. The aetiology of many salivary gland tumours is not fully determined.

By far the most frequent salivary gland neoplasm is the pleomorphic adenoma. This shows mixed patterns of

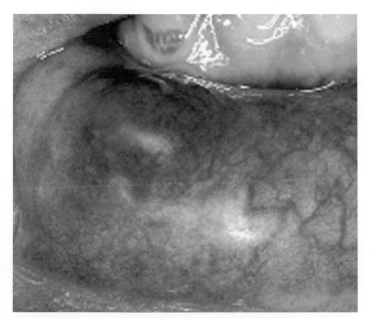

**Fig. 9.14** Mucocele of the lower lip: a bluish-grey cystic lesion immediately below the labial mucosa caused by damage to a minor salivary gland duct and escape of saliva into the loose connective tissues of the lip. Traumatic injury to the lip by the teeth after a fall is typical.

differentiation with combinations of epithelial and myoepithelial cells set in a characteristic stroma (Fig. 9.15). The tumours are variably encapsulated and, if their excision is incomplete, particularly in the parotid, residual tumour can give rise to multiple recurrences, which are very difficult to treat. A further complication is the possibility of malignant transformation (carcinoma ex pleomorphic adenoma) in longstanding pleomorphic adenoma.

The most frequent malignant salivary neoplasms are adenoid cystic carcinoma and mucoepidermoid carcinoma. Adenoid cystic carcinoma tends to occur in older individuals and often shows a distinctive cribriform or 'lace-like' growth pattern (Fig. 9.16). It has a particular tendency for perineural spread, thus making it very difficult to eradicate surgically. Mucoepidermoid carcinoma shows a variable mixture of squamoid, mucous, and intermediate cell types.

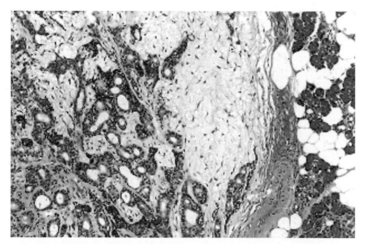

FIG. 9.15 Pleomorphic adenoma (on the left) separated from normal parotid tissue (on the right) by a thin capsule of collagenous tissue. Pleomorphic adenoma is a benign epithelial neoplasm of 'mixed patterns', here represented as fused glands (left) and spindle-celled cartilage-like tissue (centre).

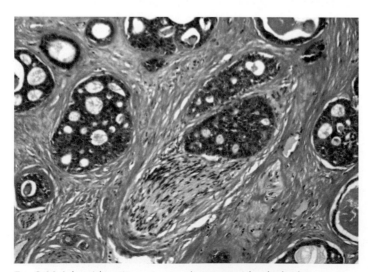

FIG. 9.16 Adenoid cystic carcinoma: the tumour islands display a characteristic 'lace-like' appearance and neural invasion is evident.

They are tumours of variable behaviour showing local invasion and sometimes spread to local lymph nodes.

## The Oropharynx

### Normal Structure and Function

The oropharynx lies behind the oral cavity, commencing at the palatoglossal arches (tonsillar pillars) and soft palate, and extending to the upper aspect of the epiglottis. It contains the palatine tonsils and the posterior third of the tongue. The major roles of the oropharnyx are in breathing, swallowing, and speech.

### Infections of the Oropharynx

The oropharynx may be affected by various bacterial and viral infections. *Streptococcus pyogenes* is a common cause of sore throat in children and streptococcal infection can precede rheumatic fever or glomerulonephritis. Diphtheria, a highly contagious infection caused by *Corynebacterium diphtheriae*, most frequently affects the oropharynx, particularly in children. The infection may have serious and not infrequently fatal complications. Immunization programmes are largely responsible for the present low incidence of diphtheria in many parts of the world. Infectious mononucleosis – 'glandular fever' – is caused by the Epstein–Barr virus and is a cause of cervical lymphadenopathy. It is infectious and can lead to a particularly troublesome sore throat in adolescents and young adults, often with persistent post-viral symptoms.

### Tumours of the Oropharynx

The most important tumours of the oropharynx are carcinomas and lymphomas. Squamous cell carcinoma is the most frequent and has similarities to oral cancer, being associated with smoking and alcohol. However, unlike oral cancer, there is recent evidence to support a causal association with HPV infection in a proportion of oropharyngeal carcinomas. The HPV-associated tumours appear to have a better prognosis. Salivary neoplasms may develop within minor salivary glands located in the oropharyngeal mucosa. Various types of lymphoma, usually non-Hodgkin's lymphoma, occur in the oropharynx.

## THE OESOPHAGUS

## Normal Structure and Function

Averaging some 25 cm in length, the oesophagus is a muscular tube with a well-defined origin at the cricoid cartilage. Its function is a simple one, namely the conduction of food from the pharynx to the stomach. This simplicity is reflected in its structure. The mucosal lining is of stratified squamous epithelium, whereas the underlying submucosa includes numbers of mucinous glands, which lubricate the lining. The muscle coat is prominent, being for the most part arranged, as in the rest of the gut, in inner circular and outer longitudinal coats. Striated (voluntary) muscle fibres are present proximally, contributing to the upper oesophageal sphincter, thus allowing voluntary initiation of swallowing. The so-called lower oesophageal sphincter is in reality the smooth muscle of the wall acting under autonomic control to prevent reflux of gastric contents. There is no clearly defined anatomical lower sphincter. Partly for this reason, the lower end of the oesophagus is much less well defined than the upper.

As a result of its simplicity of function, the oesophagus produces a relatively limited range of symptoms in disease. The retrosternal burning pain of heartburn is a common effect of reflux of gastroduodenal contents into the oesophagus. Dysphagia (difficulty in swallowing) is an important and sometimes sinister symptom (see p. 244). Oesophageal disease is also an important cause of haematemesis (vomiting of blood).

## Congenital Abnormalities, Disorders of Motility, and Vascular Abnormality

### Key Points

- Atresia, with and without tracheo-oesophageal fistula, occurs in neonates.
- Achalasia is a motor disorder of the lower oesophageal sphincter.
- Hiatus hernia is strongly associated with acid reflux.
- Oesophageal varices are an important cause of upper gastrointestinal haemorrhage in portal hypertension.

### Atresia

The oesophagus and trachea both derive from the embryonic foregut. Congenital abnormalities of the oesophagus and trachea are commonly related. Duplication cysts, lined by either squamous or respiratory epithelium, are recognized. More importantly, oesophageal atresia is a cause of neonatal dysphagia resulting from failure of canalization (luminal development) of the oesophagus. It is commonly associated with tracheo-oesophageal fistula and a high risk of neonatal aspiration pneumonia (Fig. 9.17).

### Achalasia

Achalasia is a Greek term meaning 'failure to relax'; this is a good description of this disorder, which is characterized by poor relaxation of the functional lower oesophageal sphincter. The disease is of unknown cause, and may present at any stage in life, usually with dysphagia and regurgitation of undigested food material. Aspiration pneumonia is a significant problem. Microscopically, the disease is characterized by a reduction in the numbers of neurons in the muscular (myenteric) plexus of the lower oesophagus. In advanced disease, the proximal oesophagus may show dilatation, inflammation, and ulceration. There is also a slightly

increased risk of carcinoma. Other diseases leading to loss of lower oesophageal motility include systemic sclerosis (muscle fibrosis and atrophy) and the South American trypanosomiasis (Chagas' disease, where there is direct parasitic infection of the myenteric neurons).

### Hiatus Hernia

This is an acquired abnormality defined by abnormal location of the oesophagogastric junction and (part of) the gastric cardia above the diaphragm. Formerly thought to be due to congenital shortening of the oesophagus, it is now considered to be due to a combination of diaphragmatic weakening and increased intra-abdominal pressure. It is therefore associated with the western diet, and particularly with obesity. In a less common abnormality (paraoesophageal or 'rolling' hiatus hernia), part of the stomach protrudes into the mediastinum alongside the oesophagus (Fig. 9.18).

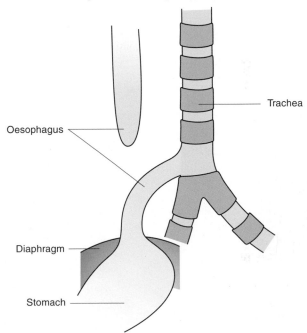

FIG. 9.17 In the most common variant of oesophageal atresia the upper oesophagus is a blind-ended tube, whereas the lower part is in communication with the trachea.

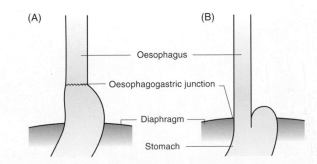

FIG. 9.18 Hiatus hernia: (A) in a sliding hiatus hernia the proximal stomach is 'pulled' into the mediastinum. (B) In the 'rolling' variant, part of the fundus of the stomach protrudes through an abnormally large diaphragmatic orifice.

The major clinical effect of hiatus hernia is loss of the lower oesophageal sphincter mechanism, leading to reflux oesophagitis.

## Diverticula

Abnormal outpouchings of the oesophageal wall can occur either by pulsion (increased intraoesophageal pressure, as may occur in achalasia) or by traction ('pulling' from an external neoplasm or inflammatory focus). Diverticula can regurgitate food and/or become distended, leading to dysphagia.

## Varices

The venous drainage of the oesophagus is through a network of veins lying in the adventitial soft tissue. At the lower end, some blood drains from this plexus into the portal venous system. In portal venous hypertension (most commonly seen in association with liver cirrhosis), backpressure in this system can lead to massive dilatation of submucosal veins (oesophageal varices; Fig. 9.19). The superficial position of the varices renders them particularly prone to rupture, often with catastrophic haemorrhage.

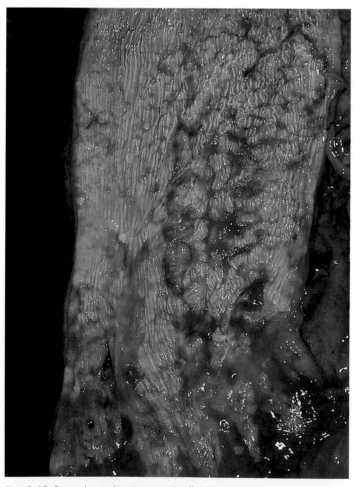

FIG. **9.19** Oesophageal varices: markedly dilated lower oesophageal veins in a patient dying from the effects of cirrhosis.

## Inflammatory Disease

Inflammation of the oesophagus, manifested endoscopically by the cardinal signs of congestion and redness of the mucosa, is usually caused by chemical irritation by refluxed gastroduodenal contents (reflux oesophagitis). A limited number of infectious agents (*Candida* spp., herpes simplex virus) may be a direct cause of oesophagitis. The oesophagus may be involved in Crohn's disease and systemic sclerosis. Oesophageal obstruction (tumour, achalasia) leads to a secondary proximal oesophagitis.

### Reflux Oesophagitis

The oesophageal squamous epithelium is not well equipped to deal with the injurious effects of gastric fluid (a potent mix of acid, pepsin, and smaller quantities of bile acids and trypsin). The main natural defence mechanism is the functional integrity of the lower oesophageal sphincter. This may be compromised by increased intra-abdominal pressure (obesity, pregnancy), and intrinsic relaxation or incompetence of the muscle sphincter (alcohol, tobacco, hiatus hernia). Other mechanisms such as acid clearance time are likely to be important in determining the severity of the disease. The issue is further complicated in that some patients with severe tissue manifestations of disease (e.g. ulceration) have no history of heartburn, whereas markedly symptomatic patients with proven reflux may show no histological evidence of inflammation.

Reflux causes cell damage to the superficial squamous epithelium. The cell loss causes compensatory basal cell hyperplasia, and this – together with some inflammatory cell exudation – constitutes the histological picture of reflux oesophagitis. More severe disease leads to complications such as oesophageal peptic ulceration and, in longstanding disease, oesophageal fibrous stricture, the latter occurring on a background of chronic ulceration. Barrett's oesophagus is a further important consequence of gastro-oesophageal reflux (see below).

### Eosinophilic Oesophagitis

Oesophageal inflammation causing symptoms of dysphagia and bolus obstruction is increasingly recognized in children and young adults. Biopsies show infiltration of the squamous epithelium by large numbers of eosinophils. These patients often have a history of atopic problems (asthma, eczema). The clinical picture can mimic reflux, but oesophageal pH studies are typically normal and the inflammatory infiltrate, in distinction to reflux disease, favours the proximal oesophagus.

### Infective Causes of Oesophagitis

The oesophagus is relatively resistant to infection, and most cases of infective oesophagitis occur in immunocompromised individuals. *Candida albicans* is a relatively common fungal cause of erosive inflammation in this situation. Viruses such as herpes simplex and cytomegalovirus may also infect the oesophagus in these individuals.

## Barrett's Oesophagus

### Key Points

- Barrett's oesophagus is an acquired glandular metaplasia of the oesophagus.
- It is caused by reflux of gastroduodenal contents.
- There is a risk of progression to adenocarcinoma.

Some individuals with long-standing reflux disease develop this condition, which is characterized by a metaplastic change in the oesophageal epithelium from stratified squamous to columnar (glandular) type (Fig. 9.20). This change, which is also known simply as columnar lined oesophagus (CLO), appears to have increased in frequency over the past 30 years. The main importance of Barrett's oesophagus is that it is undoubtedly associated with an increased risk of progression to adenocarcinoma. Microscopically, the columnar epithelium can show a range of appearances, with three basic patterns being recognized:

1. Junctional (resembling gastric cardia)
2. Gastric fundic (including acid- and pepsin-secreting cells)
3. Intestinal (with small intestinal-type goblet cells).

Clinical follow-up has shown that it is the intestinal type that is most often associated with malignancy. Dysplastic changes can sometimes be recognized in biopsy specimens as an intermediate stage between metaplastic epithelium and invasive malignancy.

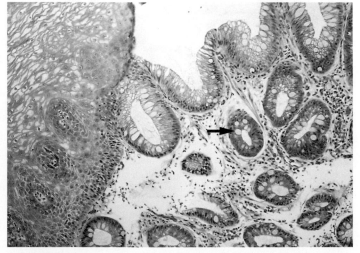

**FIG. 9.20** Biopsy of the squamocolumnar junction in an endoscopically obvious case of Barrett's oesophagus. There is glandular epithelium (right) in addition to the normal squamous mucosa (left). Intestinal metaplasia is indicated by the presence of goblet cells (arrow).

### Clinicopathological Problems in Barrett's Oesophagus

When first described (by Norman Barrett, a thoracic surgeon at St Thomas' Hospital, London during the early 1950s), columnar epithelium in the apparent oesophagus was thought to reflect a congenitally short oesophagus with 'pulling up' of the stomach into the thorax. It is now clear that this is not the case. There are two major related practical problems in the identification and management of this disorder in clinical practice.

#### Definition of the Normal Lower Limit of Squamous Epithelium

It is usually considered that the squamocolumnar junction in normal individuals is synonymous with the gastro-oesophageal junction, although some authorities state that the distal 1–2 cm of the normal oesophagus is lined by columnar epithelium of junctional type. A major source of confusion is identification of the gastro-oesophageal junction in practice. Endoscopists rely on the funnel-like appearance at the transition from the tubular oesophagus to the more capacious stomach, and also on the appearance of the beginnings of gastric mucosal folds. As these landmarks are rather fluid in life, published studies on Barrett's oesophagus have often allowed an upward margin of error of 1–5 cm before columnar epithelium on biopsy was considered abnormal. It is therefore not surprising that the reported prevalence of the condition at endoscopy has varied widely. More recently, some workers have attempted to bypass the anatomical problems by redefining Barrett's oesophagus as the presence of metaplastic intestinal epithelium in the region of the squamocolumnar junction, reasoning that it is the presence of intestinal metaplasia that defines those who are at high risk of progression to malignancy.

#### Clinical Follow-up in Barrett's Oesophagus

Patients identified as having Barrett's oesophagus are at increased risk of developing adenocarcinoma. The risk for the individual case is, however, small. Follow-up of all patients with Barrett's oesophagus (by endoscopy and multiple biopsy) has not been demonstrated to be a cost-effective measure. Often, follow-up is reserved for those patients with long segment disease or intestinal metaplasia, and particularly those with dysplasia. High-grade dysplasia carries a very high risk of progression to invasive malignancy, and may be an indicator for prophylactic oesophagectomy. Newer therapies including laser ablation of the abnormal mucosa and endoscopic mucosal resection are increasingly used, especially for dysplasia that is limited in extent.

## Oesophageal Neoplasms

### Benign neoplasms

Benign tumours of the oesophagus are uncommon. The epithelium occasionally gives rise to squamous cell papillomas, but the most frequently occurring type is of mesenchymal origin – the leiomyoma (benign smooth muscle tumour).

## *Malignant Neoplasms*

### Key Points

- Squamous cell carcinoma is related to diet and smoking, and shows a marked geographical variation.
- Adenocarcinoma is increasing in incidence, and occurs mostly in Barrett's oesophagus.
- Both types of carcinoma have a poor prognosis.

Almost all malignancies of the oesophagus are of epithelial origin (Fig. 9.21A). The clinical presentation is usually with dysphagia that often rapidly progresses to inability to swallow fluids. Of the two major histological types, squamous cell carcinoma (Fig. 9.21B) arises in the oesophageal squamous lining, whereas adenocarcinoma is mostly associated with Barrett's oesophagus (Fig. 9.21C) and is now the more common type in the western world.

Squamous carcinoma of the oesophagus shows a wide geographical variation in incidence, with particularly prominent epidemiological hotspots being sites around the Caspian Sea and in parts of China. Rare cases have a defined genetic component, being associated with a characteristic

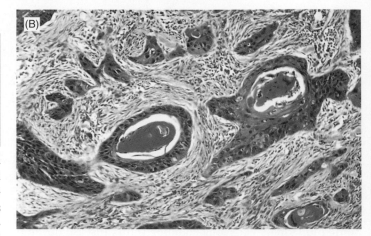

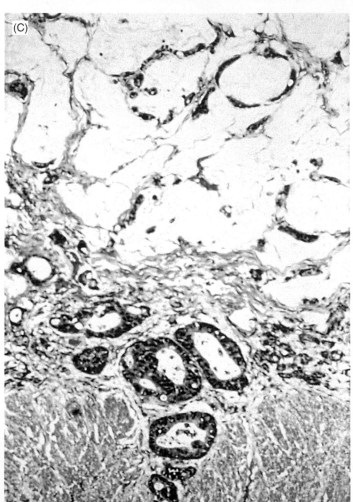

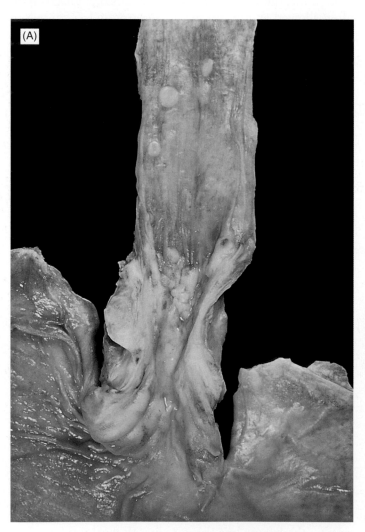

**FIG. 9.21** (A) Macroscopic view of an ulcerated, stenosing carcinoma of the lower oesophagus. (B) Squamous cell carcinoma with islands of neoplastic cells showing central keratin formation. (C) Adenocarcinoma showing obvious gland formation.

palmar and plantar hyperkeratosis (tylosis). Other cases may occur after the ingestion of corrosives, or as a result of long-standing mucosal irritation in achalasia. Macroscopically, squamous cell carcinomas present as irregular ulcerated, exophytic masses that partly or almost totally occlude the lumen. At the time of presentation, they have usually invaded through the oesophageal muscularis and, in the absence of a serosal covering, they have commonly infiltrated surrounding structures and may have spread to mediastinal or supraclavicular lymph nodes. The clinical prognosis is very poor.

Adenocarcinomas generally arise in Barrett's oesophagus. This is a disease of western society, being associated with obesity and oesophageal reflux. These tumours have shown a remarkable rise in incidence during the past 20–30 years (paralleled by the rising prevalence of Barrett's oesophagus). The reasons for this changing epidemiology are, as yet, unclear. Macroscopically, they are similar to squamous carcinomas, but the surrounding mucosa often has the velvety pink appearance of Barrett's metaplasia, as distinct from the normal silvery grey squamous mucosa. Again, the lesion is commonly at an advanced stage at presentation but, arising as it does in the lower oesophagus, the spread is more commonly to nodes along the greater and lesser curves of the stomach and the liver. The prognosis, again, is dismal.

## THE STOMACH

### Normal Structure and Function

The stomach is a roughly J-shaped dilatation of the gut, functioning as a reservoir of ingested food and controlling the release of manageable quantities into the duodenum, which has a much smaller capacity. The process of digestion is also begun in the stomach with the secretion of acid and pepsinogen. The so-called intrinsic factor required for vitamin $B_{12}$ absorption is also produced by the gastric epithelium. Both macroscopically and histologically the stomach is divided into three regions: first, the cardia is an ill-defined region lying just below the oesophagogastric junction; the mucosal crypts are relatively simple and contain mainly mucin-secreting cells; second, the body or fundic mucosa occupies most of the gastric lining, extending distally to the incisura angularis. It is in the body region that large numbers of acid-secreting parietal (or oxyntic) cells and pepsinogen-producing chief cells are located. The third major region, the antrum, extends from the incisura to the pylorus, where there is a well-defined muscular sphincter. Mucosal crypts are shorter and less densely packed in the antrum. Parietal cells are still present, but chief cells are rare in this region. Gastrin-secreting G-cells are identified in pyloric crypts. Small numbers of neuroendocrine cells may be seen throughout the stomach. The microscopic features of a gastric gland are summarized in Fig. 9.22.

### Congenital Abnormalities

Congenital defects of the stomach are uncommon. Cysts and duplications may occur. In diaphragmatic hernia there is a failure of development of part of one dome of the

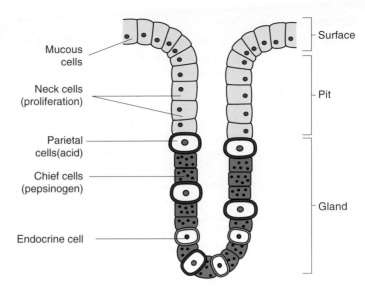

**Fig. 9.22** Schematic representation of the microscopic structure of a gastric gland. The relative proportion of different cell types varies across the stomach. In the cardia, mucous cells predominate. The body ('fundic') glands contain the great bulk of secretory parietal and chief cells. In the antrum, gastrin-producing endocrine cells are prominent.

diaphragm, with herniation of all or part of the stomach, usually together with intestine, into the thoracic cavity. The main presenting problem is respiratory embarrassment.

In congenital pyloric stenosis there is hypertrophy of the circular muscle at the pyloric sphincter, leading to gastric outflow obstruction which presents clinically with projectile vomiting. This condition is about five times more common in males than in females.

### Inflammatory Disorders

**Key Points**

- Acute gastritis is associated with alcohol and drug injury.
- Chronic gastritis may be due to bacterial infection, chemical injury, or autoimmunity.

Gastritis, in its many forms, is a source of considerable confusion to the student, clinician, and pathologist. Gastritis may be classified histologically, endoscopically, by topographic distribution in the stomach, or by aetiology. The terminologies used do not always correspond. Thus, the endoscopic appearance of 'gastritis' correlates very poorly with the biopsy appearances. The histological changes and topographical distribution of abnormality have been found to be the best markers of aetiology, and thus form the basis of a rational approach to classification and, ultimately, clinical treatment.

In the past, the causes of acute gastritis have been relatively well understood, but it is only during the past 20–30 years that the aetiology and pathogenesis of most cases of chronic gastritis have become clear.

## Acute Gastritis

Acute inflammation of the gastric mucosa has long been associated with chemical injury, particularly by alcohol and non-steroidal anti-inflammatory drugs (NSAIDs). More recently, another form of acute gastritis occurring in the early stages of *H. pylori* infection has been described. Acute gastritis may be subclinical, or present with abdominal pain, vomiting, and/or haemorrhage. Macroscopically, the mucosa is oedematous and congested, and may show superficial mucosal erosion (the site of blood loss). Histologically, there is capillary congestion and leakage of blood cells into the lamina propria. In erosive gastritis the superficial epithelium is lost. This picture of haemorrhagic, erosive gastritis is typical of chemical injury. *H. pylori* acute gastritis is characterized by a more prominent neutrophil response. Occasionally other more virulent organisms (particularly streptococci) may cause a severe, usually fatal, purulent gastritis.

## Chronic Gastritis

The discovery, usually attributed to the Australians Warren and Marshall in 1983, of *H. pylori* has radically changed our concepts of chronic gastritis. The award of the Nobel Prize for Medicine in 2005 for this discovery is a rare example of the recognition of a basic morphological observation by a practising diagnostic pathologist (Robin Warren).

In the past it was recognized that a small subset of patients with chronic gastritis had an autoimmune attack on the gastric mucosa, but most instances were put down to vague dietary or endogenous (acid, bile) agents. It is now clear that three major types exist – *H. pylori* induced, autoimmune and chemical (reactive) – with a few exceptional cases having unusual causes and often characteristic histological features.

### Helicobacter-associated Chronic Gastritis

*Helicobacter pylori* is a spiral bacterium that has become remarkably well adapted to life at the interface between the surface epithelium of the stomach and the covering layer of secreted mucus. The organism causes direct epithelial cell injury, and also excites a vigorous immune response – two mechanisms for developing a chronic inflammatory reaction. Histologically, the mucosa shows a mixed inflammatory cell response with neutrophil infiltration of the epithelium, and a lymphocyte and plasma cell infiltrate in the stroma (this mixed pattern is often referred to as 'active chronic gastritis'; Fig. 9.23). Severe, long-standing epithelial injury may lead to glandular atrophy. The epithelium may also show an adaptive response termed 'intestinal metaplasia', in which a partial or almost complete change in epithelial cell differentiation towards small intestinal type occurs. This benefits the host insofar as the intestinal mucosa is resistant to *H. pylori* infection.

Two topographic patterns of *H. pylori* infection are recognized, although the distinction may not be clear in an individual patient. Many patients have a predominantly antral

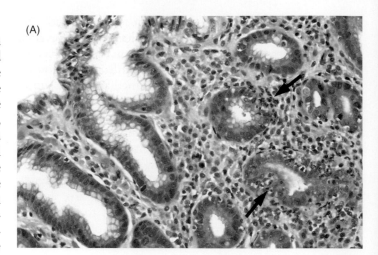

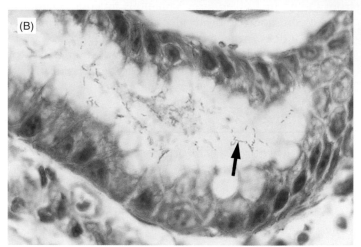

**FIG. 9.23** (A) Active chronic gastritis: chronic inflammatory cell infiltration of the lamina propria with neutrophil movement into crypts (arrows). (B) *Helicobacter pylori* organisms in the surface mucus are seen better (arrow) in a Giemsa stain.

active chronic gastritis. These are the individuals who are most at risk of developing duodenal ulceration. Somewhat less commonly infection and inflammation involve both body and antrum ('pangastritis'). This disease pattern is associated with gastric ulcer and adenocarcinoma.

### Autoimmune Chronic Gastritis

The association has long been recognized between vitamin $B_{12}$ deficiency, macrocytic anaemia, and a form of chronic gastritis. This syndrome – which is referred to clinically as pernicious anaemia – is associated with circulating antibodies to gastric parietal cells and is a good example of organ-specific autoimmunity. Histologically, there is chronic gastritis (not usually showing neutrophil 'activity') involving mainly the body of the stomach. In longstanding cases, mucosal atrophy is prominent and there is commonly extensive intestinal metaplasia. The associated anaemia is explained by gastric parietal cell loss, with consequent deficiency of intrinsic factor and inadequate vitamin $B_{12}$ absorption in the terminal ileum.

### Chemical (Reactive) Gastritis

This pattern of mucosal response is often termed 'bile reflux gastritis'. Indeed, reflux of bile and alkaline small intestinal material is a common cause of gastric epithelial cell injury in patients with gastroduodenal motility disturbances, which may be an isolated (primary) phenomenon or may follow surgery to the pyloric region. Similar patterns of mucosal change may be seen after other chemical injuries, particularly long-term NSAID ingestion, and the term 'chemical gastritis' is therefore preferred. Histologically, there is marked hyperplasia in the proliferative compartment of the gastric pits (the neck cells) with oedema of the mucosa (Fig. 9.24). A cellular inflammatory infiltrate is often remarkably absent or scant. *H. pylori* is not usually seen.

### Epidemiology, Pathogenesis, and Diagnosis of H. pylori Infection

*Helicobacter pylori* is a microaerophilic, motile, spiral bacterium which is Gram negative by conventional bacteriological analysis. These organisms can be identified in, and cultured from, the stomachs of healthy individuals. In western society, infection is more prevalent among older age groups, whereas in developing countries infection is very commonly acquired in childhood and is almost universal by middle age. Once infected, a few individuals can eliminate the organism, but the great majority develop a persisting chronic gastritis. *H. pylori* is transmitted from person to person, but the exact route (oral–oral, faecal–oral) is not clear. Infection is associated with low socioeconomic status and crowded living conditions.

Gastric mucosal colonization by *H. pylori* and the consequent superficial active chronic gastritis are not necessarily (or even commonly) associated with clinical disease. In the absence of ulceration there is a very poor correlation between infection and dyspeptic symptoms. Infection is, however, associated, with varying degrees of certainty, with a number of important conditions, ranging from peptic ulceration to atrophic gastritis, adenocarcinoma, and lymphoma (Fig. 9.25). There is also an epidemiological link with extraintestinal disease such as abnormally short stature and ischaemic heart disease, although the link in these instances is unlikely to be causal. The ability of *H. pylori* to cause disease is dependent (as in many chronic infectious diseases) on both bacterial virulence factors and variations in host response. Studies of mutant organisms have shown that bacterial motility and urease activity are essential for survival. The organism also produces adhesion factors, including a haemagglutinin that binds to sugar moieties on the gastric epithelial cell membrane. Virulent strains have also been shown to produce a number of tissue-injuring factors, including Gram-negative lipopolysaccharide and the highly antigenic CagA and VacA proteins, as well as a number of heat shock proteins. The host cell response (polymorph leukocytes, lymphocytes, and plasma cells) is characterized by high levels of proinflammatory cytokines including IL-1, IL-8, and TNF-α. Cytokine production is thought to be important in the increased gastrin secretion seen in *H. pylori* gastritis. Other physiological changes have been identified, including an increased gastrin response to infused gastrin-releasing peptide (GRP). These changes are most marked in patients with duodenal ulceration. Some individuals show a tendency to low gastric acid output, and these tend to develop a severe pangastritis, gastric ulceration, and possibly adenocarcinoma.

Diagnosis of *H. pylori* infection is not simple. Direct culture is difficult and not routinely used, although it can provide useful information on antibiotic sensitivity. Minimally invasive tests include faecal antigen testing, the urease breath test (measuring radiolabelled carbon released from ingested urea), and serology. The last is useful in epidemiological studies, but suffers from the fact that circulating antibodies can be detected after elimination of infection.

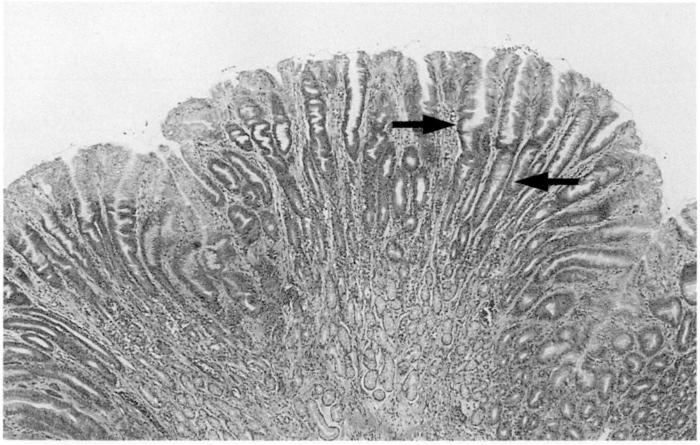

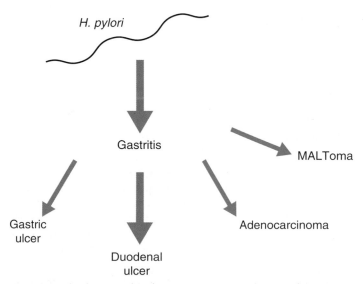

**Fig. 9.25** *Helicobacter pylori* disease associations. The size of the arrow is a rough indication of the clinical magnitude of the association. MALToma = mucosa-associated lymphoid tissue lymphoma.

**Fig. 9.24** In chemical gastritis there is striking expansion of the proliferative 'neck cell' compartment of the pits (arrows).

Endoscopy offers the most reliable diagnosis. Mucosal biopsies can be directly tested for urease activity when placed on gel-covered slides. Histological examination of specially stained sections is still the 'gold standard', and also allows assessment of inflammation, atrophy, intestinal metaplasia, and dysplasia.

### Special Forms of Gastritis

A few uncommon, but well-recognized, patterns of gastritis are worth noting. Granulomatous gastritis may be seen in the context of sarcoidosis and Crohn's disease. Although both of these diagnoses must be considered when granulomatous inflammation is identified in a gastric biopsy, a significant number of patients in this circumstance show no evidence of disease elsewhere. The cause of this isolated granulomatous gastritis is unclear.

In lymphocytic gastritis there is an increase in numbers of lymphocytes *within* the gastric mucosal epithelium. This pattern is similar to that seen in coeliac disease (see p. 256). Some cases are indeed associated with coeliac disease and some with *H. pylori* infection but, in many, the cause is unclear.

Eosinophilic gastritis is characterized by a dense infiltrate of eosinophil leukocytes in the wall of the stomach. A hypersensitivity response to ingested antigen is strongly suspected, but a specific source is not always identified.

## Peptic Ulceration

### Key Points

- Ulcers are caused by loss of balance between mucosal defence and acid attack.
- Acute ulcers are seen in chemical injury and severe stress (shock).
- Chronic ulcers are strongly associated with *Helicobacter* gastritis.
- Complications include haemorrhage, perforation, and stenosis.

Peptic ulceration is defined by the fact that it occurs only in mucosal surfaces exposed to the potentially injurious effect of gastric acid and pepsin. It is seen (in decreasing order of frequency) in the duodenum, stomach, distal oesophagus, and, after surgery, in relation to gastroenterostomy stomas. Although acid pepsin attack is a prerequisite for disease ('no acid, no ulcer' is a hallowed catchphrase), the precise pathogenesis involves consideration of a number of factors, including mucosal defence mechanisms, prostaglandin metabolism, mucosal blood flow, and, crucially, the effect of *H. pylori* infection. The relative importance of the different mechanisms is well illustrated by comparing gastric and duodenal peptic ulcers (see below and *Table 9.1*). Peptic ulcers are usually considered in separate acute and chronic categories.

### Acute Peptic Ulcers

Mucosal erosion (loss of continuity of the epithelial lining) is a common feature of acute gastritis. If the defect is severe enough to penetrate the muscularis mucosae and involve the submucosa, this becomes – by definition – an ulcer. Acute ulcers can be distinguished morphologically from chronic ones by the lack of fibrosis in the former. The importance of distinguishing between erosions and acute ulcers is that ulcers are considerably slower to heal. Acute peptic ulcers occur in acute gastritis caused by chemical injury (NSAIDs or alcohol), where severe epithelial injury is the primary cause. Acute ulcers, which are often multiple in the stomach and duodenum, can be seen in extreme hyperacidity, most often due to gastrin-secreting neuroendocrine tumours (the Zollinger–Ellison syndrome).

A particular form of acute peptic ulceration occurs in patients with a range of severe systemic illnesses. These ulcers are thought to arise as a consequence of mucosal ischaemia leading to increased susceptibility to acid pepsin attack. This complication can lead to severe blood loss in already vulnerable individuals. The ulcers have acquired a number of eponyms depending on the clinical circumstances in which they arise – thus, Cushing's ulcer in patients with

**TABLE 9.1** Comparison of important features of chronic gastric and duodenal ulcers

| Parameter | Ulcer type | |
| | Gastric | Duodenal |
| --- | --- | --- |
| Causal factor | 'Undermined mucosal defences' | 'Increased acid attack with weakened defences' |
| Epidemiology | Risk increases with age (50+ years) | Occurs at younger age than gastric ulcer (35+ years) More common than gastric ulcer (3:1) Associated with blood group O |
| Gastric acid output | Low to normal | Normal to high |
| *H. pylori* infection | Commonly involves antrum and body ('pangastritis') | Yes (90+%) Commonly confined to antrum Organisms may be seen in foci of duodenal gastric metaplasia |

severe head injury or cerebrovascular accident and Curling's ulcer in severely burned individuals.

### Chronic Peptic Ulcers

Chronic peptic ulcers tend to occur near mucosal junctions, i.e. in the first part of the duodenum, the proximal gastric antrum, and near the squamocolumnar junction in the oesophagus. In this discussion we concern ourselves principally with gastric ulcers (GUs) and duodenal ulcers (DUs). Peptic ulcers in the oesophagus are morphologically similar, but are more closely related in their aetiology to reflux oesophagitis and Barrett's oesophagus. GUs and DUs are common, and share an association with *H. pylori* infection and chronic gastritis, but they do show some important differences (see *Table 9.1*), e.g. duodenal ulcer tends to occur in a younger age group, in patients of blood group O, and in those with high normal or increased gastric acid output. GU is a disease of older individuals who have normal or low acid output. In all cases there is a persistent mucosal defect (commonly 1–2 cm in diameter) with well-defined edges (Fig. 9.26). The floor (surface) of the ulcer consists of fibrin and non-viable tissue debris. This overlies a layer of granulation tissue and a base of fibrous tissue. These changes almost always extend into the muscularis and commonly beyond, to involve surrounding tissues and organs (e.g. the pancreas) in a chronic inflammatory mass.

This process can lead to a number of complications that again are common to all peptic ulcers. The associated fibrosis can lead, by the process of contraction of collagen, to stenosis. This is particularly common in ulcers of the gastric pylorus leading to gastric outlet obstruction. Deep penetration of ulcers can expose major arteries, leading to

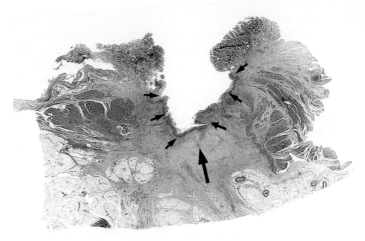

**FIG. 9.26** Whole-mount histological preparation of a chronic gastric ulcer. There is a mucosal defect (small arrows) extending through the wall of the stomach. The muscle coat is destroyed, and the base of the ulcer is made up of fibrous tissue (large arrow).

major haemorrhage. More rapidly penetrating ulcers can perforate into the peritoneal cavity, presenting as acute peritonitis.

GUs tend to occur on the lesser curve, most commonly in the antrum and pylorus. The surrounding mucosa often shows severe active chronic gastritis with intestinal metaplasia. The gastritis tends to involve the whole stomach. The gastric mucosa is also usually abnormal in patients with DUs, showing a mild-to-moderate *H. pylori*-associated gastritis that tends to be confined to the antrum. The duodenal mucosa in the vicinity of a DU commonly shows gastric metaplasia, a change in epithelial differentiation towards

## PEPTIC ULCERS IN UNUSUAL SITES

The patient, a 67-year-old man, was referred to a gastroenterologist in 1980 for an assessment in relation to a claim he was making to a War Injuries Compensation Panel. The patient had been a prisoner of war in Burma in 1945, since when he had suffered from constant diarrhoea, had always felt weak, and was very thin and underweight. On taking a careful history, the physician discovered that in 1972 the patient had suffered a perforation of the upper jejunum. Pathological examination of the resected segment of jejunum at the time of operation had revealed a perforated ulcer in the small bowel and some stunting of the villi in adjacent mucosa, but no specific diagnosis had been made. The physician therefore requested that the slides from the resection be reviewed by an expert gastrointestinal pathologist.

On review in 1980, the pathologist noted several, relatively clean, punched-out ulcers in the small bowel, involving the full thickness of the wall with complete destruction of the muscle coat, fibrous tissue in the base of the ulcer, and very little related inflammation (Fig. 9.27). One of these ulcers

was perforated. The non-ulcerated mucosa showed some shortening and broadening of the villi, mild inflammation

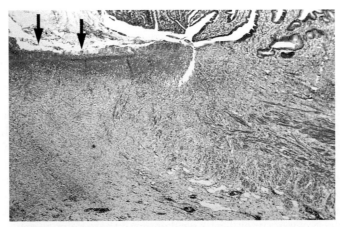

**FIG. 9.27** Base of an ulcer in the small bowel showing complete replacement of the muscle coat by fibrous tissue. The surface of the ulcer is arrowed.

of the lamina propria, but no intraepithelial lymphocytes. This picture was confirmed on repeat small bowel biopsy (Fig. 9.28A). As the ulcers had the typical appearances of peptic ulcers and the adjacent mucosa showed non-specific damage, the pathologist suggested that the patient might be suffering from the Zollinger–Ellison syndrome. (In this syndrome, a neoplasm – often benign and usually present in the pancreas – produces excess gastrin, which stimulates markedly elevated acid production by the stomach. This

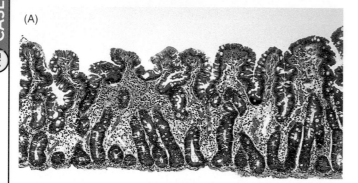

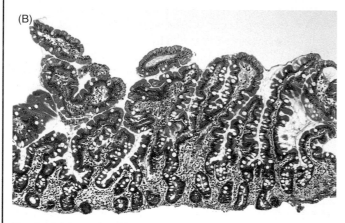

FIG. 9.28 (A) Duodenal biopsy before treatment. Note the shortened, slightly swollen villi, but no other abnormalities. (B) Jejunal biopsy after treatment; note the normal mucosa.

excessive acid passes into the small bowel, where it can cause mucosal abnormalities and peptic ulceration well into the jejunum.) Gastric acidity studies revealed very high levels of gastric acid, and serum gastrin levels were markedly raised. The patient was immediately started on the $H_2$-receptor blocker ranitidine to suppress gastric acid production. Within days he felt better, his diarrhoea stopped, and he had begun to put on weight. A follow-up biopsy of the duodenum several weeks after the patient had been started on ranitidine showed a normal small bowel mucosal appearance (Fig. 9.28B). On review 6 months later, the patient was fit and well and had put on 19 kg in weight to bring him up to normal weight for his height and age. He did not receive any compensation from the War Injuries Compensation Panel!

Lessons to be learned from this case:

- It is always worthwhile taking a careful history.
- Expert opinions – both clinical and pathological – are sometimes required.
- Peptic ulcers beyond the first part of the duodenum and certainly in the jejunum should raise suspicion of the Zollinger–Ellison syndrome.
- Patients with the Zollinger–Ellison syndrome may present without dyspepsia.

There are at least four mechanisms for the production of diarrhoea and steatorrhoea in Zollinger–Ellison syndrome:

1. Extensive gastrin causes increased gastric acid and fluid production.
2. Low pH in the small intestine causes mucosal damage.
3. Bile salts are precipitated in an acid environment, resulting in a failure of micelle production and fat emulsification.
4. Pancreatic enzymes are denatured by acid, leading to functional pancreatic insufficiency.

## Further Reading

Kingham JGC, Levison DA, Fairclough PD. Diarrhoea and reversible enteropathy in Zollinger–Ellison syndrome. *Lancet* 1981;ii:610–612.

cells of gastric lining type. This is thought to be an adaptive response to acid pepsin injury. *H. pylori* may be seen in the metaplastic epithelium.

The exact pathogenesis of peptic ulcers is not clear, although much progress has been made in recent years with the recognition of the important role played by *H. pylori*. Mucosal surfaces normally coming into contact with gastric acid and pepsin have evolved a number of defence mechanisms. These include a surface-adherent mucus/bicarbonate layer, epithelial cell defences, and mucosal blood flow. Peptic ulcers can occur either by weakening of these defence mechanisms (the most important pathway, particularly in GU) or

by increased acid attack (best illustrated by the Zollinger–Ellison syndrome but also a feature of many DUs). Surface mucus is significantly disrupted by *H. pylori*, and may also be degraded by reflux of biliary and duodenal secretions into the stomach. Epithelial cell defences are undermined by the cytotoxic effects of *H. pylori* and NSAIDs. Mucosal blood flow alterations are probably more important in acute ulcers occurring in clinical states of shock.

### Gastric Mucosal Defences: A More Detailed Survey

The surface mucus layer on the gastric epithelium is strongly adherent to the apical cell surfaces, and is important in maintaining the pH gradient between the strongly acidic gastric contents and the neutral epithelial cell layer. Experimental manipulation has shown that maintenance of this gradient is a function of mucous layer thickness. There is evidence that changes in the mucous layer occur *in vivo* in the presence of *H. pylori* infection. Reflux of bile-containing duodenal or jejunal contents into the stomach is an important cause of ulceration in the stomach in patients who have undergone a gastrojejunostomy. Bile is another agent known to be efficient in stripping the mucous layer from the surface epithelium. The importance of this mechanism in gastric ulcer occurring in the intact stomach is less well established.

Apart from mucus, gastric surface epithelial cells also secrete bicarbonate – which is a major factor in maintaining the pH gradient between the mucosa and the gastric contents. The epithelial cells themselves form a significant barrier to acid. The apical cell membranes of these cells and the tight intercellular junctions combine to effect this role. This function can be disrupted by the direct cytotoxic effect of *H. pylori*, or by the indirect damage caused by the inflammatory response to this organism. Mucosal blood flow is an important fallback mechanism for clearing up any hydrogen ions that may have escaped through the mucus/epithelial barrier. Loss of this mechanism is likely to be an important contributor to acute ulcers in shock, but there is some evidence that mucosal blood flow is also decreased in some patients with chronic peptic ulcers. Prostaglandins appear to have a protective effect against mucosal epithelial cell damage. Interference in this pathway is the probable mechanism of ulceration in NSAID patients.

A number of endogenous peptide/protein factors are important in maintaining epithelial cell integrity and, indeed, in effecting repair in areas of damage. Growth factors such as epidermal growth factor (EGF) and transforming growth factor α (TGF-α) are important in this regard, as are the trefoil peptides – a family of mucin-associated molecules that have important effects in maintaining a protective mucous layer and in stimulating motility of epithelial cells across areas of ulceration. The importance of trefoil peptides is emphasized by their close association with regeneration and repair of ulcers at a number of sites in the gastrointestinal tract (e.g. Barrett's oesophagus, peptic ulcer, and inflammatory bowel disease).

## Gastric Neoplasms and Polyps

### Polyps and Benign Tumours in the Stomach

A number of conditions give rise to mucosal elevations in the stomach, all of which are described macroscopically (and endoscopically) as 'polyps'. Many such lesions are non-neoplastic. Polyps of hyperplastic and inflammatory type occur on a background of gastritis and are of little clinical significance. Not uncommonly, multiple mucosal polyps are seen in the body and cardia of the stomach, which, histologically, are seen to be due to marked dilatation of the fundic glands (fundic cyst polyps). The pathogenesis of these is unclear, but it is interesting that they are more common in patients with familial adenomatous polyposis (FAP) of the colon and are also associated with long-term acid suppression with proton pump inhibitors. True benign neoplastic epithelial polyps are unusual. These adenomas are morphologically very similar to the much more common colorectal adenomas. Their recognition is very important because they have a very high risk of progression to invasive malignancy (adenocarcinoma).

### Malignant Neoplasms

> **Key Points**
>
> - Gastric carcinoma shows marked geographical variation in incidence.
> - Its incidence is decreasing in western populations.
> - The intestinal subtype is associated with chronic gastritis and H. pylori infection.
> - The diffuse type is not related to gastritis.

#### Adenocarcinoma

Carcinoma of the stomach is a disease notable for its variable geographical incidence. The highest incidence is seen in the Far East, notably Japan. From the pathologist's viewpoint, the disease is interesting in that the two major histological subtypes (intestinal and diffuse – see below) have quite different epidemiological and genetic profiles. Migrant studies have shown that the geographical variation in incidence of gastric cancer is largely due to environmental influences, and the consumption of smoked foods rich in nitrates has been implicated. Fresh fruit and vegetables appear to have a protective effect, possibly mediated by antioxidants such as ascorbic acid. An improved diet has been proposed as a major contributory factor in explaining the declining overall incidence of gastric cancer in western society over the past few decades.

#### Morphology

Gastric carcinomas can be classified by their site of origin (e.g. antral, fundic, cardiac). The topographical site of the tumour is of no prognostic significance, but is of considerable importance in tumour epidemiology. The recent overall decline in the incidence of gastric carcinoma appears to involve mainly tumours of the distal stomach, whereas cancers of the cardiac mucosa have actually increased in incidence. These cardiac tumours appear to share the epidemiological associations of carcinomas arising in Barrett's oesophagus.

Gastric carcinomas can be classified macroscopically as polypoid, exophytic, ulcerative, or infiltrative (Fig. 9.29). These categories are again of little independent clinical significance, but the diffusely infiltrative lesions give rise to a rigid immobile ('leather-bottle') stomach known as linitis plastica. This can give a characteristic appearance radiologically on barium meal examination.

Microscopic examination has yielded a number of classifications. The most useful is the Lauren system, which defines two major subgroups (Fig. 9.30). Intestinal carcinomas are gland-forming neoplasms which, as the term would suggest, resemble carcinomas of the large and small intestines (and indeed oesophageal adenocarcinoma). Diffuse carcinomas are characterized by non-cohesive, mucin-containing, 'signet-ring' cells that infiltrate widely through the wall of the

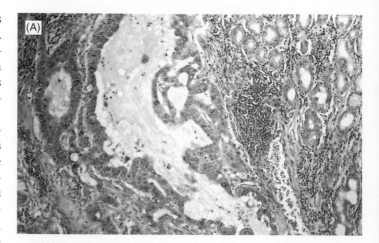

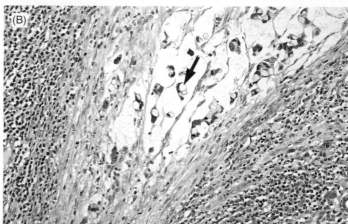

**FIG. 9.30** (A) Intestinal-type gastric adenocarcinoma with well-formed glands. (B) Diffuse carcinoma made up of dissociated mucin-producing, signet-ring cells (arrow).

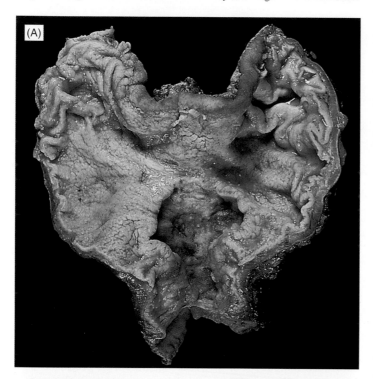

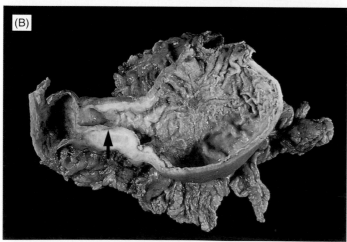

**FIG. 9.29** (A) Large ulcerated gastric carcinoma. (B) Infiltrative carcinoma showing marked thickening of the wall in the region of the antrum and pylorus (arrow).

stomach, often being associated with the macroscopic pattern of linitis plastica. This classification is of clinical use because, for tumours of equivalent stage, the prognosis is worse in diffuse cancers. These two categories are also different in epidemiology and pathogenesis. Intestinal cancers tend to occur in older individuals and have declined in incidence in recent years. Diffuse adenocarcinomas now make up about 50% of gastric cancers, and tend to occur in a younger age group.

*Aetiology and Pathogenesis*

Intestinal adenocarcinomas frequently develop on a background of chronic gastritis with atrophy. As in oesophageal adenocarcinomas, there is an association with intestinal metaplasia, and a preinvasive state of dysplasia can be recognized. Chronic gastritis of all types shows an association with carcinoma but, in view of its frequency, there has recently been a considerable focus of attention on the role of *H. pylori* as a potential carcinogenic agent.

*H. pylori* is not directly mutagenic, but infection is associated in some patients with decreased acid production. This hypochlorhydria allows the proliferation of other organisms, some of which are capable of generating mutagenic compounds from dietary nitrates. DNA damage from reactive oxygen species (generated directly by *H. pylori* and also by inflammatory neutrophils and macrophages) is an important factor, and highlights the previously mentioned protective effect of antioxidants in the diet (see p. 251). Increased epithelial cell proliferation, resulting from the cytotoxic effects of *H. pylori* and possibly also from cytokine stimulation, is important in providing the fertile ground of DNA synthesis in which mutagenic agents can operate.

Diffuse carcinomas are not associated with chronic gastritis and do not have a clearly defined precursor dysplastic lesion. At the molecular genetic level, there are also some differences between the tumour types, confirming the epidemiological differences. Intestinal cancers are characterized by upregulation of growth factor receptors such as Her2, whereas diffuse neoplasms show downregulation or mutation of the *E-cadherin* gene coding for an important epithelial cell adhesion molecule.

### Prognostic Factors in Gastric Cancer

As mentioned above, the outcome in adenocarcinoma of the stomach depends to some extent on the tumour type (intestinal or diffuse). A number of other prognostic indicators have been studied but, as in most human malignancies, tumour stage is of prime importance. Most patients in Western society present at an advanced stage of disease, when the malignant cells have invaded through the stomach wall and spread to local and regional lymph nodes and/or the liver. In Japan where, because of a high incidence, there is a screening programme for gastric carcinoma, survival following resection of 'early' gastric cancer (defined as

## 9.1 Special Study Topic

### GASTRIC LYMPHOMA: A DISEASE OF MUCOSA-ASSOCIATED LYMPHOID TISSUE

The gastrointestinal tract is the most common primary site of MALT lymphoma (also known as marginal zone lymphoma). Within the gut, the majority of such tumours arise in the stomach. Clinical presentation of gastric lymphoma is variable. Low-grade lesions present with non-specific symptoms such as dyspepsia. Higher-grade tumours may present with anorexia and weight loss, and are easily confused clinically with gastric carcinoma. Macroscopically, MALT lymphomas are often poorly defined, but higher-grade examples present as solid ulcerated tumour masses. Microscopically and immunophenotypically, these tumours are mostly low-grade B-cell lymphomas of marginal zone origin. They are made up of small- to medium-sized lymphocytes, which may show some plasma cell differentiation. They often infiltrate around reactive follicles. The most characteristic histological feature is tumour cell infiltration of the epithelium of gastric glands (the lymphoepithelial lesion – Fig. 9.31). Regional lymph nodes may be involved by tumour. Unlike other low grade B-cell lymphomas, it is unusual to have systemic disease (distant lymph node or bone marrow involvement) at presentation. High-grade MALT lymphomas are made up of larger blast-like cells. Many high-grade tumours show residual elements of lower-grade neoplasm, and it is thought that some arise by progression from these pre-existing neoplasms.

### Pathogenesis

It is now clear that MALT cells and their neoplastic equivalents comprise a distinct subset of lymphocytes that are characterized by their tendency to home in to mucosal

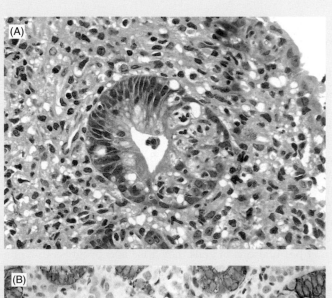

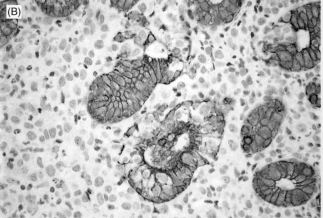

**FIG. 9.31** Gastric B-cell lymphoma of mucosa-associated lymphoid tissue (MALT) origin (marginal zone lymphoma). (A) The characteristic lymphoepithelial lesion shows atypical lymphoid cells invading a gastric gland. The extent of this process is emphasized in (B), where the glands are highlighted by the immunohistochemical demonstration of cytokeratin.

## Special Study Topic continued . . .

sites. Normal MALT is seen at a number of sites, the best example being Peyer's patches of the small intestine. It is rather paradoxical that the most common site of MALT lymphoma is the stomach, given that this organ does not have a native lymphoid population. However, epidemiological and morphological studies have shown that the presence of MALT in the stomach is, in the great majority of individuals, a reaction to *H. pylori* infection. The current concept of the development of gastric MALT lymphoma is that lymphoid cells, initially attracted to the mucosa by *H. pylori*, slowly accumulate genetic changes and eventually develop into an autonomously proliferating, monoclonal, B-cell lymphoma. Most MALT lymphomas evolve through this genetically unstable route, slowly progressing from a phase in which

lymphoid proliferation is dependent on *H. pylori*-induced T-cell help, to a phase of antigen independence and eventually, in some cases, to transformation to a more aggressive phase. A minority of gastric MALT lymphomas acquire a chromosomal translocation, t(11:18), at an early stage. Such tumours are antigen independent (and usually do not respond to antibiotic treatment), but they are relatively genetically stable and rarely transform to high-grade disease.

### Further Reading

Liu H, Ye H, Ruskone-Fourmestraux J, *et al*. t(11:18) is a marker for all stage gastric MALT lymphomas that will not respond to *H. pylori* eradication. *Gastroenterology* 2002;**122**: 1286–1294.

---

carcinoma invading no deeper than the submucosa of the stomach) is much better than in North America or Europe.

### Other Gastric Neoplasms

Endocrine cell (carcinoid) tumours of the stomach are rare and, although malignant, have a better prognosis than adenocarcinoma. Gastric malignant lymphomas are a source of considerable biological and clinical interest. These neoplasms are almost invariably of B-cell lineage. They are the best and most common example of lymphoma arising in the MALT. As with adenocarcinoma, there is a strong epidemiological link with *H. pylori* colonization. These organisms are antigenic and provoke a chronic inflammatory cell reaction in the mucosa. This is the background upon which clonal populations of cells may arise and progress to a clinical lymphoid neoplasm. Prognosis depends on the grade and stage of the tumour. The link to *H. pylori* is emphasized by regression of histologically proven neoplasms after antibiotic therapy, which is now the initial treatment for most such tumours.

### Gastrointestinal Stromal Tumours

It is an interesting paradox that, although most of the tissue of the gastrointestinal tract is mesenchymal in origin, the great majority of neoplasms are epithelial. Nevertheless, connective tissue tumours are an important clinical problem. They are seen throughout the gut, but are most common in the stomach. It was formerly thought that these were of smooth muscle origin and they were labelled leiomyomas or leiomyosarcomas to indicate their probable benign or malignant clinical course. In fact, with the exception of the oesophagus, most mesenchymal tumours show no evidence of muscle differentiation and are usually referred to as gastrointestinal stromal tumours (GISTs). The cells in GISTs resemble the pacemaker cells regulating gut motility– the interstitial cells of Cajal.

GISTs can present with ulceration and bleeding, as an obstruction, or as abdominal masses. On gross examination of resected specimens, these tumours are usually well demarcated from surrounding tissues (Fig. 9.32). Microscopically, they are usually made up of spindle-shaped cells and there may be evident necrosis. Some tumours behave in an entirely benign fashion whereas others can progress rapidly to metastatic disease. It can be difficult to predict prognosis in an individual patient, but tumour size and the frequency of mitotic figures are important (thus, for example, tumours >10 cm or showing >10 mitoses per high power microscopic field are at very high risk of malignant behaviour).

It has been shown that approximately 75% of GISTs show a mutation of the c-*kit* oncogene, and overexpress the gene product CD117 on the cell membrane. Mutations of the platelet-derived growth factor receptor α (*PDGFRA*) gene are seen in a further 10% of GISTs. Detection of these mutations in tumour tissue is useful in diagnosing these neoplasms. It is also of great therapeutic importance, because the tyrosine kinase-inhibiting drug imatinib acts directly to

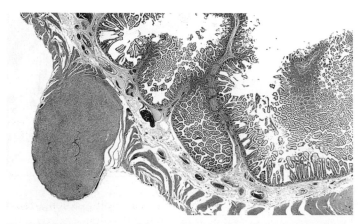

**FIG. 9.32** Stromal tumour of the small intestine manifested as a well-demarcated nodule in the muscularis.

inhibit the effect of the *c-kit* oncogene mutation. This drug can be remarkably effective in controlling inoperable and metastatic GISTs. However, efficacy is most marked in the presence of some specific mutations (e.g. in codon 11 of *c-kit*) whereas other mutations in *c-kit* and *PDGFRA* are markers of drug resistance. This story is an excellent example of how understanding tumour biology can lead to development of specific, effective, non-toxic therapy.

# THE INTESTINES

## Normal Structure and Function

### Small Intestine

The small intestine is the main site of enzymatic digestion and absorption of nutrients. In the duodenum, the gastric contents are mixed with bile and pancreatic secretions, and the main process of digestion begins. Absorption then proceeds in the jejunum and ileum. The mucosa of the small intestine provides a vast area for absorption through its villous structure. The villi are covered by specialized absorptive cells (enterocytes) that have microvilli on their luminal surfaces, further increasing the surface area. Enterocytes produce hydrolytic enzymes such as disaccharidases and peptidases.

Other cells present in the small intestinal mucosa include the following:

- Epithelial stem cells in the intestinal crypts: these can divide and differentiate into all other epithelial cell types.
- Endocrine cells: these produce a variety of hormones such as enteroglucagon, cholecystokinin, gastrin, motilin, secretin, vasoactive intestinal polypeptide (VIP), and serotonin (5-hydroxytryptamine [5-HT]).
- Paneth cells: these are present at the bases of the crypts, and contain prominent large lysozyme-rich granules. Their secretions modulate the intestinal flora.
- The mucin-producing cells of Brunner's glands: these submucosal glands are mainly present in the duodenum, and produce mucus and epidermal growth factor (EGF). They are, therefore, considered to have a role in mucosal repair.
- The cells in the lamina propria, namely lymphocytes, plasma cells, eosinophils, and mast cells. These occupy the space between the crypts and prominent lymphatics and blood capillaries. The lymphoid cells belong to the MALT. In some parts of the intestine the lymphoid cells are aggregated; this is particularly prominent in the terminal ileum, where they form Peyer's patches.

### Large Intestine

This is composed of the caecum, ascending colon, transverse colon, descending colon, sigmoid colon, and rectum. Its functions include:

- storage and elimination of food residues
- maintenance of fluid and electrolyte balance
- the large intestine being the main site for the bacterial degradation of complex carbohydrates and other nutrients.

The mucosa of the large bowel differs from that of the small in the following important respects:

- It is flat with no villi.
- It contains straight crypts lined by absorptive and mucus-producing goblet cells.
- The endocrine cells and Paneth cells are less numerous, the latter normally being found only on the right side of the colon and in very small numbers.
- The lamina propria is less prominent and contains very few lymphatics; thus, malignancy confined to the mucosa has very limited metastatic potential.

It is important to know the blood supply of the intestines, because this determines the site and pattern of ischaemic damage, and is also followed by lymphatics, thereby determining the routes of spread of carcinoma. The superior mesenteric artery supplies the entire small intestine apart from the first half of the duodenum. This artery also supplies the right side of the colon and most of the transverse colon. In the small intestine, the terminal branches of the superior mesenteric artery are end-arteries, with few anastomoses between them. In the large bowel there is a degree of distal and proximal anastomosis between all of the supplying vessels. The inferior mesenteric artery supplies the distal transverse, the descending and the sigmoid colon, and the upper part of the rectum. The middle and inferior rectal arteries, branches of the internal iliac, and internal pudendal arteries supply the remainder of the rectum. The venous drainage of the bowel, apart from the anal canal, is via the portal system to the liver. This is the reason why primary gastrointestinal malignancies frequently spread to the liver, producing hepatic metastases.

The sympathetic nervous supply to the gut originates in the coeliac and mesenteric plexus. Parasympathetic ganglia lie within the gut wall, where, together with other neurons, they form the submucosal (Meissner's) plexus and muscular (Auerbach's) plexus. Parasympathetic stimulation increases muscular contraction, blood supply, and secretory activity, whereas sympathetic activity has the opposite effect. There are also sensory receptors in the mucosa and bowel wall that respond to changes in volume and composition of bowel contents; by releasing neurotransmitters such as VIP, cholecystokinin, and somatostatin, these receptors produce motor and secretory responses.

## Congenital Disorders

### Atresia

Failure of development or canalization of part of the gut is most often described in the duodenum and the anorectal area. Duodenal atresia is strongly associated with trisomy 21 (Down's syndrome).

## Malrotation

Failure of the caecum to descend into the right iliac fossa can lead to positioning of the entire large bowel to the left side of the abdominal cavity.

## Diverticula and Duplications

Congenital diverticula of the upper small intestine may be a source of abnormal bacterial overgrowth, with consequent malabsorption (see below). Meckel's diverticulum is a well-recognized vestigial remnant of the embryological vitellointestinal duct, and is found attached to the wall of the distal ileum. It may become inflamed and mimic acute appendicitis. Occasionally, heterotopic gastric and/or pancreatic epithelium may be present in the diverticulum, leading to local ileal peptic ulceration.

## Hirschsprung's Disease

This condition is characterized by a lack of normal ganglion cells in the myenteric plexus of part of the bowel. It is due to the failure of migration of primitive neuroblasts into the developing gut. The distal large bowel is usually affected, but the abnormality may extend to involve the entire colon and even part of the small intestine. Diagnosis can be made on biopsies by demonstrating a lack of ganglia, and the associated, unchecked proliferation of parasympathetic acetylcholinesterase-producing nerves in the mucosa.

# Malabsorption

Malabsorption can be due to a range of mechanisms:

- Inadequate digestion: due to pancreatic insufficiency, hepatobiliary disease, post-gastrectomy
- Intestinal damage: causes include coeliac disease, tropical sprue, post-infective malabsorption, Crohn's disease, parasitic disease, drugs, radiation enteritis, Whipple's disease, lymphoma, immunodeficiency, amyloidosis, and intestinal resection
- Altered intestinal flora (bacterial overgrowth): jejunal diverticulosis, blind loops
- Biochemical abnormality: causes include abetalipoproteinaemia, disaccharidase deficiency, specific amino acid malabsorption (e.g. Hartnup's disease), and bile acid deficiencies
- Lymphatic obstruction: intestinal lymphangiectasia (congenital or acquired)
- Inadequate absorptive surface: intestinal resection or bypass
- Endocrine disturbances: carcinoid syndrome, Verner–Morrison syndrome (VIPoma, due to a VIP-producing tumour), diabetes mellitus, hypothyroidism
- Circulatory disturbance: mesenteric vascular insufficiency.

## Coeliac Disease

### Key Points

- Coeliac disease results from an abnormal immune response to wheat gliadin.
- Epithelial cell damage leads to small intestinal villous atrophy.
- Coeliac disease is associated with dermatitis herpetiformis and intestinal lymphoma.

Coeliac disease is the most common intestinal cause of malabsorption in the western world. It affects about 1 in 2,000 individuals in the UK, but 1 in 300 in the west of Ireland. The condition usually presents in infancy or early childhood, but may become manifest only in adult life. It is due to a genetically determined, abnormal cell-mediated immune response to gliadin, a derivative of the wheat protein gluten (hence its alternative name gluten-sensitive enteropathy). There is a strong familial tendency and an association with HLA-B8. The skin disease dermatitis herpetiformis is also associated with HLA-B8, and most patients with this skin disease appear also to have coeliac disease.

The diagnosis is usually suspected in a child who fails to thrive, and suspicion is heightened if the stools are bulky and pale due to malabsorption of fat. Serological testing usually reveals the presence of antibodies to gliadin and endomysium including tissue transglutaminase (TTG). TTG antibodies are particularly useful in diagnostic screening but the diagnosis can be firmly established only on a mucosal biopsy of distal duodenum or jejunum that reveals the typical picture of villous atrophy and crypt hyperplasia (Fig. 9.33). These features are associated with increased numbers of plasma cells and lymphocytes in the lamina propria, and increased numbers of intraepithelial, CD8-expressing, cytotoxic T lymphocytes. Absolute confirmation of the diagnosis depends on return of these features to normal on re-biopsy after several weeks on a gluten-free diet.

Villous atrophy is due to damage to the surface enterocytes brought about by the immune reaction to gliadin. This results in a marked increase in cell death among the enterocytes, which is compensated for by an increased production of enterocytes in the crypts – hence crypt hyperplasia.

The immediate effects of coeliac disease are impaired nutrition and development due to malabsorption of fats, proteins, carbohydrates, and vitamins. Long-term effects are an increased risk of T-cell lymphoma of the small intestine (enteropathy-associated T-cell lymphoma). There also appears to be an increased incidence of certain other tumours, e.g. small intestinal and oesophageal carcinoma. Splenic atrophy – the cause of which is uncertain – is also commonly observed.

Some individuals with coeliac disease develop recurrent symptoms despite adherence to a gluten-free diet. The intraepithelial T lymphocytes in these cases can sometimes be shown to have lost cell surface antigens such as CD8. This is now recognized as a marker of developing lymphoma.

## Tropical Sprue

Identical, but usually less severe, changes to those found in coeliac disease are seen in tropical sprue. This is a form of malabsorption found in the tropics and subtropics, but not in Africa. It usually presents with diarrhoea, weight loss, and a macrocytic anaemia resulting from folate or vitamin $B_{12}$ deficiency. It is not caused by gluten sensitivity, but may be relieved by broad-spectrum antibiotics, or resolve spontaneously when the patient leaves the tropics. Its aetiology is uncertain, but abnormal bacterial colonization of the upper small intestine is the probable cause.

## Giardiasis

Ingestion of water containing the encysted form of *Giardia lamblia* is the cause of giardiasis, which may give rise to mild malabsorption. Diagnosis is made by small intestinal biopsy, which reveals the trophozoite phase of the parasite close, or attached, to surface mucosa.

## Altered Intestinal Flora

This occurs in bowel stasis as in diverticula or blind loops after surgical bypass procedures. Abnormal overgrowth of organisms may compete for nutrients such as vitamin $B_{12}$, interfere with the action of bile salts, or inactivate mucosal enzymes.

## Whipple's Disease

This is a rare multisystem disease caused by infection by bacteria (*Tropheryma whippelii*, a Gram-positive actinomycete). The disease may present with symptoms due to the infection of lymph nodes, joints, heart valves, lungs, or the central nervous system, but the most common presentation is with malabsorption. The disease responds to broad-spectrum antibiotics.

## Bacterial Infections

Bacterial infection of the intestinal tract is a major cause of disease and death throughout the world. Often, infection is acquired through drinking contaminated water.

## Cholera

This is due to infection with *Vibrio cholerae*, which produces a powerful exotoxin causing enterocytes to secrete abundant fluid and sodium ions. Massive watery diarrhoea may result, with devastating fluid loss and a rapidly fatal outcome. The toxin binds to epithelial cells, causing increased adenylyl cyclase activity, which results in high cAMP levels in the intestinal mucosa. Histological changes in the mucosa are minimal.

## Salmonella spp.

Infection by *Salmonella typhi* or *S. paratyphi* causes typhoid and the milder paratyphoid fever. These diseases are seen only rarely in western countries, due largely to the availability of clean drinking water. However, food poisoning by less virulent salmonellae is becoming increasingly common in the UK. Symptoms usually relate to the upper intestinal

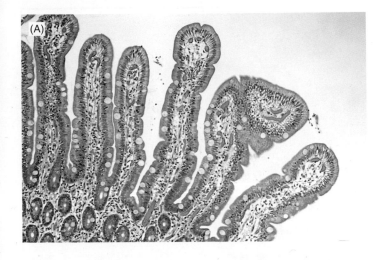

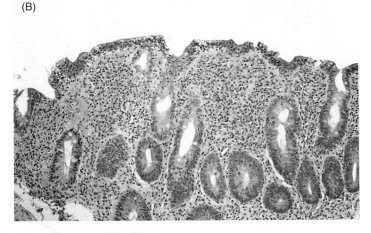

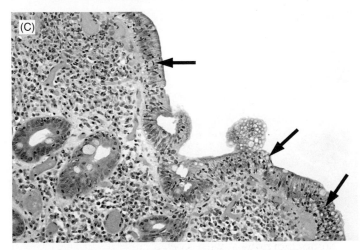

FIG. 9.33 (A) A normal duodenal biopsy, showing well-formed villi. (B) In this case of coeliac disease the villous architecture is lost ('subtotal villous atrophy') and (C) there is an increased complement of intraepithelial lymphocytes (arrows).

tract, with colicky periumbilical pain, vomiting, and watery diarrhoea, but sometimes they relate to the large intestine with frequent bloody stools and tenderness over the sigmoid colon. Sigmoidoscopy in the latter case reveals changes that are very similar, both macroscopically and microscopically, to those of ulcerative colitis (see below).

## WHIPPLE'S DISEASE

The patient, a 45-year-old male, presented with non-specific symptoms of feeling unwell, vague joint pains, and significant weight loss. A physical examination revealed the presence of generalized moderate lymphadenopathy, but no other abnormalities. The results of basic laboratory tests were all within normal ranges. A lymph node biopsy showed no evidence of malignancy, but there was a reactive picture characterized by the presence of large numbers of macrophages with prominent eosinophilic cytoplasm (Fig. 9.34). These macrophages were positive on a periodic acid–Schiff (PAS) stain, which stains for mucin, carbohydrate, and certain organisms. On the basis of these appearances and the clinical findings, a diagnosis of Whipple's disease (a rare infection due to *Tropheryma whippelii*) was suggested. As lymph node appearances are not specific in this disease, it was decided to seek confirmation of the diagnosis by performing a duodenal biopsy. This showed slight shortening and swelling of the villi, prominent dilated mucosal lymphatics, and an increased inflammatory infiltrate in the lamina propria, including large numbers of swollen pink macrophages (Fig. 9.35), confirming the diagnosis of Whipple's disease. The patient was immediately placed on the broad-spectrum antibiotic tetracycline, and within a few weeks his symptoms had disappeared, he felt much better, and he had begun to put on weight. A follow-up duodenal biopsy performed 6 months after the start of the course of tetracycline therapy revealed a nearly normal small bowel mucosa (Fig. 9.36).

The patient was then lost to follow-up for over a year, after which time he re-presented with unmistakable signs of

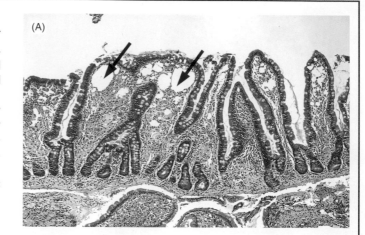

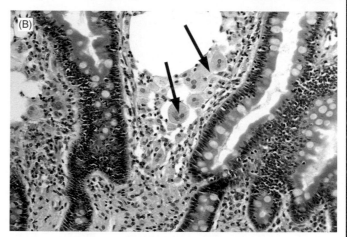

**FIG. 9.35** (A) Low-power and (B) higher-power views of duodenal biopsy, showing features described in the text. Arrows indicate dilated lymphatics in A and macrophages in B.

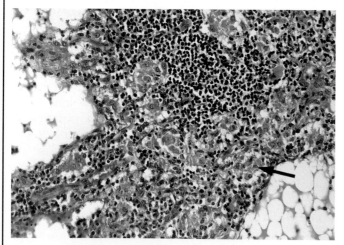

**FIG. 9.34** Haematoxylin and eosin staining of lymph node, showing fat and large numbers of pink swollen macrophages (arrow).

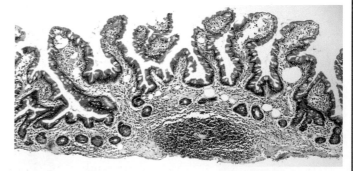

**FIG. 9.36** Duodenal biopsy after broad-spectrum antibiotic therapy. Note the normal villous architecture, no dilated lymphatics, and normal inflammatory cell component in the lamina propria.

dementia. A reappraisal of the management of the case by the physician raised the possibility that the dementia might also be due to Whipple's disease, because tetracycline does not cross the blood–brain barrier. The patient was immediately started on a prolonged course of trimethoprim, and within a few weeks the clinical signs of dementia had all but disappeared.

Lessons to be learnt from this case:

- Whipple's disease, due to an unusual bacterium capable of intracellular survival, is a relatively rare systemic infection usually affecting middle-aged men.

- Symptoms may relate to joints, lymph nodes, skin, brain, or the gastrointestinal tract.
- The diagnostic gold standard is small bowel (duodenal) biopsy.
- The condition can be fatal if not treated, but readily responds to broad-spectrum antibiotics. An antibiotic that crosses the blood–brain barrier should be used.
- Whipple's disease is a rare, but curable, cause of malabsorption.

## Bacillary Dysentery

This is an acute infection of the large bowel causing painful diarrhoea with blood and mucus in the stools. *Shigella flexneri* and *S. dysenteriae* can produce mucosal appearances very similar to those of ulcerative colitis, although the more common *S. sonnei* produces less severe pathology.

## Campylobacter Colitis

*Campylobacter jejuni* and *C. coli* are relatively frequent causes of severe gastroenteritis and colitis. Histological changes in rectal and colonic biopsies are non-specific and similar to those seen in other forms of infective colitis.

## Escherichia coli Diarrhoea

*E. coli* is associated with a variety of diarrhoeal illnesses. Most are due to toxin formation. Some bacterial serogroups, particularly O157:H7, are important causes of food-borne epidemics, associated in some individuals with development of the haemolytic–uraemic syndrome and a mortality rate of approximately 10%.

## Neonatal Diarrhoea

Specific enteropathogenic serotypes of *E. coli* cause a significant proportion of diarrhoeal illness seen in neonates and infants. The resulting diarrhoea may be so severe that it leads to dehydration and death.

## Staphylococcal Enterocolitis

This infection is relatively rare, but is a real threat among hospitalized patients receiving broad-spectrum antibiotics. These drugs alter the normal bowel flora such that infection with *Staphylococcus aureus* can occur. This may result in severe diarrhoea accompanied by shock and dehydration, and can be life threatening. The symptoms are caused by a powerful endotoxin released by the organisms. Occasionally, the disease is relatively mild and may respond to treatment, but more often it is severe and can be fatal. The small intestine is predominantly involved with ulceration.

## Tuberculosis

This usually affects the terminal ileum. The primary infection – usually caused by drinking milk infected by bovine tuberculosis (TB) – is now rarely seen in the UK following the pasteurization of milk supplies. The condition results in a trivial lesion in the ileal mucosa associated with enlarged, caseating mesenteric nodes. Secondary TB is the result of swallowing infected sputum in the presence of severe pulmonary TB. This results in deep transverse ileal ulcers, which heal by scarring and cause strictures. Sometimes the disease can involve the ileocaecal valve and cause a picture that is macroscopically indistinguishable from that of Crohn's disease. Antibiotic therapy is the treatment of choice for intra-abdominal TB, but surgery is often required for complications, or to obtain tissue for diagnosis. Complications include obstruction by adhesions, perforation of ulcers (rare), and malabsorption due to extensive mucosal damage or lymphatic obstruction.

## Actinomycosis

This usually presents as an inflammatory mass in the region of the appendix and caecum. The organism *Actinomyces israelii* – a Gram-positive filamentous bacterium normally present in the mouth – may escape acid digestion in the stomach and infect the bowel. The disease is characterized by the formation of sinuses linking the bowel lumen to the skin surface, and fistulae. Yellowish (sulphur) granules composed of colonies of the organism are often visible to the naked eye in the watery pus.

## Antibiotic-associated Colitis

This is due to overgrowth of *Clostridium difficile* in the colon after suppression of the normal bowel flora by broad-spectrum antibiotics. The disease can be mild or severe. Histologically, there is superficial loss of epithelial cells which become embedded in an exudate containing mucin, polymorphs, and abundant fibrin, forming a pseudomembrane on the surface – hence the term 'pseudomembranous colitis' (Fig. 9.37).

## Viral Infections

Most cases of acute gastroenteritis in the UK are due to viral infections. It is often not possible to confirm the diagnosis by laboratory means because of the relative insensitivity of available tests, and the fact that only tiny doses of viruses may cause illness. The main causative agents are parvoviruses and 'small round structured' viruses. These infect the small intestine, damage enterocytes, and cause mild villous atrophy and crypt hyperplasia, and inflammation of the lamina propria.

The large bowel is occasionally infected by cytomegalovirus, which can cause an acute haemorrhagic colitis. It may occur anew or complicate ulcerative colitis. The virus can be recognized due to the large intranuclear inclusions that it produces in mucosal cells, both epithelial and endothelial.

Some cases of acquired immune deficiency disease (AIDS) especially in Africa, show severe malabsorption and nutritional disturbances. Sometimes, the symptoms appear to be directly due to the effects of HIV, although often a superimposed opportunistic intestinal infection can be identified such as those due to coccidial protozoa (cryptosporidiosis) or *Mycobacterium avium-intracellulare*.

## Fungal and Chlamydial Diseases (see also Chapter 19)

Fungal infections of the alimentary tract are rare, but are being seen increasingly in immunocompromised patients.

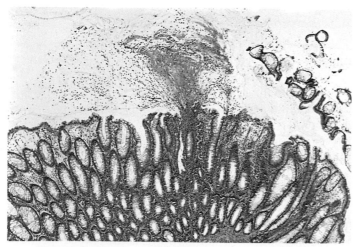

**FIG. 9.37** Pseudomembranous colitis: the colonic mucosal surface shows an erupting fibrinous 'pseudomembrane'.

In such instances, normally non-pathogenic phycomycetes are often found. Lymphogranuloma venereum is a sexually transmitted infection caused by specific serotypes of *Chlamydia trachomatis*. It is usually seen in females, and may cause rectal strictures due to spread to the rectum via the lymphatics. The histological picture is characterized by granulomas and non-specific chronic inflammation.

## Parasitic Infection (see also Chapter 19)

Giardiasis has been mentioned previously in relation to malabsorption and cryptosporidiosis in relation to AIDS. Other important protozoal parasitic diseases of the intestine are amoebiasis and schistosomiasis.

Amoebiasis affects the large intestine, and is the result of infection by the protozoan *Entamoeba histolytica*. It is more prevalent in the tropics than in temperate climates. Infection is by the faecal–oral route. Ingested as cysts, the organism is passed unharmed through the stomach, eventually reaching the large intestine where the cyst wall is dissolved, liberating active amoebae. These invade the mucosa by means of release of a cytolytic enzyme. They cause characteristic undermining 'flask-shaped' ulcers (recognizable under the microscope), or they may cause a more diffuse colitis. Organisms can be recognized in faeces or the tissues, and often contain ingested red blood cells.

Large intestinal schistosomiasis is usually due to *Schistosoma mansoni* or *S. japonicum*, but is sometimes seen with *S. haematobium*. For an account of the lifecycle of the parasites, see Chapter 19, pp. 567–569. The pathological changes in schistosomiasis are the result of the inflammatory response to the presence of eggs embedded in the wall of the intestine. Left-sided lesions are almost always due to *S. mansoni*, whereas right-sided colonic and appendiceal lesions may be caused by *S. haematobium*.

## Idiopathic Chronic Inflammatory Bowel Disease

There are two main idiopathic inflammatory bowel diseases, namely Crohn's disease and ulcerative colitis. Their main features are summarized and contrasted in *Table 9.2*. It is very important to remember that, before a diagnosis of idiopathic inflammatory bowel disease is made, infective causes of inflammation must be excluded.

### Crohn's Disease

Crohn's disease usually presents in the 20- to 60-year-old age group. It most often affects the terminal ileum, but may also involve the large bowel either alone or together with the small bowel. Less often, the disease may affect other parts of the intestine from the mouth to the anus, and also give rise to discontinuous skin lesions. The macroscopic appearances of the bowel vary according to the stage of the disease. The initial lesion is mucosal swelling

TABLE 9.2 Comparison of the main features of Crohn's disease and ulcerative colitis

| Feature | Crohn's disease | Ulcerative colitis |
|---|---|---|
| Characteristics | Chronic, relapsing, inflammatory condition of unknown aetiology | Chronic, relapsing, inflammatory condition of unknown aetiology |
| Presentation | Abdominal pain or obstruction | Bloody diarrhoea |
| Sites | Anywhere in the gastrointestinal tract Most common in distal ileum, then colon | Confined to large bowel. May be localized to rectum or, in continuity, with any length of the colon |
| Inflammation | Transmural, patchy, often partly granulomatous | Mucosal, diffuse, non-granulomatous |
| Complications | Malabsorption | Blood loss |
| | Fistula formation | Electrolyte disturbances |
| | Anal lesions | Toxic dilatation |
| | Malignancy (slight ↑ incidence of adenocarcinoma) | Malignancy (↑ incidence of adenocarcinoma in extensive colitis) |
| | Amyloidosis | Extracolonic complications: |
| | Perforation | Skin: pigmentation, erythema nodosum |
| | | Liver: sclerosing cholangitis |
| | | Eye: uveitis, particularly anterior (iritis) |
| | | Joints: ankylosing spondylitis, arthritis |

due to submucosal oedema. This obscures the normal transverse folds of the mucosa. In this setting small superficial (aphthous) ulcers develop. In turn these deepen, giving rise to fissures. In the established, more chronic, form of the disease the mucosa shows a distinct cobblestone pattern due to the oedematous swollen mucosa being divided into segments by deep fissuring ulcers. The bowel wall at this stage is thickened due to a combination of oedema, inflammation, and fibrosis, which may lead to stricture formation. Regional lymph nodes are usually enlarged. Characteristic of bowel involvement by Crohn's disease is the fact that these areas of abnormality are separated by macroscopically normal segments. These discrete, diseased areas of bowel are referred to as 'skip lesions'. Thickened segments of bowel wall can lead to narrowing of the lumen with partial obstruction (Fig. 9.38).

Histologically, Crohn's disease is characterized by inflammation of all layers of the bowel (transmural inflammation – Fig. 9.39). The submucosa is usually oedematous, and the ulcers extend from the mucosa deep into the bowel wall, forming fissures. Fibrous scarring becomes prominent with time. The full-thickness inflammation is characterized by focal aggregates of

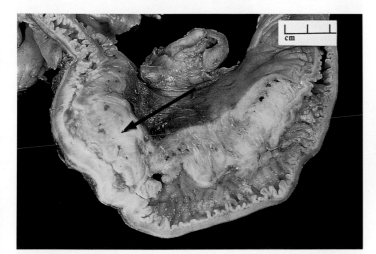

FIG. 9.38 In this case of Crohn's disease, a segment (arrow) in which the wall is thickened by inflammation and fibrosis obstructs the small intestine.

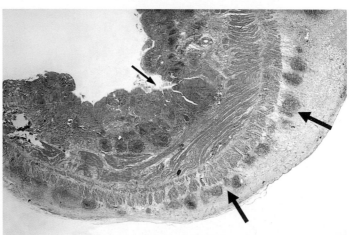

FIG. 9.39 Low-power histology of Crohn's disease. Fissures (small arrow) disrupt the mucosa, and lymphoid chronic inflammation extends through the wall to the subserosal fat (large arrows).

lymphocytes and, in many cases, non-caseating granulomas (Fig. 9.40).

Local complications of Crohn's disease include inflammatory adhesions to other loops of the bowel, the parietal peritoneum or bladder. Deep fissuring ulcers may extend through the full thickness of the bowel wall into an adjacent viscus or on to the skin (particularly in the perianal region), and cause a fistula. Other complications include intestinal obstruction due to stricture formation or fibrous adhesions, perforation of the bowel by a deep fissuring ulcer, leading to an intra-abdominal abscess, perianal fistulae, fissures and abscesses, a small increased risk of carcinoma of the bowel after many years, and occasionally heavy bleeding from ulcers. Crohn's disease usually follows a relapsing and remitting pattern, but because the scarring of the bowel wall and adhesions are permanent the likelihood of obstructive symptoms increases with time. Crohn's disease is also characterized by systemic complications (see *Table 9.2*).

### Ulcerative Colitis

Ulcerative colitis contrasts with Crohn's disease in a number of important respects (see *Table 9.2*). Patients with active ulcerative colitis typically develop diarrhoea in which faecal matter is mixed with blood, mucus, and pus. The disease

begins in the rectum; if confined to the rectum it is referred to as proctitis. It may extend proximally in continuity throughout part or the whole of the large bowel (Fig. 9.41). The term 'extensive colitis' is usually applied to disease affecting the colon proximally, at least to the hepatic flexure.

As with Crohn's disease, the appearances vary depending on the activity of the disease process. In active or early disease the mucosa appears to be congested and friable, and shows areas of shallow ulceration, which eventually become confluent. The ulceration is typically superficial, extending no deeper than the submucosa. Histology at this stage shows marked congestion and oedema of the mucosa, a diffuse increase in chronic inflammatory cells in the lamina propria, cryptitis (neutrophil polymorphs infiltrating between epithelial cells of the crypts), crypt abscesses (collections of neutrophil polymorphs in distended crypts), and a reduction in the number of mucous cells in the glands (Fig. 9.42).

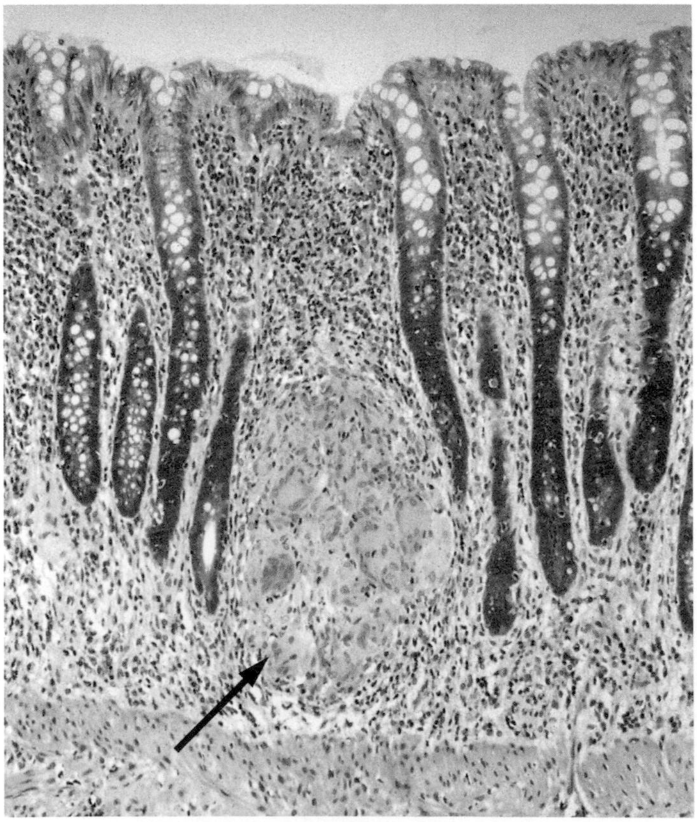

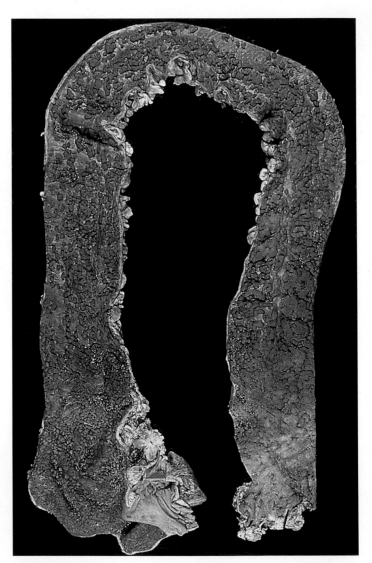

**FIG. 9.40** Inflammatory infiltration of the lamina propria and a granuloma (arrow) in a colonic biopsy from a patient with Crohn's disease.

**FIG. 9.41** Specimen from a total colectomy performed for refractory ulcerative colitis. The mucosa is diffusely red and inflamed. Many inflammatory pseudopolyps are present.

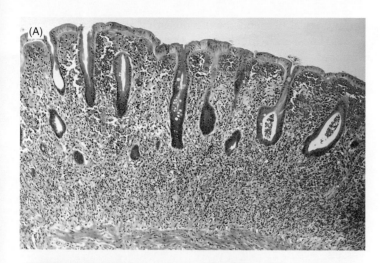

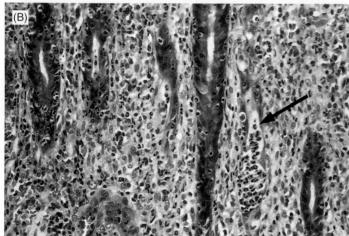

**FIG. 9.42** (A) Diffuse mucosal inflammation and crypt shortening in ulcerative colitis. (B) A higher-power view of a crypt abscess (arrow).

Such inflamed mucosa is often seen adjacent to an area of ulceration. The submucosa and deeper layers of the bowel wall are generally not inflamed.

In quiescent or treated colitis, the bowel mucosa usually appears macroscopically slightly reddened, granular, and thinned, but is not ulcerated. Histology shows mild chronic inflammation of the lamina propria, but usually no cryptitis or crypt abscesses. Glands may appear shortened or distorted but usually in inactive disease mucous cell numbers are not reduced, in contrast to the appearances in active disease.

Relatively infrequently the disease may present or relapse in a fulminant form in which the colon shows extensive confluent mucosal ulceration. This is associated with oedema and inflammation extending into the muscle layer. The damaged bowel wall progressively dilates, leading to the situation known as acute toxic megacolon. This can be life threatening due to rapid loss of fluid, blood, and electrolytes, or to perforation.

Local complications of ulcerative colitis include blood and fluid loss that may be severe, toxic dilatation, and perforation; dysplasia and carcinoma may develop in longstanding extensive disease. Systemic complications of ulcerative colitis include erythema nodosum, pyoderma gangrenosum, iritis (anterior uveitis), arthritis, ankylosing spondylitis, and chronic liver disease – particularly sclerosing cholangitis.

The natural history of ulcerative colitis is very variable, with small numbers of patients requiring early surgery and small numbers having persistent active disease despite medical treatment, but most patients are generally reasonably controlled by medical treatment although they have occasional relapses. Longstanding extensive colitis, i.e. colitis present for >10 years and extending from the rectum to at least the hepatic flexure, is associated with a significantly increased risk of the development of rectal or colonic carcinoma. The development of carcinoma in ulcerative colitis is believed usually to be preceded by a non-invasive phase, in which mucosal epithelial cells show varying degrees of dysplasia. It is suggested that patients who have had extensive colitis for >10 years should undergo regular colonoscopy with biopsy in order to try to diagnose preinvasive neoplastic lesions. Repeated biopsies showing high-grade dysplasia even without invasion are regarded as an indication for colectomy.

The aetiologies of both ulcerative colitis and Crohn's disease are unknown. Both show a familial tendency and a number of candidate genes are under investigation. Mutations in *CARD15* (*NOD2*) appear to account for 10–15% of patients with Crohn's disease. The product of this gene is involved in macrophage activation. The clinical and pathological differences between the two conditions suggest that they probably have different aetiologies, although cases in which the clinical and pathological findings overlap are not rare. The granulomatous nature of Crohn's disease has led to extensive investigations for a bacterial causative agent, particularly a mycobacterium, but so far no convincing candidate has been identified. Smoking is a significant predisposing factor for Crohn's disease. With ulcerative colitis, possible aetiological factors include stress, and infective and immunological causes. It has been suggested that some sort of infection may trigger an inappropriate autoimmune response, which leads to destruction of the colonic mucosa. Steroids and anti-inflammatory agents are usually effective in ulcerative colitis, suggesting that immune activation may be important. Smoking appears to protect against ulcerative colitis as, interestingly, does a history of appendicectomy.

## Vascular Disease of the Intestines

Intestinal ischaemia may result from sudden occlusion of vessels. This may be by thrombosis on an atheromatous plaque, or by an embolus lodging in a mesenteric vessel (see Chapter 6, pp. 112–114 for further discussion of thrombosis and embolism). Ischaemic injury may also occur in the presence of patent vessels if the blood supply is inadequate to maintain gut nutrition, e.g. in hypotensive shock or non-occlusive arterial narrowing. Venous thrombosis is a rarer cause of ischaemia, but may occur in hypercoagulable states or, locally, in an impacted hernia (Fig. 9.43). Systemic vasculitis is a further cause of ischaemia.

From a pathogenic viewpoint, ischaemia can be considered as acute or chronic in type.

### Acute Ischaemia

A sudden critical decrease in blood supply to the intestines threatens the viability of the bowel and the life of the patient. The most common cause is arterial thromboembolism, followed by *in situ* thrombus formation and non-occlusive vascular disease. Cellular injury is caused by anoxia and also often by reperfusion injury, in a manner analogous to that seen in the myocardium (see Chapter 6, pp. 138–140). The clinical features and severity of injury depend on the depth of intestinal damage. If infarction is confined to the mucosa, then complete regeneration is possible. Submucosal extension (mural infarction) can lead to fibrous stricture. Transmural infarction (gangrene) will lead to perforation if not surgically resected. Even before perforation, septicaemia may ensue as a result of unimpeded invasion by bacteria from the bowel lumen.

### Chronic Ischaemia

This condition is almost always seen in association with widespread atherosclerosis. Classically, it presents as 'mesenteric angina', i.e. postprandial abdominal pain due to an inability to increase blood supply in response to the increased physiological demands of the digestive and absorptive processes. These individuals are at extremely high risk of superimposed acute ischaemia, and frequently have areas of fibrous stricture due to previous mural infarcts. Diagnostic difficulty can arise in the investigation of patients with bloody diarrhoea, in that microscopic features of ischaemia on biopsy can be confused with inflammatory bowel disease, pseudomembranous colitis, or solitary rectal ulcer.

### Necrotizing Enterocolitis

This is a condition, mainly seen in infants, in which there is intestinal gangrene caused partly by ischaemia and partly by overwhelming bacterial infection. Vasculitis is characteristic and inflammatory changes are seen in thrombosed blood vessels.

### Vascular Malformations

A number of conditions are characterized by an abnormal proliferation of mature blood vessels in the wall of the bowel. Classification of these is complex. Some are congenital, whereas others appear to develop in adult life. Angiodysplasia is one such lesion, presenting in later life as colonic bleeding from abnormal submucosal vessels, often in the right side of the colon.

## Acquired Disorders of Gut Motility

### Diverticular Disease

Non-congenital intestinal diverticula are abnormal outpouchings of mucosa without associated smooth muscle, often extending through the bowel wall to reach mesenteric or subserosal fat (Fig. 9.44). The presence of such diverticula (diverticular disease) is common in the colon, particularly in the sigmoid colon. Diverticula occur near the taenia coli at the points of penetration of blood vessels. There is marked adjacent muscular hypertrophy, and the mucosa can be thrown up into a complex pattern of folds. Diverticular disease is a condition of older individuals, and is associated with increased intraluminal pressure, probably as a result of a low-fibre diet. Patients complain of colicky lower abdominal pain. Complicated disease occurs when diverticula become ulcerated, often due to an impacted faecolith. Bacterial infection can ensue, leading to a localized abscess or, worse, disseminated peritonitis with septicaemia. Localized disease not uncommonly leads to fistula formation, particularly to the bladder and vagina. Diverticular disease does not predispose to malignancy.

### Other Mechanical Disorders

These include strangulation of bowel in a hernia sac (see Fig. 9.43) and volvulus. The latter is an apparently spontaneous twist in a loop of bowel (often small intestine or sigmoid colon). This may occur around a congenital or acquired

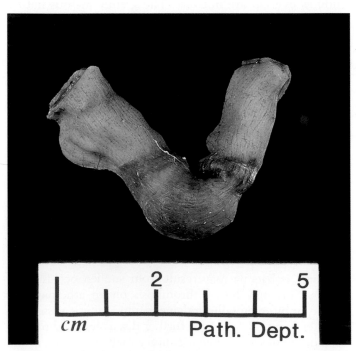

**FIG. 9.43** Dark discoloration of ischaemic small intestine removed from an inguinal hernia. Note the band-like constrictions at either side of the ischaemic segment indicating the site of constriction in the neck of the hernia sac.

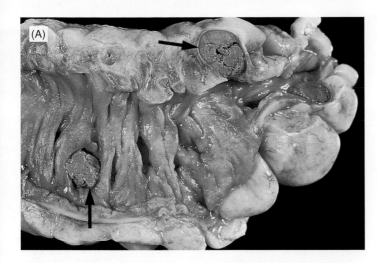

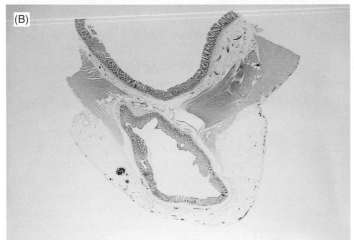

FIG. 9.44 (A) Sigmoid colon resected for diverticular disease. Multiple mucosal outpouchings are visible, some with impacted hard faeces (faecoliths; arrows). (B) A full-mount histological preparation showing a mucosal diverticulum extending through the muscle wall of the colon.

fibrous adhesion or as a result of an unusually long mesentery. Volvulus and strangulation lead to luminal obstruction and eventually to infarction by venous thrombosis. Intussusception is an invagination of one bowel segment into another. There is usually a lesion at the apex of the invaginating bowel. This may be a polyp or an intramural tumour, or something as simple as a focus of lymphoid hyperplasia. The hyperplasia is usually the case in ileocolic intussusception, the most common type seen in clinical practice.

## Intestinal Polyps and Neoplasms

As in the stomach, a number of discrete mucosal elevations ('polyps') are described in the intestines. Many are non-neoplastic, and most are more common in the large bowel. Thus, inflammatory polyps may be seen, often in association with Crohn's disease or ulcerative colitis. So-called hyperplastic (metaplastic) polyps are seen only in the large bowel, where they are the most frequently identified polyps. They

are of uncertain cause but are probably neoplastic in nature, forming the low-grade end of the serrated neoplasia spectrum (see below). Hamartomatous polyps are spread (more or less evenly) through the stomach and intestines in the autosomal dominant inherited condition of Peutz–Jeghers syndrome, the main other feature of which is a characteristic circumoral skin pigmentation.

True neoplastic polyps are far more common in the large than in the small bowel. They are most often of epithelial origin, and are therefore termed 'adenomas'. These lesions are common, being seen in about a third of individuals at age 70 years. There are two basic morphological varieties: one contains tubular crypts arising from a lobulated surface (the tubular adenoma); the other (less common) type has a small intestine-like velvety surface made up of numerous epithelium-lined projections (the villous adenoma – Fig. 9.45). In practice, many adenomas show mixtures

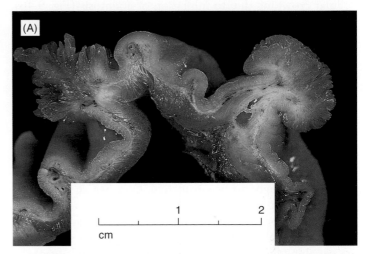

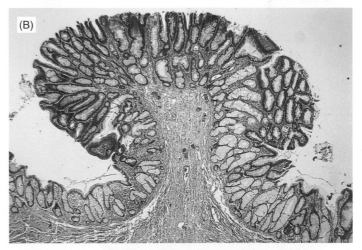

FIG. 9.45 (A) Longitudinal section through resected bowel, showing two distinct adenomas. The lesion on the left shows the frond-like architecture of a villous adenoma, and that on the right shows the smoother lobulated outline of a tubular adenoma. (B) Low-power photomicrograph of a tubular adenoma, showing that the lesion is made up of distorted, elongated crypts. Even at this power the dark ('hyperchromatic') atypical nuclei are visible. Note the raised stalk. This must be examined carefully for signs of early invasion.

of both features and are called tubulovillous adenomas. Macroscopically, tubular adenomas are rounded, usually <15 mm in diameter, and are frequently attached to the bowel wall by a definite stalk. Villous adenomas are flatter and larger (often >25 mm in diameter). In all adenomas the neoplastic cells are epithelial, and these show varying degrees of dysplasia.

Adenomatous polyps are important in their own right as causes of bleeding and anaemia due to traumatic surface ulceration by the passing faecal stream. Nevertheless, it is the association between these lesions and the development of invasive malignancy (adenocarcinoma) that is of greatest clinical concern.

Serrated epithelial lesions of the large bowel are a spectrum of lesions ranging from hyperplastic polyp through serrated adenoma to serrated adenocarcinoma. All show a characteristic 'saw-tooth' epithelial surface, thought to reflect cellular crowding due to inhibition of apoptosis (Fig. 9.46). Hyperplastic polyps are more common in the left colon but the larger lesions with a clinically significant risk of progression to cancer are more often seen in the right colon.

## Colorectal Carcinoma

Cancers of the large bowel are among the most common neoplasms in western society. There is a strong link with the lifestyle of developed countries, which is confirmed in migrant studies. Diet is strongly implicated, particularly an intake that is rich in fat and poor in fibre. Antioxidant vitamins (A, D, E) are thought to be protective. Diet has an important effect on transit time through the gut, and also in modifying the resident flora. Fat-rich diets increase the bile acid content of faeces and also favour growth of *Clostridium* spp. which are capable of generating carcinogenic compounds from the

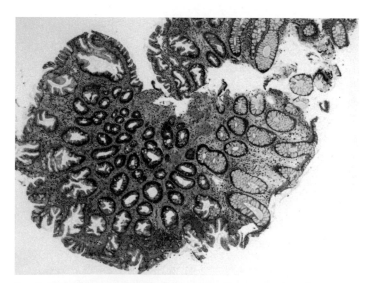

**FIG. 9.46** Rectal hyperplastic polyp showing the saw-tooth surface defining epithelial serration. There is no dysplasia. Serrated adenomas have a similar architecture, but with cytological atypia similar to that seen in conventional adenomatous polyps (see Fig. 9.45).

bile acids. There is good evidence that exercise is protective against intestinal neoplasia. Long-standing ulcerative colitis (and to a lesser extent colonic Crohn's disease) carries a significantly increased risk of colorectal cancer.

### Pathology of Large Bowel Carcinoma

The great majority of colorectal carcinomas are adenocarcinomas. About half are found in the rectum, a further third in the sigmoid colon, and the rest are spread equally across the remainder of the colon. There is some emerging evidence, however, that right-sided cancers are becoming relatively more common. There are distinct macroscopic subtypes, which show predilection for different regions of the bowel. Thus, rectal tumours are commonly ulcerated raised plaques, whereas sigmoid, descending, and transverse colon cancers most often present as a circumferential infiltrated 'napkin-ring' constriction (Fig. 9.47). Carcinomas of the right colon characteristically appear as polypoid masses growing into the capacious lumen of this part of the gut. These macroscopic features underlie differing modes of presentation, with rectal tumours often presenting with fresh bleeding, annular constricting lesions as obstructions, and right colonic tumours as insidious anaemia.

Microscopically, the great majority of colorectal carcinomas are moderately differentiated adenocarcinomas (Fig. 9.48). Some produce large amounts of mucin. By far the most important pathological parameter in clinical practice is the staging of the tumour on a surgical resection specimen using either Dukes' system (Fig. 9.49) or, increasingly, the TNM (tumour, nodes, metastasis) system which has the advantage of subdividing Dukes' stage B tumours (most of the surgically resected cases) into T3 and T4 (the latter defined as tumour invading through the bowel wall with peritoneal ulceration and/or invasion into other adjacent organs). T4 tumours have a worse prognosis and are usually considered for adjuvant chemotherapy, as are patients with node-positive disease (Dukes' C, TNM stage N1 or N2).

### Pathology in Clinical Practice

Recently, there has been considerable emphasis on assessing the completeness of excision of large bowel tumours, particularly in the case of the rectum, which, unlike most of the intestine, is largely not covered by peritoneum but lies embedded in the deep pelvic soft tissues. The emphasis on assessing completeness of excision in the circumferential (soft tissue) margin has been instrumental in changing surgical practice, encouraging wider clearance in surgical resections of the rectum ('total mesorectal excision', see Fig. 9.47B). Pathological reporting of tumour stage and completeness of excision also has important implications in deciding on the use of adjuvant chemotherapy or radiotherapy. Identification by the pathologist of tumour invasion into veins in the pericolic/perirectal soft tissues is also of clinical importance, being predictive of future systemic metastatic disease.

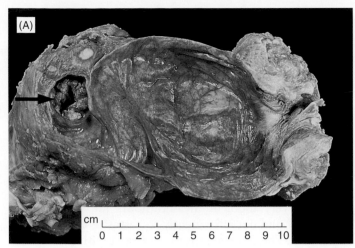

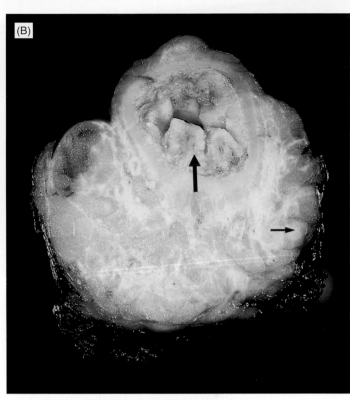

FIG. 9.47 (A) Rectum opened up to give a view of a stenosing cancer (arrow) at the rectosigmoid junction. Note the enlarged white nodes in the adjacent fat. Microscopy showed these to be largely replaced by metastatic carcinoma. (B) Transverse section through a total mesorectal excision for rectal carcinoma. The tumour presents as a raised plaque (large arrow). There is extension through the wall into perirectal fat. Margin involvement was confirmed microscopically in the region indicated by the small arrow. The patient was therefore referred to the multidisciplinary team meeting for discussion of chemotherapy and radiotherapy.

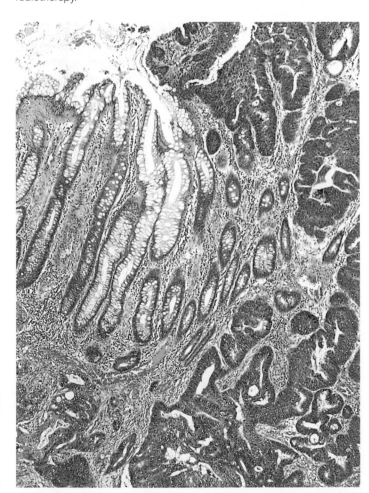

FIG. 9.48 Invasive, moderately differentiated adenocarcinoma arising in large bowel mucosa.

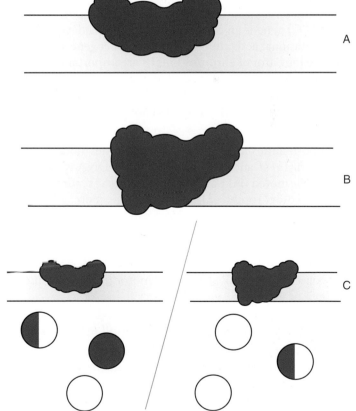

FIG. 9.49 Dukes' staging system for large bowel carcinoma. Stage A tumours are confined to the bowel muscle wall. Stage B cancers show invasion completely through the muscle wall. Dukes' stage C is defined by the presence of lymph node metastases, irrespective of the depth of invasion of the primary tumour.

### The Adenoma–Carcinoma Sequence

It is thought that most – if not all – colorectal carcinomas develop in pre-existing adenomas. The evidence for this may be summarized as follows:

- Adenomas and carcinomas share the same epidemiological spread in world populations (and the same topographical spread in the colon).
- Patients with colorectal cancer have a higher incidence of adenomas than unaffected control individuals.
- The risk of developing carcinoma increases markedly in patients with higher numbers of adenomatous polyps (e.g. FAP).
- It is common to find residual adenomatous tissue on histological examination of cancers and, conversely, focal early invasive carcinoma can be seen arising in adenomatous polyps.

### Molecular Pathology of Large Bowel Adenoma and Carcinoma

The strong clinical and epidemiological evidence in favour of a progression from normal through adenoma to carcinoma in the large bowel, together with the ready availability of tissue specimens, has made this system an ideal model for studying the genetic events involved in the development of a cancer. In this context, a number of crucial events have been defined:

- Mutation and/or loss of the adenomatous polyposis coli (*APC*) gene is an early event in adenoma development.
- Mutational activation of the K-*ras* oncogene and loss of the long arm of chromosome 18 are important events in increasing growth of the adenomas.
- Mutation and/or loss of the *TP53* tumour-suppressor gene is associated with progression from adenoma to carcinoma.

Abnormalities in a number of other genes, notably those such as *hMLH1* and *hMSH2* involved in DNA repair, have also been noted in patients with Lynch syndrome (see Special Study Topic 9.2) and in a proportion of sporadic carcinomas. Defects in these genes can be detected as alterations in non-coding DNA termed 'microsatellite' instability. This abnormality is also commonly seen in serrated neoplasms, which also show frequent increased methylation and consequent inactivation of promotor regions of tumour-suppressor genes.

### Adenoma and Carcinoma of the Small Intestine

Primary neoplasms of the small intestinal mucosa are very uncommon in comparison with the incidence of such neoplasms in the colorectum. An exception to this rule is the area of duodenum around the ampulla of Vater, where adenomatous lesions are well recognized. These may progress to invasive adenocarcinoma, and are more common in patients with FAP. Adenomas and carcinomas of the small intestine have similar microscopic appearances to their large bowel equivalents.

### Endocrine Tumours

Cells of neuroendocrine type are seen admixed throughout the epithelial cell population of the intestines (also in the stomach and lungs). These are defined by the presence of neurosecretory granules. Cells of this type produce a wide range of peptides, which may be active either locally or systemically. Neoplasms of such cells are usually called carcinoids in clinical practice but the term 'endocrine cell tumour' is now preferred. The most common site of origin of such tumours is in the midgut-derived epithelium of the ileum and appendix (see below for details of appendiceal tumours). As a rule these neoplasms all have malignant potential but many are very indolent. Ileal tumours are of low-grade malignancy, and not infrequently metastasize to local nodes or the liver. These neoplasms may present with local effects (e.g. obstruction, intussusception) or by systemic effects of active products produced by the tumour. Foregut endocrine tumours (including islet cell pancreatic neoplasms) may produce hormones such as gastrin or insulin. Midgut neoplasms more often produce smaller active products such as 5-HT. This is passed in the portal circulation to the liver where it is inactivated to 5-hydroxyindoleacetic acid (5-HIAA). Elevated 5-HIAA levels in urine can be used as an aid in diagnosing these tumours. Carcinoid syndrome is a systemic disorder characterized by flushing attacks, diarrhoea, and, occasionally, endothelial thickening of the right side of the heart, leading to tricuspid and pulmonary stenosis. This syndrome is usually seen when intestinal carcinoids have metastasized to the liver, and 5-HT is therefore released directly into the systemic circulation.

### Intestinal Lymphoma

Lymphomas (see Chapter 8) in the gastrointestinal tract are most frequently seen in the stomach (55%), with most of the remaining cases arising in the intestines. Indeed, lymphoma is the most common form of small intestinal malignancy. Most tumours are of B-cell origin. T-cell lymphomas are rarer, but show a strong association with coeliac disease and are most commonly found in the small intestine. Clinically, lymphomas may present as bowel obstruction or anaemia due to chronic blood loss. The prognosis and treatment depend on the grade and stage of tumour.

## THE APPENDIX

The appendix is a vestigial narrow outpouching of the caecum that has no important physiological utility, but is very important as a focus of intra-abdominal sepsis, being a major cause of the surgical 'acute abdomen'. It is an occasional site of primary neoplasia.

## Acute Appendicitis

Although this disease is extremely common – particularly in the second and third decades of life – its aetiology is poorly understood. It is often thought to be due to luminal obstruction by impacted hard faeces (a 'faecolith'), enterobius worms, or reactive hyperplasia of the lymphoid tissue in the wall of the appendix. However, in many cases of undoubted acute appendicitis, there is no evident obstruction. The earliest morphological change is mucosal ulceration, perhaps reflecting increased intraluminal pressure. The inflammatory infiltrate spreads through the wall (acute suppurative appendicitis), rapidly causing a localized peritonitis (Fig. 9.50). The blood vessels within the appendix become thrombosed, leading to ischaemic necrosis of the wall (gangrenous appendicitis). Unchecked, the appendix is then liable to spontaneous rupture with consequent disseminated peritonitis. This condition may be rapidly fatal through the development of septicaemia. Other complications include a localized inflammatory mass in the right iliac fossa (appendix abscess), subphrenic abscess, and (via portal blood spread) hepatic abscess.

Less common causes of appendiceal inflammation include Crohn's disease, ulcerative colitis, tuberculosis, and involvement in infection by *Yersinia pseudotuberculosis*.

## Appendiceal Neoplasms

The appendix may give rise to epithelial neoplasms, which tend to produce large amounts of mucus. Most present as a dilated appendix ('mucocele') and show no evidence of tumour invasion beyond the mucosa. These are generally cytologically low-grade neoplasms. Rupture of such a lesion can lead to peritoneal dissemination of the mucus-producing tumour cells, which turns the abdomen into a gelatinous mass – a condition known clinically as pseudomyxoma peritonei. Frankly malignant adenocarcinomas, similar to those in the colon, do occur in the appendix, but are rare. In women, mucinous tumours of the appendix may present with ovarian enlargement as a result of spread to the ovary. The possibility of a primary appendiceal tumour must therefore be considered in all patients with a mucinous ovarian tumour (see Chapter 14, pp. 432–433).

The appendix is a well-recognized site of development of endocrine tumours. Most are identified incidentally at appendicectomy and have an excellent prognosis. One subtype, the goblet cell or adenocarcinoid, is more aggressive in its course.

## THE ANUS

The anal canal is an ectodermal inpouching that typically measures 4 cm in length. It is lined by stratified squamous epithelium, and is continuous externally with the skin at the anal verge and internally with the rectum at the dentate (pectinate) line. The anus is susceptible to a number of disease conditions including fistulae and fissures. It is commonly involved in Crohn's disease. Cutaneous disease (dermatitis, psoriasis, and so on) may also involve the anal canal and perianal skin.

### Haemorrhoids

These are prominent vascular cushions straddling the anorectal junction. In association with high intraluminal pressure they may become abnormally prominent and congested, and may even prolapse and ulcerate. Bleeding from haemorrhoids is common. The mere presence of these lesions does not exclude more significant pathology because they are not uncommonly associated with neoplasms or anal fissures.

### Rectal Prolapse

Protrusion of part of the wall of the rectum into the anal canal is most commonly seen in women. If the mucosa alone is involved, the presentation may be as a solitary rectal ulcer, which can be identified on biopsy by a characteristic pattern of crypt hyperplasia and congestion, fibrosis, and muscularization of the lamina propria. These lesions may closely mimic malignant ulcers on clinical assessment.

### Anal Neoplasms

Squamous carcinoma is the most common and important anal neoplasm. This disease shows a strong epidemiological association with HPV infection and especially (as with carcinoma of the uterine cervix) with HPV types 16 and 18. Preinvasive disease can be identified as anal intraepithelial neoplasia, often in anal warts (condylomata). Much more rarely the anus may be the primary site of a malignant melanoma.

## THE PERITONEUM

The peritoneum is a serous membrane lined by mesothelial cells. Similar to the pleura and pericardium, it has a parietal

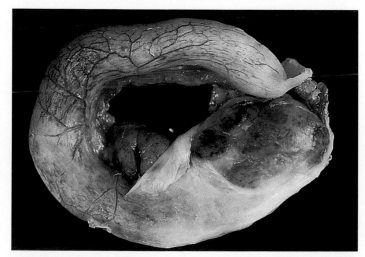

FIG. 9.50 Appendicectomy specimen: the tip of the appendix is swollen, haemorrhagic, and partly covered by a purulent white exudate, typical of acute appendicitis.

layer lining the abdominal wall and a visceral layer covering the organs (principally the gut) that protrude into the abdominal cavity.

## Peritonitis

This term is normally used to describe acute inflammation of the peritoneum. The great majority of cases are due to perforation of a viscus (e.g. perforated peptic ulcer) or extension of inflammation from transmural inflammation of the gut (appendicitis, bowel infarction, diverticulitis). Commonly, peritonitis is diffusely spread across much of the peritoneal cavity, but may become localized (as in an appendicular, subphrenic, or diverticular abscess). So-called primary bacterial peritonitis (i.e. not associated with underlying visceral disease) is rare.

## Peritoneal Neoplasms

The peritoneum is a common site of secondary spread of neoplasms, often by direct spread of neoplastic cells from underlying organs (stomach, colon, pancreas, ovary). This occurrence may give rise to fluid accumulation (ascites). Occasionally, tumour cells may appear to migrate across the peritoneal cavity, forming distinct secondary deposits in other organs. The best example of this is Krukenberg's tumour, which involves the spread of diffuse-type gastric adenocarcinoma to the ovary.

Primary malignant mesothelioma may develop in the peritoneum. Similar to the more common pleural mesothelioma, there is a strong link to asbestos exposure.

## 9.2 Special Study Topic

### FAMILIAL PREDISPOSITION TO COLORECTAL CANCER

It has long been recognized that large-bowel cancers cluster in some families. This is most clearly manifest in FAP, a condition in which numerous adenomatous polyps develop from childhood. In untreated affected individuals, carcinoma is inevitable by about age 40 years. FAP is readily recognizable in affected patients because of its obvious phenotype. Although adenomatous polyps define the clinical feature in FAP, there are a number of other associated abnormalities, including abdominal desmoid tumours, osteomas, and retinal abnormalities. Family studies showed that inheritance was clearly of the autosomal dominant type, with a high degree of penetrance. The gene responsible for the condition (called adenomatous polyposis coli, APC) was eventually mapped to a locus on the long arm of chromosome 5 (5q21). APC mutations have been identified in varying regions of this large gene, and there is a significant correlation between site of mutation and the familial phenotype. Some mutations are associated with particularly large numbers of adenomas whereas others are associated with some of the extraintestinal manifestations occasionally seen in FAP (e.g. abdominal desmoid tumours).

The protein product of APC has been characterized as a cytoplasmic protein, the main function of which is to bind β-catenin. β-Catenin is involved in cell adhesion, and also acts as a nuclear signal, switching on a number of genes involved in cell proliferation. It may have an effect in inhibiting cell death via the apoptotic pathway. Mutation of APC leads to loss of the β-catenin-binding function. It is intuitively easy to see how the consequent deregulation of cell proliferation and disruption of cell–cell adhesion can contribute to the development of epithelial neoplasms. Increasing knowledge of the genetics of FAP has made a real contribution to the screening of affected families. In the past, all family members were regularly surveyed using colonoscopy, but now only those individuals who carry the mutation need be followed up.

APC is a typical tumour-suppressor gene in that both alleles normally need to be inactivated before a neoplasm develops. FAP patients carry the 'first hit' in the genome of all of their cells, and thus require just one acquired mutation or deletion to allow for clinical progression. In fact, APC mutations are a feature of many sporadic colorectal cancers, and mutations can be detected in the earliest stages of adenoma development. Inactivation of APC is probably the key first event in a common pathway of colorectal tumorigenesis.

A further important type of hereditary colorectal cancer has been defined in recent years – Lynch syndrome or hereditary non-polyposis colorectal cancer (HNPCC). This type was identified by looking at families in which there was an excessive incidence of large bowel malignancies, particularly occurring at a relatively young age. These families were initially defined on clinical grounds by the Amsterdam criteria:

- Three or more relatives with colorectal cancer, one of whom is a first-degree relative of both the others
- At least two generations affected
- At least one case diagnosed before the age of 50 years.

It was noted that such families manifested some unusual features. Some showed an excessive incidence of certain extracolonic tumours (e.g. carcinomas of endometrium, ovary, stomach). The colonic tumours themselves have certain definable features in patients with Lynch syndrome. They tend to arise in the proximal (right) colon, and to secrete more mucus than most colonic tumours. Individual tumours also have a better prognosis than sporadic cancers. Biologically, these neoplasms are also distinct in having a low incidence of APC, ras, and p53 mutations. They are characterized by a particular abnormality defined by variability in the sequences of the microsatellite regions of DNA within the tumour cells, when compared with normal cellular DNA from the same patient (microsatellites are regions of non-coding DNA often containing long sequences of CA repeats). This 'microsatellite instability' was recognized as similar to that seen in bacteria and yeast deficient for DNA-mismatch repair

## Special Study Topic continued . . .

proteins. The genes responsible for the human condition (*hMSH2* and *hMLH1* among others) vary in different kindreds, but their products are known to be involved in this important mechanism of DNA repair.

Lynch syndrome is more difficult to recognize than FAP because affected individuals do not have numerous polyps. At present, it seems prudent to look for mutations in younger patients in whom the tumours show microsatellite instability, and then to screen family members accordingly.

Large numbers of families remain in which there is an undoubted predisposition to colorectal cancer but the genetic defect has not as yet been characterized. Ongoing developments in molecular genetics will undoubtedly increase our understanding of these issues and allow for increased opportunities for population screening.

### Further Reading

van Wenzel T, Middeldorp A, Wijnen JT, Morreau H. A review of the genetic background and tumour profiling in familial colorectal cancer. *Mutagenesis* 2012;**27**:239–245.

## SUMMARY

Gastrointestinal disease includes many of the common congenital, inflammatory, and neoplastic human disorders. In the upper gastrointestinal tract, reflux of gastroduodenal contents into the oesophagus is associated with the increasingly frequent occurrence of Barrett's oesophagus and adenocarcinoma. *Helicobacter pylori* infection of the stomach is a very significant cause of disease, including gastric and duodenal ulceration, gastric adenocarcinoma, and MALT lymphoma. Malabsorption of nutrients has numerous causes, including important small intestinal disorders, particularly coeliac disease. There are two major types of idiopathic inflammatory bowel disease: Crohn's disease is a granulomatous condition that may affect any part of the gastrointestinal tract, whereas ulcerative colitis is a mucosal disorder affecting only the large bowel. Colorectal carcinoma is one of the most common internal malignancies, arising most commonly on a background of adenomatous polyps. The prognosis is strongly dependent on tumour stage.

## ACKNOWLEDGEMENTS

The contributions of David Levison and the late D Gordon MacDonald to this chapter in the 14th edition are gratefully acknowledged.

## FURTHER READING

Odze RD, Goldblum JR, Crawford JM. *Surgical Pathology of the GI Tract, Liver, Biliary Tract, and Pancreas*, 2nd edn. Philadelphia, PA: Saunders, 2008.

Rosai J. *Rosai and Ackerman's Surgical Pathology*, 10th edn. London: Mosby, 2011: Chapters 11 and 12.

Shepherd NA, Warren BF, Williams GT, *et al. Morson and Dawson's Gastrointestinal Pathology*, 5th edn. Oxford: Blackwell Publishing, 2013.

# 10

# THE LIVER, GALLBLADDER, AND PANCREAS

Dina G Tiniakos and Alastair D Burt

## THE LIVER

### Normal Structure

> **Key Points**
>
> - The liver is a large metabolically active organ involved in homeostasis and detoxification.
> - The predominant cell type is the hepatocyte.
> - Hepatocytes can be injured by a range of insults but have remarkable capacity for regeneration.

The liver is an important, multifunctional organ with major roles in the synthesis of plasma proteins, in detoxification and excretion of potentially toxic exogenous and endogenous substances, and in digestion and absorption through the secretion of bile. It receives a dual blood supply from the hepatic artery and portal vein, and drains through the sinusoids via the hepatic veins to the inferior vena cava. The portal venous system draws blood from the intestine and therefore everything that is absorbed from the gut passes through the liver before entering the systemic circulation. Failure of this metabolic guardian function in liver disease is an important determinant of clinical symptoms.

Bile passes in the opposite direction to blood flow, from the canaliculus formed between two hepatocytes to the bile ducts. Three structures – the hepatic arteriole, portal venule, and biliary duct – form the so-called portal triad that is embedded within loose connective tissue; this is one of the key structural landmarks at a microscopic level in the liver. The boundary between the portal tract (the fibrovascular connective tissue and the portal triad) and adjacent hepatocytes is called the limiting plate.

The intrahepatic biliary tree originates from the surrounding developing liver and this process involves complex control of cell proliferation, migration, and programmed cell death. Failure of this process during intrauterine life can result in a spectrum of 'ductal plate malformations' causing failure of normal bile flow in infancy and later life, e.g. mutation of the gene *Jagged-1* is associated with the failure of differentiation or survival of bile ducts resulting in atresia of ducts seen as part of Alagille's syndrome (Fig. 10.1). Mutations in *PKD* genes encoding polycystins, proteins found in the primary cilia of bile duct cells (and renal tubule cells), result in a common hereditary disease with cysts in multiple organs including the liver.

It is convenient to think of the liver microanatomy in zones, loosely defined geographical areas corresponding to particular functions of the liver. Over the years a number of different systems have been developed, but there is still controversy over which is the best. In the older lobular concept the terminal venule, draining blood from the parenchyma and returning it to the inferior vena cava, is the focus and is at the centre of the lobule (Fig. 10.2A). Thus blood flows from the corners of the lobule through the sinusoids into the terminal hepatic venules. This model is useful in explaining the haemodynamics of portal hypertension caused by obstruction to blood flow. In the acinar model, the territory supplied by the blood vessels traversing the portal tracts is known as the acinar unit, and it in turn is divided into three zones (Fig. 10.2B,C). It is apparent that zone 1 is better oxygenated and this is where many synthetic processes, such as albumin production, occur. By contrast, zone 3 has many enzymes involved in phase 1 (oxidative) and phase 2 (conjugative) detoxification reactions. It experiences lower oxygen tensions and is thus more vulnerable to both toxic and ischaemic injury. Note that in this model some zone 3 hepatocytes actually lie very close to the portal tract.

Within the parenchyma of the liver there is a complex network of cells. Although the predominant cell type is the

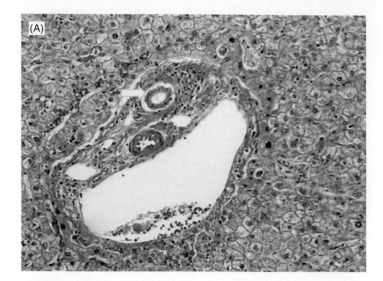

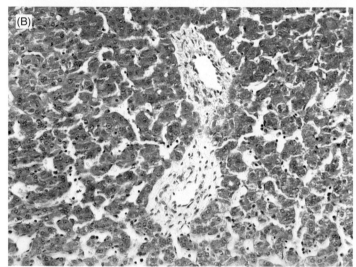

FIG. 10.1 Comparison of normal liver (A) with a biopsy from a child with Alagille's syndrome (B). In normal liver the portal tracts contain a bile duct (arrow), portal vein, and hepatic artery but in Alagille's syndrome the bile duct is missing.

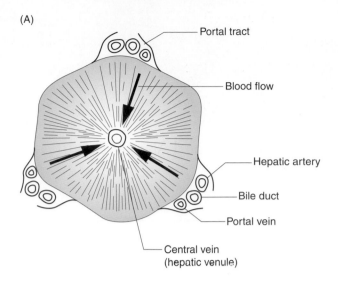

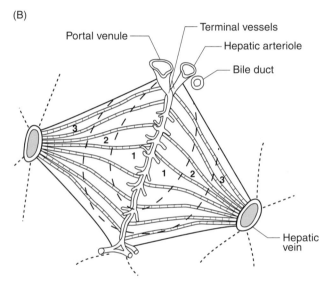

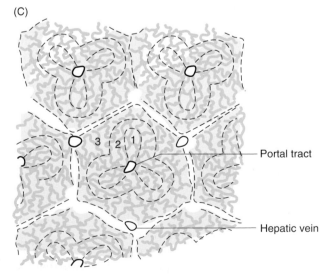

FIG. 10.2 Comparison of lobular and acinar models of the liver microarchitecture: (A) hepatic lobule arranged round a single central (hepatic) vein into which blood flows. (B) Simple acinus arranged around a hepatic artery branch. (C) Relationship between adjacent acini in the liver.

hepatocyte, a significant number of other cells, both resident and transitory, are important. Hepatocytes are arranged in plates, lining the blood-filled sinusoids. Sinusoidal endothelial cells are fenestrated, allowing direct access of hepatocytes to constituents of the blood. On the sinusoidal endothelial wall lie phagocytic Kupffer cells and within the perisinusoidal space of Disse are the hepatic stellate cells; these are myofibroblast precursors important in liver fibrosis (Fig. 10.3). Liver-specific natural killer (NK) cells are located within the space of Disse and play an important role in the innate immune system response to viral infections. When liver cells are injured, regeneration is rapid and may be complete. Proliferation of hepatocytes can occur anywhere in the acinus, although experimental studies suggest that there is a reserve of hepatic progenitor cells close to the portal tract, within the canal of Hering, the ductular compartment

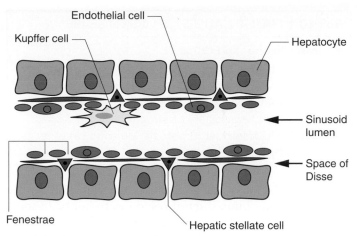

Kupffer cell — Endothelial cell — Hepatocyte — Sinusoid lumen — Space of Disse — Fenestrae — Hepatic stellate cell

FIG. 10.3 Schematic diagram of liver parenchyma and sinusoids.

connecting the bile canaliculi to the bile ductules at the limiting plate. The hepatic progenitor cells are capable of differentiating into hepatocytes and/or bile duct cells (cholangiocytes) when toxic injury or extensive hepatic necrosis precludes regeneration of mature hepatocytes.

## Liver Function Tests

A set of biochemical investigations is commonly requested as part of the initial clinical workup of all patients with suspected liver disease. Although the variables measured can give vital information to the clinician and the pathologist interpreting a biopsy, a number of important caveats need to be borne in mind to avoid over-interpretation of tests. First, the liver is frequently involved as a bystander in many cases of systemic illness. Do not assume that because liver function tests are abnormal the liver is the main site of disease. Second, the tests are a package and should not individually be regarded as specific. Thus a raised bilirubin may indicate not only failure of liver excretory function but also increased breakdown of red blood cells. *Table 10.1* shows the major liver function tests and their usefulness.

## Clinical Symptoms and Signs in Liver Disease

The liver capsule is innervated and so swelling or inflammation can cause pain. Major features alerting the clinician to the presence of significant liver disease all have a basis in pathophysiology and therefore may give important clues to the underlying liver problem. Thus itch may indicate retention of bile salts because of cholestasis, suggesting biliary disease. A tendency to bruise or bleed easily may indicate low platelet counts because portal hypertension associated with cirrhosis has caused splenic enlargement and increased destruction of platelets. Alternatively, hepatocyte necrosis caused by toxins, virus, or drugs may affect the synthetic function of the liver, which normally

TABLE **10.1** Routinely used liver function tests

| Albumin | Synthesized exclusively by hepatocytes |
| --- | --- |
| | Serum levels reduced in liver failure |
| | Low levels associated with oedema and ascites |
| Bilirubin | Serum levels increased in all forms of jaundice |
| | May be conjugated, unconjugated or mixed |
| | Normal levels <20 μmol/L |
| Aminotransferases | Aspartate and alanine aminotransferases |
| | Released by injured hepatocytes |
| | Surrogate marker of liver cell necrosis but poor prognostic indicator |
| Alkaline phosphatase | Enzyme present in bile canaliculi |
| | Elevated levels in cholestatic liver disease (impaired bile flow) |
| | Other extrahepatic sources including bone |
| γ-Glutamyl transpeptidase | Also elevated in cholestatic disorders |
| | Enzyme induced by ethanol |
| | Surrogate marker of alcohol misuse |
| Prothrombin time | Reflects changes in levels of coagulation factors |
| | Prolonged in liver failure due to decreased synthesis of several clotting factors including those that are vitamin K dependent |

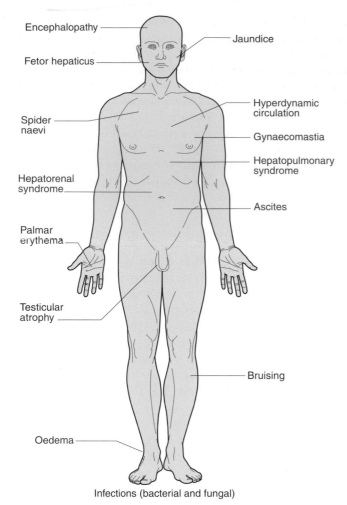

Encephalopathy

Fetor hepaticus

Spider naevi

Hepatorenal syndrome

Palmar erythema

Testicular atrophy

Oedema

Jaundice

Hyperdynamic circulation

Gynaecomastia

Hepatopulmonary syndrome

Ascites

Bruising

Infections (bacterial and fungal)

**Fig. 10.4** Features of hepatic failure.

---

produces most of the essential clotting factors (Fig. 10.4). In broad terms the serious complications of liver disease can be divided into:

- manifestations of hepatic failure
- effects of portal hypertension (e.g. bleeding oesophageal varices)
- risk of liver cancer.

## Patterns of Injury and Causes of Liver Disease

The liver is susceptible to a wide range of insults and liver disease is an important cause of morbidity and mortality worldwide. The major causes of liver disease are outlined in *Box 10.1*. In broad terms, clinical disease can be regarded as being either acute or chronic. With acute liver injury the patient will either die of liver failure if the disease process is severe (or require liver transplantation) or recover completely. By contrast, with chronic liver disease there is frequently progressive inflammation and scarring; this is accompanied by attempts at regeneration by surviving liver cells and cirrhosis develops. Patients with cirrhosis are then at risk of developing a malignant tumour, hepatocellular carcinoma.

---

> **Box 10.1** MAJOR CAUSES OF LIVER DISEASE
>
> - Toxic: alcohol and drugs
> - Viruses: hepatitis B and C
> - Autoimmune disease: primary biliary cirrhosis; autoimmune hepatitis
> - Cholestasis: e.g. biliary obstruction by gallstones
> - Metabolic: haemochromatosis; Wilson's disease; $\alpha_1$-antitrypsin deficiency

Despite the many diverse causes of liver disease, the liver has a rather limited set of responses to injury. In some conditions the injury is manifest by accumulation of lipids within the hepatocytes: this is a central theme in alcoholic liver disease and in liver injury associated with the so-called metabolic syndrome (type 2 diabetes, hypertension, obesity, and dyslipidaemia) – the fatty liver diseases. In many disorders there is irreversible liver cell injury through either necrosis or apoptosis (see Chapter 4, pp. 52–56). Inflammation is a common feature, particularly in chronic conditions. The predominant inflammatory cell type is the T lymphocyte; these cells may have a key role in liver cell apoptosis. In response to liver cell loss, there is regeneration of surviving epithelial cells as noted above. In some situations there may be massive liver cell necrosis, where most of the parenchyma is lost; in such circumstances there may then not be sufficient critical mass of surviving cells to repopulate the liver. When there is persistent injury and inflammation there is stimulation of a repair process involving the hepatic stellate cells; this leads to the development of fibrosis and is discussed more fully in Chapter 4.

## Viral Hepatitis

Most clinically significant forms of viral hepatitis are caused by a disparate group of viruses known as hepatitis viruses (A, B, C, D, E). In addition a number of other viruses including Epstein–Barr virus, cytomegalovirus, rubella, and arboviruses (causing yellow fever) may at times be responsible for liver dysfunction. By convention, hepatitis is used to refer to diffuse liver injury, although the severity of the injury may be heterogeneous within the liver. The clinical presentation is variable. Acute hepatitis A infection often presents with general malaise, anorexia, and sometimes abdominal discomfort and liver tenderness. Only after this does the patient develop jaundice; thereafter recovery tends to occur. Sometimes presentation is with florid, overwhelming liver failure. Other forms of viral hepatitis may present similarly with an acute hepatitis but more often the onset may be insidious with presentation only after evidence of chronic disease is present.

### Hepatitis Viruses

Hepatitis A virus characteristically produces a mild illness and full recovery occurs. Hepatitis B and C virus infections frequently result in chronic hepatitis, leading to cirrhosis and even hepatocellular carcinoma. Hepatitis D synergizes with hepatitis B to produce more severe disease. Hepatitis E infection generally resolves after a mild illness but pregnant women sometimes develop life-threatening liver failure. Hepatitis G virus is a more recent discovery but it is not considered a major pathogen in causing viral liver disease. A summary of the main hepatitis viruses is provided in *Table 10.2*.

## Histology

Morphologically, there is very little qualitative difference between the effects of the different hepatitis viruses, although the severity may vary and the underlying mechanisms of hepatocyte death differ. Hepatitis A virus is thought to be directly cytopathic whereas hepatitis B and C viruses destroy hepatocytes by virtue of the cytotoxic T-cell response to virally infected cells. Many hepatocytes show sublethal injury in the form of cloudy swelling or hydropic change, but there is also programmed cell death (apoptosis). Shrunken, pyknotic cells are clearly visible in biopsies (Fig. 10.5). In severe cases there may be bridging necrosis linking adjacent portal tracts and even massive widespread necrosis (Fig. 10.5). This is associated clinically with fulminant liver failure. Associated with this is a lymphoid infiltrate in the sinusoids and portal tracts. Sinusoidal Kupffer cells are activated and prominent; many contain ceroid pigment, which

**TABLE 10.2** Viral hepatitides

|  | A | B | C | D | E |
|---|---|---|---|---|---|
| Virus | RNA | DNA | RNA | Defective RNA | RNA |
| Spread | Faecal–oral | Blood products; sexually; intravenous drug use; mother to child | Blood products; intravenous drug use; sporadic | Probably as for hepatitis B | Faecal–oral |
| Incubation period | 15–40 days | 50–180 days | 40–75 days | Co-infection with B or subsequent infection | 30–50 days |
| Pathogenesis | Direct cytopathic | Triggers immune destruction | ? Immune | Synergizes with B | ? Direct |
| Chronicity | No | Yes | Yes | Yes | No |
| Geographical distribution | Worldwide | Worldwide | Worldwide | Endemic in southern Europe and the Middle East | Predominantly Asia; increasing incidence in Europe after exposure to undercooked pork |
| Diagnosis | IgM to virus | e antigen = infective; IgG to s antigen indicates previous infection | Antibody to HCV; HCV RNA detected by polymerase chain reaction | Protein present in hepatocyte nuclei | Antibody to hepatitis E virus; HEV RNA detected by polymerase chain reaction |

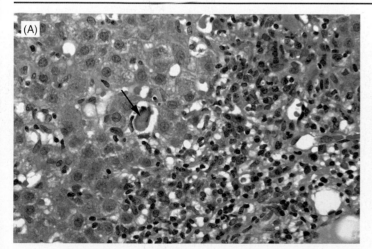
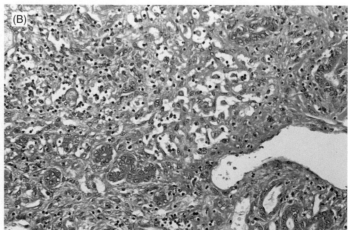

**FIG. 10.5** Liver cell necrosis in hepatitis: (A) an acidophil (apoptotic) body (arrow) – the dead hepatocyte – is surrounded by lymphocytes. (B) Massive necrosis where there are few remaining hepatocytes. The ductular structures seen here represent an attempt at regeneration.

represents phagocytosed debris from dead hepatocytes. In infection caused by hepatitis A virus plasma cells may be prominent in portal areas. Bilirubinostasis is common, with bile accumulated in hepatocytes and canaliculi.

As the liver can rapidly regenerate, evidence of hepatocyte proliferation such as mitotic figures and binucleate cells can be seen, even during acute disease. Resolution results in structurally normal liver with no fibrosis, although a mild increase in chronic inflammatory cells may persist in portal areas for more than 6 months. Sometimes the viral hepatitis enters a chronic stage and may even progress to cirrhosis. This is particularly the case with hepatitis C in which some 85% of infected individuals fail to clear the virus; many of these patients develop progressive fibrosis and cirrhosis. With hepatitis B, around 5% go on to become chronic carriers. In some parts of the world individuals are infected early in life through infected mothers; many of these go on to get chronic disease with ultimately cirrhosis and hepatocellular carcinoma. It is estimated that some 350–400 million people worldwide are chronic carriers of hepatitis B virus. Nevertheless, hepatitis B is a preventable disease and a safe and effective vaccine is available.

## Chronic Hepatitis

Liver inflammation persisting for more than 6 months without sustained improvement is defined as chronic hepatitis. However, the disease may have a fluctuating course in terms of injury, as assessed biochemically or by liver biopsy. A spectrum of biopsy changes is seen depending on disease activity which itself may be modulated by immunosuppressive drugs and the underlying cause. The pathological features are illustrated in Fig. 10.6. The hallmark of chronic hepatitis is the presence of so-called interface hepatitis. This is a process of chronic inflammation, leading to hepatocyte death and fibrosis, which occurs at the limiting plate of the portal tracts. If interface hepatitis is severe then bridging necrosis and fibrosis occur between adjacent portal regions, leading to the rapid evolution of cirrhosis.

Chronic hepatitis is often perceived as being complicated and confusing. This is in part because the causes, clinical features, biochemical and immunological findings, and morphological features overlap but are not interchangeable. In other words, every case of chronic hepatitis should be regarded as a syndrome and the task of the investigating clinician is to discern as much as possible about each of these components, e.g. clinically a patient may have signs of liver disease. Immunologically there may be evidence of autoimmunity but this does not indicate whether there is cirrhosis. A biopsy may show cirrhosis but this does not necessarily give a reason for the underlying disease, and so on. Therefore it must be stressed that the biopsy diagnosis of chronic hepatitis is a morphological statement. Further clinical, imaging, and serological investigation will be required to establish the aetiology in most cases (*Table 10.3*).

A number of attempts have been made to 'score' the severity of liver disease histologically on a liver biopsy. Each approach has its strengths and weaknesses, but it is valid and useful to comment on the amount of cell destruction and the extent of fibrosis. Both factors contribute to prognosis and inform on the benefits of therapeutic intervention. In recent years, the role of liver biopsy in chronic hepatitis has diminished due to improved therapy with novel antiviral agents and the evolution of non-invasive methods for the assessment of advanced liver fibrosis (transient elastography and/or scores based on combinations of serum biomarkers with clinical data).

## Biliary Disease (*Table 10.4*)

### Key Points

- The liver conjugates and excretes toxic substances in bile. Failure of this pathway leads to cholestasis, which in turn causes secondary damage to the hepatocytes.
- If prolonged cholestasis occurs then cirrhosis may ensue.
- Primary biliary disease (primary biliary cirrhosis and primary sclerosing cholangitis) is generally autoimmune.
- Secondary biliary disease is usually related to obstruction, either intrinsic such as tumour or gallstones or extrinsic such as liver flukes.

### Primary Biliary Disease

In primary biliary disease there is destruction of bile ducts by immunological mechanisms. Damage to hepatocytes and subsequent fibrosis combined with hepatocyte regeneration lead to cirrhosis.

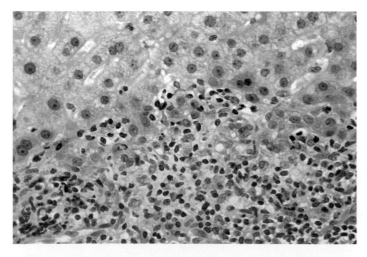

**FIG. 10.6** Chronic hepatitis: so-called interface hepatitis in which there is inflammation and death of hepatocytes at the limiting plate between the parenchyma and the portal tract.

**TABLE 10.3** Aetiology and diagnosis of chronic hepatitis

| Aetiology | Clinical features | Biochemical | Immunology | Additional biopsy features |
|---|---|---|---|---|
| Autoimmune | F > M; peak 15–20 and 45–55 years Other autoimmune diseases | – | Antinuclear antibody (Ab) Antismooth muscle Ab | May be frequent plasma cells |
| Hepatitis B | M > F; any age; more severe disease if hepatitis D virus is co-present | – | HBe and HBs Ags (antigens) present | HBsAg detected in hepatocytes by immunohistochemistry |
| Hepatitis C | Any age; often post-transfusion, homosexual, or intravenous drug use | – | Anti-HCV Abs HCV RNA present | Steatosis; lymphoid aggregates in portal tracts |
| Idiopathic and drug induced | Methyldopa; isoniazid | – | Often have autoantibodies | Similar to autoimmune |
| $\alpha_1$-Antitrypsin deficiency | Late childhood/young adult presentation; may have emphysema; defect in $\alpha_1$-antitrypsin secretion; homozygous ZZ phenotype causes disease | – | Low serum $\alpha_1$-antitrypsin abnormal phenotype | Accumulation of $\alpha_1$-antitrypsin, periodic acid–Schiff-positive globules in hepatocytes |
| Wilson's disease | Kayser–Fleischer rings in cornea Lenticular degeneration in brain | Low serum ceruloplasmin | – | Excess copper and copper-binding protein in liver |

**TABLE 10.4** Biliary disease

| Disease | Clinical features | Biochemistry | Immunology | Biopsy | Other |
|---|---|---|---|---|---|
| Primary biliary cirrhosis | F > M 9:1 Itch; xanthelasma | Very high alkaline phosphatase | Anti-mitochondrial antibodies (AMAs) | Granulomas; small bile duct destruction; chronic inflammation | Cirrhosis |
| Primary sclerosing cholangitis | M > F 3:1 Two-thirds have ulcerative colitis | Very high alkaline phosphatase | Antibodies to neutrophil cytoplasmic antigens (ANCAs) HLA-B8, -DRW52, -DR3 and -DR2 association | Fibrous obliteration of larger ducts; chronic inflammation | Risk of cholangiocarcinoma |
| Obstruction (secondary) | Any age Gallstones; tumours; parasites | High alkaline phosphatase; very high bilirubin | – | Bile lakes; acute inflammation | Risk of ascending infection |

## Primary Biliary Cirrhosis

In primary biliary cirrhosis there is a chronic inflammatory infiltrate in portal tracts, and lymphocytes can be seen migrating into the biliary epithelium which then degenerates and dies. This disease primarily affects small bile ducts and may also destroy the canals of Hering. Approximately a quarter of biopsies contain epithelioid granulomas, sometimes in the hepatic parenchyma, but often close to bile ducts (Fig. 10.7). Patients are typically women in their sixth decade who may present with jaundice or itch (pruritus), due to retention of bile salts, and a general feeling of malaise. Sometimes sequelae of cirrhosis such as ruptured oesophageal varices result in an accelerated and more dramatic presentation. The disease is often indolent and evidence may be found of abnormalities

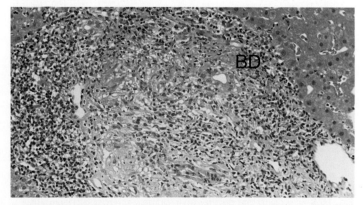

**FIG. 10.7** Primary biliary cirrhosis: an injured bile duct (BD) is surrounded by a granulomatous and lymphocytic infiltrate.

in liver function tests with the presence of anti-mitochondrial antibodies stretching back for some years if blood samples are available for testing.

### Primary Sclerosing Cholangitis

This is usually associated with ulcerative colitis. There is fibrous obliteration of bile ducts (Fig. 10.8). Larger ducts and even extrahepatic bile ducts may be affected. These patients are at risk of developing bile duct cancer – cholangiocarcinoma. In both primary biliary cirrhosis and primary sclerosing cholangitis periportal hepatocyte injury occurs and, in the early disease stages, there is often proliferation of poorly formed ductular structures (ductular reaction). This is probably a regenerative phenomenon.

### Secondary Biliary Disease

This is usually caused by bile outflow obstruction as a result of gallstones. However, bile duct carcinoma, pancreatic carcinoma, extrinsic compression of the bile duct by lymph nodes at the porta hepatis, or post-traumatic stricture may also cause obstruction. Bile accumulates in canaliculi between hepatocytes, and in Kupffer cells. It may extravasate to form bile lakes. These are more common in zone 3 perivenular hepatocytes. There is an inflammatory response, predominantly of acute inflammatory cells, which is most notable in the portal tracts. Oedema in the portal tracts is often marked and there may be a very extensive ductular reaction, irregularly dilated bile ducts, and distorted ductules with degenerative epithelial changes. Prolonged obstruction leads to bridging fibrosis between adjacent portal areas and eventual cirrhosis.

## Alcoholic Liver Disease and Other Fatty Liver Diseases

Alcohol is one of the most common causes of liver disease in developed countries. It can produce acute reversible injury (steatosis or fatty change) or irreversible changes characterized by hepatocyte death and fibrosis (alcoholic hepatitis and cirrhosis).

### Pathogenesis

Habitual alcohol intake induces the microsomal ethanol oxidizing system (particularly the cytochrome P450 CYP2E1). This, in addition to alcohol dehydrogenases, produces acetaldehyde and depletes the cell of nicotinamide adenosine dinucleotide phosphate (reduced form) (NADPH). These changes directly cause triglyceride accumulation, leading to fatty change as well as cell death. The inflammatory response to cell death includes cytokine production which triggers hepatic stellate cells to synthesize collagen.

### Steatosis

Hepatocytes become swollen as the cytoplasm accumulates globules of fat, particularly evident in zone 3 where alcohol-metabolizing enzymes predominate. Steatosis is not specific to alcohol injury: it is also seen in obesity, diabetes, drug toxicity (corticosteroids, tamoxifen, and so on), malabsorption syndromes, malnutrition, and rare metabolic diseases. It is normally reversible but can in some cases cause massive enlargement of the liver (Fig. 10.9).

### Alcoholic hepatitis

Hepatocytes lose osmotic control and become ballooned and hydropic. Occasional cells undergo necrosis and elicit a focal neutrophil response (spotty necrosis). The cytoskeleton of cells is damaged and aggregates of misfolded keratin intermediate filaments associated with ubiquitin and heat-shock proteins are visible as Mallory–Denk bodies (previously known as Mallory's hyaline) (Fig. 10.10). Although not specific this is a useful diagnostic clue.

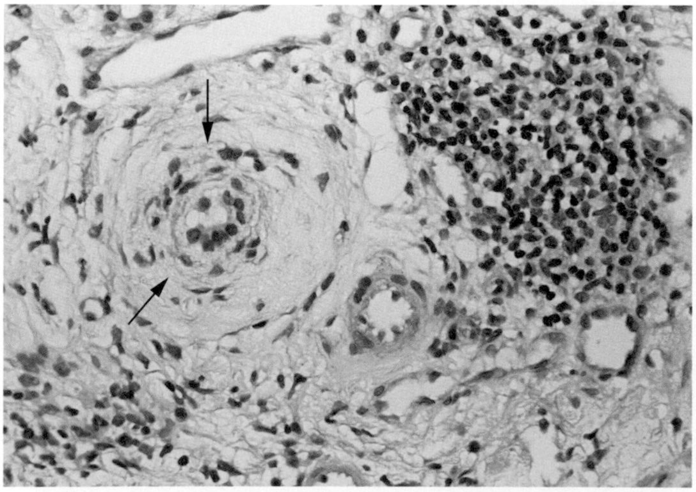

FIG. 10.8 Sclerosing bile duct lesion in primary sclerosing cholangitis. An 'onion skin'-like cuff of collagen is seen around a degenerate bile duct (arrows).

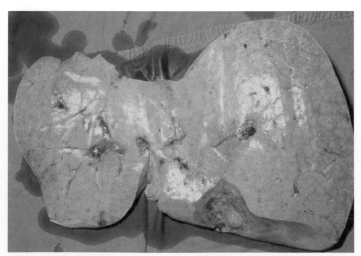

FIG. 10.9 Massive fatty liver: this was the appearance *post mortem* of the liver of a middle-aged female with an 11-year history of alcohol misuse. The liver weighed 2890 g, over twice the normal weight.

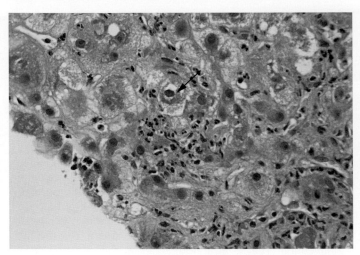

FIG. 10.10 Alcoholic hepatitis: this shows a ballooned hepatocyte (arrow) containing a large Mallory–Denk body and surrounded by polymorphs.

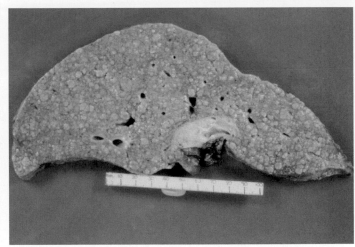

FIG. 10.11 End-stage cirrhosis in a patient with fatty liver disease.

## Cirrhosis

Progressive injury and fibrosis lead to fibrous septa, which join adjacent perivenular regions. Portal–venous bridging also occurs. Within these small delineated regions, regenerative hepatocytes form nodules (micronodular cirrhosis). In the long term a significant proportion of patients with cirrhosis may develop hepatocellular carcinoma.

## Non-alcoholic Fatty Liver Disease

A condition that is histologically similar to alcoholic steatosis and steatohepatitis is increasingly encountered in obese patients; in such patient populations there is a high incidence of type 2 diabetes mellitus and other features of the metabolic syndrome, a constellation of disorders related to adverse cardiovascular outcomes. Patients are usually discovered to have abnormal liver function tests, after blood testing for complaints of liver tenderness or tiredness without markers of other liver disease (viral, autoimmune, or drug induced). On imaging, they have evidence of fatty liver ('bright liver'). The underlying pathogenesis is thought to be related to an insulin-resistant state with oversupply of fatty acids, coupled with altered fatty acid metabolism. The accumulation of triglycerides in the fat droplets, leading to steatosis, is now considered an adaptive protective response, whereas lipotoxic metabolites of hepatocellular free fatty acids are considered major players in inducing steatohepatitis, the progressive form of non-alcoholic fatty liver disease that may lead to cirrhosis (Fig. 10.11). Steatosis usually has a benign course but there are now well-documented instances of slow progression to cirrhosis. The importance of the condition is its increasing prevalence related to the obesity 'epidemic', its relationship to treatable or preventable conditions such as diabetes and obesity, and the necessity to ensure that patients are not falsely accused of secret excessive alcohol consumption and the attendant stigma associated with it.

## Drug-induced Liver Injury

This may be a predictable, dose-related toxic injury (e.g. paracetamol/acetaminophen) or an unpredictable, idiosyncratic reaction (such as the immunological injury present in halothane hepatitis). The injury may be primarily hepatotoxic (e.g. paracetamol) or cholestatic (e.g. chlorpromazine), or mixed ('cholestatic hepatitis', e.g. amoxicillin). The possibility of an adverse drug reaction should always be considered in patients taking medication who have abnormal liver function biochemistry. Drugs may produce all forms of acute, chronic, or vascular liver disease, and have been incriminated in causing liver tumours (e.g. anabolic and contraceptive steroids). Some herbal agents may rarely be responsible for serious liver injury (e.g. germander, bush teas), so enquiries for ingestion of herbal remedies should be included routinely when taking a patient's drug history.

## Storage Diseases

$\alpha_1$-Antitrypsin deficiency and Wilson's disease have already been mentioned under chronic hepatitis. Many other lipid and glycogen storage diseases affect the liver but their precise description is beyond the scope of this book. Haemochromatosis is a condition that results in enhanced absorption of iron from the gut and a gross excess of iron stored in the liver (more than 10 times normal). It is usually autosomal recessive. The gene responsible for the most common form of the disorder, HFE, is on chromosome 6 and in linkage disequilibrium with HLA-A3. Two common mutations together explain more than 80% of cases. Recently other (non-HFE) genetic defects have been identified that may also lead to iron overload.

Michelle was an 18-year-old woman studying design technology at college. She had always been in good health. She drank alcohol at weekends and intermittently smoked cigarettes but she did not use recreational drugs. She lived in a flat with her boyfriend who was an unemployed labourer. The couple had a difficult relationship and after one serious argument Michelle deliberately took an overdose of 24 paracetamol tablets. She was drunk at the time and her boyfriend was unaware that she had taken the tablets. She woke up the following day feeling unwell but put this down to a bad hangover. She did not seek any medical advice about having taken the overdose. The next day she began to feel nauseous and sleepy and went to bed. By the next day she felt very unwell and her boyfriend noticed that she was a strange colour. She was rushed to hospital; by this stage she was semi-comatose and unable to give any history. After a detailed examination, it was established that she had no signs of chronic liver disease. She did, however, have jaundice (yellow pigmentation of the skin and sclera) and a peculiar smell to her breath (fetor hepaticus: see p. 276). Some bruising was also noted on her limbs.

The medical team involved in Michelle's care considered the possibility of an overdose and measured blood paracetamol levels; given the length of time since taking the tablets it is not surprising that the drug was undetectable in the blood. The team also used blood tests to assess liver and renal function. Serum albumin was reduced at 30 g/L. Serum aminotransferases (a measure of hepatocyte integrity – elevated levels indicate damage) were grossly elevated, serum alanine aminotransferase being 20 times the upper limit of normal, whereas serum alkaline phosphatase (an indicator of cholestasis: impairment of bile flow) was only mildly elevated. Blood tests revealed no evidence of viral hepatitis and there was no evidence of an immunological problem. Renal function blood tests showed a serum urea of 48 mg/dL and creatinine of 564 µmol/L, indicating renal failure. The precise cause of her problems remained a mystery to the medical team at this stage, but it was clear that she now had developed liver and kidney failure (so-called hepatorenal syndrome) and they suspected that the underlying problem was a toxic injury.

Further evidence that Michelle had hepatic failure could be found by assessing her clotting times; this showed prolongation of the prothrombin time (see p. 275) and a markedly reduced factor V level in the blood. This explained the bruising noted on her limbs; by now she also showed bleeding of her gums. She had developed a deep coma and the decision was taken to put her on the urgent organ transplantation list. Fortunately a donor was identified within a matter of hours and she underwent a 5-hour operation in which a cadaveric liver was engrafted and the damaged liver removed. The liver that was removed was examined by the pathologists. It weighed approximately 900 g (normal for this age and her body mass would be around 1400 g).

It had a mottled appearance but no distinct masses were seen. Microscopically, sections of liver showed large areas of coagulative necrosis; this had a geographical pattern and could be seen around hepatic veins but not around portal tracts (Fig. 10.12). This is described as zonal necrosis and is a classic appearance in toxin-induced liver injury such as that associated with paracetamol overdose. The distribution of damage can be explained by there being more drug-metabolizing enzymes found normally in hepatocytes around the veins than elsewhere; more toxic metabolites are generated in these cells, making them more susceptible to injury. After the transplantation surgery Michelle became alert again and all blood tests showed that her liver function had essentially returned to normal. Furthermore, her renal function also improved despite there being no specific intervention. The renal abnormalities in this situation were therefore secondary to the liver dysfunction and reversed when the hepatic function returned.

As noted elsewhere, the liver has a remarkable capacity for regeneration and after some acute insults can recover completely with a return to the normal structure and function. With Michelle, however, the degree of liver cell necrosis was such that it had exceeded the level beyond which such repair could occur, and secondary effects on other organ systems had occurred. Had she not received a transplant she would certainly have died; fortunately she made a good recovery after her operation. She admitted to the medical team that she had taken an overdose but she had not intended to take her life.

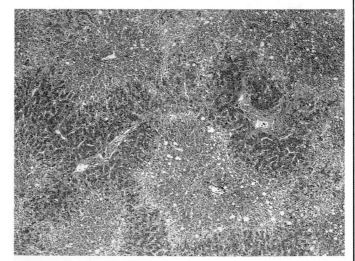

**FIG. 10.12** Histological changes in the liver removed at the time of transplantation from the patient in the case study. This shows zonal necrosis with coagulative necrosis involving all hepatocytes in the regions around hepatic veins and so-called midzones. There is some preservation of cells around the portal tracts.

The excess iron is found in hepatocytes but, as the severity of iron overload increases, it is also found in Kupffer cells and the biliary epithelium (Fig. 10.13). The presence of iron is directly fibrogenic and periportal fibrosis eventually leads to a predominantly macronodular cirrhosis. Treatment by venesection or with iron-chelating drugs such as desferrioxamine prevents disease progression. Haemochromatosis is a multisystem disease and iron is deposited in other organs.

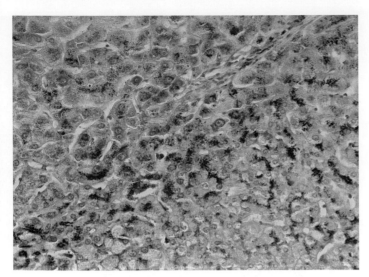

**Fig. 10.13** Genetic haemochromatosis: this shows staining of iron in hepatocytes using Perls' stain. The blue granules represent abnormal accumulation of haemosiderin; normal hepatocytes should be negative.

**TABLE 10.5** Causes of portal hypertension

| | |
|---|---|
| **Presinusoidal** | *Portal vein thrombosis* |
| | Tumour |
| | Infection |
| | *Portal tract fibrosis* |
| | Biliary cirrhosis |
| | Sarcoidosis |
| | Schistosomiasis |
| **Sinusoidal** | *Nodular regenerative hyperplasia* |
| | *Cirrhosis* |
| | *Sinusoidal fibrosis (some drugs)* |
| **Postsinusoidal** | *Veno-occlusive disease (bush teas, some drugs)* |
| | *Budd–Chiari syndrome (hepatic vein thrombosis)* |

Excess accumulation in pancreatic islets can lead to diabetes; other endocrine effects include excess melanin production, resulting in skin pigmentation – the syndrome of bronzed diabetes.

Secondary iron overload (secondary haemosiderosis) can occur in people with alcohol problems or haemoglobinopathies, and patients undergoing multiple transfusions. Iron is particularly prominent in Kupffer cells. Differentiation from primary genetic haemochromatosis may be impossible from a liver biopsy alone.

## End-stage Cirrhosis

This is the end-stage of many forms of liver injury and is defined as the presence of regenerative nodules separated by fibrous tissue septa, affecting the whole liver. Many clues to the aetiology of cirrhosis are not apparent in biopsies taken at this 'end-stage'. If serological or biochemical evidence fails to reveal a cause, then the cirrhosis is known as cryptogenic. Most cases of cryptogenic cirrhosis are probably the result of progressive non-alcoholic fatty liver disease. Patients with cirrhosis may be symptom free for long periods of time but in many there will then be decompensation with the development of hepatic failure (see Fig. 10.4).

## Portal Hypertension

This is increased blood pressure in the portal vein, >1 kPa (7 mmHg), reflecting the resistance to blood flow through grossly disturbed liver structure, as occurs in cirrhosis. It is further compounded by intrahepatic arteriovenous shunting of blood. Portal hypertension is caused by a variety of other conditions (*Table 10.5*). It leads to splenic enlargement and this may result in excessive removal of red cells and platelets from the blood – the syndrome of hypersplenism. There

is also dilatation of the plexus of venous channels around the gastric fundus and oesophagus to form varices. These varices are thin walled and bleed readily, causing torrential and life-threatening haematemesis. Portal hypertension also contributes to the development of ascites.

## Congenital Malformations

*Atresia* of the extrahepatic ducts presents in neonates with signs of biliary obstruction. It may be partial or complete. As noted above there are some inherited disorders (e.g. Alagille's syndrome) in which there is paucity or atresia of intrahepatic bile ducts. Solitary cysts, multiple cysts in association with some forms of renal cystic disease, and congenital hepatic fibrosis are part of a spectrum of abnormal duct development (ductal plate malformations). Von Meyenberg complexes (biliary microhamartomas) are small nodules, often subcapsular, formed by groups of bile duct-like structures in a fibrous stroma. Focal nodular hyperplasia is a rare tumour-like malformation most probably caused by abnormal blood flow. It is composed of nodules of regenerating hepatocytes separated by fibrous bands which often form characteristic stellate scars visible by imaging. Although this lesion is more common in females, contraceptive steroids are not implicated in its pathogenesis.

## Tumours

### Benign Tumours

Cavernous haemangiomas are found incidentally in the liver in about 2% of postmortem examinations and are considered the most common benign liver tumour. Hepatocellular adenomas are associated with the use of oral contraceptives and anabolic steroids (see Special Study Topic 10.1). They are well-defined nodules that are vascular and well differentiated. They lack biliary elements (see Fig. 10.15 in Special Study Topic 10.1).

Mucinous cystic neoplasms are rare tumours of biliary origin presenting as solitary cysts, almost exclusively in adult females. They are considered premalignant when non-invasive and should be completely excised because they may recur or develop malignancy.

## Malignant Tumours

The most common malignant tumour is metastatic carcinoma from lung, breast, gastrointestinal tract, or pancreas. About 80% of primary tumours are hepatocellular carcinomas (Fig. 10.14). Most cases arise in cirrhotic livers and may be multifocal. However, a small number arise in non-cirrhotic livers, including the fibrolamellar variant in young patients (<40 years), which has a better prognosis than the usual hepatocellular carcinoma arising in cirrhotic liver. Histologically, the tumours vary from well to poorly differentiated, but the cells often resemble hepatocytes in their polygonal shape and granular cytoplasm (see Fig. 10.15 in Special Study Topic 10.1). There may be evidence of bile secretion in well-differentiated tumours. Many less well-differentiated tumours produce and release α-fetoprotein (AFP), a useful serum marker for diagnosis and follow-up.

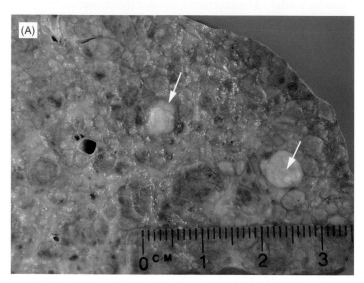

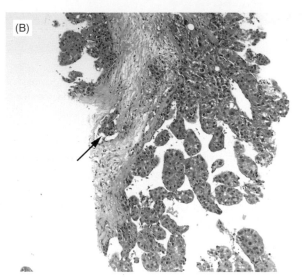

Fig. 10.14 (A) Cirrhotic liver removed at time of transplantation. Several nodules (arrows) are larger and either white or bile stained; these are small hepatocellular carcinomas. (B) Biopsy appearances in hepatocellular carcinoma. The tumour has a trabecular arrangement and there is evidence of vascular invasion (arrow).

## 10.1 Special Study Topic

### Hepatocellular Adenoma – Current Management is Based on Genotype/Phenotype Correlations

With the extensive use of abdominal imaging, and especially liver ultrasonography, the frequency of image-detected asymptomatic liver tumours has risen in recent years. Most incidentally identified liver tumours are benign, but in some cases the differentiation from those that are malignant is difficult. In addition, some benign liver neoplasms have malignant potential. Most common benign lesions such as haemangiomas, focal nodular hyperplasia, and focal steatosis may be easily diagnosed by imaging alone due to their typical ultrasound and radiological features. The less frequent hepatocellular adenomas (HCAs), however, are more difficult to diagnose by imaging and their identification relies on the appropriate clinical history and absence of typical imaging features suggestive of haemangioma or focal nodular hyperplasia. Significant bleeding, occurring in 20–25% of HCAs, and the rare (up to 7%) incidence of malignant transformation to hepatocellular carcinoma (HCC) are well-known risks for patients with HCAs.

The prevalence of an HCA is 3–4/100,000 population in Europe and North America. Most cases (85%) occur in females using oral contraceptives, but males using anabolic steroids for body-building may also be affected. Other rare causes include inherited metabolic disorders (type 1 or 3 glycogenosis [glycogen storage disease] and galactosaemia). Obesity has recently been identified as a potential risk factor for HCA development.

HCAs may be single or multiple. When more than 10 adenomas are present, the condition is termed 'adenomatosis'. The risk of haemorrhage is higher in tumours measuring >5 cm and the risk of malignant transformation depends on gender, because the prevalence of malignancy is 10 times higher in males than in females, depending

## Special Study Topic continued . . .

on HCA subtype and the underlying clinical condition. Being overweight/obese and the metabolic syndrome, a constellation of disorders associated with increased risk of cardiovascular disease (excess body fat around the waist, high blood pressure, increased fasting serum glucose levels, and abnormal serum triglyceride levels), have recently appeared as risk factors for malignant transformation of HCAs, especially in males.

Grossly, HCAs are of varying size (from a few millimetres to 20 cm in diameter) with ill-defined margins arising in a *non-cirrhotic* liver. Steatosis, congestion, or haemorrhage may be visible within the tumour parenchyma (Fig. 10.15A).

Histologically, HCAs are composed of benign hepatocytes arranged in one- to two-cell-thick plates. Their cytoplasm may be normal or clear, or contain fat. Portal tracts are not

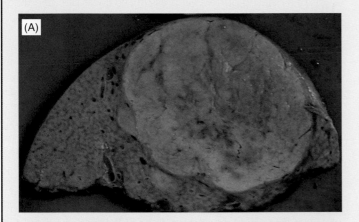

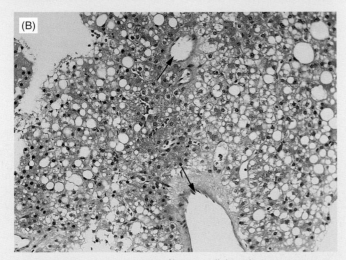

FIG. 10.15 (A) Gross appearance of hepatocellular adenoma in non-cirrhotic liver. Courtesy of Dr Christopher Bellamy, Division of Pathology, University of Edinburgh. (B) Histological appearance of a hepatocellular adenoma. This resembles non-tumorous liver and is composed of hepatocytes arranged in up to two-cell-thick plates, but there are no portal tracts. Large atypical arteries (arrows) and steatosis are present.

seen, but isolated arteries unaccompanied by bile ducts may be prevalent. Nuclear atypia and mitotic figures are unusual (Fig. 10.14B). Sometimes, histological distinction from well-differentiated HCC can be difficult.

Recent advances in basic science underlying the pathogenesis of HCA have allowed their molecular classification into distinct subgroups according to genotype with different pathological features (phenotype) and risk of transformation to HCC. Three major molecular pathways have been found to be altered in specific HCA subtypes:

1. Inactivation of hepatocyte nuclear factor 1A (*HNF1A*), a transcription factor involved in hepatocyte differentiation, which occurs in 35% of HCAs (*HNF1A-inactivated adenoma, H-HCA*)
2. Activating mutations in β-*catenin*, found in 10% of HCA (β-*catenin-activated adenoma, β-HCA*)
3. Activation of the interleukin 6 (IL-6)/signal transducer and activator of transcription 3 (STAT3) signalling pathway by somatic mutations of the *IL6ST* or *STAT3* genes, which occur in 55% of HCAs (*inflammatory adenoma, I-HCA*).

Finally, <10% of HCAs do not have any known mutation or specific histological phenotype (*unclassified HCA*).

The different HCA molecular subtypes may be identified by simple surrogate morphological features and immunohistochemical markers, enabling correct management of these tumours even if elaborate molecular techniques for their classification are not available. H-HCA displays marked steatosis and absence of liver fatty acid-binding protein (L-FABP) immunostaining. It occurs almost exclusively in females. I-HCA shows inflammatory infiltrates, sinusoidal dilatation, and thick-walled arteries. The inflammatory proteins serum amyloid protein A and C-reactive protein are strongly expressed by tumour cells. I-HCA occurs more frequently in females, particularly overweight/obese patients. β-HCA is characterized by overexpression of glutamine synthetase, a target of β-catenin, and by aberrant nuclear β-catenin immunostaining. β-HCA occurs more commonly in males and is associated with male hormone use and inherited metabolic diseases (i.e. glycogenosis). β-HCA has a greater risk of malignant transformation than the other subtypes.

The two major HCA subtypes, H-HCA and I-HCA, can now be identified by experienced radiologists using magnetic resonance imaging (MRI). Biopsy is, however, an important tool for confirmation of HCA diagnosis and subgroup classification according to phenotype, because this may affect patient management and follow-up. Large HCAs (>5 cm), which carry a high risk of bleeding, are treated by surgery, radiofrequency ablation, or embolization.

## Further Reading

Bioulac-Sage P, Balabaud C, Wanless I. Focal nodular hyperplasia and hepatocellular adenoma. In: *WHO Classification of Tumours of the Digestive System*, 4th edn. Lyon: International Agency for Research on Cancer, 2010.

## Special Study Topic continued . . .

Bioulac-Sage P, Laumonier H, Couchy G, *et al.* Hepatocellular adenoma management and phenotypic classification: the Bordeaux experience. *Hepatology* 2009;**50**:481–489.

Farges O, Ferreira N, Dokmak S, *et al.* Changing trends in malignant transformation of hepatocellular adenoma. *Gut* 2011;**60**:85–89.

Zucman-Rossi J, Jeannot E, Nhieu JT, *et al.* Genotype–phenotype correlation in hepatocellular adenoma: new classification and relationship with HCC. *Hepatology* 2006;**43**:515–524.

**CASE HISTORY 10.2**

Nigel is a 55-year-old plumber who was infected with hepatitis C virus (HCV) in 1983 after a car accident, which resulted in multiple injuries and severe blood loss requiring blood transfusion. HCV was discovered in 1989 and therefore specific testing of blood products for its presence, as is now done routinely, was not possible at that time. Nigel was diagnosed with chronic hepatitis C in 2003 when routine blood tests repeatedly showed increased values of liver enzymes (aspartate aminotransferase [AST] 130 IU/L, alanine aminotransferase [ALT] 120 IU/L) and he tested positive for anti-HCV antibodies and the presence of high values of HCV RNA in the serum. A liver biopsy performed at the time showed moderate inflammatory activity and advanced fibrosis. He was then treated with interferon-α subcutaneously but failed to show a response because HCV RNA was still detected in his serum after 24 weeks of therapy. The failure of treatment was attributed in part to the viral genotype, because he was infected with HCV genotype 1, which is more difficult to treat.

Nigel was diagnosed with HCV-related cirrhosis in 2010, but his liver function was not severely affected. He was re-offered treatment with a combination of pegylated interferon-α-2a subcutaneously once a week plus an orally administered antiviral agent, ribavirin, daily. Unfortunately, again he did not respond to therapy. He was advised to follow a healthy lifestyle and avoid alcohol, and was entered into a surveillance programme with liver ultrasonography every 6 months because he was considered at risk for developing hepatocellular carcinoma (HCC).

His most recent ultrasound examination revealed a 1.5-cm nodule in the right lobe of the liver which on a subsequent CT scan did not show typical imaging features of HCC. A firm diagnosis could not be reached non-invasively and therefore the atypical nodule was biopsied under CT guidance, with an additional core biopsy taken from the surrounding liver.

Histology of the non-tumorous liver confirmed cirrhosis. In the tissue core from the nodule, a well-differentiated hepatocellular tumour with a trabecular morphology, focal pseudogland formation, and isolated arterial branches was seen. The nuclear:cytoplasmic ratio was increased in tumour cells and some nuclei had an irregular contour. The reticulin framework was only partially preserved and in some areas three-cell-thick plates were noted. The differential diagnosis of the liver nodule included a high-grade dysplastic nodule, which is a premalignant tumour, and a well-differentiated HCC. Immunohistochemistry for three putative markers of hepatocellular malignancy – glypican 3, glutamine synthetase, and heat shock protein 70 – showed diffuse positive immunostaining and the tumour was diagnosed as HCC.

Nigel's hepatic function was well preserved and he had no signs of increased portal vein pressure, so it was decided that the best treatment for this small HCC was surgical resection. Nigel is alive and well 3 years after surgery.

With the introduction in 1992 of sensitive tests to screen blood donors for anti-HCV antibodies, transmission of HCV through blood transfusion has become very rare. Unfortunately, Nigel was transfused with HCV-infected blood almost 10 years earlier. He did not recall having been ill at the time, which is not unexpected because acute hepatitis C is known to often run a subclinical course.

Natural history studies indicate that up to 85% of patients who develop acute hepatitis C will remain HCV infected. Chronic HCV infection is dangerous for both infected individuals and their contacts because the former are at risk of progression to cirrhosis and the latter are at risk of acquiring the virus. The risk of developing cirrhosis in chronic hepatitis C ranges from 5% to 25% over a period of 25–30 years. Patients with HCV-related cirrhosis are at risk for the development of hepatic decompensation (30% over 10 years) as well as HCC (1–3% per year). Identifying individuals at risk for developing progressive disease is difficult. Currently, the best approach is to evaluate the extent of fibrosis on liver biopsy, using a validated histological staging system. Patients with no or minimal fibrosis are at low risk for liver-related complications and liver-related death over the next 10–20 years. Advanced fibrosis, as Nigel had, is a predictor of possible progression to cirrhosis and an indication for treatment.

Patients with cirrhosis should be followed up with ultrasonography for early detection of enlarged liver nodules suspicious of malignancy. HCC arising in cirrhosis is usually preceded by the appearance of non-malignant precancerous lesions, such as low-grade dysplastic nodules and high-grade dysplastic nodules. In non-cirrhotic liver, the evolution of hepatocellular neoplasia in humans has not as yet been clarified. Distinction between high-grade dysplastic nodules and well-differentiated HCC in biopsy material is challenging for pathologists.

A guided liver biopsy is needed in almost half the patients with a liver nodule measuring 1–2 cm because frequently they show atypical imaging features. Liver biopsy is a highly specific and sensitive technique for diagnosing HCC in liver tumours measuring >1 cm but less reliable for smaller tumours. The risk of needle-track seeding with malignant cells is very low (2.7%), so liver biopsy is generally considered a safe procedure. Unfortunately, up to 10% of biopsy specimens may be inadequate for histological diagnosis. Biopsy provides both architectural and cytological information, as well as material for subsequent biomarker studies; therefore it is considered superior to fine-needle aspiration for HCC diagnosis. It is hoped that, in the future, tissue biomarker information will permit a personalized approach to HCC treatment.

Worldwide the most common aetiological factors are hepatitis B virus acting synergistically with aflatoxin B$_1$, a mycotoxin product of *Aspergillus flavus*. Hepatitis C is also important and alcohol may have a promoter function, working synergistically with virus-induced damage and regeneration to promote the acquisition of mutations. Hepatocellular carcinoma may arise in a background of non-alcoholic steatohepatitis, even in the absence of cirrhosis. All forms of cirrhosis increase the risk of hepatocellular carcinoma.

Cholangiocarcinoma comprises about a sixth of primary hepatic cancers. It is an adenocarcinoma, which often spreads by ramification of portal tracts through the liver. Its incidence is high in patients with primary sclerosing cholangitis and in south-east Asia where liver flukes are prevalent. There is some evidence that the disease is more common than previously thought, perhaps due in part to better recognition but also due to an underlying real increase in incidence which some have attributed to as yet undiscovered environmental factors. Angiosarcomas are rare but important because they may be related to occupational exposure to vinyl chloride. Hepatoblastomas, although very rare, are the most frequent liver tumours in children. They occur before the age of 5, most commonly in young males and, histologically, resemble fetal or embryonal liver.

## Non-viral Infections Causing Liver Disease

Although viruses are the most common cause of inflammatory liver disease, a number of other important infections can affect the liver. Most of these are tropical but they can occur anywhere in the world in view of the increase in global travel (see also Chapter 19).

### Weil's Disease

Caused by the spirochaete *Leptospira ictohaemorrhagica*, Weil's disease is typically contracted from water contaminated by the urine of infected rats. The spirochaete penetrates the skin, particularly through skin defects such as unhealed wounds, and may cause liver cell necrosis, presenting as jaundice and an increased tendency to bleeding.

### Hydatid Disease

Caused by *Echinococcus granulosus* and contracted from a reservoir animal such as sheep, hydatid disease can result in cystic lesions within the liver. In addition to causing local problems resulting in obstruction to bile flow, the cysts may contain parasites that cause further disease if they rupture.

### Amoebiasis

Encysted infection by *Entamoeba histolytica* may cause abscesses that can compress other structures within the liver, e.g. leading to duct obstruction, or may rupture through the liver capsule.

### Flukes

Usually called liver flukes, organisms such as *Clonorchis sinensis* inhabit the bile ducts causing obstruction, inflammation, and scarring, and predisposing to cholangiocarcinoma.

### Schistosomiasis

*Schistosoma japonicum* and *S. mansoni* can migrate to the liver. An inflammatory response to ova, particularly in portal tracts, may lead to scarring, causing bile duct obstruction. Schistosome disease is a significant cause of secondary biliary cirrhosis and the most common cause of portal hypertension worldwide.

### Visceral Leishmaniasis

Parasitization of Kupffer cells may occur as part of a more generalized disease. In chronic adult cases, diffuse panacinar fibrosis may develop.

### Malaria

Replication of malarial parasites may occur within hepatocytes. Malarial dark-brown pigment accumulates within Kupffer cells and erythrocytes. Stuffing of Kupffer cells with red blood cells (erythrophagocytosis) can also be seen.

## Liver in Systemic Disease

The liver often shows non-specific reactive changes, including mild inflammation and steatosis, when intercurrent disease is present elsewhere. Other more specific abnormalities include:

- amyloidosis
- sarcoidosis, in which granulomas may be found

- malignant infiltration by metastatic carcinoma or leukaemia
- tuberculosis, in miliary cases
- fungal infection, in cases of immunodeficiency such as acquired immune deficiency syndrome (AIDS) or immunosuppressive therapy
- cardiac failure, in which perivenular congestion and atrophy may occur
- graft-versus-host disease after a bone marrow transplantation
- fatty liver of pregnancy.

## THE GALLBLADDER

### Normal Function

The gallbladder is connected to the intrahepatic and extrahepatic bile ducts by the cystic duct. It stores and concentrates bile from the liver and increases its viscosity by releasing mucus from the lining epithelium. The release of bile from the gallbladder is stimulated by food, especially fatty food, in the duodenum under the influence of cholecystokinin.

### Gallstones (Cholelithiasis)

Although rare in developing countries, gallstones are extremely common in western society. In many cases cholelithiasis remains undetected clinically and may be an incidental finding *post mortem*. The primary problem is supersaturation of bile. Bile normally contains cholesterol, held in suspension by phospholipid micelles containing lecithin, as well as bile acids and pigments derived from bilirubin. Nucleation occurs in the supersaturated, lithogenic bile and stones then enlarge (Fig. 10.16). Stones may be single or multiple, small or large (Fig. 10.17). They may be composed predominantly of cholesterol or, more commonly, have a lower cholesterol content with a greater component of bile salts and pigment (mixed stones). Pigment stones are smaller and have a higher bilirubin content, with only a minor cholesterol component. These are less common and are found typically in patients with haemolytic disorders such as hereditary spherocytosis (see Chapter 8, pp. 218–219).

In some gallbladders excess cholesterol is phagocytosed by macrophages in the lamina propria. These aggregates of foamy macrophages produce yellow stippling and protrusion of the gallbladder mucosa, an appearance known as cholesterolosis or 'strawberry' gallbladder. This is of no clinical significance.

### Cholecystitis

#### Acute Cholecystitis

Initially, acute cholecystitis is usually the result of an injury to the gallbladder mucosa caused by gallstones, perhaps by

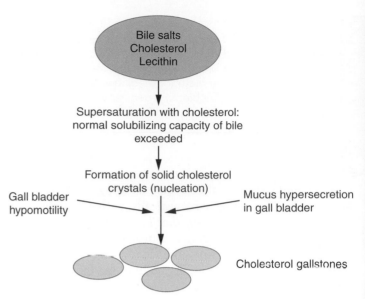

**FIG. 10.16** Mechanisms of gallstone development.

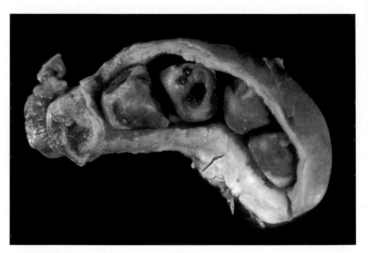

**FIG. 10.17** Macroscopic picture of gallbladder containing mixed stones.

obstruction of the cystic duct. However, in fully developed cases, there is often superimposed infection by bowel commensal bacteria, which further amplifies the acute inflammatory response. Histologically, there is ulceration of the mucosa with vascular congestion, oedema, and exudation. The neutrophil polymorph infiltrate may extend throughout the entire thickness of the gallbladder wall. A dilated, pus-filled gallbladder is known as empyema and there is a danger of rupture. Obstruction of the cystic duct with no infection may result in accumulation of sterile mucus, which distends the gallbladder to produce a mucocele.

#### Chronic Cholecystitis

This is generally associated with gallstones and may follow acute cholecystitis or develop insidiously. There may be superimposed acute cholecystitis. The gallbladder is thickened and fibrotic muscle fibres are hypertrophied. The mucosal epithelium may be atrophic or hyperplastic, sometimes forming diverticula which can reach the serosal surface (these diverticula are often called Rokitansky–Aschoff sinuses). The presence of cholesterol and bile in damaged diverticula stimulates a xanthogranulomatous response, with large numbers of foamy histiocytes and multinucleated foreign body giant cells containing cholesterol crystals. Severe chronic cholecystitis often causes fibrosis of the gallbladder bed, so that the inflamed organ is firmly adherent to the liver and difficult to remove. Diffuse calcification of the gallbladder wall, known as 'porcelain gallbladder', may rarely occur.

## Tumours

All tumours of the gallbladder are rare, but adenocarcinoma is the most frequent. This is most common in the sixth or seventh decade of life. Adenocarcinoma of the gallbladder tends to arise in the fundus and infiltrates diffusely without causing any symptoms until it is at an advanced stage. For this reason half the cases are diagnosed incidentally in cholecystectomy specimens. More than three-quarters of cases have gallstones. However, the incidence of carcinoma in the gallbladder of patients with cholelithiasis is <0.2%. In contrast, up to 10% of porcelain gallbladders may harbour a carcinoma. Occasional squamous carcinomas have been described, presumably arising from metaplastic squamous epithelium. Gallstones are invariably found in these cases.

# THE PANCREAS

## Normal Structure and Function

> ### Key Points
>
> - The exocrine pancreas secretes digestive enzymes.
> - The endocrine cells are grouped together in the islets of Langerhans.
> - The principal hormones secreted by the islets are insulin and glucagon.

The pancreas is often thought of as two separate organs – an exocrine organ concerned with digestion, and an endocrine organ concerned with the metabolism of carbohydrate, fat, and protein (see Chapter 17). Their association within one gland is simply regarded as fortuitous. However, knowledge of the anatomy, physiology, and pathology of the pancreas militates against this simplistic approach.

### Structure

Connective tissue septa divide the pancreas into lobules. Within the lobule the secretory unit is the acinus. The secretory products pass into the acinar lumen and drain to the main pancreatic duct. In 85% of cases the pancreatic duct joins the common bile duct to form the ampulla of Vater, which then enters the duodenum. In 15% of cases the two ducts do not join to form an ampulla and they enter the duodenum separately. Endocrine cells are grouped together into the islets of Langerhans. Most of the islet endocrine cells are insulin-secreting B (or β) cells and glucagon-secreting A (or α) cells. Somatostatin-secreting D (or δ) cells and pancreatic polypeptide-secreting PP cells also exist.

The anatomy of the pancreatic blood supply is significant. Within lobules, much of the circulation passes by arterioles to the islets, the exocrine tissue being supplied by a portal system of capillaries, which drains the blood from the sinusoids of the islets (Fig. 10.18). The pancreatic acini around islets are thus exposed to very high levels of islet hormones – possibly several hundred times higher than the levels in the systemic circulation.

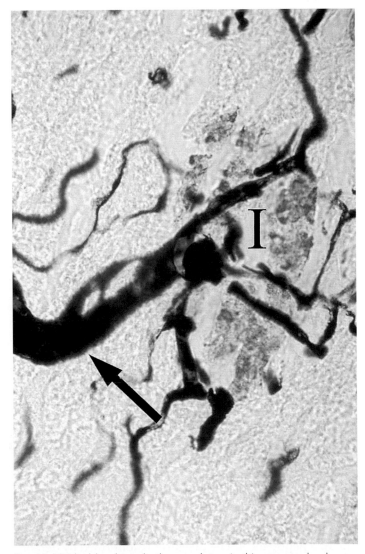

**FIG. 10.18** Islet blood supply: the vasculature in this pancreas has been injected with India ink. The islets have been immunostained to show insulin-containing B cells. An arteriole (arrowed) enters the islet (I) and divides into intra-islet sinusoids, which leave the islet and supply the surrounding exocrine tissue.

### Functional Aspects

The exocrine pancreas secretes about 1–2 L/day of an alkaline fluid containing about 20 enzymes. Bicarbonate is secreted by the duct epithelium. The enzymes include proteases – trypsin and chymotrypsin – lipases, phospholipases, elastase, and amylase. Protease inhibitors are also present within acinar cells and in the pancreatic secretion. Most enzymes are secreted in precursor forms which are activated in the duodenum, a process in which trypsin has a key role.

In addition to its anabolic systemic effects, insulin is a major trophic hormone for the exocrine pancreas, increasing the rate of DNA and protein synthesis in acinar tissue. Weight for weight the exocrine pancreas synthesizes considerably more protein (mainly enzymes) than any other tissue in the body (eight times more than the liver, for example). As one of the main actions of insulin in all cells of the body is to stimulate protein synthesis, it is interesting to speculate that the islets, with their distinct blood supply which ensures very high levels of insulin in the exocrine capillaries, have evolved to aid the massive protein-synthesizing requirements of the exocrine pancreas. Thus, the pancreas, in some respects, functions as a single organ.

## Pancreatitis

Pancreatitis is classified clinically and pathologically into acute and chronic forms.

### Acute Pancreatitis

> **Key Points**
>
> - Pancreatitis is associated most commonly with gallstones or alcohol misuse.
> - There is upper abdominal pain.
> - Serum amylase is raised.
> - There is autodigestion, causing fat necrosis.
> - Systemic complications include shock.
> - Local complications are pseudocyst and abscess formation.

Acute pancreatitis is defined as an acute inflammatory process within the pancreas usually associated with necrosis of intrapancreatic acini and adipose tissue. If there is macroscopic haemorrhage the term 'acute haemorrhagic pancreatitis' is used, but this probably simply represents the most severe form of acute pancreatitis.

#### Clinical Features

The onset is sudden with abdominal pain, vomiting, and collapse, and may easily be confused clinically with perforation of a peptic ulcer. The diagnosis is confirmed by demonstrating a serum amylase level >1,200 IU/L. Two-thirds of patients admitted to hospital have a mild illness, which settles readily with nasogastric suction and intravenous fluids.

Severe pancreatitis, characterized by shock, hypocalcaemia, hypoxaemia, and hyperglycaemia, is less common and has a 50% mortality rate.

#### Pathogenesis

The initiating event in gallstone-associated pancreatitis appears to be temporary impaction of a gallstone at the ampulla of Vater. If this results in retrograde reflux of bile into the pancreatic duct, acute pancreatitis may be triggered. Reflux will occur only if there is a common channel between the pancreatic duct and common bile duct and if the stone is of the right size (usually about 3 mm in diameter). Thus not everyone with gallstones will have acute pancreatitis.

The initial damage in the pancreas in gallstone acute pancreatitis appears to be to the pancreatic duct epithelial cells. This results in duct inflammation and periductal necrosis, seen microscopically (Fig. 10.19). Normal bile alone does not damage the pancreatic duct, but infected bile or bile preincubated with trypsin causes ductal inflammation and necrosis when infused into the pancreatic duct at physiological pressure. Both infection and trypsin convert primary bile salts into secondary bile salts, which are toxic to pancreatic duct epithelium. Bile is infected in at least 40% of cases of gallstone pancreatitis and, in the presence of an obstructing stone, bile that has refluxed into the pancreas can be altered by pancreatic trypsin. Although in alcohol-associated acute pancreatitis the pancreatic ducts are also thought to be the initial site of damage, the mechanism causing this is not known, and is likely to be different from that involved in gallstone pancreatitis.

Wherever the process starts, necrosis causes release of digestive enzymes into the substance of the pancreas. These enzymes are thought to damage further pancreatic parenchymal cells and blood vessels by a process of

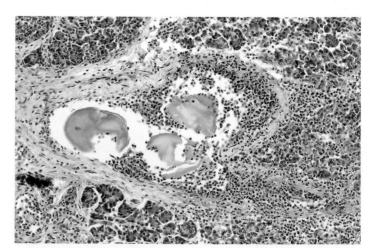

**FIG. 10.19** Duct inflammation and perilobular necrosis: an inflamed interlobular duct is present which contains proteinaceous concretions and polymorphs. An acute inflammatory infiltrate extends into the surrounding exocrine parenchyma.

autodigestion. Necrotic blood vessels, particularly veins, are liable to thrombose causing ischaemic damage to further areas of the pancreas, thus initiating a vicious cycle of further enzyme release, which may result in extensive coagulative necrosis of entire lobules and intervening ducts and blood vessels (panlobular necrosis) – this corresponds to the macroscopic appearance of acute haemorrhagic pancreatitis (Fig. 10.20). Release of pancreatic enzymes into the tissues surrounding the pancreas causes necrosis of adipose tissue in other sites (Fig. 10.21) and peritonitis, which initially is likely to be sterile.

## Defence Mechanisms

Plasma contains the anti-proteolytic enzymes $\alpha_1$-antitrypsin and $\alpha_2$-macroglobulin and pancreatic juice contains pancreatic secretory trypsin inhibitor. These combine with active proteolytic enzymes such as trypsin to inactivate them. Release and activation of these anti-proteolytic enzymes in the inflammatory exudate in acute pancreatitis may help inhibit the autodigestive process.

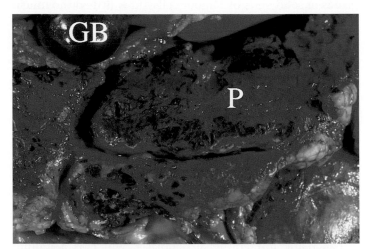

**FIG. 10.20** Acute haemorrhagic pancreatitis: in this postmortem specimen the pancreas (P) and gallbladder (GB) have been exposed. The pancreas is haemorrhagic and necrotic.

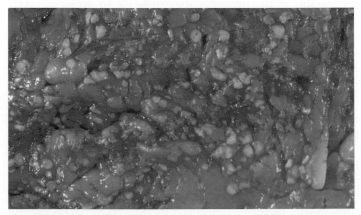

**FIG. 10.21** Fat necrosis of the omentum: dark-yellow flecks of fat necrosis can readily be seen.

## Complications of Acute Pancreatitis

### Systemic

Severe acute pancreatitis is complicated by chemical peritonitis, which, even in the absence of superadded bacterial peritonitis, can cause death from endotoxic shock due to escape of intestinal endotoxin into the circulation. Release of pancreatic enzymes into the blood may also contribute to the shock syndrome complex, in which adult respiratory distress syndrome (see Chapter 7, pp.176–177) and acute renal failure are serious, life-threatening, additional complications.

### Local

Sepsis in a necrotic pancreas may result in widespread suppuration or a pancreatic abscess. The causal organisms are *Escherichia coli* and other gut commensals. Another local effect is the formation of a pseudocyst – a localized collection of pancreatic juice and necrotic debris resulting from disruption of the pancreatic ductal drainage. It is lined by granulation tissue and commonly forms in the lesser sac.

## Chronic Pancreatitis

### Key Points

- Chronic pancreatitis is associated with alcohol misuse.
- There is severe long-lasting upper abdominal pain.
- There is pancreatic calcification.
- Eventually there is pancreatic exocrine and endocrine insufficiency.

### Clinical Features

Most patients present with episodes of severe, erratic abdominal pain, which may persist for years and lead to analgesic addiction. The pain may be exacerbated by food and thus weight loss may ensue. Some patients develop intermittent jaundice due to stenosis of the common bile duct. Steatorrhoea and diabetes (exocrine and endocrine pancreatic failure) are usually later manifestations, but may be the presenting features in the few patients in whom the disease process has been painless. Plain abdominal radiographs may show diffuse pancreatic calcification and endoscopic retrograde cholangiopancreatography (ERCP) or magnetic resonance cholangiopancreatography (MRCP) shows the presence of intraductal calculi plus areas of stenosis and dilatation of the main pancreatic duct.

### Aetiology and Pathogenesis

Most cases of chronic pancreatitis occur in patients who abuse alcohol. The disease is not associated with gallstones. Epidemiologically, it is common in countries where wine is drunk and a high alcohol intake is accompanied by a diet rich in protein. Alcohol increases the protein concentration in pancreatic juice, with subsequent precipitation of concretions in the ducts: when calcified these form stones, which

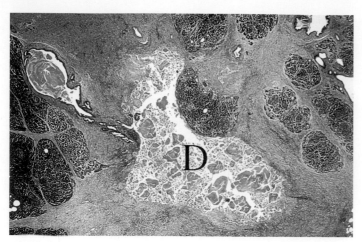

**FIG. 10.22** Chronic pancreatitis: the main pancreatic duct (D) is ulcerated and contains concretions. Fibrous tissue surrounds the duct and pancreatic lobules.

can be seen on plain abdominal radiographs. The stones ulcerate the ductal epithelium leading to periductal inflammation and fibrosis (Fig. 10.22). The fibrous tissue contracts and causes ductal strictures, with secondary dilatation of the duct behind the stricture and acinar atrophy.

Hereditary chronic pancreatitis is a rare disorder with an autosomal dominant transmission. It is caused by a mutation in the cationic trypsinogen gene and patients present before the age of 20 years. The mutation interferes with a trypsin inactivation mechanism, allowing active trypsin within the pancreatic duct to trigger pancreatic autodigestion.

It will be appreciated that the site of initial damage in the pancreas in both alcohol-related acute pancreatitis and chronic pancreatitis is the pancreatic duct. Not surprisingly, therefore, there is some overlap clinically and pathologically between these two conditions in affected people with alcohol problems. Thus, a patient may present with typical acute pancreatitis, which may be the prelude to continuing chronic pain and the development of chronic pancreatitis. In turn, patients with chronic pancreatitis may have particularly severe episodes of pain that are clinically and biochemically indistinguishable from an attack of acute pancreatitis.

## Carcinoma of the Pancreas

### Key Points

- Histologically, pancreatic carcinomas are adenocarcinomas.
- They are most common in the head of the pancreas.
- They usually present as obstructive jaundice.
- Prognosis is very poor, even in those patients treated surgically.

Carcinoma of the pancreas has doubled in incidence in the UK during the past 50 years. The increase in the USA has been even higher and there it now ranks second only to colorectal carcinoma among alimentary tract cancers. It is more common in males than in females, and increases progressively in incidence after the age of 50 years. Epidemiologically, it has been linked to smoking and a high-fat/high-protein diet. There is an increased risk of pancreatic carcinoma in patients with chronic pancreatitis and particularly those with hereditary chronic pancreatitis. Up to 10% of patients with pancreatic carcinoma have a family history of this tumour, indicating a possible genetic basis that has not as yet been clarified.

Sixty-five per cent of tumours are situated in the head of the pancreas where they usually obstruct the common bile duct, causing obstructive jaundice. Carcinoma arising in the body or tail of the pancreas is usually clinically silent until there are multiple metastases. Pancreatic cancer may also present with bizarre clinical effects due to unexplained venous thrombosis (migrating thrombophlebitis), peripheral neuropathy, or myopathy. Histologically, the tumour is an adenocarcinoma. Most ductal adenocarcinomas are fairly well-differentiated tumours. Poorly differentiated ductal adenocarcinomas, composed of densely packed tubular glands or solid nests of tumour cells, show little or no mucin production and marked nuclear pleomorphism.

Ninety per cent of tumours have K-*ras* gene mutations at codon 12, leading to activation of this oncogene. This suggests that K-*ras* mutations are an early event in the development of this cancer. Mutations of K-*ras* have been detected in stool, pancreatic juice, cytology, and/or blood samples from patients with pancreatic ductal adenocarcinoma, but the value of identifying these mutations in routine clinical practice remains uncertain. Diagnosis is made by imaging and brush cytology of the pancreatic or common bile duct at endoscopy (if the tumour is in the head of pancreas). Ultrasound-guided percutaneous fine-needle aspiration cytology or biopsy can also be performed. The most frequent precursor lesion of pancreatic ductal adenocarcinoma is pancreatic intraepithelial neoplasia, which is a minute (<5 mm) histological lesion confined to the pancreatic ducts. Less commonly, macroscopically detectable cystic tumours, such as mucinous cystic neoplasms and intraductal neoplasms of the pancreas, may progress to invasive ductal adenocarcinoma.

The prognosis in carcinoma of the pancreas is extremely poor, with 90% of patients not surviving more than 6 months. The most important factor for prognosis is resectability. However, even if successfully resected, most ductal adenocarcinomas recur within 2 years, mostly locally or in the liver, and less frequently in the peritoneal cavity or the lymph nodes. One of the strongest prognostic factors for survival after surgical resection is the ratio of the number of lymph nodes with metastasis to the total number of examined lymph nodes. Histological features, such as tumour differentiation and number of mitoses, are less significant prognostic factors. Adjuvant chemotherapy may slightly prolong patient survival. Patients with carcinoma in the immediate region of the ampulla often present relatively early with obstructive jaundice. Survival after surgery in these patients is usually better than that after surgery for carcinoma of the head of pancreas, but even here the 5-year survival rate is only approximately 25%.

## Neuroendocrine Neoplasms of the Pancreas

A neuroendocrine tumour (NET), previously known as islet cell tumour, is usually a solitary discrete nodule embedded in the pancreas. Microscopically, NETs are well differentiated and their tumour cells closely resemble normal islet cells, forming cords or clusters separated by fibrous stroma. All pancreatic NETs are regarded as having malignant potential and 65–80% of the cases show malignant behaviour with grossly visible invasion of adjacent structures or metastasis. Poorly differentiated neuroendocrine carcinomas consist of densely packed nests or diffuse sheets of tumour cells and often show extensive necrosis. They have highly aggressive behaviour and are usually at an advanced stage when detected, with survival ranging from 1 month to 1 year.

A 68-year-old woman presented with a 1-week history of epigastric pain, anorexia, and pale stools. She was noted to be jaundiced (bilirubin 270 μmol/L, alkaline phosphatase 768 IU/L, AST 116 IU/L, ALT 149 IU/L, γ-glutamyl transferase 417 IU/L). An abdominal ultrasound scan showed markedly dilated intra- and extrahepatic ducts. The common bile duct was 20 mm in diameter at its upper end. There was no evidence of gallstones. Pancreas, liver, spleen, and kidneys were unremarkable on the scan. ERCP was performed and a bulging tumour was seen at the ampulla before cannulation of the ducts. Bile drainage was achieved with a sphincterotomy and multiple biopsies were taken of the ampullary tumour. Microscopy of the biopsies showed the presence of an ulcerated, moderately differentiated adenocarcinoma (Fig. 10.23). A CT scan of the abdomen showed no evidence of tumour in the head of the pancreas or the liver. Whipple's operation was performed (removal of duodenum, common bile duct, gallbladder, and head of pancreas en bloc). There was a 15-mm diameter tumour at the ampulla (Fig. 10.24). The tumour invaded the duodenal wall, the common bile duct, and a small area of the head of the pancreas. All the resection margins were free of tumour, as were the lymph nodes in the specimen. The patient was well and tumour free 2.5 years later.

### Comment

The anatomical site of this adenocarcinoma, the ampulla of Vater, ensured a relatively early clinical presentation due to biliary obstruction that caused jaundice. Abdominal pain,

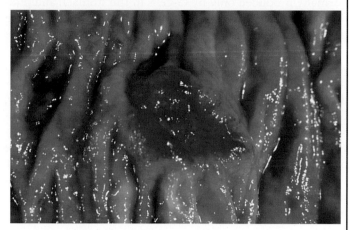

FIG. 10.24 Ampullary tumour in the duodenum: it is forming a raised ulcer, 15 mm in diameter.

pancreatitis, and weight loss may also occur in patients with ampullary adenocarcinoma. The tumour in this case appears to have been removed before it had metastasized. Carcinomas arising at clinically more silent sites, e.g. the body or tail of pancreas, have usually metastasized by the time of clinical presentation.

The ampulla of Vater may be affected by carcinomas of the duodenal mucosa, the distal common bile duct, or the head of pancreas, but only those located in the ampulla, surrounding it or completely destroying it, are regarded as 'ampullary carcinomas'. Very often, establishing the organ origin of ampullary carcinomas is very difficult, especially in large tumours (>4 cm) that involve many adjacent structures. The most common histological type is intestinal, resembling adenocarcinoma of the colon. The less frequent pancreatobiliary-type adenocarcinoma resembles pancreatic ductal or extrahepatic bile duct carcinoma. Mixed tumours may rarely occur.

Endoscopic ultrasonography, CT, and ERCP are very useful for assessing the extent of tumour spread before surgery. The prognosis of ampullary carcinoma depends on the histological type, tumour differentiation, and stage, with the stage being the best predictor. Patients with carcinomas localized in the ampulla and not extending into surrounding tissues have 45% 5-year survival rate. Intestinal-type ampullary adenocarcinomas have a better prognosis than pancreatobiliary-type tumours, and patients with well-differentiated carcinomas survive longer than those with poorly differentiated tumours.

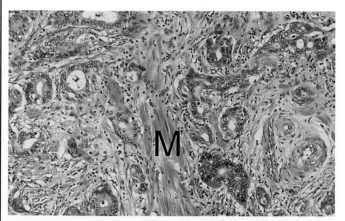

FIG. 10.23 Ampullary tumour: this is a moderately differentiated adenocarcinoma that is invading through smooth muscle (M).

### Insulinoma

This is the most common NET of the pancreas, although still very rare. It is associated clinically with recurrent attacks of hypoglycaemia, which may result in confusion, mania, dizziness, or coma. These effects are reversed by taking glucose or by excision of the tumour. Insulinomas are usually detected when very small (<1 cm) and for this reason 90% run a benign course.

### Gastrinoma

Gastrinomas are NETs that produce gastrin. Gastrin is normally produced only by G-cells in the stomach and duodenum. Most gastrinomas occur in the submucosa of the duodenum or the gastric antrum, but the pancreas is the most common site for an ectopic gastrinoma. Gastrinomas are associated with the Zollinger–Ellison syndrome in which persistent hypersecretion of acid gastric juice causes duodenal and even jejunal peptic ulceration (see Chapter 9, Case History 9.2, pp. 249–250). Most pancreatic gastrinomas are malignant.

It should be noted that the ending '-oma' after the name of a hormone (e.g. insulinoma, gastrinoma) is used for NET when there is a clinical syndrome related to the production of that specific hormone and not when this is demonstrated by immunohistochemistry only on tumour tissue sections.

## SUMMARY

- The liver is a metabolically active tissue which can be subjected to a wide range of insults including viral infections, toxins, and chemicals (in particular alcohol), autoimmune processes, and inherited metabolic diseases.
- Distinct patterns of injury are seen with different agents (e.g. viruses – chronic hepatitis; biliary disease – cholestatic injury; alcohol excess and metabolic syndrome – fatty liver disease).
- Acute liver injury is associated with hepatocyte necrosis; if extensive this may be associated with liver failure but where there is less damage the liver may undergo marked regeneration with a return to normal structure.
- Chronic liver injury is generally associated with fibrosis; when accompanied by nodular regenerative change there may be transformation of the liver architecture to cirrhosis.
- The key clinical complications of liver disease are: failure of normal liver function (synthetic, detoxifying, and so on); portal hypertension; and risk of hepatic malignancy.
- Gallstones (cholelithiasis) are common in western countries.
- Acute and chronic cholecystitis are important and sometimes serious complications of gallstone disease.
- Acute pancreatitis is a life-threatening condition which is associated with gallstone disease and alcohol excess.
- Chronic pancreatitis may be caused by excess alcohol and can lead to pancreatic exocrine and endocrine insufficiency.
- Carcinoma of the pancreas, an important form of solid organ malignancy of increasing incidence, commonly presents as obstructive jaundice.

## FURTHER READING

Bosman FT, Carneiro F, Hruban RH, Theise ND. *WHO Classification of Tumours of the Digestive System*, 4th edn. Lyon: International Agency for Research on Cancer, 2010.

Burt AD, Portmann BC, Ferrell LD. *MacSween's Pathology of the Liver*, 6th edn. Edinburgh: Churchill Livingstone, 2012.

Iacobuzio-Donahue CA, Montgomery EA. *Gastro-intestinal and Liver Pathology*, 2nd edn. Philadelphia, PA: Saunders, 2011.

Odze RD, Goldblum JR, Crawford JM. *Surgical Pathology of the GI Tract, Liver, Biliary Tract and Pancreas*, 3rd edn. Philadelphia: Saunders, 2014.

# 11

# THE NERVOUS SYSTEMS AND THE EYE

James AR Nicoll and Fiona Roberts

## NORMAL STRUCTURE AND FUNCTION

The central nervous system (CNS), i.e. the brain and the spinal cord, is composed of two types of tissue, both involved in disease processes. The first consists of the highly specialized nerve cells (neurons) and the neuroglial cells, all of which are of neuroepithelial origin. The second comprises the meninges, the blood vessels and their supporting connective tissue, all derived from mesoderm, and the microglia (phagocytic cells).

## APPLIED ANATOMY

The dura mater acts as the periosteum to the skull and spine. Extensions of the dura – the falx cerebri and the tentorium cerebelli – subdivide the cranial cavity into three spaces, two supratentorial and one infratentorial (the posterior fossa). The subdural space lies between the dura and the outer surface of the arachnoid, and blood or pus can spread widely throughout it (Fig. 11.1). The arachnoid lies in contact with the dura; the pia is closely attached to the brain. The subarachnoid space is filled with cerebrospinal fluid (CSF). It is widest in the basal cisterns and within sulci. It contains the major cerebral arteries and veins; arterial branches pass into the brain.

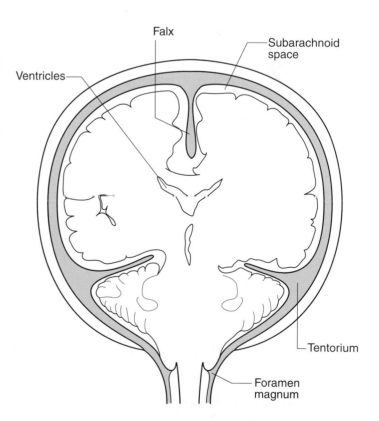

FIG. 11.1 The intracranial compartments. (From Adams JA, Graham DI. *Introduction to Neuropathology*. London: Churchill Livingstone, 1988.)

Capillaries in the brain, unlike those in other organs of the body, have circumferential tight junctions (zona occludens) between the endothelial cells. These help to prevent the passage of large and small molecules between the blood and the CSF (the blood–CSF barrier) or the interstitial space of the brain (the blood–brain barrier).

# CIRCULATION OF CEREBROSPINAL FLUID

Cerebrospinal fluid is formed mainly by the choroid plexus in the ventricles. Its total volume of 120–150 mL is renewed several times a day. CSF passes from the lateral ventricles via the foramen of Monro into the third ventricle, and then via the aqueduct of Sylvius to the fourth ventricle. More CSF is formed in the third and fourth ventricles, and it then passes through the exit foramina of Luschka and Magendie, in the fourth ventricle, to reach the subarachnoid space. Thereafter, it spreads over the surface of the brain and spinal cord and is absorbed into the blood through arachnoid granulations, which project into dural venous sinuses (Fig. 11.2).

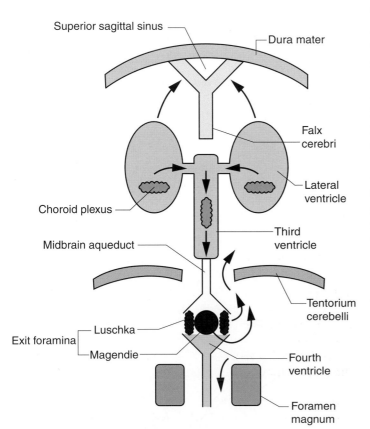

FIG. 11.2 The formation and circulation of cerebrospinal fluid. (From Adams JH and Graham DI. *Introduction to Neuropathology*. London: Churchill Livingstone, 1988.)

## Normal Cerebrospinal Fluid

### Key Points

The key features of the CSF are:
- clear and colourless
- specific gravity of 1.006
- 0.15–0.45 g/L of protein
- 2.8–4.4 mmol/L of glucose
- 128 mmol/L of sodium and 128 mmol/L of chloride
- <5 lymphocytes/mm$^3$

The main functions of the CSF are to provide mechanical protection for the brain and spinal cord, chemical homeostasis, and intracranial pressure regulation. Specimens are ordinarily obtained by lumbar puncture but ventricular CSF may sometimes be obtained via a ventricular shunt or drain. The pressure of the CSF should always be measured and fluid sent for microbiology, cytology, biochemistry, and sometimes immunological studies.

# ANATOMICAL BASIS OF CLINICAL SIGNS AND SYMPTOMS

The anatomical localization of symptoms and signs is based on clinicopathological correlation. Functional and structural imaging (positron emission tomography [PET], magnetic resonance imaging [MRI], and computed tomography [CT]) have shown that traditional concepts of localization are not always correct; some tasks have such a complex functional integration that precise clinical localization is not possible. A summary of the principal functions of the different regions of the brain follows.

The cerebral hemispheres are divided into frontal, parietal, temporal, and occipital lobes. The left cerebral hemisphere is dominant in right-handed and most left-handed individuals. Verbal, linguistic, calculating, and analytical functions reside in the dominant hemisphere whereas visual, spatial, and perceptual skills are located in the non-dominant hemisphere.

## Frontal Lobe

Movements of the face, arm, and trunk are represented on the lateral surface of the hemisphere and movements of the leg on the medial surface. Functions such as hand or lip movements have the greatest area of representation. Symptoms and signs of frontal lobe disease include:

- contralateral monoplegia or hemiplegia
- alterations in higher functions (e.g. disinhibition, reduced motivation, and mood changes)
- expressive dysphasia if dominant hemisphere affected (Broca's area)

- primitive reflexes (grasp, pouts, and so on)
- apraxia of gait
- loss of cortical inhibition resulting in incontinence of urine and faeces.

## Parietal Lobe

The main sensory cortex lies behind the central sulcus and has a similar topography and representation to the motor cortex. Symptoms and signs of parietal lobe disease include:

- contralateral disturbance of cortical sensation
- dominant lobe involvement which may result in acalculia, dysgraphia, and dyslexia.
- non-dominant lobe involvement which may result in loss of spatial orientation and body image.

## Temporal Lobe

The temporal lobe is made up of the lateral cortex, buried insular cortex, and the deep limbic lobe, which includes part of the rhinencephalon, hippocampus, and associated structures. Symptoms and signs of temporal lobe disease include:

- memory loss (hippocampus and limbic system)
- receptive dysphasia if dominant hemisphere affected (Wernicke's area)
- epilepsy with memory disturbance, déjà-vu, hallucinations of smell and taste, complex partial seizures
- upper homonymous quadrantanopia if optic radiation is damaged.

## Occipital Lobe

The visual cortex lies on the medial surface of the occipital lobe. Symptoms and signs of occipital lobe disease include:

- unilateral cortical lesion producing homonymous hemianopia
- cortical blindness occurring with extensive bilateral lesions of striate cortex
- visual hallucinations
- visual agnosia.

## Thalamus

The thalami are a pair of masses of grey matter, lying in the lateral walls of the third ventricle. Each thalamus has four regions: anterior, posterior, medial; and lateral; these cause the characteristic thalamic syndromes.

## Hypothalamus

The hypothalamus lies in the lateral walls of the third ventricle and is connected to the reticular formation in the midbrain, the limbic system, and the autonomic nuclei of the brain stem and spinal cord. It largely controls the release of hormones from the anterior pituitary gland, body temperature, fluid balance, circadian rhythm, and reproductive function.

## The Basal Ganglia

These are masses of grey matter that lie anterior to the thalami and include the corpus striatum (putamen and caudate nucleus), substantia nigra, globus pallidus, and subthalamic nuclei. The basal ganglia are responsible for the control and modulation of movements and the maintenance of posture.

## The Cerebellum

The cerebellum is connected to the pons and medulla by the cerebellar peduncles. It consists of two large hemispheres and a small midline vermis. The cerebellum controls and coordinates movements and maintains stance, posture, and gait. Symptoms and signs of cerebellar syndromes include:

- anterior syndromes in which the patient walks with a broadened gait but with coordinated limbs and without speech disturbance or abnormal ocular movements
- posterior syndromes in which the gait is profoundly disturbed with an inability to stand without swaying
- hemispheric syndrome in which unilateral disease results in the lack of coordination of ipsilateral limbs, unsteadiness of gait, slurring of speech or dysarthria, and nystagmus
- pancerebellar syndromes in which there is marked disturbance of gait and balance, ataxia in all limbs, altered ocular movements, and dysarthria.

## The Brain Stem

The brain stem is divided into the midbrain, pons, and medulla. Each region contains cranial nerve nuclei and ascending and descending pathways. The principal structures of the midbrain include the colliculi, cerebral peduncles, third and fourth cranial nerve nuclei, and medial longitudinal fasciculus. The principal symptoms and signs are of contralateral spastic hemiplegia, diplopia, and impairment of vertical eye movements and convergence. Syndromes due to disease in either the pons or the medulla oblongata reflect the involvement of sensory and motor long tracts, cranial nerve nuclei, and vital centres involved in respiration and control of the heart; if there are bilateral paramedian lesions the patient may become 'locked in'.

## The Spinal Cord

The spinal cord extends from the base of the skull to the first lumbar vertebra. The major ascending tracts carry sensation to the cerebellum or thalamus and then on to the cerebral cortex. Some of the fibres terminate in the dorsal horn before crossing over to form the lateral and anterior spinal thalamic tracts which carry the sensations of pain, temperature, and light touch. Other fibres of the dorsal roots pass into the dorsal horns and then ascend in the posterior column to end in the nucleus gracilis and nucleus cuneatus: they carry the sensations of vibration, weight, proprioception, and pressure. The major descending pathway is the corticospinal tract, which arises from the primary cortex and passes down through the internal capsule into the cerebral peduncle and midbrain, and into the base of the pons. It then descends into the pyramidal decussation and on to the ventral horn cells within the spinal cord. Spinal cord disease tends to result in a combination of motor, sensory, and autonomic dysfunction.

## CELLS OF NEUROEPITHELIAL ORIGIN

As the mature neuron is essentially incapable of dividing after the first few days of life, loss of neurons is structurally irreversible. Immunocytochemistry for neurotransmitters has defined various functional types but all have a perikaryon or cell body, dendrites, and an axon. The perikaryon of large neurons contains stacks of rough endoplasmic reticulum and free ribosomes known as Nissl granules. Neurons also contain microtubules and neurofilaments.

Neuroglia – astrocytes, oligodendrocytes, and ependymal cells – are also of neuroepithelial origin. Astrocytes are stellate cells with branching processes that contain intracellular filaments composed mainly of glial fibrillary acidic protein (GFAP). Astrocytes are attached to the walls of blood vessels by one or more swellings – so-called foot processes. Oligodendrocytes, small cells with short processes, are associated with the formation and maintenance of myelin. These various cell types can be seen residing in the cerebral cortex and white matter (Fig. 11.3). A single layer of ependymal cells lines the ventricular system and central canal of the spinal cord.

## THE REACTIONS OF THE CNS TO DISEASE

### Reactions of the Neuron

#### Structural Changes Result from Hypoxia

Without a constant supply of oxygen and glucose neurons undergo ischaemic cell change (Fig. 11.4A). The cell body becomes contracted and triangular and the cytoplasm becomes intensely eosinophilic, with disappearance of Nissl granules. The nucleus becomes triangular and pyknotic. Changes in the neuroglia and blood vessels are proportional to the severity of neuronal destruction and evolve with time.

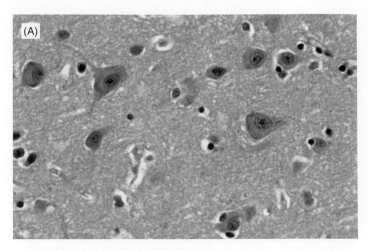

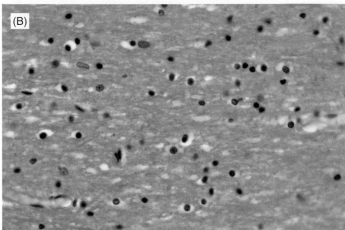

**Fig. 11.3** Normal brain: (A) neocortex: triangular cells are neurons; their cytoplasm contains Nissl granules. The background is neuropil. (B) White matter: myelinated white matter within which are oligodendrocytes and a few astrocytes.

### Reactions to Axonal Transection

After axonal transection, changes take place proximally in the cell body – central chromatolysis (Fig. 11.4B) – and in the distal axon – wallerian degeneration.

Central chromatolysis occurs between 5 and 8 days after transection, and is characterized by swelling of the cell body and displacement of the nucleus to the periphery of the cell. The cytoplasm becomes pale and homogeneous and there is dispersion of the Nissl substance – chromatolysis – accompanied by increased synthesis of RNA and protein. This reaction occurs in central and peripheral neurons, but particularly the latter. It may be followed by recovery with or without axonal regeneration, or may proceed to degeneration and ultimate death of the neuron. Effective regeneration is limited to the peripheral nervous system (PNS). In contrast, those neurons with projections lying entirely within the CNS tend to undergo retrograde degeneration and die. However, there is evidence of continuing neurogenesis from a population of stem cells residing in the subventricular zone of the basal ganglia and hippocampi.

Wällerian degeneration describes the series of changes that take place in the axon after transection. Within 2–3 hours, swellings and bulbs develop at the severed ends of the proximal and distal stumps due to alterations in axoplasmic flow. They are frequently seen adjacent to infarcts and haematomas as well as in certain types of head injury, where they may form part of the complex of diffuse traumatic axonal injury. If regeneration does not occur then the distal portion of the axon undergoes progressive degeneration. Changes also take place within the terminal innervation fields of the axons: axonal debris and the degenerating terminals are removed by phagocytosis. If a motor nerve is involved the muscle undergoes neurogenic atrophy (see Chapter 12, p. 388).

The process occurs more quickly in the PNS than in the CNS. The axon breaks up into fragments and the myelin sheath is broken down, ultimately into neutral fat. Within the PNS most breakdown products are removed by macrophages within weeks and the Schwann cells proliferate to form cords of cells within neural tubes. In contrast, the process within the CNS is much slower, macrophages remaining for many months and even years.

After damage to neurons, some function may recover due to 'plasticity', as surviving neurons form new contacts with neurons that have lost their afferent connections.

### Inclusion Bodies (Box 11.1)

A variety of structural abnormalities occur within neurons and some are characteristic of specific diseases.

### Astrocytes

Damage to the CNS is invariably accompanied by hypertrophy and hyperplasia of astrocytes, a process known as astrocytosis or gliosis (Fig. 11.5), in which numerous intracellular fibres of GFAP are laid down in an irregular manner.

## Microglia

These cells of the mononuclear–phagocyte system are normally present throughout the CNS and perform homeostatic functions, reacting to any pathological process

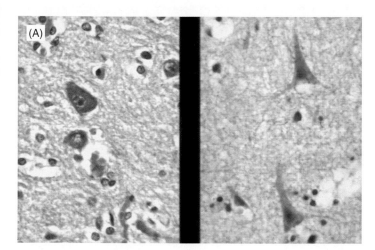

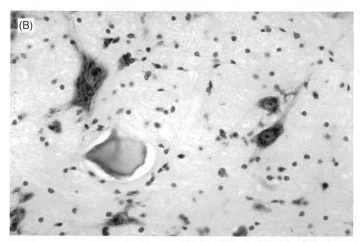

FIG. 11.4 Neurons: (A) left panel: normal motor neuron in ventral horn of spinal cord. The dark granules are the Nissl granules. The pale area is the region occupied by lipofuscin. Right panel: neurons showing the features of ischaemic cell change. They are shrunken and contain hyperchromatic nuclei, have intensely eosinophilic cytoplasm, and may be decorated by incrustations. (B) A neuron (left of centre) showing the features of central chromatolysis. Note the pale homogeneous cytoplasm and displaced nucleus.

---

**Box 11.1** EXAMPLES OF NEURONAL INCLUSION BODIES

*Cytoplasmic*
- Neurofibrillary tangles (tau) in Alzheimer's disease
- Lewy bodies (α-synuclein) in Parkinson's disease and dementia with Lewy bodies
- 'Storage' product in metabolic disorders (peroxisomal and lysosomal disorders)

*Nuclear*
- Huntington's disease (huntingtin)
- Viral inclusions in viral encephalitis

---

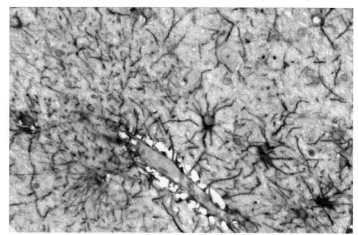

FIG. 11.5 Astrocytes: reactive fibre-forming astrocytes that are both hypertrophied and hyperplastic (immunohistochemistry of glial fibrillary acidic protein [GFAP]).

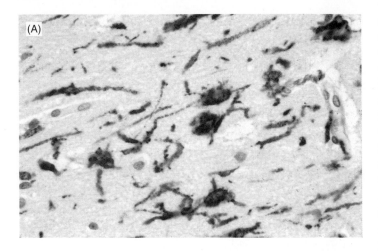

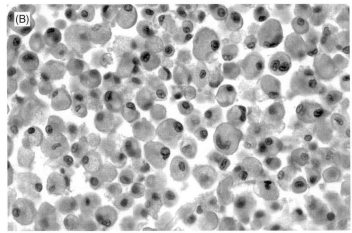

**FIG. 11.6** Microglia: (A) they have short processes that become progressively shorter, with more perinuclear cytoplasm, as the cells react (immunohistochemistry CD68). (B) Lipid-laden macrophages in a cerebral infarct.

(Fig. 11.6A). They are particularly noticeable where there is tissue destruction, e.g. in an infarct, when microglia become enlarged and laden with tissue breakdown products to appear as macrophages (Fig. 11.6B). When neurons are killed selectively, they become surrounded by enlarged microglia and undergo phagocytosis, a process known as neuronophagia.

## Blood Vessels

Proliferation of capillaries is seen around infarcts and abscesses, and in relation to rapidly growing cerebral tumours. Dysfunction of the blood–brain barrier may result in vascular oedema and swelling of the brain (see below).

## RAISED INTRACRANIAL PRESSURE, BRAIN SWELLING AND OEDEMA, AND HYDROCEPHALUS

After the fontanelles close in late infancy, the intracranial contents of the brain (about 70% of the intracranial volume), CSF (about 15%), and blood (about 15%) are enclosed in a rigid bony container. Any increase in the volume of one component will lead to an increase in intracranial pressure (ICP) unless compensated by a corresponding reduction of the others. Thus, pathological processes such as tumour, haematoma or a massive recent cerebral infarct ultimately cause an increase in ICP (*Box 11.2*). There is, however, a period of spatial compensation during which the ICP remains within normal limits, brought about principally due to a reduction in both the volume of CSF within the ventricles and the subarachnoid space, and the volume of blood within the intracranial veins. When all available space has been used a critical point is reached, beyond which a further slight increase in the volume of the intracranial contents will cause an abrupt increase in ICP and rapid deterioration in the patient's condition. Arteriolar vasodilatation due to increased arterial $PCO_2$ ($PaCO_2$), or the use of some anaesthetic agents, may be sufficient to produce this effect. The compensatory

---

**Box 11.2 DEFINITIONS OF RAISED INTRACRANIAL PRESSURE (ICP)**

- Normal upper limit of ICP is about 2.7 kPa (20 mmHg)
- High ICP is >5.4 kPa (40 mmHg)
- Raised ICP is usually due to an intracranial expanding mass
- A pressure gradient forms between supratentorial and infratentorial compartments, or between the intracranial and spinal subarachnoid spaces

---

**Box 11.3 NEUROLOGICAL FEATURES ASSOCIATED WITH PROGRESSIVE ELEVATION OF INTRACRANIAL PRESSURE DUE TO A UNILATERAL, SUPRATENTORIAL, INTRACRANIAL, EXPANDING LESION**

- Reduction in level of consciousness
- Dilatation of pupil ipsilateral to mass lesion and papilloedema
- Bradycardia, increase in pulse pressure, and increase in mean arterial blood pressure
- Cheyne–Stokes respiration

---

**Box 11.4 PRINCIPAL CHANGES IN THE INTRACRANIAL COMPARTMENT DUE TO A UNILATERAL MASS LESION**

- Narrowing of sulci and flattening of gyri
- Reduction in size of the ipsilateral ventricle
- Midline shift
- Supracallosal (subfalcine) hernia
- Tentorial hernia
- Compression of the ipsilateral oculomotor nerve
- Tonsillar hernia
- Brain-stem haemorrhage/infarction including Kernohan's notch
- Calcarine infarction

mechanisms fail more quickly when the lesion is expanding rapidly. Intracranial expanding lesions (*Boxes 11.3* and *11.4*) also cause distortion and displacement of the brain, and the associated increase in ICP is often of greater prognostic significance than the nature of the lesion itself.

In a tentorial hernia the medial part of the ipsilateral temporal lobe is squeezed through the tentorial opening (Fig. 11.7), and compresses and displaces the midbrain against the contralateral rigid edge of the tentorium (Fig. 11.8). This pressure may produce a distinct groove on the contralateral surface of the midbrain: Kernohan's notch. The tentorial opening is plugged, CSF is continuously produced, and a pressure gradient develops, the supratentorial pressure exceeding the infratentorial pressure. This is associated with a rapid deterioration in the patient's conscious level.

A tonsillar hernia (cerebellar cone), i.e. impaction of the cerebellar tonsils in the foramen magnum, is most common with infratentorial expanding lesions. The tonsils compress the medulla and produce apnoea by distorting the respiratory centre. By obstructing the flow of CSF through the fourth ventricle, such herniation may further increase the ICP, so that a vicious circle is set up.

In a patient with an intracranial expanding lesion, lumbar puncture can precipitate internal herniation with serious consequences. Even if only a small amount of CSF is withdrawn, more may leak into the spinal extradural space via the puncture wound in the meninges. Lumbar puncture

is therefore contraindicated in a patient thought to have a raised ICP until the presence of an intracranial expanding lesion has been excluded by CT or MRI.

## Brain Swelling and Oedema

An increase in the volume of the brain due to oedema or increased cerebral blood volume contributes to raised ICP. Vasodilatation leading to an increase in cerebral blood volume may occur due to hypoxia or hypercapnia, or as a result of loss of vasomotor tone which may complicate acute brain damage.

Cerebral oedema is classified as vasogenic or cytotoxic. The vasogenic type corresponds to oedema elsewhere in the body resulting from an increased filtration pressure and/or increased permeability of the capillaries and venules. It is often prominent in the tissue around cerebral contusions, recent infarcts, a brain abscess. and very frequently in association with a brain tumour. In the less common cytotoxic oedema, usually seen in some metabolic derangements, intracellular fluid accumulates. This is a disturbance of

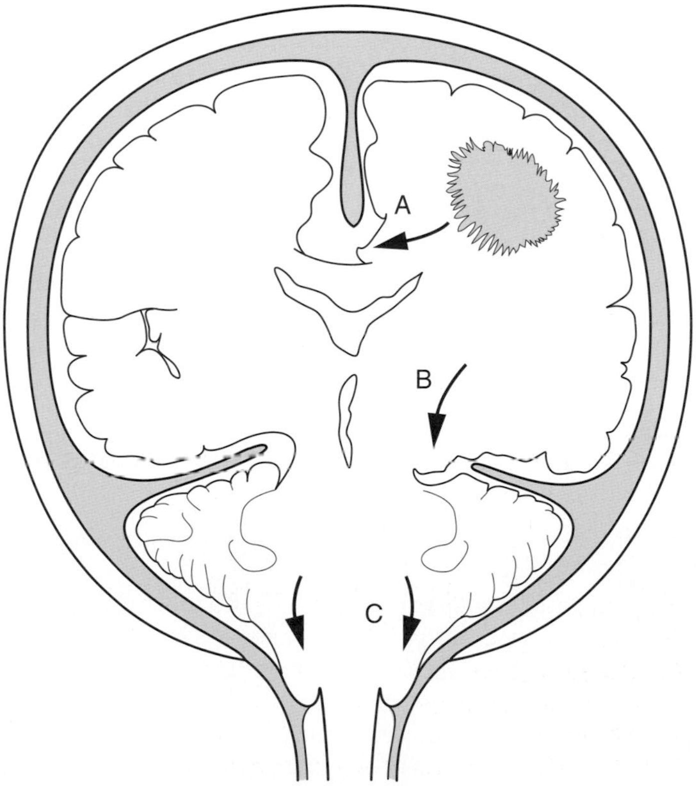

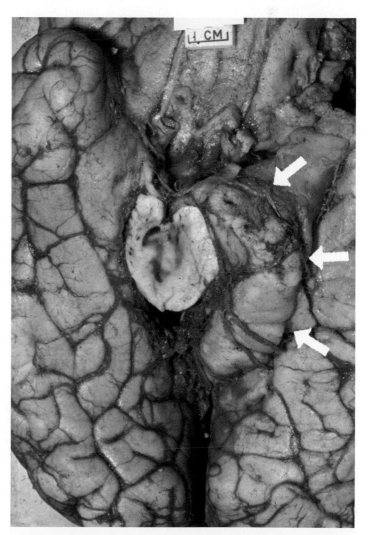

**FIG. 11.7** Raised intracranial pressure, showing the intracranial compartments and the result of a mass lesion on the right-hand side. In addition to a shift of the midline structures and distortion of the ventricular system, there is (A) a supracallosal (subfalcine) hernia, (B) a tentorial hernia, and (C) a tonsillar hernia.

**FIG. 11.8** Raised intracranial pressure: the medial part of the temporal lobe has pushed medially and downwards to form a tentorial hernia. The deep groove (arrows) indicates the position of the edge of the tentorium. There is also secondary haemorrhage into the brain stem.

cellular osmoregulation, the blood–brain barrier to proteins remaining intact.

## Hydrocephalus

The term hydrocephalus means an increased volume of CSF within the cranial cavity (*Box 11.5*). The most common cause of enlargement of the ventricles is cerebral atrophy (see p. 319) in which the ICP is not increased. Acute hydrocephalus with increased ICP is most often due to obstruction to the free flow of CSF. The ventricles enlarge and there is a reduction in the bulk of the white matter in the cerebral hemispheres. In obstructive hydrocephalus it is the site of the lesion rather than its nature that is of importance. Thus, even a small lesion in a critical site adjacent to an interventricular foramen of Monro or the aqueduct in the midbrain will rapidly produce hydrocephalus. Any process such as previous meningitis or subarachnoid haemorrhage which results in partial obliteration of the subarachnoid space will also obstruct the flow of CSF.

The ventricular system proximal to the obstruction enlarges. If it is at a foramen of Monro, one lateral ventricle enlarges: if it is in the third ventricle or the aqueduct, both lateral ventricles enlarge; if it is at the exit foramina of the fourth ventricle, the entire ventricular system enlarges; if the obstruction is in the subarachnoid space, the entire ventricular system enlarges but on this occasion the hydrocephalus is communicating in type because CSF can flow out of the exit foramina in the fourth ventricle into the subarachnoid space.

## Normal Pressure Hydrocephalus

This is characterized by ventricular enlargement and a clinical syndrome of progressive dementia, disturbance of gait, and urinary incontinence or urgency. Routine measurements of CSF pressure may be normal but continuous monitoring of ICP can demonstrate episodes of moderate intracranial hypertension. It has been suggested that a more appropriate term might be 'intermittent hydrocephalus'. A ventriculoperitoneal shunt may result in clinical improvement. In most cases the cause is not known, but there may be a history of previous subarachnoid haemorrhage after a head injury or a previous haemorrhagic stroke, leading to partial obliteration of the subarachnoid space.

# HEAD INJURY

There are two principal types of head injury: missile and blunt. In blunt head injury the two main causes of damage to the brain are acceleration/deceleration and contact. Sudden deceleration or acceleration of the head causes the brain to move within the cranial cavity, producing shear strains within the brain or contact between brain and the bony irregularities at the base of the skull. Damage is particularly severe when there is a rotational element in the acceleration/deceleration. Nothing needs to strike the head nor does the head need to strike anything to produce brain damage – what matters is the acceleration/deceleration conditions that exist at the moment of injury. The various features of brain damage are classified as primary and secondary according to whether they occur at the moment of injury or as a subsequent reaction to the injury, and therefore potentially preventable.

Missile injuries are produced by various types of objects that fall or are propelled through the air. The object often enters the cranial cavity, producing focal brain damage. See *Box 11.6* for a summary of the key epidemiological features of head injury.

## Blunt Injury: Primary Damage

The major elements in blunt injury are fracture of the skull, contusions/lacerations usually with subarachnoid haemorrhage, intracranial haematomas, and diffuse traumatic axonal injury.

### Fracture of the Skull

Many patients with a fracture do not sustain significant brain damage although about 25% of fatal head injuries are not associated with a fracture; in patients with a fracture, however, there is a high incidence of intracranial haematoma. The fracture may be depressed causing local pressure on the

---

**Box 11.5** MAJOR FORMS OF HYDROCEPHALUS

- Internal hydrocephalus: increased volume of cerebrospinal fluid (CSF) within the ventricular system
- External hydrocephalus: an excess of CSF in the subarachnoid space
- Communicating hydrocephalus: when CSF can flow freely from the ventricular system to the subarachnoid space
- Non-communicating hydrocephalus: when CSF cannot flow from the fourth ventricle to the subarachnoid space
- Compensatory hydrocephalus: an increased volume of CSF after loss of brain tissue

---

**Box 11.6** EPIDEMIOLOGY OF TRAUMATIC BRAIN INJURY

- Trauma is the most common cause of death under age 45 years
- Brain damage after head injury is the most important factor contributing to death or serious incapacity
- About 300 per 100,000 of the population require hospital admission per year
- Principal causes of head injury include road traffic accidents, falls, assaults and injuries at work, in the home, and during sports
- Head injuries from road traffic accidents are most common in young males; alcohol is frequently involved

brain. If there is a scalp laceration the fracture is compound and a potential source of intracranial sepsis. Any fracture of the base of the skull provides a potential source of infection from the nose, paranasal sinuses, or middle ear; there may be CSF rhinorrhoea or otorrhoea. Tearing of a meningeal artery may produce an extradural haematoma.

## Cerebral Contusions and Lacerations

These are the most common form of brain damage directly attributable to injury. They may occur at the site of contact, particularly if there is a depressed fracture, but in any blunt head injury they tend to involve the frontal poles, orbital gyri, temporal poles, and inferior and lateral surfaces of the anterior halves of the temporal lobes (Fig. 11.9).

## Intracranial Haematoma

This is a frequent complication of a head injury and is the most common cause of deterioration and death in patients who have been conscious immediately after their injury. The incidence of haematoma is high in patients with a fracture of the skull. Traumatic intracranial haematomas may be extradural, subdural, subarachnoid, or intracerebral.

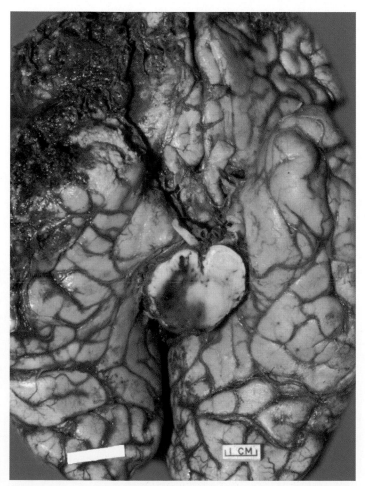

**FIG. 11.9** Cerebral contusions: the frontal and temporal lobes are affected by haemorrhagic contusions.

### Extradural Haematoma

This is caused by haemorrhage from a meningeal blood vessel, usually the middle meningeal artery, damaged by a skull fracture. The haematoma gradually strips the dura from the skull to form a large ovoid mass that progressively compresses the adjacent brain. The initial injury may seem mild as the patient experiences a lucid interval of some hours before developing a headache and becoming drowsy. As the haematoma enlarges, the ICP increases, and the patient lapses into coma and may die unless the haematoma is evacuated.

### Subdural Haematoma

A subdural haematoma results from rupture of bridging veins, which drain into the superior sagittal sinus, or from haemorrhage into the subdural space from severe surface contusions. The blood spreads diffusely throughout the subdural space.

#### Acute subdural haematoma

This is a common postmortem finding if death has occurred soon after the injury. The haematoma may be large and act as an acute intracranial expanding lesion, or it may only be a thin film of blood. Some patients with acute subdural haematoma experience a lucid interval similar to that associated with extradural haematoma.

#### Chronic subdural haematoma

Chronic subdural haematoma presents weeks or months after an apparently trivial head injury; some patients deny any history of injury. The haematoma is organized and becomes encapsulated in a fibrous membrane. Chronic subdural haematoma is particularly common in old people who already have some cerebral atrophy; as the haematoma expands very slowly, probably as the result of repeated small haemorrhages into it, it may become quite large before symptoms appear. In untreated cases, however, death is usually attributable to brain damage secondary to a high ICP. Chronic subdural haematoma is frequently bilateral.

### Intracerebral Haematoma

Intracerebral haematoma tends to be associated with contusions and occurs principally in the frontal or temporal lobe. The term 'burst lobe' is used to describe the combination of an intracerebral haematoma in continuity with a subdural haematoma through surface contusions. Small, deeply seated intracerebral haematomas – often referred to as 'basal ganglia haematomas' – also occur and have a higher incidence in patients with diffuse traumatic axonal injury (see below).

## Diffuse Traumatic Axonal Injury

Nerve fibres are torn at the moment of injury as a result of shear strains produced by acceleration/deceleration forces, particularly rotational. This may occur in the absence of contusions and the only abnormalities observed *post mortem* may be haemorrhagic lesions in the corpus callosum (Fig. 11.10) and the rostral brain stem: the diagnosis can be made only after histological examination. The striking abnormality is the presence of axonal varicosities and bulbs in many regions of the brain (Fig. 11.11). In patients who survive for weeks or months – usually in a severely disabled or vegetative state – there is enlargement of the ventricular system due to a reduction in the bulk of the white matter. There are often also small, shrunken, cystic lesions in the corpus callosum and the rostral brain stem. Microscopy at this stage shows widespread wällerian degeneration secondary to the axonal disruption. Axonal damage in a patient dying from a head injury may also be a consequence of ischaemia and internal herniations, therefore representing a secondary complication.

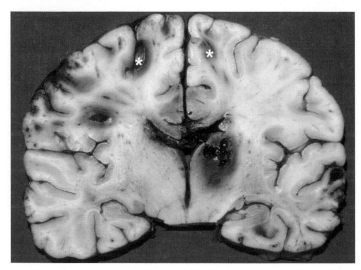

FIG. 11.10 Diffuse traumatic axonal injury: there is a haemorrhagic lesion in the corpus callosum to the right of the midline. There are also gliding contusions (*) in the dorsomedial sectors of the hemispheres and a haematoma in the right thalamus. Note the relative absence of superficial contusions.

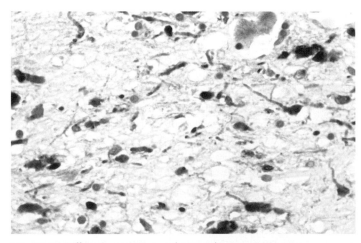

FIG. 11.11 Diffuse traumatic axonal injury: there are many irregularly shaped axons and some bulbs in the corpus callosum (immunohistochemistry of β-amyloid precursor protein [APP]).

## Blunt Injury: Secondary Damage

The main features are raised ICP, ischaemia, and infection. Secondary damage after a head injury with brain swelling often causes an increase in ICP and distortion and herniation of the brain (see p. 300). Particularly in children there may be acute swelling of both hemispheres soon after injury.

### Ischaemic Brain Damage

This is a frequent occurrence. Some of the causes are recognized, e.g. cardiorespiratory arrest or status epilepticus. The pathogenesis of other types of ischaemic damage is not understood but is probably attributable to acute haemodynamic instability soon after injury. Raised ICP after head injury reduces cerebral perfusion, resulting in ischaemia with consequent oedema, further compromising the ICP; in this way a vicious cycle may be initiated with fatal results.

### Infection

Infection brought about by bacteria entering the skull through a compound fracture of the vault or a basal skull fracture usually presents as meningitis, mainly in the early post-traumatic period. A small traumatic fistula from the subarachnoid space to one of the sinuses may result in late-onset sepsis. An intracranial abscess is rare and usually secondary to a penetrating injury.

### Clinical Aspects

Clinical aspects of the pathogenesis of brain damage due to a head injury are complex and the primary damage may be the beginning of an evolving process which may range from progressive improvement – as in most patients with so-called concussion – to death. Diffuse brain damage is probably the most important with regard to the clinical outcome because, unlike intracranial haematoma, much of it is not amenable to treatment. The Glasgow Coma Scale (GCS) is an internationally recognized method of assessing the conscious state and monitoring changes over time; the lowest score (3/15) represents deep coma and the highest (15/15) a fully awake person. The Glasgow Outcome Scale (GOS) allows objective assessment of the degree of subsequent recovery.

Head injury is a major cause of disability and death. Of patients who survive the initial injury and remain in a coma for at least 6 hours, a third die within 6 months, a third recover, and a third are moderately or severely disabled; around 3% are vegetative. Residual disabilities include mental (impaired intellect, memory, and behavioural problems) and physical defects (hemiparesis and dysphasia). Most recovery occurs within the first 6 months after injury. There is an accumulating population of disabled survivors from head injury, 1 in 300 families having a member with such a disability.

Head injury is an important cause of epilepsy. About 5% of patients admitted to hospital after blunt head injury develop seizures. These tend to occur in the first week after injury (early epilepsy) or are delayed for 2–3 months (late epilepsy). With penetrating head injuries the incidence of epilepsy is about 45%.

# CIRCULATORY DISTURBANCES: VASCULAR DISEASE AND HYPOXIC BRAIN DAMAGE

Cerebrovascular disease can result in a sudden disturbance of brain function (stroke). The annual incidence in western countries varies between 150 and 200 per 100,000 population. Strokes account for 10% of all deaths; about 50% of new strokes are fatal and of those who survive about 50% are permanently disabled and only 10% return to normal activity. A distinction is made between transient ischaemic attacks – a fully reversible neurological deficit usually lasting for a few minutes, but occasionally up to 24 hours in which it is assumed that no structural brain damage has occurred – and a completed stroke in which permanent brain damage of varying severity has developed. The numerous risk factors for strokes due to infarction and haemorrhage include those for atheroma (see Chapter 6, pp. 133–137) and hypertension.

## Arterial Supply to Brain

The arterial supply to the cerebral hemispheres is derived from branches of the circle of Willis, an anastomotic channel between the major cerebral arteries at the base of the brain (Fig. 11.12). Potential anastomoses between the vertebral and internal carotid arteries are important if the blood flow through the internal carotid or vertebral arteries is compromised. There is an increased risk of infarction if these potential anastomoses are deficient due to an anomaly in the circle of Willis or acquired disease such as atheromatous stenosis.

The spinal cord is supplied from the spinal branches of the vertebral, deep cervical, intercostal, and lumbar arteries; they arise from the aorta in a segmental manner and feed into the anterior spinal artery which supplies the anterior two-thirds of the spinal cord and two smaller posterior spinal arteries. Structural damage resulting from ischaemia usually takes the form of an infarct but in less severe ischaemia only neurons undergo necrosis (selective neuronal necrosis).

## Cerebral Infarction

Cerebral infarction is the cause of about 85% of strokes. After a local arrest or reduction of cerebral blood flow (CBF) cellular elements of an area of brain may undergo necrosis. Infarcts range from small discrete lesions to necrosis of large parts of the brain: they may occur in any part of the brain but are most common in the distribution of the

middle cerebral artery. All or only part of the arterial territory may be affected (Fig. 11.13).

The structural changes depend upon the size of the lesion and the survival time. A cerebral infarct may be pale or haemorrhagic. An intensely haemorrhagic infarct

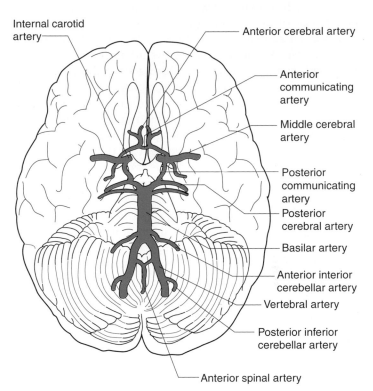

**FIG. 11.12** Circle of Willis: the anterior part of the circle is derived from the internal carotid arteries which divide into the proximal portions of the paired middle and anterior cerebral arteries, and the posterior part from the vertebral and basilar system which is the origin of the paired posterior cerebral arteries. The circle is completed anteriorly by the anterior communicating artery, which joins the anterior cerebral arteries, and posteriorly by the posterior communicating arteries, which join the posterior cerebral and internal carotid arteries.

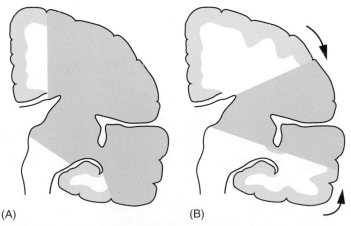

**FIG. 11.13** Diagrammatic representations of infarcts in the territory supplied by a middle cerebral artery. (A) Infarct involving the entire territory and (B) infarct restricted to the central territory. Arrows in (B) indicate collateral flow from the anterior and posterior cerebral arteries. (From Adams JH, Graham DI. *Introduction to Neuropathology*. London: Churchill Livingstone, 1988.)

may resemble a haematoma, but the architecture of the necrotic tissue is preserved (Fig. 11.14). A pale infarct less than 24 hours old is difficult to identify macroscopically, but thereafter the dead tissue becomes soft and swollen and there is a loss of the normal sharp definition between the grey and white matter. Swelling of the necrotic tissue and oedema of the surrounding brain may cause a large infarct to act as an acutely expanding mass lesion with raised ICP (Fig. 11.15). Within a few days the infarct becomes soft as the dead tissue disintegrates. During the following weeks the dead tissue is removed by macrophages and there is gliosis. The lesion ultimately becomes shrunken and cystic and, if there has been haemorrhage, brown due to haemosiderin within the macrophages. Shrinkage of a cerebral infarct is usually accompanied by enlargement of the adjacent ventricle (Fig. 11.16). Wällerian degeneration of the interrupted nerve fibres occurs; thus, if the infarct involves the internal capsule, there is progressive shrinkage of the corticospinal tract in the brain stem and spinal cord.

The pathogenesis of cerebral infarction includes embolism, atheroma, and many other causes. Cerebral embolism accounts for between 30% and 60% of strokes. Most emboli pass into the middle cerebral artery, and many produce only transient occlusion. The major sources are the heart (see Chapter 6, pp. 112–114), and atheroma of the extracranial neck arteries and arch of aorta. Atheromatous narrowing or occlusion may occur in any part of the carotid or vertebral arteries. Stenosis does not necessarily lead to infarction because, at normal blood pressure, the internal cross-sectional area of an artery must be reduced by up to 90% before blood flow is significantly impaired; a combination of systemic circulatory insufficiency and stenosis results in many cases of infarction. The most common site is at the origin of an internal carotid artery, but infarction results only if the collateral circulation is inadequate. In some cases, thrombosis extends along the internal carotid artery into the middle and anterior cerebral arteries to produce infarction of a large part of the cerebral hemisphere. The most common intracranial site of thrombosis is a middle cerebral artery, usually due to embolism, thrombosis formed on atheroma, or basal vasospasm after rupture of an adjacent saccular aneurysm. Occlusion of the extracranial neck arteries may also follow embolism, dissecting aneurysm, and trauma. The vertebral artery may be occluded due to deformation by osteophytes, certain neck movements, e.g. hyperextension during intubation for anaesthesia, or rheumatoid arthritis with subluxation of the atlanto-occipital joint.

Primary thrombosis of the veins and venous sinuses (noninfectious or marantic) occurs most frequently in poorly nourished and dehydrated children during the course of acute infections; it may occur in adults with congestive

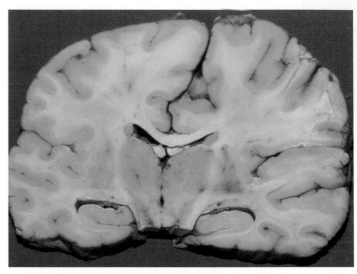

**FIG. 11.15** Cerebral infarction: there is a large infarct in the right cerebral hemisphere due to occlusion of the ipsilateral internal carotid artery. There are internal herniae and some asymmetry of the ventricles due to midline shift.

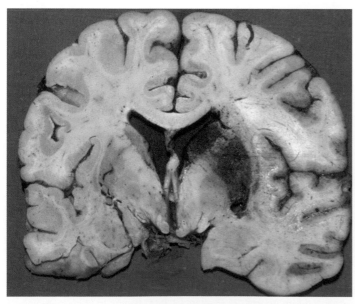

**FIG. 11.14** Recent infarct in the right cerebral hemisphere. The basal ganglia show the features of haemorrhagic infarction (reperfusion injury).

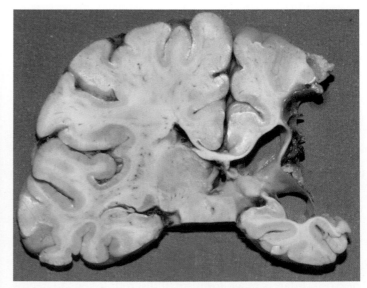

**FIG. 11.16** Cerebral infarction of several years' duration. The necrotic tissue has been removed and the ipsilateral lateral ventricle is enlarged (compensatory hydrocephalus).

cardiac failure, or during pregnancy and the puerperium. Thrombosis may be secondary to pyogenic infection (septic thrombosis).

## Brain Damage due to Cardiac Arrest

Neurons require a continuous adequate supply of oxygen and glucose which depends on cardiorespiratory function and CBF; this is determined by the cerebral perfusion pressure (the difference between the systemic arterial blood pressure and the cerebral venous pressure). An autoregulatory mechanism maintains a relatively constant CBF in spite of changes in perfusion pressure even when systemic arterial pressure falls as low as 6.65 kPa (50 mmHg) provided that the patient is in the horizontal position. At arterial pressures lower than this, CBF falls rapidly. Autoregulation may be impaired in hypertension, hypoxia, or hypercapnia, or in many acute conditions producing brain damage, e.g. head injury and strokes.

Patients who sustain severe diffuse brain damage after cardiac arrest often die within a few days. The brain may appear normal macroscopically, but, if the patient has survived for more than 12 hours, microscopy shows widespread and severe neuronal necrosis with a distinctive pattern of selective vulnerability. Worst affected are the neocortex and hippocampus, with the greatest involvement of the CA1 sector. There is diffuse necrosis of the Purkinje cells of the cerebellum and loss of the sensory nuclei of the brain stem.

## 11.1 Special Study Topic

Written by I Bone, Emeritus Professor of Neurology, University of Glasgow.

### THROMBOLYTIC THERAPY IN ACUTE ISCHAEMIC STROKE

The management of patients with ischaemic strokes in specialized stroke units has greatly improved outcomes. In part this has been through good general management of blood pressure (avoiding hypotension), maintaining adequate oxygenation, anticipating dysphagia with the risk of aspiration, prophylaxis of venous thrombosis in immobile patients, and suppressing fever, if present.

An increasing part of acute management involves the consideration of methods that may re-canalize the occluded blood vessel, thus permitting reperfusion and salvage of ischaemic non-necrotic tissue. Natural fibrinolysins normally released by the injured endothelium may not work sufficiently quickly to be clinically effective. Thrombolytic agents speed up the conversion of plasminogen to plasmin, a potent natural fibrinolytic, thus promoting early clot lysis. Several different thrombolytic agents have been developed and trialled in ischaemic stroke.

### Streptokinase

Clinical trials of intravenous streptokinase have failed to show benefit in patients with acute ischaemic stroke, although it is uncertain whether this difference from tissue plasminogen activator (tPA) trial results (see below) reflects a longer time window from onset (<6 hours), the dose used, or the specific properties of streptokinase itself. Intra-arterial streptokinase, urokinase, and pro-urokinase are undergoing clinical trials.

### Tissue Plasminogen Activator

The results of the National Institute of Neurologic Disorders and Stroke (NINDS) tPA trial were published in December 1995 and resulted in approval by the US Food and Drug Administration (FDA) for clinical use. The NINDS study showed that the use of intravenous tPA within 3 hours of ischaemic stroke onset substantially improved long-term functional outcome compared with placebo, even when including the risk of symptomatic intracerebral haemorrhage. The trial showed that, for every 100 patients given IV tPA, 12 more experience complete neurological recovery compared with placebo. Symptomatic intracranial haemorrhage occurred in 6%. The risk of intracerebral haemorrhage increased significantly in patients treated with tPA in whom the CT scan showed obvious evidence of early infarction as well as in those with more marked clinical deficit (as measured by the National Institutes of Health (NIH) Stroke Scale) at baseline.[1]

The European Cooperative Acute Stroke Study (ECASS) randomized trial of intravenous tPA[2] with a 6-hour time limit to treatment, and using a higher dose of tPA, did not demonstrate benefit, largely due to the high rate of brain haemorrhage. A follow-up trial from the European investigators (ECASS II) tested a lower dose of intravenous tPA (0.9/kg) in the 3- to 6-hour window and excluded patients with early extensive infarction visible on CT. This study showed no significant benefit.[3]

From these studies a maximum time of 3 hours from stroke onset to treatment is recommended. A CT scan must be carried out before treatment to exclude intracranial bleeding or extensive infarction evidenced by sulcal effacement, mass effect, and oedema. Caution is advised before giving intravenous tPA to patients with severe stroke (NIH Stroke Scale >23)[4]. This treatment should not be given to those who are severely hypertensive (systolic pressure >185 mmHg or diastolic pressure >110 mmHg), have a recent history of head injury or blood loss, are rapidly recovering, or have experienced a seizure at presentation. Treating patients who do not fulfil the protocol guidelines results in excessive risk with no observable benefit. Debate persists as to how specialist the provisions of a stroke centre offering such treatment should be. Combined intravenous and intra-arterial regimens remain under study, as do other modes of clot lysis (glycoprotein IIb/IIIa inhibitors) and fragmentation (ultrasound).

## Special Study Topic continued . . .

### References

1. Adams HP Jr, Brott TG, Furlan AJ, *et al*. Guidelines for thrombolytic therapy for acute stroke: a supplement to the guidelines for the management of patients with acute ischemic stroke. A statement for healthcare professionals from a Special Writing Group of the Stroke Council, American Heart Association. *Circulation* 1996;**94**:1167.
2. Hacke W, Kaste M, Fieschi C, *et al*. Intravenous thrombolysis with recombinant tissue plasminogen activator for acute hemispheric stroke. The European Cooperative Acute Stroke Study (ECASS). *JAMA* 1995;**274**:1017–1025.
3. Hacke W, Kaste M, Fieschi C, *et al*. Randomised double-blind placebo-controlled trial of thrombolytic therapy with intravenous alteplase in acute ischaemic stroke (ECASS II). Second European-Australasian Acute Stroke Study Investigators. *Lancet* 1998;**352**:1245–1251.
4. The NINDS t-PA Stroke Study Group. Intracerebral haemorrhage after intravenous t-PA therapy for ischemic stroke. *Stroke* 1997;**28**:2109–2118.

In postmortem cases, brain damage is generally more severe in young children than adults. A similar pattern of damage may be seen in carbon monoxide intoxication and status epilepticus. Severe hypoglycaemia may also cause widespread brain damage.

Brain damage due to hypotension is concentrated in the boundary zones between the main cerebral and cerebellar arterial territories (Fig. 11.17). The lesions tend to be largest in the parieto-occipital regions where the territories of the anterior, middle, and posterior cerebral arteries meet. There is variable involvement of the basal ganglia. The hippocampi, despite their vulnerability to cardiac arrest, are usually not involved. This type of brain damage is seen most commonly in shock and fatal head injury, and is caused by a major episode of hypotension; autoregulation fails and CBF falls most in the boundary zones, those regions most remote from the parent arteries.

## Spontaneous (Non-traumatic) Intracranial Haemorrhage

Haemorrhage is the cause of about 15% of strokes. The major types are intracerebral and subarachnoid haemorrhage.

Intracerebral haematomas develop in late middle age due to rupture of one of the numerous microaneurysms found in hypertensive individuals, most commonly in the basal ganglia and the internal capsule (Fig. 11.18); other sites are the pons and cerebellum. The haematoma rapidly increases in size and produces a sudden rise in ICP, with distortion and herniation of the brain. Blood may rupture into the ventricles or the subarachnoid space. The onset is sudden, and patients with large haematomas rarely survive for more than a day or two.

The postmortem appearances vary with time; a recent haematoma is composed of dark-red clot, but after a week the periphery is brownish and there are early reactive changes in macrophages, astrocytes, and capillaries. Gliosis leads eventually to the formation of a poorly defined capsule, and the clot is ultimately completely removed by macrophages and replaced by yellow fluid to form a cyst.

Another common cause of spontaneous intracranial haemorrhage is rupture of a vascular malformation which may range from a small capillary angioma to a massive arteriovenous malformation composed of large, often thick-walled vascular channels (Fig. 11.19). Many of these lesions are compatible with long survival, sometimes punctuated by

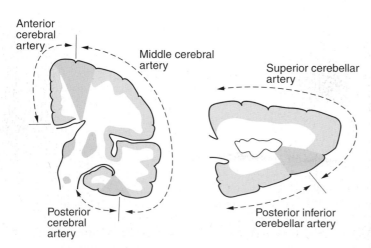

FIG. 11.17 Diagram to show arterial boundary zones in the cerebral and cerebellar hemispheres. They lie between the territories supplied by the major arteries.

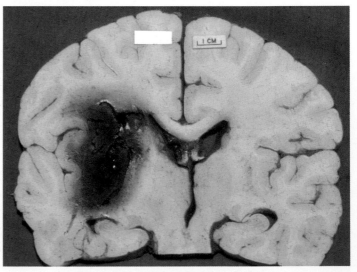

FIG. 11.18 Intracerebral haemorrhage: there is a large haematoma in the basal ganglia due to chronic hypertension.

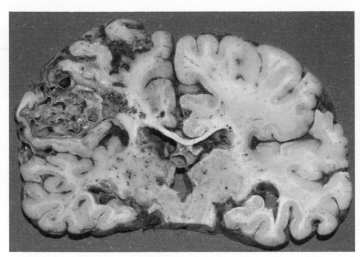

FIG. 11.19 Arteriovenous malformation: there is a large plexus of vascular channels of varying size in the upper part of the left cerebral hemisphere. (Reproduced from Graham DI, Nicoll JAR, Bone I. *Adams & Graham's Introduction to Neuropathology*, 3rd edn. London: Hodder Arnold, 2006.)

episodes of haemorrhage. Spontaneous intracranial haemorrhage may be due to bleeding into a tumour or to haemorrhagic diseases, e.g. acute leukaemia or coagulation disorders.

### Subarachnoid Haemorrhage

In most patients with spontaneous (non-traumatic) subarachnoid haemorrhage this is due to rupture of a saccular aneurysm on one of the major cerebral arteries, and in about 5% of patients is due to rupture of a vascular malformation. In a further 10–15% it is due to some other disease, such as a blood dyscrasia or extension of either an intracerebral or an intraventricular haemorrhage into the subarachnoid space. In up to 5% of patients a cause is not found.

Saccular aneurysms occur on the arteries of the base of the brain and rupture occurs in 6–12/100,000 population per year. About 10–15% of patients are found to have multiple (usually two or three) aneurysms. The common sites are the upper end of the internal carotid artery (40%), the anterior communicating artery (30%), the middle cerebral artery (20%), and the basilar and vertebral arteries (5–10%). Aneurysms occur more commonly in women, and between age 40 and 60 years. Although often called congenital aneurysms, the developmental abnormality is a defect in the media of the artery at a division. Early atheroma and hypertension probably contribute to the development of the aneurysm. Most aneurysms that rupture measure 5–10 mm in diameter. Some 10% of patients die before reaching hospital, and a further 30% within the next few days. A further 35% re-bleed and die within the first year, most within the first 2 weeks.

When a saccular aneurysm ruptures, the haemorrhage may be limited to its immediate vicinity, but more often it spreads extensively through the CSF in the subarachnoid space (Fig. 11.20). Blood may track into the brain to produce an intracerebral haematoma as an acute expanding

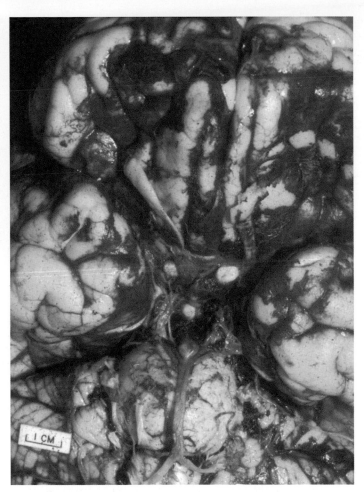

FIG. 11.20 Subarachnoid haemorrhage: there is a large amount of recent haemorrhage in the basal cisterns due to rupture of an aneurysm at the upper end of the basilar artery.

lesion. If the aneurysm is embedded in brain tissue, intracerebral haemorrhage may occur without subarachnoid haemorrhage. Anterior communicating artery aneurysms tend to burst into the frontal lobe, posterior communicating aneurysms into the temporal lobe. Late complications include cerebral infarction in the distribution of the affected artery, attributable to arterial vasospasm, and hydrocephalus.

Fusiform atheromatous aneurysms of major cerebral arteries occur, but rarely rupture. Mycotic aneurysms produced by infected emboli may also occur. Dissecting aneurysms may affect the carotid or vertebral arteries thus restricting blood flow.

## INFECTIONS OF THE NERVOUS SYSTEM

The brain and spinal cord are relatively well protected against invasion of microorganisms by the bone of the skull and spine, the dura, the blood–brain barrier, the microglia, and the systemic immune system. However, microorganisms that have gained access may spread rapidly, particularly via the CSF pathways, and many relatively non-pathogenic microorganisms can in various circumstances cause serious infections of the nervous system (*Box 11.7*).

Clinical features of acute CNS infection include headache, neck stiffness, photophobia, pyrexia, malaise, and impaired consciousness. Relevant enquiries include the patient's occupation, recent travel, and risk factors for HIV infection. Investigation includes examination of the CSF, usually by lumbar puncture, although the risks of this procedure in the presence of raised ICP must be borne in mind. The key features of the CSF in infections and opportunistic infections of the brain are summarized in *Tables 11.1* and *11.2*.

---

**Box 11.7** RISK FACTORS FOR INFECTION OF THE NERVOUS SYSTEM

- Trauma (particularly with compound fractures)
- Congenital malformations (e.g. spina bifida)
- Iatrogenic (e.g. neurosurgical procedures or lumbar puncture)
- Local foci of infection, e.g. mastoid and middle ear
- Blood-borne infection
- Immunodeficiency states

---

**TABLE 11.1** Cerebrospinal fluid in infections

|  | Glucose (mmol/L) | Protein (g/L) | Cells |
|---|---|---|---|
| Normal | 2.7–4.1 | 0.15–0.45 | <5 lymphocytes/mm$^3$ |
| Bacterial meningitis | Decreased | Increased | +++ polymorphs |
| Abscess | Normal | Increased | + polymorphs and lymphocytes |
| Viral meningitis | Normal | Increased | ++ lymphocytes |
| Tuberculosis | Decreased | Increased | ++ polymorphs early, lymphocytes late |

**TABLE 11.2** Opportunistic infections affecting the central nervous system

| Viruses | Papovavirus (progressive multifocal leukoencephalopathy) |
|---|---|
|  | Cytomegalovirus encephalitis/myelitis/retinitis |
|  | Herpes simplex (type 2) meningitis or myelitis |
|  | Herpes simplex (type 1) encephalitis |
|  | Immunosuppressive measles myelitis or encephalitis |
|  | Varicella-zoster encephalitis/myelitis |
| Bacteria | *Mycobacterium avium-intracellulare* |
|  | *Nocardia* sp. (abscesses) |
|  | Syphilis |
| Fungi | *Cryptococcus neoformans* |
|  | *Candida albicans* |
|  | *Aspergillus fumigatus* |
|  | Mucormycosis |
|  | Coccidioidomycosis |
|  | Histoplasmosis |
| Protozoa | Toxoplasmosis (*Toxoplasma gondii*) |

## Bacterial Infections

---

**Key Points**

- Spread to the CNS may be haematogenous, from bone infection, or as a result of trauma.
- Bacterial infections cause meningitis and brain abscess.
- In bacterial meningitis the CSF is turbid and contains polymorphs and bacteria.
- Brain abscess presents as a space-occupying lesion.
- Tuberculosis causes a subacute meningitis or abscess (tuberculoma).

---

### Acute Bacterial Meningitis

Bacterial meningitis, characterized by spread of bacteria and inflammatory cells through the subarachnoid space, is an emergency requiring rapid diagnosis and treatment. The most common causative organisms are *Escherichia coli* in infants, *Haemophilus influenzae* in children, *Neisseria meningitidis* in young adults, and *Streptococcus pneumoniae* in elderly people.

Most cases of meningitis are of haematogenous origin. Infection with *N. meningitidis* (meningococcal meningitis) is spread by droplet infection from nasopharyngeal carriers and may occur as an epidemic. The meningococci pass to the meninges via the bloodstream and fatal meningococcal septicaemia can occur before meningitis develops; a purpuric rash is an important early sign. Early antibiotic therapy may be given on clinical suspicion but the precise diagnosis depends on examination of the CSF (see *Table 11.1*). The causal organisms are often apparent in stained films but sometimes they can be detected only by culture. Immunization reduces the risk of infection.

Meningitis may also be brought about by spread from infection in the bones of the skull or after a compound fracture of the skull. Iatrogenic infection occasionally follows surgery or lumbar puncture. In meningitis, pus is found in the intracranial and spinal subarachnoid spaces, and is thickest at the base of the brain. In rapidly fatal cases there may be no more than an excess of turbid fluid in the sulci and histological examination is required to confirm the presence of acute inflammation. The ventricles may contain turbid CSF. Mild hydrocephalus is common because the exudate interferes with the flow of CSF.

Long-term effects are common in survivors and include hydrocephalus due to obliteration of the exit foramina of the fourth ventricle and/or subarachnoid space. Involvement of the cranial nerves traversing the subarachnoid space may result in cranial nerve palsies.

### Brain Abscess

The clinical features include fever and those of raised ICP. The abscess consists of pus surrounded by oedematous brain containing reactive astrocytes and, within 2–3 weeks, a collagenous capsule. The causative organisms include streptococci, *Bacteroides* spp., *Proteus* spp., staphylococci,

*E. coli* and *H. influenzae*, and there may be mixed infections. There are several possible routes of infection. Local spread from infection in the skull (chronic otitis media, chronic mastoiditis, penetrating injury, or surgery) usually results in a single abscess (Fig. 11.21), whereas multiple brain abscesses often follow haematogenous spread from infection in the lung (bronchiectasis, pneumonia, empyema) or heart (infective endocarditis). Haematogenous spread is also associated with congenital heart disease with a right-to-left shunt.

Clinical diagnosis is by recognition of a focal lesion in the brain with a necrotic centre by CT or MRI scan, and by aspiration of abscess contents and microbiological culture. Treatment is antibiotic therapy and may include therapeutic aspiration of pus.

## Tuberculosis

Infection of the CNS by *Mycobacterium tuberculosis* is always secondary to disease elsewhere; its frequency is therefore related to the incidence of tuberculosis in a given population. There are two principal forms: tuberculous meningitis and tuberculomas.

### Tuberculous Meningitis

The bacilli almost always reach the subarachnoid space via the bloodstream, either as a component of miliary tuberculosis or spread from a tuberculous focus elsewhere in the body. Occasionally infection spreads to the subarachnoid space from tuberculosis of a vertebral body. Tuberculous meningitis has a subacute or chronic course. A gelatinous or caseous exudate, which is most abundant in the basal cisterns (Fig. 11.22A), within sulci, and around the spinal cord obstructs the flow of CSF, with almost invariable hydrocephalus. Small tubercles measuring 1–2 mm in diameter may be seen in the pia arachnoid. Lymphocytes, plasma cells, and macrophages are seen but Langhans-type giant cells are uncommon (Fig. 11.22B). Obliterative endarteritis causes small infarcts in the brain or the cranial nerve roots, leading to focal neurological signs. Mycobacteria are rarely seen on examination of the CSF (Ziehl–Neelsen stain) but may be demonstrated by culture, fluorescence of rhodamine auramine, or polymerase chain reaction (PCR).

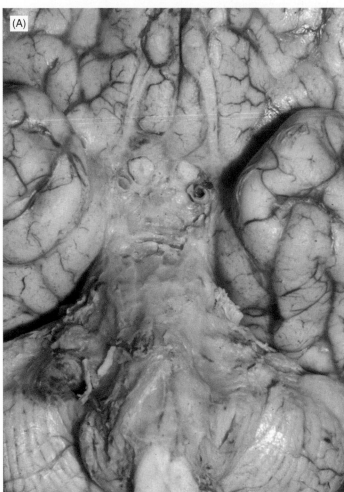

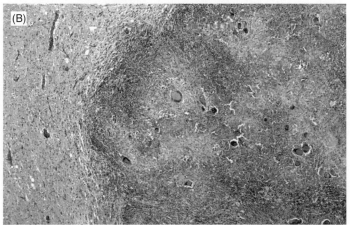

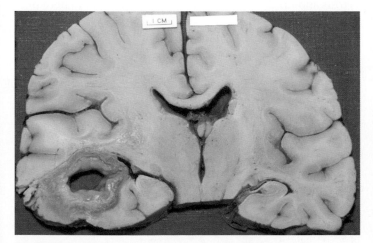

**FIG. 11.21** Cerebral abscess: there is an encapsulated abscess in the left temporal lobe secondary to chronic suppurative otitis media. (Reproduced from Graham DI, Nicoll JAR, Bone I. *Adams & Graham's Introduction to Neuropathology*, 3rd edn. London: Hodder Arnold, 2006.)

**FIG. 11.22** Tuberculous meningitis: (A) there is thick exudate at the base of the brain. (B) Within the meninges is a caseating granulomatous inflammatory process with Langhans' giant cells.

### Tuberculoma

In countries where tuberculosis is rife, tuberculoma (tuberculous abscess) is a common cause of an intracranial expanding lesion. In adults tuberculomas usually occur in the cerebral hemispheres but in children they particularly affect the cerebellum. A tuberculoma has a core of caseous material surrounded by granulomatous inflammation with lymphocytes, epithelioid histiocytes (macrophages), and Langhans-type giant cells.

### Syphilis

Syphilis, caused by *Treponema pallidum*, is now uncommon. It may cause a transient meningoencephalitis (secondary stage), subacute meningitis (tertiary stage) with cranial nerve palsies, gummas in the meninges, and subacute encephalitis, causing progressive dementia many years after the primary infection (general paralysis of the insane). Degeneration of the posterior spinal columns results in the syndrome of tabes dorsalis.

## Fungal Infections

Fungal infections of the CNS are uncommon and usually arise by haematogenous spread from the lungs or direct spread from the nose and sinuses. As lesions at the portal of entry may be small and readily overlooked, the brain may appear to be the only organ involved. In other cases infection of the nervous system may be a manifestation of generalized infection. Immunocompromised patients are particularly vulnerable to fungal infections.

Brain abscesses, often multiple, may be caused by *Aspergillus*, *Candida*, and *Histoplasma* spp. Accurate identification depends on culture. Colonization of the walls of blood vessels by fungi and the associated thrombosis result in infarction. The inflammatory response is predominantly chronic. Mucormycosis, a rare opportunistic infection with a particular predilection for patients with poorly controlled diabetes, starts in the paranasal regions and spreads directly into the anterior fossa of the skull to produce selective involvement of the frontal lobes. Cryptococcosis infection usually presents as a subacute meningitis; the exudate in the subarachnoid space is gelatinous and contains masses of encapsulated cryptococci.

## Viral Infections

### Key Points

- Spread of virus to the CNS is usually via the haematogenous route.
- Viral meningitis is usually mild.
- Viral encephalitis (e.g. due to herpes simplex virus) is uncommon but severe.
- Persistent viral infections occur (subacute sclerosing panencephalitis and progressive multifocal leukoencephalopathy).

- In acquired immune deficiency syndrome (AIDS), the CNS is affected by human immunodeficiency virus (HIV) encephalitis, opportunistic infection, and lymphoma.

Patients with acute viral infections present with aseptic meningitis or encephalitis. Most viruses reach the nervous system via the bloodstream, often after primary replication of the virus in lymphoid tissue. The viruses enter the body by various routes, e.g. infections of the skin or mucous membranes (herpes simplex virus), via the alimentary tract (enteroviruses), or by the bite of an arthropod (arboviruses). The rabies virus reaches the CNS by travelling along the peripheral nerves.

### Aseptic Meningitis

This common but usually not severe acute infection of the CNS occurs particularly in children and is most often due to enteroviruses or the mumps virus. As aseptic meningitis is rarely fatal, little is known about its pathology, which probably amounts to infiltration of the subarachnoid space by lymphocytes, plasma cells, and macrophages.

### Acute Viral Encephalitis

Many types of acute viral encephalitis have similar histological features with lymphocytes forming cuffs around blood vessels and extending into the brain parenchyma (Fig. 11.23). Viral inclusion bodies may be seen (Fig. 11.24) in neurons or glial cells and viral antigens can be demonstrated by immunocytochemistry. The causal virus can usually be isolated from brain tissue (biopsy or necropsy) or identified in CSF by polymerase chain reaction. There may be necrosis, ranging from selective neuronal necrosis in poliomyelitis to frank infarction of grey and white matter in herpes simplex encephalitis. After tissue destruction astrocytosis and lipid-containing macrophages appear. There may

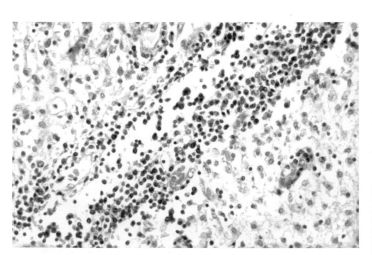

**FIG. 11.23** Acute viral meningitis: the inflammatory cells (mainly around small blood vessels) are lymphocytes and plasma cells.

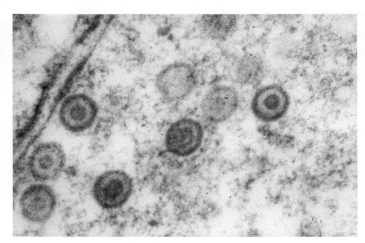

FIG. 11.24 Acute viral encephalitis: intracellular herpes simplex viral particles (electron microscopy).

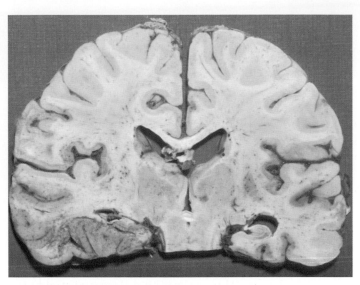

FIG. 11.26 Encephalitis due to herpes simplex virus. This patient survived for several weeks, severely brain damaged. The affected regions are now shrunken and focally cystic. The left temporal lobe is more severely affected than the right.

be a diffuse hyperplasia of microglia with the formation of rod cells and small clusters of microglia.

## Herpes Simplex Encephalitis

This necrotizing encephalitis, which is often rapidly fatal if untreated, is almost always due to herpes simplex type I and is the most common viral encephalitis encountered in western Europe. There is extensive asymmetrical necrosis in the temporal lobes, the insulae, and the cingulate gyri. Swelling of the more severely affected temporal lobe is often sufficient to produce a shift of the midline structures and a tentorial hernia (Fig. 11.25). If the patient survives the acute stage, the necrotic tissue becomes shrunken and cystic (Fig. 11.26). Despite the selective distribution of the necrosis, histological examination discloses a diffuse meningoencephalitis. Appropriate antiviral treatment should be given as soon as

the diagnosis is considered. Confirmatory biopsy from the temporal lobe is now rarely performed because drug therapy is relatively non-toxic.

## Varicella-zoster

Asymptomatic latent infection is established in sensory ganglia after chickenpox in childhood. Re-activation of the virus occurs episodically with ageing and in immunosuppressed individuals. There is inflammation of the ganglion and a painful cutaneous rash in the appropriate dermatome, most commonly in the thoracic and trigeminal distribution.

## Cytomegalovirus

Cytomegalovirus CNS infection may be acquired *in utero*. In the neonate it presents as an acute disseminated necrotizing encephalomyelitis with selective involvement of periventricular tissue. Cytomegalic inclusions ('owl's eye' inclusions) may be found in various types of cell. Survivors almost always have learning difficulties, the principal abnormalities in the brain being hydrocephalus and periventricular calcification. Infection early in pregnancy may lead to malformations such as microgyria. Periventricular encephalitis is also seen in opportunistic infection with cytomegalovirus in patients with AIDS.

## Infections with Enteroviruses

Polioviruses, Coxsackievirus, and echoviruses (echo: enteric cytopathic human orphan) are small RNA viruses that are frequent causes of aseptic meningitis. Enteroviruses are ingested and then multiply in the pharynx and gastrointestinal tract. Within a few days, virus is present in adjacent lymphoid tissue and, if the antibody response is inadequate,

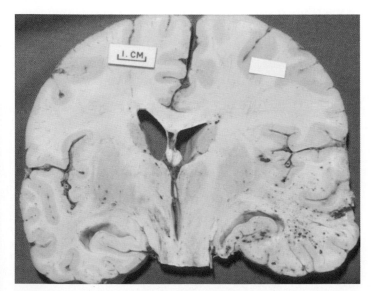

FIG. 11.25 Encephalitis due to herpes simplex virus. Within the swollen right temporal lobe there are many small haemorrhagic foci. There is also a shift of the midline structures to the left.

virus reaches the CNS via the bloodstream. Faecal excretion of virus continues long after the acute infection.

### Acute Anterior Poliomyelitis

This disease is classically due to polioviruses but is occasionally caused by other enteroviruses. The virus selectively attacks neurons in the ventral horns of the spinal cord, particularly in the lumbar and cervical enlargements, leading to paralysis of the limb muscles. If the motor nuclei in the brain stem are affected – bulbar polio – there may be involvement of the respiratory centre. In the acute stage the CNS usually appears normal macroscopically but there may be foci of haemorrhage in the brain stem and ventral horns. Microscopy discloses the typical features of a generalized acute viral encephalitis with selectively severe involvement of the spinal cord or brain stem. After the acute stage of the disease, there is loss of neurons in the affected ventral horns, atrophy of the related nerve roots and neurogenic atrophy of the affected muscles (see Chapter 12, p. 388).

### Infections with Arboviruses

These RNA viruses are transmitted from host to host by bloodsucking insects and multiply in both vertebrate and invertebrate hosts. Humans are not a natural host for any arbovirus but may become infected during periods of epizootic spread among the natural hosts (usually wild birds and small mammals). Severe forms of encephalitis in humans include St Louis encephalitis, which is mosquito borne, and louping ill, due to a tick-borne virus.

### Rabies

Rabies remains a major problem in many countries. Most human cases follow the bite of a rabid dog although the major reservoirs are the fox, skunk, and jackal. The rhabdovirus enters the body from the saliva and reaches the CNS by retrograde transport along peripheral nerves from the bite. The incubation of the disease varies according to the distance of the bite from the CNS; sometimes it is as short as 2 weeks but more commonly is 13 months or even longer. As the old name of hydrophobia implies, spasm of the muscles of swallowing on attempting to drink water may be an early symptom. The pathognomonic histological feature is the Negri body, an intracytoplasmic inclusion 1–7 μm in diameter, within which virus can be identified.

### Persistent Virus Infections

#### Subacute Sclerosing Panencephalitis

This rare form of encephalitis occurs mainly between the ages of 4 and 20 years and has a prolonged clinical course. It occurs some years after an apparently uncomplicated bout of measles and appears to be due to re-activation of latent measles virus. There are high levels of both IgM and IgG antibodies in the blood and CSF. Microscopic examination shows a subacute meningoencephalitis. Neuronophagia is

common, and residual neurons may contain intranuclear and/or cytoplasmic inclusion bodies. There is considerable gliosis in the white matter.

#### Progressive Multifocal Leukoencephalopathy

This disease, caused by viruses of the polyoma subgroup of papovaviruses, is virtually restricted to immunocompromised patients. Distributed throughout the white matter are multiple small grey foci of demyelination which can coalesce to form large, often cystic, areas. Demyelination is accompanied by large bizarre astrocytes, macrophages, and abnormal oligodendrocytes, the large nuclei of which contain inclusion bodies consisting of pseudocrystalline arrays of virions.

#### Acquired Immune Deficiency Syndrome (AIDS)

> **Key Points**
>
> - About 60% of patients with AIDS have clinical neurological abnormalities.
> - Neuropathological abnormalities are identified *post mortem* in almost 90% of cases.
> - The CNS may be affected in three ways: direct effects of HIV itself, opportunistic infection secondary to the immunosuppression, and lymphoma.
> - Often a patient with AIDS may have more than one CNS pathology.
> - Antiretroviral treatment enables patients to live relatively healthy lives.

A mild self-limiting meningitis is common in early HIV infection. An encephalitis occurring in later stages in 15–60% of patients is thought to underlie the clinically defined AIDS-related dementia; it is characterized by multinucleated giant cells seen particularly around blood vessels (Fig. 11.27) in the white matter, often associated with diffuse degeneration of the white matter. Replication of HIV occurs within these

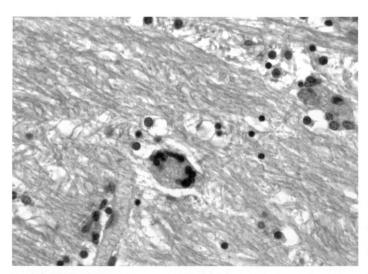

**FIG. 11.27** HIV encephalitis: multinucleated giant cells are a characteristic feature.

giant cells. Some patients develop HIV-associated myelopathy ('vacuolar myelopathy'), analogous to HIV encephalitis.

### Opportunistic infections

The more common opportunistic infections to involve the CNS in AIDS include toxoplasmosis, progressive multifocal leukoencephalopathy (PML), cryptococcosis, cytomegalovirus encephalitis, and fungal infections. These are described in more detail in Chapter 19.

### Lymphoma

Primary or secondary lymphomas may occur in patients with AIDS. Most are high-grade, B-cell, non-Hodgkin's lymphomas. Many are associated with Epstein–Barr virus infection.

### Opportunistic Infections in Immunocompromised Patients

Immunocompromised patients, including those with AIDS, transplant recipients, patients with haematological or lymphoid disorders, or diabetes, and patients undergoing chemotherapy or radiotherapy, are particularly vulnerable to infection. They are at risk of severe disease from organisms that often result in only mild or asymptomatic infection in the immunocompetent (see *Table 11.2*); these are described in Chapter 19.

## DEMYELINATING DISEASES

Myelin is formed from the cell membrane of oligodendrocytes and wraps axons to facilitate saltatory conduction of action potentials. Demyelinating disorders of the CNS are characterized by destruction of the myelin sheaths with relative preservation of the axons (primary or selective demyelination). They are distinct from genetic disorders of myelin formation (dysmyelination) and diseases causing breakdown of myelin secondary to neuronal destruction (wällerian degeneration). See *Table 11.3* for a classification of demyelinating diseases.

## Multiple Sclerosis

### Key Points

- Multiple sclerosis (MS) is the most common demyelinating disorder.
- It is a chronic disease with onset in early adulthood.
- There are usually multiple focal lesions in the brain and spinal cord.
- There is selective loss of myelin with preservation of the axons.

### Clinical Features

Multiple sclerosis is the most common demyelinating disorder and is characterized by multifocal demyelination and gliosis in the brain and spinal cord. It is slightly more

**TABLE 11.3** Classification of demyelinating diseases

| Primary | Multiple sclerosis |
| | Acute disseminated (perivenous) encephalomyelitis |
| | Acute haemorrhagic leukoencephalitis |
| **Secondary** | |
| Viral | Progressive multifocal leukoencephalopathy |
| Toxic/metabolic | Central pontine myelinolysis |
| | Marchiafava–Bignami disease |

common in females than males, and the peak age of onset is in the 20s and 30s. Clinical signs and symptoms reflect the distribution of demyelination in the brain and spinal cord. Presentation is usually with a focal neurological deficit such as optic neuritis, limb weakness, diplopia, paraesthesia, bladder dysfunction, vertigo, and nystagmus; these often resolve spontaneously. The disease is characterized by relapses and remissions in the early years, but recurring episodes tend to result in increasing disability. The intervening periods of remission may extend over years, and the rate of progress and severity vary considerably. In some cases, the disease becomes relentlessly progressive in the later stages, often leading to paraplegia due to extensive involvement of the spinal cord. Occasionally the presentation is acute and rapidly progressive, or there is slow chronic progression from the start. Clinical diagnosis may be difficult especially in the early stages (*Box 11.8*). The lifespan may be normal, but severely disabled patients are at risk from bronchopneumonia, urinary tract infections, and bed sores.

### Pathology

In MS foci of primary demyelination (plaques) are distributed widely throughout the CNS. These well-circumscribed, firm, grey lesions vary greatly in number, size, and location. They are commonly found in cerebral white matter, especially adjacent to the lateral ventricles, optic nerves and chiasma, brain stem, cerebellar white matter, and spinal cord. The appearances of the plaques vary with their age.

In acute plaques, in which there is a substantial amount of active demyelination, there is selective destruction of myelin sheaths with sparing of axons. A prominent inflammatory cell infiltrate of lipid-laden macrophages, containing myelin breakdown products, lymphocytes, and plasma cells,

### Box 11.8 DIAGNOSIS OF MULTIPLE SCLEROSIS

- Clinical evidence of lesions disseminated in space and time
- MRI showing multiple focal CNS lesions, particularly in white matter
- Visual-evoked responses – electrophysiological evidence of slowed conduction
- Oligoclonal bands of IgG in cerebrospinal fluid

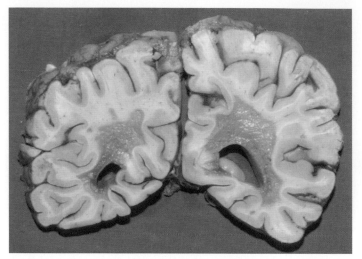

**FIG. 11.28** Multiple sclerosis: there are large grey plaques of demyelination in relation to the occipital horns of the ventricles.

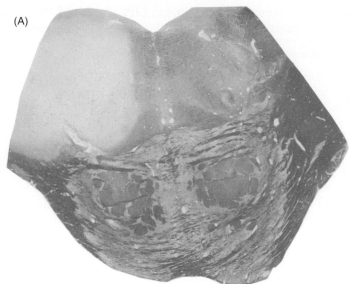

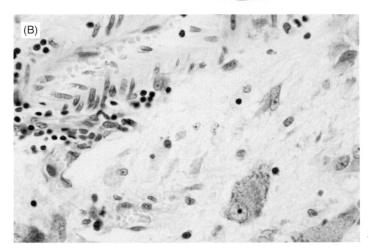

**FIG. 11.29** Multiple sclerosis: (A) there is a plaque of demyelination in one dorsolateral sector of the pons. (B) Within the area of demyelination there is preservation of neurons and variable cuffing of blood vessels by lymphocytes. (Stain: luxol fast blue/cresyl violet.)

is seen. MRI studies suggest that localized breakdown of the blood–brain barrier is a very early, possibly initiating, event in the formation of a plaque. Chronic plaques, in which the demyelination occurred many years before, are commonly seen at *post mortem* (Fig. 11.28). Histologically there is complete loss of myelin (Fig. 11.29), with a reduction in the number of oligodendrocytes. Axons in the lesion, which are normal or only slightly reduced in density, therefore have no myelin sheaths. Astrocytes are increased in numbers and hypertrophic. There is often a scanty infiltrate of T lymphocytes. Remyelination sometimes occurs in MS and is recognized by areas of myelin staining intermediate in intensity between normal white matter and complete demyelination (shadow plaques). Electron microscopy demonstrates axons with abnormally thin myelin sheaths characteristic of remyelination.

The pathological basis of clinical remission in multiple sclerosis is not known but may include re-myelination, resolution of oedema, and restoration of conduction in demyelinated axons, e.g. by redistribution of the membrane ion channels on which the action potential relies.

## Aetiology

Familial aggregation of multiple sclerosis and twin studies, which show a higher level of concordance among monozygotic than dizygotic twins, suggest that genetic factors may be important. MS is not inherited in a simple genetic fashion, but patients have over-representation of certain histocompatability antigens, suggesting that genetic variation in control of the immune response may be important. The variation in the prevalence of MS with latitude is unexplained: there is a gradient in each hemisphere with high disease rates at high latitudes, e.g. in north-east Scotland (1 in 500 of the population) and virtual absence at the equator. Environmental factors, particularly in childhood, appear to be important. People who migrate from one area to another after the age of 15 years retain the incidence of their childhood locality. Before the Second World War, MS was unknown in the isolated communities of the Faroe islands but, with increased contact with the rest of the world, it has a high prevalence of MS. Although these studies suggest an infective aetiology, none of the numerous candidate organisms studied has been consistently implicated. Oligoclonal bands of IgG in CSF indicate that IgG is produced by plasma cells derived from a small number of B-lymphocyte clones. These observations may indicate a reaction to an infective agent or an autoimmune response to a neural component (e.g. myelin). Demyelinating antibodies have been detected in the serum of patients with MS, but these are not specific because they are found in patients with other disorders.

This evidence can be combined into a hypothesis: immune-mediated demyelination is triggered in genetically susceptible individuals by an infective organism acquired in childhood. Despite our ignorance about the pathogenesis of multiple sclerosis, drugs that target specific facets of the immune system (e.g. interferon-β) appear to reduce the number of relapses in some cases.

## Other Demyelinating Disorders

### Acute Disseminated (Perivenous) Encephalomyelitis

This self-limiting disease of older children and young adults is an unusual sequel to various acute viral diseases such as mumps, measles, chickenpox, or rubella (post-infectious encephalitis) and primary immunization against smallpox and rabies (post-vaccinial encephalitis). Onset is rapid, occurring between 5 and 14 days after the start of the initial infection or immunization. Diffusely distributed throughout the brain and spinal cord are characteristic areas of perivenular demyelination associated with inflammatory oedema and infiltrated mainly by neutrophil polymorphs in the acute state and later by lymphocytes and macrophages. The disease is due to an autoimmune response directed against CNS antigen such as myelin basic protein.

### Acute Haemorrhagic Leukoencephalitis

This uncommon disease has a rapid onset, a short clinical course, and usually a fatal outcome. It may occur as a sequel to viral infections, septic shock, drug treatment, and hypersensitivity reactions. *Post mortem* the brain is swollen and there are numerous petechial haemorrhages, particularly in the white matter. Microscopic examination shows focal necrosis of the walls of venules and arterioles, perivascular haemorrhages, and perivascular demyelination, often with infiltration first by neutrophil polymorphs and later by lymphocytes and macrophages. The condition is thought to be a hyperacute variant of acute disseminated perivenous encephalomyelitis and be caused by the deposition of immune complexes and the activation of complement.

Progressive multifocal leukoencephalopathy is described on p. 314.

### Central Pontine Myelinolysis

This is characterized by a symmetrical area of demyelination in the centre of the pons. It occurs most often in middle-aged or elderly people with alcohol problems and seems to be associated with rapid therapeutic correction of hyponatraemia.

# METABOLIC DISORDERS

## Primary Metabolic Disorders

The disorders in this group usually develop in early life; although uncommon, they make a considerable contribution to morbidity and mortality in children. They may present with neurological symptoms alone or with other systemic abnormalities. Different diseases may share a common phenotype such as a cherry-red spot of the macula. Many are inherited as autosomal recessive diseases and a few show X-linked recessive inheritance. In most a critical enzyme system is absent or inactive. Many of these disorders are due to deficiencies

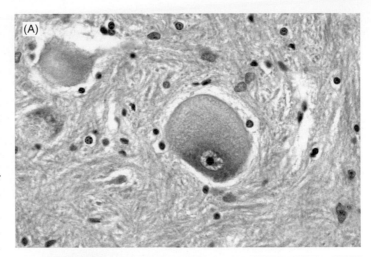

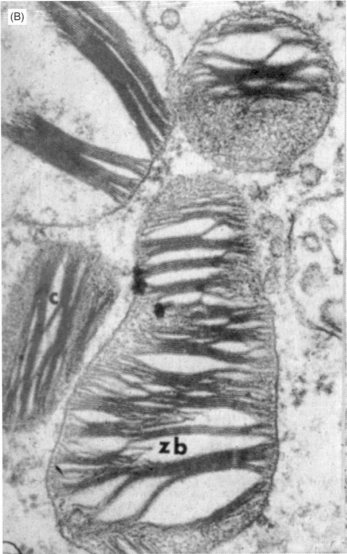

FIG. 11.30 Mucopolysaccharidosis – Hurler's disease: (A) enlarged neurons due to accumulation of PAS-positive cytoplasmic material that has displaced the nucleus. (B) Membrane-bound collections of lipid lamellae (electron microscopy). PAS = periodic acid–Schiff; zb = zebra bodies. (Reproduced from Graham DI, Nicoll JAR, Bone I. *Adams & Graham's Introduction to Neuropathology*, 3rd edn. London: Hodder Arnold, 2006.)

of particular lysosomal enzymes, which play an essential role in the degradation of normal metabolites or cell-breakdown products, e.g. lipids, carbohydrates, mucopolysaccharides (Fig. 11.30), or amino acids. As a result the undegraded material accumulates in and enlarges the lysosomes of certain cells, the distribution depending on the particular enzyme deficiency. Some disorders affect neurons which become enlarged with a ballooned appearance (neuronal storage disorders); others affect white matter (leukodystrophies). Diagnosis by assay of the relevant lysosomal enzymes in blood, urine, leukocytes, or cultured fibroblasts is now often possible and increasingly genetic tests are available. The lipid storage disorders (sphingolipidoses) are probably the most important group. The sphingolipids include gangliosides, cerebrosides, sulphatides, and sphingomyelins. One of the most common storage disorders affecting especially the neurons is Tay–Sachs disease, in which there is deficiency of hexosaminidase A, resulting from a mutation in the *HEXA* gene on chromosome 15 and causing abnormal accumulation (i.e. 'storage') of its substrate ganglioside.

The leukodystrophies, a complex group of uncommon disorders, have in common diffuse symmetrical demyelination and astrocytosis of the white matter of the cerebral hemispheres, and sometimes also of the cerebellum, brain stem, and spinal cord. Most types are genetically determined and occur in childhood. They are therefore regarded as dysmyelinating diseases because it is thought that the myelin is biochemically abnormal before it degenerates, in contrast to the primary demyelinating disorders in which myelination is thought to be normal before the onset of the demyelination.

### Other Inborn Errors of Metabolism

Neonatal hypothyroidism, phenylketonuria, and galactosaemia are the most important of these because they can be detected by screening tests in infants, and brain damage can be prevented or reduced by either replacement therapy or exclusion of the precursor substances from the diet.

### Hepatolenticular Degeneration

Hepatolenticular degeneration (Wilson's disease) is an autosomal recessive disorder of copper metabolism in which cirrhosis of the liver is accompanied by brain changes, mainly in the putamen and caudate nucleus, which become soft, shrunken, and ultimately cystic. Neuronal loss is accompanied by large astrocytes with strikingly vesicular swollen nuclei (Alzheimer's type II astrocytes). A greenish-brown discoloration of the cornea near the limbus (known as the Kayser–Fleischer ring) is also due to the deposition of copper.

## Secondary Metabolic Disorders

The metabolic complexity of the CNS makes it dependent on the functional integrity of other systems in the body. Therefore, it is not surprising that secondary metabolic effects on the CNS are an early manifestation of systemic disease. In many instances the clinical features are reversible and there are minimal morphological changes. It is only when the metabolic disorder has been profound and prolonged that structural changes occur.

These disorders include brain damage due to hypoxia after cardiac arrest, carbon monoxide poisoning, and hypoglycaemia.

### Hepatic Encephalopathy

Hepatic encephalopathy invariably accompanies severe liver failure. In massive hepatic necrosis acute hepatic encephalopathy is characterized by rapidly developing coma. In cirrhosis, particularly when there is portal systemic shunting of blood, chronic hepatic encephalopathy develops. Hepatic encephalopathy is due to an accumulation of neurotoxic substances in the blood, which originate in the gastrointestinal tract and are normally metabolized from the portal vein by the liver.

### Kernicterus

Kernicterus is a metabolic disorder in the perinatal period also known as bilirubin encephalopathy. Severe jaundice in infancy carries the risk of brain damage, particularly when the plasma level of unconjugated bilirubin exceeds 250 μmol/L. In premature infants functional immaturity of the liver is responsible, but in full-term infants haemolytic anaemia due to fetal–maternal rhesus (Rh) incompatibility or glucose 6-phosphate dehydrogenase (G6PD) deficiency are important causes.

# DEFICIENCY DISORDERS AND INTOXICATIONS

Deficiencies of vitamins and protein are responsible for various neurological disorders. In developed countries many cases of vitamin deficiency are due to alcohol misuse, less commonly to malabsorption from gastrointestinal tract disease, and rarely to food fads. In contrast, the deficiency syndromes that are common in developing countries are usually due to an inadequate food supply. Malnutrition may cause irreparable brain damage at critical periods of prenatal and postnatal development.

## Deficiency Disorders

### Vitamin B₁ (Thiamine) Deficiency

Vitamin B₁ deficiency, in addition to causing a peripheral neuropathy, sometimes presents as the Wernicke–Korsakoff syndrome (Wernicke's encephalopathy). The deficiency may be chronic as in alcoholism or prolonged malnutrition, or acute, e.g. as a complication of persistent vomiting. The clinical onset is acute or subacute: features include disturbances of consciousness, ophthalmoplegia, nystagmus, and ataxia and, if untreated, terminal coma. The blood pyruvate level is raised. In acutely fatal cases there are petechial haemorrhages in the mamillary bodies, the floor and walls of the third ventricle, and the thalami, around the aqueduct in the midbrain, and in the floor of the fourth ventricle. Improvement after administration of the vitamin B group may be dramatic, but a full recovery is unlikely if structures are already damaged before treatment is started. Such patients usually have a persistent psychosis of Korsakoff's type.

Ethanol consumption during pregnancy can cause a variety of CNS abnormalities; these range from macroscopic changes with mental impairment (fetal alcohol syndrome) to more subtle cognitive and behavioural disorders (fetal alcohol effects).

### Vitamin B$_{12}$ (Cyanocobalamin) Deficiency

Vitamin B$_{12}$ deficiency particularly affects haematopoietic tissue, epithelial surfaces, and the nervous system, with structural abnormalities in the spinal cord and the optic and peripheral nerves. In subacute combined degeneration of the spinal cord there are degenerative changes in the lateral and posterior columns, particularly in the thoracic region (Fig. 11.31).

## Intoxications

> **Key Points**
>
> Key neurological features of alcohol misuse are:
> - increased incidence of head injury
> - withdrawal-induced epilepsy (this is the most common cause of late-onset epilepsy)
> - cerebral atrophy, particularly of the frontal lobes
> - delerium tremens; Wernicke's encephalopathy/ Korsakoff's psychosis
> - partial atrophy of the superior vermis of the cerebellum
> - peripheral neuropathy
> - fetal alcohol syndrome
> - muscle disease
> - central pontine myelinolysis.

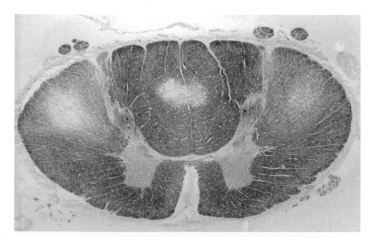

**FIG. 11.31** Subacute combined degeneration of the spinal cord: there is vacuolar degeneration in the posterior and lateral columns. (Stain: luxol fast blue/cresyl violet.) (Reproduced from Graham DI, Nicoll JAR, Bone I. *Adams & Graham's Introduction to Neuropathology*, 3rd edn. London: Hodder Arnold, 2006.)

Interest in the effect of toxins on the nervous system has been growing rapidly. Some disorders may occur after exposure to substances including alcohol/ethanol, therapeutic drugs, pest control products, industrial chemicals, chemical warfare agents, food additives, heavy metals, and narcotics.

# AGEING AND DEMENTIA

## Ageing and the Brain

The mean adult brain weight is 1450 g for males and 1350 g for females, with a range of ±100 g about these means, in keeping with differences in body mass between the sexes. After about the age of 65 years the brain becomes smaller as a result of atrophy, losing up to 100 g in weight, and the cerebral hemispheres shrink away from the skull. Atrophy of the brain is shown by narrowed gyri and widened sulci, particularly at the frontal and temporal poles. The cerebral cortex is thinned, and there is a reduction in the amount of white matter and compensatory enlargement of the ventricular system. Microscopic changes may include gliosis, a slight loss of neurons, and a few senile plaques in the cerebral cortex. Mild cerebrovascular pathology is very common, including arteriosclerosis in the basal ganglia and cerebral white matter, and amyloid deposition in the walls of small cortical and meningeal blood vessels; these changes are not necessarily associated with any intellectual impairment. The ageing brain is vulnerable to neurodegenerative diseases.

> **Key Points**
>
> Features of neurodegenerative diseases:
> - Their prevalence increases with ageing.
> - They are progressive, ultimately fatal disorders.
> - They are chronic debilitating diseases so are a major social and economic burden.
> - Dysfunction and degeneration of neurons may be widespread within the cerebrum causing dementia (e.g. Alzheimer's disease) or localized causing specific neurological syndromes (e.g. Parkinson's disease, motor neuron disease).
> - Different neurodegenerative diseases are characterized by extracellular, cytoplasmic, or intranuclear accumulation of specific proteins leading to the concept of 'proteinopathies'.
> - Rare familial examples may be caused by mutation of the gene encoding the accumulating protein.
> - Experimental therapeutic strategies target accumulating proteins.

## Dementia

Dementia can be defined as an acquired and persistent generalized disturbance of higher mental functions in an otherwise alert person. Dementia is rare before the age of 60 years, but becomes increasingly common with age, affecting 5% of those over 65 years and 20% of those over 80 years. The most common causes of dementia are Alzheimer's disease, cerebrovascular disease, and Lewy body disease; there are many rarer causes. It is important to establish the underlying cause of the dementia because effective treatment is available for some of the disorders, and may be soon for others as our knowledge is rapidly increasing. Counselling is appropriate for those disorders with a genetic component, e.g. Huntington's disease. The causes of dementia are summarized in *Table 11.4*.

**TABLE 11.4** Causes of dementia

| | |
|---|---|
| **Neurodegenerative disorders** | |
| Common | Alzheimer's disease |
| | Dementia with Lewy bodies |
| Rare | Frontotemporal lobar degeneration |
| | Huntington's disease |
| | Creutzfeldt–Jakob disease |
| | Progressive supranuclear palsy |
| **Cerebrovascular disease** | Multi-infarct dementia |
| | Subcortical arteriosclerotic dementia |
| | Global hypoxia/hypoperfusion |
| | Vasculitis |
| **Infections** | HIV/AIDS |
| | Neurosyphilis |
| | Herpes simplex encephalitis |
| | Subacute sclerosing panencephalitis |
| | Progressive multifocal leukoencephalopathy |
| **Trauma** | Traumatic brain damage |
| | Chronic traumatic encephalopathy/Dementia pugilistica |
| | Chronic subdural haematoma |
| **Metabolic, toxic, and nutritional deficiency** | Chronic alcoholism |
| | Hepatic failure |
| | Renal failure |
| | Hypothyroidism |
| | Vitamin deficiencies: thiamine (Wernicke–Korsakoff syndrome) |
| **Myelin disorders** | Multiple sclerosis |
| | Leukodystrophy |
| **Neoplasia** | Primary or secondary tumours (especially frontal lobe) |
| | Paraneoplastic syndromes |
| **Miscellaneous** | Hydrocephalus |

## Alzheimer's Disease

### Key Points

- Alzheimer's disease is a progressive condition that is fatal within 5–15 years.
- It is usually sporadic; rarely there is autosomal dominant inheritance.
- Apolipoprotein E (apoE) ε4 allele is a genetic risk factor.
- There is cerebral atrophy.
- Histological features include plaques, neurofibrillary tangles, and loss of neurons and synapses.

Alzheimer's disease accounts for about 70% of cases of dementia and is the fourth most common cause of death in developed countries after heart disease, cancer, and stroke. There are over 5 million people with the disease in the USA, with an annual cost of $US200 billion; the figures for the UK are 800,000 patients and £23 billion annual cost. Most patients are cared for in the community within families or in nursing homes. This represents an enormous social and economic burden, which will increase in the coming decades with the predicted increasing lifespan in most countries throughout the world. Some liken Alzheimer's disease to an acceleration of the normal ageing process; others consider it to be a separate entity. Presentation is frequently with memory impairment due to involvement of the temporal lobes. The course is invariably progressive and fatal, typically within 5–15 years. Most patients die from bronchopneumonia or inanition. In a very small proportion of cases (<1%), the disease is inherited in an autosomal dominant manner.

### Pathology

*Post mortem* the brain is atrophied, sometimes weighing <1000 g. The atrophy is accentuated in the frontal and temporal lobes and there is compensatory enlargement of the ventricles (Fig. 11.32). A definite diagnosis of Alzheimer's disease requires histological examination of the brain. The microscopic features found in the cerebral cortex are as follows:

- *Plaques:* small focal deposits in the cerebral cortex of amyloid β-protein. Some plaques contain dystrophic neuronal processes (neuritic plaques) (Fig. 11.33).
- Neurofibrillary tangles: abnormal aggregates of cytoskeletal filaments within a neuron (termed 'paired helical filaments' and largely composed of tau protein) (Fig. 11.33).
- Amyloid angiopathy: accumulation of amyloid β-protein in the walls of cerebral and meningeal blood vessels.
- Activation of microglia and astrocytes.
- Loss of neurons.
- Loss of synapses.

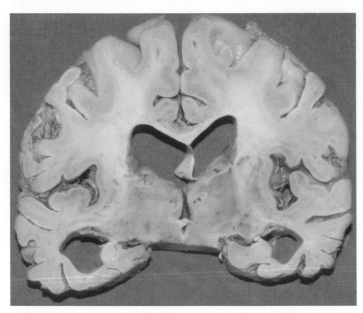

FIG. 11.32 Alzheimer's disease: there is selective atrophy of the medial parts of each temporal lobe with associated compensatory hydrocephalus.

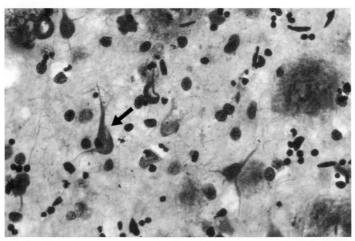

FIG. 11.33 Alzheimer's disease: there is a typical senile plaque composed of filamentous and granular material. A neurofibrillary tangle is seen in a neuron (arrow). (Stain: King's amyloid.)

## Aetiology

The pathogenesis of Alzheimer's disease is still unclear, although there has been intense focus on the deposition of amyloid β-protein in the cortex as a putative initiating event. A small number of familial cases have a point mutation in the amyloid precursor protein (APP) gene (located on chromosome 21), from which amyloid β-protein is derived. Additional autosomal dominant, disease-causing point mutations include presenilin 1 and 2. Individuals with Down's syndrome, who have trisomy 21 and therefore three copies of the *APP* gene, all develop Alzheimer's disease by the age of 40 years. Deposition of amyloid β-protein has been identified as one of the earliest features of Alzheimer's disease pathology to appear in those with Down's syndrome

dying at a younger age. However, a causal role for abnormal aggregation of amyloid β-protein in the pathogenesis of the common form of sporadic Alzheimer's disease has not yet been established with certainty. There is also evidence for mechanisms involving intraneuronal aggregation of the cytoskeleton-associated tau-forming tangles. Recent genome-wide association studies point to important roles for lipid metabolism and inflammation in the pathogenesis of Alzheimer's disease.

Neurochemical studies have shown impairment of the cholinergic system, with decreased choline acetyltransferase activity in the cerebral cortex. Although this is not the only neurotransmitter system affected, current therapies aim to reverse this deficit. There is also interest that anti-inflammatory medication and immunization against amyloid β-protein may influence the course of the disease.

## Dementia with Lewy Bodies

This disorder is now known to account for 10–20% of all cases of dementia. Clinical distinction from other forms of dementia is challenging but characteristic features include fluctuating cognitive function, visual hallucinations, and a parkinsonian movement disorder. Indeed, there is a considerable overlap with Parkinson's disease. Macroscopically, there is atrophy of the cerebrum similar to that seen in Alzheimer's disease but, in addition, there is loss of pigmentation of the substantia nigra. Microscopically, in addition to depletion of pigmented dopaminergic neurons in the substantia nigra and Lewy bodies in residual neurons, as seen in Parkinson's disease, Lewy bodies are also present in the cerebral cortex. There is a poorly understood overlap with Alzheimer's disease because many of the patients also have plaques and tangles. The synapse-associated protein α-synuclein is a major component of both cortical and brain-stem Lewy bodies in dementia with Lewy bodies.

## Vascular Dementia

The brain is crucially reliant on a continuous supply of blood delivering oxygen and nutrients and removing waste products in order to maintain its normal functions. Cerebrovascular disease is very common in elderly people, including atherosclerosis affecting arteries supplying the brain and arteriosclerosis affecting smaller vessels within the brain. Although the relationship between cerebrovascular disease and dementia is poorly understood, the term 'vascular dementia' implies that the cognitive dysfunction is due to cerebrovascular disease. Clinical clues to a vascular cause for dementia include abrupt onset and a stepwise deterioration, a history of stroke, and imaging evidence of cerebrovascular pathology. There is increasing recognition that dementia may have mixed causes, in particular vascular pathology may contribute to the dementia associated with Alzheimer's disease and dementia with Lewy bodies. Large regional cerebral infarcts are unlikely to present with dementia.

### Multi-infarct Dementia (Large-vessel Disease)

This is dementia associated with multiple small infarcts, typically scattered widely throughout the cerebral hemispheres. It is relatively common, accounting for 10–15% of all cases of dementia. Most patients are elderly and hypertensive. Widespread atheroma of the major cerebral arteries results in repeated cerebral infarction, often due to thromboembolism. Some studies have suggested that there is a critical volume of infarction (50–100 mL) that acts as a threshold above which the development of dementia is likely. Assessment of the distribution of the infarcts has not clearly demonstrated specific brain regions implicated in this disorder. However, it seems likely that cognitive function is associated with involvement of the limbic system and association cortex.

### Subcortical Vascular Dementia (Small-vessel Disease)

There is diffuse ischaemic degeneration of the cerebral white matter associated with small-vessel disease in the form of arteriosclerosis, in which there is collagenous thickening of the walls of small arteries. The basal ganglia are often affected by 'lacunes' – small cavitated lesions that may be either small infarcts or greatly enlarged perivascular spaces. Lesser degrees of these forms of pathology are very common in elderly, cognitively normal people. Lacunes and cerebral white matter degeneration may be detected during life by brain imaging and are strongly associated with longstanding hypertension.

## Other Causes of Dementia

### Frontotemporal Dementia

Frontotemporal dementia (FTD) is relatively rare but is increasing in recognition particularly as the cause of a significant proportion of dementia in those aged <65 years. It is more likely than other dementias to be familial with a single gene mutation as the cause, resulting in an autosomal dominant pattern of inheritance. Presentation is often with behavioural or language problems. There is marked relatively selective atrophy of the frontal and or temporal lobes (frontotemporal lobar degeneration – FTLD) which may be asymmetrical. Microscopically, in affected areas there is severe degeneration of the cortical neuropil and neuronal loss. The classification is complex and changing rapidly with increasing understanding of the subtypes, e.g. in FTLD-tau there is accumulation of tau protein in neurons and glia, associated with mutations in the gene encoding tau. In FTLD-TDP-43 there is accumulation of TAR DNA-binding protein (TDP-43) in neurons, associated with mutations in the TDP-43 gene and other genes. FTLD-TDP-43 is linked with motor neuron disease in which there is accumulation of TDP-43 in motor neurons.

### Huntington's Disease

In this autosomal dominant disorder progressive dementia is accompanied by involuntary choreiform movements. Huntington's disease (HD) usually begins in the 40s or 50s and has an incidence of about 47 per 100,000 population. The cause of Huntington's disease is an increased number of trinucleotide repeats (CAG), which encode the amino acid glutamine, in the *huntingtin* gene on chromosome 4. The normal gene contains 9–37 CAG repeats, whereas in patients with HD there may be in the region of 37–100. This knowledge allows prediction of susceptibility in as yet unaffected family members and antenatal testing. The mutation is unstable and the phenomenon of anticipation may occur: in succeeding generations the disease occurs with an earlier age of onset and increasing severity as the number of CAG repeats increases. On examination of the brain the most striking feature is selective atrophy of the caudate nucleus (Fig. 11.34). There may also be cortical atrophy. Histological examination reveals loss of small neurons and gliosis in the caudate nuclei with variable involvement of other nuclei in the basal ganglia and the cerebral cortex. The huntingtin protein produced in HD is abnormal, containing a long chain of glutamine amino acid residues as a consequence of the CAG repeats in the huntingtin gene, and accumulates as dot-like intranuclear inclusions.

### AIDS Dementia

AIDS dementia is discussed in Chapter 19 (p. 547).

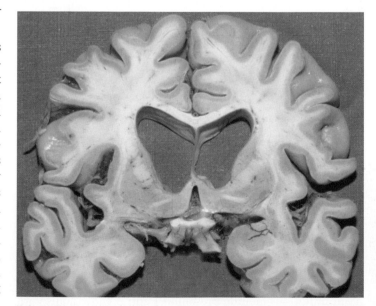

**Fig. 11.34** Huntington's disease: the basal ganglia are markedly atrophied with a flattened outline compared with age-matched control. The cerebral cortex is also atrophied and compensatory hydrocephalus is a feature.

### Creutzfeldt–Jakob Disease

Creutzfeldt–Jakob disease (CJD) is unusual in that it may be acquired by transmission, inherited as an autosomal dominant trait (about 10% of cases), or occur sporadically. Iatrogenic transmission has rarely occurred via contaminated neurosurgical instruments, cadaveric dural and corneal grafts, and cadaveric pituitary extracts (used for growth hormone and gonadotrophin replacement). It can also be transmitted to experimental animals. The incubation period may vary from several years to decades. The incidence of CJD in most countries is about 1 case/million per year. It is characterized clinically by rapidly progressive dementia, myoclonus (repeated jerking movements of the limbs), and a typical appearance on an electroencephalogram (EEG). Macroscopically, the brain appears normal with little or no atrophy. At present the diagnosis can be made with certainty only by histological examination. The microscopic features are vacuolation of grey matter (spongiform encephalopathy) with neuronal loss and gliosis (Fig. 11.35) and demonstration of prion protein (PrP) accumulation by immunohistochemistry.

Creutzfeldt–Jakob disease is due to an unconventional transmissible agent that is very resistant to normal disinfecting procedures such as standard autoclaving. It appears to have no nucleic acid but to be composed only of protein, hence the term prion. The disease process is characterized by the conversion of a normal cellular protein (PrP$^c$) into an abnormal isoform (PrP$^{sc}$) by a change in conformation. The PrP$^{sc}$ that accumulates in affected tissue is derived from the host *PrP* gene and can be detected by immunohistochemistry. The relationship between transmissibility and genetic factors is not yet entirely clear. However, there are thought to be three ways in which PrP$^{sc}$ can form: first, by a point mutation in the *PrP* gene rendering the protein more likely to misfold to form PrP$^{sc}$ and initiate the disease – this occurs in the familial form of CJD. Second, the presence of PrP$^{sc}$ induces the conversion of PrP$^c$ into more PrP$^{sc}$ – this occurs when the disorder is transmitted. Third, sporadic CJD occurs, presumably, when PrP$^{sc}$ is formed from PrP$^c$ as a chance event in the aged brain. Homozygosity at codon

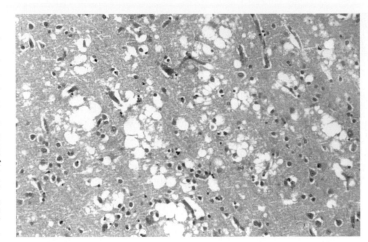

**Fig. 11.35** Creutzfeldt–Jakob disease: there is spongiform change in the cortex that is characterized by many vacuoles, which become coalescent. Neuronal loss and astrocytosis are accompanying features.

129, which codes for either methionine or valine, of the host *PrP* gene appears to represent a genetic susceptibility factor.

### Variant CJD

This disorder, described almost exclusively in the UK, is thought to be caused by ingestion of products from cattle infected with bovine spongiform encephalopathy (BSE) after an epidemic of BSE in cattle in the late 1980s and early 1990s. Presentation is with psychiatric symptoms (anxiety and depression), cerebellar ataxia, and dementia in patients mainly aged <40. The clinical time course is more protracted than for classic CJD. Pathologically, there is abundant deposition of PrP with numerous 'florid plaques', composed of amyloid cores surrounded by vacuoles, in the cerebral cortex and cerebellum. About 170 people in the UK have been affected by variant CJD (vCJD) since it was first described in the early 1990s and the disease now seems to be well past its peak. A very few cases are thought to have been acquired by blood transfusion from patients incubating the disease. The BSE/vCJD event has had a major impact on healthcare, particularly in relation to blood transfusion and sourcing of blood products.

---

## ALZHEIMER'S DISEASE

**CASE HISTORY 11.1**

A 78-year-old female, Mrs AD, attended her general practitioner, accompanied by her daughter with whom she had lived for 2 years. The complaints were that she had become increasingly confused over the past 6 months, had got lost several times in the last few weeks on the way back from the local shops, and wandered the house at night looking for her husband who had died 3 years previously. It was clear to the general practitioner that she was suffering cognitive impairment with pronounced failure of memory and he referred her to a memory clinic at the local hospital. Assessment at the clinic confirmed these problems, which were progressive in nature, and a Mini-Mental State Examination (MMSE) resulted in a score of 20/30, indicating moderate cognitive dysfunction.

Initial investigations excluded readily treatable causes of cognitive impairment in elderly people. There were no clinical features to suggest dementia with Lewy bodies or vascular dementia. There was no family history. MRI of the brain showed mild generalized cerebral atrophy, with more marked atrophy affecting both medial temporal lobes and mildly enlarged lateral ventricles. Mrs AD's cognitive function continued to decline slowly over the coming months. A clinical diagnosis of Alzheimer's disease was made. Treatment with a cholinesterase inhibitor was commenced and seemed to be of some benefit for about a year but Mrs AD's condition then continued to deteriorate.

During a visit to the memory clinic Mrs AD was given the opportunity to enrol in a clinical study, which involved some additional investigations and the possibility ultimately of brain donation to a brain bank. Mrs AD and her daughter were both keen to agree to this. Additional investigations included: a PET scan with an amyloid ligand, which showed evidence of extensive amyloid deposition throughout the cerebral cortex; a lumbar puncture to obtain CSF, analysis of which showed an abnormally low level of amyloid β-protein and a high level of tau protein; and genetic testing performed on a blood sample, which showed that Mrs AD was heterozygous for apolipoprotein E (apoE) ε4. These findings supported the diagnosis of Alzheimer's disease.

Unfortunately, Mrs AD's cognitive function continued to decline over the next 3 years. Her daughter was no longer able to cope with her at home and Mrs AD was admitted to a local nursing home. Five years later Mrs AD was mute and bedbound and developed bronchopneumonia from which she died.

Mrs AD's brain was donated to a nearby brain bank as had been consented to previously. The brain weight was 1030 g and macroscopic examination revealed severe symmetrical cerebral atrophy affecting in particular the frontal, temporal, and parietal lobes with corresponding dilatation of the lateral ventricles. Histological examination of sections of cerebral cortex stained with a silver stain showed the presence of numerous plaques and tangles (Fig. 11.36). Immunohistochemistry for amyloid β-protein confirmed the presence of plaques and demonstrated moderately severe cerebral amyloid angiopathy (Fig. 11.37). Immunohistochemistry for tau confirmed the presence of numerous neurofibrillary tangles and dystrophic neurites within the plaques (Fig. 11.38). The clinical diagnosis of

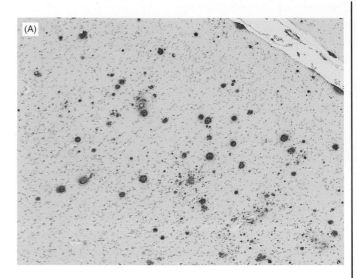

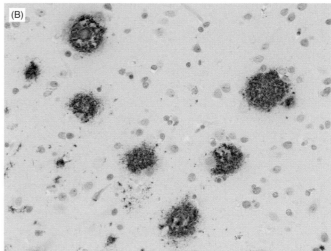

FIG. 11.37 (A) The cerebral cortex is extensively peppered with plaques; (B) these are composed predominantly of amyloid β-protein (Aβ) (Aβ immunohistochemistry).

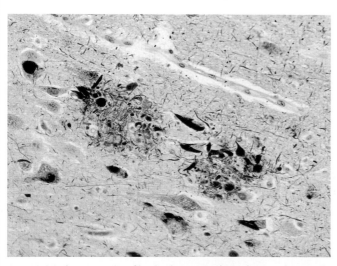

FIG. 11.36 The presence of both plaques and tangles in substantial numbers indicates a diagnosis of Alzheimer's disease (modified Bielschowsky's stain).

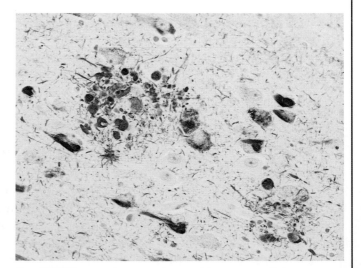

FIG. 11.38 Tau protein accumulates within neurons to form tangles in the cell bodies and also within neuronal cell processes, particularly those associated with plaques (dystrophic neurites) (tau immunohistochemistry).

Alzheimer's disease was therefore confirmed. Additional investigations showed no evidence of concomitant vascular dementia, dementia with Lewy bodies, or frontotemporal lobar degeneration.

## Learning Points

- Alzheimer's disease is the most common cause of dementia, resulting in a social and economic burden often lasting over many years.
- Most cases of AD are sporadic, i.e. without a genetic cause, although there are genetic risk factors (apoE ε4).
- Currently, there is not complete correlation between the clinical diagnosis during life of the cause of dementia and postmortem neuropathology. However, the development of new investigations is taking place rapidly. In particular, scans to detect amyloid protein in the brain and examination of amyloid β-protein and tau levels in the CSF are currently being transferred from their use as research tools to the clinic to increase diagnostic accuracy during life.

- Nevertheless, histological examination, usually performed only *post mortem* in selected cases, is still considered the 'gold standard'.
- There is a national registration system for potential brain donors operating through a network of brain banks (Brains for Dementia Research).
- Although there is currently no therapy that affects the underlying progressive nature of the disease, intense efforts are being made around the world in clinical trials of new potential therapies.

## Further Reading

Alzheimer Research Forum: www.alzforum.org

Alzheimer's Research UK: www.alzheimersresearchuk.org

Brains for Dementia Research: www.brainsfordementiaresearch .org.uk

Lowe J, Mirra SS, Hyman BT, Dickson DW, *et al*. Ageing and dementia. *In*: Love S, Louis DN, Ellison DW (eds), *Greenfield's Neuropathology*, 8th edn. London: Hodder Arnold, 2008: 1031–1152.

# DISORDERS OF MOVEMENT

This diverse group of disorders is characterized by a progressive degeneration of neurons and their associated pathways within anatomically or functionally defined regions or systems. Patients may therefore present with the clinical features of dysfunction of the motor or sensory systems, cerebellar ataxia, or involuntary movements, alone or in combination with other neurological abnormalities. Dementia may be a feature if neuronal degeneration is widespread. These disorders can occur in isolation or there may be overlap, both clinically and pathologically. The conditions described here are relatively discrete and well-defined examples of this group of disorders and are summarized in *Table 11.5*.

## Parkinsonism

Parkinsonism refers to the clinical syndrome of disturbed motor function characterized by tremor, rigidity, and slowing of movement (bradykinesia). It is brought about by damage to, or malfunction of, the nigral system which may have many causes including drugs and toxins (e.g. phenothiazines, manganese), vascular disease, viral infections (e.g. encephalitis lethargica), trauma (e.g. dementia pugilistica), and multiple system atrophy (striatonigral degeneration). Most cases are idiopathic, known as Parkinson's disease. It occurs most often in elderly patients with a prevalence of about 1% over the age of 60 years.

The clinical syndrome is caused by selective and progressive destruction of the pigmented neurons in the substantia

**TABLE 11.5** Principal disorders of movement

| Disorder | Location of neurodegeneration | Clinical features |
|---|---|---|
| Parkinson's disease | Substantia nigra | Parkinsonism: tremor, rigidity, bradykinesia |
| Motor neuron disease | Lower and/or upper motor neurons | Weakness, atrophy of muscles, fasciculation |
| Multiple system atrophy | Variable including: cerebellum and connections, autonomic neurons of spinal cord, striatonigral system | Cerebellar and autonomic dysfunction, parkinsonism |
| Friedreich's ataxia | Posterior columns of the spinal cord and spinocerebellar tracts | Ataxia, dysarthria, sensory abnormalities |

nigra, accompanied by deposition of granules of neuromelanin pigment. Residual pigmented neurons contain large intra-cytoplasmic inclusions known as Lewy bodies (Fig. 11.39). In advanced cases, depigmentation of the substantia nigra is readily apparent macroscopically (Fig. 11.39A). The neurons of the substantia nigra project to the corpus striatum (globus pallidus and putamen) where they release the neurotransmitter dopamine. Treatment with a dopamine precursor (L-dopa) may relieve the symptoms of the disease but does not slow the progress of the underlying neuronal degeneration. Most cases of Parkinson's disease occur sporadically but, rarely, it is inherited as an autosomal dominant trait with mutations in the *park 1* gene on chromosome 4 encoding α-synuclein, a component of Lewy bodies, among many other mutations that have been identified. There is a poorly understood overlap with dementia with Lewy bodies.

## Motor Neuron Disease

In this disorder there is a relentless and progressive degeneration of motor neurons. It tends to occur in middle and late adult life, is more common in males, and is usually fatal in 4–5 years from respiratory failure. Motor neuron disease (MND) occurs worldwide and accounts for approximately 1/1,000 deaths. It is usually sporadic and the aetiology is unknown. However, some pedigrees have been identified in

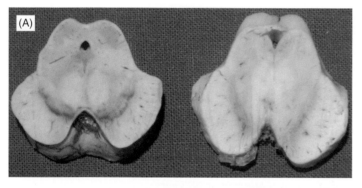

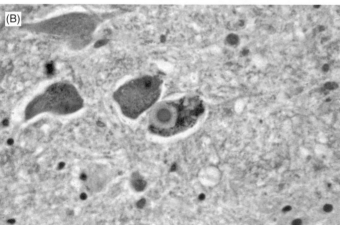

FIG. 11.39 Parkinson's disease: (A) compared with the normally pigmented substantia nigra on the left there is depigmentation of the substantia nigra on the right. (B) The Lewy body consists of a rounded eosinophilic inclusion, which classically comprises a dense core surrounded by a pale halo.

which MND is inherited as an autosomal dominant trait due to mutations in the gene encoding superoxide dismutase, a free radical scavenger on chromosome 21. Among the many other MND-causing genetic mutations that have been identified, *C9ORF72* mutations seem particularly associated with MND, occurring together with frontotemporal dementia. Three variants of MND are recognized according to the distribution of the disease process:

- Progressive muscular atrophy: selective involvement of the lower motor neurons of the spinal cord (anterior horn cells) results in weakness, fasciculation, and atrophy affecting limb muscles.
- Progressive bulbar palsy: selective involvement of the cranial nerve motor nuclei in the brain stem causes wasting and fasciculation affecting the tongue, dysarthria, and dysphagia.
- Amyotrophic lateral sclerosis: upper motor neurons are affected, leading to degeneration of the corticospinal tracts and a spastic paraparesis.

No sharply dividing line can be drawn between these variants and their names merely emphasize that, in any one case, the early stages of the disease may have a particular distribution. In the terminal stages there is often widespread involvement of motor neurons in the brain stem and spinal cord.

Pathologically, there is atrophy of the anterior horns with loss of motor neurons and astrocytosis, particularly in the cervical and lumbar segments of the spinal cord. In sporadic MND, residual motor neurons usually have inclusions containing TDP-43. There may be degeneration of the pyramidal tracts resulting from involvement of the primary motor cortex. The hypoglossal nuclei in the brain stem are usually conspicuously involved by neuronal depletion. Affected muscles show severe neurogenic atrophy.

## DEVELOPMENTAL ABNORMALITIES

Serious developmental abnormalities affect between 2% and 3% of all infants at birth, and of these approximately a third are malformations of the CNS. In over half, the aetiology remains undetermined, but genetic factors, maternal infections such as rubella and cytomegalovirus, the fetal alcohol syndrome, and exposure to pharmaceutical drugs, tobacco, and possibly vitamin deficiencies are implicated. The teratogenic effects of an agent depend on its nature, the gestational stage at which it acts and the genetic background of the individual.

The clinically important disorders in which there are chromosomal abnormalities include trisomy 21, 18 and 13, Klinefelter's syndrome (XXY), and Turner's syndrome (XO). Down's syndrome (trisomy 21) has an incidence of 1.4/1,000 livebirths. The incidence in babies born to women aged >40 is about 1% and increases with age. The brain is usually small and the characteristic feature in cases of mothers aged >40 years is the presence of a large number of Alzheimer's neurofibrillary tangles and plaques.

## Defects in the Neural Tube

These are among the most common congenital malformations. The incidence in the UK varies from 0.1% to 1% of livebirths: there is a familial tendency and the risk of recurrence after one affected child is about 5%. Defects of the neural tube may be diagnosed prenatally in 90% of cases by the presence of raised α-fetoprotein levels in blood and amniotic fluid and by ultrasonography. Defects arise from failure of closure of the neural tube and are induced by damage occurring during week 4 of fetal development from a combination of genetic and environmental factors.

Anencephaly is more common in female than in male infants. The head is retroflexed, the cranial vault is missing, and the base of the skull is flattened. The brain is represented by a small disorganized mass of glia, malformed brain, and choroid plexus which sits on the base of the skull and is usually covered by a thin smooth membrane.

### Spina Bifida

Spina bifida is a result of failure of fusion of the neural arches (Fig. 11.40). Most cases occur in the lumbosacral region.

#### Spina Bifida Cystica

Some 80–90% of cases have a myelomeningocele in which the abnormal cord is exposed by a defect in the skin, vertebral arches, and meninges: there are often associated abnormalities such as syringomyelia or diastematomyelia. In the remaining 10–20% of cases, the lesion is a meningocele that involves only meninges, the vertebral arches, and skin. The cord is virtually normal. Most patients who survive with myelomeningocele are paraplegic, with absence of sphincter control; many have learning disabilities. There is an increased risk of meningitis and urinary tract infections. Hydrocephalus occurs in cases with an associated Arnold–Chiari malformation.

#### Spina Bifida Occulta

This is said to occur in around 10% of normal adults as determined by the absence of one or more spinous processes within the lumbosacral region on radiology. The overlying skin may be abnormally pigmented or there may be a hairy patch or dermal sinus. It is normally asymptomatic but neurological disturbances may develop in adult life.

### Hydrocephalus

Hydrocephalus is commonly seen in severe abnormalities. The principal causes are spina bifida, Arnold–Chiari malformation, aqueduct stenosis, intrauterine infections, and intrauterine CNS haemorrhage.

### Chiari Malformations

Chiari malformations affect the cerebellum, brain stem, and base of the skull. The most common malformation (Arnold–Chiari malformation) is second in frequency to anenceph-

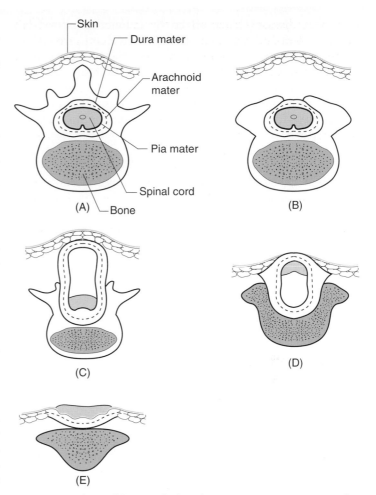

**FIG. 11.40** Defects of the neural tube: diagrammatic representation of spina bifida. (A) Normal; (B) spina bifida occulta; (C) meningocele; (D) myelomeningocele; and (E) myelocele. (From Adams JH, Graham DI. *Introduction to Neuropathology.* London: Churchill Livingstone, 1988.)

aly among severe CNS malformations. In the Arnold–Chiari malformation, an abnormality of the hindbrain and cerebellum is associated with a lumbar myelomeningocele and hydrocephalus.

### Microcephaly

Microcephaly denotes a brain that weighs <1,000 g in adults and more than two standard deviations below the mean normal weight for the age and sex of the patient.

## Phakomatoses

This group of mainly familial disorders is characterized by malformations of the neuraxis, together with multiple small tumours that involve neuroectodermal structures. The skin, eyes, and some internal organs such as the kidneys are also commonly involved.

### Neurofibromatosis

Type 1 (neurofibromatosis 1 [NF1], von Recklinghausen's disease) is a relatively common (1 in 3,000) autosomal dominant disease characterized by cutaneous café-au-lait pigmentation and neurofibromas. NF1 is due to mutations in *neurofibromin 1*, a tumour-suppressor gene. In the central form of the disease (NF2) tumours are common, the most characteristic being bilateral schwannomas of cranial nerve VIII and tumours of the spinal nerve roots. NF2 is due to mutation of the *merlin* gene, also a tumour-suppressor gene.

### Tuberous Sclerosis (Bourneville's Disease)

This is a mendelian dominant condition that occurs in 1/100,000 and is caused by mutations in the *TSC1* or *TSC2* gene. It is characterized by seizures, learning difficulties, and various skin manifestations. Rhabdomyomas of the heart occur in a third of cases. The brain may be small, normal, or increased in size, the most characteristic feature being the presence of pale, firm tubers in the cerebral cortex.

## THE SPINAL CORD

The spinal cord extends from the base of the skull where it is continuous with the medulla to the first lumbar vertebra, below which it becomes the filum terminale. The major ascending tracts carry sensation to the cerebellum, thalamus, and cerebral cortex.

The tissue of the spinal cord is similar to that of the brain, but the relative frequencies of various lesions are very different. Specific diseases of the spinal cord are described elsewhere, but so-called transverse lesions, various types of spinal injury, and the consequent ascending and descending wällerian degeneration within the cord, and vascular lesions are dealt with here. Spinal cord disease tends to result in a combination of motor, sensory, and autonomic dysfunction.

## Applied Anatomy

The spinal cord in transverse section is shown in Fig. 11.41. Descending fibres are motor, ascending fibres sensory. The descending fibres associated with higher control of sphincter function are in the lateral white matter of the cord just in front of the lateral corticospinal tracts. Ascending fibres associated with bladder function are in the more superficial part of the lateral white columns.

## Transverse Lesions

These occur when partial or complete interruption of the cord is produced by local disease or trauma.

### Causes of Slowly Progressive Effects

- Extrinsic tumours in the extradural space, e.g. metastatic carcinoma (Fig. 11.42) or lymphoma, or in the subdural space, e.g. meningioma or schwannoma.
- Intrinsic tumours, e.g. astrocytoma or ependymoma, are rarer causes.
- Tuberculosis is still a common cause in various parts of the world. It leads to angular curvature of the spine, 'cold' abscesses, and granulomatous masses, any of which can cause pressure on the cord; this may be so severe that infarction of the cord may occur at this level.
- Lesions in the vertebral column, e.g. prolapsed intervertebral disc, cervical spondylosis, kyphoscoliosis.

### Causes of Acute Transverse Lesions

- Trauma, usually a fracture dislocation of the vertebra
- Infarction when the circulation of the anterior spinal artery is impaired

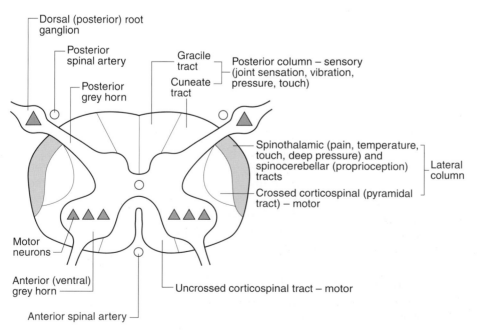

FIG. 11.41 Normal spinal cord.

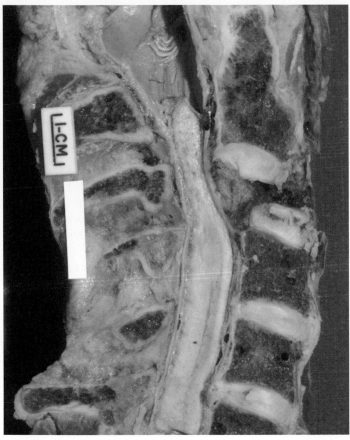

**FIG. 11.42** Compression of the spinal cord: metastatic carcinoma in the vertebral bodies (right) is compressing the spinal cord.

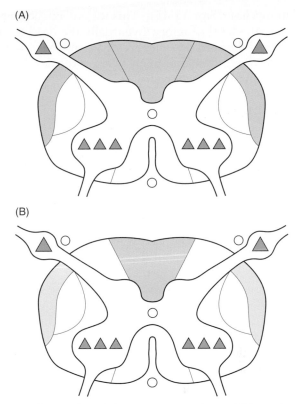

**FIG. 11.43** The spinal cord above a transverse lesion. (A) Immediately above there is degeneration of the posterior columns and the spinocerebellar and the spinothalamic tracts. (B) Well above there is preservation of the cuneate tracts and less severe degeneration of the spinothalamic and spinocerebellar tracts.

- Haemorrhage, usually from a vascular malformation
- Transverse myelitis: this is a clinical rather than a pathological term and is used to describe an acute transverse lesion in the spinal cord in the absence of a compressive lesion. Causes include infarction, demyelination, caisson disease (decompression sickness), infection, or haemorrhage
- Acute demyelination.

The inevitable consequence of a total or partial transverse lesion of the cord, besides the local damage, is the development of ascending (Fig. 11.43) and descending (Fig. 11.44) wällerian degeneration in the interrupted tracts of the spinal cord. Degeneration occurs in those fibres that are separated from their cell bodies by the lesion.

## Spinal Injury

Non-missile injuries result from subluxations and fracture/dislocations of the vertebral column, and are usually brought about by acute flexion or extension. Missile injuries are caused by bullets or stab wounds. The clinical outcome depends on the severity of irreversible damage at the level of injury where there are varying degrees of haemorrhagic necrosis. The affected cord is soft and swollen, and there is often a haematoma within the cord (traumatic

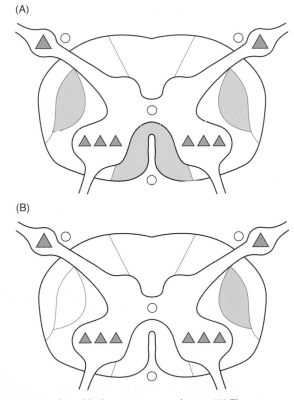

**FIG. 11.44** Spinal cord below a transverse lesion. (A) There is degeneration in the corticospinal tracts. (B) There is degeneration in one corticospinal tract due to an old infarct in the internal capsule.

haematomyelia) (Fig. 11.45). This often extends above and below the level of injury. Eventually the dead tissue is removed and the cord becomes greatly narrowed. A delayed result of trauma, often after many years, is the development of post-traumatic syringomyelia.

## Spina Bifida

See p. 327.

## Syringomyelia

Syringomyelia is a cyst-like space (syrinx) that develops within the cervical cord (syringomyelia) or lower brain stem (syringobulbia). The cavity usually extends through several segments of the cervical cord and, as it enlarges, the cord becomes swollen and soft. Occasionally, syringomyelia occurs in association with tumours affecting the spinal cord. The effects are due to destruction of the cord by the enlarging cavity. The first fibres to be affected are the decussating sensory fibres conveying the sensations of heat and pain: the resulting defect, known as dissociated anaesthesia, is a selective insensitivity to heat and pain in the region corresponding to the involved segments of the spinal cord.

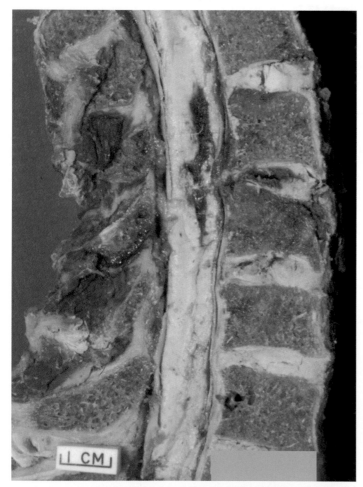

**FIG. 11.45** Fracture dislocation of spine: note haemorrhage into the intervertebral disc and associated spinal cord.

A neuropathic arthritis affecting the joints of the upper limbs often occurs.

## Prolapsed Intervertebral Disc

This is a common cause of compression of the nerve roots and more rarely causes compression of the cord. The intervertebral disc consists of a central nodule of semifluid matrix, the nucleus pulposus, surrounded by a ring of fibrous tissue and fibrocartilage, the annulus fibrosus. The posterior segment of the annulus is thinner and less firmly attached to bone and, after unusual stress, part of the matrix of the nucleus pulposus may herniate through it. This lesion, often termed a 'slipped disc', usually tracks posterolaterally and compresses the nerve root in the intervertebral foramen (Fig. 11.46). Disc protrusions almost always occur in the lumbar spine and L5–S1, L4–5, and L3–4 discs are affected in that order of frequency; they also occur occasionally in the cervical spine. A small protrusion may produce localized pain by irritation of the posterior longitudinal ligament; a larger one may give sciatica root pain due to pressure on nerves leaving the spinal column. The rarer central protrusions may compress the cauda equina, causing paraparesis and sphincter dysfunction.

## Cervical Spondylosis

Cervical spondylosis results from degeneration of intervertebral discs in the cervical region. The disc spaces are narrowed, osteophytes form, and, in addition to compression of nerve roots, there may be interference with the blood supply to the spinal cord where the vertebral canal is narrowest. The importance of cervical spondylosis is uncertain because it can be demonstrated radiologically in some 50% of adults aged >50 and in some 75% > 65. It may therefore be that secondary ischaemic damage in the spinal cord – cervical myelopathy – occurs only in individuals with congenital narrowing of the vertebral canal.

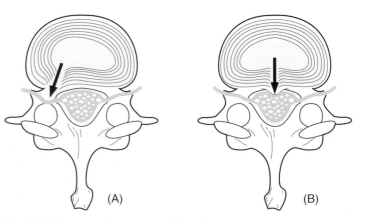

**FIG. 11.46** Prolapsed intervertebral disc: (A) posterolateral protrusion compressing a nerve. (B) Central protrusion compressing the cauda equina. (From Adams JH, Graham DI. *Introduction to Neuropathology.* London: Churchill Livingstone, 1988.)

## Vascular Damage to the Spinal Cord

This is usually due to pathology in the anterior spinal artery. The blood supply to the ventral portion of the cord may be affected in neurosyphilis, collagen disorders, compression of the segmental artery by tumour, dissecting aneurysm of the aorta, and surgery on the aorta.

# TUMOURS OF THE NERVOUS SYSTEM

### Key Points

- CNS tumours may be intrinsic (neuroepithelial) or extrinsic to the neuraxis, or metastatic.
- Metastatic tumours, in adults, are far more common than primary tumours.
- Most patients present with headache, seizures, or focal neurological deficits.
- Most intrinsic tumours are derived from glial cells ('gliomas').
- Gliomas are regarded as low or high grade rather than truly benign or malignant.
- The most common primary brain tumour is glioblastoma – a rapidly growing high-grade tumour.

Primary brain tumours are uncommon with an annual incidence of 5–10/100,000 of the population. Although rare in childhood, in this age group they are the second most common form of neoplasm, exceeded only by leukaemia. Intracranial tumours behave as expanding intracranial lesions leading to raised ICP. The effective size of the tumour is frequently contributed to by oedema in the adjacent brain; this usually responds dramatically to corticosteroid therapy. MRI or CT allows the tumour to be located and biopsied to provide a histological diagnosis. Treatment options include surgery, radiotherapy, and chemotherapy.

The aetiology of primary CNS tumours is largely unknown. Immunosuppression, whether due to AIDS, drug therapy (e.g. in patients who receive renal transplants), or leukaemia is associated with the development of lymphomas. Development of neoplasms is increasingly recognized to be associated with specific genetic alterations in the tumour cells, e.g. *p53* and *IDH1* mutations and *PDGFR* gene amplification in low-grade astrocytomas; *EGFR* gene amplification, loss of one copy of parts of chromosomes 10 and 19, and *MGMT* promotor methylation in glioblastomas; loss of heterozygosity of 1p and 19q in oligodendrogliomas; and chromosome 22 alterations in meningiomas. Increasingly, specific genetic profiles of individual tumours are being associated with differences in tumour progression and response to therapy. A number of genetic syndromes, although rare, have a well-documented association with CNS tumours (*Table 11.6*).

An abbreviated version of the current World Health Organization (WHO) classification of tumours of the nervous system is given in *Table 11.7*. The classification is

**TABLE 11.6** Familial tumour syndromes

| Genetic syndrome | Associated tumours |
|---|---|
| Neurofibromatosis type 1 | Neurofibromas, gliomas, malignant peripheral nerve sheath tumours |
| Neurofibromatosis type 2 | Schwannomas, meningiomas, gliomas |
| Von Hippel–Lindau syndrome | Haemangioblastoma |
| Li–Fraumeni syndrome (*TP53* germline mutations) | Gliomas |
| Tuberous sclerosis | Subependymal giant cell astrocytoma |

**TABLE 11.7** Simplified World Health Organization classification of tumours of the central nervous system

| | |
|---|---|
| Astrocytic tumours | Astrocytoma |
| | Anaplastic astrocytoma |
| | Glioblastoma |
| | Pilocytic astrocytoma |
| | Pleomorphic xanthoastrocytoma |
| | Subependymal giant cell astrocytoma |
| Oligodendroglial tumours | Oligodendroglioma |
| | Anaplastic oligodendroglioma |
| Ependymal tumours | Ependymoma |
| | Anaplastic ependymoma |
| | Myxopapillary ependymoma |
| | Subependymoma |
| Mixed gliomas | |
| Choroid plexus tumours | Choroid plexus papilloma |
| | Choroid plexus carcinoma |
| Neuronal and mixed neuronal-glial tumours | Gangliocytoma |
| | Ganglioglioma |
| Primitive neuroectodermal tumours | Medulloblastoma |
| | Neuroblastoma |
| Tumours of cranial and spinal nerves | Schwannoma |
| | Neurofibroma |
| | Malignant peripheral nerve sheath tumour |
| Tumours of the meninges | Meningioma |
| | Anaplastic meningioma |
| | Haemangioblastoma |
| | Hemangiopericytoma |
| Haematopoietic neoplasms | Primary lymphoma |

(*Continued*)

**TABLE 11.7** (*Continued*)

| | |
|---|---|
| Germ cell tumours | Germinoma |
| | Embryonal carcinoma |
| | Yolk sac tumour (endodermal sinus tumour) |
| | Choriocarcinoma |
| | Teratoma |
| | Mixed germ cell tumours |
| Cysts and tumour-like lesions | Epidermoid cyst |
| | Dermoid cyst |
| | Colloid cyst of the third ventricle |
| Tumours of the sellar region | Pituitary adenoma |
| | Pituitary carcinoma |
| | Craniopharyngioma |
| Local extensions from regional tumours | Paraganglioma |
| | Chordoma |
| Metastatic tumours | Focal deposits |
| | Malignant meningitis |

based mainly on the histological appearance of the tumour. Diagnosis is often facilitated by immunocytochemistry, e.g. glial tumours express GFAP and neuronal tumours express specific neuronal antigens. Tumours may be conveniently categorized as intrinsic when arising in the substance of the brain or spinal cord, extrinsic when arising in adjacent structures and compressing the brain or spinal cord, or metastatic.

## Intrinsic Tumours

Most primary brain tumours, known collectively as 'gliomas', resemble specific types of glial cells, i.e. astrocytes, oligodendrocytes, and ependymal cells. The corresponding tumours are astrocytoma, oligodendroglioma, and ependymoma. Some are low grade and composed of well-differentiated cells without mitotic figures. High-grade glial tumours are composed of poorly differentiated pleomorphic cells; features including mitoses, endothelial cell hyperplasia, and tumour necrosis are likely to be present. As in other tissues, the general rule usually applies that the more primitive or undifferentiated the cells, the more rapid the tumour growth. The terms 'benign' and 'malignant' do not readily apply to glial tumours. No matter how well differentiated or benign a glioma appears, it almost invariably infiltrates into the adjacent brain, rendering complete surgical excision impossible and recurrence almost certain. On the other hand, no matter how rapidly growing and poorly differentiated the glioma appears, metastasis outside the CNS is very unlikely. Occasionally, glial tumour cells spread diffusely throughout the subarachnoid space (meningeal gliomatosis).

### Astrocytoma

Astrocytoma is a low-grade tumour that occurs most frequently in the cerebrum of young adults. CT or MR scans show an ill-defined low-density lesion without contrast enhancement. Macroscopically, the tumour may be difficult to distinguish from the surrounding brain. It is homogeneous, abnormally firm, may contain cysts, and diffusely infiltrates surrounding brain structures. Histologically, the tumour is composed of cells resembling astrocytes. Mitoses, endothelial cell hyperplasia, and necrosis are not present. The mean survival is 8 years, most eventually transforming to a high-grade tumour (anaplastic astrocytoma or glioblastoma). The rare pilocytic variant occurs in children and young adults, typically in the cerebellum or optic nerves; unusually among gliomas it is very low grade and may be regarded as benign. Anaplastic astrocytoma has a peak incidence in the fifth decade. Mitotic figures are identified but there is no endothelial hyperplasia or necrosis. Mean survival is 2–3 years.

### Glioblastoma

Glioblastoma is by far the most common glial tumour and usually arises in patients aged >50 years. It may derive by evolution of an astrocytoma or arise anew as a glioblastoma. Imaging typically shows a central low-density area with a ring of surrounding enhancement. Macroscopically it is firm, white or yellow in colour, with areas of haemorrhage and necrosis; although it may appear well circumscribed, histologically there is infiltration of surrounding brain structures by tumour cells (Fig. 11.47). Mitoses, endothelial cell hyperplasia and tumour necrosis are present. The prognosis is very poor with a mean survival of less than a year.

### Oligodendroglioma

This is a slowly growing, relatively circumscribed, and commonly calcified tumour. The cells are uniformly small and round, resembling normal oligodendroglial cells, with clear cytoplasm and distinct cell membranes. Anaplastic change is less common than in astrocytomas. In comparison with astrocytic tumours there is a poor correlation between the histological features and biological behaviour. Prolonged survival may occur.

### Ependymoma

Ependymoma occurs in relation to the ventricles, the central canal of the spinal cord, or the filum terminale, in keeping with its resemblance to ependymal cells. A common site is in the fourth ventricle in children. The tumour cells are characteristically orientated around small blood vessels to form perivascular pseudo-rosettes. A high-grade variant (anaplastic ependymoma) has a marked tendency to seed through the CSF pathways. Myxopapillary ependymoma arises at the lower end of the spinal cord from the filum terminale. It is a very slowly growing, gelatinous tumour that ensheathes the nerve roots of the cauda equina. The tumour

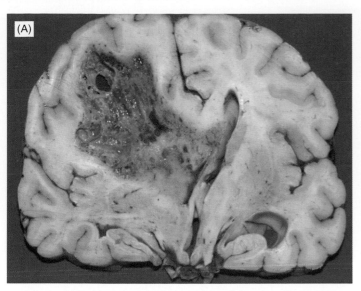

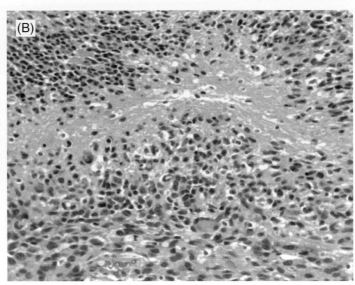

**Fig. 11.47** Glioblastoma: (A) there is a partly cystic necrotic tumour in the posterior frontal lobe that has remarkably well-defined margins. Associated brain swelling has produced internal herniation, ventricular asymmetry, and a shift of the medial structures. (B) There are serpiginous foci of necrosis with surrounding nuclear pseudopalisading. The tumour is pleomorphic and multinucleate tumour giant cells, vascular endothelial cell hyperplasia, and mitotic figures are present.

consists of papillary structures comprising a central vascular core surrounded by mucoid connective tissue and covered by ependymal cells.

### Choroid Plexus Tumour

Choroid plexus tumour is most often seen in children, forming a cauliflower-like tumour within a ventricle. The papillary structures have a vascular connective tissue core covered by columnar epithelium, very similar in appearance to normal choroid plexus. Most choroid plexus tumours are benign (papillomas) although malignant examples may occur (carcinomas).

### Medulloblastoma

This primitive neuroectodermal tumour of the cerebellum occurs most often in childhood but sometimes in young adults. Poorly differentiated and rapidly growing, this tumour tends to spread throughout the subarachnoid

---

## GLIOBLASTOMA

### Presentation

A 65-year-old female presented with a history in recent weeks that her family had complained that her driving had become quite erratic and, on occasions, she had been unable to change lanes when driving on the motorway. More recently, she described a 'heavy feeling in her head' when waking up in the morning, which would clear after a few hours. This 'headache' had become more intense in the past few days, and she had vomited on one occasion. She had a history of previous surgery for breast carcinoma some 15 years earlier. On examination, she was found to have bilateral papilloedema, a homonymous left hemianopia, and slightly increased tone on the left side. There was also a degree of left-sided inattention.

### Investigations

A CT scan was performed and this showed a large space-occupying lesion in the right hemisphere, extending from the temporal lobe into the parietal lobe (Fig. 11.48A,B). There was significant mass effect, with distortion and effacement of the

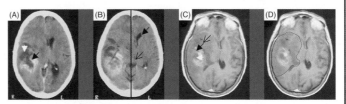

**Fig. 11.48** Glioblastoma: (A) post-contrast CT scan, showing enhancement (black arrows), necrotic centre (white arrow), and mass effect. (B) Post-contrast CT scan, showing midline shift (black line is the midline of the cranial cavity, with the right frontal horn (black arrow) and the third ventricle (open arrow) on the left of the midline. (C) Post-contrast MR scan, showing enhancement (black arrow), necrosis (white arrow), and oedema (open arrow). (D) Post-contrast MR scan, showing the probable extent of the tumour. (Courtesy of Mr Papanastassiou, Department of Neurosurgery, Southern General Hospital, Glasgow.)

ventricular system on that side and midline shift from right to left (Fig. 11.48B). After the administration of contrast, there was irregular, inhomogeneous enhancement (black arrow), with areas of hypodensity within the lesion (white arrow), probably representing necrosis, and surrounding vasogenic oedema (Fig. 11.48C). An MRI scan was also performed, partly in view of her previous history of breast carcinoma, to exclude the presence of multiple lesions. The post-gadolinium-enhanced T1-weighted images demonstrate rather better the features of this tumour (Fig. 11.48C,D). There were no other visible lesions.

Her family's comments about her driving are typical of somebody with peripheral hemianopic visual field loss, which initially goes unnoticed until a traffic accident or near miss occurs. Her headaches were indicative of raised ICP with their diffuse, 'heavy' nature and their early morning occurrence. This was confirmed by the presence of papilloedema on fundoscopy. The scan appearances are those of an intra-axial malignant brain tumour, most likely primary (intrinsic), but in view of her previous history of breast carcinoma a secondary or metastatic lesion could not be totally excluded.

## Management

The patient was started on corticosteroids,, which helped reduce cerebral oedema and resolved her headaches within a few days. She then underwent craniotomy and tumour resection, as the most efficient way of reducing the tumour mass effect as well as obtaining tissue for histological diagnosis. The tumour was confirmed as a primary brain tumour and classified as a glioblastoma, grade IV (WHO classification). This is the most aggressive malignant brain tumour, with a median survival of 9–12 months despite maximum therapy involving surgery, radiotherapy, and often chemotherapy. She received postoperative external beam radiotherapy and remained well and active for the next 8 months, until she had signs of tumour recurrence. She received no other therapy and she died 10 months after diagnosis.

Despite the often clear delineation of the enhancing part of the tumour on imaging, glioblastoma is a diffuse tumour with malignant cells spreading out from the main tumour mass, usually along white matter pathways. Biopsy and postmortem studies have shown that the extent of tumour cell spread will quite often include the area of surrounding oedema (open arrow in Fig. 11.48C and outlined in Fig. 11.48D) and on occasions even spread to the other hemisphere through the corpus callosum.

---

space, and it frequently seeds into the ventricular system and the spinal subarachnoid space. The tumour is composed of closely packed cells which express neuronal antigens and have fine cytoplasmic processes. Mitotic figures are numerous. Although it is a high-grade tumour, current therapy is curative in about half the cases. Tumours of similar morphology occasionally occur in the cerebral hemispheres in children, when they are referred to as neuroblastoma.

## Extrinsic Tumours

### Meningioma

Meningiomas are attached to the meninges and probably originate from arachnoidal granulations. They account for between 15% and 20% of primary intracranial tumours, occurring mainly in adults. Meningiomas are solid, lobulated tumours, well demarcated from the brain tissue into which they project, forming a depression (Fig. 11.49A). They tend to arise adjacent to the major venous sinuses, commonly parasagittally or from the base of the skull, often in the region of the olfactory groove or the sphenoidal ridge. Spinal meningiomas are intradural tumours which may cause cord compression. Most meningiomas are benign and can often be successfully removed. Some, however, infiltrate the overlying bone which may be greatly thickened. There are various histological types, the most common having a somewhat whorled appearance owing to the concentric arrangement of the cells. Many meningiomas contain numerous spherical calcified particles – psammoma bodies (Fig. 11.49B). Only rarely do meningiomas become anaplastic.

### Lymphoma

Primary cerebral lymphomas are almost exclusively diffuse large B-cell lymphomas. There is an increased incidence of

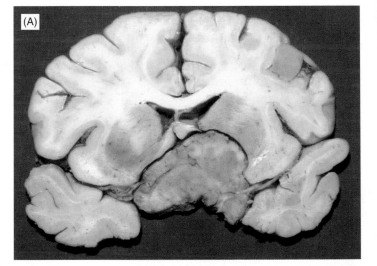

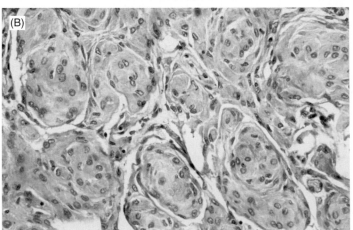

**FIG. 11.49** Meningioma: (A) the tumour arising from the base of the skull has produced a depression in the undersurface of the frontal lobes from which it can be readily withdrawn. (B) Histology of the tumour shows whorls of cells. These can calcify to produce psammoma bodies.

lymphomas in immunocompromised individuals, including in patients with AIDS. Lymphomas arising elsewhere in the body may involve the CNS.

## Germ Cell Tumours

Primary germ cell tumours tend to arise in the midline, particularly in the suprasellar and pineal regions. Such tumours are classified in a similar way to germ cell tumours arising in the testis or ovary.

## Craniopharyngioma

This tumour characteristically occurs as a suprasellar mass projecting upwards into the hypothalamus and the third ventricle, and downwards into the pituitary fossa. It is an encapsulated, sharply circumscribed tumour, which is often cystic. There is usually considerable calcification that can be seen on plain radiographs of the skull or CT scans. The solid parts of the tumour are composed of sheets of epithelial cells showing squamous differentiation with foci of keratinization.

## Epidermoid and Dermoid Cysts

These are the same as similar cysts that occur elsewhere in the body (see Chapter 18). They occur particularly in the posterior fossa and the vertebral canal, when there may be a fistula connecting the cyst with the overlying skin. They also occur within the diploë of the skull.

## Colloid Cyst of the Third Ventricle

This type of cyst develops in the third ventricle, usually contains green gelatinous fluid, and is lined by a flat cuboidal or stratified epithelium. A colloid cyst may have an intermittent ball–valve effect on the interventricular foramina, leading to episodes of acute hydrocephalus that result in severe headache or sudden death.

## Haemangioblastoma

This tumour occurs most frequently in the cerebellum in adult life. The classic type consists of a large cyst containing a mural nodule of tumour, but sometimes the tumour is solid. It is basically benign but recurrence is not uncommon. Some patients have polycythaemia due to production of erythropoietin by the tumour. The tumour consists of a closely packed network of vascular channels of varying size and large polygonal cells that are usually distended with lipid. Haemangioblastomas may be solitary lesions but they may also be a component of the von Hippel–Lindau syndrome in which there may be multiple haemangioblastomas, similar tumours in the retinas, congenital cysts in the pancreas and kidneys, and renal cell carcinoma.

## Schwannoma

This slowly growing encapsulated tumour arises from the Schwann cells of cranial, spinal, or peripheral nerves. A common site is the vestibular portion of the acoustic nerve (often referred to as an 'acoustic neuroma') which takes its origin just within the internal auditory meatus; enlargement of this is usually visible radiologically. The patient usually presents

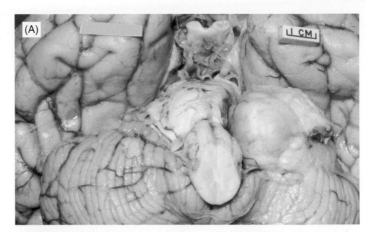

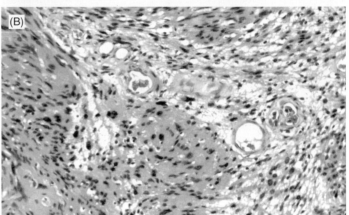

FIG. 11.50 Schwannoma: (A) a cerebellopontine angle mass that has distorted nearby structures and induced a degree of obstructive hydrocephalus. (B) Histologically, in addition to closely packed elongated cells, there are more loosely arranged cells.

with deafness and the tumour may fill the cerebellopontine angle (Fig. 11.50). Bilateral acoustic schwannomas are a feature of NF2. In the spinal canal, schwannomas occur as intradural tumours almost invariably on dorsal nerve roots, where their main effect is compression of the spinal cord. They may extend through an intervertebral foramen to produce a 'dumb-bell' tumour. Nerve fibres are spread over the surface and are not incorporated into the tumour. On histological examination the cells are elongated and arranged in ill-defined fascicles. In areas the nuclei may form parallel rows ('palisading').

## Neurofibroma

This usually presents as a fusiform swelling on a single nerve. Sometimes a group of nerves is affected by numerous oval and irregular swellings, this being referred to as a plexiform neurofibroma. Such lesions tend to occur in the scalp and neck, when the overlying skin becomes firm and nodular. On histological examination the nerve is expanded by elongated cells, often separated by a mucoid matrix. In contrast to schwannomas, residual axons can be identified in a neurofibroma. Multiple neurofibromas are the hallmark of NF1. Unlike schwannomas, a small but significant proportion of neurofibromas undergo malignant transformation.

### Malignant Peripheral Nerve Sheath Tumour

These sarcomas often result from malignant transformation of a neurofibroma in patients with NF1, but may arise anew.

### Pituitary Tumours

These are described in Chapter 17.

## Metastatic Tumours

These are more common than gliomas. Most metastatic tumours are carcinomas, commonly from the lung, breast, and gastrointestinal tract, but a wide range of other tumours may metastasize to the CNS, including melanoma, lymphoma, sarcoma, and germ cell tumour (Fig. 11.51). Metastases are characteristically multiple, rounded, and well-circumscribed lesions, with central necrosis and surrounding oedema. Deposits of tumour in the vertebrae or spinal extradural space lead to compression of the spinal cord.

### Malignant Meningitis

Tumour cells may spread through the subarachnoid space, sometimes without an associated deposit of solid tumour in the brain or spinal cord. Patients often present with cranial nerve palsies. Malignant cells may be identified in the CSF (Fig. 11.52). The neoplastic cells may be secondary (e.g. carcinoma, melanoma) or primary (e.g. medulloblastoma, ependymoma, glioblastoma).

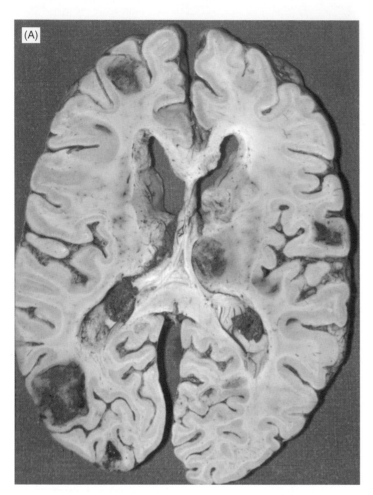

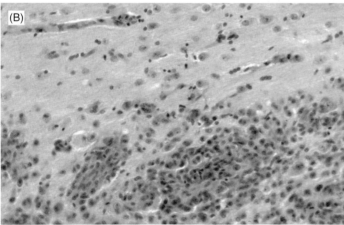

**Fig. 11.51** Metastatic tumour: (A) horizontal slice of brain in which there are multiple metastases. (B) Interface between brain tissue (top) and a deposit of metastatic melanoma (bottom).

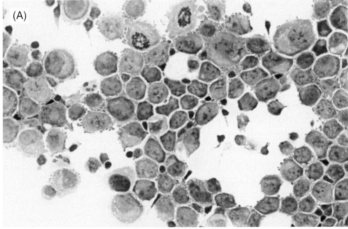

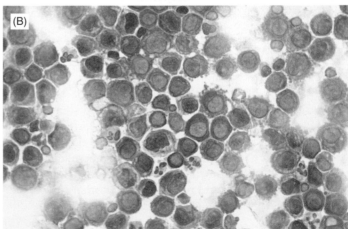

**Fig. 11.52** Malignant meningitis: (A) cytospin preparation showing many large malignant cells with nuclear pleomorphism, multiple nucleoli, and mitosis (Leishman stain). (B) These cells stain with an epithelial marker confirming metastatic carcinoma (same case as A) (immunohistochemistry for cytokeratin).

### Non-metastatic (Remote Paraneoplastic) Effects of Carcinoma

Various indirect neurological syndromes develop in about 3% of all patients with carcinoma, without a constant relationship between the course of the neurological disorders and that of the carcinoma (*Box 11.9*). They may develop concurrently or the neurological disorder may antedate evidence of tumour. The commonest disorders are peripheral neuropathy, a myasthenic syndrome (see Chapter 12, p. 389), encephalomyelitis and subacute atrophy of the cerebellum.

The pathogenesis of these syndromes is incompletely understood. A likely explanation is that of an antigen–antibody reaction after the discovery of specific circulating antibodies against neural tissue, anti-Yo (paraneoplastic cerebellar degeneration) and anti-Hu (paraneoplastic encephalomyelitis/sensory neuropathy) being the best characterized.

## THE PERIPHERAL NERVOUS SYSTEM

## Normal Structure and Function

The PNS comprises the paired cranial nerves, with the exception of the olfactory and optic nerves, which join the CNS at different parts of the brain stem, the 31 pairs of spinal nerves and their endings, the fibres of the autonomic nervous system (sympathetic and parasympathetic), and the associated ganglia.

Most peripheral nerves are mixed, comprising somatic motor and sensory, visceral sensory, and autonomic fibres. The nerve fibres are either myelinated (3–12 μm in diameter) or unmyelinated (average diameter of 1.5 μm). Fibre density alters with disease and decreases with age.

Histologically, a peripheral nerve consists of longitudinally orientated nerve fibres running in a fascicle. Each fibre is surrounded by collagenous tissue called the endoneurium, each fascicle by perineurium, and all the fascicles in a given nerve by the epineurium. Within the endoneurium the myelinated axons are supported by Schwann cells which manufacture and maintain the myelin sheaths between the nodes of Ranvier. Unlike the oligodendrocyte of the CNS, which supports the internodal myelin of many axons, the Schwann cell supports the internodal myelin of only one segment of an axon. The thickness of the myelin sheath is proportional to the diameter of the axon.

By electron microscopy (EM) an axon of the PNS consists of a plasma membrane, the axolemma, and axoplasm which contains 25-nm microtubules and 10-nm neurofilaments, mitochondria, and various types of vesicles and granules. There is continuous movement of the various components of the axon both away from (anterograde transport) and towards (retrograde transport) the neuronal cell body. The speed of transport varies between 4 and 400 mm/day.

## Applied Anatomy and Nerve Conduction

Biopsy of a peripheral nerve is an invasive procedure and therefore it is undertaken only after full consideration of the clinical history, including information about family, occupation, drugs, systemic disease, the physical examination, electrophysiology, and the results of any laboratory tests.

Nerve conduction studies consist of placing a bipolar stimulator to measure latency, amplitude, and speed of the electrical impulse along a sensory or motor nerve. Slowing of conduction is indicative of a demyelinating disorder, whereas the amplitude of the electrical response indicates the number of functioning axons in the nerve. Conduction studies can also be used to investigate nerve function of the brachial and lumbosacral plexus or nerve roots, and the neuromuscular junction in myasthenia gravis and the Eaton–Lambert syndrome (see Chapter 12, pp. 388–389).

The sural nerve, which is purely sensory, is usually chosen for biopsy; if a motor nerve is required then the musculocutaneous nerve and associated muscle are sampled. In the laboratory routine examination includes paraffin histology, resin-embedded semi-thin sections, and EM. Morphometry and teasing after osmification may also be carried out.

## Reactions to Injury and Disease

Peripheral nerves undergo three main types of degeneration: axonal (wällerian) degeneration, distal axonal degeneration, and segmental demyelination. They are also capable of regeneration. Features of more than one of these changes may be seen in an individual case, although one type tends to predominate. Determining the nature of the change is important because recovery is quicker if Schwann cells can remyelinate a fibre rapidly, whereas recovery would be greatly delayed if wällerian degeneration occurred.

### Axonal (Wällerian) Degeneration

The changes in this degeneration are similar to those seen in the CNS (see pp. 298–299). They may follow death of neuronal cell bodies in the spinal cord, or injury to nerve roots or peripheral nerves. Distal to the site of injury there is degeneration of the axon and its myelin sheath. The debris is removed by macrophages and Schwann cells proliferate to form new myelin if axonal regeneration (i.e. sprouting) has occurred. If the continuity of the endoneurial tubes is preserved, the chance of recovery is greater. Axons regenerate at the rate of about 2 mm/day. However, many sprouts may not reach the distal stump, and will proliferate in the dense tissue scar to form a painful swelling called an amputation or traumatic neuroma. Proximal to the lesion the neuronal cell body may undergo central chromatolysis, a feature that is now recognized as a metabolic response to the attempt at regeneration.

### Distal Axonal Degeneration

In the 'dying back' of distal neuropathies, which present typically with sensory loss in a 'glove-and-stocking' distribution, degeneration of axons occurs first, the process then extending back towards the neuronal cell body; this in turn results in secondary loss of myelin.

### Segmental Demyelination

This occurs when there is damage to Schwann cells and the myelin sheath of a previously healthy myelinated nerve. The result is an axon that shows patchy loss of internodal myelin. With recovery the damaged internodal myelin is usually replaced by the myelin from several adjacent Schwann cells, leading to a decrease in the internodal length. In a segment with repeated demyelination and attempts at healing, there is hyperplasia of Schwann cells with concentric wrapping of their cell processes and the formation of 'onion bulbs' along the nerve fibres. This type of change is typically seen in the chronic neuropathies.

## Clinical Presentation and Classification of Peripheral Neuropathies

Patients may present with sensory, motor, or mixed features depending on the cause, the diameter of the affected fibres, and whether the fibres were myelinated. In general there are two broad categories of neuropathy, namely the polyneuropathies, which may be acute or chronic in onset and manifest as widespread symmetrical involvement, and the plexus syndromes and mononeuropathies.

Classification may be by: (1) speed of onset (acute, subacute, or chronic); (2) functional disturbance (motor, sensory, autonomic, or mixed); (3) distribution (proximal, distal, symmetrical, or asymmetrical); (4) pathological process (axonal degeneration, 'dying back', or segmental demyelination); or (5) causation (infections, metabolic, inflammation, vascular, carcinomatous, and so on) – see *Table 11.8*. Disease of a single peripheral nerve is termed a 'mononeuropathy'. When many single nerves are damaged one after the other, this is referred to as mononeuritis multiplex. A knowledge of the anatomy and muscle innervation of the plexus and peripheral nerves is essential to localize the site of the lesion and deduce its likely cause.

## Polyneuropathies

### Guillain–Barré syndrome

This is the most common cause of acute onset neuromuscular paralysis starting within 1–2 weeks of a febrile illness; there is also an association with immunization, surgery, and malignancy. It has an incidence of about 2/100,000 and presents with rapid onset of numbness, paraesthesiae, and an ascending paralysis. There may be involvement of cranial nerve III, and autonomic involvement may present as sphincter disturbance and cardiac arrhythmia. CSF changes are typical with a high protein in the absence of or with few lymphocytes.

There is a severe inflammatory polyneuropathy with a mortality rate of 5–10%; ventilation is required in up to 20% of cases. Most cases recover over many months/years: however, a few develop a chronic relapsing–remitting disease with 'onion bulb' thickening of peripheral nerves.

The principal pathology is segmental demyelination secondary to a T-cell-mediated immune response. There is a strong relationship with *Campylobacter jejuni* (about 25% of UK-based cases), *Mycoplasma pneumoniae*, and HIV, all of which have ganglioside-like epitopes as the postulated mechanism initiating the autoimmune response.

### Diabetes Mellitus

This is the most common metabolic cause of a neuropathy which may present as a symmetrical predominantly sensory polyneuropathy occurring in some 10–30% of all individuals with diabetes, and autonomic neuropathy, proximal painful motor neuropathy, or cranial mononeuropathy affecting principally the cranial nerves III, IV, and VI. All types and sizes of nerve may be affected. The sensory and autonomic neuropathies are due to axonal and segmental demyelinative changes, whereas the motor and cranial neuropathies are probably vascular in origin because many of the perineurial and endoneurial capillaries are narrowed by thickened basal lamina.

### Uraemia

Symptoms and signs parallel renal function, tending to resolve as kidney function improves.

### Paraneoplastic

This is one of the remote effects of malignancy on the nervous systems. Usually there is a sensory or mixed sensorimotor neuropathy in association with small-cell carcinoma of the bronchus, but also with lymphoma. There may be anti-Hu antibodies in the serum.

### Paraproteinaemia

This may occur in association with myeloma, lymphoma, and Waldenström's macroglobinaemia. In about 10% of the late-onset chronic cases there is a specific IgM antibody to myelin-associated glycoprotein. There is both axonal loss and demyelination.

TABLE **11.8** Principal features of the neuropathies

| Onset | Cause | Clinical | Pathology |
|---|---|---|---|
| Acute (days to weeks) | **Inflammatory** | | |
| | Post-infectious (Guillain–Barré) | Motor, distal, autonomic | Demyelination |
| | Vasculitis | Multiple mononeuropathy | Axonal |
| | **Infections** | | |
| | Herpes zoster | Dermatomal | Axonal |
| | Herpes simplex | Oral/genital | Axonal |
| | HIV | Variable | Variable |
| | Diphtheria | Mixed cranial nerve | Demyelination |
| | **Metabolic** | | |
| | Porphyria | Motor, autonomic | Axonal |
| Subacute (weeks) | **Drugs** | | |
| | Isoniazid | Sensorimotor | Axonal |
| | Vincristine | Sensorimotor, distal | Axonal |
| | cis-Platinum | | |
| | **Environmental** | Usually sensory | Axonal |
| | Lead | Motor | |
| | Solvents | | |
| | Acrylamide | | |
| | **Nutritional** | Distal sensory | Axonal, demyelination |
| | Alcohol abuse | | |
| | Vitamin B deficiency | | |
| Chronic (months to years) | **Infection** | | |
| | Leprosy | Distal | Axonal |
| | HIV | Variable | Variable |
| | **Malignancy** | | |
| | Paraneoplastic | Sensory or sensorimotor | Axonal |
| | **Connective tissue disorders** | Often multiple mononeuropathy | Vascular |
| | **Metabolic** | Variable | Axonal |
| | Diabetes mellitus | | |
| | Uraemia | | |
| | **Chronic inflammatory demyelinating polyneuropathy (CIDP)** | Sensorimotor | Demyelination |
| | **Hereditary motor and sensory neuropathy (HMSN)** | Variable, distal | 'Onion bulbs' |

## Toxins

There are many substances that may damage either the neuronal cell body or its myelinated axon. Principal among these are alcohol abuse and the associated nutritional and vitamin B deficiencies, recreational (e.g. heroin) and prescription drugs (e.g. isoniazid, vinca alkaloids, dapsone), and occupational exposure to chemicals such as lead, arsenic, solvents, and acrylamide. Characteristically cases present with a 'dying-back' neuropathy.

## Infections

The two most common causes are herpes zoster and leprosy. In zoster the virus lies dormant in the dorsal root ganglia and, if reactivated, passes down the nerve to the associated sensory dermatome manifesting as shingles. In the tuberculoid form of leprosy there is destruction of the peripheral nerves by granulomatous inflammation, resulting in skin ulceration and loss of digits.

## Hereditary Diseases

The hereditary motor sensory neuropathies (HMSNs) are a heterogeneous group of disorders with a prevalence of about 1/2,500 characterized clinically by distal wasting, the lower limbs having an 'inverted wine bottle' appearance. Principal among this group is HMSN-1 (Charcot–Marie–Tooth disease), which is an autosomal dominant disorder, with about two-thirds of patients having a duplication of PMP-22 (17p11.2) which encodes a Schwann cell protein. Histologically, a characteristic feature of the pathology is demyelination, with thickened 'onion bulbs' reflecting repeated remyelination.

### Vascular Disease

Atheroma and arteriosclerosis are common causes of peripheral neuropathy. The result is ischaemia which may amount to infarction of nerve roots or peripheral nerve. Involvement of the lower limbs is common especially in individuals with diabetes. Multiple mononeuropathy due to vasculitis may also be a presenting feature of polyarteritis nodosa, systemic lupus erythematosus (SLE), and rheumatoid arthritis.

### Plexus Syndromes and Mononeuropathies

Patients with brachial plexus involvement may present with a thoracic outlet syndrome, brachial 'neuritis', or with Pancoast's tumour. Lumbosacral plexus syndromes usually result from surgical trauma after hysterectomy, lumbar sympathectomy from compression by an abdominal mass, infiltration by tumour, or radiotherapy.

Trauma with fractures, compression, and entrapment are common causes of a mononeuropathy. There is also an association with certain systemic diseases, including diabetes mellitus, vasculitis, sarcoidosis, and leprosy. Commonly affected sites are the nerve roots compressed in intervertebral foramina of the spine by intervertebral disc prolapse or osteophytes, the median nerve in the carpal tunnel at the wrist, the ulnar nerve in the flexor carpal tunnel at the elbow, and the common peroneal nerve at the neck of the fibula. The nerve distal to the site of injury undergoes axonal (wällerian) degeneration.

## Disorders of the Neuromuscular Junction

These include myasthenia gravis and the Eaton–Lambert syndrome, both of which are described elsewhere (see Chapter 12, pp. 388–389).

## Nerve Sheath Tumours

Schwannomas and neurofibromas may develop anywhere in the PNS, including within the cranial cavity or spinal canal (see p. 335). Similar lesions are also seen in the skin.

# THE EYE

The pathological changes that occur in the eye and the orbit are in many respects identical to those described in other systems of the body. However, owing to the particular anatomical and functional properties of the eye, there are some

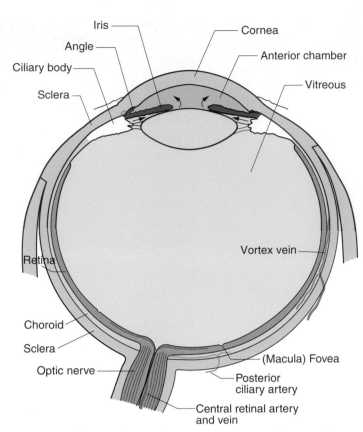

**FIG. 11.53** Schematic diagram showing the structure of the eye. The arrows in the anterior segment show the principal route of aqueous flow.

important specific disease processes. The structure of the eye is shown in Fig. 11.53.

## Genetic Disease

### Retinitis Pigmentosa

This is a group of inherited diseases (autosomal dominant, autosomal recessive, or X linked) in which there is progressive loss of photoreceptors from the peripheral retina to the macula, resulting in tunnel vision. This is associated with secondary proliferation of the retinal pigment epithelium, causing scattered pigmentation of the fundus. Autosomal dominant forms of the disease are associated with mutations in the gene coding for rhodopsin, the rod photoreceptor pigment, and peripherin, a photoreceptor cell-specific glycoprotein.

## Ocular Inflammation

### Inflammation of the Conjunctiva and Cornea

Conjunctivitis is commonly associated with allergies. However, there are several other causal agents including bacterial and viral infections, *Chlamydia trachomatis*, and dry eyes (conjunctivitis sicca). Adenoviruses of various types cause hyperplasia of lymphoid tissue – follicular conjunctivitis. Adenovirus type 8 causes epidemic haemorrhagic conjunctivitis.

Both adults and neonates may develop conjunctivitis caused by *C. trachomatis* (types D–K). In neonates the infection may be severe and is contracted on passage through the birth canal. On microscopy characteristic intracytoplasmic inclusions are seen in smears of conjunctival epithelium. Infection caused by *C. trachomatis* (types A–C) is the most common cause of blindness in tropical zones due to conjunctival scarring, eyelid distortion, and abrasion of the cornea by in-turned lashes.

Ulceration of the cornea is common and is usually viral or bacterial. The cornea is particularly involved in herpes simplex infection, the epithelium being destroyed in a finger-like or dendritic pattern. Herpes simplex keratitis is often recurrent and the resulting corneal scarring may require corneal transplantation.

### Intraocular Infections

#### Pyogenic Bacterial Infection

Traumatic penetration of the cornea or sclera leads to the introduction of bacteria, usually staphylococci, streptococci, or Gram-negative rods. Alternatively organisms may reach the eye via the bloodstream from a distant source of infection – *metastatic endophthalmitis*. Abscesses may form in any chamber of the eye.

#### Other Infections

*Candida* spp. are the most common fungal pathogen in the eye and are most frequently reported in immunosuppressed patients and intravenous drug users in whom they cause metastatic endophthalmitis. Herpes simplex and cytomegalovirus attack the retina and lead to haemorrhagic necrotizing retinitis, particularly in immunocompromised patients.

The protozoan parasite *Toxoplasma gondii* is acquired by eating poorly cooked meat or from soil contaminated by cat faeces. It causes a progressive, recurring retinochoroiditis, particularly in congenitally infected individuals. Dogs are the natural host for the nematode worm *Toxocara canis*. Contamination of soil and grass by ova can result in accidental ingestion, particularly in young children. The ocular manifestations include a unilateral granulomatous endophthalmitis.

### Granulomatous Inflammation

Tuberculosis, syphilis, and brucellosis are rare ocular infections that result in granulomatous inflammation, usually located in the uveal tract (iris, ciliary body, and choroid). The ocular manifestations of sarcoidosis include non-caseating granulomas in the iris, choroid, retina, and optic nerve.

Sympathetic ophthalmitis, a bilateral granulomatous uveitis, can occur after injury to one eye. The injury usually

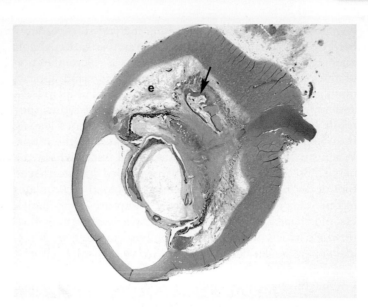

**Fig. 11.54** Shrinkage and disorganization of the eye after inflammation (phthisis bulbi). The retina is detached and entrapped within fibrous tissue. There is osseous metaplasia (arrow). Low pressure has resulted in an exudate (e) in the suprachoroidal space.

includes uveal incarceration within the sclera. Sympathetic ophthalmitis is considered an autoimmune disease, induced by exposure of previously sequestered ocular antigens to the immune system, mediated by MHC (major histocompatibility complex) class 2-restricted CD4+ T cells. It can usually be prevented if the injured eye is enucleated within 3 weeks.

### Rheumatoid Disease

The ocular complications of this connective tissue disease include corneal ulceration and spontaneous perforation (rheumatoid melt), and a necrotizing scleritis. Severe collagen destruction in the sclera may result in perforation (scleromalacia perforans).

### Non-specific Non-granulomatous Uveitis

In many cases the cause of chronic uveitis is unknown, despite intense investigation. In the early stages there is lymphocytic infiltration of the uveal tract. However, in most cases of uveitis the globe is enucleated during the chronic stage of the disease, when the inflammatory process is complicated by loss of vision and pain. The end-stage of any chronic inflammatory disease is a striking shrinkage of the eye with massive subretinal fibrosis and secondary ossification – phthisis bulbi (Fig. 11.54).

## Vascular and Degenerative Diseases

### Retinal Vascular Disease

Important changes occur when there is focal occlusive disease (diabetes, malignant hypertension) in the retinal arterioles: the subsequent ischaemia leads to exudation through damaged capillary endothelium. The clinical and pathological changes of retinal ischaemia include soft exudates, hard exudates, haemorrhage, and neovascularization. A soft exudate or cotton-wool spot represents a microinfarction of the retina due to acute arterial occlusion and appears rapidly. Conversely, hard exudates take several years to form and appear as discrete pale yellow areas in the retina; they result from accumulation of plasma-rich exudates leaking from capillaries in the outer plexiform layer of the retina. When small arterioles rupture, the blood tracks within the nerve fibre layer to produce flame-shaped haemorrhages. Blot or dot haemorrhages are seen when blood accumulates in the outer plexiform layer after the rupture of capillaries. Haemorrhages are most prominent when the venous outflow is partially impaired by thrombosis in the central retinal vein. Circular haemorrhages with white centres (Roth's spots) are classically seen in bacterial endocarditis.

One of the most important responses to focal retinal ischaemia is the release of vasoformative factors (including vascular endothelial growth factor – VEGF) from surviving neural tissue: this causes proliferation of endothelial cells into the ischaemic area – neovascularization. Although this process is potentially beneficial, the delicate, newly formed vessels tend to penetrate the vitreous where they stimulate the formation of membranes that cause retinal detachment and blindness. Vasoproliferative retinopathy is a common complication of the later stages of diabetes mellitus, so-called diabetic retinopathy; this can now be controlled by laser treatment or with injections of anti-VEGF antibodies.

### Age-related Macular Degeneration

Age-related macular degeneration is the most important cause of untreatable visual loss in the ageing western population. The pathogenesis is poorly understood but recent studies have implicated local inflammation and activation of complement among the processes involved. In particular, a specific polymorphism (Y402H) in the gene encoding complement factor H is strongly associated with disease susceptibility. The disease results in atrophy of photoreceptors at the macula and is accompanied by degenerative changes in the retinal pigment epithelium (RPE) (senile macular degeneration). This degeneration in the RPE may be complicated by haemorrhage and fibrosis (senile disciform degeneration of the macula). The overlying photoreceptor tissue is destroyed with loss of central vision. Early senile disciform degeneration may now be successfully treated by intraocular injection of anti-VEGF antibodies.

### Cataract

The biconvex lens substance is formed by cells that contain transparent crystalline lens proteins. A cataract is any opacity of the crystalline lens. The cells of the lens are enclosed in an elastic membrane, the lens capsule. Metabolism of the lens is maintained by diffusion of nutrients from the aqueous. Any change in the biochemical composition of the aqueous fluid, as occurs in metabolic diseases, e.g. diabetes mellitus

or hypocalcaemia, may result in the formation of abnormal opaque proteins in the damaged lens cells. Other insults such as uveitis, ionizing radiation, or trauma may also result in opacities. Congenital cataracts may form if there is damage to the developing lens fibres *in utero*, e.g. as a result of rubella infection. The most common form of cataract, however, is senile cataract, which is due to degradation of lens proteins in the oldest, central part of the lens. Most cases of cataract are treated by removal of the opaque lens matter by 'phakoemulsification' and the insertion of a plastic lens implant into the residue of the lens capsule behind the iris.

### Glaucoma

Glaucoma is a generic name for a group of diseases in which the intraocular pressure increases to a level that impairs the vascular perfusion of the neural tissue and causes blind-

(A)

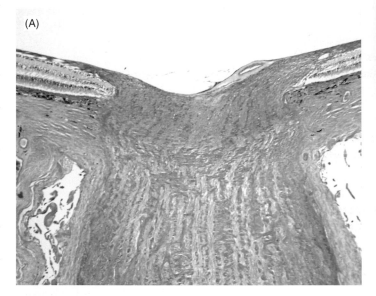

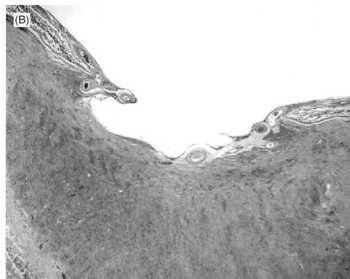

(B)

**FIG. 11.55** Optic nerve in glaucoma: (A) normal optic disc for comparison. (B) Atrophic nerve head giving rise to the 'cupping' seen in advanced glaucoma.

ness. The most serious effects on visual function are due to ischaemic atrophy of the axons in the nerve fibres of the disc, and secondary atrophy of the nerve fibre layer of the retina. Excavation or cupping of the disc may become so advanced that it extends into the optic nerve (Fig. 11.55). The rise in pressure is due to obstruction to the outflow of aqueous, which can occur as the result of: (1) closing off the chamber angle; (2) an abnormality within the outflow system; or (3) a developmental failure in modelling of the trabecular meshwork and the chamber angle.

### Closed-angle Glaucoma

In the primary form the iridocorneal angle is narrow and the anterior chamber shallow, such that the iris and lens may come into contact when the iris is in mid-dilatation; this prevents the flow of aqueous through the pupil and pressure builds up behind the iris, which becomes further bowed anteriorly and causes further occlusion of the angle. This form of glaucoma is of acute onset, with ocular congestion, corneal oedema, and severe pain. If untreated, blindness occurs due to pressure on the blood vessels in the optic disc. Predisposing factors include race (Eskimos and East Asians), female gender, hypermetropia, and predisposing anatomy (narrow angle or plateau iris).

Secondary closed-angle glaucoma has many causes, but the most common is fibrovascular adhesion between iris and cornea after ischaemic retinal disease and uveitis.

### Open-angle Glaucoma

The primary type is an insidious disease of elderly people and the condition may go unnoticed in the early stages. It is presumed that the abnormally high intraocular pressure is the result of an abnormal resistance in the outflow system. However, no cause for this has yet been established. In secondary open-angle glaucoma there is mechanical obstruction of the outflow system by inflammatory cells, tumour cells, or particulate matter from a degenerative lens cortex.

### Congenital Glaucoma

In infants and children, glaucoma can result from developmental abnormalities in which there is a failure in the modelling of the trabecular meshwork and the chamber angle in the early stages of intrauterine life. Increasing intraocular pressure causes the malleable infant eye to expand uniformly, and it may become so large that it resembles an ox's eye – buphthalmos.

## Tumours

The tumours of the eyelid, conjunctiva, and orbital tissues do not differ significantly in morphology and behaviour from those occurring elsewhere. Intraocular tumours are rare, but are important because of the serious effect on vision and their unusual patterns of behaviour. The most

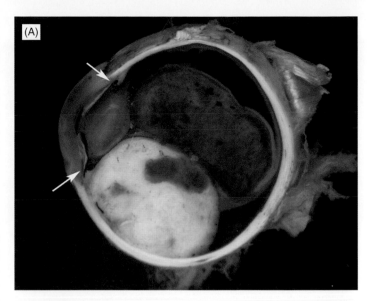

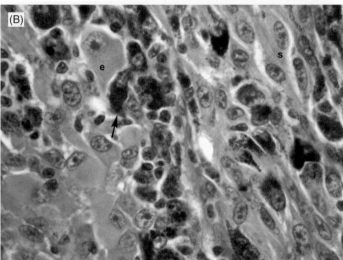

**FIG. 11.56** Malignant melanoma of the choroid: (A) this large tumour shows both pigmented and non-pigmented areas and has pushed the lens forward, causing closure of the chamber angle (arrow) with secondary glaucoma. (B) Histology of this tumour shows large epithelioid cells (e) and spindle cells (s). Some of the cells contain brown melanin pigment (arrow).

common intraocular tumours are malignant melanoma and metastases in adults, and retinoblastoma in children.

### Malignant Melanoma

Malignant melanoma may occur in any part of the eye, but is most common in the choroid. The tumour adopts a collar-stud or nodular mass and may be pigmented or non-pigmented (Fig. 11.56A). Microscopically the tumour cells are either spindle shaped or round epithelioid (Fig. 11.56B). Growth within the eye can lead to retinal detachment, cataract, and secondary closed-angle glaucoma due to lens–pupil block or neovascularization. Extension outwith the eye usually takes place through intrascleral vascular and neural channels and the choroidal (vortex) veins.

The prognosis is best for small tumours (<7 mm in diameter) of spindle cell type which carry a 95% 5-year survival rate. Conversely, large tumours (>15 mm in diameter) of epithelioid cell type have a 50% 5-year survival rate. The clinical course is not always predictable and this tumour is notorious for producing multiple, rapidly enlarging liver metastases as long as 20 years after enucleation of the affected eye (the big liver and glass-eye syndrome). More recently certain cytogenetic abnormalities, including monosomy 3, have been shown to be better predictors of metastatic disease than clinical or histological criteria.

### Retinoblastoma

This is a malignant tumour of the retina, which occurs in infants and children: the incidence is approximately

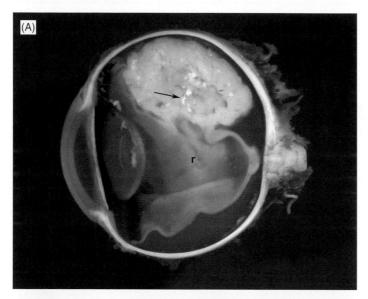

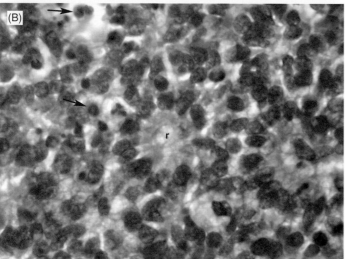

**FIG. 11.57** Retinoblastoma: (A) this large white tumour is in continuity with the retina (r). There is focal calcification within the tumour (arrow). (B) Histology of this tumour shows typical rosettes (r) as well as numerous apoptotic bodies (arrows).

1:23,000 livebirths. It affects both sexes equally and in 40% of cases other relatives are affected. The familial cases are inherited in an autosomal dominant manner, although penetrance is variable. These familial cases are at an increased risk of a second malignancy, especially in bone or soft tissue. Spontaneous, non-familial tumours are usually unilateral and present at a later age.

The retinoblastoma gene occurs on the long arm of chromosome 13 (13q14). It codes for the RB nucleoprotein, which normally suppresses cell division. For a tumour to develop, both copies of the retinoblastoma gene must be lost (the 'two hit' hypothesis). In familial cases the first hit occurs through inheritance of a mutant allele and affects every cell in the body. The second hit occurs as a somatic mutation. In non-familial cases two acquired somatic mutations occur such that these tumours are usually unilateral and unifocal. Clinically the child may present with a squint due to poor vision in the affected eye. When the tumour is large and fills the vitreous or detaches the retina, a white mass is seen behind the lens giving a white pupil (leukocoria).

A retinoblastoma forms a solid white, partially calcified, and partially necrotic mass (Fig. 11.57A). The tumour is composed of small, round cells with scanty cytoplasm and a high mitotic rate. Differentiation is seen as circular rosettes of tumour cells (Fig. 11.57B). Extraocular extension occurs by spread either along the optic nerve into the brain or through the sclera into the orbit. Involvement of the choroid may result in metastases to visceral organs. With modern forms of management including surgery, systemic chemotherapy, and radiotherapy cure rates in excess of 90% are the rule.

## SUMMARY

- Cerebrovascular disease is the third most common cause of death.
- Disease of the CNS is a major cause of mortality and morbidity in childhood.
- Of patients who die in a neurosurgical intensive care unit, 75% do so as a result of an expanding intracranial mass lesion.
- Head injury is the most common cause of death in patients aged <30 years.
- Infections of the CNS are not uncommon and, even in the context of AIDS and other diseases in which the immune system is impaired, they are treatable.
- Neurodegenerative diseases are usually progressive, associated with ageing, and characterized by abnormal accumulation of proteins which result in dysfunction and cell death. The causes of some rare familial types are known, but the great majority are considered to be due to an interaction between genetic susceptibility and environmental factors.

- Most cases of dementia result from neurodegenerative disease.
- Alzheimer's disease is the most common cause of dementia, being responsible for about 70% of cases; dementia with Lewy bodies accounts for 15%.
- Several years after the peak of BSE, cases of vCJD were identified in the UK.
- Myelin is unique to the nervous system (CNS and PNS) and in health is required for normal saltatory conduction of action potentials. MS (of the CNS) and neuropathy (of the PNS) are common forms of demyelination.
- Intrinsic tumours of the brain are uncommon; more common are metastatic tumours from the bronchus, breast, and gastrointestinal tract.
- Corneal ulceration is usually caused by viruses or bacteria.
- After injury to one eye, both eyes may be affected by sympathetic ophthalmitis.
- Intraocular vascular proliferation is a common complication of late-stage diabetes mellitus.
- Age-related macular degeneration is an important cause of untreatable blindness in the western world.
- Primary open-angle glaucoma is a common cause of insidious visual loss in elderly people.
- Malignant melanoma is the most common primary intraocular tumour in adults.
- Retinoblastoma is the most common primary intraocular tumour in children.

## ACKNOWLEDGEMENT

The authors acknowledge the contribution of David I Graham to this chapter.

## FURTHER READING

Ellison D, Love S, Chimelli L, *et al. Neuropathology. A Reference Text of CNS Pathology*, 3rd edn. London: Mosby, 2013.

Graham DI, Nicoll JAR, Bone I. *Adams & Graham's Introduction to Neuropathology*, 3rd edn. London: Hodder Arnold, 2006.

Gray F, de Girolami U, Poirier J. *Escourolle and Poirier. Manual of basic neuropathology*, 4th edn. Philadelphia, PA: Butterworth Heinemann, 2004.

Lee WR. *Ophthalmic Histopathology.* Berlin: Springer-Verlag, 2002.

Lindsay KW, Bone I, Callendar R. *Neurology and Neurosurgery Illustrated*, 4th edn. Edinburgh: Churchill Livingstone, 2004.

Love S, Louis DN, Ellison DW, eds. *Greenfield's Neuropathology*, 8th edn. London: Hodder Arnold, 2008.

Spencer WH, ed. *Ophthalmic Pathology*, Vols 1–4. Philadelphia, PA: WB Saunders, 1996.

# 12

# THE LOCOMOTOR SYSTEM

Elaine MacDuff

## INTRODUCTION

Disorders of the locomotor system are not among the most important diseases in terms of mortality, but they are of enormous social and economic significance in terms of their morbidity. They are responsible for around 20% of general practitioner consultations. Osteoporosis, rheumatoid arthritis, osteoarthritis, and backache are particularly important in this regard.

## NORMAL BONE STRUCTURE AND FUNCTION

Bone has two main functions: it forms a rigid endoskeleton and has a central role in mineral homeostasis, principally of calcium and phosphate, but also of sodium and magnesium.

Bone is composed of cells, a protein matrix, and mineral. There are two main cell types: bone-forming cells, principally osteoblasts, and bone-resorbing cells called osteoclasts (Fig. 12.1). Osteoblasts are derived from primitive bone marrow stromal cells known as osteoprogenitor cells under the influence of growth factors such as bone morphogenic proteins (BMPs). Osteoblasts lie in sheets on the surface of bone trabeculae. Their cytoplasm contains abundant rough endoplasmic reticulum and Golgi apparatus for protein synthesis and processing, and is rich in alkaline phosphatase for mineralization of the matrix. They express numerous receptors including those for oestrogen and androgens, vitamin D, parathyroid hormone (PTH), growth factors, and cytokines. After completing a cycle of activity, osteoblasts undergo apoptosis or mature into osteocytes, which are relatively inactive cells lying in lacunae within bone. Long cytoplasmic processes run within canaliculi through bone and interconnect osteocytes and osteoblasts by intercellular junctions. Osteocytes may be sensitive to electric currents produced by deformation of crystals in bone (piezo-electricity), and so may be involved in control of bone remodelling in response to mechanical stress.

Osteoclasts lie in the shallow depressions (Howship's lacunae) on the surface of bone. They are large multinucleated cells derived from haematopoietic stem cells of granulocyte–macrophage lineage under the influence of colony-stimulating factors and tumour necrosis factor (TNF). Stimulated by interleukins such as interleukin 1 (IL-1) and IL-6, they closely attach to bone at their periphery (sealing zone), and secrete acid, generated by carbonic anhydrase, and lysosomal enzymes, including acid phosphatase and collagenase, to remove mineral and matrix simultaneously. Measurement of urinary collagen degradation products such as deoxypyridinoline (DPD) and terminal peptide fragments from type I collagen provides an indication of osteoclastic activity. Their plasma membrane is thrown into folds forming a 'ruffled border' with abundant surface area adjacent to bone.

The protein matrix of bone consists largely of type I collagen produced by osteoblasts. There are, in addition, small amounts of non-collagenous proteins including calcium-binding proteins such as osteonectin and bone sialoprotein and those involved in mineralization such as osteocalcin. Cell adhesion proteins, including osteopontin and growth factors including transforming growth factor (TGF), are also present.

Bone is initially laid down as a non-mineralized protein-rich form known as osteoid. Over the next 10 days or so, osteoid becomes mineralized to form bone. The mineral matrix accounts for two-thirds of bone mass; its main component

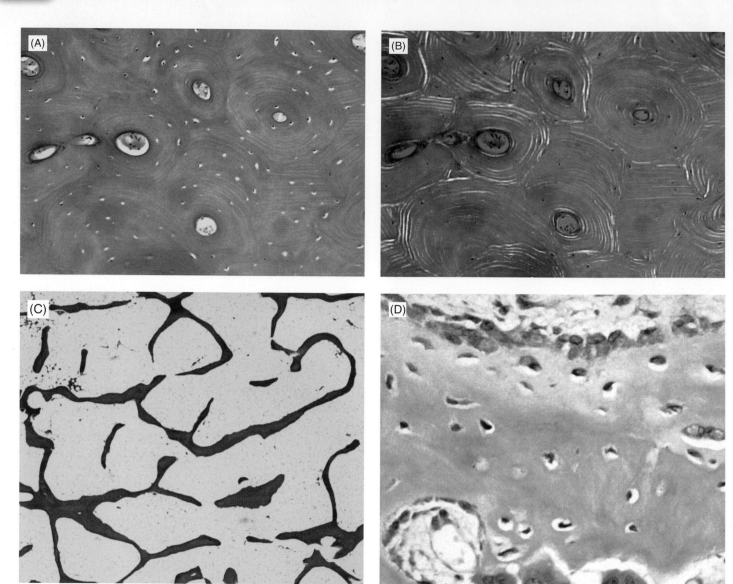

**Fɪɢ. 12.1** Normal bone structure and function: (A) cortical bone is arranged in concentric cylindrical structures – haversian systems – seen here in cross-section. (B) Polarization microscopy shows the lamellar structure well. (C) Bone within the medulla forms a meshwork of trabeculae, known as cancellous bone; this is also lamellar in type. (D) The cellular composition of bone shown in this photomicrograph is of rapidly formed woven bone with a random arrangement of the collagen fibres. A row of osteoblasts covers the upper surface of the bone: the perinuclear vacuoles are the prominent Golgi apparatus of cells that synthesize and export protein. Osteocytes are seen in their lacunae within the bone trabeculae. Three active multinucleated osteoclasts lie within resorption cavities on the lower surface.

is hydroxyapatite ($Ca_{10}[PO_4]_6[OH]_2$). Substantial amounts of sodium, potassium, magnesium, carbonate, and citrate are also present.

## Types of Bone

Bone is found in two patterns, woven and lamellar (see Fig. 12.1). Woven bone is formed where bone is laid down rapidly, as in fetal growth, during healing of a fracture, and in bone-forming tumours. It contains numerous plump osteocytes and collagen fibres are arranged randomly.

Lamellar bone, in contrast, is laid down slowly, is structurally strong, and forms the adult skeleton. The collagen lies in parallel sheets, the fibres of which run in different directions, resulting in a laminated structure. The osteocytes are

small and relatively sparse. Adult lamellar bone is arranged in two forms: compact and cancellous. Compact bone forms the cortex of bones. Its basic unit is the haversian system (osteon) (see Fig. 12.1A), each consisting of a concentric array of bone surrounding a central artery and vein. Cancellous (spongy) bone is found between the cortices of bones and at the ends of long bones. It is composed of plates or trabeculae separated by marrow spaces. Compact bone accounts for about 80% of the adult skeleton and cancellous bone about 20%.

## Bone Turnover

Bone is constantly being formed and resorbed; approximately 10% of the adult skeleton is replaced annually. Bone remodelling is carried out by osteoclasts and osteoblasts coupled together by chemical mediators in bone modelling units (BMUs), so that adult bone mass is kept fairly constant. Imbalance of formation and resorption can cause disease: it may lead to a decreased bone mass, e.g. in osteoporosis (pp. 350–352). Bone turnover is a complex process, which is gradually becoming understood, and is illustrated in Fig. 12.2 and discussed in more detail in Special Study Topic 12.1.

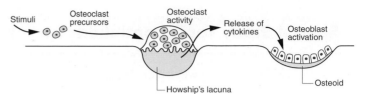

**FIG. 12.2** The cycle of bone turnover: various agents promote bone resorption by stimulating osteoclast formation and maturation. As these cells resorb bone, cytokines are released, which in turn promote osteoblastic activity, thus completing the cycle.

# 12.1 Special Study Topic

## CONTROL OF BONE TURNOVER

In recent years, considerable advances have been made in our understanding of the mechanisms that control bone turnover and, in particular, of the factors regulating osteoclast formation and bone destruction. This may lead to targeted therapies for the common metabolic bone disorders of osteoporosis and Paget's disease, and the bone destruction that is a feature of metastatic tumours in the skeleton.

## Osteoclast Formation

As indicated earlier, osteoclasts are multinucleated cells derived from precursors of monocyte/macrophage lineage. These precursor cells fuse to form non-functioning osteoclasts (Fig. 12.3), which are then activated. They resorb bone and eventually undergo apoptosis, thus stopping the phase of

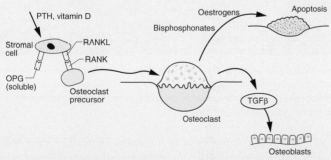

**FIG. 12.3** Osteoclast precursors (monocyte/macrophage lineage cells) are stimulated to become osteoclasts by receptor activator of nuclear factor B ligand (RANKL). This molecule is upregulated on the surface of marrow stromal cells by vitamin D (Vit D), parathyroid hormone (PTH), and other factors. Overactivity of RANKL is normally prevented by the soluble protein osteoprotegerin (OPG). In the process of removing bone, osteoclasts produce cytokines such as transforming growth factor (TGF) which both stimulate osteoblasts to produce new bone and inhibit osteoclasts. Unwanted osteoclasts undergo apoptosis under the influence of oestrogens and bisphosphonates.

bone resorption. The cycle of bone turnover starts with the activation of bone resorption.

Osteoclast formation is promoted by two main substances. The first is macrophage colony-stimulating factor (M-CSF), which is derived from bone marrow stromal cells and osteoblasts. The second is RANKL (receptor activator of nuclear factor B ligand) – a molecule produced by and expressed on the surface of marrow stromal cells. RANKL acts through a cell surface receptor, RANK, on the surface of osteoclast precursors. Most factors that stimulate osteoclast formation, such as vitamin D, PTH-related peptide (PTHrP), and IL-11, do so by up-regulating RANKL expression.

As in any biological system, there is an antagonistic mechanism, which in health ensures homeostasis. This inhibitory substance is known as osteoprotegerin (OPG) and is a soluble protein that competes with the cell-bound RANKL. OPG is a member of the TNF superfamily and is produced by a wide variety of cell types. Effectively, the ratio RANKL:OPG at any site will determine the extent of bone resorption. As osteoclastic activity removes bone, in the process cytokines such as TGF are released that both inhibit osteoclasts and stimulate osteoblasts. Thus, when the phase of resorption ceases, osteoblasts start to synthesize newly formed uncalcified matrix (known as osteoid), which becomes mineralized approximately 7 days later. A very thin layer of osteoid covering up to 20% of the trabecular surface area is therefore a normal finding.

Much work has been carried out in animal models. Transgenic mice deficient in RANKL and those overexpressing OPG both develop osteopetrosis (p. 357); in contrast, animals lacking OPG develop osteopenia (osteoporosis).

## Regulation of Bone Destruction in Malignant Disease

Bone destruction is a major problem in patients with metastatic carcinoma and those with myeloma. Although cancer cells can resorb bone directly in tissue culture, there is no doubt that *in vivo* bone destruction is primarily due to the action of osteoclasts. Thus anti-osteoclast therapies such as bisphosphonates are often effective. It appears that PTHrP is the most important of the many factors produced by tumour cells that can stimulate osteoclastic activity. Growth factors such as TGF, fibroblast growth factor, and insulin-like growth factors are released as the bone matrix is resorbed, and these

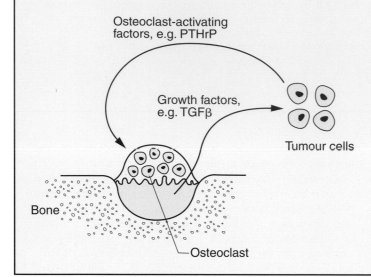

in turn promote further tumour growth. In this way a vicious cycle is established (Fig. 12.4). TNF appears to be the major osteoclast-stimulating factor in multiple myeloma.

## Further Reading

Graham R, Russell G, Espina B, Hulley P. Bone biology and the pathogenesis of osteoporosis. *Curr Opin Rheumatol* 2006;18(suppl 1):S3–S10.

**FIG. 12.4** The vicious cycle of bone destruction: osteoclasts produce growth factors that stimulate tumour cells in the marrow to grow and proliferate. More tumour cells produce more osteoclast-activating factors and the vicious cycle is completed. TGF-β = transforming growth factor β; PTHrP = parathyroid hormone-related peptide.

# DISEASES OF BONE

## Metabolic Bone Disease

Metabolic bone diseases are a group of generalized skeletal disorders that result from abnormal formation, resorption, or mineralization of bone.

### *Osteoporosis*

**Key Points**

- Bone mass is reduced, but chemical composition remains normal.
- Symptoms are most common in postmenopausal females, but may also occur in elderly males and all age groups.
- It may result in fractures of long bones and vertebral collapse (Fig. 12.5).

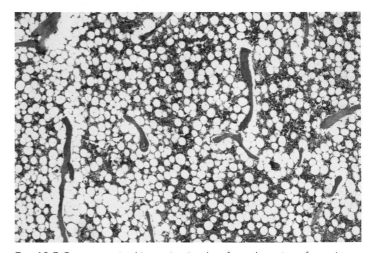

**FIG. 12.5** Osteoporosis: this section is taken from the spine of a patient with steroid-induced osteoporosis. The bone trabeculae are thinned and some appear disconnected from each other. It is easy to see why vertebral collapse has occurred.

Osteoporosis occurs when bone strength is reduced below the level required for its normal structural function. Bone strength is determined by two factors: bone mass and bone quality. The term 'osteoporosis' is usually applied to the common generalized disorder that predisposes to fractures, especially in elderly people. The localized form that occurs after immobilization is a form of disuse atrophy. In both forms of osteoporosis the bone, although reduced in amount, is of normal chemical composition and fully mineralized.

The concept of osteoporosis has changed greatly in recent years. Traditionally, it had been viewed as a disorder of postmenopausal females with fractures. Now, it is regarded as a clinically silent disorder that affects all ages. Furthermore, it is now possible to detect pre-symptomatic osteoporosis and prevent its progression. Generalized osteoporosis has three main subgroups:

- Primary type 1 (postmenopausal) osteoporosis: occurs in females after the menopause
- Primary type 2 (senile) osteoporosis: this occurs after the age of 75 and affects females and males with a ratio of 2:1
- Secondary osteoporosis: when the reduced bone mass is caused by other diseases or drug effects.

## Definition

Osteoporosis has been defined as: 'a systemic skeletal disease characterized by low bone mass and microarchitectural deterioration of bone tissue, with a consequent increase in bone fragility and susceptibility to fracture'. Although this is a useful conceptual definition, the World Health Organization has defined quantitative criteria for osteoporosis and osteopenia (low bone mass) in comparison with the mean of young adult females (*Table 12.1*). Bone density is usually measured by dual-energy radiograph absorptiometry (DXA) of the spine or hip.

## Clinical Features

Osteoporosis can be regarded as a subclinical and clinical disease; the clinical consequences are typically seen in postmenopausal females, but are increasingly recognized in males. Rare cases of juvenile osteoporosis are described. Symptomatic osteoporosis develops when bone loss is sufficiently severe that mechanical failure occurs with two main manifestations:

- Vertebral crush fractures, which may lead to severe back pain and loss of height. If the fracture wedges anteriorly, kyphosis may result.
- Long bone fractures, which may follow minor injury. The common sites are the neck of femur and distal radius (typically Colles' fracture). Forearm fractures are often the first sign of osteoporosis. Femoral neck fractures are a major cause of morbidity and mortality in elderly people.

In the UK, over 70,000 hip, 50,000 wrist, and 120,000 vertebral fractures occur each year; hip fractures alone cost the health service more than £1.73 billion per year.

## Pathological Findings

The changes of osteoporosis are seen in both cancellous and cortical bone. In cancellous bone, the trabeculae are thinned (see Fig. 12.5) and some appear disconnected. Within the vertebral bodies, for example, the number of horizontal trabeculae is reduced; this reduces the amount of support for the weight-bearing vertical trabeculae, which therefore tend to fracture. Similar changes are seen in the cancellous bone found towards the ends of long bones. Within the cortex, the porosity is increased by enlargement of haversian canals due to central osteoclastic activity, whereas the cortex is thinned by endosteal bone resorption. In both sites, the bone is of normal composition.

## Pathogenesis of Osteoporosis

Recent research in bone biology has helped to clarify the pathogenesis of osteoporosis. The major determinants of osteoporosis are peak bone mass and rate of bone loss with age. Bone mass increases throughout childhood and in early adult life after linear growth ceases, so that peak bone mass is achieved by 30 years of age. The most important factors determining peak bone mass are as follows:

- Genetic potential: this appears to be responsible for 75–80% of variation. There is considerable interracial variation, low bone mass being more common in Anglo-Saxon, Japanese, and Indian individuals. A number of candidate genes is being studied including the vitamin D and oestrogen receptor genes and the gene for type I collagen A1 (*CollA1*).
- Adequate nutrition, especially calcium and vitamin D intake.
- Physical activity, especially weight-bearing exercise.

Skeletal mass in both sexes diminishes from the fourth decade onwards (Fig. 12.6), initially at a low rate of <1% per year. Bone loss occurs earlier in women, in whom there is a marked acceleration at the time of the menopause to between 3% and 5% per year. This is due to falling oestrogen levels, which lead to reduction in osteoclast apoptosis and therefore to increased activity. Loss of bone is most marked at sites of rapid turnover such as the cancellous bone of the vertebrae, ribs, pelvis, and ends of long bones, which have a much higher surface area than dense cortical bone. This explains the frequency of fractures at the ends of long bones.

**TABLE 12.1** Osteoporosis defined by bone mass

| | |
|---|---|
| Normal | Bone mass 1 standard deviation (SD) below young normal mean |
| Osteopenia | Bone mass >1 SD but <2.5 SD below young normal mean |
| Osteoporosis | Bone mass ≥2.5 SD below young normal mean |
| Established osteoporosis | Bone mass ≥2.5 SD below young normal mean + fracture |

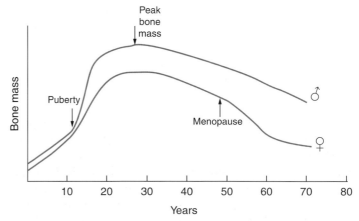

**FIG. 12.6** Changes in bone mass with age. This line diagram shows the rapid acceleration in bone growth during puberty to reach peak bone mass. This is followed by a slow decline in both sexes, the more rapid fall in postmenopausal females accounting for the greater risk of osteoporosis than in males.

There are many risk factors for the development of osteoporosis (*Box 12.1*) and there are a large number of disorders that may cause secondary osteoporosis (*Box 12.2*).

### Treatment

It is now recognized that prevention is the best management for osteoporosis, with emphasis on lifestyle measures to maximize peak bone mass and reduce rates of bone loss. Bisphosphonates, selective oestrogen receptor modulators, such as raloxifene, and human PTH are successful in treating established osteoporosis. Testosterone replacement therapy is indicated in males with osteoporosis due to hypogonadism. Coexisting osteomalacia should be treated.

## *Osteomalacia*

### Key Points

- Osteomalacia occurs due to failure of bone mineralization.
- There is bowing or fracture of abnormally soft bones.
- Histologically there are thickened osteoid seams.
- It is usually due to vitamin D deficiency.

In this disorder, failure of mineralization leads to bones that are abnormally soft, resulting in deformity or fracture. This is shown histologically by the accumulation of excessive amounts of osteoid (unmineralized bone) on the surface of bone trabeculae. Rickets is the equivalent disorder in childhood and is more severe than osteomalacia because there is also defective mineralization of epiphyseal cartilage, which leads to growth disturbance and skeletal abnormalities. The causes of osteomalacia and rickets are summarized

**Box 12.1** FACTORS IMPLICATED IN DEVELOPMENT OF PRIMARY OSTEOPOROSIS

- Female sex
- Body size: thin boned
- Age
- Racial factors: white people and Asians at highest risk
- Family history
- Early menopause
- Inactive lifestyle
- Excessive alcohol and smoking
- Amenorrhoea, e.g. in anorexia nervosa

**Box 12.2** CAUSES OF SECONDARY OSTEOPOROSIS

- Endocrine causes
- Glucocorticoid excess (iatrogenic or endogenous)
- Hyperthyroidism
- Hyperparathyroidism
- Hypogonadism
- Nutritional causes
- Malabsorption
- Chronic liver disease
- Inflammatory disorders
- Rheumatoid arthritis
- Crohn's disease

in *Table 12.2*. Most cases are due to abnormalities of vitamin D, usually deficiency or impaired metabolism, as is seen in liver disease or renal failure (see Chapter 13, p. 393). In the UK, osteomalacia occurs particularly in elderly people.

**TABLE 12.2** Major causes of osteomalacia and rickets

| | |
|---|---|
| **Vitamin D deficiency** | |
| Dietary insufficiency | |
| Malabsorption | Coeliac disease, gastric and bowel surgery, biliary disease |
| Reduced skin synthesis | Low UV light exposure, skin pigmentation, low skin exposure |
| **Abnormal vitamin D metabolism** | |
| Increased degradation | Drugs, e.g. anticonvulsants |
| Diminished 25-hydroxylation | Chronic liver disease |
| Decreased 1-hydroxylation | Renal failure, type 1 vitamin D-dependent rickets |
| **Normal vitamin D levels** | |
| End-organ resistance | Type 2 vitamin D-dependent rickets |
| Low serum phosphate | Renal tubular disorders, e.g. Fanconi's syndrome, X-linked hypophosphataemic rickets |
| **Abnormal bone mineralization** | |
| Low bone alkaline phosphatase | Hypophosphatasia |
| Chemicals, drugs | Aluminium toxicity |

## Clinical Features

Patients with osteomalacia usually complain of bone pain and tenderness, with weakness of proximal muscles often resulting in a waddling gait. Pathological fractures may occur. In children with rickets there is retarded growth. There may be bowing of the long bones and pelvic deformity, resulting in a narrowed or flattened pelvic outlet, which may lead to difficulties in childbirth for females. The epiphyseal plate is widened and the costochondral junctions are swollen, giving rise to the so-called 'rickety rosary'. Radiological examination shows a loss of normal bone density (osteopenia), particularly in the long bones. The radiological hallmark of osteomalacia is the pseudofracture or Looser's zone, a transverse linear lucency perpendicular to the bone surface, typically of a rib, pubic ramus, inner scapular border, and the long bones. In rickets the epiphyseal plate is widened with an irregularly cupped metaphysis. The appearance of epiphyseal centres of ossification may be delayed.

## Pathology

The delay in mineralization of bone matrix leads to an increase in osteoid, which covers over 25% of the trabecular surface area and forms thickened seams (Fig. 12.7). In addition, the calcification front is deficient. An increase in osteoid may occur in many conditions where there is rapid new bone formation such as fracture healing, Paget's disease, and hyperparathyroidism, but in these conditions there is no mineralization defect.

In rickets, failure to mineralize the matrix of the epiphyseal cartilage prevents osteoclastic resorption of cartilage, and leads to a thickened and irregular hypertrophic zone. The woven bone laid down on the surface of cartilage is also not mineralized, so there is failure to remodel the metaphysis.

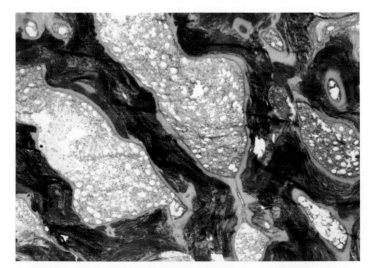

**Fig. 12.7** Osteomalacia: histological examination of undecalcified sections shows that most of the bone (purple) surfaces are covered by a thick layer of unmineralized osteoid (pale blue), reflecting the delay in mineralization. (Stain: toluidine blue.)

Treatment of the underlying cause (e.g. oral vitamin D in dietary deficiency) is rapidly followed by mineralization of matrix and the radiological appearances of the epiphyses revert to normal, but bone deformity may remain.

## Hyperparathyroidism

### Key Points

- Hyperparathyroidism may be primary, secondary, or tertiary.
- There is increased bone resorption with osteoporosis and fractures.
- It has renal, muscular, and gastrointestinal effects.

Parathyroid hormone is important in the regulation of calcium metabolism and bone turnover, and has effects on both osteoblastic and osteoclastic activity. Overactivity of the parathyroid glands is classified as primary, secondary, or tertiary (see Chapter 17, p. 493). Primary hyperparathyroidism is usually due to the presence of a parathyroid adenoma but in <5% of cases there is diffuse hyperplasia of all four glands, or a parathyroid carcinoma. Primary hyperparathyroidism affects 1 in 1,000 people and is the most common cause of hypercalcaemia in asymptomatic individuals. Early diagnosis due to routine measurement of serum calcium means that bone disease is now found in <5% of cases. Secondary hyperparathyroidism refers to the parathyroid hyperplasia and increased PTH secretion that occur as a physiological response to hypocalcaemia. The most common cause is chronic renal failure, the bone changes of which are discussed below. Tertiary hyperparathyroidism may occur in longstanding secondary hyperparathyroidism when an autonomous nodule develops in a hyperplastic gland, resulting in hypercalcaemia.

## Clinical Features

The bone changes are the same in each form, but depend on the duration and severity of the hyperparathyroidism. Some patients complain of bone pain. Radiographs may be normal or show generalized osteopenia. There may be subperiosteal cortical resorption, particularly affecting the phalanges and sometimes the outer ends of the clavicles. Rarely, especially in secondary hyperparathyroidism, there is an increase in bone density (osteosclerosis). Occasionally, one or more localized areas of radiolucency, so-called brown tumours, are seen. In hyperparathyroidism there is an increased incidence of pseudogout and gout (pp. 376–378). Surgical removal of a parathyroid adenoma or of hyperplastic glands is followed by a rapid fall in serum levels of PTH. Normal bone structure is usually rapidly restored.

## Pathology

Due to increased PTH levels, there is increased bone resorption produced by increased numbers of osteoclasts

(Fig. 12.8A). These are seen on the surface of and within trabeculae of cancellous bone and in haversian systems of cortical bone. As resorption is accompanied by increased bone formation, osteoblasts are found lined up on the surfaces, but overall there is loss of bone. As the disease progresses, much bone may be resorbed and replaced by small irregular trabeculae of woven bone, with loss of the normal bony architecture. Fibrous tissue forms around sites of resorption and in longstanding cases the marrow spaces become filled with fibrous tissue, in which cystic degeneration occasionally occurs. In the past, these features led to the descriptive term 'osteitis fibrosa cystica'. In 'brown tumours' (Fig. 12.8B), bone is replaced by numerous osteoclasts, fibrous tissue,

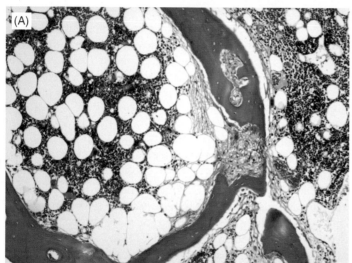

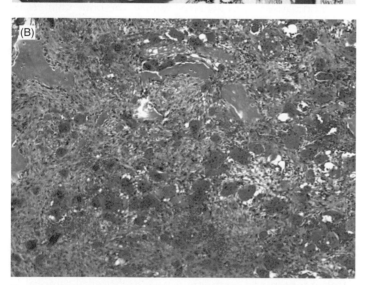

**FIG. 12.8** (A) Hyperparathyroid bone changes: there are increased osteoclasts on the bone surface forming intra-trabecular tunnels. The resorbed bone is replaced by fibrous tissue. (B) Brown tumour of hyperparathyroidism. The patient was a middle-aged female with a past history of two malignant tumours who developed a destructive lesion of the distal humerus. Biopsy shows numerous osteoclasts among fibrous stroma and some reactive new bone formation. She was also known to have chronic renal failure. The lytic lesion rapidly filled in after removal of an enlarged parathyroid gland.

and haemorrhage with abundant haemosiderin, resulting in a destructive lesion that may simulate giant cell tumour of bone (p. 364).

### Renal Osteodystrophy

> **Key Points**
>
> - This is a bone disorder resulting from the electrolyte and endocrine derangements that accompany chronic renal failure.
> - It includes hyperparathyroidism, osteomalacia, and adynamic bone disease.

Renal osteodystrophy refers to the complex group of bone changes seen in patients with chronic renal failure (see Chapter 13, pp. 392–394). It is a combination of secondary hyperparathyroidism and osteomalacia, although the latter is less common. In the past 20 years new treatments have emerged that have altered the pattern of disease seen.

Pathophysiology

The pathophysiology of renal osteodystrophy is summarized in Fig. 12.9. Diminished glomerular filtration and reduced tubular excretion lead to retention of phosphate, which causes a reciprocal fall in serum calcium and also impairs renal $1\alpha$-hydroxylase, causing a reduction in vitamin D synthesis. Both of these factors stimulate PTH secretion and parathyroid hyperplasia so that serum calcium and phosphate levels return to normal. The lower renal mass produces less $1\alpha$-hydroxylase, and less synthesis of 1,25-dihydroxy-vitamin $D_3$ (1,25$(OH)_2D_3$) results, leading to osteomalacia. In the past a severe form of osteomalacia, seen in dialysis patients with bone pain, pathological fracture, and muscle weakness, was shown to be due to inhibition of normal mineralization by deposition of aluminium derived from

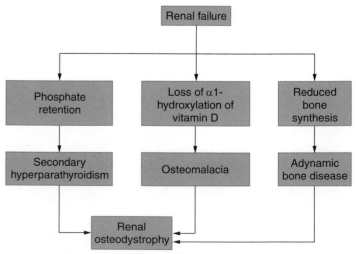

**FIG. 12.9** Pathophysiology of renal osteodystrophy.

dialysis fluid or orally administered aluminium-containing, phosphate-binding gels.

The aim of modern treatment is to maintain normal serum calcium and phosphate levels, lower PTH levels, and correct any vitamin D deficiency. Hyperparathyroid bone disease has become less frequent and less severe, although osteomalacia is now uncommonly seen. As these forms decrease, there has been an increase in adynamic bone disease, a state of low bone turnover leading to reduced bone mass and an increased risk of fracture. This is seen especially in those on continuous peritoneal dialysis. It is thought to be due to inhibition of osteoblastic activity.

## Pathology

The histological changes vary between high and low turnover forms. In the former, the appearances include those of hyperparathyroidism as described above. In keeping with a high turnover state there is frequently an increase in trabecular surface area covered by osteoid, but the seams are of normal thickness and the mineralization front is normal. When coexistent osteomalacia develops, there are thickened osteoid seams and a reduced mineralization front. In adynamic bone disease the bone surfaces are inactive with little osteoblastic or osteoclastic activity.

Osteosclerosis, increased density of bone due to extensive formation of woven bone, may be seen, usually in the axial skeleton. Areas of sclerosis adjacent to the vertebral endplates give a striped radiological appearance known as a 'rugger-jersey spine'. In patients undergoing long-term haemodialysis, accumulation of $\beta_2$-microglobulin leads to deposition of amyloid especially in the bones, joints, and periarticular structures.

Renal transplant recipients are at risk of developing osteonecrosis, particularly of the femoral heads and condyles (see p. 358), and osteoporosis. As steroid therapy is implicated in both conditions, the use of ciclosporin as an immunosuppressive agent and consequent reduction of steroid dosage resulted in a lower incidence of these complications.

## Paget's Disease of Bone

### Key Points

- Paget's disease is a common disease in elderly people, especially among those of Anglo-Saxon origin.
- Increased bone resorption leads to increased turnover.
- The abnormal bone is structurally weak.
- The thickened bone may compress nerves or the spinal cord.

Paget's disease is a disorder of excessive turnover of bone that results in disorganization of bone architecture. Although commonly discussed with metabolic bone diseases, it is not a generalized skeletal disorder, but may affect part or all of one, several, or many bones. Most frequently, the vertebrae, pelvis, skull, and femur, tibia, and humerus are involved. The incidence of Paget's disease shows considerable geographical variation. Almost unknown in Japan and rare in Scandinavia and the tropics, it is common in Britain and in people of Anglo-Saxon origin. Occasionally found in young adults, Paget's disease can be detected *post mortem* or by radiology in about 3% of patients aged >40 years, rising to 10% of those > 80. There is a slight male preponderance and a significant hereditary predisposition.

### Clinical Features

Of the large number of people with Paget's disease only about 5% have symptoms. The common complaints are as follows:

- Bone pain.
- Deformity: even when thickened, the bone in Paget's disease is structurally weak due to destruction of cortical haversian systems; this leads to bowing of the long bones.
- Pathological fractures, often transverse, result from structurally weakened bone.
- Osteoarthritis occurs more commonly due to stresses placed on the joints by bone deformity.
- Deafness is caused by compression of the eighth cranial nerve, the exit foramen of which is narrowed through the thickened skull.
- Spinal cord compression may follow enlargement, or less commonly collapse, of an involved vertebra.
- Paget's sarcoma: this most serious complication is fortunately rare, affecting <1% of patients. The sarcoma usually arises in long bones, especially the femur and humerus, and is usually an osteosarcoma or high-grade undifferentiated sarcoma. The prognosis in Paget's sarcoma is poor; most patients develop early pulmonary metastases and die within 2 years.
- Rarely, patients with extensive Paget's disease have high cardiac output and compromised cardiac function (high output cardiac failure) due to increased blood flow through the affected bones.

### Pathology

Paget's disease starts at one site in a bone and gradually extends with a lytic advancing front. In early Paget's disease there is intense activity of very large osteoclasts. In response, plump osteoblasts rapidly lay down new bone, some of which is woven rather than lamellar. The marrow spaces contain vascular fibrous tissue. As the disease progresses, resorption lessens and bone formation becomes more prominent with increasing sclerosis. The shafts of the long bones are thickened on the periosteal and endosteal surfaces, so that the bone is enlarged and the marrow cavity narrowed. The weakened bones may be bowed. The skull enlarges and is sometimes three to four times thicker than

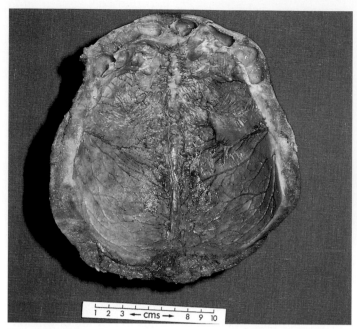

FIG. 12.10 Paget's disease of bone: characteristic thickening of the skull with loss of distinction between the tables.

normal (Fig. 12.10). Histologically, the trabeculae become thickened, and show a 'mosaic' or 'jigsaw' pattern of cement lines, indicating previous phases of bone resorption and formation (Fig. 12.11). Normal cortical haversian systems are replaced by irregularly arranged trabeculae. Eventually the marrow becomes densely fibrosed and the bone surfaces become inactive. Radiographs of the long bones may show a sharply defined flame-shaped area of bone resorption. Localized rarefaction of the skull is known as osteoporosis circumscripta.

### Aetiology

The aetiology is uncertain. One theory is that Paget's disease is due to viral infection of osteoclasts and their precursors. Intranuclear inclusions found in the osteoclasts of patients with Paget's disease resemble those of paramyxoviruses, and immunohistochemical techniques and some nucleic acid hybridization studies support this theory. As indicated above, there is a genetic predisposition to Paget's disease. Mutations of the sequestosome 1 gene (*SQSTM1*) are found in some cases. This gene appears to be involved in the RANK-NFκB signalling pathway.

## Generalized Developmental Abnormalities of Bone

### Key Points

- Generalized developmental abnormalities of bone are rare conditions, usually presenting in childhood.
- There is an abnormal growth or structure of bone.
- The underlying molecular mechanisms are increasingly understood.
- There is the potential for genetic screening.

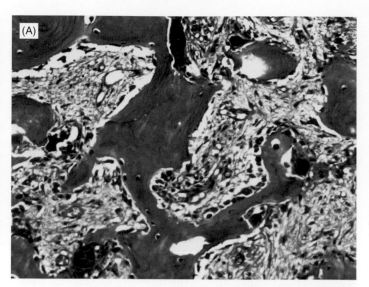

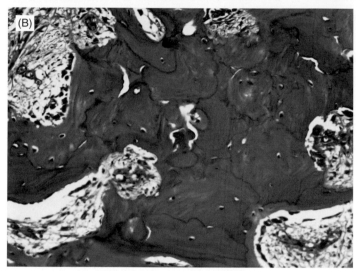

FIG. 12.11 Paget's disease of bone: (A) the active phase is characterized by numerous large osteoclasts eroding bone, followed by new bone formation by sheets of osteoblasts. The marrow is replaced by vascular fibrous tissue. (B) Repeated episodes of irregular resorption and synthesis result in a jigsaw or mosaic pattern of cement lines.

## Osteogenesis Imperfecta (Brittle Bone Syndrome)

This is a rare (1–5 in 100,000 births) inherited disease characterized by bone fragility and repeated fractures. There are several subtypes, which vary in the disease's severity and the age of onset. In some there are extraskeletal abnormalities, such as abnormal dentine (dentinogenesis imperfecta), cardiac valvular disease, and blue sclerae (the choroid pigment may be seen through the thinned sclerae). The current classification and the underlying molecular mechanisms that explain the clinical variations are summarized in *Table 12.3*.

### Pathogenesis

Osteogenesis imperfecta results from mutations in the structural genes for type I collagen. Type I collagen is composed of two proteins – pro-$_1$ and pro-$_2$ – encoded by two genes *COL1A1* and *COL1A2*, which are located on chromosomes

TABLE 12.3 Osteogenesis imperfecta: major subtypes

| Type | Clinical features | Inheritance |
|---|---|---|
| I | Mild: fractures, little deformity, normal stature, blue sclerae, joint laxity, deafness, dentinogenesis imperfecta | Autosomal dominant |
| II | Perinatal lethal: severe disease, usually lethal in perinatal period, short limbs | New dominant mutations |
| III | Progressive deforming: severe progressive disease, short stature, deformity, sclerae blue in infancy, white later | Heterogeneous: majority autosomal dominant |
| IV | Moderate deformity, short stature, normal sclerae, dentinogenesis imperfecta (intermediate between I and III) | Autosomal dominant |

17 and 7, respectively. Two pro-$_1$ and one pro-$_2$ chains twist together to form a triple helix. Numerous mutations including gene deletions, insertions, and duplications have been described, but most cases are caused by single-point mutations. In the mild form of osteogenesis imperfecta (type 1) the collagen is of normal type, but is present in reduced amounts. This is often due to mutations that knock out one copy of the COL1A1 gene, leading to diminished production of the collagen $\alpha_1$ chain. Thus, although the amount of bone is reduced, it is structurally normal. In contrast, in the more severe forms, mutations within the collagen genes result in abnormal collagen protein chains, which combine to form an abnormal triple helix. The resulting collagen is structurally weaker, and also turns over more rapidly. In the more severe forms the most common defects are single-base mutations that result in substitution of a glycine amino acid by a larger amino acid such as asparagine. Glycine is essential in the formation of the collagen triple helix. The closer the mutation is to the carboxy-terminal end of the chain, from which the helix winds up, and the larger the substituting amino acid, the more badly affected is the collagen formed.

The pathological appearances vary depending on the severity of the clinical disease. In general, osteoblast activity is defective with a reduction in bone formation, so that osteocytes appear crowded. The more severely affected the patient, the higher the proportion of woven to lamellar bone. The shafts of long bones are thin whereas the epiphyses are broad and often disorganized. Multiple fractures may result in bowing of limb bones.

The radiological appearance of multiple healing fractures of varying ages may be misinterpreted as evidence of 'non-accidental injury', with serious medicolegal implications for the parents.

## Achondroplasia

Achondroplasia is the most common skeletal dysplasia (1 in 15,000–40,000 livebirths) and is characterized by short stature. There is failure of enchondral ossification leading to diminished growth of the limbs. Achondroplasia is inherited in an autosomal dominant manner, and is due to a mutation of the fibroblast growth factor receptor 3 (FGFR3) gene on chromosome 4. This gene has a very high mutation rate, so >80% of affected children are born to normal parents. The mutation causes the receptor to be switched on, suppressing cartilage growth. Other mutations of this gene give rise to other rarer bone dysplasias. Patients with achondroplasia have distinctive features: the head appears large, the forehead bulging, and the root of the nose sunken. The limbs are disproportionately short compared with the trunk and cranium. The hands are broad with fingers of equal length (trident hands). The spinal canal is narrowed and spinal cord compression is common in adults. These changes are a consequence of the abnormal enchondral ossification. At the epiphyseal line the cartilage cells form short rows or are irregularly arranged, with little or no ossification, resulting in reduced bone growth.

Some affected infants die, usually from neurological complications such as hydrocephalus as a result of maldevelopment of the skull base, but most survive into adult life with normal intellect.

## Osteopetrosis (Marble Bone Disease, Albers–Schönberg Disease)

### Key Points

- In osteopetrosis there are dense bones due to reduced osteoclastic activity.
- There are pathological fractures.
- There is obliteration of the marrow cavity leading to anaemia.
- There is nerve compression leading to blindness and deafness.

Osteopetrosis is a heterogeneous group of disorders characterized by increased bone density due to defective osteoclastic activity. Broadly, there is a severe form in infancy, usually inherited as an autosomal recessive condition, in which there is failure of resorption of the fetal cartilaginous model of bones, so that the marrow cavities fail to form. Severe anaemia with a peripheral blood leukoerythroblastic reaction develops which, with infections due to leukopenia, may be life threatening. The bones are radio-opaque and show evidence of abnormal remodelling. Despite the increased bone density the bones are structurally abnormal and subject to pathological fracture. Skull involvement with narrowing of exit foramina may result in deafness or blindness. Patients with severe disease may be treated by bone marrow transplantation. Donor osteoclasts derived from marrow precursors resorb the cartilaginous matrix and allow remodelling. Milder forms inherited as autosomal dominant traits are often not recognized until adult life, typically after a fracture. The precise pathogenic mechanisms in humans remain uncertain in most cases. In one mild form, an absence of osteoclast carbonic anhydrase activity is responsible.

## Osteonecrosis

> ### Key Points
>
> - Osteonecrosis is death of bone due to loss of its blood supply.
> - The major causes are trauma, metabolic disorders, and steroids.
> - Juxta-articular osteonecrosis leads to secondary osteoarthritis.

Osteonecrosis (aseptic necrosis, avascular necrosis) refers to death of bone as a result of interference with its blood supply, by definition not associated with infection. The most common cause is a fracture that disrupts the major blood supply to an area of bone. The femoral head and scaphoid are two sites where the distribution of vessels is especially likely to cause clinically important osteonecrosis.

A large number of non-traumatic conditions are associated with osteonecrosis (*Box 12.3*) and sometimes no clear cause can be found (idiopathic). In some cases the pathogenesis seems clear: in compressed-air workers, nitrogen bubbles form during decompression and block small blood vessels, whereas in sickle cell anaemia sludging of red cells has the same effect. In contrast, the mechanisms responsible for the osteonecrosis complicating steroid therapy and alcohol excess are speculative.

Necrosis may involve the cancellous bone of the shaft of a long bone. The resulting infarct is sometimes seen as an area of increased density on radiographs due chiefly to calcification of dead marrow. Such lesions are asymptomatic, although rarely they may be complicated by a sarcoma. In contrast, in juxta-articular sites such as the femoral head (Fig. 12.12) or condyles, a wedge-shaped segment of necrotic bone may eventually collapse with deformity of the joint surface and secondary osteoarthritis. The histological features are of necrosis of haematopoietic marrow followed by loss of osteocytes from their lacunae. Initial steps in repair consist of revascularization of dead marrow followed by deposition of live bone on the surface of necrotic trabeculae (appositional new bone).

---

### Box 12.3 CAUSES OF OSTEONECROSIS

- Trauma, e.g. fracture of neck of femur
- Dysbarism (caisson disease)
- Sickle cell disease
- Gaucher's disease
- Alcohol excess
- Steroid therapy
- Radiotherapy
- Connective tissue disorders, e.g. systemic lupus erythematosus

---

Osteonecrosis is seen in several disorders of childhood. Perthes' disease affects the hips in children, particularly males, who present with pain and a limp. About 10% of cases are bilateral. Pathologically there is osteonecrosis of the femoral epiphysis, which may heal without significant deformity or collapse, often resulting in osteoarthritis in later life. In other conditions bone necrosis follows an episode of trauma. In osteochondritis dissecans, a wedge-shaped area of bone and its attached articular cartilage separate from the articular surface leaving a well-demarcated defect. The bone undergoes necrosis. This commonly involves the lateral aspect of the medial femoral condyle. The loose body formed (see p. 379) may cause locking and damage to the articular cartilage. Similar conditions may affect the tarsal

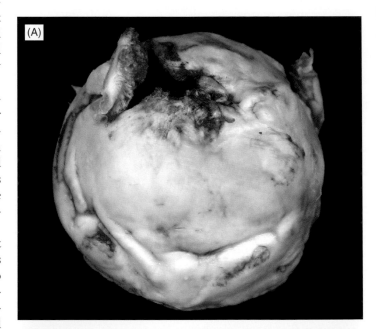

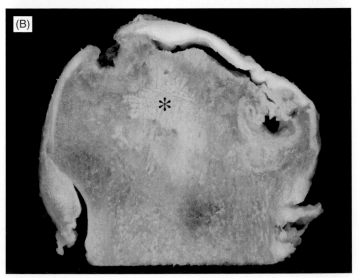

**Fig. 12.12** Osteonecrosis (avascular necrosis) of the femoral head: the articular surface of the femoral head shows a crescent-shaped depression (A) which, on the cut section (B), is seen to be due to a subchondral fracture. The yellow tissue (*) is necrotic bone.

navicular (Köhler's disease), lunate (Kienböck's disease), and second metatarsal (Freiberg's disease).

## Infection of Bone and Joints

### *Osteomyelitis*

**Key Points**

- Osteomyelitis may be due to infection by blood-borne microorganisms or through direct inoculation.
- Causative organisms are pyogenic organisms, especially *Staphylococcus aureus*.
- It is characterized by bone necrosis and reactive bone formation.
- There is a risk of chronic osteomyelitis.
- Early diagnosis is important.

Osteomyelitis occurs in several circumstances. Classic acute osteomyelitis mainly affects children and adolescents. The organisms reach the bone by blood, spread from a focus elsewhere in the body such as a boil. Frequently, no source can be found and it is assumed that there is a minor lesion that is clinically inapparent or has healed. Any bone may be affected but the metaphyses of long bones (distal femur, proximal tibia, and humerus) adjacent to actively growing epiphyses, and the vertebral column, are most often involved. The incidence of this disease has fallen in recent decades. Intravenous drug users and those with genitourinary infections are at risk of haematogenous osteomyelitis, often due to coliforms. More common is spread from an adjacent site of infection. Examples of this include compound fractures or after orthopaedic surgery, especially where metallic implants such as nails, plates, and screws, and prosthetic joints, are inserted. Another important cause is diabetes mellitus, particularly with peripheral vascular disease and skin ulcers. Awareness of the disease is important because delay in diagnosis and failure to institute antibiotic treatment may lead to considerable morbidity.

The causative organism of most serious infections is coagulase-positive staphylococci, although streptococci, coagulase-negative staphylococci, Gram-negative bacilli, and anaerobes are sometimes isolated. Sickle cell anaemia predisposes to infection by salmonellae.

Typically, the patient with acute osteomyelitis is unwell with a high fever, and complains of severe pain and tenderness aggravated by any movement. The erythrocyte sedimentation rate, white blood count, and acute phase reactants such as C-reactive protein are usually elevated. Changes on conventional radiographs frequently do not appear for 7 days or so, but magnetic resonance imaging (MRI) shows an abnormal signal much earlier. If acute osteomyelitis is suspected, blood cultures should be taken and large doses of antibiotics given immediately to prevent septicaemia. A high index of suspicion is required to make the diagnosis in immunosuppressed patients who frequently have few symptoms or signs.

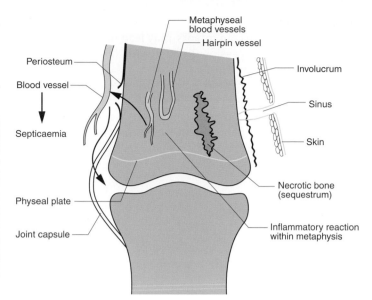

**FIG. 12.13** Osteomyelitis is often due to haematogenous spread from foci elsewhere. The bacteria lodge within metaphyseal (hairpin) blood vessels and set up an inflammatory reaction in the medullary canal. This spreads through the cortex, elevates the periosteum, and may spread locally into an adjacent joint, causing septic arthritis, or into blood vessels, leading to bacteraemia or septicaemia. Interference with the blood supply leads to bone death, with formation of a sequestrum; meanwhile, the periosteum lays down a shell of new bone, the involucrum. Pus may track to the skin surface forming a discharging sinus.

### Pathology

The following description refers to untreated acute haematogenous osteomyelitis (Fig. 12.13). Most cases involve the metaphysis of long bones, in which dilated vascular sinusoids with sluggish blood flow provide an ideal site for multiplication of bacteria. Bacteria pass into the marrow spaces and provoke an acute inflammatory response. Pus spreads rapidly throughout the medullary cavity and cortex, elevates the periosteum, and forms a subperiosteal abscess. Pus may track into the surrounding soft tissues, ultimately reaching the skin surface to form a sinus. Vascular thrombosis leads to bone necrosis, the piece of dead bone being known as a sequestrum. Meanwhile cytokines released by the inflammatory cells activate osteoclasts, causing bone destruction. As infection becomes less acute, subperiosteal new bone may form an incomplete shell (involucrum) around the dead bone.

### Complications

- Septicaemia: spread of infection, particularly when due to staphylococci, may lead to septicaemia with abscesses in the lung, kidney, or myocardium and acute endocarditis. This accounted for a mortality rate of 25% before antibiotic therapy was available.
- Septic arthritis: direct spread of infection occurs in joints such as the hip and shoulder, in which the metaphysis lies within the joint capsule.

- Alteration in growth rate: damage to the epiphyseal plate, particularly in infants, may lead to growth retardation, whereas occasionally increased blood flow causes accelerated growth.
- Chronic osteomyelitis: acute osteomyelitis, particularly in adults, may become chronic with recurrent exacerbation of infection with abscesses, discharging sinuses, and increasing patchy bone sclerosis. Secondary amyloidosis and occasionally squamous carcinoma arising in a sinus may complicate longstanding chronic osteomyelitis.

### Subacute Pyogenic Infection

Many patients develop a subacute pyogenic infection with an insidious onset and little fever or malaise. Most cases affect the spine, but other bones may be involved.

#### Vertebral Osteomyelitis

Infection of the vertebral column occurs mainly in adults. Bacterial spread is usually haematogenous, either arterial or by retrograde spread through the vertebral venous plexus, which communicates directly with pelvic veins. In about two-thirds of patients the lumbar spine is involved. *Staphylococcus aureus* is the most common organism. Infection with coliforms may follow genitourinary surgery. In most patients the onset is insidious with intermittent attacks of backache and little fever. The initial focus is in or close to the vertebral endplate. Infection spreads to involve the adjacent disc and cancellous bone of the vertebral body, both of which undergo necrosis. Pressure on the spinal cord may lead to paraplegia. Some collapse of bone occurs with loss of the disc space. Reactive new bone formation may cause spontaneous fusion of adjacent vertebrae.

#### Brodie's Abscess

This is a form of localized subacute or chronic osteomyelitis that is usually situated in the metaphysis of a long bone, especially the upper end of the tibia. It usually occurs in adolescents. A central cavity containing pus, which may be sterile, is lined by granulation tissue and surrounded by reactive bone sclerosis.

### Septic Arthritis

#### Key Points

- Septic arthritis may be caused by haematogenous spread or direct inoculation.
- *Staphylococcus aureus* is the main causative organism.
- There is rapid destruction of joints unless treated early.

Joint infection may result from haematogenous spread to the synovium or direct extension from acute osteomyelitis, or follow penetrating injury or surgery, especially joint replacement or arthroscopy. *S. aureus* is the most common causative organism, but *Neisseria gonorrhoeae* (see Chapter 19, p. 538) is a common cause in young adults and *Haemophilus influenzae* in infancy. Patients with rheumatoid arthritis and those on steroid therapy are at increased risk of joint infection, which often gives rise to a few local symptoms. Classically, children and young adults present with high fever and a swollen, hot, painful joint. Although an inflamed knee is obvious clinically, inflammation of the hip, common in infancy, may be readily missed. Elderly patients frequently show few signs of systemic upset.

Gonococcal arthritis is now a major cause of bacterial arthritis, especially in healthy young adults. Most patients complain of flitting pain in many joints particularly the knees, ankles, wrists, and elbows. Tenosynovitis and a skin rash are often present. It is thought that joint involvement follows a bacteraemic phase after genital infection. Culture of gonococci from inflamed joints is often difficult. Permanent joint damage rarely results.

#### Pathology

The synovium is acutely inflamed with large numbers of neutrophils, which cause destruction of the articular cartilage (Fig. 12.14). Secondary osteoarthritis may ensue.

### Tuberculosis of Bone and Joints

In recent years the overall incidence of tuberculosis (TB) in developed countries has risen due to acquired immune deficiency syndrome (AIDS), immigration from developing countries, and emergence of drug-resistant strains. Skeletal TB is almost always due to haematogenous spread from infection elsewhere, usually the lung or urinary tract. *Mycobacterium tuberculosis* is responsible for most infections but atypical mycobacteria are important in immuno-compromised individuals. Early diagnosis and treatment are important to minimize tissue destruction.

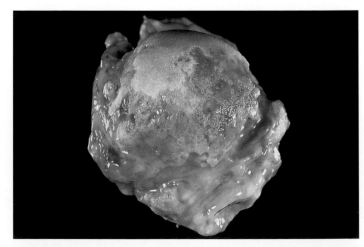

**FIG. 12.14** Septic arthritis: humeral head showing marked destruction of the articular cartilage by acute inflammation.

About half the infections involve the spine (tuberculous spondylitis, Pott's disease), usually the lower thoracic and lumbar vertebrae (Fig. 12.15). Initially one vertebral body is affected with early involvement of the intervertebral disc. Bone destruction leads to vertebral collapse. A local paraspinal abscess develops and infection may extend along the anterior spinal ligaments to other vertebrae, or track anteriorly along tissue planes. In the lumbar spine infection may spread along the sheath of the psoas muscle to point in the groin as a 'cold' or 'psoas' abscess. Angulation of the spine may occur with a severe kyphosis (tuberculous gibbus). Patients with vertebral TB may develop spinal cord compression. This may occur early in the disease due to pressure from an extradural abscess or bone or disc material, or late when the cord may be stretched over the apex of a severe kyphosis.

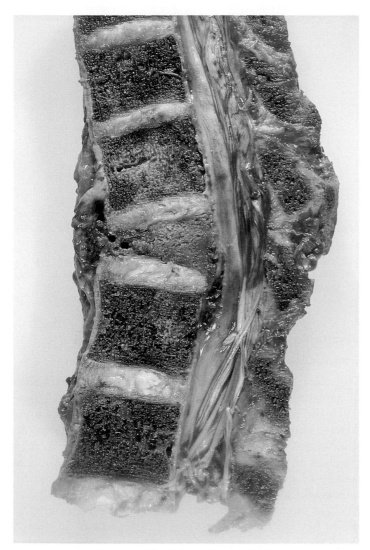

**Fig. 12.15** Tuberculosis of the spine: there is involvement of at least two vertebrae, one of which has collapsed. The discs are better preserved than is typically seen. The differential diagnosis includes metastatic carcinoma.

Tuberculous arthritis results from haematogenous spread of infection to the synovium or by extension from an affected intracapsular portion of bone. The hip and knee are most commonly involved. Inflammation of the synovium invades the subchondral bone and dissects it from the articular cartilage, leading to destruction of the joint surface. Less commonly, bone involvement occurs in the absence of joint disease, typically with destructive lesions in the metaphysis of long bones, e.g. the knee, femoral neck, and greater trochanter. The tubular bones of the hands may be affected (dactylitis).

The histological appearances are typical of TB elsewhere: alcohol- and acid-fast bacilli may be identified in histological sections, but are often difficult to find; for this reason, tissue should also be submitted for bacteriological examination including culture. Polymerase chain reaction to detect the bacterial DNA is a rapid and sensitive technique.

## Other Infections of Bone and Joints

### Brucellosis

Brucellosis is transmitted to humans from infected animals or animal products. Infection of bone and joints is more common in chronic brucellosis than in the acute form. Typically one or a few peripheral joints, especially the hip and knee, are involved. Sacroiliitis is also seen. The organism is difficult to culture but positive serological tests allow diagnosis. Histologically the synovium or bone contains non-caseating granulomas.

### Lyme Disease

This is a multisystem infection caused by the spirochete *Borrelia burgdorferi*, which is transmitted by ticks of the genus *Ixodes*, particularly in areas with large deer populations. (The name derives from Lyme, Connecticut, where a cluster of children with arthritis led, in 1975, to recognition of the disease.) A skin rash (erythema chronicum migrans), and cardiac, nervous system, and osteoarticular involvement have all been described.

Joint manifestations include migratory joint pains, intermittent attacks of acute arthritis, and chronic erosive arthritis, which, in about 10% of patients, may cause permanent disability. Large joints, particularly the knee, are affected. Lyme arthritis responds to treatment with high-dose penicillin, although irreversible damage may have occurred.

### Viral Arthritis

Many common viral infections, e.g. hepatitis C, mumps, rubella and its vaccine, and parvovirus are associated with transient arthritis or arthralgia. In all instances the arthritis is non-destructive and does not lead to chronic joint disease.

Infections related to prosthetic joint replacements are discussed on p. 379.

# TUMOURS IN BONE

> ## Key Points
>
> - Metastatic carcinoma is far more common than primary bone tumours.
> - The breast, lung, prostate, kidney, and thyroid are the most common primary sites.
> - Myeloma is by far the most common primary tumour (see Chapter 8, pp. 227–228).
> - Osteosarcoma and Ewing's sarcoma particularly affect adolescents and are highly malignant.
> - Chondrosarcoma is usually a tumour of middle-aged and elderly people, and is of fairly low grade.

## Metastatic Tumours

Metastatic tumours far exceed primary bone tumours in frequency, and may be found *post mortem* in at least 50% of patients who have died with disseminated tumour. Almost all are carcinomas, particularly those arising from the lung, breast, prostate, kidney, and thyroid, and they account for 80% in adults. In children neuroblastoma and rhabdomyosarcoma often spread to bone. Metastases occur most commonly in areas where haematopoietic marrow is present. In adults this is the vertebral column, ribs, proximal femur, and humerus (Fig. 12.16). Retrograde spread to the spine occurs along the prevertebral venous plexus. Metastatic tumours in bone occasionally present as solitary lesions, but usually multiple further metastases rapidly develop. However, surgical removal of a primary renal or thyroid carcinoma and a solitary metastasis may result in long survival.

Many bone metastases are asymptomatic. The clinical effects are principally of pain and bone destruction (osteolysis), which leads to pathological fracture of the long bones, vertebral collapse, or spinal cord compression. Rarely carcinomas, typically of the prostate and sometimes of the breast, may induce reactive new bone formation, giving rise to osteosclerotic metastases. Hypercalcaemia may occur and is usually due to the production by tumour cells of PTHrP, which has functional similarity to PTH and induces humoral hypercalcaemia of malignancy. The mechanisms of bone destruction are discussed in Special Study Topic 12.1.

## Primary Bone Tumours

Although much less common than metastases, primary bone tumours are an important cause of disability and death, particularly in young people. As they are rare, expertise in management is concentrated in regional centres. A summary of the typical anatomical locations and age ranges is given in *Table 12.4*.

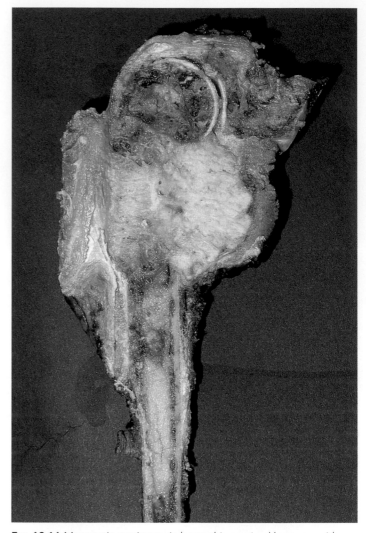

**FIG. 12.16** Metastatic carcinoma in bone: this proximal humerus with adjacent shoulder joint and glenoid was resected for metastatic renal carcinoma. A large tumour mass occupies the medulla and has extended into the adjacent soft tissue, particularly medially.

### Benign Bone Tumours

#### Osteoid Osteoma

This lesion commonly occurs in the shafts of long bones of adolescents and young adults, who complain of persistent pain, worse at night, often relieved by aspirin or non-steroidal anti-inflammatory drugs (NSAIDs). Lesions in the spine often cause scoliosis, whereas those close to joints may simulate arthritis. Radiographs show a small lucent nidus, usually <1 cm in diameter, which is often surrounded by a mass of sclerotic bone. Computed tomography (CT) and MRI are superior to plain radiographs in demonstrating the nidus. Isotope bone scans show a 'hot' area of increased uptake.

Histologically osteoid osteoma consists of a well-defined, highly vascular nidus of trabeculae of woven bone and benign osteoblasts. The nidus is surrounded by a variable

**TABLE 12.4** Primary bone tumours

| Tumour | Main age group (years) | Major site(s) |
|---|---|---|
| Osteoma | Adults | Skull, sinuses |
| Osteoid osteoma | 10–30 | Long bones, spine |
| Osteoblastoma | 10–30 | Spine, long bones |
| Enchondroma | Wide range | 50% hands, feet |
| Osteochondroma | 10–20 | Metaphysis of long bones |
| Chondroblastoma | 10–20 | Epiphysis of long bones |
| Chondromyxoid fibroma | 5–30 | Metaphysis of long bones |
| Aneurysmal bone cyst | 5–20 | Spine, metaphysis of long bones |
| Simple bone cyst | 5–15 | Metaphysis of long bones |
| Fibrous dysplasia | 5–30 | Any, especially femur, ribs, skull |
| Non-ossifying fibroma | 5–15 | Metaphysis of long bones |
| Adamantinoma | 10–50 | Diaphysis of tibia |
| Giant cell tumour | 20–45 | Epiphysis of long bones |
| Osteosarcoma | 10–25 | Metaphysis of long bones, knee |
| Parosteal osteosarcoma | 20–50 | Surface, metaphysis of long bones, 60% femur |
| Chondrosarcoma | 40–70 | Pelvis, femur, humerus, rib |
| Malignant fibrous histiocytoma | Adults | Metaphysis of long bones |
| Chordoma | 40–70 | Sacrum, skull base, spine |
| Ewing's tumour | 5–20 | Long bones, pelvis |

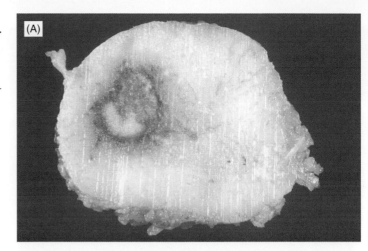

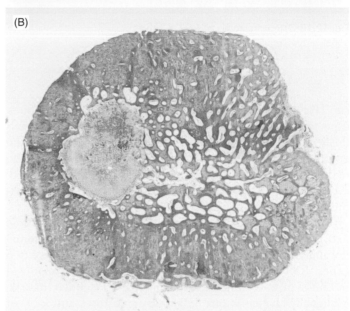

**FIG. 12.17** Osteoid osteoma: this shows a transverse section of an excised length of fibula containing a nidus of an osteoid osteoma, on both naked eye inspection (A) and histology (B). The nidus is well defined and surrounded by sclerotic bone.

amount of reactive bone (Fig. 12.17). Symptoms may recur if the lesion is incompletely removed. Most cases are now treated by radiofrequency ablation. Benign bone-forming lesions >1 cm are known as osteoblastomas, and commonly affect the spine. They tend not to be surrounded by sclerotic bone and pain is less of a feature than with osteoid osteoma. Large lesions may cause spinal cord compression.

### Enchondroma

This is a benign tumour of cartilage found within the medullary cavity. Over half of enchondromas occur within the tubular bones of the hands and feet, although the long bones such as the humerus and femur may also be affected. Many enchondromas are asymptomatic incidental radiological findings of lytic lesions with spotty calcification. Lesions in the hand may cause swelling or pain after injury, sometimes with a pathological fracture. Histologically they are composed of lobules of cartilage, consisting of a hyaline matrix containing uniform chondrocytes with small darkly staining nuclei. Ollier's disease is a disorder of multiple enchondromas, which are predominantly unilateral. The combination of multiple enchondromas and soft-tissue haemangiomas is known as Maffucci's syndrome. Both conditions are usually not inherited.

Malignant transformation of solitary enchondromas is rare. In contrast, 20% of patients with Ollier's disease develop chondrosarcomas. The risk is higher still in those with Maffucci's syndrome. In addition these patients appear to be at increased risk of non-skeletal malignancies such as primary brain tumours and pancreatic carcinoma.

### Osteocartilaginous Exostosis

Osteocartilaginous exostosis (osteochondroma) is a common bony outgrowth covered by a proliferating cartilage

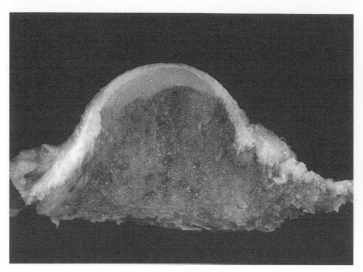

Fig. 12.18 Osteocartilaginous exostosis: this small exostosis consists of a thin cartilaginous cap with underlying cancellous bone.

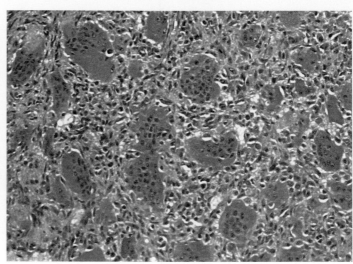

Fig. 12.19 Giant cell tumour of bone: the tumour consists of large multinucleated osteoclasts of reactive nature interspersed with ovoid mononuclear tumour cells.

cap (Fig. 12.18) attached to the metaphyses of long bones, especially the femur, humerus, and tibia. Although previously regarded as a developmental anomaly arising from the epiphyseal growth plate, it is now thought to be a benign neoplasm. The lesions are usually noticed in childhood. Growth commonly ceases in adult life where the cartilaginous cap is completely replaced by bone.

Exostoses are usually single. Hereditary multiple exostoses (diaphyseal aclasis) is inherited as an autosomal dominant trait and is usually due to mutation of one of two genes, *EXT1* and *EXT2*, which encode enzymes involved in the synthesis of the cartilaginous extracellular matrix. Malignant change is rare in solitary exostoses and <2% of those patients with multiple lesions develop chondrosarcoma, which is usually of low grade. Pain, not associated with fracture of the stalk of the exostosis or with bursitis, or resumption of growth, raises a suspicion of malignancy.

Subungual exostosis is a painful mass of bone and cartilage, which usually involves the distal phalanx of the great toe and commonly arises as a reaction to infection or trauma. It never becomes malignant.

### Giant Cell Tumour

Giant cell tumour principally affects individuals aged between 20 and 40 years. Most tumours occur in the long bones with half in the distal femur and proximal tibia. Almost all arise in the bone end, although extension into the metaphysis is often seen. Radiologically, a giant cell tumour is a lytic lesion that often causes eccentric expansion, and may be covered by a shell of subperiosteal bone or extend into the soft tissue. Pathological fracture often occurs. Grossly the tumour is soft and red with areas of haemorrhage and necrosis. On microscopy, ovoid mononuclear

tumour cells are interspersed with very large reactive osteoclasts (Fig. 12.19).

A giant cell tumour is a benign but locally aggressive tumour. The incidence of local recurrence depends on the extent of surgery. Around 20% of cases treated by curettage recur locally, often with soft-tissue involvement. A very small number metastasize or undergo sarcomatous transformation.

### *Malignant Primary Bone Tumours*

#### Osteosarcoma

> **Key Points**
>
> - Osteosarcoma is a malignant tumour, the cells of which form bone.
> - Peak age is 10–25 years.
> - Over half arise around the knee.
> - There is early blood-borne metastasis.

Other than multiple myeloma (see Chapter 8, pp. 227–228), osteosarcoma is the most common primary malignant tumour of bone, with approximately 150 new cases (3/1,000,000 population) diagnosed in Britain each year. Three-quarters of patients are aged between 10 and 25 years old with males more frequently affected. In more than half the patients aged >40 years the tumour complicates Paget's disease or occurs in previously irradiated bone. Patients present with increasing pain and swelling. Most osteosarcomas arise in the medullary cavity of the metaphysis of long bones, with over half occurring around the knee. The proximal humerus and distal radius are other common sites. Most osteosarcomas arise sporadically, but some occur in families with the Li–Fraumeni syndrome or familial retino-blastoma (see Chapter 5, pp. 96–99). Parosteal osteosarcoma is a low-grade tumour that forms a well-defined lobulated mass, often on the posterior aspect of the distal femur. Metastatic spread is less frequent and the prognosis is much better than in conventional osteosarcoma.

### Pathology

By definition, osteosarcoma is a malignant tumour in which osteoid or bone is formed directly by the tumour cells (Fig. 12.20). The gross appearances vary greatly. Some tumours are densely sclerotic, whereas others are fleshy. Telangiectatic osteosarcomas contain large blood-filled spaces. The naked eye appearances are modified by the response to preoperative chemotherapy which gives rise to large areas of necrosis and haemorrhage. The histological appearances also vary. Some tumours contain abundant 'tumour bone'. In others, only small foci of bone or osteoid are present and much of the tumour consists of malignant cartilage or sheets of malignant spindle-shaped cells.

Osteosarcoma spreads within the medulla, then penetrates and partially destroys the cortex to extend beneath the periosteum and eventually into the surrounding soft tissue (Fig. 12.21). In rapidly growing tumours the periosteum is raised and lays down spicules of new bone perpendicular to the cortex (sunray spiculation). At the junction between raised and normal periosteum, Codman's triangle of reactive bone may develop.

### Prognosis and treatment

Osteosarcoma is an aggressive tumour with early blood-borne pulmonary metastases, which are evident at presentation in 15% or so of cases. In most patients undetectable pulmonary micrometastases are also already present when the primary tumour is discovered. In an attempt to deal with these silent metastases modern therapy combines preoperative and postoperative chemotherapy with surgery. Many patients can be treated by local resection and endoprosthetic replacement, rather than by amputation. Only 20% or so of patients treated by surgery alone survived 5 years. With modern combination chemotherapy approximately 65% of patients survive for 5 years. Osteosarcoma arising in Paget's disease has a worse prognosis.

### Chondrosarcoma

Chondrosarcoma usually arises anew, although about 10% of cases are due to malignant change in a pre-existing benign cartilage tumour. The tumour may occur within the medullary cavity (central) or on the surface of bone (peripheral), usually in a pre-existing exostosis. Chondrosarcoma normally affects middle-aged and elderly people. Most tumours

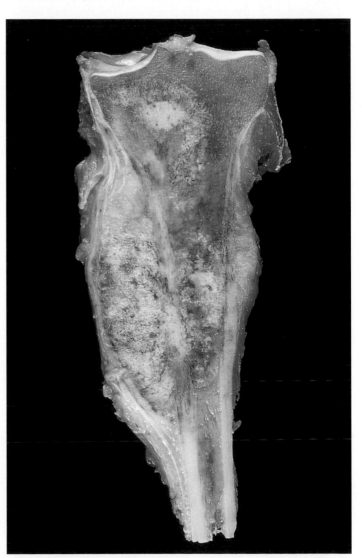

**FIG. 12.21** Osteosarcoma: this large tumour has arisen in the metaphysis of the proximal tibia and has penetrated the cortex to extend through the periosteum, forming a circumferential soft-tissue mass. The growth plate is closed, but the tumour has penetrated through its scar to involve the epiphysis.

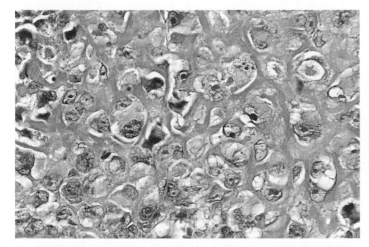

**FIG. 12.20** Osteosarcoma: a delicate meshwork of eosinophilic osteoid matrix has been formed directly by large ovoid malignant cells.

A 13-year-old girl complained of increasing pain in her left knee over a 3-month period. In the past month she had also been aware of the development of swelling in her distal thigh. A radiograph (Fig. 12.22) showed a destructive lesion in the metaphysis of the distal femur with periosteal reaction and MRI confirmed the presence of a large tumour with soft-tissue extension. A needle biopsy was carried out and showed a highly malignant tumour (Fig. 12.23). Despite the poorly differentiated nature of this tumour, the presence of a small amount of osteoid formation in this clinical and radiological context helped to establish a diagnosis of osteosarcoma. A chest radiograph and CT scan showed no evidence of metastases.

The patient was treated with three courses of neoadjuvant (preoperative) chemotherapy (doxorubicin and platinum based). After this, the distal femur was excised with insertion of a custom-made prosthesis. The resected femur was examined pathologically (Fig. 12.24) and it was noted

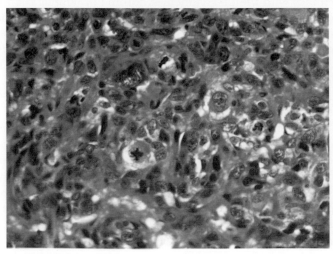

**FIG. 12.23** Biopsy of femur: the tumour shows large cells with pleomorphic nuclei, and numerous mitotic figures including one abnormal one. Although osteoid is not present in this biopsy, it was seen elsewhere and the features are those of an osteosarcoma.

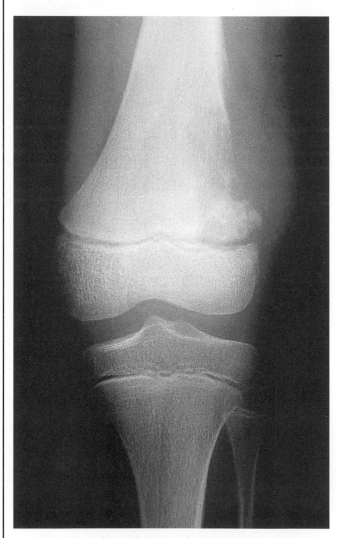

**FIG. 12.22** This radiograph shows a destructive lesion in the distal femoral metaphysis with cortical destruction and soft-tissue extension. A periosteal reaction is present (Codman's triangle). The features are of a malignant tumour and in this age group osteosarcoma is the most likely diagnosis.

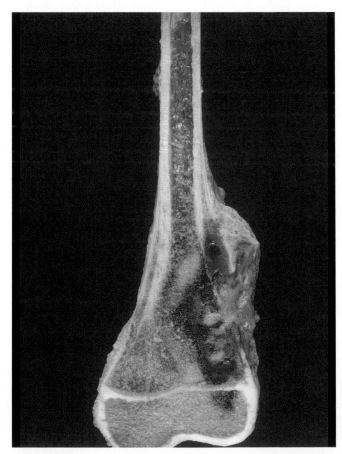

**FIG. 12.24** Resection of distal femur: the gross appearances reflect those of the radiograph in Fig. 12.22. There is a large tumour occupying much of the medullary canal; it has penetrated through the cortex into soft tissue. This extraosseous mass has shrunk, representing a good response to preoperative chemotherapy. Tumour has also penetrated the physeal plate to extend into the epiphysis, indicating that this is an incomplete barrier to tumour spread.

that almost all the tumour had undergone necrosis, with only small areas containing damaged tumour cells (Fig. 12.25).

Three more courses of chemotherapy were given, and the patient remains well several years later.

The main learning points from this case are as follows:

- This is the typical age and a typical site for an osteosarcoma.
- Osteosarcomas can be histologically highly malignant and are usually clinically aggressive.
- Such tumours respond well to chemotherapy, which permits limb-sparing surgery.
- The diagnosis of bone tumours requires their discussion at multidisciplinary team meetings where clinical, radiological, and histopathological evidence is correlated.

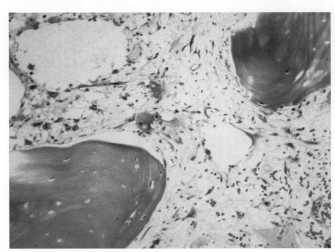

FIG. 12.25 This section from the medullary canal shows two large bony trabeculae separated by loose fibrovascular tissue. Compared with Fig. 12.23 almost all the tumour cells have been killed and there are only occasional residual cells, which have been severely damaged by chemotherapy.

arise in the axial skeleton, especially the pelvis, shoulder girdle, and ribs, or in the proximal femur and humerus (Fig. 12.26). It is rare in the tubular bones of the hands and feet. Most patients with chondrosarcoma complain of swelling or pain. Indeed, pain associated with a cartilage tumour in the absence of pathological fracture or other mechanical cause is highly suggestive of malignancy.

*Pathology*

Central tumours consist of lobules or sheets of cartilage, which may permeate throughout the marrow spaces and erode the bone cortex. More aggressive tumours destroy the cortex and form a subperiosteal mass. A greatly thickened cartilaginous cap with nodules of proliferating cartilage on the surface indicates that malignant change in an exostosis has occurred.

Most chondrosarcomas do not show the classic cytological features of malignancy. The finding of many chondrocytes with a plump nucleus and moderate numbers of binucleate cells in a cartilage tumour of the axial skeleton allows a diagnosis of malignancy if the clinical and radiological features are also compatible. Only rare high-grade chondrosarcomas contain pleomorphic cells and moderate numbers of mitoses (Fig. 12.27).

*Prognosis and treatment*

Most chondrosarcomas are slow-growing tumours, which often run a prolonged course with repeated local recurrences. Tumours of the pelvis or chest wall may be surgically irresectable and eventually lead to death by involvement of vital structures. Only around 15% of chondrosarcomas metastasize, usually to the lungs. Successful management

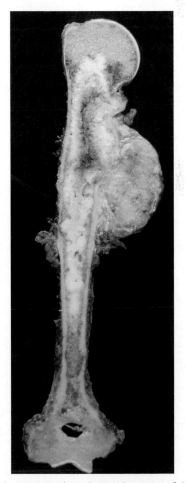

FIG. 12.26 Chondrosarcoma: this advanced tumour of the proximal humerus has arisen within the medullary canal, but has extended through the medial humeral cortex to form a large soft-tissue mass.

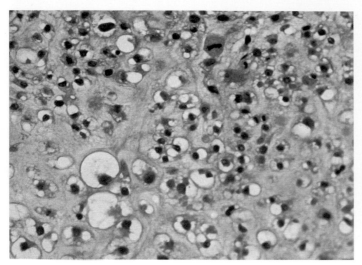

FIG. 12.27 Chondrosarcoma: this tumour is clearly cartilaginous as the cells lie within lacunae in a chondroid matrix, but there is considerable variation in nuclear size and three mitotic figures are present. This is therefore a high-grade tumour.

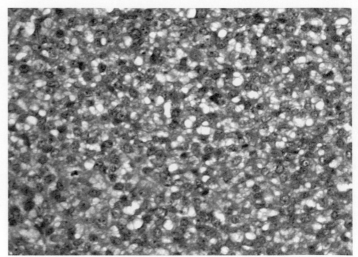

FIG. 12.28 Ewing's sarcoma: this is a malignant round cell tumour, the cells of which have clear cytoplasm due to the presence of glycogen. The nuclei are regular and mitotic figures are sparse for such an aggressive tumour.

of chondrosarcoma is best achieved by adequate wide surgical excision at the first operation; chondrosarcoma is rarely sensitive to chemotherapy or radiotherapy.

## Ewing's Sarcoma

This highly malignant tumour typically affects the long bones and flat bones of the pelvis, scapulae, and ribs of children and adolescents. The tumour originates within the medullary cavity but rapidly penetrates the cortex, elevates the periosteum, and forms a large soft-tissue mass. Radiographs show a moth-eaten pattern of bone destruction, often with parallel layers of reactive periosteal new bone, giving a so-called onion skin appearance. Patients present with pain and swelling. In some, fever, and elevation of the white cell count and erythrocyte sedimentation rate, may simulate osteomyelitis.

### Aetiology

Ewing's sarcoma is a primitive tumour of neuroectodermal origin. Cytogenetic analysis has shown a characteristic rearrangement of the *EWS* gene on chromosome 22 with the *FLI-1* gene on chromosome 11 in a reciprocal translocation t(11; 22)(q24;q12). This hybrid gene produces a chimaeric protein that acts as an activated transcription factor. Other translocations have been found in a minority of Ewing's tumours.

### Pathology

Ewing's sarcoma consists of sheets of small round cells with uniform pale nuclei and sparse mitotic activity (Fig. 12.28). There is often intracellular glycogen and the cells usually express the cell surface antigen CD99. Ewing's tumour must be distinguished from other round cell tumours, e.g. lymphoma of bone and metastatic neuroblastoma in young children, in which urinary catecholamine levels are usually elevated.

### Prognosis and treatment

Ewing's tumour is highly aggressive with early metastases to lung and other bones. The prognosis is especially poor in those patients with systemic symptoms and large tumours, especially those in the pelvis. Similar to osteosarcoma, combined therapy with chemotherapy and surgery or radiotherapy has significantly improved the prognosis, so that over 50% of patients now survive.

## Malignant Fibrous Histiocytoma

This group of tumours includes spindle cell tumours of bone with cells that do not form bone. These affect a wide age range of patients who usually present with pain, swelling, or pathological fracture. Typically a destructive lesion is seen in the metaphysis of a long bone. About a third of cases arise in association with pre-existing lesions such as Paget's disease or previous irradiation. Malignant fibrous histiocytoma is an aggressive tumour. Early blood-borne metastases are common. The cells of malignant fibrous histiocytoma are typically arranged in short bundles radiating from a central point – a 'storiform' pattern similar to the spokes of a wheel. The tumour is probably best regarded as a primitive sarcoma of fibroblast origin. Metastatic carcinoma, especially from the lung and kidney, may have a spindle cell appearance, which can be confused with malignant fibrous histiocytoma.

## Non-Hodgkin Lymphoma of Bone

Although disseminated non-Hodgkin lymphoma commonly involves bone, primary malignant lymphoma is relatively rare. Most tumours are diffuse non-Hodgkin lymphomas of large B-cell type. In contrast with disseminated lymphoma involving bone, primary bone lymphoma has a relatively good prognosis. Between 50% and 80% of patients survive 5 years, especially those who are young.

### Chordoma

This rare tumour arises from notochordal remnants and affects the sacrum, base of skull, and less commonly the vertebrae of middle-aged or elderly people. Chordomas are slow-growing tumours with symptoms due to pressure on adjacent organs. Sacrococcygeal tumours give rise to the symptoms of sacral nerve compression. A large palpable mass may be felt on rectal examination. Chordomas tend to kill by local invasion, but around 10% eventually metastasize. They are lobulated gelatinous tumours that infiltrate bone and extend into adjacent tissues. Microscopy shows cords of vacuolated (physaliferous) cells that express epithelial antigens such as cytokeratin, which helps in the distinction from chondrosarcoma.

## Tumour-like Lesions of Bone

### Fibrous Dysplasia

This benign abnormality of bone may affect one or several bones. Most patients present in childhood, although new lesions may develop after puberty. The ribs, jaw, femur, and tibia are common sites. Increasing deformity and multiple fractures may occur, although lesions usually cease to grow at puberty. Malignant change is rare in the absence of radiation therapy. Fibrous dysplasia often expands the bone and consists of white gritty fibrous tissue, occasionally with cysts and nodules of cartilage. Histologically, loose, spindle-celled, fibrous stroma contains scattered curving 'lobster-claw' trabeculae of woven bone (Fig. 12.29). These are not arranged along stress lines and sometimes give rise to a 'ground-glass' appearance on radiology. Osteoblasts are not present on the surfaces of trabeculae, which are formed by metaplasia from the stroma. The triad of polyostotic fibrous dysplasia (multiple bone involvement), patchy skin pigmentation, and precocious puberty is referred to as Albright's syndrome, a condition more common in females. It is due to mutation of the *GNAS1* gene, which codes for an ADP-dependent G protein.

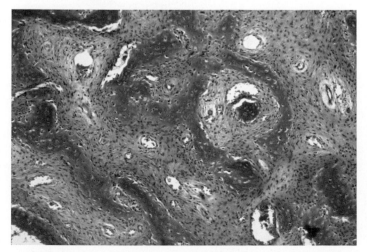

**FIG. 12.29** Fibrous dysplasia: irregularly orientated trabeculae of woven bone are formed from a vascular fibroblastic stroma.

### Langerhans' Cell Histiocytosis (Eosinophil Granuloma)

Langerhans' cell histiocytosis may occur at any age or site, but most commonly arises in children and young adults with one or more lesions in skull, long bones, vertebrae, and pelvis. Well-defined lytic lesions are seen, although in long bones cortical erosion and pathological fracture may occur, suggesting malignancy. Vertebral involvement may lead to bony collapse and a flat dense vertebra (vertebra plana). Histologically, groups of pale-staining Langerhans' cells are mixed with numerous eosinophils. Patients with solitary or few lesions may be cured by surgery or low doses of radiotherapy, or the lesions may heal spontaneously. It is important to ascertain whether there is systemic involvement because this worsens the prognosis.

### Metaphyseal Fibrous Defect

This is a common developmental abnormality with a distinctive radiological appearance. There is a scalloped radiolucent area with a sclerotic margin in the metaphyseal cortex of long bones of children. These lesions may disappear spontaneously or enlarge to involve the medullary cavity, when they are known as non-ossifying fibromas. There may be pathological fracture. The lesion has a bright orange colour due to the presence of many lipid-laden macrophages, which lie in whorled fibrous tissue containing small osteoclasts.

### Cysts of Bone

Aneurysmal bone cyst may affect any bone but typically occurs in the posterior elements of vertebrae and the metaphysis of long bones. Patients, usually children and young adults, complain of pain and swelling which often increases rapidly. Radiographs show a well-circumscribed area of bone lysis, often with very marked eccentric expansion and sometimes described as a 'blow-out'. Anastomosing blood-filled spaces are seen (Fig. 12.30), separated by fibrous septa containing bony trabeculae and osteoclastic giant cells.

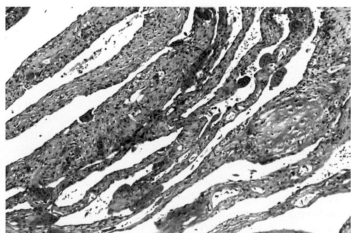

**FIG. 12.30** Aneurysmal bone cyst: the lesion consists of septa containing osteoclasts, fibroblasts, and osteoid. Importantly, there is no endothelial lining, indicating that this is not a haemangioma.

Although aneurysmal bone cysts may simulate a malignant tumour clinically and radiologically, they are benign. Recent evidence indicates that they are benign neoplasms and not simply reactive conditions. A variety of benign and malignant tumours may contain areas of secondary aneurysmal bone cyst change, so the pathologist must examine the entire specimen for any pre-existing lesion.

Simple (unicameral) bone cysts are common findings in children and adolescents, and typically affect the metaphyses of the humerus, femur, and tibia. The patient usually presents with a pathological fracture. Radiological examination shows a slightly expanded cyst with a thinned cortex. The cyst is smooth walled and contains clear fluid unless there has been a fracture. The wall consists of a thin layer of fibrous tissue, sometimes containing osteoclasts and haemosiderin. Injection of steroids into the cyst promotes healing.

Subchondral cysts are frequently seen in osteoarthritis. Similar fibrous-walled cysts containing mucoid fluid may occur near the bone end in the absence of degenerative joint disease and are referred to as intraosseous ganglia. Hydatid cysts (see Chapter 19, pp. 569–570) may occur in bone.

# DISEASES OF JOINTS

## Normal Joint Structure

There are two main types of joint. Synovial (diarthrodial) joints have a synovial lining and usually allow large amounts of movement. Synarthroses are joints in which the bones are joined by fibrous tissue, e.g. the cranial sutures, or by cartilage, e.g. the pubic symphysis. In these, movement is very limited. They are not discussed further.

The basic structure of a synovial joint (Fig. 12.31) is that the two bone ends are covered by articular cartilage and that there is a synovial lining, which produces fluid to nourish and lubricate the cartilage. Joint stability is maintained by the joint capsule, a dense fibrous sheath that encloses the joint, and ligaments, localized bands of fibrous tissue that limit joint movement.

### Articular Cartilage

The hyaline cartilage (Fig. 12.31B) that covers the bone ends is an avascular tissue that provides a smooth, low-friction surface. It resists compressive forces by deforming under mechanical loading but recovers its shape on removal of the load. Normal articular cartilage is a smooth, bluish, translucent material composed of chondrocytes, proteoglycans, collagen, and water.

Collagen is responsible for much of the tensile strength of cartilage. Around 90% of collagen in articular cartilage is type II, whereas other types (V, VI, IX, X, XI) are also found in specific zones, e.g. type VI collagen is located chiefly around chondrocytes. Other proteins such as chondronectin and anchorin may link collagen and chondrocytes. In the deep

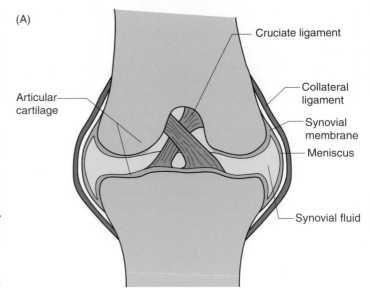

(A)

Cruciate ligament

Articular cartilage

Collateral ligament

Synovial membrane

Meniscus

Synovial fluid

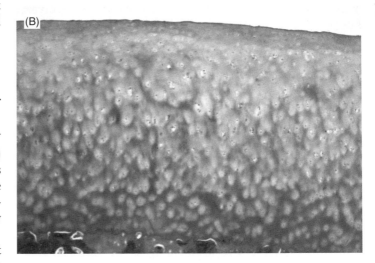

(B)

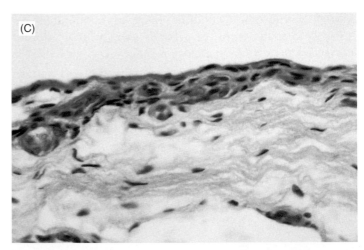

(C)

**FIG. 12.31** Normal joint structure: (A) structure of a synovial joint (knee). (B) Articular cartilage is a smooth-surfaced material covering the bone ends. Small uniform chondrocytes lie in lacunae within a hyaline matrix. (C) In health, the synovial membrane consists of fibrovascular tissue covered by a thin layer of flattened cells, which can be shown to be a mixture of fibroblast-like and macrophage-like cells.

and intermediate zones, collagen fibres are orientated perpendicular to the articular surface, whereas in the superficial zone the fibres lie parallel to the surface forming the 'lamina splendens', a poorly cellular layer. The extracellular matrix of cartilage contains proteoglycan core proteins, link proteins, hyaluronic acid, and glycosaminoglycans (largely keratan sulphate and chondroitin sulphate). These macromolecules are capable of binding large amounts of water. The numerous anionic groups on glycosaminoglycan chains cause mutual repulsion. Together these factors endow cartilage with the ability to resist compression. Proteoglycans are not evenly distributed in cartilage, being present in larger amounts in deeper zones and around chondrocytes.

Chondrocytes are responsible for the continuing turnover of the extracellular matrix of articular cartilage. They synthesize matrix components (e.g. collagen, proteoglycans) as well as enzymes capable of degrading them (e.g. collagenase). The 'lacunae' seen around chondrocytes by light microscopy are artefacts caused by shrinkage of cytoplasm during fixation.

Joint motion and mechanical loading appear to be essential for the maintenance of normal articular cartilage. Immobilization rapidly leads to atrophy.

## Synovium

The synovial membrane (Fig. 12.31C) covers all intra-articular structures except articular cartilage and fibrocartilaginous menisci. It consists of a layer of fibrous or adipose tissue supporting the intima, a surface of synovial lining cells, which broadly fall into two subtypes: macrophage-like cells that are phagocytic and fibroblast-like cells that secrete hyaluronic acid into the synovial fluid. In health this viscous fluid is present in small amounts, acts as a lubricant, and is of importance in the nutrition of articular cartilage.

# Arthritis

Disorders of the joints are disabling conditions that cause serious morbidity. They are of major economic importance both to the patients, who may have long periods off work, and to society as a whole. Joint replacement is very common. It is an expensive operation in terms of professional time, bed occupancy, and prosthetic materials. Over 160,000 total hip and knee replacements are carried out each year in the UK, mostly for osteoarthritis and rheumatoid arthritis.

## Osteoarthritis (Degenerative Joint Disease)

### Key Points
- Osteoarthritis is the most common form of arthritis.
- It mainly affects middle-aged and elderly people.
- Weight-bearing joints are worst affected.
- It is a disorder of articular cartilage.

Osteoarthritis is the most common chronic joint disease, affecting over 2 million people in the UK. It is largely a disease of elderly people affecting at least one joint in two-thirds of the population aged >75. It principally affects the large weight-bearing joints (hip, knee) and the joints of the cervical and lower lumbar spine. Osteoarthritis in young people is usually seen only when there is a predisposing cause (Table 12.5). Primary generalized osteoarthritis, often familial and more common in females, affects multiple joints including the interphalangeal joints of the hands.

### Clinical Features

Patients complain of pain, relieved by rest, stiffness, and sometimes crepitus on movement. Osteoarthritis of the hip often results in a characteristic limp (antalgic gait). Spinal involvement, principally of the intervertebral discs and the posterior apophyseal joints, is very common, and gives rise to stiffness and pain due to compression of nerve roots, particularly in the cervical spine. Bony spurs may compress the vertebral arteries, compromising cerebral blood flow.

### Pathology

In osteoarthritis, changes are seen within the articular cartilage, the underlying bone, and, secondarily, within the synovium. An early change is loss of proteoglycan from the superficial zone of articular cartilage. Disruption of the smooth surface of cartilage follows, initially tangential to the surface (flaking) and then extending vertically into the deeper zones (fibrillation). Proliferation of chondrocytes, forming clusters around fissures, and increased proteoglycan synthesis may be regarded as unsuccessful attempts at healing. Progressive loss of articular cartilage occurs by abrasion, with eventual exposure of the underlying bone. The bone becomes greatly thickened and the surface

**TABLE 12.5** Conditions that predispose to osteoarthritis

| Underlying joint disorders | Metabolic/endocrine |
|---|---|
| Intra-articular fracture | Ochronosis (alkaptonuria) |
| Previous septic arthritis | Haemochromatosis |
| Rheumatoid or other inflammatory arthritis | Gout |
| Osteonecrosis including Perthes' disease | |
| Congenital dislocation of the hip | |
| Intra-articular corticosteroids in excess | |

| Abnormal stresses | Neuropathic disorders |
|---|---|
| Malaligned fracture | Peripheral neuropathy |
| ? Chronic overuse | Spinal cord disorders, e.g. syringomyelia |

polished (eburnation – Fig. 12.32). Cystic spaces containing loose fibrous tissue appear in the subchondral bone. Bone remodelling alters the shape of the joint surface. This is particularly obvious in osteoarthritis of the femoral head in which the superior weight-bearing surface is flattened. At the margin of the articular cartilage, outgrowths of cartilage develop and undergo ossification to become osteophytes. These may cause deformity and limitation of movement. Palpable osteophytes of the distal and proximal interphalangeal joints are known as Heberden's and Bouchard's nodes respectively.

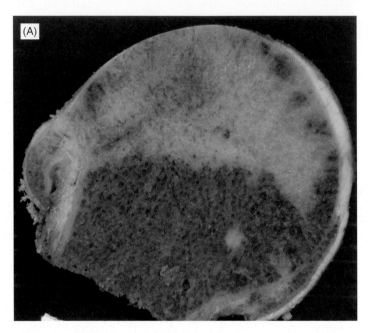

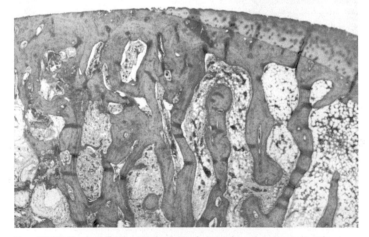

**FIG. 12.32** Osteoarthritis: (A) the articular cartilage has been lost from the weight-bearing surface of this femoral head. The underlying bone so exposed becomes thickened and polished. Osteophytes, protruding pieces of cartilage, and bone have formed at the joint margin. (B) The articular cartilage is progressively thinned from right to left and is finally lost completely. To the left of this, bone provides the articular surface and it is noticeably thicker (sclerotic) in this area.

The synovium may be normal, but is often hypertrophied with mild chronic inflammation. Abraded fragments of bone and cartilage become embedded in the synovium.

### Aetiology and Pathogenesis

Osteoarthritis is not a single disease, but the end-result of joint damage from many causes. In the past, osteoarthritis was considered to be a degenerative disease. A more modern approach is to regard it as an active disease process – as the response of a joint to injury. There is both synthesis of new components and loss of existing tissue in the process of remodelling. It is most likely that the primary change in osteoarthritis is an alteration in chondrocyte activity, with a resultant change in the composition of the articular cartilage, in particular of proteoglycans. Local low-grade inflammation appears to be important and there is evidence that cytokines such as IL-1 and TNF act on the chondrocyte, causing it to release metalloproteases, which degrade the matrix. Genetic factors are also important. Mutations of type II collagen genes are found in some families with osteoarthritis and mutation of the *ADAM12* gene (encoding a protease enzyme) also appears to be important.

The reasons for joint destruction in many of the secondary forms of osteoarthritis are easy to understand. Thus, loss of articular cartilage due to previous septic or rheumatoid arthritis, or an incongruity of the articular surface due to an intra-articular fracture, can readily be accepted as leading to further cartilage damage. Chronic overuse, e.g. in the knees and ankles of footballers, does appear to contribute to the subsequent development of osteoarthritis.

### Neuropathic Arthropathy (Charcot's Joint)

This accelerated form of osteoarthritis occurs in a joint that has lost proprioceptive and pain sensation, e.g. in diabetes or similar sensory neuropathy, syphilis, and syringomyelia (see Chapter 11, p. 330). The cartilage is destroyed and the bone ends become distorted with formation of very large osteophytes. These and the joint surface may fracture with hyperplastic callus formation. Progressive disorganization of the joint results. The florid changes contrast with the relative lack of pain.

### Rheumatoid Arthritis

#### Key Points

- Rheumatoid arthritis is an autoimmune disorder.
- Genetic and environmental factors are involved in its aetiology.
- It particularly affects young to middle-aged females.
- It is a multisystem disease.
- It involves primary inflammation of the synovium with secondary joint damage.

In contrast with osteoarthritis, rheumatoid arthritis is a systemic inflammatory disease, the brunt of which usually falls on the joints. It is common, affecting 1% of the adult population, and occurs more often in females. People of any age may be affected, but the onset is typically in the fourth to sixth decades.

Rheumatoid arthritis may involve any synovial joint, but is usually a symmetrical polyarthritis affecting principally the metacarpophalangeal and proximal interphalangeal joints, wrist, shoulder, and knee. Patients complain of pain and stiffness, especially in the morning. The affected joints are warm and swollen due to joint effusion and synovial hyperplasia. The onset is usually insidious over weeks or months, but rarely symptoms may develop more acutely over days. In most cases the disease follows a course of repeated, partial, or complete remissions and relapses, with further loss of function during each relapse. Less commonly, the disease progresses rapidly with joint destruction and severe disability. Some patients have one episode of arthritis, which resolves, and no further problems.

In 75% of patients, rheumatoid factors can be identified in the serum and synovial fluid. These are antibodies, usually of IgM, IgG, and IgA type, which react with the Fc compartment of IgG to form immune complexes. Patients whose serum contains these antibodies are known as seropositive. This is associated with more aggressive disease than those without rheumatoid factors (seronegative). More recently, antibodies against cyclic citrullinated proteins (CCPs) appear to be equally sensitive but far more specific than rheumatoid factors for the diagnosis of rheumatoid arthritis.

### Pathology

Joint involvement in rheumatoid arthritis is characterized by inflammation and hyperplasia of the synovium followed by destruction of articular structures (Fig. 12.33). The synovium is thrown into villous folds with hyperplasia of synovial lining cells. The synovium is infiltrated by lymphocytes and plasma cells. Lymphoid aggregates with germinal centres are often seen. Fibrin exudes onto the synovial surface, sometimes forming loose bodies known as rice bodies. Neutrophil polymorphs are present in the superficial synovium in significant numbers during acute exacerbations.

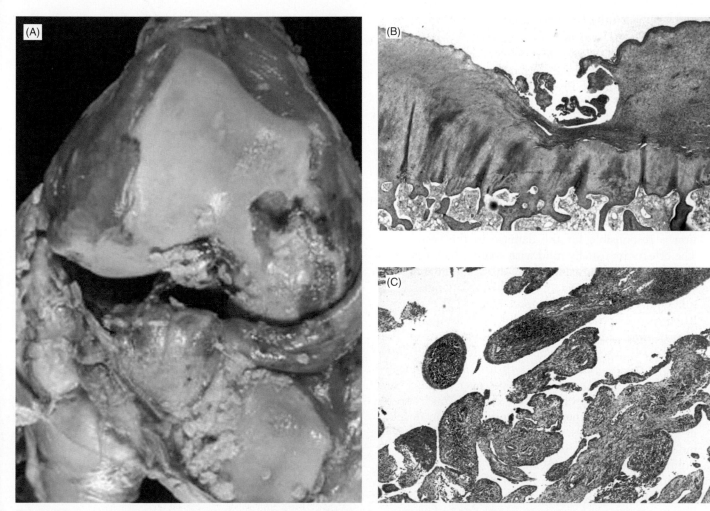

**FIG. 12.33** Rheumatoid arthritis: (A) the knee joint has been opened to show the distal femur, the articular cartilage of which has been eroded from the periphery by haemosiderin-stained pannus (granulation tissue). (B) Low-power microscopy demonstrates that the pannus grows over and erodes the cartilage. (C) The synovium shows a villous architecture, the villi are densely infiltrated by chronic inflammatory cells, and there is fibrinous exudate.

These changes in the synovium are reversible. With time, granulation tissue (pannus) grows over the surface of the articular cartilage, interferes with its nutrition, and causes degradation of its matrix. Permanent joint damage now results. Resorption of the subchondral bone gives rise to radiological 'erosions'. If much articular cartilage is lost, granulation tissue from both sides of the joint forms adhesions, followed sometimes by fibrous union (fibrous ankylosis).

Destruction of the joint capsule and tendons, which are eroded by inflamed synovium of tendon sheaths, leads to striking deformities. Ulnar deviation of the fingers is common and dislocation and subluxation lead to characteristic boutonnière and swan-neck deformities. There is atrophy of muscles surrounding the joints (e.g. interossei in the hand), whereas a combination of disuse atrophy and local hyperaemia leads to loss of bone close to the bone ends (juxta-articular osteoporosis). Involvement of the cervical spine may lead to atlantoaxial subluxation and spinal cord compression. Hyperextension during intubation for general anaesthesia may precipitate neurological damage.

### Extra-articular Manifestations

It must be re-emphasized that rheumatoid arthritis is a multisystem disease. Although its effects on the joints give rise to much morbidity, there are many extra-articular complications, which may be severe and life threatening:

- Vascular and cardiac disease: patients with rheumatoid disease are at much increased risk of vascular disease including atheroma and ischaemic heart disease. Myocarditis and endocarditis can also occur.
- Vasculitis: arteritis with fibrinoid necrosis of the vessel wall (see Chapter 6, p. 124) may occur and usually affects seropositive patients with severe disease. Immune complex deposition with complement activation is responsible for the damage to the vessel wall. The effects are usually mild with splinter haemorrhages in the nail folds, but gangrene of digits and infarction of viscera occasionally occur. Vasculitis may lead to peripheral neuropathy (see Chapter 11, p. 339).
- Rheumatoid nodules: these nodules consist of a central area of fibrinoid necrosis surrounded by macrophages (Fig. 12.34). Rheumatoid nodules are found in 20–35% of patients with rheumatoid arthritis and are typically located in the subcutaneous tissues over extensor surfaces such as the olecranon process. They may also be seen in the viscera. Rheumatoid nodules usually develop in patients who are seropositive. Their presence often indicates a more aggressive course.
- Pulmonary disease (see Chapter 7, p. 177): diffuse pulmonary fibrosis may occur in rheumatoid arthritis. Rheumatoid nodules are occasionally found in the lung. Rarely, patients with rheumatoid arthritis and pneumoconiosis develop large rheumatoid nodules with central breakdown and widespread fibrosis. This is known as

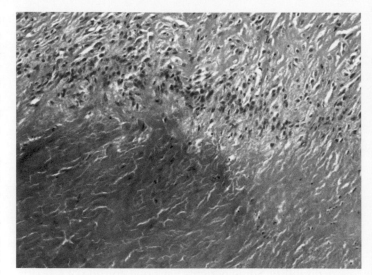

FIG. 12.34 Rheumatoid nodule. The lower half of the illustration consists of necrobiotic collagen with basophilic (blue) staining. Above, and surrounding this, is a reaction of macrophages, the nuclei of which are orientated in a parallel manner known as palisading.

Caplan's syndrome. The incidence of this complication has diminished with that of pneumoconiosis.
- Serosal inflammation: pericarditis and pleurisy are common.
- Amyloidosis: rheumatoid arthritis is one of the most common causes of secondary amyloidosis (see Chapter 13, p. 407).
- Anaemia: similar to many chronic diseases, rheumatoid arthritis is often complicated by microcytic/hypochromic anaemia (anaemia of chronic disease, see Chapter 8, p. 217), whereas NSAIDs may produce acute erosive gastritis with resultant gastrointestinal blood loss and iron deficiency.
- Felty's syndrome: this is splenomegaly with hypersplenism and leukopenia, which may lead to infections.
- Eye involvement: keratoconjunctivitis sicca as part of Sjögren's syndrome (see Chapter 9, p. 239) is the most common ocular complication of rheumatoid arthritis. Inflammation of the sclera (scleritis) may lead to perforation of the globe (scleromalacia perforans). Histologically, this is characterized by fibrinoid necrosis of collagen with surrounding histiocytes, a reaction similar to rheumatoid nodules (see above).

### Aetiology and Pathogenesis

Despite much research, the cause of rheumatoid arthritis remains unknown. Rheumatoid arthritis is an autoimmune disorder that affects individuals with a genetic predisposition who are exposed to an appropriate antigenic stimulus. Once initiated, the disease appears to be self-perpetuating, usually resulting in joint destruction. A summary of the mechanisms thought to be responsible is given in Fig. 12.35.

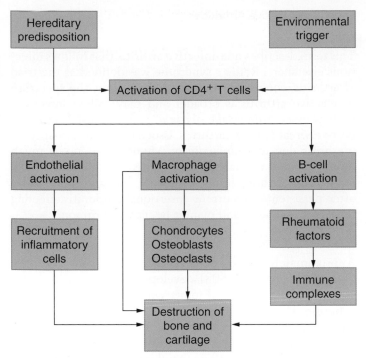

**FIG. 12.35** Pathogenesis of rheumatoid arthritis.

### Genetic Predisposition

It has long been known that rheumatoid arthritis has a familial tendency, but that not all members of a family are affected. Susceptibility to rheumatoid arthritis is associated with certain alleles of the class II major histocompatibility complex (MHC) (see Chapter 2, p. 23) particularly human leukocyte antigen (HLA)-DRB1 and HLA-DR4. Class II MHC molecules are expressed on the surface of antigen-presenting cells and are essential for recognition of antigen by T cells.

### Initiating Factors

The trigger for the development of rheumatoid arthritis has not been identified. It is possible that a variety of different antigenic stimuli may be responsible. The prime suspects have been infective agents, in particular viruses such as Epstein–Barr virus and human parvovirus B19, and bacteria including *E. coli*, but evidence that rheumatoid arthritis is started by an infection is circumstantial. Endogenous antigens may be responsible for triggering rheumatoid arthritis. Autoantibodies directed against IgG (rheumatoid factors) and type II collagen are found in the serum and synovial fluid of many patients with rheumatoid arthritis, but there is no convincing evidence that these initiate the disease.

### Development of Synovitis

The earliest pathological change found in rheumatoid synovium is a perivascular accumulation of T lymphocytes (principally CD4 positive). Synovial lining cells and macrophages process antigen and present it to T lymphocytes, which then proliferate. T cells activate macrophages, stimulate proliferation of endothelial cells (angiogenesis), and also activate B cells. These differentiate into plasma cells, which produce antibodies including rheumatoid factors. In this way the synovial membrane mass is greatly increased with an extensive network of new blood vessels and accumulation of T cells, B cells, plasma cells, and macrophages.

### Destruction of Joint Structures

Irreversible destruction of the joint occurs when the proliferating synovium invades articular cartilage, subchondral bone, tendons, and joint capsule. Synovial cells and macrophages produce proteolytic enzymes such as collagenase and stromelysin, which are capable of destroying the matrix proteins of cartilage and bone. They also produce cytokines such as TNF and IL-1, which appear to be particularly important in joint damage. Anti-cytokine therapies are now widely used. Under the influence of cytokines, chondrocytes reduce their production of extracellular matrix and secrete enzymes that break down existing matrix. Immune complexes formed by rheumatoid factors and IgG activate complement (see Chapter 2, p. 22), which contributes to tissue damage. Chemotactic factors such as C5a and leukotriene $B_4$ attract neutrophil polymorphs into the synovial fluid. These cells degranulate with the release of proteases, which participate in the destruction of articular cartilage. Erosion of subchondral bone is largely attributable to activation of osteoclasts by cytokines such as RANKL (p. 349) rather than by direct proteolytic action.

### *Juvenile Rheumatoid Arthritis (Still's Disease)*

This disease differs in several ways from adult rheumatoid arthritis. By definition the disorder commences before the age of 16, most commonly between 1 and 3 years. Patients often present with involvement of a few joints, or with severe systemic disease, which may precede development of arthritis. These patients have a high spiking fever accompanied by a distinctive macular rash seen on the trunk, proximal limbs, and over pressure areas. There may be hepatosplenomegaly, lymphadenopathy, or serosal inflammation, especially pericarditis.

Juvenile rheumatoid arthritis generally involves the knees, wrists, elbows, and ankles. Involvement of the cervical spine and sacroiliac joints is common. Most patients are seronegative. Other features include growth retardation and chronic uveitis, which may lead to blindness. The pathological features resemble those seen in adult rheumatoid arthritis. The disease often persists into adult life or it may go into spontaneous remission.

### *Seronegative Arthritis*

#### Key Points

- Seronegative arthritis involves the sacroiliac joints and the spine as well as peripheral joints.
- Patients often have uveitis and aortitis.
- There is a strong association with HLA-B27.

This term is applied to a group of inflammatory polyarthritides in which tests for rheumatoid factor are negative and that tend to involve the sacroiliac joints and the spine (spondylitis), as well as peripheral joints. This group includes ankylosing spondylitis, psoriatic arthropathy, reactive arthritis, and arthritis associated with Crohn's disease and ulcerative colitis. It excludes cases of seronegative rheumatoid arthritis.

## Association with HLA-B27

There is a strong association between seronegative arthritis with sacroiliac involvement and the histocompatability antigen HLA-B27. About 8% of a general white population possess this antigen, whereas over 90% of patients with ankylosing spondylitis, 70–90% with Reiter's syndrome, and 50–70% with psoriatic arthropathy are HLA-B27 positive. Patients homozygous for HLA-B27 tend to have more severe disease.

## Ankylosing Spondylitis

This is now recognized to be a common disorder with a prevalence of 0.5–1% in western populations, although in many cases, especially in females, symptoms are mild and recognition depends on radiological changes. Patients are typically in their early 20s, and complain of persistent sacroiliac and lumbar pain with limitation of movement. The onset is usually insidious. Patients may also complain of pain and swelling related to asymmetrical involvement of the peripheral joints, especially the lower limbs. The condition is usually self-limiting but in a minority progresses until the spine is fused (bamboo spine). When the cervical spine is involved, atlantoaxial dislocation may occur and care must be exercised during anaesthesia.

### Pathology

Ankylosing spondylitis is characterized by inflammation at the sites of insertion of ligaments into bone, the joint capsule and fibres of the annulus fibrosus of the intervertebral discs. The site of ligamentous insertion is the enthesis, and the resultant disease is known as enthesopathy. Inflammation is followed by fibrosis and ossification, particularly around intervertebral discs, with the formation of bridging spurs of bone (syndesmophytes). The synovitis histologically resembles that seen in rheumatoid arthritis. Bony ankylosis is more common than in rheumatoid arthritis, and may affect large joints, particularly the hips.

### Extra-articular manifestations

Patients with ankylosing spondylitis may lose weight and develop low-grade fever with a high erythrocyte sedimentation rate (ESR). Uveitis (see Chapter 11, p. 341) occurs in a quarter of cases, and a similar proportion develop aortitis with aortic incompetence (see Chapter 6, p. 146). Although chest expansion is often restricted, pulmonary ventilation is usually well maintained. Diffuse bilateral upper lobe fibrosis, of uncertain aetiology, is a well-recognized late complication.

## Other Seronegative Arthritides
### Reactive arthritis

This term describes non-infective arthritis that follows infections elsewhere. Reiter's syndrome was defined as the triad of arthritis, conjunctivitis. and urethritis, but the spectrum of reactive arthritis is broader and may follow infections with *Shigella*, *Salmonella*, *Yersinia*, and *Campylobacter* spp. Post-venereal reactive arthritis associated with non-specific urethritis due to *Chlamydia* or *Mycoplasma* spp. is much more common in males. The arthritis typically affects the large weight-bearing joints, the hands, feet, and spine, and is often persistent or recurrent. Insertional tendonitis affecting the Achilles tendon and plantar fascia are common.

### Psoriatic arthropathy

Approximately 10% of patients with psoriasis (see Chapter 18, pp. 506–508) develop an associated arthritis, typically affecting several joints with an asymmetrical distribution. The distal interphalangeal joints of the hands and feet, knees, hips, ankles, and wrists are commonly involved. The inflammation is sometimes restricted to the distal interphalangeal joints and is associated with pitting of the nails. Rarely this progresses to osteolysis of the affected phalanges (arthritis mutilans). Sacroiliac and spinal involvement occurs in up to 40% of patients. Pathologically the changes in the synovium resemble those of rheumatoid arthritis.

### Arthritis in inflammatory bowel disease

Peripheral and spinal arthritis can be found in patients with Crohn's disease and ulcerative colitis.

## Haemophilic Arthropathy

Patients with haemophilia (see Chapter 3, p. 39) are at risk of repeated episodes of intra-articular haemorrhage (haemarthrosis) and ultimately chronic destructive arthritis. The knees, ankles, elbows, shoulders, and hips are most often affected. The joint becomes chronically swollen, with limitation of movement.

Pathologically, the synovium becomes grossly hyperplastic and laden with haemosiderin. There is erosion of articular cartilage from the margin, with eventual development of osteoarthritis. Many chondrocytes contain haemosiderin. The accumulation of iron is of major importance in the pathogenesis of haemophilic arthropathy, both by its effect on chondrocyte metabolism and by stimulating synovial proliferation.

## Arthritis due to Deposition of Crystals
### Gout

### Key Points

- Gout is caused by excess levels of uric acid.
- There may be acute or chronic arthritis.
- Crystals are identified on joint aspiration.
- There is accumulation of urates in tissues to form deposits known as tophi.

Gout is an arthritis resulting from deposition of uric acid crystals. Gout particularly affects middle-aged males. It is usually associated with hyperuricaemia, defined as an elevated serum urate concentration >7 mg/dL (0.5 mmol/L). Occasionally the serum urate level may be normal during an attack. Most hyperuricaemic patients remain asymptomatic; the proportion developing clinical gout increases with the serum urate level. Gout may cause an acute arthritis, or in longstanding cases lead to a chronic destructive arthritis. Asymptomatic hyperuricaemia is strongly associated with hypertension, cardiovascular disease, and the insulin resistance syndrome.

### Acute gout

One or more joints are affected and are exquisitely painful, red, and swollen. In over half the patients the metatarsophalangeal joint of the big toe is the first joint to be affected (podagra). This is probably explicable on the grounds that the lower temperature of the extremities reduces the solubility of urates. Dietary or alcoholic excess, drugs, trauma, and surgery often precipitate attacks. An attack usually starts at night and lasts for a few days or weeks. Examination of fluid aspirated from an involved joint shows many inflammatory cells, particularly neutrophil polymorphs and large numbers of needle-shaped crystals within and outside cells. Neutrophils phagocytose urate crystals and release lysosomal enzymes. Complement is activated and other mediators of inflammation such as leukotrienes and prostaglandins are released, with further chemotaxis for neutrophils. Macrophages are also involved. They release cytokines such as I-L1, TNF, and IL-8.

### Chronic 'tophaceous' gout

Chronic 'tophaceous' gout is associated with the formation of crystalline deposits (tophi) of sodium biurate, particularly in fibrous tissue, hyaline cartilage, and fibrocartilage (Fig. 12.36). Microscopy shows aggregates of urate crystals surrounded by foreign body giant cells and histiocytes. When viewed in polarized light they are strongly negatively birefringent. Tophi are found in the pinna of the ear, articular cartilage with associated degenerative changes, and periarticular structures. Subchondral and subperiosteal deposition gives rise to punched-out lytic erosions in bone.

### Aetiology

Hyperuricaemia is due to increased production of uric acid or decreased urinary excretion, or both. Gout may be classified as primary or secondary.

Primary gout represents those patients who do not have another disorder causing hyperuricaemia. It is clear that there is a genetic predisposition. In most cases decreased urinary excretion is responsible. Even in this group there are predisposing factors including obesity, hypertriglyceridaemia, a diet rich in purines, and excessive alcohol consumption. In a few cases specific enzyme disorders have been recognized. Increased activity of 5-phosphoribosyl-1-pyrophosphate

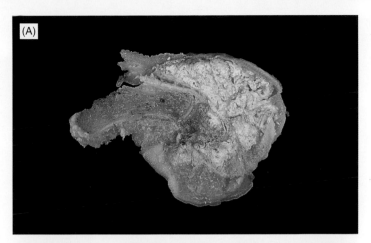

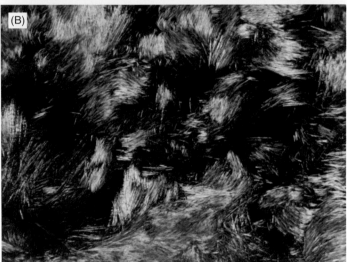

**Fig. 12.36** Gout: (A) this small toe was amputated for persistent pain. The cut section shows extensive deposition of chalky, white crystalline material within the distal phalanx and in adjacent soft tissue. (B) On polarization microscopy, large numbers of brilliantly birefringent crystals are seen.

synthetase (PRPP) and decreased hypoxanthine–guanine phosphoribosyl transferase (HGPRT) activity (Lesch–Nyhan syndrome) both result in increased urate production. Both of these extremely rare disorders are X linked.

Secondary gout refers to those cases that develop during the course of another disease. Patients with malignancy, particularly leukaemia or myeloproliferative disorders treated by chemotherapy, may develop gout as a consequence of increased purine catabolism. Many drugs including thiazide diuretics interfere with renal excretion of uric acid and cause gout.

### Calcium Pyrophosphate Deposition Disease (Pseudogout)

Calcium pyrophosphate crystals are commonly deposited in the cartilage and juxta-articular tissues of elderly people. At least a third of those aged >80 are affected. Calcium pyrophosphate deposition disease may be sporadic or familial. It may also be secondary to underlying conditions including hyperparathyroidism, hypothyroidism, and

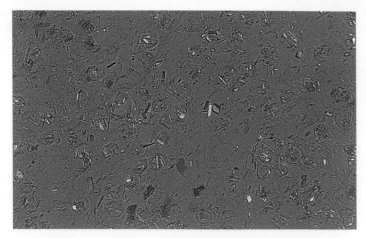

FIG. 12.37 Pseudogout: numerous rod-shaped crystals can be seen on polarization microscopy in fluid aspirated from the knee of an elderly male.

haemochromatosis. When the condition develops in younger patients a cause should be sought. Mutations of the *ANKH* gene have been found in some patients with sporadic and familial disease. Calcium pyrophosphate deposition disease and osteoarthritis often coexist.

Both acute crystal synovitis and chronic deposition may occur. Acute attacks (pseudogout) lasting days to weeks may affect one or several joints, most commonly the knee. Surgery or illness may precipitate an attack. Synovial fluid contains abundant neutrophils and rhomboid and rod-shaped crystals (Fig. 12.37), which show weak positive birefringence in polarized light.

Chronic deposition within the menisci, articular cartilage, ligaments, tendons, and joint capsule is detectable on plain radiographs as small calcified foci, an appearance known as chondrocalcinosis. The knees, hips, symphysis pubis, and intervertebral discs are often affected. Although usually asymptomatic, some individuals develop subacute or chronic synovitis with morning stiffness. A white chalky precipitate is seen, whereas microscopy shows clusters of rhomboid-shaped crystals.

### Basic Calcium Phosphate (Calcium Apatite) Crystal Deposition Disease

Acute and chronic syndromes such as tendonitis and bursitis may occur in response to deposition of calcium apatite crystals. An erosive arthritis has also been described affecting various joints. Crystals may be identified in the synovial fluid. A rapidly progressive destructive arthritis of the shoulder (so-called 'Milwaukee shoulder'), particularly affects elderly females.

## Other Joint Disorders

### *Pathology of Joint Replacement*

The management of patients with arthritis was revolutionized in the early 1960s by the development of low-friction arthroplasties (artificial joints), which can restore mobility

and give pain relief. Most prostheses are manufactured from largely inert metallic alloys and high-molecular-weight polyethylene, and are anchored to the skeleton by acrylic cement aided by ingrowth of bone or fibrous tissue into the prostheses. Implants made from silicone polymers are often used to replace small joints in the hands, usually in rheumatoid arthritis.

Unfortunately, in some patients the prosthesis becomes loose. This is often due to mechanical loosening in which friction between the components of the prosthesis results in fine wear products of metal or polyethylene. These, along with fragments of acrylic cement, induce a reaction of macrophages and foreign body giant cells (Fig. 12.38), which stimulate osteoclasts to resorb bone. As the prosthesis loosens, a vicious cycle is established. Patients may experience considerable pain and insertion of a larger prosthesis (revision arthroplasty) is often required. Recently a

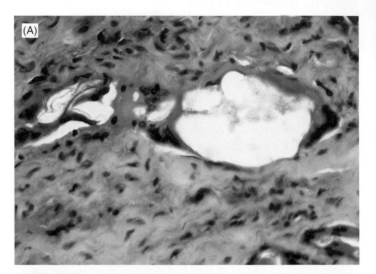

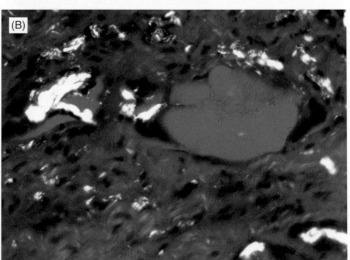

FIG. 12.38 Reaction to a joint prosthesis: (A) foreign body giant cells surround a pool of acrylic cement (right) and fragments of high-molecular-weight polyethylene (left). (B) On polarization, the cement is not birefringent, but unsuspected large amounts of polyethylene are revealed.

specific complication relating to metal-on-metal prostheses has been described. This is called aseptic, lymphocyte-dominated, vasculitis-associated lesion (ALVAL). It is thought that metal ions are released from the prosthesis and elicit a type IV hypersensitivity reaction in surrounding tissues. Histologically there is a dense perivascular lymphocytic infiltrate.

Infection remains an important complication. It may occur in the first few months after surgery due to wound contamination, or may appear insidiously years later due to haematogenous spread of organisms. Once established, deep infection is very difficult to eradicate and it may be necessary to remove the prosthesis. Coagulase-positive and -negative staphylococci and coliforms are often responsible, and organisms of low virulence, including anaerobes, may be cultured.

## Intra-articular Loose Bodies

Multiple soft loose bodies (rice or melon-seed bodies) formed from fibrin or necrotic synovium are found in tuberculous or rheumatoid arthritis. Hard loose bodies may cause repeated episodes of locking of the joint, and damage to the articular cartilage, resulting in osteoarthritis. In synovial chondromatosis multiple nodules of cartilage form by metaplasia in the synovial membrane and may become ossified. Some nodules become detached and lie free in the synovial fluid. In osteochondritis dissecans (see p. 358), the loose body consists of articular cartilage and underlying necrotic bone. Fracture of marginal osteophytes in osteoarthritis may occur, particularly in neuropathic joints. Rarely intra-articular fractures may result in loose bodies.

## Tenosynovial Giant Cell Tumour (Pigmented Villonodular Synovitis)

This benign proliferative lesion of synovium occurs in two distinct clinical settings. Localized nodular synovitis presents as a firm, nodular swelling on the finger, often in women aged between 30 and 50 years. It consists of a lobulated nodule arising from a tendon sheath or joint and contains giant cells and groups of histiocytes (tissue macrophages) containing abundant haemosiderin and lipid, which impart a tan colour. The lesion occasionally recurs. It may erode bone.

Diffuse pigmented villonodular synovitis most often involves the knee or hip joint, causing pain, blood-stained effusion, or locking of the joint. The synovium forms hyperplastic pigmented villi, which become matted together to form solid nodular masses. The enlarged villi are covered by hyperplastic synovial cells and have numerous macrophages containing haemosiderin and lipid. The diffuse form of pigmented villonodular synovitis is more difficult to eradicate, and tends to recur. Bone may be eroded especially in cases involving the hip joint (Fig. 12.39).

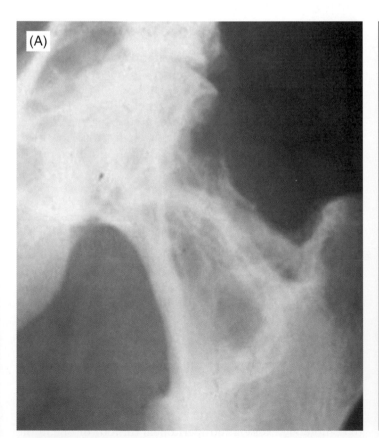
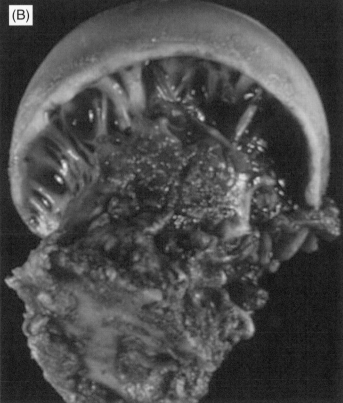

**Fig. 12.39** Tenosynovial giant cell tumour (pigmented villonodular synovitis): (A) the radiograph of the left hip and (B) the gross photograph of the resected specimen show extensive erosion of the bone of the neck and inferior surface of the head of the femur. The lesional tissue is brown/tan and multinodular.

In the past, pigmented villonodular synovitis was thought to be an inflammatory or reactive condition, but it is now more commonly regarded as a neoplasm. Very rare malignant forms are seen, supporting this view.

### Ganglia

These common lesions occur in the soft tissue around joints or tendon sheaths, most often on the dorsum of the wrist. They develop by myxoid change in fibrous tissue with formation of thin-walled cysts containing clear fluid. Sometimes there is a communication between the ganglion and an adjacent joint. Similar lesions may occur within the periosteum and sometimes within bone (intraosseous ganglion).

### Meniscal cyst

Myxoid change may occur in the loose fibrous tissue adjacent to the lateral meniscus or in the meniscus itself, resulting in a lesion histologically identical to a ganglion.

### Bursitis

A bursa is a synovium-lined sac, and is found chiefly over bony prominences. It may communicate with a joint and is subject to the same disorders. Repeated mild trauma may result in inflammation (as, for instance, in prepatellar bursitis – housemaid's knee).

### Amyloidosis

Deposition of amyloid is commonly found in the synovium and degenerate articular cartilage in elderly patients who do not have systemic amyloidosis. It is of little significance. The amyloid appears to be derived from the plasma protein transthyretin. Deposition of amyloid of $\beta_2$-microglobulin origin within the synovium, articular cartilage, and adjacent bone may be found in patients on long-term haemodialysis.

## SOFT-TISSUE TUMOURS AND TUMOUR-LIKE LESIONS

Soft-tissue tumours arise from skeletal muscle, fat, and fibrous tissue, as well as the blood vessels and nerves supplying them. They are classified on the basis of the adult tissue that they resemble, although they arise not from differentiated tissues but from primitive mesenchymal cells.

Most soft-tissue tumours are benign, and usually small, superficially situated lesions such as lipomas. In contrast, soft-tissue sarcomas are typically large tumours within the deep soft tissues of the limbs and retroperitoneum. Soft-tissue sarcomas are a heterogeneous group of tumours of varying histological type and biological behaviour. Although uncommon they cause considerable morbidity and mortality.

Fibromatoses are a group of infiltrative and recurrent lesions that do not metastasize. A small but important group of benign reactive conditions tends to grow rapidly and may be confused histologically with sarcomas. Tumours of peripheral nerve are discussed in Chapter 11 (see p. 340), those of blood vessels in Chapter 6 (see pp. 128–129), and fibrous histiocytoma and dermatofibrosarcoma protuberans in Chapter 18 (see pp. 531–532).

## Benign Tumours

### Lipoma

This common, slowly growing tumour is typically found in the subcutaneous tissues of the back, shoulder, and neck, and the proximal parts of the limbs in patients aged >40. Less commonly, lipomas of deep soft tissue grow to considerable size and cause symptoms due to pressure. The pathologist must examine these tumours very carefully as some well-differentiated liposarcomas with locally aggressive behaviour closely resemble lipomas histologically. Lipomas are lobulated, encapsulated masses of mature adipose tissue. There are a number of histological variants, e.g. angiolipomas, which contain numerous thin-walled capillaries and may be painful, especially when microthrombi form within their rich vascular network.

### Leiomyoma

There are three main types of benign smooth muscle tumour in soft tissue. Cutaneous leiomyomas arise from erector pili muscles and are usually multiple and painful. Genital leiomyomas, e.g. those arising from the dartos muscle in the scrotum, are usually solitary and painless, whereas vascular leiomyomas originate from abnormal thick-walled veins and typically form painful lumps in the legs of middle-aged patients, particularly females. Leiomyomas consist of spindle-shaped cells that closely resemble normal smooth muscle cells.

## Malignant Tumours

### General Features

Most soft-tissue sarcomas are well-circumscribed masses in deep soft tissue (Fig. 12.40). Although they may appear to be encapsulated, there is microscopic invasion of the surrounding tissues. Surgical 'shelling out' of the tumour is almost inevitably followed by local recurrence. The prognosis depends on several factors. The risk of local recurrence is largely related to the adequacy of surgical removal, which itself depends on the anatomical site and the skill of the surgeon. Thus, a tumour confined to a single muscle compartment in the thigh may be completely removed by a 'compartmental excision'. It may be impossible, however, to completely excise a retroperitoneal tumour or one in the

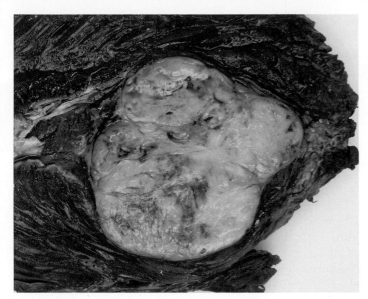

Fig. 12.40 High-grade sarcoma: this tumour arising in the right vastus intermedialis was resected *en bloc*. The apparent degree of circumscription is deceptive because the tumour had an infiltrative pattern on histology.

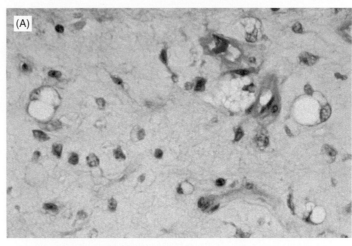

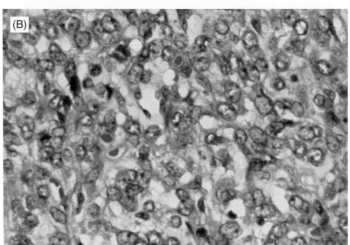

Fig. 12.41 Myxoid/round cell liposarcoma: (A) myxoid liposarcoma consists of small cells in a loose myxoid background, with occasional cells that have vacuolated cytoplasm containing lipid. (B) Round cell liposarcoma consists of closely packed and more hyperchromatic cells, some showing vacuolation. These two patterns may be seen within one tumour, as in this case. The round cell component confers a much worse prognosis.

popliteal fossa. Factors influencing the risk of metastases include the histological grade, size, and anatomical location. There are several different histological grading systems. High-grade tumours tend to metastasize early, whereas low-grade lesions give problems largely from local recurrence or extension. In general the more superficial a tumour and the smaller it is, the better the prognosis.

Even with modern techniques such as immunocytochemistry, electron microscopy, and molecular and cytogenetic analysis, precise histological typing of sarcomas is often difficult. Around 5% of tumours can be reported only as 'sarcoma of uncertain histogenesis'. With few exceptions the grade of a tumour is more important than its histological type in determining prognosis. The value of cytogenetic analysis is discussed below.

### Liposarcoma

Liposarcoma occurs mainly in the deep soft tissue of the limbs or in the retroperitoneum in patients aged >50. There are several histological subtypes that show varying degrees of differentiation towards adipose tissue. A well-differentiated liposarcoma is a low-grade tumour, which rarely metastasizes unless it becomes associated with a high-grade non-adipose component, so-called dedifferentiated liposarcoma. Myxoid and round cell liposarcomas form a spectrum from low-grade to high-grade tumours (Fig. 12.41). They share the same chromosomal translocation (see p. 383). Pleomorphic liposarcomas are highly malignant tumours that are associated with early pulmonary metastases.

### Rhabdomyosarcoma

Although rhabdomyosarcoma is the most common soft-tissue tumour of childhood and adolescence, it is rare in older patients. Three main histological types are recognized: embryonal, alveolar, and pleomorphic.

Embryonal rhabdomyosarcoma occurs mainly in children, in the head and neck, genitourinary tract, and retroperitoneum. Tumours occurring in the vagina or bladder project as grape-like gelatinous masses and are known as 'botryoid' (grape-like) sarcomas. They consist of spindle-shaped cells and show varying degrees of skeletal muscle differentiation. An embryonal rhabdomyosarcoma usually responds well to combined chemotherapy, radiotherapy, and surgery.

Alveolar rhabdomyosarcomas occur in adolescents, particularly arising in skeletal muscle of the limbs. Tumour cells adhere to fibrous septa, which divide the cells into clumps. Loss of cohesion in the centre of the groups produces an alveolar pattern (Fig. 12.42). Many cases are associated with a t(2;13) or t(1;13) translocation. The prognosis of this group of tumours remains poor.

Pleomorphic rhabdomyosarcomas are very rare and occur chiefly in the skeletal muscles of older people. It is often difficult to separate this group from other pleomorphic sarcomas.

Immunohistochemical staining for muscle specific proteins, e.g. the intermediate filament desmin, myo-$D_1$, a nuclear protein expressed early in skeletal muscle differentiation, and myogenin (Fig. 12.42), helps establish the diagnosis.

## Leiomyosarcoma

This tumour usually affects middle-aged and elderly people. About half of soft-tissue leiomyosarcomas arise in the retroperitoneum and have a poor prognosis, with less than 30% of patients surviving 5 years. Of the remainder, most are found in the dermis or subcutaneous tissue. In keeping with other superficially situated sarcomas the prognosis for these tumours is better, with over 90% of patients with dermal tumours and 65% with subcutaneous lesions surviving 5 years. Histologically, leiomyosarcomas consist of spindle-shaped cells resembling normal smooth muscle cells, which are arranged in long interlacing fascicles. Many tumours express desmin and smooth muscle actin. The principal criterion in distinguishing malignant and benign smooth muscle tumours is the number of mitotic figures. Nuclear pleomorphism without mitotic activity may be found in leiomyomas.

## Malignant Fibrous Histiocytoma (Undifferentiated High-grade Pleomorphic Sarcoma)

This is an aggressive tumour with a high risk of recurrence and metastasis, and a poor prognosis, particularly when sited in the retroperitoneum. The distinctive histological feature is a 'storiform' pattern in which cells are arranged in short bundles from a central point, likened to a cartwheel. There are several subtypes. Its histogenesis is uncertain, but it is best regarded as an undifferentiated high-grade sarcoma as is its counterpart in bone (see p. 368).

## Synovial Sarcoma

Despite its name this tumour is not a tumour of the synovium. It is typically found adjacent to, but not in, large joints of adolescents and young adults. Sometimes the lesion has been present for many years and may have recently increased in size. Historically, the entity was defined by a biphasic pattern of a spindle cell sarcoma with groups of epithelial cells arranged in acini and tubules (Fig. 12.43). Later it was recognized that some tumours consisted of spindle cells alone. These are known as monophasic synovial sarcoma. A characteristic translocation, t(X;18), has been found in synovial sarcoma. It is an aggressive tumour, with metastases in 50–70% of patients, often many years after diagnosis.

## Fibromatosis

This term includes several fibrous lesions that have a tendency to infiltrate adjacent tissues and recur, but do not metastasize.

Palmar fibromatosis (Dupuytren's contracture) begins as a firm nodule in the palm of middle-aged and elderly

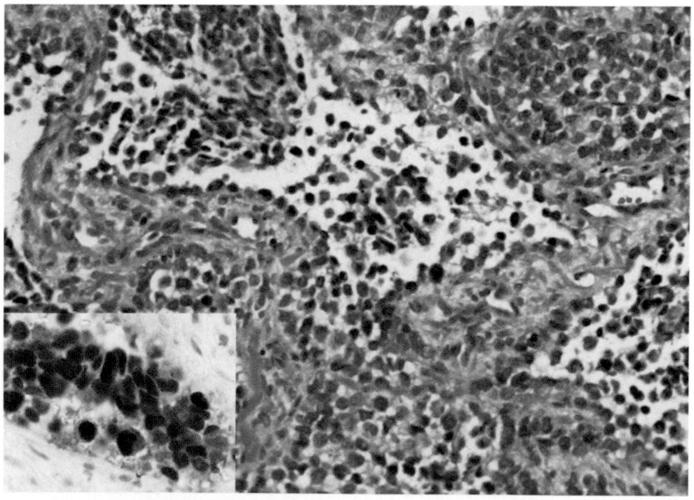

FIG. 12.42 Alveolar rhabdomyosarcoma: the tumour is composed of sheets of round cells, which show central discohesion with the formation of an alveolar or honeycomb pattern. The insert (lower left) shows that the nuclei stain with an antibody directed against myogenin, a nuclear regulatory protein involved in skeletal muscle differentiation, helping to confirm the diagnosis.

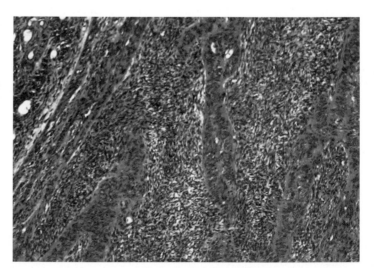

FIG. 12.43 Biphasic synovial sarcoma: as the name suggests, there are two patterns to this tumour, namely well-differentiated glandular structures and closely packed spindle-shaped cells.

patients and in time extends to form subcutaneous bands, which produce flexion contractures, especially of the fourth and fifth fingers. Histologically, the palmar aponeurosis is expanded by multiple nodules of proliferating myofibroblasts. In time these nodules become heavily collagenized and poorly cellular. Similar lesions may occur in the sole of the foot, usually without contracture (plantar fibromatosis) or in the penis (Peyronie's disease).

Musculoaponeurotic fibromatosis is seen typically in the muscles of the shoulder and pelvic girdles and in the thigh, where it forms a firm mass, which infiltrates widely through muscle, often further than can be identified at surgery.

For this reason complete excision is difficult and repeated recurrences are common, sometimes with involvement of major structures such as the brachial plexus. Recently, it has been suggested that conservative surgery, perhaps supplemented by low-dose chemotherapy or radiotherapy, is as successful as attempts at radical surgery. Abdominal desmoids are similar lesions seen in rectus abdominis of females during or after pregnancy but tend to be smaller, less aggressive, and less likely to recur. Abdominal desmoid tumours also occur in association with familial adenomatous polyposis (FAP) (see Chapter 9, p. 270).

## 12.2 Special Study Topic

### CHROMOSOMAL REARRANGEMENTS IN SARCOMAS

Over the past two decades, it has emerged from cytogenetic analysis of tumour specimens that many soft-tissue sarcomas have characteristic chromosomal rearrangements. This finding is important for several reasons:

- Detection of a known translocation, either by cell culture and examination of chromosomes (karyotyping) or by molecular genetic techniques, may establish or confirm a precise histological diagnosis in a case where there may be diagnostic difficulty.
- More accurate staging is made possible by the identification of small numbers of occult tumour cells, e.g. in bone marrow biopsies or pleural fluids by molecular techniques such as reverse transcriptase polymerase chain reaction (RT-PCR), which are much more sensitive than light microscopy.
- Some translocations found in a given tumour type appear to be associated with a better prognosis than examples of the tumour with a different rearrangement. For example, within synovial sarcomas, the translocation involving the *SSX1* gene correlates with a worse outcome than that with the *SSX2* gene (*Table 12.6*).
- A more robust classification of tumours is possible. Demonstration that two histologically different tumours share the same translocation indicates that they may be part of a single biological entity, e.g. the myxoid and round cell forms of liposarcoma have a very different prognosis. The demonstration of t(12;16)(q13;p11) in examples of both of these tumours, together with the long-known phenomenon of round cell transformation affecting myxoid liposarcoma, indicates that the two represent the opposite ends of a spectrum. Conversely, if two tumours thought to be closely related, e.g. clear cell

sarcoma and malignant melanoma, do not share the same translocation, then their postulated relationship can be refuted.

- Through detection of these abnormalities, much can be learned about the underlying molecular oncogenic mechanisms in these tumours.
- Finally, it is likely that, through understanding of these mechanisms, new targeted therapies can be designed that may have greater anti-tumour effects than conventional cytotoxic therapies.

*Table 12.6* details some of the better-recognized tumours, their translocations and the associated genetic effects. A characteristic feature is the production of hybrid genes, which encode fusion protein products. These typically act as aberrant transcriptional regulators, and promote tumour cell growth.

**TABLE 12.6** Common sarcomas with characteristic translocations

| Tumour | Translocation | Fusion product |
|---|---|---|
| Alveolar rhabdomyosarcoma | t(2;13)(q35;q14) | PAX3-FKHR |
| Alveolar soft part sarcoma | t(X;17)(p11;q25) | ASPL-TFE3 |
| Clear cell sarcoma | t(12;22)(q13;q12) | ESW-ATF1 |
| Dermatofibrosarcoma protuberans | t(17;22)(q22;q13) | COL1A1-PDGFb |
| Desmoplastic small round cell tumour | t(11;22)(p13;q12) | EWS-WT1 |
| Ewing's sarcoma | t(11;22)(q24;q12) | EWS-FLI1 |
| Extraskeletal myxoid chondrosarcoma | t(9;22)(q22;q12) | EWS-CHN |
| Myxoid liposarcoma | t(12;16)(q13;p11) | TLS-CHOP |
| Synovial sarcoma | t(X;18)(p11;q11) | SYT-SSX1 or -SX2 |

## Special Study Topic continued . . .

### Ewing's Sarcoma and the *EWS* Gene

The first consistent translocation demonstrated in a sarcoma was t(11;22)(q24;q12) in Ewing's tumour (Fig. 12.44). This was important because it established that a group of malignant tumours composed of small round blue cells, namely Ewing's tumour of bone and soft tissue, so-called Askin tumour of the chest wall, and primitive neuroectodermal tumours of bone and soft tissue were all variants of the same tumour type. This kinship also established that Ewing's tumour, the histogenesis of which was unknown, was a neuroectodermal tumour showing varying degrees of differentiation.

The translocation t(11;22) is found in 85% of cases of Ewing's tumour. In this rearrangement the 5'-end of the *EWS* gene on chromosome 22 fuses with the 3'-end of the *FLI1* gene on chromosome 11. *FLI1* encodes a transcription factor. The hybrid gene produces a chimaeric protein, which functions as an aberrant transcription factor with effects on a number of downstream genes, including some involved in apoptosis. In this way, the hybrid gene can be regarded as an oncogene. Subsequently, a number of other genes related to *FLI1* (members of the ETS group of transcription factors) have been shown to be involved in variant translocations in Ewing's tumour, e.g. the translocation t(11;22)(q24;q12) leads to the production of an EWS–ERG fusion product.

Perhaps more interestingly, the *EWS* gene has been shown to be a partner in rearrangements with other genes in four further soft-tissue tumours, including extraskeletal myxoid chondrosarcoma (the *CHN* gene on chromosome 9) and some examples of myxoid liposarcoma (the *CHOP* gene on chromosome 12). The *EWS* gene is a member of the TET group of genes, the products of which have RNA-binding functions. It seems likely that this gene, the function of which is not yet fully understood, is important in the genesis of several forms of soft-tissue sarcoma

Much current research is directed towards fuller understanding of the functions of the genes involved in these translocations. As has already been shown in chronic myeloid leukaemia (see Chapter 8, p. 226), identification of a characteristic molecular abnormality may allow specific therapies to be devised.

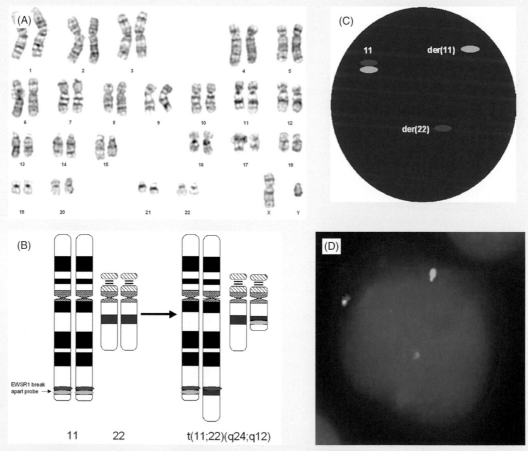

**FIG. 12.44** (A) Karyotype showing a reciprocal translocation between chromosomes 11 and 22 as seen in Ewing's sarcoma. (B) Chromosome ideograms showing the t(11;22) translocation with chromosome 11 in black and 22 in blue. The red and green regions represent the EWSR1 break-apart probe (Vysis) for Ewing's gene. (C) Diagram showing interphase fluorescence *in situ* hybridization (FISH) pattern with the split signal indicating a translocation involving Ewing's gene. (D) Interphase FISH image showing the pattern illustrated in C.

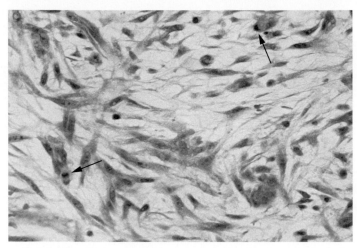

FIG. **12.45** Nodular fasciitis: loosely arranged fibroblasts lie randomly like cells in tissue culture. Although there are two mitotic figures (arrows) these are of normal appearance and, although the cells vary in size, the nuclei are not hyperchromatic.

### Reactive Tumour-like Lesions of Soft Tissue

The clinical history in nodular fasciitis is usually of a rapidly growing tender nodule in the upper limb, especially the forearm of a young adult. Most often the lesion is subcutaneous, but sometimes muscle or deep fascia is involved. Microscopy shows loosely arranged fibroblasts randomly arranged like cells in tissue culture, with frequent mitotic figures of normal morphology (Fig. 12.45). There is a prominent vascular pattern with scattered chronic inflammatory cells. This entirely benign lesion must not be misdiagnosed as a sarcoma.

Myositis ossificans occurs mainly in the muscles of the limbs of young people. Patients complain of a rapidly growing soft-tissue swelling, sometimes after trauma. Many patients have low-grade fever and an elevated white blood count, suggesting infection. On microscopy there is a characteristic zoning pattern, a central zone of proliferating fibroblasts merging with areas of primitive bone formation, which may mature to form a well-defined peripheral shell of woven bone in 4–6 weeks. There is a danger that myositis ossificans is misdiagnosed as osteosarcoma, particularly in the early stages, before 'zoning' has developed.

## SKELETAL MUSCLE

## Normal Muscle Structure

The largest tissue within the body, muscle, accounting for 40% of an average male's weight, is highly organized to contract, produce movement or stability, and do work. Skeletal muscle consists of long multinucleated syncytia formed by fusion of columns of single cells. The cytoplasm contains bundles of myosin and actin filaments forming contractile myofibrils. The individual subunit is the sarcomere and these are arranged end to end to form muscle fibres. The parallel alignment of actin and myosin bundles gives a characteristic band-like appearance on light microscopy and alternating dark (A, anisotropic) and light (I, isotropic) bands are seen on electron microscopy. A variety of other proteins including α-actinin and dystrophin are found within muscle cells. The individual muscle fibre is surrounded by the endomysium. Fibres are bound into fascicles by the perimysium, whereas the muscle itself is sheathed by the epimysium.

Muscle contracts when the relevant motor neuron is stimulated to release acetylcholine (ACh) into the cleft at the neuromuscular junction. Binding of ACh to the motor endplate results in altered permeability, and an action potential is conducted over the entire surface of the membrane and into its interior through transverse tubules, which dip perpendicularly into the fibre. Muscle fibres share motor nerve twigs, forming groups known as motor units, based on a single anterior horn cell and the fibres that it supplies. In general, the more delicate the muscle function, the fewer the muscle fibres that each nerve fibre innervates.

The two major proteins, actin and myosin, interact with each other in a sliding manner, akin to a rower; myosin slides past actin, binds to it, pulls back, releases, and then repeats the cycle. This so-called sliding filament mechanism requires continual energy provided by the breakdown of adenosine triphosphate (ATP). This reaction occurs before myosin and actin bind and energy is stored in the crossbridge which is cocked like a gun. A fresh molecule of ATP is required to release the linkage, explaining the phenomenon of rigor mortis, where after death muscle contraction continues until proteolysis occurs.

### Fibre Types

Muscle fibres are divided into two main groups according to the type of work that they are required to do. Type 1 (slow twitch, aerobic, red) fibres contain much myoglobin to provide increased oxygen uptake and are capable of continuous endurance activity, unlike type 2 (fast twitch, anaerobic, white) fibres, which respond rapidly but quickly become fatigued (Fig. 12.46). Type 2 also includes some fibres with

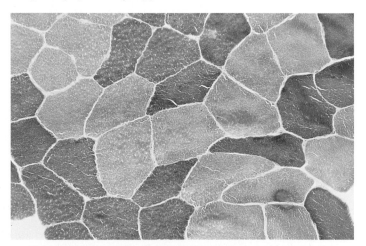

FIG. **12.46** Normal muscle stained to show ATPase activity at pH 9.4. Type 1 fibres are pale staining and type 2 are dark.

characteristics of each. The proportions vary between individuals and this may explain ability as a sprinter or marathon runner.

## Diseases of Muscle

Most patients with muscle symptoms, usually undue fatigue or weakness, do not have specific muscle diseases (myopathies). Myopathies have characteristic presenting complaints, which allow their classification when combined with laboratory investigations such as electromyography (EMG), estimation of serum levels of creatine kinase (which is released from the cytoplasm of damaged muscle cells), and muscle biopsy. Recently, DNA analysis and genetic assessment have changed the approach to muscle disease.

### Indications for Muscle Biopsy

> **Key Points**
>
> Muscle biopsy is used:
> - to establish the diagnosis in an inflammatory myopathy before treatment
> - to establish the diagnosis in weakness of unknown cause
> - to establish the diagnosis in hereditary myopathies and dystrophies
> - to identify a treatable disorder
> - to evaluate carrier status in a female relative of a boy with Duchenne muscular dystrophy.

Muscle biopsies are usually taken from a large proximal limb muscle, e.g. quadriceps, because these are most often affected. Severely affected muscles should be avoided because they may show only the features of 'end-stage' muscle disease and it may therefore be impossible to determine the cause of the process. Needle biopsies, taken under local anaesthetic, are usually adequate when specialized histochemical stains are available, especially in suspected metabolic disorders. The specimen is snap frozen and stored at −70°C before cutting frozen sections as required.

The main changes seen in muscle biopsies are as follows:

- Necrosis: usually of a segment of a muscle fibre, e.g. in inflammatory myopathies, but large areas of necrosis may be seen if the blood supply is affected.
- Atrophy: of either fibre type. Type 2 atrophy is seen whenever muscle is damaged in systemic disease or during steroid therapy. Neurogenic atrophy follows loss of nerve supply to a muscle fibre.
- Hypertrophy: a compensatory response to loss of fibres in many muscle diseases, especially dystrophies and in denervation.
- Regeneration: occurs if the basement membrane and endomysium remain intact. Regenerating fibres are basophilic due to increased cytoplasmic RNA.

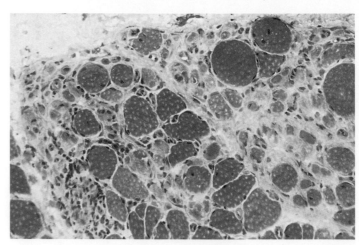

**FIG. 12.47** Polymyositis: necrosis and regeneration of muscle fibres are accompanied by focal chronic inflammation and fibrosis.

### Myopathies

#### Inflammatory Myopathies

This group includes polymyositis (Fig. 12.47) and dermatomyositis, disorders thought to have an autoimmune aetiology. In polymyositis cytotoxic T cells attack the muscle fibre, whereas in dermatomyositis autoantibodies are deposited in intramuscular blood vessels. Both conditions may affect adolescents or adults and usually have a slow onset over weeks to months, so that the patient often notices the weakness only when it is sufficiently severe that climbing stairs or lifting the arms above the head is difficult. In dermatomyositis there is a rash over the eyelids, cheekbones, sternum, elbows, knees, and small joints of the hand. In severe cases, especially in adolescents, calcific deposits may affect damaged muscles. In some patients cardiac involvement, especially of the conducting system, may cause sudden death; others develop pulmonary fibrosis. About a fifth of patients have a connective tissue disorder such as systemic lupus erythematosus, systemic sclerosis, or Sjögren's syndrome. The incidence of common malignancies is slightly increased in middle-aged patients with these myopathies.

Muscle biopsy shows necrosis of muscle fibres with subsequent phagocytosis and regeneration and focal chronic inflammation. EMG shows 'myopathic' changes and muscle fibre necrosis leads to an increase in serum creatine kinase.

Viral infections, notably influenza and Coxsackievirus, may very rarely cause inflammatory myositis and the damage may be severe with rhabdomyolysis.

#### Metabolic Myopathies

Muscle symptoms in these disorders are related to exercise intolerance. Defects in glycogen, lipid, purine nucleotide, and mitochondrial pathways can all lead to metabolic myopathies. McArdle's disease, the most common disorder of glycogen metabolism, is an inherited recessive disorder due to lack of myophosphorylase (Fig. 12.48). Exercise intolerance with stiffness is found, symptoms usually being precipitated by brief bursts of high intensity activity. Severe

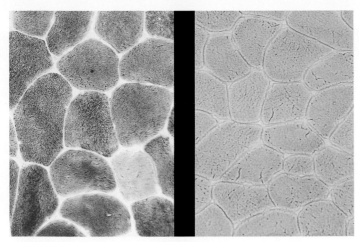

**Fig. 12.48** McArdle's disease: muscle stained for the presence of myophosphorylase activity. Normal (left) shows abundant dark blue reaction product, which is absent in the biopsy from an affected individual (right).

attacks may involve rhabdomyolysis with myoglobinuria and hence renal failure.

Mitochondrial myopathies have only relatively recently been characterized. Deficiencies in oxidative enzymes are now known to be responsible. They are of interest because many are due to mutations in mitochondrial rather than genomic DNA and are therefore inherited through the maternal line. Many patients present with chronic progressive external ophthalmoplegia, with paralysis of external ocular muscles and mild limb weakness. Cardiac conduction defects, retinopathy, and seizures may also be present.

### Periodic Paralysis (Channelopathies)

Ion channels (see cystic fibrosis transmembrane conductance regulatory chlorine channel, Chapter 7, p. 171) are crucial components of cell membranes, allowing ions to flow rapidly while maintaining extracellular and intracellular concentrations. They are selective for different ions and controlled by specific stimuli, such as neurotransmitters. Several hereditary muscle disorders are due to mutations in ion channel proteins. They are frequently autosomal dominant in inheritance and usually characterized by episodic symptoms of muscle weakness and cramps, e.g. hyperkalaemic periodic paralysis. Malignant hyperpyrexia is a serious ion-channel disorder characterized by an abnormal response to general anaesthetics, especially halothane. Intense muscle contraction starts after anaesthesia and is followed by a rapid rise in body temperature. Release of calcium from the sarcoplasmic reticulum causes massive muscle necrosis (rhabdomyolysis). The muscle relaxant dantrolene stops the symptoms and prevents terminal shock.

### Myopathies Associated with Systemic Disease

Many systemic diseases, e.g. chronic heart, respiratory, liver, and renal disease, cause muscle weakness. Although muscles are not primarily affected, patients may complain of muscle weakness, serum creatine kinase may be elevated, and EMG may show myopathic changes. Muscle biopsy may be normal or show mild-to-moderate atrophy of type 2 fibres, because these are susceptible to muscle damage of any kind. An exception is diabetes in which neurogenic atrophy is usually seen. Muscle disease usually responds to treatment of the underlying condition.

### Muscular Dystrophies

Muscular dystrophies are a group of inherited conditions with an intrinsic defect of muscle and are characterized by progressive muscle wasting and weakness.

Duchenne muscular dystrophy is the most common dystrophy of childhood and affects 1 in 3,500 male births. An X-linked recessive condition, it affects boys who present before 5 years with delayed motor function, a waddling gait, and an inability to run. Due to weakness of the pelvic girdle muscles they find difficulty in rising from the floor without the help of their arms. Most are confined to a wheelchair by 12 years of age and die due to cardiomyopathy or respiratory failure by the late teens or early 20s. About a third have intellectual impairment. Becker muscular dystrophy is a clinically similar but milder form with onset in the teens and early 20s, and many patients survive into middle age and beyond.

Mutations in the dystrophin gene on the short arm of chromosome X cause both disorders and its protein product, dystrophin, has been characterized. Normal dystrophin is a large molecular component of the sarcolemmal plasma membrane. When the gene is mutated, dystrophin is either absent or undetectable as in Duchenne dystrophy, or of abnormal constitution as in Becker dystrophy. The clinical phenotypes correlate well with the quantity and quality of dystrophin (Fig. 12.49). In Duchenne dystrophy two-thirds of mutations are inherited from the mother. The remaining third of mutations are new mutations, reflecting the large size of the gene, which contains several hot spots. Most patients with Duchenne dystrophy have a deletion or duplication resulting in truncation of translation and a small unstable molecule. The muscle biopsy shows a characteristic appearance with variation in muscle fibre size, some showing necrosis. In the later stages muscle is replaced by fat and fibrous tissue (Fig. 12.50).

Myotonic dystrophy, an autosomally inherited progressive neuromuscular disorder, is characterized by failure of muscle to relax after contraction (myotonia) and progressive weakness. It involves other systems, with cardiac conduction defects, cataracts, premature balding, reduced fertility, and mental impairment. It is caused by an increased number of cytosine–thymidine–guanine (CTG) trinucleotide repeats in an untranslated region of the dystrophica myotonia protein kinase gene. The normal gene has between 5 and 30 such repeats, whereas affected alleles have from 50 to several thousand. An interesting feature is the phenomenon of 'anticipation' – the clinical symptoms increase

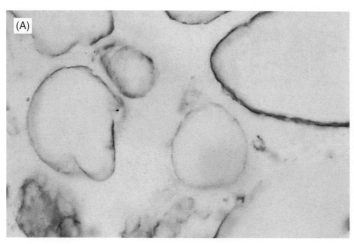

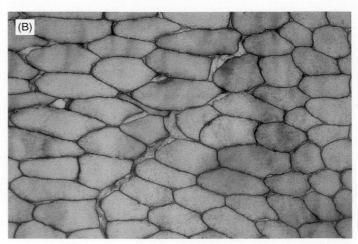

FIG. 12.49 Becker-type muscular dystrophy: staining for dystrophin shows patchy and variable staining at the periphery of the fibres (A) compared with the regular pattern of normal muscle (B). Staining is typically absent in Duchenne dystrophy.

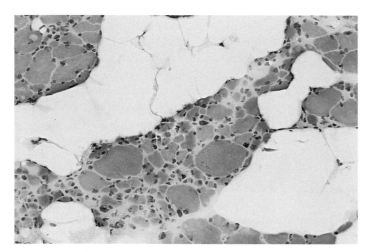

FIG. 12.50 Duchenne muscular dystrophy: this biopsy from advanced disease shows muscle fibres, many of which are atrophic, lying among adipose tissue.

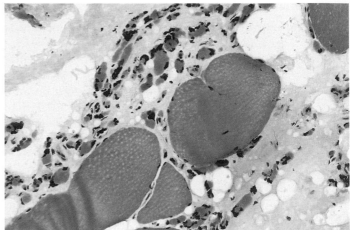

FIG. 12.51 Neurogenic atrophy: the majority of muscle fibres are denervated and have atrophied to small fibres with nuclei that appear large. A few large hypertrophied fibres are present.

with successive generations. EMG and muscle biopsy show characteristic features.

A variety of other much rarer dystrophies has been described, and the mutations characterized.

### Neurogenic Disorders

As muscle fibre function depends on the integrity of the whole motor unit, disorders that produce lesions in the motor neuron, peripheral motor nerves, and neuromuscular junction may all result in atrophy of the muscle with shrinkage of fibres. Diagnostic problems can arise because these disorders may simulate myopathies, especially dystrophies. Among these are hereditary disorders such as spinal muscular atrophies (SMAs), which fall into three broad categories: severe infantile SMA causing death from respiratory failure in infancy; milder juvenile cases with scoliosis; and adults with a better prognosis. The biopsy appearances (Fig. 12.51) depend on the rate and degree of denervation. Initially,

atrophic muscle fibres are scattered at random through the fascicles, but later small clusters of tiny fibres can be identified followed by large group atrophy as more neurons fail.

Motor neuron disease (see Chapter 11, p. 326) affects upper and lower motor neurons and causes severe generalized atrophy, leading to death within 3 years or so. Similar features are seen in hereditary peripheral neuropathies, diabetes, and the post-polio syndrome.

## Disorders of Neuromuscular Transmission

There are two major disorders, each with an immunological basis.

### Myasthenia Gravis

This disease occurs predominantly in young females and middle-aged males, who present with abnormal fatigue of skeletal muscles and weakness on exercise and recovery after rest. The external ocular and facial muscles are usually affected causing ptosis and diplopia. There may be difficulty in swallowing, speaking, and chewing. Symptoms may be restricted to the eyes but more often generalized weakness with respiratory symptoms develops, particularly in exacerbations (crises). There is often pathology within the thymus – thymic hyperplasia in young females and thymoma in older individuals.

Antibodies to ACh receptors are present in 90% of patients, providing a diagnostic test. The antibody titre does not correlate with the severity of the disease. In pregnant patients the antibody may cross the placenta, causing transient neonatal myasthenia gravis.

### Eaton–Lambert Syndrome

Unlike myasthenia gravis, in this syndrome muscle weakness improves with repeated exercise. An antibody to presynaptic structures prevents release of ACh at the nerve terminal. There is a strong association with malignancy, notably small cell carcinoma of the lung.

## SUMMARY

- Locomotor diseases, principally osteoporosis and arthritis, are a major source of morbidity, especially in middle-aged and elderly individuals, and thus have an economic cost for society.
- Recent scientific studies have done much to elucidate the mechanisms that control bone turnover in metabolic diseases such as osteoporosis and Paget's disease, and this will open avenues for new targeted therapies.

- Similar advances are being made in the biology of inflammatory joint diseases such as rheumatoid arthritis, again with prospects for treatment.
- Infections of bone and joint are far less common than in the past but awareness is important to allow early diagnosis and treatment, which remain the key to preventing the tissue destruction and loss of function that characterize these diseases in the later stages.
- Metastatic carcinomas are common in bone and cause bone destruction and major symptoms, especially in those patients in the later stages of malignancy.
- In contrast, primary sarcomas of bone are rare, but those affected experience considerable morbidity and mortality.
- Most soft-tissue tumours are benign, but those that are deeply situated, larger than 5 cm, and symptomatic should be regarded as malignant until proven otherwise.
- Muscle disorders are uncommon conditions that fall into several groups including inflammatory myopathies and muscular dystrophies. For the latter, the molecular mechanisms are increasingly understood, thus offering opportunities for genetic screening and, potentially, novel therapies.

## FURTHER READING

Athanasou NA. *Colour Atlas of Bone, Joint and Soft Tissue Pathology*. Oxford: Oxford University Press, 1999.

Fletcher CDM, Bridge JA, Hogendoorn P, Mertens F. *World Health Organization Classification of Tumours of Soft Tissue and Bone*. Lyon: IARC Press, 2013.

Goldblum JR, Weiss SW, Folpe AL. *Enzinger and Weiss's Soft Tissue Tumors*, 6th edn. St Louis, MO: Mosby, 2013.

# 13

# THE KIDNEYS AND URINARY TRACT

Stewart Fleming

## CLINICAL FEATURES OF RENAL DISEASE

### Key Points

- Renal diseases are common and account for a considerable amount of morbidity and mortality.
- The main manifestations can be divided into several distinct types of clinical presentation.

The diseases of the kidney are complex but illustrate many of the principles of inflammatory disease, immunologically mediated disease, genetically determined disease, vascular disease, and malignancy.

Heavy proteinuria in excess of 3 g/24 h (urine albumin:creatinine ratio >300 mg/mmol) results in hypo-albuminaemia and generalized oedema; these three features together constitute the *nephrotic syndrome*. Hyperlipidaemia is an almost invariable accompaniment and hypertension and impaired renal function may be present. The proteinuria is due to increased glomerular permeability resulting from a variety of glomerular diseases. In addition to generalized oedema there may be ascites and pleural effusions. There is increased susceptibility to infection and thrombosis including a risk of renal vein thrombosis.

The *acute nephritic syndrome* is most frequently seen in acute proliferative glomerulonephritis. The clinical features are diffuse oedema including the facial region, hypertension, and oliguria. Urinary examination reveals proteinuria, haematuria, and the presence of red cell casts.

*Asymptomatic proteinuria* may result from the same diseases that cause the nephrotic syndrome, the main difference being that the proteinuria is of insufficient severity to cause hypoalbuminaemia and oedema. It is usually detected during a routine medical examination.

*Painless haematuria* may result from intrinsic renal disease, diseases of the collecting system and bladder, and malignancy in the urinary tract. Microscopic examination of the urine, renal imaging, and cystoscopy may be helpful in localizing the site and cause of blood loss.

*Hypertension* (see Chapter 6, pp. 129–133) is usually idiopathic or essential in type but in a significant proportion of cases it is due to underlying parenchymal renal disease. The prevalence of hypertension varies among the different types of primary renal disease, and in advanced renal failure it may be as high as 80%. Hypertension is not only a consequence of renal disease but also a major cause of the progression of renal damage in a variety of different forms of intrinsic renal disease.

*Renal failure*, classified as either acute or chronic, has a large number of causes. In acute renal failure there is an abrupt deterioration in renal function occurring over a period of hours or days. It may be classified as:

- prerenal – due to inadequate perfusion after circulatory collapse
- renal – due to renal parenchymal disease/damage
- postrenal – due to obstructive disorders of the urinary tract.

Chronic renal failure develops over a period of weeks, months, or years. The consequences of a reduction in adequate renal function are a variety of complications due to the retention of waste products, impaired water, electrolyte and acid–base balance, loss of erythropoietin production, impaired vitamin D metabolism, activation of the renin–angiotensin system, and the development of hypertension.

# PROGRESSION OF RENAL DISEASE

## Key Points

- Progression of renal disease is associated with a number of factors.
- Reduced renal mass may lead to hyperfiltration injury in the remaining glomeruli.
- Tubulointerstitial damage may be due to proteinuria and local ischaemia.
- Chronic renal failure is a gradual reduction in the glomerular filtration rate.
- An international classification describes five stages of chronic kidney disease.

A number of factors may be important in the progression of renal disease from acute presentation to chronic renal disease, chronic renal impairment, and end-stage renal failure. Coexisting arterial disease, hypertension, persistent activity of the original disease, and some genetic factors may be important in determining the rate of progression. A reduction in nephron mass that reduces the glomerular filtration of the blood to about 30–50% of normal may result in progressive renal damage independent of continuing activity of the underlying disease. The secondary factors leading to progression are of major clinical interest because they may provide an opportunity to interrupt the cycle, which leads to established renal failure. Two main histological characteristics are seen, namely focal glomerulosclerosis and tubulointerstitial inflammation, and fibrosis (Fig. 13.1).

Glomerulosclerosis appears to develop as part of the response to glomerular hyperfiltration, which occurs as a compensatory response to maintain renal function. The consequence of this glomerular hyperfiltration is compensatory hypertrophy and haemodynamic changes leading to endothelial and epithelial cell injury, with increasing glomerular permeability to protein and increasing deposition of mesangial matrix. Many mediators of chronic inflammation

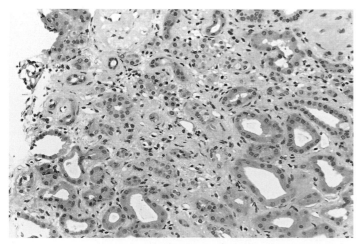

**Fig. 13.1** The renal parenchyma in end-stage renal failure is characterized by extensive glomerulosclerosis, tubular atrophy, and hypertrophic and hyaline changes in the arteries and arterioles. Virtually no functioning renal parenchyma remains.

and fibrosis, particularly transforming growth factor β (TGF-β), are thought to have a role in the progressive glomerular damage and loss. There is convincing evidence that a protective effect may be obtained by reducing intraglomerular pressure with angiotensin-converting enzyme inhibitors or angiotensin receptor blockade. Tubulointerstitial damage, as evidenced by tubular atrophy, interstitial inflammation, and interstitial fibrosis, is now recognized to be a major prognostic factor in the progression of a variety of different renal diseases. Many factors may lead to tubular injury, including urinary protein, urinary complement, and immunoglobulins, cytokines liberated into the urinary filtrate or the interstitium, or local haemodynamic factors leading to relative ischaemia. The end-result of expansion of the interstitial fibroblast population, and in particular expansion of the interstitial extracellular matrix, is a feature of the irreversible progression of renal disease.

## Chronic Renal Failure

Chronic renal failure results when the functions of the kidneys have been so reduced by a chronic disease process that there is retention of nitrogenous waste products normally excreted in the urine. This reduction in glomerular filtration rate can be detected by measurement of urea and creatinine in the blood or creatinine clearance from analysis of blood and 24-hour urine samples.

The estimated glomerular filtration rate (eGFR), a laboratory calculation taking into account the serum creatinine, age, sex, and race of the individual, is now the most common method of reporting renal function in adults. Using eGFR there are five recognized stages of chronic kidney disease (CKD) ranging from CKD 1 (in which eGFR is normal but there is other evidence of kidney disease such as proteinuria, chronic glomerulonephritis, calculi, scarring, or polycystic kidneys) to CKD 5 (in which eGFR <15 mL/min per 1.73 m$^2$ or the patient is undergoing chronic dialysis or has received a kidney transplant) (*Table 13.1*). Patients with stage 5 CKD are said to have 'established renal failure', a term that has replaced 'end-stage renal failure'. Patients with stage 5 CKD who are being treated by dialysis or have a functioning kidney transplant are said to be on 'renal replacement therapy'.

CKD is common, being present in as many as 10% of the population, and the incidence increases with increasing age.

**TABLE 13.1** Classification of chronic kidney disease (CKD) by estimated glomerular filtration rate (eGFR)

| CKD stage | eGFR (mL/min per 1.73 m$^2$) |
|---|---|
| 1 With another abnormality (e.g. proteinuria) | >90 |
| 2 With another abnormality (e.g. proteinuria) | 60–89 |
| 3 | 30–59 |
| 4 | 15–29 |
| 5 | <15 |

The most common cause of CKD, particularly in elderly people, is ischaemic nephropathy due to hypertension or vascular disease. The identification of ischaemic nephropathy is important because, even in its milder stages, it is associated with an increased risk of cardiovascular death. As renal function deteriorates further the toxicity of nitrogenous waste products, the loss of homeostasis of fluid, electrolyte and acid–base balance, and disturbances in the endocrine functions of the kidney all result in important effects. Many disease processes may lead to chronic renal failure (*Box 13.1*) and their pathological characteristics are described in the appropriate sections of this chapter. The biochemical, clinical, and morphological changes that accompany chronic renal failure, irrespective of the underlying primary renal disease, are described below.

## Nitrogenous Waste Products

The clinical features of waste product retention are those of chronic poisoning; they become more pronounced as renal function declines. Patients with CKD 4 and 5 complain of non-specific symptoms such as tiredness, lethargy, and anorexia. Platelet function is abnormal, leading to easy bruising and bleeding from the gastrointestinal tract, and disturbances of the immune system predispose to infection. In advanced renal failure fibrinous pericarditis and pneumonitis, consisting of a serofibrinous exudate in the alveolar spaces, may be present. The pulmonary changes resemble those of neonatal hyaline membrane disease, but there is often partial organization of the exudate. The effects on the nervous system include peripheral neuropathy, poor concentration, sleep disturbance, and ultimately coma, but there are few obvious pathological changes in the brain.

## Sodium and Water Balance

In chronic renal failure the kidney's inability to control salt and water balance can lead to either overhydration or dehydration. In most patients, sodium and fluid retention occur, leading to hypertension and peripheral and pulmonary oedema. Less commonly, but particularly where the primary renal disorder is tubular or interstitial (e.g. calculus disease), sodium and fluid depletion will occur unless a high salt and

---

**Box 13.1** CAUSES OF CHRONIC RENAL FAILURE

- Diabetes mellitus
- Glomerulonephritis
- Renovascular disease/hypertension
- Reflux nephropathy
- Renal calculi
- Obstructive uropathy
- Polycystic kidney disease
- Systemic vasculitis (e.g. systemic lupus erythematosus, Henoch–Schönlein purpura)
- Myeloma
- Amyloidosis
- Other diseases

---

fluid intake is maintained. Loss of urinary-concentrating function due to tubular damage, combined with the osmotic diuretic effect of high concentrations of nitrogenous waste products such as urea, explains the relatively fixed output of dilute urine occurring in chronic renal failure.

## Acid–Base Balance and Electrolyte Disturbances

To conserve acid–base balance the kidneys must excrete 40–60 mmol of acid ($H^+$) daily. In chronic renal failure total ammonia production and acid secretion into the tubules are reduced and there is also some urinary loss of bicarbonate, which is normally completely reabsorbed. As a result of these changes the patient with chronic renal failure is prone to develop acidosis. In renal failure, chronic acidosis may cause tissue catabolism, which results in deterioration of nutritional status and may aggravate renal bone disease.

Excessive potassium and phosphate, generated by dietary intake or protein breakdown, are normally excreted by the kidney. In chronic renal failure potassium retention may occur and be exacerbated by acidosis, resulting in the exchange of intracellular potassium for hydrogen ions. Hyperkalaemia may cause muscle stiffness and abdominal pain but is often asymptomatic until potentially fatal cardiac arrhythmias develop. Hyperphosphataemia occurs in later renal failure resulting in calcium phosphate deposition (metastatic calcification) in the soft tissues, particularly in the arterial wall, periarticular tissues, and conjunctivae. Pruritus is a frequent symptom in patients with advanced renal failure and calcium phosphate deposition in the skin is thought to contribute to this. These abnormalities in calcium phosphate balance are compounded by impaired activation of 25-hydroxy-vitamin D in the kidney (see below) and lead to secondary hyperparathyroidism.

## Endocrine Disturbances

The principal endocrine functions of the kidney concern bone metabolism, erythropoiesis, and blood pressure control. Renal bone disease or renal osteodystrophy describes the various bone changes occurring in renal failure as a result of impaired activation of vitamin D, altered calcium phosphate balance, and secondary hyperparathyroidism. These include osteitis fibrosis cystica, osteomalacia, and osteoporosis (see Chapter 12).

Anaemia is a common feature of chronic renal failure and occurs principally as a result of a lack of adequate production of erythropoietin from the peritubular cells of the renal cortex. This secondary anaemia contributes to the symptoms of tiredness and poor exercise tolerance in renal failure and can be corrected by subcutaneous or intravenous recombinant erythropoietin treatment.

In chronic renal failure the renin–angiotensin–aldosterone system is inappropriately activated, resulting in hypertension. The renal changes resulting from hypertension cause further injury to the already damaged kidneys and hasten the onset of renal failure. Hypertension may also contribute to left ventricular hypertrophy and vascular disease with resultant cardiac failure, and the risk of serious cardio-vascular events. Effective antihypertensive drug therapy can protect against this damage and extend the longevity of the failing kidney.

## GENETICALLY DETERMINED RENAL DISEASE

The two main groups of genetically determined renal disease of note are polycystic kidney disease and genetic abnormalities of the glomerular basement membrane. Polycystic kidney disease occurs in two main forms. Autosomal dominant polycystic kidney disease (ADPKD) is the most common form of cystic renal disease and one of the most common genetic diseases in the community, affecting approximately 1:500 to 1:1,000 individuals. It accounts for about 10% of patients requiring renal replacement therapy. The disease is genetically heterogeneous and is caused by germline mutation in one of three separate genes: the *polycystin 1* gene, which is located on the short arm of chromosome 16 and accounts for 85% of cases; the *polycystin 2* gene on the long arm of chromosome 4 (10–14% of cases); and a third polycystic kidney disease gene, the location of which has yet to be identified, and that is responsible for a minority of cases. These genes regulate the action of the primary cilium and cell polarity. The cysts sometimes cause pain and haematuria but many of the patients with ADPKD remain asymptomatic until adult life. Then there may be a progressive deterioration in renal function, usually during the third or fourth decade, leading to established renal failure, particularly in those with untreated hypertension. The kidneys contain large numbers of cysts and may expand to weigh more than 1 kg (Fig. 13.2). The cysts may be several centimetres in diameter and contain serous or blood-stained fluid. Cysts are present throughout the nephron (Fig. 13.3).

Autosomal recessive polycystic kidney disease (ARPKD) is much less common but leads to renal failure in infancy or early childhood. ARPKD is caused by a genetic mutation in the *PKHD1* gene, which encodes the protein fibrocystin. In ARPKD there is less severe renal enlargement and the cysts are limited to dilatation of the collecting ducts. Those patients who survive infancy develop hepatic fibrosis and, with age, the liver complications become more significant.

The major genetically determined abnormality of the glomerular basement membrane is Alport's syndrome. This disease usually shows an X-linked pattern of inheritance and is associated with mutation in the type IV collagen genes responsible for encoding the proteins that make up the glomerular basement membrane. Alport's syndrome may present in the first and second decades with proteinuria, haematuria, and progressive renal failure but this may be delayed until later life. Males are often more severely affected than females. The disease is diagnosed by characteristic electron microscopic appearances of the glomerular basement membrane (Fig. 13.4), but can also be confirmed

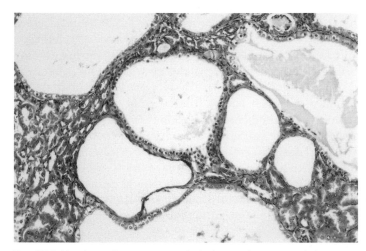

**FIG. 13.3** Histological examination of a kidney with autosomal dominant polycystic kidney disease shows cysts developing from all parts of the nephron. Intervening parenchyma is compressed and shows progressive ischaemia and hypertensive damage.

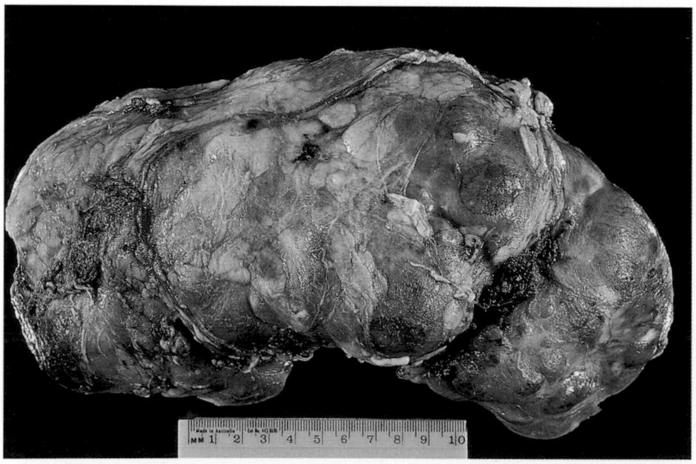

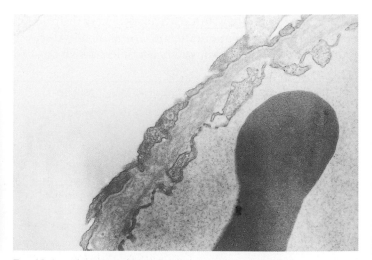

**FIG. 13.2** Autosomal dominant polycystic kidney disease: in this disease the kidney is enormously enlarged with cysts throughout the renal parenchyma. Many of these cysts will be up to several centimetres in diameter. Haemorrhage and infection within cysts is common.

**FIG. 13.4** In Alport's syndrome there is a genetic abnormality of type IV collagen, which is an essential part of the glomerular basement membrane. As a consequence there is a failure of basement membrane assembly with the appearance of multilayering and fragmentation.

by genotyping. It is usually accompanied by high-frequency nerve deafness and sometimes ocular abnormalities.

# GLOMERULAR DISEASE

## Glomerulonephritis

### Key Points

- Glomerulonephritis encompasses a group of renal diseases in which the lesions are primarily glomerular, other changes in the kidney being secondary to glomerular injury.
- When the mononuclear phagocyte system is not able to remove circulating immune complexes, some will deposit in the glomerular capillaries.
- Glomerular subendothelial immune complexes damage the glomerulus in at least two ways.
- The major histological features of immune complex glomerular injury are hypercellularity, thickening of the glomerular wall, and crescent formation.

### *Pathogenesis*

Most cases of glomerulonephritis are due to injury caused by the presence of antigen–antibody complexes in the glomeruli. These immune complexes may localize within the glomeruli in the following ways:

- Circulating immune complexes may be filtered out in the glomerular capillaries.
- Antibodies may form to constituents of the glomerular basement membrane, to which such antibodies become bound.
- Circulating antibodies may react with non-basement membrane glomerular antigens, or antigens from the plasma that have become trapped within the glomerulus to form immune complexes *in situ*.
- In some instances non-antibody substances within the glomeruli may activate complement via the alternative pathway and cause glomerular damage without antibody deposition.

### Factors Influencing Deposition of Immune Complexes within Glomeruli

The kidney receives a relatively large blood supply and the glomeruli are unusual in that their capillaries lie between two arterioles; as a consequence, the glomerular capillary pressure is much greater than in most other capillary beds. In addition, the normal glomerular capillary wall acts as a progressive sieve: very small molecules and ions pass freely through the endothelial layer, basement membrane, and epithelial slit pores to appear in the glomerular filtrate, but cells and very large molecular aggregates are kept within the vascular tree by the pore size of the endothelial cells. Between these two extremes, macromolecules and antigen–antibody

complexes can penetrate into the glomerular capillary wall (Fig. 13.5). The depth of such penetration depends not only on molecular size, but also on their shape and charge.

The mononuclear phagocyte system removes foreign material and large protein aggregates from the blood. In normal circumstances it may remove most of the circulating immune complexes. If the system is presented with an excess of such complexes or if its activity is depressed, e.g. by infections, drugs, or neoplasia, then it may be incapable of clearing the blood of circulating immune complexes and some will deposit in the glomerular capillaries. Other factors include the release of vasoactive agents, which increase the permeability of the glomerular (and other) capillaries, and treatment with glucocorticoids, which, by contrast, impede the transfer of macromolecules across the basement membrane.

### Mechanisms of Glomerular Injury by Immune Complexes

The presence of glomerular subendothelial immune complexes causes damage in at least two ways. The immune complexes activate the complement cascade, with production of the C5–9 lytic complex, which damages the adjacent cells and basement membranes. In addition, products of complement activation, notably C5a, increase capillary permeability and are chemotactic for neutrophil polymorphs and monocytes, which in consequence accumulate in the lesion. These cells phagocytose immune complexes but, in doing so, secrete numerous lysosomal enzymes, some of which can degrade cell and basement membranes. There may be local activation of the coagulation cascade, either secondary to complement activation or by cell damage, with the release of various enzymes and protein breakdown products. This leads to deposition of fibrin in the lumen and walls of the glomerular capillaries. Early administration of anticoagulants in experimental immune complex nephritis has been shown to prevent some of the glomerular injury. If the injury to the glomerular capillaries is severe, components of the clotting

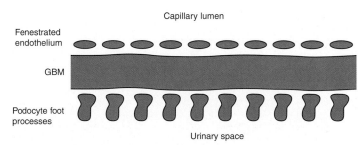

**FIG. 13.5** The glomerulus is a specialized capillary bed with close approximation of the endothelium and the epithelium (podocytes) separated only by a thin glomerular basement membrane (GBM). The endothelium is fenestrated to allow the free passage of macromolecules. The GBM is a product of both the endothelial and epithelial cells. The podocytes have specialist filtration structures called foot processes, which align themselves on the GBM. This specialized capillary bed is supported by modified smooth muscle cells called mesangial cells. The latter are also phagocytic and have a major role in determining the intraglomerular pressure. Filtration occurs from the capillary lumen into the urinary filtration space.

system may escape into Bowman's space where deposition of fibrin promotes the formation of cellular aggregates or crescents, which further impair glomerular function.

## Glomerular Manifestations of Immune Complex Injury

The major histological features of immune complex glomerular injury can be explained by the pathogenic mechanism:

● Hypercellularity is due to an increase in the number of glomerular cells, and the arrest and emigration of neutrophil polymorphs and monocytes in response to immune complex deposition, activation of complement, and endothelial injury (Fig. 13.6).

● Thickening of the glomerular capillary wall as seen by light microscopy (Fig. 13.7) has a variety of causes. Large subepithelial, intramembranous, or subendothelial deposits of immune complexes, swelling of the damaged epithelial or endothelial cells, or prolongation of long mesangial cell processes between the endothelium and basement membrane secondary to immune complex deposition can all give rise to a thickened capillary wall. Production of the basement membrane material by endothelial and epithelial cells may also be stimulated by the presence of immune complexes.

● Crescent formation: the escape of fibrin into Bowman's space stimulates the lining epithelial cells to divide and this, together with mononuclear phagocytes, produces a crescent-shaped mass of cells that compresses the glomerular tuft – hence the name of the lesion (Fig. 13.8).

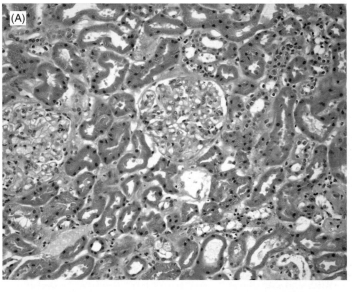

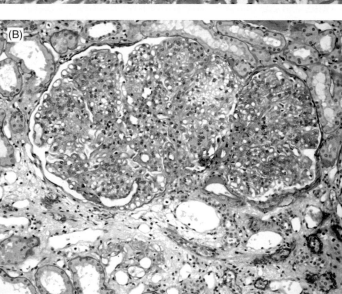

FIG. 13.6 (A) Normal glomeruli; (B) these glomeruli show an increase in cellularity due to proliferation of endogenous glomerular cells, predominantly mesangial cells, and infiltration of the glomerulus by inflammatory cells.

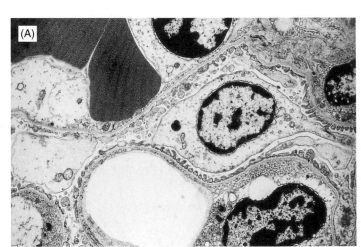

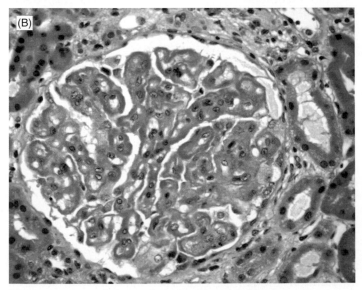

FIG. 13.7 (A) Normal glomerular basement membrane shown by electron microscopy. (B) The glomerular basement membrane here shown by light microscopy is markedly thickened, a feature seen in a variety of diseases including membranous glomerulonephritis and diabetic nephropathy.

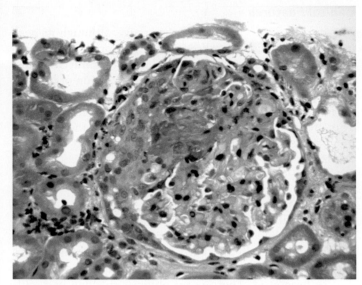

FIG. 13.8 A crescent is a proliferation of macrophages and epithelial cells within Bowman's space but outwith the glomerular capillary bed.

The above changes may affect all glomeruli (diffuse) or only some glomeruli (focal) and they may involve the whole glomerulus (global) or part of the glomerulus (segmental).

## Classification

Although the following description is not comprehensive it covers the major clinically important glomerulonephritides. Certain systemic diseases, e.g. systemic lupus erythematosus (SLE), diabetes mellitus, and amyloidosis, can give rise to glomerular lesions resulting in clinical syndromes resembling one or other type of glomerulonephritis.

## Minimal-change Nephropathy

### Key Points

- Minimal-change nephropathy is the most common cause of the nephrotic syndrome in children but it can also occur in adults.
- Spontaneous remission and recurrences are common.
- Hypertension and renal impairment are usually absent.
- There are a few histological changes.

### General Features

Minimal-change nephropathy has a peak incidence in children aged between 1 and 5 years, but occurs in children and adults of all ages. As usual, in the nephrotic syndrome, there is a rise in the level of blood lipids, including cholesterol, and a predisposition to infection, thrombosis, and thromboembolism. The proteinuria is due to increased glomerular capillary permeability, and is usually highly selective, albumin being accompanied by much smaller amounts of the plasma proteins than the less-selective proteinuria observed in most renal diseases, with or without the nephrotic syndrome. A short course of high-dose glucocorticoid therapy will usually induce remission of the nephrotic syndrome and, although further relapses may occur, this form of glomerulonephritis does not progress to renal failure.

### Pathological Changes

Microscopically, the glomeruli look normal apart from an appearance of dilatation of the capillaries; there is no thickening of the capillary walls and no increased cellularity of the glomerular tufts. The most conspicuous glomerular change on electron microscopy is effacement of the foot processes of the epithelial cells, the basement membrane being covered externally by a layer of epithelial cell cytoplasm; the epithelial cells also show an increase in surface activity with the production of microvillous processes (Fig. 13.9).

### Aetiology

The nature of this disease remains unknown. Immunofluorescence studies on the glomeruli are negative for immunoglobulins and complement. The disease is occasionally associated with routine prophylactic immunization, with hypersensitivity reactions (bee stings and asthma) and there is evidence that defects in T-cell function may be involved; this is supported by the occasional occurrence of the disease in patients with Hodgkin's disease or non-Hodgkin's lymphoma. It can also be associated with morbid obesity and a familial form has been described. Foot process effacement has been associated with loss of polyanion from the glomerular basement membrane, consequent change in electrical charge, and hence altered basement membrane permeability.

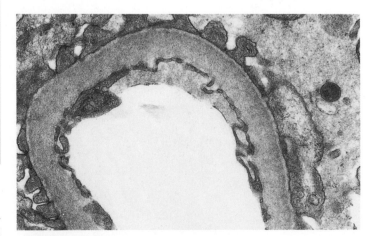

FIG. 13.9 In minimal-change nephropathy the light microscopic appearance of the glomerulus is normal. On examination by electron microscopy there is loss of the normal glomerular epithelial foot processes, known as foot process fusion, and there may be some vacuolation of the epithelium. No other abnormalities are seen in this disease.

## Focal Glomerulosclerosis

At one time thought to be a variant of minimal-change glomerulonephritis, focal glomerulosclerosis is now regarded as a distinct entity. The clinical features at presentation are similar to those of minimal-change glomerulonephritis, but proteinuria is *less selective* and *red cells* are more commonly present in the urine. Although most of the glomeruli appear normal, those close to the medulla show sclerosis, consisting of deposition of hyaline material with consequent obliteration of capillaries (Fig. 13.10). This change is at first segmental but gradually destroys the whole glomerulus and extends peripherally to involve more glomeruli. There is associated tubular atrophy. An unusual collapsing variant is seen in HIV infection.

Renal biopsy is diagnostic only if it includes some of the deeper, affected glomeruli. The condition is resistant to steroid therapy, although in some cases there may be an initial response. The prognosis is poor, many cases progressing to renal failure, although this may take a number of years, and the disease tends to recur in renal transplant recipients. Some patients in whom a diagnosis of minimal-change glomerulonephritis is made based on a superficial renal biopsy and who eventually develop chronic renal failure are really missed cases of focal segmental glomerulosclerosis.

## Diffuse Membranous Glomerulonephritis

### Key Points

- Diffuse membranous glomerulonephritis is more common in males than in females.
- It usually presents as the nephrotic syndrome with non-selective proteinuria and the urine often contains small numbers of red cells.
- The main histological change is diffuse hyaline thickening of the walls of all the glomerular capillaries.

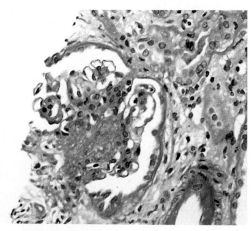

**FIG. 13.10** Focal segmental glomerulosclerosis is a disease in which there is fibrosis of part of the glomerular tuft, with only a proportion of the glomeruli affected. Within the affected segment there is obliteration of the capillary spaces, extracellular matrix accumulation, and sometimes the presence of foamy macrophages.

### Clinical Features

This disease occurs over a wide age range, although its peak incidence is in middle age. Idiopathic membranous glomerulonephritis shows a variable clinical course. Some cases may remit spontaneously but a significant proportion of patients pursue an indolent course for many months or years, ending in chronic renal failure. Treatment remains controversial. The effects of steroids and cytotoxic drugs on the course of the disease are uncertain and are still the subject of clinical trials.

### Pathological Changes

The essential change is in the glomerulus, and consists of a diffuse hyaline thickening of the walls of all the glomerular capillaries. In the early stages this is minimal and hard to detect, but it becomes increasingly obvious as the disease progresses. There is no obvious swelling or proliferation of endothelial or mesangial cells, and no leukocytic infiltration. By light microscopy the capillary walls appear thickened and eosinophilic, and hyaline and silver staining techniques give an appearance of spikes on the basement membrane. Immunofluorescence staining reveals immune complexes on the capillary wall. Electron microscopy shows irregular deposition of dense amorphous material in the outer subepithelial part of the glomerular basement membrane (Fig. 13.11). The laying down of new basement membrane between the deposits corresponds to the spikes seen by light microscopy of silver preparations. Eventually the basement membrane spikes thicken and unite to envelop the deposits and these are gradually replaced by basement membrane, which, in consequence, is considerably thickened and irregular.

In the chronic stage of the disease, the thickening of the glomerular capillary walls results in narrowing of the lumina; renal blood flow and glomerular filtration rate are seriously diminished, and uraemia and hypertension develop. Proteinuria diminishes, polyuria often develops, and the oedema tends to subside and may disappear. Microscopy of the kidneys at this stage shows gross diffuse thickening of glomerular capillary walls, some glomeruli being almost solid eosinophilic hyaline material, whereas others are less severely affected and still have some patent capillary lumina. Tubular atrophy secondary to ischaemia accompanies the glomerular hyalinization, and interstitial fibrosis occurs, but lipid deposits, indicative of the preceding nephrotic stage, may persist. The kidneys may be slightly shrunken and show the superadded changes of hypertension.

### Aetiology

Examination of renal biopsies by immunofluorescence microscopy shows deposition of immunoglobulin, usually mainly IgG, along the walls of the glomerular capillaries. The deposition is diffuse throughout all the capillaries and at an early stage appears granular. As the disease progresses the deposits increase in size and number and tend

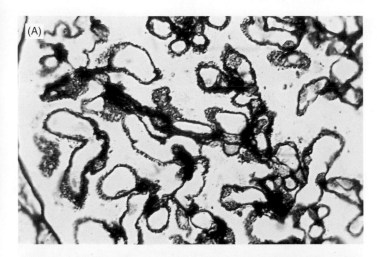

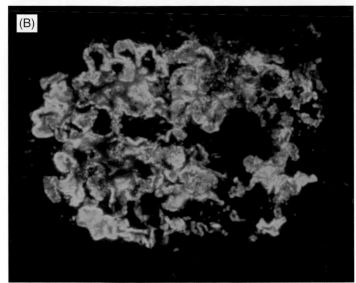

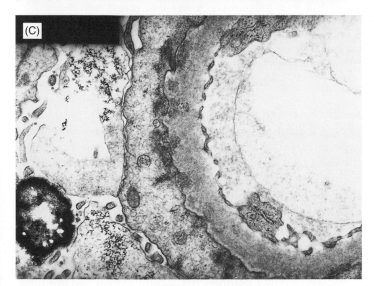

**FIG. 13.11** Membranous nephropathy is characterized by thickening of the glomerular capillary walls but with normal cellularity. (A) The thickened capillary walls exhibit a spiky appearance on silver-stained preparations. (B) Immunofluorescence staining reveals the presence of immune complexes, in this case IgM, within the capillary walls as granular deposits. (C) Electron microscopic examination reveals the presence of subepithelial electron-dense immune complexes.

to become confluent. Deposition of complement is also usually demonstrable by immunofluorescence, its distribution being the same as that of the immunoglobulin(s), but it is deposited in smaller amounts and in some cases is not detectable. The low level of complement deposition may be equated with the absence of inflammatory features (by contrast with acute post-infectious glomerulonephritis). There is evidence to suggest *in situ* formation of immune complexes in some types of membranous glomerulonephritis.

Autoantibodies directed against the podocyte membrane M-type phospholipase $A_2$ receptor ($PLA_2R$) are present in most cases of primary membranous glomerulonephritis. These antibodies are absent in secondary membranous glomerulonephritis, which may be associated with infections, such as malaria, syphilis, and hepatitis B, and their corresponding (microbial) antigens have been demonstrated in the glomerular deposits in such cases. There is also an association with malignant tumours, and the possibility of a lymphoma or carcinoma should be borne in mind in any middle-aged or elderly patient presenting with 'idiopathic' membranous glomerulonephritis. Membranous glomerulonephritis may also occur in patients treated with certain drugs, notably penicillamine and gold salts, and is also one of the renal manifestations of SLE. In all of these associations, the glomerular deposition of immunoglobulin suggests the involvement of immune complexes, the antigens being assumed to be derived from tumours, drugs, and so on. In patients with SLE, the deposits have been shown to consist of autoantigens complexed with autoantibodies (see Chapter 2, pp. 26–27).

## Mesangiocapillary (Membranoproliferative) Glomerulonephritis

This condition occurs at all ages but particularly in older children. Its presenting features may be those of the acute nephritic syndrome, nephrotic syndrome, or asymptomatic proteinuria and haematuria. Overall the prognosis is poor and most patients go on to develop chronic renal failure. The response to immunosuppression is poor, and if renal transplantation is performed the condition tends to recur in the graft.

### Pathological Changes

At an early stage the glomeruli show diffuse proliferative change with increase in size and number of mesangial and endothelial cells; the mesangia in particular show increased cellularity and the lobular architecture of the glomeruli is accentuated (Fig. 13.12). The capillary lumina are reduced and there is irregular thickening of the capillary walls. Silver stains may show a double basement membrane. Two main types are discernible by electron microscopy:

1. In type I, discrete irregular deposits are found on the inner, subendothelial, side of the (original) basement

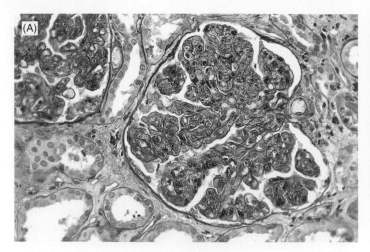

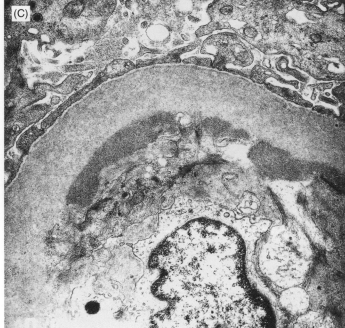

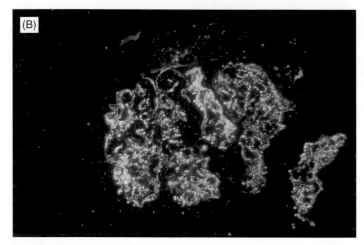

**FIG. 13.12** Mesangiocapillary glomerulonephritis, also known as membranoproliferative glomerulonephritis, is characterized by a combination of hypercellularity and capillary wall thickening. (A) At the light microscopy level the hypercellularity is seen clearly with accentuation of the glomerular lobular architecture and a reduction in the capillary luminal space. Thickening of the glomerular capillary wall is also evident. (B) Immunofluorescence staining in cases of mesangiocapillary glomerulonephritis reveals the deposition of granules of immune complexes within capillary walls and mesangial regions in most cases. In the example illustrated here the immunofluorescence reactivity demonstrates IgG deposition within the glomerulus. (C) Examination of cases of mesangiocapillary glomerulonephritis by electron microscopy reveals different patterns of deposition. In one form there is electron-dense thickening of the glomerular basement membrane itself. This form is known as dense deposit disease. The presence of focal electron-dense deposits in the subendothelial space as shown here is the much more common form.

membrane, and there is extension of the cytoplasm of mesangial cells between the endothelium and the basement membrane (mesangial interposition). A second layer of basement membrane is laid down between the endothelium and the mesangial cytoplasmic extension, thus accounting for the double contour seen in some silver-stained preparations.

2. In type II, dense material is deposited within the lamina densa, causing a more diffuse thickening of the basement membrane. This has sometimes led to the use of the term 'dense deposit disease' (Fig. 13.12).

A type III form of mesangiocapillary glomerulonephritis, with both subendothelial and subepithelial deposits, has also been described but is regarded as a variant of type I. The two patterns of deposition are sometimes distinguishable by light microscopy of very thin sections but are seen more

readily by electron microscopy. In some cases, particularly of type II disease, there is formation of small crescents in the capsule of occasional glomeruli. As the disease progresses the mesangial cells diminish in number and hyaline material accumulates, while the capillaries become progressively thickened so that glomerulosclerosis and chronic renal failure usually result.

## Aetiology

The aetiology of mesangiocapillary glomerulonephritis is unknown. In type I, components of complement and immunoglobulin (IgG and/or IgM) are detectable in the capillary walls (see Fig. 13.12) and it is likely that the disease is of an immune complex nature. Associations with subacute bacterial endocarditis, sickle cell disease, and hepatitis B have been described. In type II there is little evidence of immune complex deposition, although C3 may be found in the mesangium and around the tubules. In both types, there may be depression of C3 in the plasma and activation of the alternative pathway of complement is involved. A factor that activates C3 (the C3 nephritic factor) has been detected in the serum in some cases. It appears to be an autoantibody to the C3bBb complex of the alternative pathway (see Chapter 4, pp. 66).

A familial predisposition is likely in mesangiocapillary glomerulonephritis and, in particular, there is a syndrome linking partial lipodystrophy and type II disease.

## Focal Glomerulonephritis, including IgA Nephropathy

This may be defined as a glomerulonephritis affecting only a proportion of the glomeruli. The lesions usually involve only part of the glomerular tuft, and can therefore be described as focal and segmental. In most patients this will be due to IgA nephropathy and the clinical features are usually microscopic or macroscopic haematuria with or without asymptomatic proteinuria. In these patients with intermittent macroscopic haematuria, episodes may be precipitated by upper respiratory tract infections, heavy exercise, or certain foods/alcohol. This disease usually affects children and young adults, and for many the prognosis will be good, but long-term follow-up is advised to identify the subgroup of patients who go on to develop chronic renal failure. There is no proven specific effective treatment for this form of glomerulonephritis, although many studies have suggested that a variety of agents might be beneficial.

Focal glomerulonephritis may also accompany a number of other systemic diseases, notably subacute bacterial endocarditis (SBE), SLE, Henoch–Schönlein purpura, the microangiopathic form of polyarteritis, Wegener's granulomatosis, and Goodpasture's syndrome. It must be emphasized that focal glomerulonephritis is not the only renal lesion that occurs in these conditions: crescentic glomerulonephritis may develop in any of them, and is the usual lesion in Goodpasture's syndrome and the vasculitides.

### Pathological Changes

The glomerular lesion consists of a cellular proliferation, probably of mesangial cells, affecting the peripheral part of one or more lobules (Fig. 13.13), and in some cases accompanied by fibrinoid necrosis of capillary loops. Within the lesions, individual capillary lumina may be obliterated by eosinophilic thrombus, which blends with the necrotic capillary walls. Red cells may be present in the capsular space and the tubules, and there may also be some proliferation of the epithelial lining of Bowman's capsule, i.e. formation of small crescents. Lesions may occur in only a small proportion of glomeruli, or involve the majority. In patients with a long history, old scarred glomerular lesions are usually seen, often adherent to the capsule. In IgA nephropathy and Henoch–Schönlein purpura nephritis there is

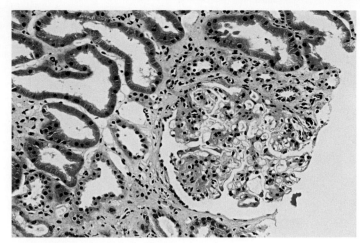

**FIG. 13.13** On occasion, proliferative glomerulonephritis is focal and segmental. In these instances the hypercellularity is limited to a portion of the glomerular tuft with obliteration of capillaries and occasionally foci of necrosis.

characteristic mesangial deposition of IgA on immunofluorescence staining.

## Acute Diffuse Proliferative Glomerulonephritis

### Clinical Features and Course

This type of glomerulonephritis occurs at all ages, although it is more prevalent in children than in adults, but it is now uncommon in developed countries. It usually follows an acute infection with group A haemolytic streptococci – most often pharyngitis (including scarlet fever), but sometimes infections of the middle ear or skin. Glomerulonephritis develops 1–4 weeks after the onset of the streptococcal infection, which has usually already resolved. Other infections, e.g. with *Staphylococcus aureus* and *Streptococcus pneumoniae*, have occasionally been implicated and acute glomerulonephritis may also complicate falciparum malaria, toxoplasmosis, schistosomiasis, and some acute viral infections.

The presenting features are usually those of an acute nephritic syndrome. Hypertension, moderate proteinuria, and mild renal impairment are usually present and urine microscopy reveals many red cells, neutrophil polymorphs, and hyaline, granular, and cellular casts. During the acute phase serious complications include acute renal failure and cardiac failure due to hypertension and fluid retention. In childhood the disease has a good outcome with complete recovery in over 90% of cases, but in adults the outcome is less favourable, a significant proportion developing chronic glomerulonephritis which leads to chronic renal failure.

### Pathological Features

Microscopically, the most conspicuous changes are diffuse enlargement and increased cellularity of the glomeruli

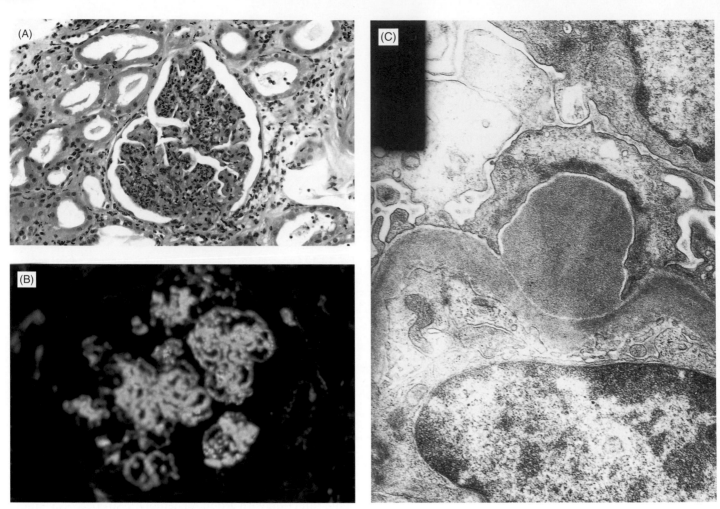

**FIG. 13.14** (A) In diffuse proliferative glomerulonephritis there is marked hypercellularity, often with an influx of neutrophil polymorphs and obliteration of the capillary spaces. The glomerular capillary walls are difficult to identify within this hypercellular glomerulus. (B) Immunofluorescence in these instances reveals the granular deposition of immune complexes in the capillary walls. (C) The electron microscopic findings in diffuse proliferative glomerulonephritis are highly characteristic. In the subepithelial space there are large 'hump'-shaped electron-dense deposits.

(Fig. 13.14A). The enlargement results in narrowing or obliteration of the capsular space and part of the glomerular tuft can often be seen to have herniated into the lumen of the proximal tubule. The capillary lumina appear narrowed, and the endothelial cells are swollen. Electron microscopy shows the hypercellularity to be the result of an increase of mesangial and endothelial cells; neutrophil polymorphs and macrophages are also seen but vary greatly in number from case to case.

An additional change in the glomerular tufts is an increase in the number of strands of basement membrane-like material demonstrable by electron microscopy in the mesangial regions. These strands are normally present between mesangial cells and are made more conspicuous by oedema. In cases that fail to resolve, the material increases in amount and contributes to the hyaline appearance of the glomeruli in the chronic stage of glomerulonephritis. Electron microscopy shows the presence of subepithelial 'humps' – deposits of electron-dense material that are indicative of immune complex formation (Fig. 13.14C). Smaller deposits may be seen on the endothelial surface of the basement membrane.

The epithelial cells do not show widespread effacement of foot processes, although this may occur focally. Some proteinaceous debris, and occasionally red cells, may be seen in the narrowed capsular spaces. In most cases, the epithelium of Bowman's capsule appears normal, but some proliferation may be seen. Epithelial crescents are few or absent in typical cases. Changes in the rest of the kidney are secondary to the glomerular lesion: there is diffuse oedema, seen as an increase in the loose interstitial tissue between the tubules, and often accompanied by a light scattering of neutrophil polymorphs or mononuclear cells. The tubules contain protein and cellular casts, including red blood cell casts, and the epithelial cells of the proximal convoluted tubules contain hyaline droplets. Occasionally there are foci of disruption of tubular epithelial cells, possibly attributable to ischaemia secondary to the glomerular changes. Hypertension is not usually sufficiently severe or prolonged to produce changes in the heart and blood vessels.

With recovery from the disease the glomeruli return to normal, although increased numbers of cells in the mesangial zones of the glomerular lobules may persist for months, and are regarded as a retrospective diagnostic feature. After acute diffuse glomerulonephritis, increase in the size and number of mesangial cells may persist for weeks or even months without serious sequelae. Increase in basement membrane-like material in the mesangial areas is, however, a more serious feature; it is seen together with persistent cellular increase in those few cases that, after a latent period, develop chronic glomerulonephritis.

### Pathogenesis

Immunofluorescence microscopy of renal biopsy material in cases of acute diffuse glomerulonephritis typically reveals granular deposition of immunoglobulin (usually mainly IgG) and components of complement in the glomerular capillary walls (see Fig. 13.14B). These findings, together with the detection by electron microscopy of dense subepithelial deposits, are strongly suggestive of the deposition of immune complexes. As acute glomerulonephritis usually follows a streptococcal infection it is likely that antibodies to streptococcal products, appearing a week or so after the infection, combine with streptococcal antigens still present in the plasma, thus providing immune complexes that would, at first, be formed in the presence of antigen excess. In keeping with this there are usually low levels of serum complement components, consistent with activation of complement by an antigen–antibody reaction, and serum antistreptolysin O (ASO) titres are usually high, indicating previous streptococcal infection. It is not understood why certain types of group A streptococci, notably Griffiths types 12, 4, 1, 25, and 49, are nephritogenic, whereas other types and other microorganisms are not.

## Crescentic Glomerulonephritis (Rapidly Progressive Glomerulonephritis)

This may develop without known predisposing cause, or follow a streptococcal infection. It can also supervene in patients with the focal glomerulonephritis associated with certain diseases, particularly vasculitis and Goodpasture's syndrome (see below). It can occur at any age, but is more common in elderly people. The clinical features and urinary changes may be indistinguishable at first from those of acute diffuse glomerulonephritis but, instead of regressing after a week or two, they become progressively more severe, leading to advanced renal failure after a period of days or weeks. Rarely, proteinuria may be severe enough to give rise to the nephrotic syndrome, whereas other cases may present in acute renal failure. Crescentic glomerulonephritis is uncommon but if diagnosed promptly immunosuppressive therapy can reverse or prevent renal failure.

### Pathological Changes

Microscopy shows the most important changes to be glomerular. As in acute diffuse glomerulonephritis, there is proliferation of both endothelial and mesangial cells, with narrowing of the capillary lumina, and variable polymorph infiltration of the tuft. Although all the glomeruli are affected, some glomerular lobules may be more severely involved than others, and there may be areas of basement membrane rupture with foci of haemorrhage and fibrinoid necrosis, and thrombi in some capillary lumina. Blood products may therefore escape into Bowman's space.

A characteristic histological feature is proliferation of the parietal epithelium of Bowman's capsule to form 'epithelial crescents' (see Fig. 13.8), which occupy the capsular space and surround the tuft. In time, the epithelial crescents are usually replaced by fibrous tissue. Immunofluorescence studies have failed to demonstrate immunoglobulins in crescents, but deposits of fibrin are present and have been shown experimentally to stimulate crescent formation.

The tubules may be dilated and usually contain hyaline and cellular casts and red cells, and proteinaceous droplets are present in the cells of the proximal convoluted tubules. There may be focal necrosis or irregular tubular atrophy and increase of intertubular connective tissue, presumably due to ischaemia resulting from the glomerular changes. In some cases hypertension is severe, and the changes of malignant hypertension become superadded. There may also be left ventricular hypertrophy and changes associated with uraemia, e.g. fibrinous pericarditis, anaemia, and superadded infections.

A surprising feature of the disease is the rapidity with which glomerular scarring may occur: thus in cases with a history of only 2 weeks or so, biopsy may reveal sclerosis of lobules or whole glomeruli, and also fibrous adhesions between the tuft and Bowman's capsule. There is thus a combination of glomerular proliferation, necrosis, thrombosis, and scarring, amounting to severe glomerular injury.

### Aetiology

The most common cause of crescentic glomerulonephritis is anti-neutrophil cytoplasmic antibody (ANCA)-associated vasculitis including microscopic polyangiitis and Wegener's granulomatosis. Renal biopsies show no evidence of immune complexes in the glomeruli but there is fibrin deposition within the necrotic glomerular segments. Patients with autoantibodies to the glomerular basement membrane (anti-GBM antibodies) develop Goodpasture's syndrome (see below), which is mostly frequently seen as a crescentic glomerulonephritis on renal biopsy. In the minority of cases, crescentic glomerulonephritis follows a streptococcal infection and these represent the severe end of the spectrum of acute diffuse proliferative glomerulonephritis. They show granular deposition of Ig and complement, and subepithelial deposits on electron microscopy.

## Subacute Bacterial Endocarditis

Renal lesions are common in SBE, but in most cases they do not lead to serious impairment of renal function and their practical importance lies mainly in the resulting haematuria, either gross or microscopic, which is of diagnostic value.

As in other organs, infarcts are common in the kidneys in SBE and are usually non-suppurative. Focal glomerulonephritis occurs in about 50% of cases, and tends to develop after some months. Most of the cases have been caused by *Streptococcus viridans* or *Haemophilus influenzae* but now *S. aureus* is a recognized cause of a more acute endocarditis, particularly in intravenous drug abusers. Microscopically, a minority of the glomeruli are usually affected, and the focal lesions show capillary thrombosis, fibrinoid necrosis, and proliferative changes. Blood is often seen in the capsular space and tubules, and there may be epithelial crescents. In keeping with an immune complex-mediated lesion, the serum complement levels are depressed, electron microscopy shows the presence of subendothelial and mesangial deposits, and immunofluorescence studies confirm the presence of immunoglobulin. Circulating immune complexes have been demonstrated by some workers. In a minority of patients with SBE, diffuse proliferative glomerulonephritis develops, and may progress to renal failure.

## Henoch–Schönlein Purpura

Henoch–Schönlein purpura occurs mainly in children, and gives rise to a skin rash, joint pains, and colic with bloody diarrhoea due to a haemorrhagic exudate into the gut. In some cases there is a focal glomerulonephritis, with haematuria and proteinuria, and this is associated with the mesangial deposition of IgA (these histological appearances are indistinguishable from IgA nephropathy). Renal failure is either absent or mild and transient, and the kidneys usually recover completely, even after recurrent attacks. Crescentic glomerulonephritis may, however, supervene, particularly in older patients, and in some other cases chronic renal failure develops after some years. Immunosuppression is of doubtful value in this form of focal nephritis except in those cases presenting with a rapidly progressive glomerulonephritis.

## Goodpasture's Syndrome

In this uncommon condition (see Special Study Topic 13.1), there is haematuria and proteinuria attributable to a focal glomerulonephritis. This is accompanied by haemorrhage from the alveolar capillaries which gives rise to haemoptysis and dyspnoea. The glomerular and pulmonary injuries are caused by autoantibodies to basement membrane collagen IV, which, in the kidney, produce a necrotizing and crescentic glomerulonephritis (Fig. 13.15A) with linear deposition of immunoglobulin on the basement membrane (Fig. 13.15B). The prognosis is poor without early treatment with plasma exchange and cytotoxic drugs.

## Systemic Lupus Erythematosus

Clinically apparent renal disease occurs in up to 50% of patients with SLE (see Chapter 2, pp. 26–27), and carries a poor prognosis. The nephrotic syndrome may develop when

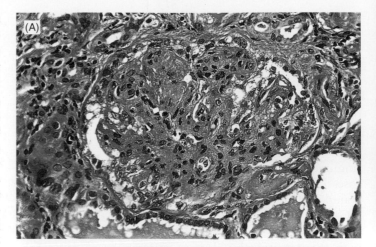

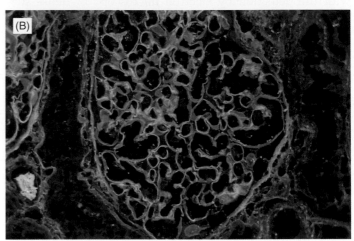

**FIG. 13.15** (A) In Goodpasture's syndrome there is a focal proliferative and necrotizing glomerulonephritis usually accompanied by crescent formation. (B) Immunofluorescence staining of renal biopsies demonstrates a linear pattern of deposition of IgG and C3 diagnostic of anti-glomerular basement membrane antibodies.

proteinuria is heavy, and uraemia, with or without hypertension, is an important cause of death. The essential changes are in the glomeruli, which show a great variety of lesions. These include:

- focal glomerulonephritis, which is indistinguishable from the proliferative and necrotizing lesions described above, except that haematoxyphil bodies are sometimes apparent
- a focal thickening of the capillary walls with a refractile eosinophilic appearance, known as the wire-loop lesion
- hyaline thrombi in individual glomerular capillaries
- various combinations of diffuse proliferative and irregular membranous change
- diffuse membranous change resembling that seen in idiopathic membranous glomerulonephritis.

Lupus nephropathy is classified on the basis of the glomerular morphology according to well-established World Health Organization (WHO) criteria (*Table 13.2*). The duration of these various lesions, and thus the degree of

## 13.1 Special Study Topic

### GOODPASTURE'S SYNDROME

Goodpasture's syndrome is a clinical syndrome involving acute renal failure, often with pulmonary haemorrhage. It is therefore one of the so-called pulmonary–renal syndromes. The acute renal failure is usually seen in association with proteinuria and haematuria. The disease is more common in elderly people. Renal biopsy shows a proliferative necrotizing glomerulonephritis usually with a high proportion of crescents. When renal biopsy material is stained by the immunofluorescence technique to demonstrate immune complexes, a linear pattern of IgG and staining for the C3 component of complement are seen on the GBM. Patients with Goodpasture's syndrome also have antibodies within their circulation that react with the GBM. These observations have led to the hypothesis that Goodpasture's syndrome is an autoimmune disease in which the patient mounts an antibody response to the constitutive components of the GBM. The GBM is an extracellular matrix comprising a number of collagens and non-collagenous glycoproteins. The autoantibodies from patients with Goodpasture's syndrome react with the type IV collagen within the basement and specifically the non-collagenous domain of the $\alpha_3$ chain of type IV collagen. The autoantibodies bind to the extracellular matrix and, within the glomerulus, activate complement leading to a localized type II hypersensitivity reaction. The disease is therefore an example of an antibody-mediated autoimmune disease that causes tissue damage through a type II hypersensitivity reaction.

Genetic factors play an important role in the aetiology of Goodpasture's syndrome and there is a strong association between the formation of anti-GBM antibodies and human leukocyte antigen (HLA)-DR2 alleles. During the induction of immune responses, antigens are presented to immunocompetent cells on the surface of macrophages in association with HLA molecules. In Goodpasture's syndrome, it has been suggested that antigenic fragments from type IV collagen presented by individuals with the appropriate HLA-DR2 alleles differ from those presented by individuals who are not susceptible to the disease. Goodpasture's syndrome is therefore a good model of antibody-mediated autoimmune disease in which there is an HLA association that determines the pattern of presentation of the autoantigen. Precisely what triggers this immune response is unclear but there is an association with hydrocarbon exposure and hydrocarbon-induced damage to the GBM.

**TABLE 13.2** WHO classification of lupus nephritis

| I | No lesion by light microscopy |
|---|---|
| II | Mesangial proliferation |
| III | Focal (<50%) proliferation |
| IV | Diffuse (>50%) proliferation |
| V | Membranous |
| (VI) | Chronic renal damage |

glomerular sclerosis, also varies greatly. Immunofluorescence and electron microscopy provide strong evidence that these glomerular changes represent the spectrum of immune complex injury, e.g. the focal lesion is accompanied by deposition of immunoglobulin and complement in the mesangium and focally in the inner parts of the capillary walls; more extensive deposition of complexes in the inner parts of the capillary walls is seen in the combination of diffuse proliferative and patchy membranous change, whereas the diffuse granular pattern of deposition, much of it along the outer part of the basement membrane, is seen in the diffuse membranous lesion. Antibodies to DNA, histones, and DNA–histone complexes have been eluted from the kidney tissue in SLE. Curious tubuloreticular structures are sometimes seen by electron microscopy in the endothelial cells. Originally thought to be viral, they are now considered to represent a response to injury by various agents, including virus infection. They are found most commonly in SLE although they have been described in other conditions, e.g. in HIV-associated nephropathy.

## Chronic Glomerulonephritis

It is apparent from the preceding descriptions of the various types of glomerulonephritis that an end-stage may be reached in which total glomerular function is so reduced that chronic renal failure develops. The time taken to reach this stage, and the rate of progression once it has developed, varies with the type of preceding glomerulonephritis. Hypertension, sometimes of the malignant type, usually develops and if untreated aggravates the renal tissue destruction. In cases where hypertension is absent or less severe, renal failure may progress more slowly. Chronic renal failure usually occurs because most of the nephrons have been so severely damaged by the causal disease that they are no longer functional. The remaining functioning glomeruli not only become hypertrophied but also filter off a relatively high proportion of the fluid passing through them. This hyperfunctioning state may itself cause further glomerular injury and consequently further deterioration of renal function.

In most patients with chronic glomerulonephritis, there is no history to suggest preceding renal disease, and the renal lesions have progressed silently until chronic renal failure develops. In such cases, it is often not possible to decide, even by histological examination of the kidneys, what type of glomerulonephritis has led to the chronic stage. In other cases, there is a history of previous glomerulonephritis: this may have been an acute attack of post-streptococcal glomerulonephritis years before, or the patient may have had membranous, mesangiocapillary or recurrent focal glomerulonephritis, which has progressed to the stage of chronic renal failure.

### Pathological Changes and Pathogenesis

Both the kidneys are uniformly and equally reduced in size, sometimes only slightly so, but often to about a third of normal. In those kidneys that are greatly shrunken, the capsule is often firmly adherent and the subcapsular surface uniformly and finely irregular. There is diffuse thinning of the cortex, which accounts largely for the reduction in kidney size, while the medullary pyramids are also, although less markedly, shrunken. The amount of fatty tissue around the renal pelvis is increased. In contrast to chronic pyelonephritis, the calyces and renal pelvis are not distorted.

The renal arteries and their major branches show arteriosclerotic thickening, and in cases complicated by malignant hypertension the cortical mottling and haemorrhages of this condition are superimposed on the changes described above. The other organs and tissues show the changes of chronic renal failure.

Microscopically, in the small granular kidneys, it is common to find all degrees of hyalinization of glomeruli. Many are completely hyalinized and some show partial destruction. A small percentage is normal or nearly so, and may be hypertrophied. In cases in which the kidneys are not greatly shrunken the glomeruli are usually more uniformly damaged: this is seen in the chronic end-stages of membranous and mesangiocapillary glomerulonephritis. The arcuate and interlobular arteries, and the afferent arterioles, show hypertensive changes. Where malignant hypertension has supervened the secondary glomerular changes are seen in those glomeruli not already destroyed by the glomerulonephritic process.

The tubules show extensive atrophy, many being completely lost, and there is an increase in the intertubular connective tissue and the irregular interstitial aggregation of lymphocytes and small numbers of plasma cells. In cases with some near-normal hypertrophied glomeruli, the corresponding tubules are enlarged and conspicuous, and account for the elevations that give the subcapsular surface its granular appearance. These surviving functioning tubules may show hyaline droplets in the epithelial cytoplasm and frequently contain protein casts, features that relate to the proteinuria. When malignant hypertension has supervened, there may be blood in the capsular spaces and in functioning tubules.

In cases of chronic glomerulonephritis preceded by the nephrotic syndrome, the kidneys may still be enlarged, and lipid deposits may still be visible in the cortex to the naked eye. Although the glomeruli show advanced sclerosis, their appearance may still suggest the type of glomerulonephritis responsible. All the glomeruli are affected to some extent, and the tubular atrophy is accordingly more uniform, without prominent enlarged tubules; for this reason, the surface of the kidney is often smooth and does not exhibit the granularity usually found in other forms of chronic glomerulonephritis.

### Clinical Features

The clinical features and changes in other organs and tissues are those of chronic renal failure and are attributable to uraemia and, usually, hypertension.

## Diabetic Glomerulosclerosis

Diabetes mellitus is one of the major causes of chronic renal disease leading to chronic renal failure and resulting in a requirement for renal replacement therapy. Several different abnormalities may be encountered in the kidneys of diabetic patients; these are known collectively as 'diabetic nephropathy'. Diabetic glomerulosclerosis is the most common pathology and may be associated with proteinuria, nephrotic syndrome, and chronic renal failure. Although diabetic glomerulosclerosis usually develops in patients with long-standing diabetes, on occasion it may present early in the clinical course and, rarely, may precede the recognition of clinical diabetes mellitus. There are three different morphological features within the diabetic glomerulus: capillary basement membrane thickening, diffuse glomerulosclerosis, and nodular glomerulosclerosis. Capillary basement membrane thickening is common but requires detailed morphometric assessment to confirm its presence. Diffuse glomerulosclerosis consists of a diffuse increase in the mesangial matrix, possibly with mild proliferation of mesangial cells. This is usually also associated with thickening of the GBM. As the disease progresses, continuing mesangial expansion and obliteration of the entire glomerulus occur. In nodular glomerulosclerosis the glomerular lesions take the form of nodular expansions of the mesangial matrix surrounded by patent peripheral capillary loops (Fig. 13.16). The expansion of the nodules with progression of diabetic

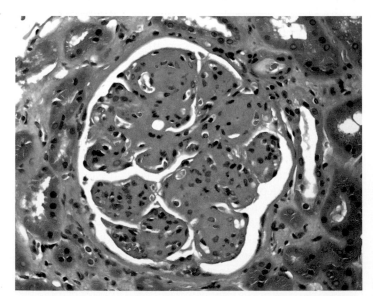

**Fig. 13.16** In diabetic nephropathy there is nodular expansion of the mesangial matrix and thickening of the glomerular capillary walls but no hypercellularity. Immunofluorescence staining in diabetic nephropathy is negative.

## 13.2 Special Study Topic

### GENE POLYMORPHISMS AND THE PROGRESSION OF DIABETIC RENAL DISEASE

The pathology of diabetic nephropathy is well established. Hyperglycaemia contributes to non-enzymatic glycosylation of glomerular extracellular matrix, increasing its stability and leading to altered charge and permeability of the GBM and glomerulosclerosis. However, not all diabetic patients will develop diabetic nephropathy and although good glycaemic control reduces the risk it is now clear that genetic factors also influence the development and progression of diabetic renal disease.

There are marked differences in the risk of end-stage renal disease (ESRD) among patients with diabetes from different racial groups. Studies from the USA have shown that people of African–Caribbean origin with diabetes are up to four times more likely to develop ESRD than patients of white European origin living in the same geographical area. Further evidence for genetic modification of diabetic nephropathy comes from the demonstration of familial clustering of diabetic nephropathy. The earliest studies from the USA and Europe showed that diabetic patients are five times more likely to develop diabetic nephropathy if they have a diabetic sibling with ESRD than if their diabetic sibling has no renal disease. Other studies have shown broadly similar results with only a variation in the quantitative value of the relative risk. More recent studies have also incorporated renal biopsy data and found a correlation between mesangial matrix and risk of diabetic nephropathy within families.

Physiological and pathological features, including blood pressure, body fat mass, and cardiovascular disease, influence diabetic nephropathy. These factors have been investigated in the attempt to identify the genetic basis of familial clustering of diabetic nephropathy. Candidate genes for which there is good evidence of involvement include those influencing blood pressure, cardiovascular function, and inflammatory response (Table 13.3).

**TABLE 13.3** Candidate genetic modifiers of diabetic nephropathy

| Pathophysiological system | Candidate gene |
| --- | --- |
| Metabolism and cardiovascular function | Apolipoprotein E |
| Renin–angiotensin system | Angiotensin converting enzyme |
| | Angiotensin receptor 1 |
| Inflammation | Interleukin 1 |
| | Transforming growth factor β |
| Glucose metabolism | Aldose reductase |
| | Glucose transporter GLUT 1 |

nephropathy leads to obliteration of the capillary tuft. This nodular diabetic glomerulosclerosis is pathognomonic of diabetes.

Diabetic nephropathy may also include hyaline arteriolosclerosis, and increased susceptibility to pyelonephritis and papillary necrosis. Diabetic nephropathy is a progressive disease, the rate of progression being influenced by coexisting hypertension, the activity of the local renin–angiotensin system, and the degree of hyperglycaemia. Recent studies have confirmed that inhibition of angiotensin generation by angiotensin-converting enzyme inhibitors or angiotensin receptor blockade has a beneficial effect on the progression of diabetic renal disease superior to that of other antihypertensive agents. Progression is less influenced by strict diabetic control.

## Amyloidosis

The kidneys are one of the most frequently involved organs in amyloidosis. Renal amyloid can be of either AA or AL type. There is deposition of amyloid proteins around glomerular capillary basement membranes (Fig. 13.17), leading to increased permeability, proteinuria, and progressive renal disease. As the deposition of amyloid increases capillaries become obliterated and glomeruli extensively

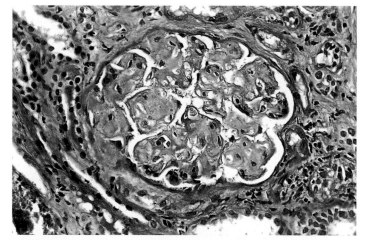

**FIG. 13.17** In amyloidosis there is marked expansion of the extracellular matrix of the glomerulus with obliteration of the capillary spaces – these features may also affect the larger blood vessels, tubules, and interstitium of the kidney. The amyloid material stains with the Congo red.

replaced by amyloid protein. There is secondary atrophy of tubules with interstitial fibrosis. The renal arterioles are also frequently involved in the deposition of amyloid leading to secondary ischaemic changes.

# DISEASES AFFECTING TUBULES

Two main groups of diseases affect the renal tubules:

1. Ischaemic or toxic injury leading to acute tubular necrosis
2. Inflammatory reactions involving the tubules and interstitium, known as tubulointerstitial nephritis.

## Acute Tubular Necrosis

### Key Points

- Acute tubular necrosis (ATN) is caused by ischaemic or toxic injury and regeneration of the tubular epithelium usually occurs.
- Arteriolar vasoconstriction, increased glomerular permeability, tubular obstruction, and back-leak of tubular fluid are all involved in the pathogenesis of ATN.
- Tubulointerstitial nephritis may be due to an acute hypersensitivity reaction to drugs.
- Chronic tubulointerstitial nephritis may occur with long-term use of non-steroidal anti-inflammatory drugs (NSAIDs) and excessive use of simple analgesics.

In ATN the kidney is injured by ischaemia (prerenal failure) or toxins, or a combination of these factors, resulting in cell injury and death of the tubular epithelium. The tubules are the most metabolically active part of the nephron and therefore most vulnerable to these insults. The tubular epithelium is capable of regeneration and, if the factors leading to acute tubular necrosis are corrected, complete recovery of renal function can be expected. However, if the exposure is prolonged irreversible damage may occur and the outcome will be chronic renal failure or established renal impairment. Examples of ischaemic and toxic causes of acute tubular necrosis are shown in *Box 13.2*.

### Box 13.2 CAUSES OF ACUTE TUBULAR NECROSIS

**Ischaemic**
- Massive haemorrhage
- Gastroenteritis
- Cardiogenic shock

**Toxic**
- Drugs (e.g. aminoglycosides)
- Heavy metal poisoning
- Rhabdomyolysis

**Both**
- Septicaemia
- Hepatorenal syndrome
- Pancreatitis

Patients with established ATN are usually oliguric although in some cases urine output is maintained despite a marked reduction in glomerular filtration rate (non-oliguric acute renal failure). During this phase there is a progressive rise in urea, creatinine, and other nitrogenous waste products, a failure to excrete acid and potassium, and retention of sodium and water. Without dialysis these abnormalities are likely to be fatal within 2–3 days. The oliguric phase of ATN may last from several hours up to several weeks and is followed by a 'diuretic phase' when urine volume increases, occasionally excessively. During this period, which seldom lasts for more than a few days, glomerular and tubular functions start to recover and dialysis can be stopped. Finally, during the 'recovery phase', sometimes lasting many weeks, renal function returns to normal or near normal.

### Pathological Changes

In fatal cases, the kidneys are usually enlarged and the cut surface bulges, due mainly to dilatation of tubules and interstitial oedema. The cortical vessels contain little blood, and the cortex appears pale, with blurring of the normal radial pattern, whereas the medulla is often dark and congested. Occasionally there are petechial haemorrhages in the cortex.

Microscopically, the glomerular tufts appear normal. Usually there is some granular debris in the capsular space and the parietal cells lining Bowman's capsule may be unduly prominent and cuboidal. The tubular changes are variable and depend on the severity and duration, and on the particular causal agents involved. In many cases, however, the aetiology is complex, and specific changes cannot readily be attributed to particular causal agents. Also, it is often difficult to identify, in histological sections, which parts of the tubules have been damaged. *Post mortem*, the lesion is often obscured by terminal ischaemic changes and postmortem autolysis.

In cases resulting from ischaemia, both the proximal and the distal convoluted tubules are commonly dilated, and the epithelial lining is flattened with basophilia of the cytoplasm and mitotic activity (Fig. 13.18). These changes, which are seen as early as 3 days after the onset, appear to be sequelae to loss of tubular epithelium; the remaining cells become flattened and undergo proliferation, thus restoring epithelial continuity. In the distal tubules proliferation may be pronounced, the cells sometimes forming syncytial masses, particularly around casts. An early change seen by electron microscopy is the loss of the normal brush border from the proximal tubular cells. The time at which these cells regain their brush border correlates well with the return of renal function.

In most cases, tubular necrosis is not seen; rather there is a simplification of the renal tubular epithelium, dilatation of the lumen, and interstitial oedema. In a minority of cases there are foci of necrosis, most numerous in the distal convoluted tubule but also occurring in the proximal tubule. This change, which is described as tubulorrhexis, may be accompanied by disruption of the tubular basement membrane and an inflammatory reaction in the adjacent inter-

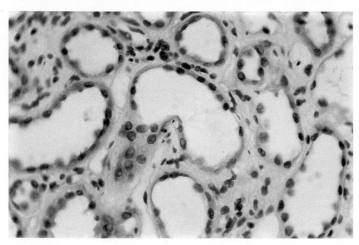

FIG. 13.18 In acute tubular necrosis there is a flattening of the epithelial cells and many of the tubules contain cellular or acellular debris. The interstitium is oedematous but there is no significant inflammatory infiltrate.

stitial tissue. This may progress to scarring and in the event of recovery lead to tubular obstruction and so to loss of function of the affected nephrons.

From the ascending limb of Henle's loop onwards, the tubules contain proteinaceous and brown granular casts, and in cases associated with haemoglobinuria or myoglobinuria brown pigment casts and rounded granules of pigmented material are particularly prominent. Distension of the inter-tubular connective tissue by oedema fluid is conspicuous in some cases, but almost absent in others. The vasa recta of the medulla usually contain groups of nucleated cells, which appear to represent erythropoietic foci, a feature that may be analogous to that seen in the hepatic sinusoids in liver cell necrosis.

The changes described above are seen in acute renal failure resulting from shock, trauma, and so on. They also occur in cases resulting from administration of the nephro-toxic poisons listed above but, in the poisoning cases, there is, in addition, more extensive necrosis affecting mainly the proximal convoluted tubules of all or most of the nephrons, resulting from the direct effect of the toxic compounds or their metabolites. This nephrotoxic change is often con-spicuous but, unlike tubulorrhexis, it does not involve rup-ture of the tubular basement membrane, and if the patient survives it is often repaired by epithelial regeneration with-out leaving any residual damage or scarring.

Some variation is observed in the nephrotoxic lesions brought about by different chemicals, e.g. mercuric chloride tends to affect the whole of the proximal convoluted tubule, and in some instances the necrotic part of the tubule rapidly becomes calcified, resulting in permanent injury. Carbon tetrachloride causes necrosis especially of the terminal part of the proximal tubule, and also perivenular hepatic necro-sis. If ethylene glycol is ingested, a small proportion of it is converted into oxalate, crystals of which form in the tubular lumina; in addition to tubular necrosis it may cause death from liver or brain injury or from acute heart failure.

## Pathogenesis of Renal Failure in Acute Tubular Necrosis

Currently, four factors are thought to be implicated in the renal failure of ATN: arteriolar vasoconstriction, increased glomerular permeability, tubular obstruction, and the back-leak of tubular fluid.

### Arteriolar Vasoconstriction

The reduction in renal blood flow in ATN is largely confined to the renal cortex. It has been suggested that disruption in the tubular transport of sodium or chloride stimulates renin release and the renin–angiotensin system mediates the observed vasoconstriction. This mechanism cannot, how-ever, fully explain the facts because angiotensin promotes arteriolar vasoconstriction whereas the cortical ischaemia in ATN is due in part to constriction of the arcuate or inter-lobular arteries of the kidney.

### Increased Glomerular Permeability

This is associated with swelling of the glomerular epithel-ial cells, best seen by scanning electron microscopy, in early post-ischaemic acute renal failure. This process can be mimicked by incubating glomeruli in solutions containing angiotensin, and is a second possible effect of the renin–angiotensin system. There is certainly a correlation between the extent of these glomerular epithelial cell changes and the eventual severity of post-ischaemic acute renal failure in humans.

### Tubular Obstruction

Microdissection studies have shown the presence of long hyaline tubular casts, consisting largely of Tamm–Horsfall protein, which must restrict tubular flow. This is associated with raised intratubular pressure and dilated tubular lumina. The diuretic phase of acute tubular necrosis is associated with a great increase in Tamm–Horsfall protein in the urine and may indicate the flushing out of these casts. Tubular constriction also leads to afferent arteriolar vasoconstric-tion, which further lowers the filtration pressure gradient. Protein casts and dilated tubules are, however, found in the recovery phase of ATN and hence tubular obstruction can-not be the whole story.

### Back-leak of Tubular Fluid

This can occur through the areas of basement membrane denuded of epithelial cover in ATN, and any rise in intra-tubular pressure due to obstruction by casts distal to the epithelial loss will increase the amount of such a fluid leak. Tubular obstruction also reduces glomerular filtration, but dextran-clearance studies suggest that this can explain only about 20% of the observed reduction.

It is obvious that the above-postulated mechanisms are to some extent interdependent, and it is likely that they all contribute to the observed renal failure. The more extensive necrosis of the proximal tubules, which occurs in cases attributable to various toxins, is more uniform and explicable as a direct toxic effect on the tubular epithelium.

## Tubulointerstitial Nephritis caused by Drugs and Toxins

In modern medical practice, drug-induced tubulointerstitial nephritis is one of the common clinical problems facing nephrologists. Drugs may act in two main ways: first as a tubular toxin resulting in the changes of ATN as discussed above; alternatively, they may elicit an acute hypersensitivity reaction within the renal parenchyma.

### Drug-induced Interstitial Nephritis

This is a well-documented form of iatrogenic disease being described in association with an increasing number of drugs, most commonly antibiotics, NSAIDs, diuretics, and more recently proton pump inhibitors. The disease usually begins about 2 weeks after exposure to the drug and may be characterized by systemic illness such as fever and eosinophilia with or without a skin rash. In many patients acute renal impairment is the only abnormality. On histological examination of renal biopsies performed in patients with drug-induced interstitial nephritis there is pronounced oedema and infiltration of the tubules and interstitium by lymphocytes and macrophages. Eosinophils and neutrophils may be present in significant numbers. Plasma cells are found in more longstanding cases. There is a variable degree of tubular damage and regeneration is usually evident. The glomeruli are, for the most part, normal in acute tubulointerstitial nephritis. The clinical features and morphology suggest a hypersensitivity reaction that is not dose related but is rather idiosyncratic. It is important to recognize drug-induced interstitial nephritis because it responds satisfactorily to withdrawal of the offending drug, and the patient should be made aware of the risk of recurrence on subsequent exposure to the drug.

In addition to an allergic-type pathogenesis, nephropathy associated with NSAIDs may involve local interstitial ischaemia because of the inhibition of the synthesis of vasodilatory prostaglandin. This is particularly important in patients who have coexisting renal disease or volume depletion. A more chronic form of drug-induced nephropathy is due to excessive long-term analgesic use. This is a disease of worldwide distribution but it appears to be more common in Australia and Scandinavia. Chronic analgesic nephropathy is characterized by a chronic tubulointerstitial nephritis with tubular atrophy, interstitial fibrosis, chronic inflammatory cell infiltrate, and, frequently, accompanying papillary necrosis. In countries with a high intake of simple analgesics it is an important cause of chronic renal failure.

### Cast Nephropathy

This is a special form of toxic tubular injury. Multiple myeloma, a neoplasm of immunoglobulin-secreting plasma cells (see Chapter 8, pp. 227–228), may involve the kidney without direct invasion. The high level of circulating immunoglobulins and particularly immunoglobulin light chains predisposes the kidney to the development of cast

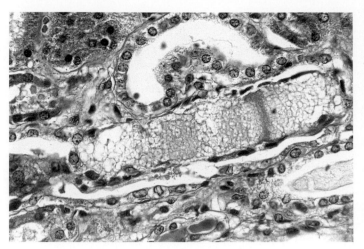

**FIG. 13.19** Patients with myeloma excrete large amounts of immunoglobulin light chains in their urine. These light chains may precipitate as casts, eliciting a tubular epithelial response and inflammation in the adjacent renal parenchyma – so-called cast nephropathy. This cast nephropathy is one of the forms of kidney involvement in multiple myeloma.

nephropathy. The main cause of this renal pathology is related to Bence Jones proteinuria. Immunoglobulin light chains are filtered into the urinary filtrate. During the tubular reabsorption of fluid the resultant high concentrations of immunoglobulins can cause precipitation of these proteins in the tubular lumen. The protein casts thus formed damage the tubular epithelium, sometimes with tubular rupture and an adjacent interstitial inflammatory cell infiltrate (Fig. 13.19). In addition, patients with multiple myeloma may be hypercalcaemic and hyperuricaemic, resulting in nephrocalcinosis and gouty nephropathy respectively. They may also develop renal amyloid or severe pyelonephritis. Renal insufficiency occurs in approximately half the patients with multiple myeloma and renal failure due to cast nephropathy is a relatively common mode of presentation of multiple myeloma.

## VASCULAR DISEASES OF THE KIDNEY

### Key Points

- Hyaline arteriosclerosis of the interlobular arteries and afferent glomerular arterioles is typical in benign or essential hypertension, whereas fibrinoid necrosis extending into the glomerular tuft is seen in the malignant phase.
- Systemic diseases causing vasculitis in the kidney are rare but important causes of renal failure.
- Thrombotic microangiopathies are characterized by thrombocytopenia, renal failure, and haemolytic anaemia.
- Atheromatous renovascular disease is common in patients with peripheral and other vascular disease.

## The Kidney and Hypertension

The kidney is centrally involved in blood pressure regulation through the control of salt and water balance, the production of renin, and possibly other mechanisms. The kidney is also unusual in possessing a microcirculation that can autoregulate blood flow. Thus, over a range of systemic blood pressures, glomerular capillary blood flow and pressure remain constant. Disturbances in renal function are often accompanied by a rise in blood pressure and thus kidney disease is the most common cause of secondary hypertension. Secondary hypertension in patients with renal disease is important because, if untreated, it accelerates the progression of renal damage that is already occurring due to the primary kidney disorder itself; this leads to more rapid development of renal failure.

The arterial tree of the kidney is usually affected more than other organs by hypertension and this results in varying degrees of renal damage. Chronic benign essential hypertension in patients without other underlying kidney disease only occasionally causes advanced renal failure despite the development of widespread arteriosclerosis. Hyaline arteriosclerosis is usually prominent in the interlobular arteries and afferent glomerular arterioles, which become tortuous, thick walled, and extremely narrowed (Fig. 13.20). These arterial and arteriolar changes tend to cause ischaemia and, because the most important lesion is the hyaline arteriosclerosis of the afferent arterioles, individual nephrons are affected. The capillary tuft of the affected glomerulus shrinks, with wrinkling of its basement membrane. The collapsed capillary tuft later becomes hyalinized and Bowman's capsule becomes filled with collagen, leading to the formation of a solid fibrous ball. The tubule atrophies and is replaced by fibrous tissue, often containing some lymphocytes. This piecemeal loss of individual nephrons occurs slowly, so that in the early stages of hypertension the kidney appears normal, but with prominent arteries visible on the cut surface. As more nephrons are lost there is diffuse thinning of the renal cortex and the kidneys become moderately reduced in size. The contraction of the small scars that replace the lost nephrons causes fine depressions on the kidney surface, which becomes finely granular in appearance. If enough nephrons are lost there may be hypertrophy of the surviving nephrons, which accentuates the roughening of the surface, giving rise to the so-called granular contracted kidney although the kidneys are seldom very small.

Malignant hypertension can cause acute renal failure and may arise anew or supervene after a period of chronic hypertension. In contrast to benign hypertension, further investigation will often reveal an underlying cause such as glomerulonephritis. In the most acute cases the surface of the kidney is smooth and spotted with tiny petechial haemorrhages. The cut surface may show mottling due to multiple tiny infarcts. The interlobular arteries often show a proliferative myointimal thickening. Fibrinoid necrosis affects mainly the distal portions of the interlobular arteries and the afferent arterioles (Fig. 13.21), but may extend into the glomerular tuft. Other glomeruli show

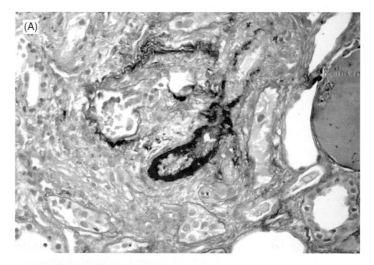

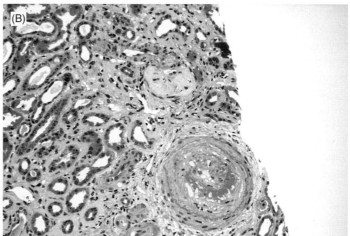

**FIG. 13.21** (A) In malignant hypertension, more severe and acute vascular changes are seen in the arterioles. (B) This is characterized by fibrin deposition, platelet activation, and transmural necrosis of the arteriolar wall, a constellation of features known as fibrinoid necrosis, which is stained red in this trichrome stain. There is little inflammatory infiltrate in fibrinoid necrosis.

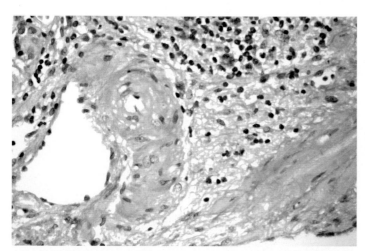

**FIG. 13.20** Hypertension affects the small arteries and arterioles of the kidney. There is a marked hyaline deposition within arteriolar walls with loss of smooth muscle cells. This leads to progressive glomerular ischaemia and glomerular fibrosis.

thickening of the capillary walls with reduplication of basement membrane, congestion, and capillary dilatation. There is often blood or proteinaceous fluid in Bowman's space and proliferation of the capsular epithelium may give rise to occasional crescents. Unlike glomerulonephritis, only a minority of the glomeruli are affected and the severe impairment of renal function is due to ischaemia caused by the arterial damage and superimposed thrombosis. The tubules may be atrophied or enlarged and usually contain proteinaceous or blood casts. There is hyperplasia of the renin-secreting cells of the juxtaglomerular apparatus and this morphological change correlates with the very high levels of renin and angiotensin II that invariably occur in malignant hypertension.

## Vasculitis and the Kidney

The intrarenal vessels may be involved in a variety of vasculitides, particularly polyarteritis nodosa, microscopic polyarteritis, and Wegener's granulomatosis. Although these are uncommon conditions, their recognition is important because of their response to immunosuppression, without which they carry a poor prognosis.

Polyarteritis nodosa is a systemic vasculitis characterized by transmural necrotizing inflammation of medium-sized or small muscular arteries. The disease typically involves the kidney but may involve other vascular beds. The involvement of the renal arteries is focal and random, but there is relative sparing of the glomeruli and the afferent arterioles. These may show, at most, ischaemic changes. At a later stage the acute inflammatory infiltrate disappears and there is transmural fibrous thickening of the artery wall with occasional microaneurysm formation.

Microscopic polyarteritis or polyangiitis differs from polyarteritis nodosa. This disease affects arterioles, capillaries, and venules, so in the kidney there tends to be a necrotizing glomerulonephritis with frequent crescent formation (Fig. 13.22). The afferent arterioles are affected but larger vessels are relatively spared. More than 90% of the patients have antibodies to the myeloperoxidase (MPO) component of neutrophil cytoplasmic antigen (ANCA). This disease is treated by immunosuppression and plasma exchange.

Wegener's granulomatosis is a similar necrotizing vasculitis affecting arterioles, venules, and capillaries, although there is a tendency also to involve medium-sized arteries. The disease characteristically includes lesions affecting the nose, sinuses, and lung, with focal necrotizing vasculitis involving the kidney. Morphologically there is a necrotizing glomerulonephritis with crescent formation and necrotizing lesions affecting the blood vessels. On renal biopsy the distinction between microscopic polyarteritis and Wegener's granulomatosis may not be possible and the categorization into these two diseases is based largely on the pattern of clinical involvement supported by the type of ANCA detected. More than 90% of patients with Wegener's granulomatosis have protease 3 (PR3) ANCA antibodies, the titres of which correlate with disease activity.

## Thrombotic Microangiopathies

In this group of disorders there is a combination of so-called malignant vascular injury, microangiopathic haemolytic anaemia, and renal failure. Malignant vascular injury is a descriptive term for severe vascular lesions characterized by fibrinoid necrosis and myointimal proliferation, with a sparse inflammatory cell infiltrate (Fig. 13.23).

The haemolytic uraemic syndrome may be of the childhood or adult type. It may be sporadic or occur in an epidemic form, in which case it is particularly associated with diarrhoeal illness caused by verocytotoxin-producing *Escherichia coli* (*E. coli* O157). In childhood the onset often

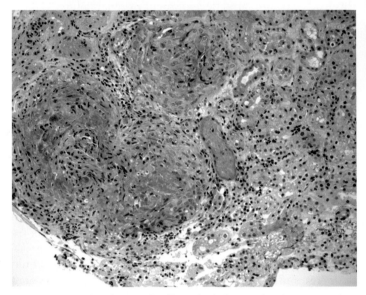

**FIG. 13.22** Vasculitis frequently affects the kidney and is characterized by a transmural inflammatory infiltrate causing localized damage with focal cellular necrosis in the blood vessel wall. Eventually this leads to ischaemia of the renal parenchyma and scarring in the blood vessel wall.

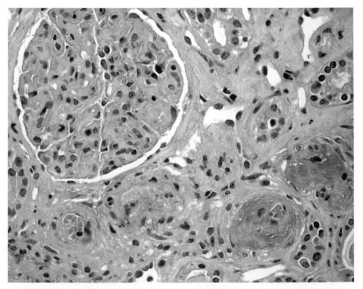

**FIG. 13.23** In the haemolytic uraemic syndrome there is fibrinoid necrosis of arterioles with fibrin and platelet deposition within glomeruli.

follows an upper respiratory tract or diarrhoeal illness of ill-defined aetiology. The main features of the disease are acute renal failure, thrombocytopenia, confusion, and microangiopathic haemolytic anaemia. In adults the disease may also follow an episode of diarrhoea but other causes include HIV infection, malignancy, and drugs such as ciclosporin and cisplatin. Mutations in complement genes (e.g. factor H; see Chapter 4, pp. 66–67) have been shown to predispose to haemolytic uraemic syndrome in those cases that are familial. Haemolytic uraemic syndrome has a significant mortality in elderly people; however, most children and young and middle-aged adults survive although the recovery of renal function may be incomplete.

Thrombotic thrombocytopenic purpura (TTP) is a rarer idiopathic condition related to the haemolytic uraemic syndrome. It has many of the above features but neurological involvement is more frequent and severe, and the extent of the renal failure tends to be more profound with higher mortality.

Progressive systemic sclerosis is a connective tissue disease with renal involvement. The renal manifestations include acute renal failure (scleroderma renal crisis), often irreversible, with severe hypertension. The disease occurs in a patient with the otherwise typical features of systemic sclerosis.

A syndrome resembling the haemolytic uraemic syndrome may occur in late pregnancy, sometimes in association with pre-eclampsia, but also seen after an uneventful pregnancy. The disease is of acute onset with renal failure, platelet consumption, and a haemolytic anaemia.

The long-term outcome for renal function from all of these disorders is variable, but the renal vasculature is scarred by malignant vascular injury and many patients will have residual renal impairment and hypertension.

## Renal Cortical Necrosis

Bilateral diffuse cortical necrosis with sparing of the medulla is an uncommon condition but when present leads to renal failure, often with incomplete recovery. It is most frequently associated with pregnancy, particularly those complicated by pre-eclampsia or placental abruption, but it may occur in other disorders such as haemolytic uraemic syndrome, septic shock, or disseminated intravascular coagulation.

## Other Vascular Diseases

Atheroma is not uncommon in the main renal arteries of patients with generalized atherosclerosis. This often occurs due to encroachment of aortic atheromatous plaque(s) into the ostium of the renal artery, and may also be present more distally. Renal ischaemia due to atherosclerotic stenosis of the renal arteries is an important cause of renal failure in elderly people and may also cause hypertension and cardiac failure. In some cases these features can be improved by relief of the stenosis by surgery, or more often by radiologically guided angioplasty.

The kidney may also be affected in the cholesterol emboli syndrome; multiple cholesterol microemboli from atheromatous plaques in the aorta become lodged in the renal vasculature, causing renal failure. Other clinical features due to cholesterol emboli occur in the skin, gastrointestinal tract, and the lower limbs. In younger patients, hypertension may result from fibromuscular dysplasia of the renal arteries. Senile arteriosclerosis in the kidneys of elderly normotensive people presents features similar to those of benign essential hypertension and does not seriously impair renal function.

# RENAL TRANSPLANTATION

Renal transplantation is the optimum renal replacement therapy for most patients with ESRD. Transplants may come from cadaveric, living related, or living unrelated donors. Effort is made to match the donor and recipient's major histocompatibility complex (MHC) antigens as closely as possible, because transplant survival is enhanced by good matching, particularly at MHC class II antigens. Advances in immunosuppressive drugs and immunosuppression protocols have reduced the incidence of transplant rejection but pathological assessment of transplant dysfunction is an important part of clinical care. The four main types of rejection and the features found in renal transplant biopsies are summarized in *Table 13.4*.

Further pathology related to drug toxicity, opportunistic infection, recurrent primary disease, or new renal disease may also be identified in renal transplants.

**TABLE 13.4** Renal transplant pathology

| Category of rejection | Pathological features |
|---|---|
| Hyperacute rejection | Early onset |
| | Rare |
| | Extensive interstitial haemorrhage |
| | Endothelial necrosis |
| **Acute cellular rejection:** | Common |
| Tubulointerstitial | Lymphocytic tubulitis, extent determines severity |
| Arterial | Lymphocytic endothelialitis |
| | Fibrinoid necrosis |
| Acute antibody mediated rejection | Neutrophils in peritubular capillaries |
| | C4d complement component on capillary endothelium |
| | Fibrinoid necrosis |
| Chronic rejection (chronic allograft nephropathy) | Arterial intimal thickening |
| | Arteriolar hyalinosis |
| | Glomerulosclerosis |
| | Tubular atrophy with interstitial fibrosis |

A 32-year-old male presented with established renal failure secondary to glomerulonephritis and hypertension. He was managed on chronic ambulatory peritoneal dialysis. He had anaemia due to defective erythropoietin production by the kidney and was treated with recombinant erythropoietin (EPO). His blood pressure was controlled with antihypertensive agents, including angiotensin-converting enzyme inhibitors. He underwent a rigorous medical examination but no other significant abnormalities were found. He was placed on the waiting list for a renal transplantation.

Six months later a kidney became available for transplantation which showed a perfect blood group match and a good MHC match. Crucially his MHC class II antigens were fully matched. He underwent renal transplantation, the new kidney being anastomosed to his iliac vessels and placed in his right iliac fossa. He was treated with conventional immunosuppressive drugs, a combination of tacrolimus, azathioprine, and corticosteroids. The graft functioned well by day 5 after surgery, but at day 10 there was a reduction in his renal function. A renal biopsy was performed which showed an acute rejection episode (Fig. 13.24). This was treated by increasing his dose of steroids and the graft function returned to normal. He remained well for the next 2 months until he developed a pyrexial illness with relatively normal graft function but mild liver dysfunction. He was found to have cytomegalovirus infection, a viral infection to which patients on long-term immunosuppression are more susceptible,

which had been transmitted in the transplanted kidney. He was treated with ganciclovir and recovered. He remains well with a functioning graft 5 years after transplantation, continuing on a maintenance dose of immunosuppressive drugs.

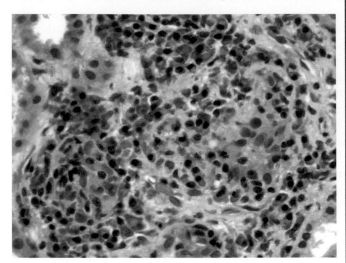

**FIG. 13.24** Biopsy of a renal transplant showing lymphocytic tubulitis characteristic of acute cellular rejection. The tubules are infiltrated by lymphocytes with additional lymphocytes and macrophages in the adjacent interstitium.

## DISEASES OF THE URINARY TRACT

### Key points

- Obstruction, vesicoureteric reflux, diabetes, pregnancy, neurogenic bladder, and calculi predispose to pyelonephritis.
- Urinary infection in childhood is often due to reflux nephropathy, which can lead to chronic pyelonephritis if unrecognized.

## Urinary Tract Obstruction

Obstruction in the urinary tract may be acute or insidious in onset and, if unrelieved, will cause significant renal damage resulting in acute or chronic renal failure. It may be intermittent or complete and may be unilateral or bilateral. Urinary

**Box 13.3** MAIN CAUSES OF URINARY TRACT OBSTRUCTION

- Developmental anomaly
- Renal stones
- Renal pelvic or ureteric tumour
- Retroperitoneal fibrosis
- Enlarged lymph nodes
- Pelvic malignancy (e.g. cervical carcinoma)
- Prostatic enlargement

tract obstruction can occur at any level of the urinary tract from the urethra to the renal pelvis and may be caused by either lesions intrinsic to the urinary tract or by extrinsic lesions causing compression. The most common causes of urinary tract obstruction are summarized in *Box 13.3*. Urinary tract obstruction predisposes to urinary tract infection and to urinary calculus formation (see below).

### Hydronephrosis

The dilatation of the renal pelvis and calyces that occurs due to obstruction of urinary outflow is termed hydronephrosis and can lead to progressive renal atrophy with fibrosis. Urinary tract obstruction with continuing glomerular filtration leads to an increase in pressure within the renal pelvis, which is transmitted back through the collecting duct into the renal parenchyma. This causes atrophy of the renal parenchyma, with tubular loss occurring as an early event. The increased pressure compresses the renal vasculature, altering the intrarenal blood flow and further exacerbating tubular atrophy and interstitial fibrosis. Only in the later stages does the glomerular filtration rate begin to diminish. These events may be accelerated by coexisting infection or calculus formation. As distension of the renal pelvis and calyces increases, the calyces become flattened and the underlying renal parenchyma progressively thins, ultimately forming a rim of mostly fibrous tissue surrounding the dilated pelvis and calyces. The atrophy of the renal parenchyma may be diffuse or focal so that some areas may be relatively spared whereas the remainder shows severe atrophy.

The clinical features of urinary tract obstruction depend to a large extent on the site and cause of the obstruction. Acute obstruction may give rise to pain resulting from rapid distension of the urinary tract proximal to the obstruction. Unilateral hydroureter and hydronephrosis may be clinically silent because renal function can be adequately maintained by the other kidney. Bilateral complete obstruction will result in renal failure. Bilateral incomplete obstruction, most commonly seen in elderly males with prostatic enlargement, results initially in tubular dysfunction with an impairment of the urinary-concentrating capacity. This results in polyuria, urinary frequency, and nocturia. Superimposed urinary tract infection may produce additional symptoms, mainly dysuria, fever, and abdominal or loin pain.

## Urinary Tract Infection

Urinary tract infection may involve either the bladder or the kidneys and renal pelvis, or both. The single most important criterion for the diagnosis of urinary tract infection is the presence of bacteria in the urine, called bacteriuria. In urine obtained through a bladder catheter the presence of an organism is significant whereas in the commonly used midstream sample there may be some contamination by urethral or perineal organisms. In these latter samples a bacterial count of $\geq 10^5$/mL is accepted as definitive of infection. Bacteriuria in the absence of symptoms is termed 'asymptomatic bacteriuria' and is of importance under two circumstances:

1. In infancy, where, in the presence of ureteric reflux, it can lead to ascent of infection to the kidney
2. In pregnancy, where it may be followed by symptomatic infection predisposing to hypertension, pre-eclampsia, and prematurity.

A urinary tract infection occurring without preceding catheterization or obstruction is usually due to bacteria normally present in the faeces. The most frequently encountered organism is *E. coli* but sometimes *Klebsiella*, *Proteus*, or *Pseudomonas* spp. are responsible. Infection complicating obstruction or instrumentation is commonly of a mixed bacterial type with *E. coli*, *Proteus* spp., and staphylococci being most often present. Haematogenous spread is a less frequent occurrence but may be seen in the course of acute pyaemia or septicaemia complicating staphylococcal infections or infective endocarditis.

By far the most common route of infection is via the lumen of the urethra. The incidence of infection is highest in females throughout all age ranges with a female:male ratio of 20:1 in children and young adults. This sex ratio falls in old age as prostatic hyperplasia contributes to an increased incidence of urinary tract infection in elderly males (see Chapter 16). The female preponderance is due mainly to the ease with which endogenous infections can ascend the short female urethra. Precipitating factors include trauma to the perineum during sexual intercourse or childbirth. Most urinary infections in females occur in anatomically normal urinary tracts and most of these are confined to the bladder (cystitis). In a small percentage of females and relatively more often in males, stagnation of urine resulting from urinary tract obstruction or dysfunction is the main aetiological factor. This is caused by urethral obstruction (due to scarring or congenital urethral valves), urinary calculi, diverticula, tumours of the bladder, congenital malformations such as double ureters, and neurological disorders such as paraplegia or multiple sclerosis leading to bladder dysfunction. In males, prostatic enlargement secondary to hyperplasia is the most common cause of urinary tract infection.

Cystitis is characterized by dysuria, increased frequency of micturition, and sometimes haematuria. The ascent of infection to the kidneys from the bladder is usually due to vesicoureteric reflux, urinary tract obstruction, or pregnancy. Vesicoureteric reflux consists of retrograde flow of bladder urine up the ureters during micturition. Reflux is normally prevented by the oblique course of the ureter through the wall of the bladder exerting a valve-like action during bladder contraction. In infancy this mechanism is less well developed and ureteric reflux is more frequent. In older children and adults reflux is less common unless associated with pregnancy or urinary tract obstruction. Vesicoureteric reflux may be demonstrated by a micturating cystogram, in which dye instilled into the bladder by catheter is examined radiologically during micturition. Reflux may be seen by dye passing into the ureters or ascending to the kidney. The main importance of reflux is that it allows infected bladder urine to reach the kidneys. Bladder infection also tends to be perpetuated by reflux, because the refluxing urine returns to the bladder after micturition and there is therefore incomplete bladder emptying.

In severe reflux urine may re-enter the renal parenchyma, especially at the upper and lower poles of the kidney where the papillae are compound. In such papillae the mouths of the collecting ducts are held open and refluxing urine may flow into them. These then tend to be the sites of intrarenal reflux and scarring in reflux nephropathy or chronic pyelonephritis (see below).

## Pyelonephritis

Pyelonephritis is inflammation of the renal pelvis, calyces, and renal parenchyma induced by bacteria. It can occur in both acute and chronic forms, and may affect one or both kidneys. Most cases are due to ascending infection often associated with vesicoureteric reflux, obstructive uropathy, or calculi. The predominant organisms are those that also cause cystitis.

### *Acute Pyelonephritis*

#### Clinical Features

This condition is less common than acute cystitis. The symptoms of acute pyelonephritis in adults are loin pain, usually with a high fever and often rigors. There may be accompanying symptoms of cystitis. Children with acute pyelonephritis may be less unwell with fewer localizing symptoms, making the condition more difficult to diagnose. In uncomplicated cases acute episodes resolve within a few days of instituting appropriate antibiotic therapy.

### Pathological Changes

These comprise acute inflammation of the pelvis, calyces, and renal parenchyma, which, in severe cases, may progress to suppuration and abscess formation. There is purulent urine with congestion and inflammation of the pelvicalyceal mucosa. Pale linear streaks of pus may extend radially from the tip of the papilla to the surface of the cortex where adjacent lesions may fuse to produce abscesses. There may be considerable destruction of the cortex although there tends to be relative sparing of glomeruli and blood vessels. When severe there may be almost total or complete obstruction and pus may accumulate in the pelves and calyces to produce a pyonephrosis. Extension of this through the renal capsule may produce a perinephric abscess.

## Chronic Pyelonephritis

Recurrent or protracted episodes of acute pyelonephritis may lead to renal parenchymal scarring. Once established this scarring causes progressive renal damage over many years, even in the absence of further infection. Chronic pyelonephritis is an important cause of established kidney disease and accounts for about 15% of the European population requiring renal replacement therapy.

### Clinical Features and Course

There may be a history of recurrent urinary infection, failure to thrive in early childhood, or nocturnal enuresis. In bilateral cases the condition usually presents with the features of chronic renal failure or hypertension. The diagnosis of chronic pyelonephritis is most easily confirmed radiologically, with typical findings comprising asymmetrical shrinkage of the kidney, irregularity of the renal outlet due to cortical scarring, and dilatation or disturbance of the calyces adjacent to the scarred areas. In some patients, heavy proteinuria approaching that seen in the nephrotic syndrome may develop. These patients show secondary focal segmental glomerulosclerosis and its presence suggests the likelihood of a more rapid deterioration of renal function.

### Pathological Changes

The macroscopic appearances of the kidney are important in differentiating chronic pyelonephritic scarring from other types of renal scarring. Unlike other forms of chronic tubulointerstitial disease the pelvic and calyceal walls are thickened and distorted, their mucosa is granular or atrophic, with scarring of the pyramids and usually calyceal dilatation. In contrast to chronic glomerulonephritis the renal parenchyma shows asymmetrical scarring and shrinkage, these scars being close to the deformed calyces and found mainly at the upper and lower poles of the kidney. Microscopically the pelvic and calyceal mucosa may be thickened by granulation tissue. There is often submucosal fibrosis and an intense chronic inflammatory cell infiltrate, sometimes with lymphoid follicle formation. In the parenchymal scars there is tubular atrophy with thickening of the basement membranes, and the interstitium is infiltrated by inflammatory cells, mostly lymphocytes and plasma cells. In the late stages of the disease there is dense fibrosis with little active inflammation. The glomeruli in the scarred areas may appear normal but show a spectrum of abnormalities with concentric periglomerular fibrosis, ischaemic injury, fibrous obliteration, and hyalinization of glomerular tufts. Obliterative endarteritis affects the blood vessels. In non-scarred areas there may be compensatory hypertrophy, and vascular changes resulting from hypertension.

Rarer forms of urinary tract infection may be encountered such as tuberculosis, schistosomiasis, fungal infection, or, more rarely, viral infection.

## Urinary Calculi

Urinary calculi are formed by the precipitation of inorganic urinary constituents, with a small amount of organic material also being incorporated. Deposition is favoured by highly concentrated urine, and hence is more frequently seen in dehydrated patients, in warm climates, or at high altitude. Deposition is also increased in metabolic disorders accompanied by excretion of excess amounts of the major constituents of urinary calculi. Changes in urinary pH and the presence of urinary tract infection may also enhance calculus formation. Calculi may develop in the renal pelvis, ureter, or bladder, although some bladder calculi probably originate in the kidney and are passed down the ureter into the bladder. At this site they may enlarge by the incorporation of additional inorganic material.

The main types of urinary calculi are as follows:

- Calcium-containing stones, the calcium salt being predominantly oxalate with lesser amounts of calcium phosphate. These comprise more than 75% of all urinary calculi and are characteristically laid down in an acid urine.
- Complex triple phosphate stones including magnesium, ammonium, carbonate, and calcium components. These comprise 15% of urinary calculi and are laid down in alkaline urine. They may form an outer laminated deposit on other stones and are strongly associated with urinary tract infection.
- Uric acid and urate–uric acid stones comprise 5% of urinary calculi but affect up to 20% of patients with gout. Similar to calcium-containing stones they are typically laid down in an acid urine. Pure uric acid stones are radiolucent, rendering their detection on a plain abdominal radiograph virtually impossible.
- Cystine stones occur in primary cystinuria, a rare but important renal disease in childhood.

The precise mechanisms of stone formation are complex and rather poorly understood. It requires both nucleation, a process whereby the stone deposition is initiated, and aggregation, whereby the stone grows in size. Some urinary constituents can promote the nucleation of others (e.g. urates can nucleate oxalate precipitates) and this explains why many urinary stones are mixed in composition. An increase in the urinary excretion of a particular substance is usually an important factor, typically in hypercalciuria in which the increased excretion of calcium and phosphate leads to the formation of calculi. Hypercalciuria occurs in hyperparathyroidism, chronic resorptive bone disease, prolonged immobilization in bed, sarcoidosis, and the milk alkali syndrome, but in most cases it is idiopathic.

Stones in the renal pelvis may be single or multiple and in some instances a single calculus may grow to occupy the entire pelvicalyceal system, resulting in a so-called 'staghorn' calculus. Small calculi may pass down the ureter to the bladder, giving rise to the clinical syndrome of renal colic with haematuria. They may arrest temporarily, usually at the narrower lower end of the ureter. When impaction is permanent, this occurs at one of three sites: the upper end of the ureter at the pelviureteric junction; the level of the pelvic brim; or the lower end of the ureter. This impaction and renal obstruction lead to hydronephrosis. When there is a urinary tract infection by urea-splitting bacteria such as *Proteus* spp., ammonia is produced and calculi or softer deposits composed of phosphates form within the resultant alkaline urine. These may be precipitated within the inflamed pelvicalyceal system. This combination of infection and calculus may result in pyonephrosis and ulceration. The chronic inflammation and epithelial regeneration resulting from calculi may give rise to squamous metaplasia of the lining of the renal pelvis, with a subsequent increase in the risk of development of squamous carcinoma.

Stones in the bladder may be solitary or multiple and can grow to several centimetres in diameter. As with stones elsewhere in the urinary tract, they increase the risk of urinary tract infection, chronic inflammation, and squamous metaplasia. They characteristically give rise to symptoms such as pain and irritation with haematuria, intermittent obstruction, frequency, and dysuria.

## TUMOURS OF THE KIDNEY AND URINARY TRACT

### Key points

- The kidney is among the 10 sites most frequently involved by malignancy, accounting for 2.5% of human cancers.
- Renal cancer is associated with smoking, obesity, hypertension, and exposure to petroleum vapours and possibly to a high-protein diet.
- It is more common in males than females.

## Malignant Tumours

There are three main types of malignant tumour in the kidney and urinary tract. Nephroblastoma or Wilms' tumour occurs in children, whereas in adults renal cell carcinoma is the major malignancy of the renal parenchyma and urothelial carcinoma, the major malignancy of the renal pelvis, ureters, and bladder.

### Nephroblastoma (Wilms' Tumour)

This affects about 1 in 10,000 children, a figure that remains uniform across different geographical regions, and usually presents between age 2 and 5 years. Most cases of nephroblastoma are solitary and sporadic but up to 10% may be multifocal or bilateral at the time of diagnosis. Occasionally, nephroblastoma is encountered as a feature of one of three different multisystem disorders (*Box 13.4*). These associations have revealed a lot about the genetics of Wilms' tumour and particularly the role of tumour-suppressor genes such as *WT1*, which is located on chromosome 11p13.

Histologically these tumours are characterized by three elements (i.e. they are triphasic): blastema, stroma, and immature tubules resembling the tissues found within the nephrogenic zone of fetal kidney (Fig. 13.25). It is known that Wilms' tumour arises from oncogenic events within the metanephric blastema of the fetal kidney and the tumour cells retain the capacity for partial differentiation

---

**Box 13.4** MULTISYSTEM DISORDERS ASSOCIATED WITH WILMS' TUMOUR

- Denys–Drash syndrome
- WAGR (**W**ilms' tumour, **a**niridia, **g**enital abnormalities, or **g**onadoblastoma, learning disability [mental **r**etardation]) syndrome
- Beckwith–Wiedemann syndrome

---

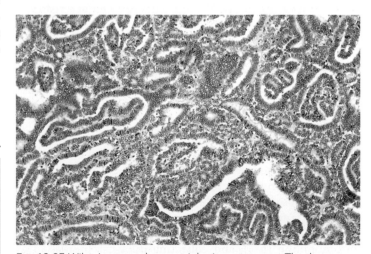

FIG. **13.25** Wilms' tumour shows a triphasic appearance. The three histological elements comprise the undifferentiated blastema, immature tubules, and stromal connective tissue. The relative contribution of these elements varies enormously between individual cases of Wilms' tumour.

into both the stromal and the epithelial elements, similar to the differentiation capacity of the normal metanephric blastema. The relative amounts of these different elements within the tumour vary. In about 5% of Wilms' tumours extreme pleomorphism may be noted and this is termed 'anaplasia', which is a poor prognostic feature. Nowadays, >85% of children with Wilms' tumour are cured by the combination of surgical and non-surgical management. This compares favourably with the position 30 years ago when the cure rate was between 10% and 30%.

### Renal Cell Carcinoma

Renal cell carcinomas account for more than 95% of renal malignancies in adults, with a median age at presentation between 55 and 60 years. The tumours are usually sporadic but rarely familial cases may be encountered, particularly as part of the von Hippel–Lindau syndrome. This association has revealed that mutation and subsequent loss of the second (normal) copy of the *VHL* gene is a key event in the development of renal carcinomas of either the sporadic or familial type. These observations also confirm the importance of the *VHL* gene as a tumour-suppressor gene. The risk factors for the development of renal cell carcinoma are rather poorly understood; the tumour is more frequently encountered in males than females and there is a moderate association with a smoking history and hypertension. There is an association with abdominal obesity and the rising prevalence of obesity in the population is predicted to lead to a 40% increase in renal carcinoma over the next decade. Recent work has identified germline mutations that predispose to renal carcinoma in the succinate dehydrogenase and fumarate hydratase genes, which encode mitochondrial enzymes of the tricarboxylate cycle.

Renal cell carcinoma is usually a solitary and large tumour at the time of presentation, although the development of newer imaging techniques has led to an increase in the number of small asymptomatic renal cell carcinomas being detected and removed. The tumours are characteristically soft and yellow, frequently with areas of haemorrhage and necrosis. Invasion of the renal vein or extension beyond the renal capsule are frequent and are important measurements in defining the stage or extent of disease at the time of surgery. Blood-borne metastases to the lungs and other tissues such as bone and brain are seen at the time of presentation in up to 20% of patients.

Histologically the most common variant (conventional or clear cell type) is composed of uniform clear cells, which are rich in glycogen and lipid (Fig. 13.26). Mitoses are infrequent suggesting slow, but nevertheless relentless, tumour growth. These tumour cells are arranged in acini, cords, or sheets, and renal cell carcinomas are typically richly vascular tumours. Other histological types such as papillary (15%), chromophobe (5%), and collecting duct carcinomas (1%) may be seen. Progression to spindle-cell or sarcomatoid variants may be encountered from any of these histological

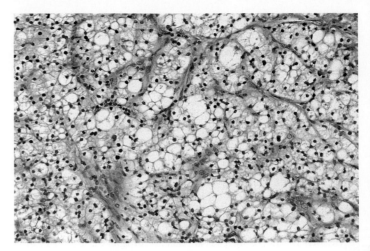

**FIG. 13.26** The most common form of renal cell carcinoma is characterized by a solid architecture composed of clear cuboidal cells supported by a rich vascular stroma. Other variants include the papillary, chromophobe, and collecting duct types.

types and is a very bad prognostic feature. The major prognostic feature in renal cell carcinoma is the stage of tumour at the time of surgical resection. Extrarenal spread either by direct infiltration of perirenal fat or by invasion of the renal vein is strongly associated with the concurrent or subsequent development of metastatic renal cell carcinoma. The tumours often present with a triad of loin pain, haematuria, and an abdominal mass, but renal cell carcinoma is notorious for the frequency of paraneoplastic syndromes associated with increased production of erythropoietin (polycythaemia), parathyroid hormone-related peptide (hypercalcaemia), and renin (hypertension).

### Transitional Cell Carcinoma

This, the third of the major renal and urinary tract malignancies, constitutes 90% of the tumours of the renal pelvis, ureter, and bladder. They cover the full spectrum from small, relatively benign tumours to highly aggressive malignancies. They are frequently multifocal, an observation that influences the extent of surgical management of these tumours. The risk of developing urothelial carcinoma has been shown to be increased in certain industries such as dye workers and workers in the rubber industry. These tumours are also associated with cigarette smoking, analgesic use, long-term cyclophosphamide therapy, and bladder infestation by *Schistosoma haematobium*. The last is more typically associated with squamous cell carcinoma, rather than transitional cell carcinoma (see Chapter 19, pp. 567–568)

The tumours may be papillary or flat and may be non-invasive or invasive. Histologically, these tumours are composed of multilayered sheets of ovoid cells exhibiting a variable degree of pleomorphism and mitotic activity. The severity of the pleomorphism and frequency of the mitotic figures are used to grade the tumour as an indication of its likely behaviour.

## Benign Tumours

### Oncocytoma

These constitute about 5% of renal tumours in surgical series. They are, however, frequently asymptomatic, being detected as in incidental observation during the investigation for other abdominal disease. They are large brown tumours with a central scar and difficult to distinguish from malignant renal tumours using imaging techniques, so therefore they are resected. They have a typical gross and microscopic appearance. They are composed of nests of intensely eosinophilic granular cells with a minor degree of pleomorphism of the nuclei and a low mitotic rate.

### Angiomyolipoma

These are rare tumours in the general population but are a common finding in patients with tuberous sclerosis (see Chapter 11, p. 328). As the name suggests they are composed of vascular smooth muscle and fat cells. They are benign and usually encountered after nephrectomy for either an asymptomatic or a symptomatic renal mass.

### Papillary Adenomas

These are small (<5 mm), usually incidental findings in the kidney. They are frequently multifocal but rarely give rise to symptoms.

---

**13.2 CASE HISTORY**

A 56-year-old male presented to his GP with microscopic haematuria that had been identified during an insurance medical examination. The GP took a careful history, did a thorough examination, and checked the patient's renal function. No other abnormalities were noted. Urine microscopy showed no evidence of red cell casts and there was no proteinuria or infection. The patient was referred to a urologist for further investigation who confirmed the haematuria and arranged a cystoscopy. At cystoscopy no abnormalities were noted in the bladder but blood was seen coming from the left ureter. Magnetic resonance imaging showed a 4-cm-diameter mass in the left kidney. No other abnormalities were noted. The patient was admitted for surgery and at operation the mass was well circumscribed and confined to the lower pole. The surgeon decided to perform nephron-sparing surgery, and carried out a partial nephrectomy. Histological examination of the 4-cm tumour showed that it was a benign oncocytoma (Fig. 13.27) and that it had been completely excised by the surgery. The patient required no further treatment. He remains alive and well 4 years later with no evidence of renal impairment.

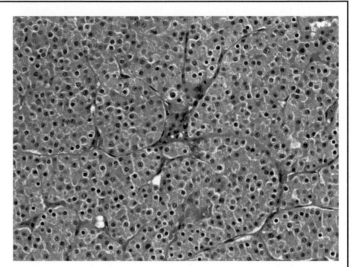

**FIG. 13.27** Renal oncocytoma is characterized by a packeted architecture of strongly eosinophilic granular cells with a cuboidal shape and central non-pleomorphic nuclei.

---

## SUMMARY

- After reading this chapter you should understand that kidney failure leads to a number of clinically significant complications and, if untreated, may lead to the patient's death.
- You should also understand that there are a number of well-established factors involved in the progression of renal disease.
- You should know the major forms of immune complex-mediated glomerular disease and how these arise.
- You need to know thoroughly the importance of the kidney as a site of injury in systemic diseases, including diabetes, hypertension, and SLE.
- There are identifiable causes and mechanisms for acute renal failure in most clinical cases.
- You must appreciate the significance of the anatomy of the urinary tract in relation to urinary tract infection.
- You should know the main types of tumour affecting the kidney and the likely outcomes after the diagnosis of these tumours.

## FURTHER READING

Fogo AB, Kashgarian M. *Diagnostic Atlas of Renal Pathology.* Philadelphia, PA: WB Saunders, 2011.

Jennette JC, Olson JL, Schwartz MM, Silva FG. *Heptinstall's Pathology of the Kidney*, 6th edn. Philadelphia, PA: Lippincott Williams & Wilkins, 2007.

Petersen RO, Sesterhenn IA, Davis CJ. *Urologic Pathology.* Philadelphia, PA: Lippincott Williams & Wilkins, 2008.

Taal MW, Chertow GM, Marsden PA, Skorecki K, Yu ASL, Brenner BM. *Brenner and Rector's The Kidney*, 9th edn. Philadelphia, PA: WB Saunders, 2011.

# 14

# THE FEMALE REPRODUCTIVE SYSTEM

C Simon Herrington

## DEVELOPMENT OF THE FEMALE GENITAL TRACT

### Key Points

- The ovary forms from the indifferent gonad.
- Development proceeds along female lines in the absence of a Y chromosome.
- The internal female genitalia form from the fused paramesonephric ducts and the urogenital sinus.

All fetuses have both 'male' and 'female' internal genitalia. Subsequent development depends upon the influence of hormones derived from the gonads as they develop into testis or ovary. The testis produces Müllerian inhibitory hormone, which leads to regression of the Müllerian (paramesonephric) ducts, and androgens, which lead to persistence of the wolffian (mesonephric) ducts. Conversely, neither of these substances is produced by the ovary; therefore, the Müllerian ducts persist and the wolffian ducts regress. The corollary of this reciprocal arrangement is that, in the absence of a Y chromosome – and hence testicular tissue – differentiation proceeds along female lines. This explains the female pheno-type of patients with, for example, 45,XO (Turner's syn-drome) or 47,XXX genotypes and the male phenotype of patients with Klinefelter's syndrome (47,XXY). Androgen insensitivity syndromes (e.g. testicular feminization) are an exception to this and occur when the androgens produced by normal testes in patients with a 46,XY genotype are ineffective as a result of end-organ insensitivity. Müllerian hormone is, however, produced and therefore both wolf-fian and Müllerian ducts regress, leading to the absence of both male and female internal genitalia. These disorders are examples of disorders of gender identity (intersex). A clas-sification of intersex is given in *Box 14.1*.

During fetal development, the germ cells migrate from the yolk sac through the dorsal mesentery to lie within the indifferent gonads, which differentiate in the female to form the ovaries. In the absence of surviving germ cells, e.g. in Turner's syndrome, the gonads fail to differentiate but rather form 'streak' gonads. In the absence of regressive

---

**Box 14.1** DISORDERS OF GENDER IDENTITY

**Normal chromosome constitution**

*Female pseudohermaphrodite (46,XX but with male development)*
    Adrenogenital syndrome
    Treatment of mother with progestogens or androgens

*Male pseudohermaphrodite (46,XY but with female development)*
    Primary gonadal defect (e.g. defects of testosterone metabolism)
    End-organ defect (e.g. testicular feminization)

**Abnormal chromosome constitution**

*Sexual ambiguity infrequent*
    Klinefelter's syndrome (47,XXY)
    Turner's syndrome (45,XO)
*Sexual ambiguity frequent*
    Mixed gonadal dysgenesis
    True hermaphrodite (both ovarian and testicular tissue present)

stimuli, the paired paramesonephric (Müllerian) ducts form the fallopian tubes and, by fusion, the uterus, cervix, and upper vagina. The lower vagina is derived from the urogenital sinus. If the process of paramesonephric duct fusion is abnormal, a variety of fusion defects can occur; these are important because they are associated with infertility and obstetric complications.

# THE VULVA

> ### Key Points
>
> - Any disorder of the skin can occur on the vulva; this includes inflammatory dermatoses and tumours.
> - Vulval intraepithelial neoplasia (VIN) is the vulval equivalent of cervical intraepithelial neoplasia (CIN) (see pp. 423–425).
> - Almost all invasive tumours of the vulva are squamous cell carcinomas.

## Inflammatory Vulval Disease

Inflammation may be either infective or non-infective. The most common vulval infection is candidiasis, which is particularly common in patients with diabetes and during pregnancy. Viral infections include human papillomavirus (HPV) infection, which can cause vulval warts, and is associated with vulval neoplasia (see below). Non-infective inflammation occurs in a wide variety of disorders, including contact dermatitis, lichen sclerosus, and lichen planus (see Chapter 18, p. 508).

## Benign Lesions of the Vulva

As in other cutaneous sites, the most commonly identified benign lesions include skin tags, melanocytic naevi (moles), and epidermal (sebaceous) cysts, most of which are removed for cosmetic reasons. Bartholin's gland cysts may become infected, form abscesses, and need to be drained.

## Non-neoplastic Epithelial Disorders

Epithelial disorders of the vulva used to be called vulval 'dystrophy', but more recently this spectrum of disease has been simplified into non-neoplastic and neoplastic forms. The non-neoplastic lesions comprise squamous hyperplasia, lichen sclerosus, and lichen planus (see Chapter 18, p. 508). Squamous hyperplasia consists of thickened squamous epithelium which may be associated with underlying inflammation. Lichen sclerosus is a specific disorder characterized by sclerosis of the upper dermis with associated chronic inflammation. The overlying squamous epithelium can be normal, atrophic, or hyperplastic. This disorder

causes significant morbidity, and there is debate about whether it is premalignant. Lichen planus shows some similarities to lichen sclerosus because they are both associated with band-like (lichenoid) inflammation at the epidermal–dermal interface. Lichen planus is not, however, associated with dermal sclerosis.

## Neoplastic Epithelial Disease

VIN is the vulval equivalent of CIN (see pp. 423–425 for a full discussion) and is premalignant. Almost all invasive tumours of the vulva are squamous cell carcinomas (Fig. 14.1), and they occur in two distinct clinicopathological groups. The first, and more common, group occurs in postmenopausal women who develop well-differentiated invasive squamous cell carcinomas, which may be associated with a poorly defined premalignant epithelial abnormality known as 'differentiated type' VIN; this is not associated with HPV infection. Some patients have surrounding lichen sclerosus, but the association between this disorder and invasive malignancy is the subject of debate. Younger women typically develop 'basaloid' or 'warty' carcinoma, which is associated with HPV infection and surrounding VIN of 'undifferentiated' (synonyms 'usual' or 'warty') type. VIN of this type is associated with an increased risk of having or developing intraepithelial (and hence invasive) disease at other anogenital sites, particularly the cervix, but including also the vagina (VaIN) and perianal region. This is an example of a field effect. Treatment of vulval carcinoma is by surgical excision, which, if the tumour is of low stage, may be curative.

Extramammary Paget's disease, which is analogous to Paget's disease of the nipple (see Chapter 15, p. 453), may involve the vulva.

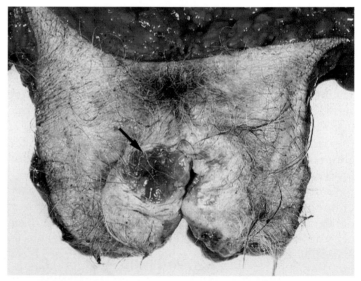

**FIG. 14.1** Macroscopic photograph showing an ulcerating vulval tumour (arrow). Histologically, this was an invasive squamous cell carcinoma.

# THE VAGINA

Atrophic vaginitis, caused by a lack of trophic (oestrogen) support for the vaginal epithelium, is a common cause of postmenopausal bleeding. As for the vulva, polyps and cysts are relatively common and most often removed for cosmetic reasons, or as a result of sexual dysfunction. An important vaginal abnormality, which occurred in female infants born to mothers treated in pregnancy with diethylstilbestrol (DES), is vaginal adenosis. Inappropriate hormonal stimulation during development led to extension of glandular epithelium from the cervix on to the vagina. Patients with this disorder are at high risk of developing clear cell carcinoma of the vagina in the abnormal epithelium. Fortunately, identification of the association between DES and this abnormality has led to its virtual disappearance.

Almost all primary tumours of the vagina are now squamous in type. These are rare tumours and, before this diagnosis can be made, the possibility of extension of either a vulval or a cervical carcinoma on to the vagina must be excluded.

This zone may also be the seat of acute inflammation, particularly if a large volume of endocervical tissue is everted into the vagina (cervical ectropion or 'erosion'). This may also be complicated by superimposed infection. The two most common specific infections are herpes simplex virus (type 2) infection (Fig. 14.2), which causes epithelial ulceration, and HPV infection, which is now recognized as the major aetiological factor for cervical cancer (see Special Study Topic 14.1).

## Neoplastic Disease of the Cervix

As at other sites, neoplastic disease of the cervix may be either epithelial or non-epithelial, and benign or malignant. If malignant, tumours may be primary or secondary (metastatic). Non-epithelial tumours (e.g. leiomyomas and leiomyosarcomas) do occur – as do metastatic carcinomas – but the vast majority of neoplasms of the cervix are epithelial, malignant (or premalignant), and primary. Neoplastic epithelial disorders may be intraepithelial, i.e. confined to the epithelial surface, or invasive, i.e. they show evidence of stromal invasion and/or metastasis. Clearly, these differ fundamentally in terms of the effect on the patient because the former is cured by simple removal. However, at many sites, these two forms are really part of a spectrum of disease, with normality at one end and metastatic cancer at the other. This is exemplified by neoplastic disorders of the cervix, for which there is a relatively well-defined morphological spectrum.

# THE CERVIX

## Non-neoplastic Disorders of the Cervix

Most non-neoplastic disorders of the cervix are inflammatory. Non-infective inflammation is extremely common – if not universal – in the transformation zone (see below).

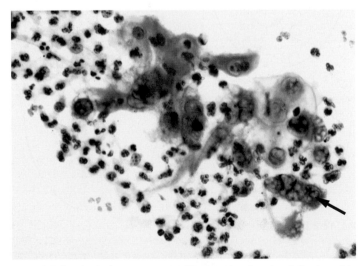

**Fig. 14.2** Cytological appearances of herpes simplex virus infection with formation of multinucleated cells (arrow).

## Squamous and Glandular Intraepithelial Neoplasia of the Cervix

Knowledge of the series of changes that the cervix undergoes throughout reproductive life is central to the understanding of cervical neoplasia (Fig. 14.3). Before puberty, the cervix is an inactive organ; the ectocervix is lined by squamous epithelium and the endocervix by columnar epithelium. After puberty, hormonal stimulation causes cervical enlargement with eversion of the squamocolumnar junction into the vagina. Exposure to the vaginal environment leads to metaplasia whereby the columnar epithelium changes into first immature and then mature squamous epithelium as a protective response. This zone of metaplastic squamous epithelium is known as the 'transformation zone', and is the region where almost all neoplasia of the cervix arises. After the menopause, the cervix shrinks and the transformation zone returns to within the endocervical canal.

CIN is defined as replacement of the normal squamous cervical mucosa by neoplastic cells, but with an intact basement membrane. The neoplastic cells are identified by the presence of classic morphological features of malignancy, i.e. nuclear hyperchromasia, pleomorphism, abnormal mitoses, and loss of epithelial polarity (see Chapter 5, p. 80). The lesion is then graded on the basis of the proportion, in thirds, of the epithelium that is occupied by abnormal 'basaloid' cells showing no evidence of cytoplasmic maturation to give grades 1, 2, and 3 (Figs 14.4 and 14.5). It should be noted that nuclear abnormality is present throughout the epithelial thickness in all grades of CIN. An alternative grading system, used particularly in the USA, divides these lesions into low- and high-grade squamous intraepithelial lesions (SILs),

with low-grade SIL corresponding approximately to CIN 1 and high-grade SIL to CIN 2 and 3.

In the UK, approximately 5–6% of the cervical smears generated by the cervical screening programme (see below) show cytological changes suggestive of CIN. A further 2–4% show abnormalities that are less well defined but carry a risk of either the presence or development of CIN. As a general rule, the higher the grade of CIN present, the greater the risk of invasive carcinoma. This forms the basis of the current recommendation in the UK that patients with CIN 2 and 3 be treated by excision of the lesion (usually by diathermy loop excision). As the risk of progression is less for patients with CIN 1, and there is greater subjectivity in the diagnosis of this lesion, many clinicians follow up patients with CIN 1 rather than excising the lesion. The principle behind this approach is that removal of an intraepithelial lesion will prevent the subsequent occurrence of an invasive one.

A less common but increasingly important group of abnormalities includes those that affect the glandular epithelium of the cervix. These abnormalities are being increasingly identified in cervical smears and, similar to squamous lesions (CIN), most neoplastic glandular lesions

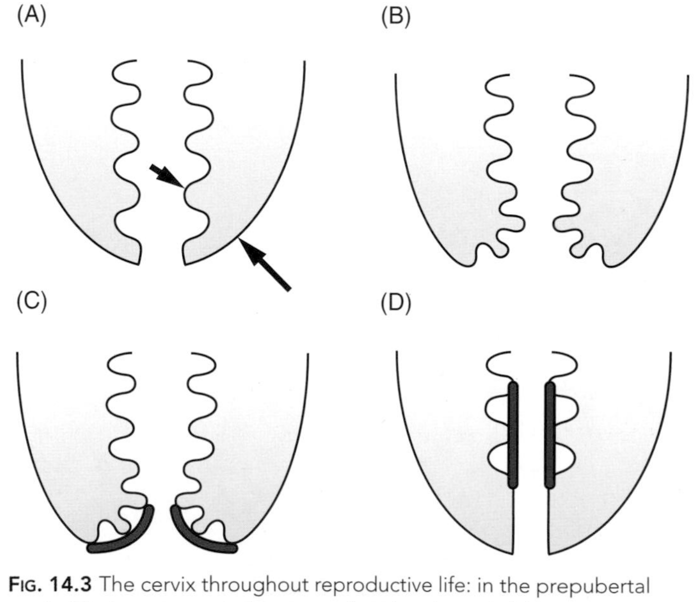

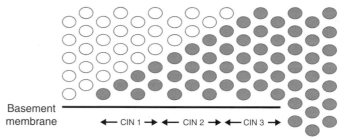

**Fig. 14.4** The spectrum of squamous neoplasia of the cervix: the grade of CIN is defined by the proportion of the epithelium occupied by immature 'basaloid' cells (dark). Invasive carcinoma occurs when the abnormal cells invade through the basement membrane. An alternative, two-tier, grading system is in increasing use and sub-divides preinvasive lesions into low-grade squamous intraepithelial lesions (SILs) and high-grade SILs: these correspond approximately to CIN 1 and CIN 2/3 respectively.

**Fig. 14.3** The cervix throughout reproductive life: in the prepubertal cervix (A), the ectocervix (long arrow) and endocervix (short arrow) meet at the external cervical os. With the onset of puberty, the endocervix everts (B) and undergoes squamous metaplasia (thick red line) (C). This area of metaplasia defines the transformation zone. (D) After the menopause, the transformation zone recedes into the endocervical canal.

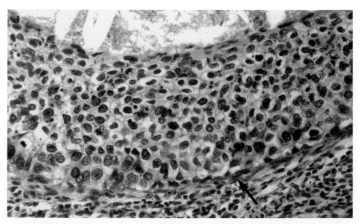

**Fig. 14.5** Cervical intraepithelial neoplasia (CIN) grade 3. Note that the basement membrane is intact (arrow).

## ABNORMAL CERVICAL SMEAR

A 24-year-old woman had a normal cervical smear after the birth of her first child. Three years later, a further routine cervical smear was taken as part of the national cervical screening programme. This contained severely dyskaryotic (a cytological term equivalent to dysplastic) cells, both singly and in groups (Fig. 14.6), suggestive of CIN 3 and raising the possibility of invasive carcinoma. She was therefore referred to her local hospital where the cervix was examined using a colposcope. Application of an acetic acid solution to the cervix revealed

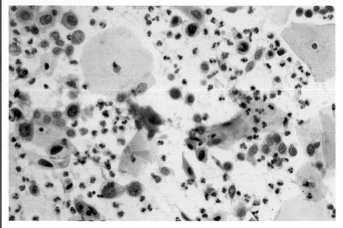

**FIG. 14.6** A cervical smear showing severe dyskaryosis. This finding suggests the presence of CIN 3. In addition, small, abnormally shaped, keratinizing (dark pink) cells are present, raising the possibility of invasive carcinoma.

an aceto-white area, which also contained prominent blood vessels. A biopsy was taken and confirmed the presence of CIN 3, which could be seen growing down into the endocervical crypts but without invasion. As the upper limit of the lesion was not visible at colposcopy, a large loop excision of the transformation zone (LLETZ) was performed in order to both excise the lesion and assess it further histologically. Histopathological examination confirmed the presence of extensive CIN 3 involving endocervical crypts, and also identified an area of early invasion of the stroma measuring 2 mm in width and 2 mm in depth. No invasion of lymphatic or vascular channels was identified, and the lesion did not extend to any of the limits of the biopsy. As the whole of the lesion had been excised, the final diagnosis was extensive CIN 3 with a focus of microinvasive squamous cell carcinoma (FIGO stage Iai). No further treatment was required, but careful follow-up with repeated cytological assessment is essential.

This case is a good example of the success of the cervical screening programme. Early detection allowed excision of this patient's invasive carcinoma while it was small enough to be cured by surgical removal. Moreover, as hysterectomy was not required, fertility was preserved.

### Key Points

- Cervical screening can detect early cervical cancer.
- Prompt referral of patients with significant cervical smear abnormalities is essential.

---

of the cervix are related to infection with HPV (see Special Study Topic 14.1). Cervical glandular intraepithelial neoplasia (CGIN) is associated with squamous CIN, which can be found in approximately 50% of cervices bearing CGIN. Most cases of CGIN are high grade (which is equivalent to adenocarcinoma *in situ*). The management of these lesions is – as for squamous CIN – excision in order to prevent progression to invasion.

### Invasive Tumours of the Cervix

#### Epidemiology and Predisposing Factors

The vast majority of invasive tumours of the cervix are primary epithelial tumours (carcinomas). The mortality from invasive cervical carcinoma is falling in the UK and, in 2010, there were 936 deaths. Cervical carcinoma has traditionally been a disease of older women, but the age-specific incidence is rising in younger women. The reasons for this are unclear, although the increase in adenocarcinoma may be one part of the explanation. Although the incidence of invasive cervical carcinoma is falling in the UK, it is important to remember that there is marked geographical variation in the incidence of this tumour. Particularly in developing countries, cervical carcinoma is a leading cause of death in women and, in 2008, over 520,000 cases of cervical cancer were

recorded worldwide. Epidemiological studies have identified several factors that are associated with an elevated risk of developing invasive cervical carcinoma. These include:

- early age at first intercourse
- number of sexual partners
- low socioeconomic status
- HPV infection.

#### Macroscopic and Microscopic Pathology

The majority of cervical carcinomas are exophytic, and present as ulcerating masses protruding into the vagina (Fig. 14.7). The cervical smear technique is therefore ideal for the detection of exfoliated cells from these tumours. This also explains why many of these tumours present with vaginal bleeding, either spontaneous or postcoital. Some tumours, however, are endophytic, i.e. they grow inwards. These may be squamous in type, but are more frequently adenocarcinomas. This pattern of growth classically leads to a 'barrel-shaped' cervix, and such tumours may not be detectable by cervical smear until they are relatively advanced.

The main tumour types that occur in the cervix are:

- squamous cell carcinoma
- adenocarcinoma of usual type
- adenosquamous carcinoma.

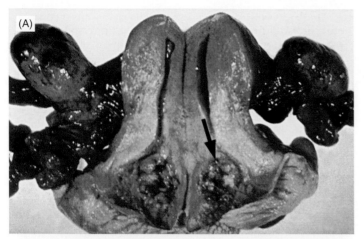

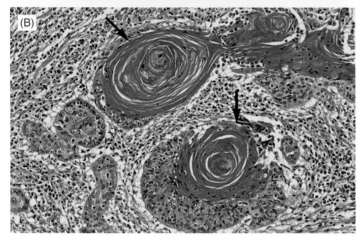

**FIG. 14.7** Invasive cervical carcinoma: (A) macroscopic appearance (arrow); (B) microscopic features of invasive squamous cell carcinoma. Note the presence of keratin pearls (arrows).

**TABLE 14.1** The FIGO (International Federation of Gynaecology and Obstetrics)(2009) staging system for cervical tumours.

| Stage | Definition |
|---|---|
| I | Confined to the cervix |
| | A. Microscopic invasion (≤5 mm deep and ≤7 mm wide) |
| | (1) ≤3 mm deep |
| | (2) >3 mm, ≤5 mm deep |
| | B. Clinically visible or dimensions greater than IA |
| II | Tumour invades beyond the uterus but not to the pelvic wall or lower third of the vagina |
| III | Tumour extends to the pelvic wall and/or involves the lower third of the vagina and/or causes hydronephrosis or non-functioning kidney |
| IV | Involves (biopsy proven) the mucosa of the bladder or rectum and/or extends beyond the true pelvis (including metastasis) |

Most cervical carcinomas are squamous in type and arise in the transformation zone, often associated with CIN. A minority of tumours are adenocarcinomas of usual type or adenosquamous carcinomas. These tumour types are all associated with HPV infection, as are neuroendocrine carcinomas. A number of rarer cervical carcinomas, e.g. gastric type adenocarcinoma, are not associated with HPV infection and are therefore not preventable by HPV vaccination.

As at other sites, carcinomas are graded according to how closely they resemble their tissue of origin because, to some extent, this can be used to predict clinical behaviour: poorly differentiated tumours tend to behave more aggressively. The staging of tumours is more important, because stage is generally a more powerful prognostic factor. The principle is that the further a tumour has spread from its site of origin, the more likely it is to kill the patient, and the more quickly that is likely to occur. The staging of cervical carcinoma differs from many other tumours in that 'microinvasive' carcinomas are recognized. These are diagnosed microscopically and must conform to predetermined size limits (*Table 14.1*). Part of the success of the cervical screening programme is that, when invasive carcinoma is identified, it is now more likely to be microinvasive – and hence curable. The more advanced stages are judged clinically, using a combination of clinical examination (often under anaesthesia) and radiological techniques. Most cervical carcinomas spread at least initially by direct extension into pelvic tissues. The mainstay of treatment of early (predominantly stage 1) carcinoma is therefore surgical excision by either cone biopsy or radical hysterectomy and pelvic lymphadenectomy (Wertheim's hysterectomy). More advanced stages are not surgically resectable and are treated with combined chemotherapy and radiotherapy (chemo-radiation).

### Prevention and Screening

The spectrum of neoplastic cervical disease exemplifies the principle behind the role of screening in the prevention of malignant disease. If intraepithelial disease is the precursor of invasive cancer, then detection and treatment of intraepithelial lesions will prevent the development of invasive disease. Cervical smears are taken every 3–5 years from the age of 20 to 64 years. Cells are scraped from the surface of the cervix using a wooden spatula, and then spread onto a glass slide. The smear is stained using the Papanicolau stain, which allows the cells to be examined under the microscope for features suggestive of malignancy. These include:

- high nucleus:cytoplasm ratio
- nuclear hyperchromasia
- abnormalities of nuclear chromatin pattern
- nuclear pleomorphism.

The presence of these features indicates the presence of dyskaryosis, which suggests a CIN (or more rarely a CGIN) lesion, and usually prompts referral to a colposcopy clinic for further investigation. Given the strong link between

HPV infection and cervical neoplasia, HPV testing is currently being incorporated into the screening programme. This is discussed further in Special Study Topic 14.1 at the end of the chapter.

# THE UTERINE BODY

## The Endometrium

### Key Points

- Dysfunctional uterine bleeding (DUB) is commonly due to functional disturbance of the menstrual cycle.
- Endometrial polyps may be malignant.
- Postmenopausal bleeding is never normal.
- Endometrial carcinoma may arise from endometrial hyperplasia.
- Endometrial carcinoma tends to present early with vaginal bleeding.
- Endometrial carcinoma is curable by early surgical intervention.

### Overview of the Normal Menstrual Cycle

To understand the abnormalities that underlie menstrual disturbances, it is important to have a basic concept of the menstrual cycle (Fig. 14.8). The first (follicular) phase involves development of ovarian follicles as a result of stimulation by follicle-stimulating hormone (FSH). The fundamental features of this development are proliferation of granulosa cells, followed by formation of a space (antrum), thinning of the overlying ovarian cortex, and then – as a result of a surge in luteinizing hormone (LH)

secretion – ovulation. The granulosa cells secrete oestrogen which stimulates proliferation of the endometrium (proliferative phase). After ovulation, the follicle collapses and the granulosa cells transform into luteal cells (luteal phase). The structure formed from this transformation is the corpus luteum, which secretes progesterone, leading to secretory transformation of the endometrium (secretory phase). This phase starts with subnuclear vacuolation of endometrial epithelial cells. This is followed by supranuclear vacuolation and then the appearance of intraluminal secretion. The corpus luteum has a finite lifespan and, after approximately 14 days, begins to degenerate. Progesterone support is therefore removed from the endometrium, which undergoes necrosis. The superficial endometrium is shed, leading to menstrual flow (menstrual phase). The basal endometrium, which does not respond to oestrogen and progesterone, remains and forms the base for the next menstrual cycle.

In the event of implantation of a conceptus into the endometrium, the corpus luteum does not degenerate but becomes a corpus luteum of pregnancy under the influence initially of LH and then human chorionic gonadotrophin (hCG), which is secreted by the placenta. Continued progestogen secretion leads to decidualization of the endometrium. It is important to appreciate that implantation does not always occur in the endometrium but may occur at other sites (ectopic pregnancy), particularly the fallopian tube. Under these circumstances, stimulation of the endometrium continues and decidualization occurs, as in normal pregnancy.

After the menopause, endocrine stimulation of the endometrium largely ceases. The endometrium therefore ceases to cycle and persists only as the basal endometrium. Many women have continued low levels of oestrogen present after the menopause (as a result of aromatization of adrenal androgens to oestrogen in peripheral fat), and hence

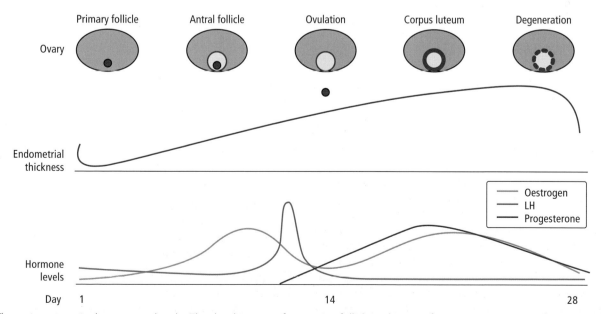

**Fig. 14.8** The major events in the menstrual cycle. The development of an ovarian follicle and its transformation into a corpus luteum are shown together with the endometrial thickness and the pattern of hormone secretion. LH = luteinizing hormone.

weak proliferation may continue. This can cause postmenopausal bleeding related to either withdrawal bleeding or the formation of endometrial polyps. This scenario is becoming increasingly common due to the high prevalence of obesity.

## Dysfunctional Uterine Bleeding

This disorder may be defined as bleeding at an inappropriate time of the cycle in the absence of an anatomical cause. Patients present with a variety of menstrual disturbances, notably intermenstrual bleeding and menorrhagia (heavy periods). There are three main groups of functional abnormality that lead to DUB:

1. Anovulatory cycles
2. Luteal phase defects
3. Irregular shedding.

Anovulatory cycles typically occur at the menarche and around the menopause (perimenopausal bleeding). Failure of ovulation leads to continued endometrial proliferation. Withdrawal bleeding then occurs either when the endometrium becomes too thick to be supported by its blood supply, or as a result of fluctuation in oestrogen levels. If ovulation continually fails to occur, then endometrial proliferation may be marked, leading to simple hyperplasia of the endometrium and, in some patients, atypical hyperplasia and invasive carcinoma. This is particularly true in patients with the polycystic ovary syndrome (PCOS), one of the hallmarks of which is failure of ovulation (see p. 431). In another group of patients, ovulation occurs but the secretory phase is abnormal. This may take the form of a coordinated delay in secretory transformation, asynchrony between glands and stroma, and, perhaps most commonly, irregular ripening when only some glands develop secretory changes. Various physiological defects – both ovarian and endometrial – are involved in this group of abnormalities. Irregular shedding occurs when fragments of endometrium do not shed during menstruation but persist into the next cycle.

It must be remembered that a significant proportion of patients who present with menstrual abnormalities will have a physical explanation for the bleeding. The presence of fibroids (see p. 430) is a good example of this, and therefore it is important that causes other than physiological abnormalities be considered when assessing the patient.

## Endometrial Polyps

Endometrial polyps are common and may present in a variety of ways, including abnormal vaginal bleeding and as an incidental abnormality identified either when a cervical smear is taken or during curettage. Endometrial polyps are most commonly benign and composed of endometrial glands and stroma with a fibrovascular core. Many are related to minor endocrine abnormalities such as anovulatory cycles. However, endometrial hyperplasia and invasive carcinoma may present as a polyp, and it is therefore important that all endometrial polyps be submitted for histological examination.

**TABLE 14.2** Gross and microscopic features of endometrial hyperplasia

|  | Simple | Complex | Atypical |
|---|---|---|---|
| **Distribution** | General | Focal | Focal |
| **Component** | Glands and stroma | Glands | Glands |
| **Glands** | Dilated, not crowded | Crowded | Crowded |
| **Cytology** | Normal | Normal | Atypical |

## Endometrial Hyperplasia

Endometrial hyperplasia occurs in three forms: simple hyperplasia (which is typically generalized), complex hyperplasia, and atypical hyperplasia (*Table 14.2*). Morphologically, there are two main features of hyperplasia, namely architectural abnormality and cytological abnormality. Those forms that show only architectural abnormality (simple and complex hyperplasia) have little or no malignant potential, whereas those that show cytological abnormality (atypical hyperplasia) are associated with a risk of having or developing invasive endometrial carcinoma. The cause of endometrial hyperplasia is often unknown, although some cases are associated with persistent oestrogen stimulation. This may simply be the result of anovulatory cycles, such as in the perimenopausal period or in patients with polycystic ovaries, or due to abnormal oestrogen secretion by, for example, an ovarian tumour such as a fibrothecoma or a granulosa cell tumour (see p. 434).

## Endometrial Carcinoma

Endometrial carcinoma occurs typically in women aged >50 and is uncommon in those aged <40. There are two main groups of patients with endometrial carcinoma: the first includes older women in whom the tumours are not associated with surrounding endometrial hyperplasia; the second comprises younger women in whom the tumours tend to arise on a background of atypical endometrial hyperplasia. The latter group may have evidence of oestrogen excess such as the PCOS (particularly in women aged <40 years) or an oestrogen-secreting tumour, e.g. ovarian fibrothecoma or granulosa cell tumour. Endometrial carcinoma is also associated with obesity and nulliparity, and may occur in the setting of Lynch syndrome, which is due to germline mutation of mismatch repair genes (see Chapter 3, pp. 42–44 and Chapter 9, pp. 270–271). Lynch syndrome should be considered in patients with a family history of endometrial or colorectal cancer, particularly when this has occurred at a young age.

Most endometrial carcinomas present non-specifically with abnormal vaginal bleeding. In younger women, most patients with such bleeding have DUB but, in older women – and particularly those who are postmenopausal – any bleeding should be considered suspicious and endometrial curettage performed. Hence, the adage PMB (postmenopausal bleeding) = D&C (dilatation and curettage). More recently, D&C has been replaced by pipelle endometrial biopsy.

Most endometrial carcinomas are exophytic tumours (Fig. 14.9) and, as they tend to grow into the endometrial cavity and cause vaginal bleeding, they present relatively early. As a result, many endometrial carcinomas are stage I at presentation (*Table 14.3*), and hence are curable by surgical resection. Microscopically, most endometrial tumours are adenocarcinomas that morphologically resemble proliferative endometrium (endometrioid adenocarcinomas); some also show mucinous differentiation. These are termed type I endometrial carcinomas and are graded (1, 2, and 3) according primarily to the proportion of tumour that exhibits solid growth. A minority of tumours differentiate along other lines to resemble, for example, tubal epithelium (serous adenocarcinoma). Serous carcinomas belong to the group of type II endometrial tumours, are considered grade 3 by definition, are characterized by mutation of the *TP53* gene, and behave more aggressively, with more frequent spread outside the uterus.

Endometrial carcinoma invades directly into the underlying myometrium (see Fig. 14.9), where it can gain access to myometrial and hence adnexal lymphat-ics. By this route, the tumour can spread to the ovaries. Surgical resection should ideally therefore include removal of the ovaries. Haematogenous spread may also occur. The prognosis of endometrial carcinoma depends on the grade, stage, and depth of myometrial invasion. Treatment is by surgical excision and adjuvant radiotherapy if there are adverse prognostic factors.

## The Myometrium

### Key Points

- Painful periods that are refractory to treatment may be due to adenomyosis.
- The most common tumour of the myometrium is the leiomyoma (fibroid).
- Leiomyomas are benign, smooth muscle tumours.
- Primary malignant tumours of the myometrium are uncommon.

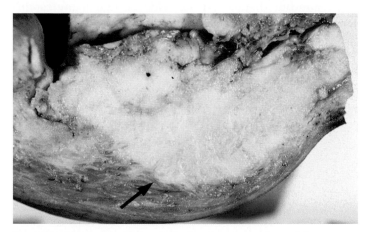

FIG. 14.9 Macroscopic photograph of an invasive endometrial carcinoma (white). Note that the tumour is invading deeply into the myometrium (arrow).

**TABLE 14.3** The FIGO (2009) staging system for endometrial carcinoma

| Stage | Definition |
|---|---|
| I | Confined to the uterine corpus[a] |
| II | Invades the cervical stroma, but does not extend beyond the uterus |
| III | Any of the following: <br> – invades uterine serosa <br> – invades adnexae <br> – invades vagina <br> – pelvic or para-aortic lymph node metastasis |
| IV | Invades bladder and/or bowel mucosa <br> Distant metastases (including intra-abdominal metastases or inguinal lymph nodes) |

[a]Stage I is separated into two substages (IA and IB), depending on the proportion of the myometrium infiltrated (confined to the endometrium or the inner half of the uterine wall, and invading into the outer half of the uterine wall respectively).

## CASE HISTORY 14.2

### POSTMENOPAUSAL BLEEDING

A 75-year-old woman who had her last menstrual period 20 years previously had two episodes of vaginal bleeding. Pelvic examination showed no abnormality. Endometrial curettage was performed, and histopathological examination of the curettings obtained showed a grade 1 endometrioid adenocarcinoma. Surgical resection was therefore performed by total abdominal hysterectomy and bilateral salpingo-oophorectomy. Pathological examination of the resected uterus showed that the endometrial cavity was filled by a polypoid tumour mass (see Fig. 14.9). Histological analysis confirmed invasion of the outer myometrium and cervix, and also identified lymphatic invasion. A small tumour deposit was present in the hilum of the right ovary. These features indicated a diagnosis of grade 1, stage III endometrioid adenocarcinoma of the endometrium. As the tumour was of high stage, the patient was treated with postoperative chemotherapy and radiotherapy.

This case illustrates that, although many endometrial carcinomas present at low stage, high-stage tumours may present in an identical way. This may occur as an unexpected finding, and demonstrates the need for careful pathological assessment in all cases.

### Key Points

- Endometrial biopsy is an important part of the investigation of postmenopausal bleeding.
- Clinical assessment may underestimate the pathological stage of endometrial tumours.

### Adenomyosis

This disorder is sometimes referred to as 'diverticular disease' of the endometrium, by analogy with diverticular disease of the colon. The normal endometrial–myometrial junction is irregular but, in some women, endometrial glands and stroma extend more deeply into the myometrium and can, occasionally, be seen extending throughout the entire myometrial thickness. The degree to which these adenomyotic foci respond to hormonal stimulation is variable, and tends to be less than the lining endometrium, but this disorder is associated with both disturbances of the menstrual cycle and painful periods (dysmenorrhoea). If adenomyosis extends deeply into the myometrium, endometrial curettage or resection may not ameliorate the patient's symptoms. This disorder should therefore be considered in patients with continuing symptoms after curettage.

### Leiomyomas

Tumours may arise from any of the tissue elements of the uterus, such as smooth muscle, blood vessels, and nerves. By far the most common of these lesions is the leiomyoma (fibroid), which is a benign tumour arising from smooth muscle. These lesions are to some extent oestrogen dependent and usually multiple. They present in a variety of ways, including abnormal vaginal bleeding, a pelvic mass, or pelvic pain. The pain may occur as a result of 'red degeneration' which typically occurs during pregnancy but may also be seen as a consequence of progestogen therapy. Macroscopically, the tumours are well circumscribed and may be submucosal (Fig. 14.10), intramural or subserosal. Submucosal and subserosal fibroids are often polypoid: submucosal fibroids may present as a polyp within the endometrial cavity. Microscopically, leiomyomas are composed of interlacing fascicles of smooth muscle cells. There is debate about whether leiomyomas ever become malignant, forming a leiomyosarcoma, or whether leiomyosarcomas are malignant from the start. From a practical point of view, it is important to identify leiomyosarcomas because they have metastatic capability.

A variety of uncommon and rare tumours occurs in the uterus. Perhaps the most important of these is the carcinosarcoma (malignant mixed Müllerian tumour), so called because of the presence of a combination of epithelial and stromal elements presumed to be derived from the Müllerian duct system. Current evidence suggests that these tumours are 'metaplastic' carcinomas, i.e. the stromal elements (sarcoma) are derived from the epithelial elements (carcinoma) by a process termed 'epithelial–mesenchymal transition'. These tumours are highly malignant with a poor prognosis. Finally, metastatic tumours must not be forgotten.

## THE FALLOPIAN TUBE

The major disorders of the fallopian tube are salpingitis, endometriosis, and ectopic pregnancy. These are dealt with elsewhere in this chapter. Primary carcinomas of the fallopian tube have traditionally been considered to be rare but there is recent evidence that many carcinomas of the ovary may originate in the fallopian tube (see pp. 432–433)

## THE OVARY

> ### Key Points
>
> - Many ovarian cysts are not malignant.
> - Ovarian tumours may be benign, borderline, or malignant.
> - Most ovarian tumours are non-functioning and tend to present late, i.e. at high stage.
> - Some ovarian tumours (e.g. thecoma, granulosa cell tumour) secrete oestrogens or androgens, and present relatively early with endometrial abnormalities or virilization respectively.

### Non-neoplastic Cysts

Non-neoplastic cysts of the ovary can be divided into three broad categories:

1. Functional
2. Inclusion
3. Endometriotic.

Endometriosis is discussed on pp. 435–436, and will not be considered further at this point.

Inclusion cysts are generally found within the superficial ovarian cortex, and probably arise either as a result of inclusion of surface mesothelium, with epithelial metaplasia,

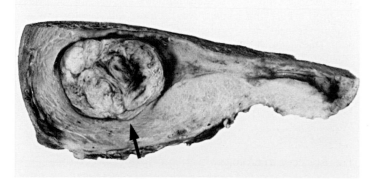

**FIG. 14.10** A submucosal uterine leiomyoma (arrow) which protrudes into the endometrial cavity. Lesions in this position may be associated with abnormal vaginal bleeding and infertility.

or by adherence of tubal epithelium at the time of ovulation. Most of them are of serous type, i.e. they are lined by epithelium that resembles the epithelium lining the fallopian tube.

Functional cysts are related to the cyclical development and atresia of ovarian follicles. Among functional cysts, *follicular cysts* are the most common type, and small cystic follicles are found in virtually all premenopausal ovaries. *Luteal cysts*, or cystic corpora lutea, are less common. Finally, follicular cysts may become luteinized during pregnancy to form luteinized follicular cysts.

## Polycystic Ovary Syndrome

A specific situation in which multiple cystic follicles are present in the ovaries is the PCOS (also known as Stein–Leventhal syndrome). The clinical syndrome comprises oligomenorrhoea, infertility, hirsutism, and obesity. From an endocrine point of view, there is disordered secretion of LH and FSH, leading to ovulation failure. The ovaries become enlarged and contain multiple cystic follicles. The capsule of the ovary is thickened, and there are usually no stigmata of ovulation, i.e. corpora lutea and corpora albicantes are absent. It is important to appreciate that a diagnosis of PCOS cannot be made on morphological grounds alone, and both clinical and endocrine data are required. However, the identification of patients with this syndrome is important in view of its association with endometrial hyperplasia and carcinoma (see p. 428). This complication may be preventable by treatment of the underlying endocrine disorder.

## Ovarian Tumours

### General Features

Ovarian tumours are relatively common, with the majority (approximately 80%) being benign and occurring in women of reproductive age. Malignant tumours occur in older women, most commonly aged 40–65 years, although certain uncommon tumour types do occur at a younger age. Many ovarian tumours – particularly of epithelial type – are bilateral: it is not clear whether these represent synchronous primary tumours or the spread of a single original tumour from one ovary to the other. Most ovarian tumours are non-functional and, in view of their relatively hidden anatomical location, tend to present late, usually as abdominal swelling due to the presence of a mass or associated ascites. Predisposing factors include nulliparity and gonadal dysgenesis. Patients with a strong family history of breast and/or ovarian cancer can now be screened for specific inherited molecular abnormalities, e.g. *BRCA1* gene mutations (see Chapter 15, pp. 459–460).

Primary ovarian tumours arise from three distinct cell types, and are classified according to the scheme presented in *Table 14.4*. However, it must be remembered that, whenever a malignant ovarian tumour is encountered, the possibility that it is a metastasis should be considered, particularly if it is of an unusual histological type and is bilateral.

**TABLE 14.4** Classification of ovarian tumours

|  | Cell of origin | Type | Proportion (%) |
|---|---|---|---|
| **Primary** | | | |
| Epithelial | Not entirely clear. The different histological types have different origins and arise through different molecular pathways (see text and see Fig. 14.13) | High-grade serous<br>Low-grade serous<br>Mucinous<br>Endometrioid/clear cell<br>Brenner/transitional<br>Carcinosarcoma<br>Undifferentiated | 65–70 |
| Germ cell tumours | Germ cells | Teratoma<br>Dysgerminoma<br>Yolk sac tumour<br>Embryonal carcinoma | 15–20 |
| Sex cord/stromal tumours | Ovarian sex cords and stroma | Granulosa cell tumours<br>Thecoma/fibroma<br>Sertoli/Leydig's tumours | 5–10 |
| Miscellaneous | Various | For example, lymphoma | |
| **Secondary** | | | |
| Metastases | – | – | 5–10 |

### Epithelial Ovarian Tumours

Macroscopically, epithelial ovarian tumours may be smooth-walled cystic lesions (Fig. 14.11) or contain a mixture of solid and cystic areas (Fig. 14.12). Papillary tumours are also relatively frequent and tend to be of serous type (see below). Each category of epithelial tumour is divided into three subcategories, based on a combination of cytological and architectural features (*Table 14.5*). This distinction is of fundamental importance, because the clinical behaviour of the tumour depends almost entirely on the presence of stromal invasion. Benign tumours effectively have no malignant potential. Invasive tumours are by definition malignant. Borderline tumours, which are most commonly serous (low-grade) or mucinous in type, are not clearly malignant but, in a small proportion of patients, may be associated with malignant features at a later date. The distinction between benign and borderline tumours is made microscopically. Although invasive carcinomas are often identifiable macroscopically, formal diagnosis requires histological examination. It is important to appreciate that the defining features of invasive carcinoma are stromal invasion and metastasis. Invasive tumours are staged according to the extent of spread as shown in *Table 14.6*. Note that this staging system also applies to fallopian tube and primary peritoneal

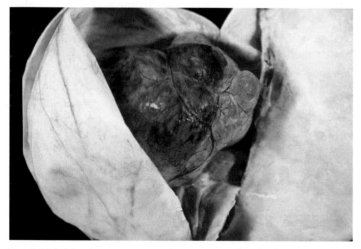

**FIG. 14.11** A benign serous cystadenoma: note that the lesion is cystic and has smooth external and internal surfaces.

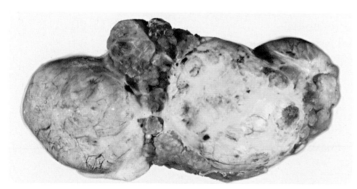

**FIG. 14.12** An invasive ovarian carcinoma: note the presence of both solid and cystic areas. Histologically, this lesion was a high-grade serous carcinoma.

**TABLE 14.5** The diagnostic criteria for epithelial ovarian tumours

| Tumour | Cytological appearance | Stromal invasion |
|---|---|---|
| Benign | Normal | No |
| Borderline | Abnormal | No |
| Invasive | Abnormal | Yes |

**TABLE 14.6** The FIGO (2013) staging system for ovarian, fallopian tube and primary peritoneal carcinomas

| Stage | | Tumour extent |
|---|---|---|
| I | | Tumour limited to the ovaries or fallopian tubes |
| | IA | One ovary (capsule intact) or fallopian tube; no tumour on surfaces, no malignant cells in ascites or peritoneal washings |
| | IB | Both ovaries (capsules intact) or fallopian tubes; no tumour on surfaces; no malignant cells in ascites or peritoneal washings |
| | IC | One or both ovaries or fallopian tubes with any of the following: capsule ruptured; tumour on surface; malignant cells in ascites or peritoneal washings |
| II | | Tumour involves one or both ovaries or fallopian tubes with pelvic extension; or primary peritoneal carcinoma |
| III | | Tumour involves one or both ovaries or fallopian tubes, or primary peritoneal carcinoma, with microscopically confirmed peritoneal spread outside the pelvis and/or retroperitoneal lymph node metastasis |
| IV | | Distant metastasis (excludes peritoneal metastasis) |

carcinomas, reflecting the fact that pelvic serous carcinomas are now staged and managed similarly irrespective of their apparent site of origin (see below).

The major types of ovarian carcinoma show histological patterns reminiscent of tubal epithelium (serous tumours), endocervical or intestinal epithelium (mucinous tumours), and endometrium (endometrioid and clear cell tumours). Other less common tumour types are also found, such as the Brenner tumour; this has a transitional morphology similar to that of the epithelium lining the urinary tract. The origin of epithelial ovarian tumours is not entirely clear, although there is increasing evidence that many high-grade serous tumours arise from the fallopian tube. High- and low-grade serous carcinomas are now recognized to represent distinct entities, with a *TP53* mutation being present in almost all high-grade serous carcinomas. Low-grade serous carcinomas are associated with *KRAS* or *BRAF*, but not *TP53*, mutations. Endometrioid and clear cell tumours often arise from ovarian endometriosis. Mucinous tumours may arise from Brenner tumours or teratomas but many mucinous ovarian

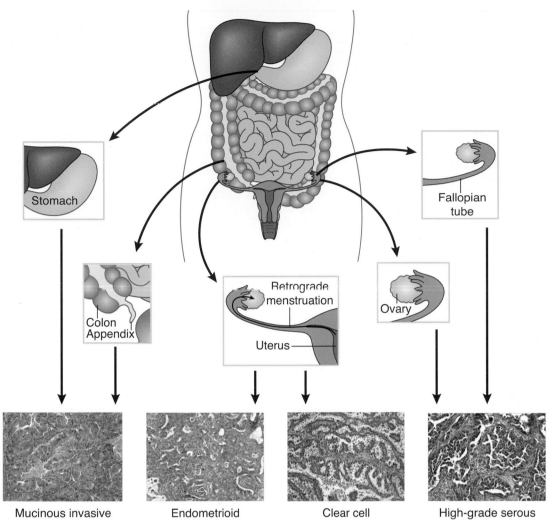

**FIG. 14.13** The origins of the different types of ovarian cancer. (Figure reproduced from Vaughan S, Coward JI, Bast RC, *et al*. Rethinking ovarian cancer: recommendations for improving outcomes. *Nature Reviews Cancer* 2011;**11**:719–725.)

tumours represent metastases from gastrointestinal, pancreatic, or biliary sites (Fig. 14.13).

Serous tumours are the most common type, are usually cystic, and may appear papillary. Low-grade (but not high-grade) serous carcinomas are often associated with benign or borderline components. A characteristic microscopic feature is the presence of psammoma bodies (Fig. 14.14), which may be present in benign, borderline, or malignant tumours, particularly if papillary. Primary mucinous tumours are uncommon and the possibility of metastasis, particularly from the gastrointestinal tract, biliary tree, or pancreas, must be excluded in all patients with these tumours, even those that appear borderline histologically. The presence of small bilateral mucinous ovarian tumours should prompt a particularly high index of suspicion because true primary ovarian mucinous tumours tend to be unilateral and larger than metastatic tumours. One important complication of mucinous tumours (particularly borderline tumours) is pseudomyxoma peritonei, which occurs as a result of mucin secretion by the tumour. This mucin, and associated neoplastic mucinous epithelium, can spread throughout the peritoneal cavity

where it may be associated with intestinal obstruction and other anatomical complications. It is now recognized that the vast majority of tumours associated with pseudomyxoma

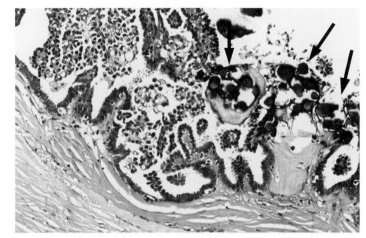

**FIG. 14.14** Microscopic appearance of a borderline serous tumour. The cells lining this cyst show cytological abnormalities, and numerous psammoma bodies are present (arrows).

## ABDOMINAL SWELLING

A 54-year-old postmenopausal woman presented with a 6-month history of gradual increase in her waist size. This had been accompanied by mild constipation, but no other significant symptoms. Clinical examination of the abdomen showed 'shifting dullness', indicating the presence of ascites, whereas pelvic examination suggested a mass in the right adnexal region. Ultrasound examination of the abdomen and pelvis confirmed the presence of ascites and showed a 60-mm mass in the right ovary, with a possible second mass in the left ovary. The ascitic fluid was drained and a sample sent for cytological assessment. This demonstrated clusters of adenocarcinoma cells. A laparotomy was performed and total abdominal hysterectomy, bilateral salpingo-oophorectomy and omentectomy carried out. Pathological examination of the specimens showed bilateral high-grade serous carcinoma of the ovary (see Fig. 14.12). The tumour in the right ovary extended through the capsule, and there were scattered tumour deposits within the omentum. A diagnosis of stage III serous carcinoma of the ovary was made. The patient was treated with adjuvant carboplatin and paclitaxel, and remained well and in remission 6 months later.

### Key Points

- Ovarian carcinoma often presents late.
- Chemotherapy is an important component of the management of patients with ovarian carcinoma.

peritonei are of appendiceal origin, with secondary spread to involve the ovaries. Endometrioid and clear cell tumours are associated with ovarian endometriosis, are typically unilateral, and tend to present at a low stage.

### Germ Cell Tumours of the Ovary

Around 95% of these tumours are mature cystic teratomas ('dermoid cysts'). The characteristic of these tumours is that mature elements derived from all three embryonic germ layers are present. The most common elements are ectodermal (skin, hair, teeth, and so on), but endodermal (intestinal, respiratory epithelium) and mesodermal (fat, muscle) elements are also present (Fig. 14.15). Rarely, malignant transformation has been described in these tumours, most commonly squamous cell carcinoma. Immature teratomas are related to mature teratomas, but contain immature neuroectodermal elements and behave in a malignant fashion. The importance of these is that they constitute 85% of ovarian teratomas in children.

All other types of germ cell tumours can occur in the ovary, but are uncommon. Dysgerminoma – which is the ovarian counterpart of testicular seminoma – occurs in young females and is an important diagnosis to make because the tumour is radiosensitive. Yolk sac tumours and embryonal carcinomas are rare and highly malignant.

### Ovarian Sex Cord/Stromal Tumours

These tumours differentiate along female (granulosa and theca cell tumours) or male (Sertoli/Leydig's cell tumours) lines. Granulosa cell tumours are fairly common, especially in postmenopausal women; these lesions behave in a low-grade malignant fashion and may secrete oestrogens. As a result of their oestrogen secretion, the tumours are associated with endometrial hyperplasia and endometrial carcinoma (see pp. 428–429). Ovarian fibromas and thecomas (Fig. 14.16) are also fairly common, but are usually benign. They too may secrete oestrogens (particularly thecomas) and may be associated with endometrial neoplasia.

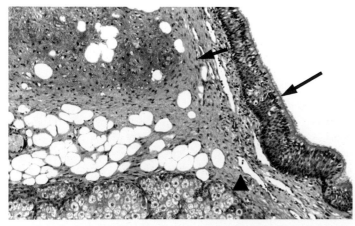

**FIG. 14.15** Microscopic appearance of a dermoid cyst showing elements from all three germ cell layers. Note the presence of cartilage (mesoderm – short arrow), respiratory epithelium (endoderm – long arrow), and sebaceous areas (ectoderm – arrow head).

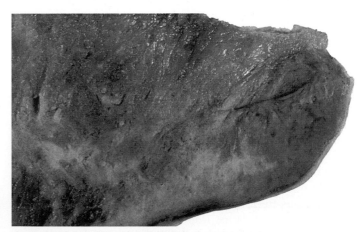

**FIG. 14.16** Macroscopic appearance of an ovarian thecoma. Note the yellow appearance, which is due to the presence of steroid hormone within the tumour cell cytoplasm.

Sertoli/Leydig's cell tumours are uncommon and reflect the pluripotential nature of ovarian stromal cells. They may be non-functioning, but may also secrete androgens, leading to virilization. Occasionally, they may secrete oestrogens.

### Metastases to the Ovary

Some non-primary ovarian tumours reflect transcoelomic spread from pelvic tumours, e.g. from a colorectal carcinoma. Others are haematogenous or lymphatic metastases from distant sites, e.g. other parts of the gastrointestinal and female genital tracts. It is important to consider this possibility when assessing patients with ovarian tumours, particularly when they are mucinous in type and bilateral, because identification of the primary site affects both staging and clinical management. One specific example of ovarian metastasis is Krukenberg's tumour, which is usually bilateral and associated with diffuse ovarian enlargement and the presence of signet-ring tumour cells. These tumours are characteristically of gastric origin.

# PELVIC INFLAMMATORY DISEASE

### Key Points

- Pelvic inflammatory disease affects the whole female genital tract.
- It is associated with intrauterine contraceptive devices.
- It may be complicated by infertility and ectopic pregnancy.
- Commonly associated organisms include *Chlamydia* spp. and actinomycetes.

Inflammation and consequent functional disturbance due to sexually transmitted infections frequently affect the whole female genital tract, even when the clinical manifestations are restricted to one region. Various aetiological agents are important, including *Neisseria gonorrhoeae*, *Actinomyces israelii*, and particularly *Chlamydia* spp. These infections have a variety of clinical consequences, including abnormal vaginal bleeding, infertility, and the formation of tubo-ovarian abscesses. The clinical pattern depends upon the anatomical distribution of the inflammatory process.

Inflammation of the endometrium occurs physiologically as part of the late secretory and menstrual phases of the menstrual cycle. Endometritis is therefore defined as endometrial inflammation that is not part of the normal menstrual cycle. As with inflammation elsewhere, endometritis may be infective or non-infective, and acute or chronic.

- Acute endometritis is uncommon, and is usually bacterial. Classically, this disorder was associated with instrumentation, such as during abortion, but this is fortunately now rare.

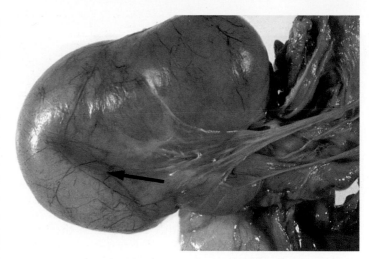

**FIG. 14.17** Resolution after adnexal inflammation has led to the formation of adhesions and a hydrosalpinx. Note that the dilated fallopian tube is 'kinked' (arrow).

- Chronic endometritis is more common, and is characterized by the presence of plasma cells within the endometrium. Acute inflammatory cells may also be present (active chronic endometritis), as may macrophages. When macrophages form aggregates (i.e. granulomas), a specific cause should be sought: possible causes include tuberculosis, fungal infection, and sarcoidosis. Granulomas are also found after transcervical resection of the endometrium, which is a procedure used for the treatment of DUB.

The most common clinical situation in which chronic endometritis is encountered is in patients with intrauterine contraceptive devices (IUCDs). It is also associated with chronic pelvic inflammatory disease. In most cases no organisms are identified, although it is important specifically to exclude actinomycosis and tuberculosis, if appropriate. Many cases of chronic endometritis are related to chlamydia infection, which is a common cause of inflammatory damage to the fallopian tube (salpingitis) and hence infertility.

Inflammation of the fallopian tube occurs predominantly by ascending infection from the uterine cavity, and is generally accompanied by infection of other parts of the female genital tract. It may be confined to the fallopian tube (salpingitis), but often involves the adjacent ovary (salpingo-oophoritis), with adhesion of fimbriae to the ovarian surface. Such an inflammatory process can extend to the peritoneal cavity (peritonitis) and may become 'sealed off' by these adhesions, leading to the formation of a tubo-ovarian abscess. Resolution of inflammation in this site usually leaves adhesions and, if these obstruct the fallopian tube, hydrosalpinx may ensue (Fig. 14.17). Interference with fallopian tube function often leads to reduced fertility and predisposes to ectopic pregnancy.

# ENDOMETRIOSIS

### Key Points

- Endometriosis is the presence of endometrial glands and stroma outside the uterine body.
- The pathogenesis is unknown.
- Endometriosis of the ovary frequently forms 'chocolate' cysts.

Endometriosis is the presence of endometrial glands and stroma outside the uterine body (Fig. 14.18). It occurs in a wide variety of different sites (*Table 14.7*), but most often affects the ovaries and other sites within the pelvis,

**TABLE 14.7** Anatomical sites of endometriosis

| Common | Uncommon | Rare |
|---|---|---|
| Ovary (80%) | Cervix | Lung |
| Uterine ligaments | Vagina | Pleura |
| Pouch of Douglas | Bladder | Skeletal muscle |
| Fallopian tube | Skin[a] | Small bowel |

[a]Cutaneous involvement occurs characteristically in scars, particularly those from caesarean sections.

particularly the pouch of Douglas and the posterior pelvic peritoneum. Note that involvement of the serosa of the uterus is included in the definition.

The pathogenesis of endometriosis is unknown, but there are several hypothesized mechanisms, including regurgitation of menstrual endometrium (retrograde menstruation), metaplasia of surface epithelia, and vascular or lymphatic spread of normal endometrium. The first is consistent with the anatomical distribution, but it is difficult to explain the presence of endometriosis in distant sites on this basis. This is also true of the metaplasia theory.

Macroscopically, endometriosis forms multiple peritoneal nodules and, within the ovary, 'chocolate' cysts. The inflammation associated with the presence of endometriosis leads to the formation of adhesions which may cause secondary anatomical abnormalities, particularly of the fallopian tubes; this may lead to a reduction in fertility and predisposes to ectopic pregnancy.

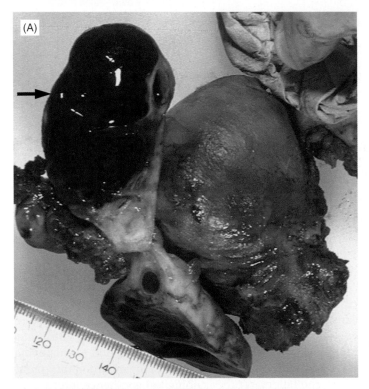

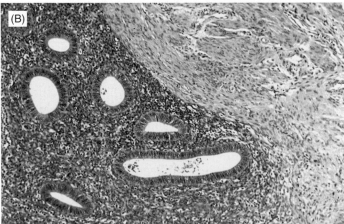

**FIG. 14.18** Endometriosis: (A) Macroscopic involvement of the ovary often takes the form of 'chocolate cysts' (arrow). (B) Microscopically, both endometrial glands and stroma are present, often with associated inflammation.

# PREGNANCY

### Key Points

- The placenta is formed from maternal and fetal elements.
- Abnormal vascularization of the placental bed is associated with pregnancy-associated hypertension (pre-eclampsia).
- Both maternal and fetal factors predispose to spontaneous miscarriage.
- Ectopic pregnancy may occur in any site accessible to the fertilized ovum.
- Ectopic pregnancy is an important gynaecological emergency.
- Patients with hydatidiform mole should be followed up carefully in specialist centres.

## Placental Pathology

The placenta is formed from both maternal and fetal components: the decidua is formed by alteration of the maternal endometrium, and the chorionic villi and fetal membranes (including the chorion) are derived from fetal tissues. Formation of the placenta involves alteration of the maternal vascular bed within the endometrium and myometrium to support placental function and fetal demand. It is now thought that abnormality of this vascularization is the fundamental abnormality in pregnancy-associated hypertension (pre-eclampsia). Further details of placental pathology are beyond the scope of this text, but can be found in textbooks of obstetric and gynaecological pathology (see Further Reading).

## Spontaneous Miscarriage and Intrauterine Fetal Death

A significant proportion of all pregnancies end in fetal loss, which occurs most frequently in the first trimester. A variety of maternal and fetal factors are involved in the maintenance of pregnancy. Therefore, pregnancy can fail as a result of a number of abnormalities; some of these are presented in *Box 14.2*.

Fetal chromosome abnormalities are the most common cause of early fetal loss (Fig. 14.19) that occurs up to 12 weeks of gestation. Many abnormalities have been described, including triploidy and specific trisomies. Maternal factors tend to be associated with later fetal loss. Physical abnormalities, such as uterine anomalies (e.g. uterus didelphys) and the presence of submucosal fibroids, interfere with placental and fetal growth within the uterine cavity, and loss tends to occur in the second trimester. It should be remembered that these abnormalities are also associated with reduced fertility. Intrauterine death in the third trimester (stillbirth) is often of unknown cause, although evidence of ascending infection is sometimes identified. It is also associated with maternal diabetes mellitus.

## Ectopic Pregnancy

Ectopic pregnancy occurs when the blastocyst implants and develops outside the endometrial cavity (Fig. 14.20). This may occur in any site accessible to the fertilized ovum (i.e. pelvic peritoneum, ovary), but by far the most common site is the fallopian tube. Underlying aetiological factors that increase the chances of this happening include any fallopian

Box 14.2 CLASSIFICATION OF PREDISPOSING
FACTORS FOR SPONTANEOUS FAILURE OF
PREGNANCY

Maternal
    Endocrine
    Physical
    Immunological
Fetal
    Chromosome abnormalities
Maternofetal
    Infection (STORCH; *Listeria* sp.; parvovirus)

STORCH = syphilis, toxoplasmosis, rubella, cytomegalovirus, herpes virus infections.

tube pathology such as: current or previous salpingitis (usually as part of pelvic inflammatory disease); endometriosis; and distortion of the fallopian tube by adhesions (e.g. those related to previous appendicectomy). The developing conceptus invades into the supporting tissues, irrespective of the anatomical site. As the fallopian tube is a thin structure with limited smooth muscle within its wall, the conceptus quickly erodes through the wall (often at around 6 weeks' gestation), with consequent intraperitoneal haemorrhage. This can be a catastrophic event because blood loss may be massive. This diagnosis should therefore be considered in

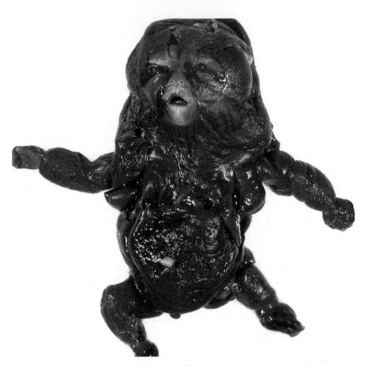

FIG. 14.19 A spontaneously aborted fetus showing hydropic changes. Cytogenetic analysis showed a karyotype of 45,XO, indicating Turner's syndrome.

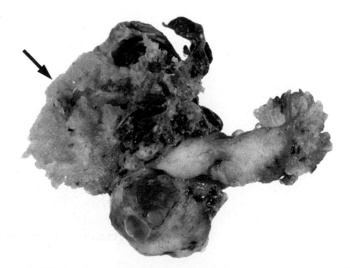

FIG. 14.20 Ectopic pregnancy: in this case, the conceptus has developed in the lumen of the fallopian tube, which has consequently ruptured. Note the presence of early placental tissue (arrow).

any woman of child-bearing age who presents with abdominal pain or circulatory collapse. Suspicion should be even greater if there is a history of amenorrhoea. The diagnosis can often be confirmed by carrying out a pregnancy test and performing an ultrasound scan of the lower abdomen. Ectopic pregnancy can sometimes be treated by 'milking' the fallopian tube or by salpingotomy, but often excision of part or all of the tube (salpingectomy) is required: this is now often performed laparoscopically.

## Gestational Trophoblastic Disease

This is a spectrum of tumours and tumour-like conditions characterized by the proliferation of trophoblastic tissue.

### Hydatidiform Mole

The most common example of this group of disorders is the hydatidiform mole, which has an incidence of approximately 1 in 2,000 pregnancies in the western world. However, it is significantly more frequent in some other parts of the world, notably Indonesia, where the incidence is as high as 1 in 80 pregnancies. Moles classically present with uterine enlargement, which is 'large for dates' and may be associated with excessive vomiting (hyperemesis), related to high levels of hCG. However, most patients with a hydatidiform mole now do not present in this way, primarily because of the increasing use of ultrasound in the monitoring of pregnancy and the submission of most evacuated products of conception for histological examination. The classic macroscopic appearance of hydatidiform mole is a large, fleshy mass of thin-walled, translucent grape-like chorionic villi (Fig. 14.21). Again, most moles do not have this appearance because the hydropic changes do not occur at early gestation. Therefore, the diagnosis is most commonly made by identifying the histological hallmark of hydatidiform moles, which is trophoblastic proliferation (Fig. 14.22). The fundamental cause of this is an excess of paternal chromosomes within the fertilized ovum. Hydatidiform

moles are divided into two main groups: partial and complete (*Table 14.8*). The most likely mechanism for the occurrence of partial mole is dual fertilization of a single ovum by two separate spermatozoa to produce a triploid conceptus that contains twice as much paternal as maternal DNA. Interestingly, maternal triploidy, in which the extra set of chromosomes is of maternal origin, does not cause a partial mole, although it is associated with early fetal loss. Complete mole contains only paternal chromosomes. The precise mechanism by which this arises is not understood but this feature underlies the absence of expression of the paternally imprinted and maternally expressed gene $p57^{KIP2}$ in complete moles. This can be used to aid the diagnosis of molar pregnancies, because complete moles lack $p57^{KIP2}$ protein expression, whereas expression is retained in partial moles. Genetic approaches, based on the identification of maternal and paternal genetic components, can also be used to investigate and classify hydatidiform moles.

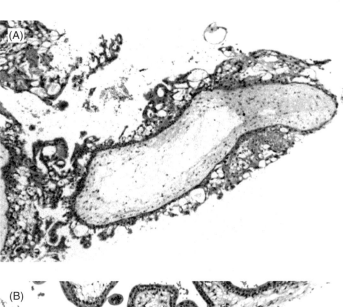

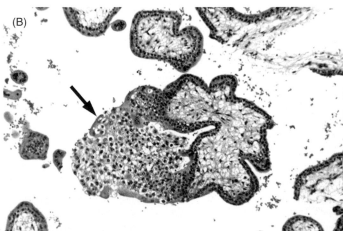

**FIG. 14.21** Macroscopic appearance of a classic hydatidiform mole.

**FIG. 14.22** Microscopic appearance of (A) a hydatidiform mole showing circumferential trophoblastic proliferation. There is early stromal degeneration. This contrasts with the appearance of normal chorionic villi (B) which have polar trophoblast (arrow).

**TABLE 14.8** Characteristics of complete and partial hydatidiform mole

| Characteristic | Complete | Partial |
| --- | --- | --- |
| Hydropic villi (if later in gestation) | All | Some |
| Fetus | Absent | Present |
| Trophoblastic hyperplasia | Marked | Minimal to moderate |
| Ploidy | Diploid | Triploid |
| Genetic content | Paternal DNA only | Paternal and maternal DNA (ratio 2:1) |
| Expression of p57$^{KIP2}$ | Absent | Present |
| Sex chromosomes | 85% XX, 15% XY | Most XXY |

Most moles do not have adverse consequences. However, some recur, become invasive, or develop into choriocarcinoma. The natural history is not predictable from the histological appearance, and therefore all patients with a diagnosis of mole should be followed up by repeated measurement of serum hCG levels. If the hCG level falls to normal, then no further treatment is required. If the level remains static or rises, then a diagnosis of persistent trophoblastic disease is made. This can be due to any of the three outcomes given above, but patients are generally managed as if they have choriocarcinoma because this is extremely responsive to treatment with chemotherapeutic agents, e.g. methotrexate.

### Choriocarcinoma

Choriocarcinoma is rare in the western world, occurring as a complication of approximately 1 in 20,000–30,000 pregnancies. However, as with hydatidiform mole, it is significantly more common in south-east Asia (up to 1 in 2,500 pregnancies). This disorder is characterized by malignancy of trophoblastic cells. Chorionic villi are never produced. The tumour is very aggressive and frequently metastasizes, but is highly responsive to chemotherapy. Choriocarcinoma is most commonly preceded by hydatidiform mole, but may also occur after an abortion, normal pregnancy, and even an ectopic pregnancy.

## 14.1 Special Study Topic

### HUMAN PAPILLOMAVIRUSES AND CERVICAL NEOPLASIA

#### Introduction

It is now recognized that virtually all (>99%) invasive cervical carcinomas are associated with HPV infection. The precise part played by HPV in this process is not completely understood, and the sequence of events is unclear. However, the pathological definition of various grades of intraepithelial neoplasia, and the epidemiological evidence that these are precursors of invasive disease, makes this pathological spectrum an ideal model for the study of virus-associated tumorigenesis.

#### Human Papillomaviruses

Papillomaviruses are small DNA viruses composed of a double-stranded DNA genome approximately 8 kb in length surrounded by capsid protein. These viruses have a simple structure, but their complexity arises from the tremendous variation in viral DNA sequence. This has led to the definition of almost 150 HPV types. This is not only of biological importance but is also of clinical relevance, because different HPV types are associated with different forms of squamous epithelial disease (see below).

All HPV types contain the same viral genes. These are divided into two groups – early and late – based on the time of the life cycle at which they are expressed. The late genes (L1 and L2) encode the capsid proteins, and the early genes encode a variety of proteins that have the common property of binding to many cellular proteins with different functions. The E1 and E2 proteins are involved in viral DNA replication, the E2 protein also being involved in regulation of the other viral genes. The E6 gene encodes a protein that not only has oncogenic properties but is also capable of binding to and inactivating the p53 protein. This has an effect equivalent to inactivating mutation or deletion of both TP53 genes. Similarly, the E7 protein can bind to the retinoblastoma gene product and several other cell cycle regulatory proteins. One of the main functions of E7 seems to be to induce the cellular machinery required for DNA synthesis, and hence pave the way for the action of the E1 and E2 proteins. It is becoming increasingly clear that HPVs, similar to many other DNA viruses, achieve their replication by interference with normal cell cycle control mechanisms. It is likely that the oncogenic potential of papillomaviruses lies at least in part in their ability to alter cell cycle checkpoints, thereby leading to accumulation and transmission of genetic abnormalities.

# Special Study Topic continued . . .

## Pathology of HPV Infection

It is thought that HPVs infect the cervical epithelium through small epithelial abrasions, although a distinct population of susceptible junctional cells has recently been identified at the squamocolumnar junction in the cervix. The viral life cycle is then closely linked to keratinocyte differentiation, with viral DNA replication, capsid protein production, and release of intact virions occurring in a coordinated fashion with maturation up to the squamous epithelium. This process leads to the cytopathic effect of HPV infection (koilocytosis), and such lesions may regress, persist, or progress.

If viral replication and production of virions do not occur, the viral DNA can persist within the cell either as an extrachromosomal molecule or by integration into the host cellular DNA. It is thought that continued early gene expression under these circumstances may be related to neoplastic progression. This is consistent with the fact that HPV DNA, particularly the *E6* and *E7* genes, can immortalize primary cervical cells in culture. Other oncogenic sequences are, however, required to effect full transformation.

## Clinical Associations of HPV Genotypes

HPV types can be subdivided into groups on the basis of their DNA sequence. They can also be grouped according to their association with clinical disease. Thus, low-risk HPVs (e.g. HPV-6, -11) are usually associated with benign exophytic genital warts. These types are only rarely found in CIN 2 and 3 and invasive carcinomas. By contrast, high-risk (especially HPV-16 and -18) HPV types are associated with all grades of CIN, but particularly CIN 2 and 3 and invasive carcinoma. Careful analysis of large numbers of invasive cervical carcinomas has identified HPV DNA in over 99% of tumours. The most common type was HPV-16 (50%), with HPV-18 being identified frequently but less commonly. HPV-16 is associated particularly with squamous cell carcinomas, but several studies have consistently shown that HPV-18 is the most common type in adenocarcinomas. The biological reasons for this are unclear. This finding has significant implications not only for the biology of cervical cancer but also for the potential value of HPV testing in the cervical screening programme, and the potential efficacy of HPV vaccination strategies.

There is current interest in using HPV testing to improve the cervical screening programme. This has been prompted by epidemiological studies that have shown not only that HPV typing can have a higher sensitivity than cytology for the detection of CIN 2, CIN 3, and invasive carcinoma, but also that the risk of progression to a high-grade lesion is greater in patients with persistent HPV infection. HPV testing has recently been introduced into the cervical screening programme in the UK and it is possible that it may replace cytology as the primary screening test. One possibility is that women would be screened using HPV testing and investigated further by cervical cytology if HPV positive.

The efficacy of prophylactic HPV vaccines has been demonstrated in several clinical trials and HPV vaccination has now been introduced in many developed countries. The two most widely used vaccines protect against HPV-16 and -18 (± HPV-6 and -11), which is likely to prevent the development of both squamous cell carcinoma and adenocarcinoma. However, this will not prevent all cervical cancer because those due to other HPV types will continue to occur. The inclusion of further HPV types in future vaccines may address this issue.

## Cofactors in the Evolution of Cervical Neoplasia

Only a small proportion of HPV infections progresses to either high-grade CIN or invasive cervical cancer. Progression of lesions is likely to involve further steps either related to continued viral gene expression (possibly as a result of persistent viral infection) or to the action of other carcinogenic factors. This concept is consistent with current multistep models of carcinogenesis (Fig. 14.23), such as that proposed for colorectal carcinogenesis (see Chapter 9). A variety of factors have been proposed to interact with HPV, and these are summarized in *Table 14.9*.

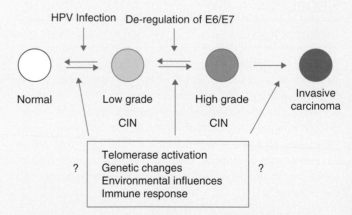

**Fig. 14.23** Schematic representation of the putative molecular events involved in cervical human papillomavirus (HPV)-associated squamous carcinogenesis. Low grade refers to low-grade squamous intraepithelial lesions, which encompass HPV effect and cervical intraepithelial neoplasia (CIN) 1. High grade refers to high-grade squamous intraepithelial lesions, which encompass CIN 2 and CIN 3.

## Special Study Topic continued . . .

**TABLE 14.9** Cofactors involved in human papillomavirus (HPV)-associated cervical neoplasia

| Factor | Effect |
|---|---|
| Secondary genetic changes | Activation of oncogenes |
| | Loss of tumour-suppressor gene function |
| Smoking | Formation of adduction products |
| | Local immunosuppression |
| Herpes simplex virus infection | Possible contribution of oncogenic factor |
| HIV infection | Immunosuppression |
| | Direct effect on HPV gene expression |
| Immunosuppression | Persistent HPV infection |
| Hormonal effects | Up-regulation of HPV early gene expression |

### Conclusions

HPV infection is the major aetiological factor for cervical neoplasia. However, it is clear that progression from infection to neoplasia requires secondary changes. These may occur partly as a result of persistent HPV gene expression with consequent production of cell cycle control defects, but other factors such as immunosuppression and smoking are also important in some patients. The strong association between HPV infection and cervical neoplasia underpins the concept, supported by clinical trial data, that vaccination against HPV will prevent many cases of cervical cancer.

## SUMMARY

The female reproductive tract is, due to its cyclical functions and ease of access of pathogens, at risk of a variety of neoplastic (often due to viral or hormonal causes) and inflammatory conditions. The role of HPV in cervical neoplasia is especially noteworthy and the prevention of this disease by cervical cytology, and hopefully by HPV vaccination, is an indication of the potential of screening and prevention programmes. Finally, the placenta and developing fetus are also at risk of developmental abnormalities, inflammation, and, rarely, neoplasia.

## FURTHER READING

Fox H, Wells M, eds. *Haines and Taylor: Obstetrical and Gynaecological Pathology*, 5th edn. Edinburgh: Churchill Livingstone, 2003.

Mutter G, Prat J, eds. *Pathology of the Female Reproductive Tract*, 3rd edn. Edinburgh: Churchill Livingstone, 2014.

Vaughan S, Coward JI, Bast RC, *et al.* Rethinking ovarian cancer: recommendations for improving outcomes. *Nature Reviews Cancer* 2011;11:719–725.

# 15

# THE BREASTS

Sarah E Pinder, Andrew HS Lee, and Ian O Ellis

## INTRODUCTION

The female breast is in the unique position of being a gland that is non-functional except during lactation. It is, nevertheless, subject to hormonal influences, particularly throughout reproductive life, and this probably accounts for most of its pathological changes, which rarely affect the male. By far the most important disease is carcinoma, which usually presents as a palpable lump. Other lesions are mostly of significance because they may produce a lump or lumpiness of the breast or other symptoms raising the suspicion of carcinoma, and must therefore be investigated. The most common of these are fibroadenomas, which are most frequent in the third decade, and fibrocystic change, which presents particularly in the premenopausal decade. As a result of the liability of the breast to injury, traumatic fat necrosis is another cause of a firm lump. Duct ectasia (dilatation of ducts) and duct papilloma may each, similar to carcinoma, cause a discharge from the nipple. Infection of the breast is rare except during lactation or associated with duct ectasia, and most congenital abnormalities are also uncommon.

## THE NORMAL BREAST

The breasts consist of a group of modified sweat glands, which develop from 15–25 downgrowths of the epidermis. At first solid cords, they develop a lumen and become the major (segmental) ducts, each of which opens separately at the nipple. Each segmental duct gives rise to the branching duct system of a segment of breast tissue. Before puberty the structure of male and female breast tissue is identical. In the female, under the hormonal stimulation of puberty, the duct system proliferates. Lobules, composed of acini

and intralobular stroma, bud from subsegmental ducts to form physiologically functional terminal duct lobular units (Fig. 15.1). Apart from duct ectasia and duct papilloma, most lesions in the breast are believed to arise from the terminal duct lobular unit. The connective tissue between the terminal duct lobular units (i.e. interlobular and segmental) is less cellular and more densely collagenous, and during puberty becomes infiltrated with fatty tissue; this

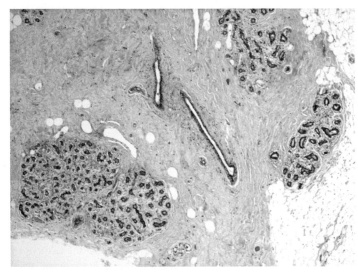

**FIG. 15.1** Normal breast: most of the breast is composed of stromal tissue, largely mature adipose and fibrous tissue. Within this lie the physiologically and pathologically important breast epithelial structures, from which most breast lesions are derived. The lobules form well-defined islands of small tubular structures (acini) (e.g. lower left) surrounded by intralobular stroma. The ducts are lined by a double layer of inner cuboidal or columnar-shaped epithelium over a layer of myoepithelial cells (centre).

accounts for most of the enlargement of the female breast at this time. Apart from a stratified squamous epithelial lining close to the nipple, the ducts and ductules are lined by a two-layered epithelium, an inner layer of cuboidal or columnar epithelial cells, and an outer discontinuous layer of smaller, contractile, myoepithelial cells. These two layers are invested in a continuous basement membrane and the duct system is ensheathed in a layer of loose connective tissue that is rich in lymphatics. There is little or no elastic tissue in the lobules, but an elastic layer surrounds the larger ducts.

The ductal epithelium of the mature female breast has some minor secretory activity, but the secretion is normally reabsorbed. During pregnancy, proliferation increases and secretory acini develop from the terminal ductular alveoli (Fig. 15.2). After the menopause, the breast epithelium atrophies and the lobular connective tissue changes to less cellular hyaline collagen; the terminal ductules may virtually disappear, but sometimes become dilated, forming microcysts lined by flattened, attenuated epithelium.

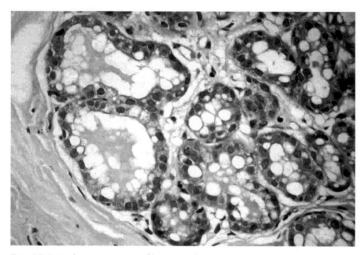

**Fig. 15.2** High-power view of lactating breast. During later pregnancy and lactation, the epithelium of the lobules becomes vacuolated with lipid-rich material, which is secreted into the lumen.

## DEVELOPMENTAL ABNORMALITIES

Congenital abnormalities of the breast are rare and relatively unimportant clinically (although potentially distressing for the female concerned), with the exception of polymastia (accessory breast parenchyma) and polythelia (accessory nipples). These may occur anywhere along the 'milk line' from the axilla to the groin and are subject to the same disorders as normally situated breasts. Failure of development of the breast at puberty is uncommon and usually associated with ovarian agenesis, as in Turner's syndrome. Precocious development may also occur, occasionally related to the presence of an ovarian granulosa cell tumour (see Chapter 14, p. 434), but usually for unexplained reasons. Adolescent or juvenile hypertrophy is the most common developmental abnormality seen. At the onset of puberty the breasts grow rapidly and out of proportion, so that they become a severe

physical and psychological burden. Rarely, the hypertrophy is unilateral. The cause is unknown and the only effective treatment is surgical reduction. Microscopically, no specific abnormality is seen and the enlargement appears to be due to an overgrowth of adipose and connective tissue.

## BENIGN BREAST LESIONS

The term 'benign breast disease' is sometimes used clinically to imply a specific pathological entity. This is clearly an oversimplification and there are a number of distinct lesions (*Table 15.1*) that merit discussion and separate nomenclature.

**TABLE 15.1** The most common benign breast lesions

| | |
|---|---|
| Non-neoplastic | Fibrocystic change |
| | Fibroadenoma |
| | Hamartoma |
| | Sclerosing lesions including sclerosing adenosis and radial scar/complex sclerosing lesion |
| Benign tumours | Papilloma |
| | Phyllodes tumour |
| Infections | Acute pyogenic mastitis/abscess |
| Non-infectious inflammatory lesions | Duct ectasia |
| | Fat necrosis |

## Infections

> **Key Points**
>
> - Breast infections are rare.
> - Breast abscesses occur mainly in association with breastfeeding or duct ectasia.

Acute pyogenic mastitis occurs mainly during lactation and is the result of infection via the ducts or through an abrasion of the nipple. It is most often caused by staphylococci acquired in hospital from the mouth of the suckling infant, which has been colonized by the prevalent strain of *Staphylococcus aureus*. Unless effectively treated, staphylococcal mastitis may cause a breast abscess; abscess formation may also occur superficial, or uncommonly deep, to the mammary gland. Acute pyogenic mastitis may become chronic if not treated adequately, or infection with pyogenic bacteria may start insidiously and persist, but these events are rare. Recurrent or chronic low-grade infection of the subareolar tissue occurs in some women, with scarring, distortion, and sometimes fistula formation.

Tuberculosis of the breast is rare in developed countries. It may arise by haematogenous, lymphatic, or direct spread, usually from the lungs or pleura. It may remain localized as a single caseating lesion, which sometimes discharges through the skin, or it may spread extensively through the breast. In view of its rarity and the occurrence of other lesions with similar histological appearances, a definite diagnosis of tuberculosis of the breast should not be made unless *Mycobacterium tuberculosis* has been detected in the lesion.

## Non-infective Inflammatory Lesions

### Duct Ectasia

> **Key Points**
> - Duct ectasia is of uncertain aetiology.
> - It usually presents with nipple discharge.
> - Microscopically, dilatation of ducts containing foamy macrophages with a surrounding chronic inflammatory infiltrate and periductal fibrosis is seen.

Duct ectasia consists of progressive dilatation of the large or intermediate ducts with surrounding chronic inflammatory change. It affects one or more segments of the breast and very rarely is palpable, similar to a 'bag of worms'. The dilated ducts contain inspissated material and their walls are thickened. Microscopically the duct epithelium appears thinned, with an underlying thickened fibrous wall that is usually infiltrated with plasma cells and lymphocytes. Foamy macrophages are often present in the lumen of the ducts and in the nipple discharge.

Duct ectasia is often symptomless, but there may be a nipple discharge. Less commonly, contraction of the periductal fibrosis may cause retraction of the nipple and raise the suspicion of carcinoma. Occasionally a dilated duct ruptures into the surrounding stroma, where its lipid contents promote a persistent inflammatory reaction with accumulation of foamy macrophages and giant cells, and fibrosis; the microscopic appearances resemble those of traumatic fat necrosis and the lesion may become palpable as a firm lump. The term 'plasma cell mastitis' is sometimes applied to cases of duct ectasia that bear an unusually heavy plasma cell infiltrate, but in essence these are the same lesion. The aetiology of duct ectasia is uncertain; it tends to occur most often in multiparous females who have not breastfed, but also occurs in nulliparous females. There is increasing evidence that the underlying mechanism for the duct dilatation is periductal inflammation, leading to destruction of the elastic network with fibrosis. Periareolar abscess or fistula formation may complicate duct ectasia, particularly in younger females.

### Granulomatous Mastitis

Granulomatous mastitis is a rare condition in which the terminal duct lobular unit is the site of an intense granulomatous and chronic inflammatory process with conspicuous giant cells. Terminal duct dilatation may be present, with associated foamy macrophages and, on occasion, actual abscess formation. The condition is often associated with a recent pregnancy but has also been described in nulliparous females. It should properly be termed 'idiopathic' granulomatous mastitis because the aetiology is unknown. In particular, no infectious cause has been identified, but tuberculosis should always be excluded in such a granulomatous inflammatory process because the microscopic appearances are essentially similar. Sarcoidosis may also be associated with granulomas in the breast, but these are not confined to lobular structures, unlike idiopathic granulomatous mastitis.

### Traumatic Fat Necrosis

> **Key Points**
> - Traumatic fat necrosis may be mistaken clinically for carcinoma.
> - It is caused by injury to the fatty breast parenchyma.
> - Microscopically, a granulomatous response to the released lipid is seen, with subsequent fibrosis.

Traumatic fat necrosis (Fig. 15.3) arises in the fatty tissue of the breast and may present as a hard lump mimicking cancer. It is caused by injury to the fat cells, although this may be relatively minor particularly in the obese or pendulous breast, and in many instances no history of trauma is obtained. The initial necrosis is accompanied by haemorrhage and followed by an acute inflammatory reaction. The lesion becomes heavily infiltrated by foamy macrophages containing lipid and often haemosiderin, and crystals of lipid may be deposited stimulating a foreign-body giant cell reaction. Granulation tissue forms around the lesion and gradually matures into a thick layer of fibrous tissue which,

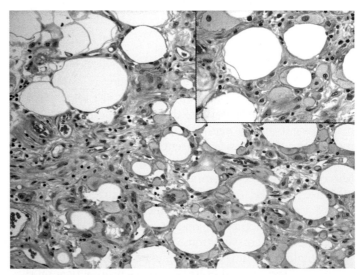

**FIG. 15.3** Fat necrosis: the main picture and higher-power inset both show fat spaces surrounded by an inflammatory response of swollen macrophages, which have taken up lipid released from the damaged adipocytes.

often together with calcification, accounts for the presentation as a firm or hard lump. The fibrous reaction may result in retraction of the nipple or fixation to the skin, features that increase the clinical resemblance to breast carcinoma.

### Reaction to Foreign Material

Leakage from silicone breast implants used either for breast augmentation or as a breast reconstruction procedure after surgery for carcinoma is usually without harmful effect but may induce a granulomatous giant-cell reaction and cause tenderness or nodularity. This was more common historically when silicone or paraffin was injected directly into the breast tissues. Microscopically, fragments of the 'inert' material may be seen, surrounded by macrophages and multinucleated giant cells.

### Galactocele

This is a cystic swelling of a lactiferous duct that develops during lactation, apparently due to obstruction of the duct. Initially it contains creamy, lipid-rich fluid that gradually becomes watery. Leakage of duct contents may induce a granulomatous reaction, or potentially become infected.

## Fibroadenoma

### Key Points

- Fibroadenoma is one of the most common breast lesions.
- It represents a localized hyperplasia rather than development of a true neoplasm.
- It presents as a well-defined mass, often in young females.
- Microscopically there is proliferation of the intralobular stroma with interspersed epithelial tubules or clefts.

Although it has previously been the convention to regard fibroadenomas as benign tumours, there is considerable evidence to support the view that they are focal areas of lobular hyperplasia rather than true neoplasms. They may present at any age after puberty but are most common in the third decade, presenting as well-defined mobile lumps, which may occasionally be multiple and bilateral. Microscopically, the dominant element is a proliferation of loose, cellular, intralobular stroma that is associated with a variable number of tubular structures (Fig. 15.4). The tubular structures appear as either elongated clefts or tubules cut in cross-section. The previous designation of 'intracanalicular' and 'pericanalicular' types, based on these patterns of stroma and epithelium, has no practical or clinical significance, and can be abandoned. Fibroadenomas are usually well-circumscribed lesions, but although they are

easily enucleated at surgery they are not truly encapsulated. Occasionally, small foci of fibroadenomatous hyperplasia are found; these are small, microscopic, lobulated areas resembling fibroadenomas, but not forming well-defined masses. Both fibroadenomatous hyperplasia and fibroadenomas may present through mammographic breast screening programmes, because associated microcalcification can form in the stroma (Fig. 15.5).

Fibroadenomas are entirely benign lesions that confer no significant predisposition to subsequent carcinoma. Indeed, many surgeons now avoid surgical excision, as long as the

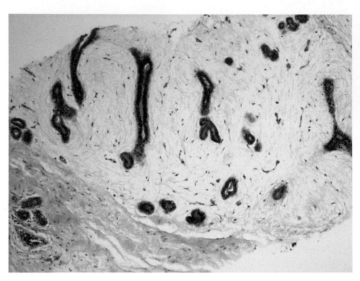

**FIG. 15.4** Fibroadenoma: a core biopsy of a fibroadenoma seen as a well-defined mass of loose myxoid connective tissue bearing ductal structures resembling tubules. A very small portion of adjacent normal breast is present (bottom left).

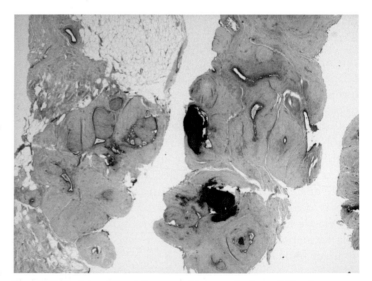

**FIG. 15.5** Hyalinized fibroadenoma with stromal microcalcification. Core biopsies from a fibroadenoma with a more hyalinized fibrous stroma than seen in Fig. 15.4, with compressed ductal structures. Large foci of microcalcification are seen in the core on the right as irregular haematoxyphilic (blue/purple) islands.

diagnosis has been established based on clinical grounds with confirmation of the nature of the lesion either cytologically or histologically by needle core biopsy. Rarely, carcinoma *in situ*, mainly of the lobular type, may develop within a fibroadenoma, but this simply reflects the fact that the epithelium, similar to that of normal breast, is not immune to carcinogenic agents.

## Phyllodes Tumour

### Key Points

- Phyllodes tumours usually present in middle-aged or elderly females as a well-defined mass.
- Microscopically, they are composed of cellular stroma with compressed 'leaf-like' clefts of epithelium.
- The majority are benign, although less common borderline and malignant forms may occur.

These uncommon tumours were historically referred to, entirely erroneously, as 'giant fibroadenomas' or 'cystosarcoma phyllodes'. It is also depressingly common for these lesions to be incorrectly spelled (and pronounced) as 'phylloides' tumours. They occur predominantly in middle-aged or elderly females and are rarely seen below the age of 40. They form large, lobulated, circumscribed masses that may grow relatively rapidly and can cause unilateral breast enlargement or even skin ulceration. Grossly, they have a whorled cut surface that resembles a compressed leaf bud (Greek *phyllo* = leaf) with visible clefts and cystic spaces. Microscopically, the stroma is cellular and surrounds elongated cleft-like spaces lined by benign epithelial cells. The stromal cells are plump and may be densely packed; nuclear abnormalities are rare and mitoses variable in number. Most phyllodes tumours are benign and complete excision is curative. Approximately 10% will recur locally, the most important predictor of which being incomplete excision. It is not, however, always easy to predict the behaviour of these tumours; those with a mitotic count above that seen in clearly benign lesions may be classified as 'borderline'. True malignant change occurs in about 5% of cases: the stroma becomes overtly sarcomatous and metastases, typically blood borne, may develop.

## Hamartoma

Breast hamartomas are relatively uncommon and formed from a disordered collection of lobules, stroma, and fat. They may occur at any age but are predominantly seen in pre- or perimenopausal females, who present with a well-defined mass. They are, however, often impalpable and may be detected only mammographically. Hamartomas vary in size from 1 cm to 25 cm at presentation. They have a fleshy cut surface and are composed microscopically of a mixture of morphologically normal, but disordered, fat, fibrous tissue, and breast epithelial structures including lobules and ducts. Smooth muscle may be present. Although occasionally large, these masses are entirely benign and, if required for cosmetic reasons, treatment is by local excision.

## Adenoma

Most lesions previously termed 'adenomas' were really examples of cellular fibroadenomas. Tubular adenomas are sharply circumscribed nodules measuring between 5 mm and 40 mm. Microscopically they are composed of closely packed ductular structures with little intervening stroma. They are entirely benign and regarded as a subtype of fibroadenoma. The status of the so-called lactational adenoma is also questionable; in the vast majority of cases they are in reality areas of lobular proliferation that become prominent and palpable as part of the physiological hyperplasia of the breast during pregnancy.

Nipple adenoma is a rare lesion that presents as a reddened rounded nodule, sometimes mimicking Paget's disease of the nipple. It is composed of proliferating ductal-type epithelium that often has a papillary structure and these lesions may indeed be a form of retroareolar benign papilloma (see below). The presence of two layers of epithelium and myoepithelium distinguishes the lesion from a carcinoma.

## Fibrocystic Change

### Key Points

- Fibrocystic change is the most common breast lesion.
- It is due to changes in hormone levels/sensitivity.
- It presents as ill-defined thickening or lumpiness in the breast in females usually aged 40–55 years.
- Microscopically, a combination of cyst formation, apocrine metaplasia, fibrosis, and/or epithelial proliferation is present.

A large number of terms have been used as synonyms for a group of changes that present clinically as a lump or lumpiness in the breast during the reproductive decades. They include fibroadenosis, cystic hyperplasia, cystic mastopathy, mammary dysplasia, and fibrocystic disease. None is entirely satisfactory but fibrocystic change is probably the most appropriate because the process is so common that it should not be regarded as a true 'disease'. The condition is the most common of all breast lesions, but produces clinical symptoms in only up to 10% of women. The peak incidence is in the premenopausal decade. After the menopause there is a sharp decline in symptomatic cases. Microscopically, a range of appearances is seen and the components described below are present in variable amounts from case to case.

Cyst formation (Figs 15.6 and 15.7) results from localized dilatation of lobular and terminal ductules, and is presumably due to obstruction. Cysts are usually multiple and mostly <10 mm in diameter, although occasional larger ones are not unusual. They are thin walled and may appear blue when seen close to the cut surface of biopsy material. The lining epithelium often becomes flattened and may be lost entirely in larger cysts. It may also undergo apocrine metaplasia (Fig. 15.8), the cells becoming larger and columnar with a convex free margin and abundant strongly eosinophilic cytoplasm. A layer of myoepithelium can usually be detected, at least in places, under the inner apocrine epithelium of the cyst. Similar to the ductules from which they

develop, the cysts are not ensheathed in elastic tissue. Unless haemorrhage has occurred, the cysts contain clear watery or mucinous fluid. Occasionally a cyst ruptures and causes an inflammatory reaction in the adjacent stroma, which may then become tender or painful.

An increase in fibrous stroma (fibrosis) occurs in most cases of fibrocystic change, but quantification of this process is difficult. In thin females, the normally fibrous breast stroma of young adult life persists with little change even after the menopause, but in obese females there is normally a progressive replacement of fibrous by fatty tissue, particularly after the menopause. With an increase in age, the fibrous stroma becomes hyaline and relatively acellular, whereas the epithelial elements atrophy. It is this collagenization of pre-existing stroma, without obvious reactive fibroblastic proliferation, that is responsible for the fibrosis of the breast seen in fibrocystic change.

Epithelial hyperplasia (Fig. 15.9) of significant degree occurs in approximately a quarter of cases of fibrocystic change. In the past the nomenclature has been confusing; European pathologists used the term 'epitheliosis' whereas in the USA 'papillomatosis' was preferred. Epithelial hyperplasia is now classified as being either of usual type or atypical. In epithelial hyperplasia of usual type several layers of epithelial cells line the ductules and the lumen may be obliterated by a solid proliferation. Nuclei are not increased in size or pleomorphic, and although occasional mitoses may be present they are of normal configuration.

Atypical ductal hyperplasia (ADH) is a specific entity diagnosed when a small area of proliferation of epithelial cells shows features distinct from usual epithelial hyperplasia and indeed resembling low-grade ductal carcinoma

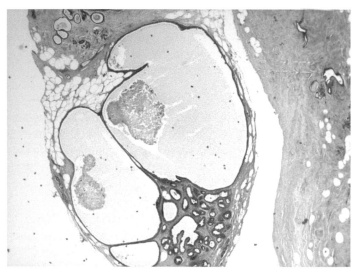

FIG. 15.6 Fibrocystic change: cysts arise from the terminal duct lobular unit and bear secretions. Most are <10 mm in diameter.

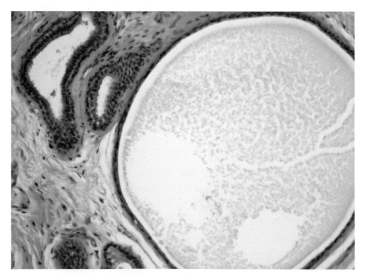

FIG. 15.7 Small cysts are common in fibrocystic change. The epithelium is flattened (compare with adjacent normal epithelial lined ducts, top left). The lumen bears flocculent secretions.

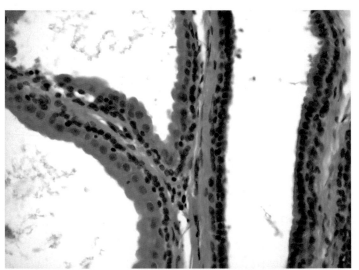

FIG. 15.8 Apocrine metaplasia in fibrocystic change. Breast cysts in fibrocystic change are commonly lined by apocrine epithelium (seen in the left of this photomicrograph). The cells in apocrine metaplasia are larger than normal epithelium (compared with the normal epithelial cells on the right), and have abundant eosinophilic (pink) cytoplasm.

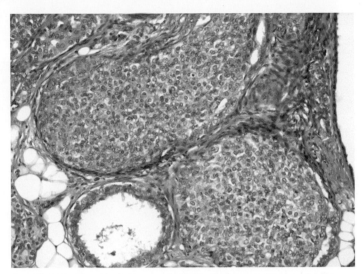

**Fig. 15.9** Florid epithelial hyperplasia of usual type in fibrocystic change. The duct space is no longer lined by a single layer of luminal epithelial cells but by a hyperplastic proliferation, which almost fills the ducts in this case. The cells, however, do not show significant pleomorphism or increase in size, and mitoses are not prominent.

*in situ* (DCIS). This term is not used when there is simply some degree of cytological atypia on a background of usual epithelial hyperplasia. The degree of atypia and the overall size of the process are, however, insufficient for diagnosis of DCIS; ADH is by definition a small, microfocal lesion.

Epithelial proliferation may also take the form of lobular *in situ* neoplasia, a term used to encompass the entities of both atypical lobular hyperplasia (ALH) and lobular carcinoma *in situ* (LCIS). Lobular *in situ* neoplasia is usually an incidental finding in breast tissue removed for fibrocystic change. As with the intraductal proliferations (ADH vs DCIS), the extent of this intralobular proliferation of cells within the lobules is less marked in ALH than in LCIS. Microscopically, small, regular, epithelial cells expand the acini of the lobules. Mitoses are few but the nuclear:cytoplasmic ratio is increased. Basement membranes remain intact. In contrast to DCIS, LCIS is often multifocal and bilateral involvement is reported to occur in up to 30% of cases.

### Epithelial Proliferation and Risk of Subsequent Breast Cancer

The relationship between benign breast lesions and subsequent breast carcinoma has in the past been the subject of great controversy. Many older studies have been seriously flawed, and it is only more recently, in studies employing careful histopathological review, that a degree of clarity has been achieved. Patients whose biopsy specimens show no epithelial hyperplasia have no increased risk of developing breast cancer; as this category accounts for approximately 70% of benign biopsies, the great majority of females who have a breast biopsy can be reassured, and do not require follow-up.

Hyperplasia of usual type (see above) gives an increased risk of carcinoma of about 1.5–2 times that of females whose breasts are 'normal'. The most significant risk, up to fourfold, occurs in women whose biopsy specimens show atypical hyperplasia (either ductal [ADH] or lobular [ALH]), and this is doubled to approximately eightfold if there is also a family history of breast cancer. However, it is important to remember that such atypia are found in less than 4% of biopsies and atypia with a family history in less than 1%. Follow-up studies have also suggested that LCIS is not generally a true obligate precursor of invasive cancer. However, affected women have a tenfold increased risk of developing breast carcinoma and recent analyses have shown that carcinoma develops more commonly in the ipsilateral than in the contralateral (other) breast, implying that a small subset of lobular *in situ* neoplasia may be a true precursor of invasive breast cancer.

Long-term follow up is advisable for the small group of women with atypical epithelial hyperplasia (ADH or ALH or LCIS); many departments now run 'high-risk' clinics for these females (as well as those with a family history of breast carcinoma), where they can be counselled, clinically examined, and offered regular radiological investigation.

### Aetiology of Fibrocystic Change

It is assumed that fibrocystic change is caused by the influence of hormones on the female breast throughout reproductive life, but this does not entirely explain why the changes are patchy within the breast. An association with menstrual irregularities has been noted, but only in some females, and there is also a relatively higher incidence in nulliparous females. Cystic changes in the breast can be produced in animals by administration of oestrogen, but most females have no evidence of hormonal imbalance. Furthermore, postmortem studies have shown that asymptomatic fibrocystic change of variable degree is present in a very large percentage of both pre- and perimenopausal females, so that its status as a disease entity has been questioned and, as described, the term 'fibrocystic disease' has been abandoned for the name fibrocystic change.

## Sclerosing Lesions

### Sclerosing Adenosis

**Key Points**

- Sclerosing adenosis is a benign disorderly proliferation of acini and stroma.
- It most commonly presents as mammographic microcalcifications, rarely as a mass.
- It may be mistaken radiologically or histopathologically for invasive carcinoma.

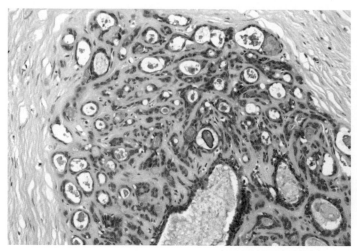

FIG. 15.10 Sclerosing adenosis is a proliferation of the terminal duct lobular unit seen as a disorderly proliferation of acinar/small tubular structures along with the intralobular stromal cells. This disorganized lobular proliferation may be mistaken by the unwary for invasive carcinoma.

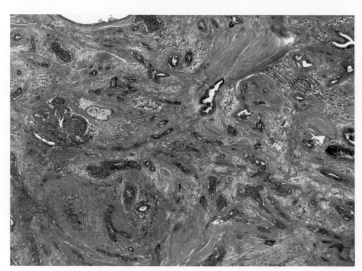

FIG. 15.11 The central portion of a radial scar, with fibrosis and elastosis bearing entrapped ductal structures. Some of these show usual type epithelial hyperplasia.

Sclerosing adenosis is a specific proliferation of the terminal duct lobular unit (Fig. 15.10). The changes may be present in association with fibrocystic change, as tiny microscopic foci in otherwise normal breast tissue, as microcalcification identified on breast screening, or, particularly in younger females, as palpable nodules mimicking tumour masses. Histologically, the normal configuration of a lobule or group of lobules is distorted by a disorderly proliferation of acini and intralobular stromal cells. A whorled pattern of microtubules may be seen but luminal structures are often small and indistinct. Microscopically it is usually possible to distinguish, at least focally, a normal two-layered epithelium. Nuclei are regular, without atypia, and mitoses are infrequent. Sclerosing adenosis is a benign condition that carries only a negligible risk of subsequent carcinoma. Its main importance stems from the fact that it may be mistaken both radiologically and pathologically for carcinoma. Fine speckled calcification is frequently found in the small luminal spaces and this may occasionally mimic the calcification of DCIS mammographically. Microscopically, the disorderly tubular structures may be misinterpreted by inexperienced pathologists as invasive carcinoma, especially in poorly prepared sections or in needle-core biopsies. Extension of sclerosing adenosis into perineural spaces also occurs in very rare cases, and care must be taken not to mistake this for evidence of malignancy.

### Radial Scar/Complex Sclerosing Lesion

#### Key Points

- Radial scar/complex sclerosing lesion is a benign lesion with central fibrous scarring and entrapped tubular structures.
- It is often detected mammographically as spiculate masses.
- It may be mistaken for carcinoma both radiologically and histopathologically.

These distinctive sclerosing lesions of the breast have previously been called 'sclerosing papillary proliferations', 'benign sclerosing ductal proliferations', and 'infiltrating epitheliosis', but the terms 'radial scar' and 'complex sclerosing lesion' are preferred. Morphologically, they are composed of radiating stellate connective tissue with a dense fibroelastic core (Fig. 15.11). Radial scars vary between 1 mm and 10 mm in diameter and are termed 'complex sclerosing lesions' when larger (>10 mm in size), but these represent the same process. Within the arms of the stellate configuration, ductules appear drawn in to the centre. A variable degree of epithelial proliferation is present. Foci of sclerosing adenosis may also be found. These lesions were initially thought to be uncommon, but as mammography has become more widely used, especially in population-based screening programmes, they are now recognized to occur relatively frequently. The precise pathogenesis is unclear, but most evidence suggests that they have a close association with fibrocystic change. Although rare, cases of both carcinoma *in situ* and invasive carcinoma arising in radial scars have been described. However, the great majority of radial scars are entirely benign. The risk of subsequent malignancy appears to be related to the degree and type of epithelial hyperplasia, as outlined above and in *Box 15.1*.

## BENIGN TUMOURS OF THE BREAST

### Papilloma

#### Key Points

- Papilloma of the breast is a benign neoplasm.
- It often presents with nipple discharge, less commonly a lump in the breast, in a middle-aged female.
- Microscopically, it is composed of fronds of benign epithelium over a fibrovascular core within a duct.

**Box 15.1** FACTORS AFFECTING THE RISK OF BREAST CARCINOMA

**Personal risk factors**
*Generic*
- Female
- Older age

*High risk*
- Strong family history of breast cancer, e.g. relative with cancer at young age or with bilateral carcinoma

*Moderate risk*
- Born in the USA, northern Europe

*Lower risk*
- Any first-degree relative with breast cancer
- Postmenopausal obesity/significant weight gain in adult life
- Early menarche (before age 12)
- Late menopause
- Late first pregnancy (after age 28)/nulliparity
- Prolonged use of hormone replacement therapy (particularly historical combined oestrogen and progesterone preparations)
- Prolonged oral contraceptive use
- Moderate alcohol intake

**Histological risk factors**
- Atypical hyperplasia – either ductal or lobular (see text) – moderate risk (four times)
- Usual epithelial hyperplasia (see text) – low risk (two times)

Papillomas are true benign neoplasms, occurring predominantly in middle-aged females. In many cases the presenting symptom is single duct discharge from the nipple; the discharge may be blood stained. Microscopically, a mass is seen lying within a breast duct, formed from fronded fibrovascular cores covered by benign bilayered epithelium and myoepithelium. This bilayer is not seen in papillary carcinoma *in situ* (see below). Duct papillomas can be separated into two main groups, central and peripheral types. Central papillomas are usually larger, single and occur in the main nipple ducts. They appear to carry no risk of subsequent carcinoma. Peripheral papillomas are smaller, more usually multiple and are often associated with other proliferative epithelial changes, including usual and atypical hyperplasia. In such cases there appears to be an increased risk of subsequent carcinoma (associated with the epithelial proliferation, as described above).

# MALIGNANT TUMOURS OF THE BREAST

**Key Points**

- By far the most common malignant tumour of the breast is an adenocarcinoma, generally referred to simply as breast carcinoma, arising from the glandular epithelial component of the breast.
- Other breast malignancies such as sarcoma and lymphoma are rare.

## Carcinoma

With the exception of skin cancers, breast cancer is the most common of human female cancers throughout the world. During the mid-1980s, mortality from cancer of the breast overtook that of every other female cancer to become the most common cause of cancer death. Mortality from lung cancer is now overtaking that from breast cancer in some countries but, importantly, nearly twice as many individuals develop breast cancer as die of it. Of note, the incidence and mortality of breast cancer are high and remarkably constant in most developed countries; the incidence is increasing, especially in younger females, and this is not entirely due to an increase in the 'at-risk' population. It is more than 200 times more common in women than in men.

Carcinoma of the breast may occur at any age, but is rare before age 25 years and most common in the developed world in those aged between 40 and 70 years. About 50% of invasive carcinomas occur in the upper outer quadrant of the breast (where there is the greatest proportion of breast parenchymal tissue), the remainder being distributed equally throughout the rest of the breast. The main presenting symptom is a palpable mass and for this reason all lumps in the breast, whatever the age of the patient, must be regarded clinically as possibly malignant until proved otherwise. A cancer arising in the axillary tail may be mistaken clinically for an enlarged lymph node.

In practice, all breast masses should be investigated and a definitive diagnosis made by fine-needle aspiration cytology or, now more commonly, needle-core biopsy. In this way women with breast cancer can have preoperative counselling, discussions about appropriate treatment options can take place, and surgeons can plan operations and operating time. Perioperative frozen section should be avoided (except in exceptional circumstances), particularly in small impalpable (screen-detected) lesions that may then be unavailable for full paraffin histology and assessment of prognostic factors. In the UK, women aged 50–70 years are routinely invited for 3-yearly mammography as part of the UK National Health Service Breast Screening Programme (NHS BSP); in this service, lesions are most commonly detected as microcalcifications, masses, distortions, or parenchymal deformities on mammography and are often impalpable.

### Carcinoma in situ and Invasive carcinoma

Carcinoma of the breast arises from the lining epithelium of the duct system. Previously it was thought that in some cases the origin was ductular and in others lobular, but it is now accepted that virtually all cancers are related to the terminal duct lobular unit. For a variable length of time, the tumour cells remain confined within the duct system, in the form of DCIS, before breaching the basement membrane and invading the breast stroma. Further research is required to define predictors of the risk of progression to invasion accurately, because it is clear that not all cases of DCIS will develop invasive carcinoma within the patient's

# 15.1 Special Study Topic

## MAMMOGRAPHIC BREAST SCREENING

Although trials of the effect of tamoxifen have been reported, there is no unequivocal way at present of preventing breast cancer. Attempts to reduce the mortality from this common malignancy have therefore concentrated on early identification. Tumour size and lymph node spread of invasive breast cancer are, at least to some extent, time dependent; small tumours (e.g. those <10 mm in size) are less likely to have lymph node metastases.

Although there has been intermittent disagreement over the efficacy of population-based breast screening programmes, randomized controlled trials and multiple reviews of the data from these, including the Marmot review in the UK in 2012, have indicated a reduction in mortality of approximately 20% in those invited for mammographic screening. The NHS BSP in the UK began in the late 1980s. Women aged 50–70 are invited for 3-yearly mammography. If an abnormality is detected the woman is invited back for additional assessment, which includes clinical examination and further breast imaging, such as additional mammography with magnification views and ultrasound examination.

Mammographic abnormalities that may be identified include well-defined, ill-defined, or spiculate masses, architectural distortions, asymmetrical densities, or microcalcifications. None of these abnormalities is specific for malignancy, e.g. microcalcification is often seen in DCIS (see main text), but can also be associated with benign changes. Invasive carcinoma is most often seen as a spiculate or ill-defined mass. At the time of assessment, fine-needle aspiration cytology or, now more commonly, core biopsy samples may be taken. The aim is to obtain a preoperative diagnosis of cancer so that one-step surgery can be performed, and to be able to diagnose benign lesions definitively. If these latter lesions are impalpable it may be appropriate to leave them in the breast and thus to avoid unnecessary benign biopsies in well women.

Core biopsy (usually with a 14- or 16-gauge needle) takes a small histological sample and requires less specific expertise in preparation and histological interpretation than cytological assessment. Occasionally, however, specific diagnosis is not possible. Core biopsy samples are reported using histological categories: B1 – normal tissue; B2 – benign lesion; B3 – lesion of uncertain malignant potential; B4 – suspicious of malignancy; or B5 – malignant. In the few cases where definitive diagnosis is not possible on core biopsy (B3 and B4 categories) either repeat sampling, e.g. with a wider bore needle (e.g. 11 or 8 gauge), or diagnostic surgical biopsy may be necessary to make a definitive diagnosis.

In general, screen-detected cancers are more often lymph node negative and smaller than symptomatic cancers. In addition they are more often of a less aggressive morphological type and of lower histological grade (Table 15.2).

**TABLE 15.2** Screen-detected and symptomatic carcinomas

|  | Proportion of screen-detected carcinomas (%) | Proportion of symptomatic carcinomas (%) |
|---|---|---|
| **Histological type** | | |
| No special type (ductal) | 28 | 47 |
| Tubular and tubular mixed | 49 | 16 |
| Lobular | 13 | 15 |
| Medullary like | 2 | 5 |
| Mucinous | 1 | 1 |
| Others | 7 | 16 |
| **Lymph node negative** | 80 | 63 |
| **Histological grade** | | |
| Grade 1 | 45 | 19 |
| Grade 2 | 40 | 34 |
| Grade 3 | 15 | 47 |

lifetime. However, as elsewhere, the distinction between *in situ* and infiltrating carcinoma is extremely important.

### Carcinoma *in situ*

By definition the cytological changes of malignancy are present in the epithelial cells of a carcinoma *in situ*, but the basement membrane remains intact and no invasion is seen. Although carcinoma *in situ* of the breast is now known to arise from the terminal duct lobular unit, it has become conventional to recognize two types: ductal and lobular. There are significant morphological, prognostic, and therefore subsequent therapeutic differences between the two, which justify subdivision into the two different types. In addition, however, the name lobular carcinoma *in situ* is somewhat misleading, because it is now generally accepted that this is not an invariable precursor of invasive cancer. Some pathologists now use the term 'lobular *in situ* neoplasia' to indicate the process of either ALH or LCIS (see Epithelial hyperplasia above).

### Ductal Carcinoma *in situ*

In symptomatic series of patients with *in situ* or invasive disease, the frequency of DCIS is approximately 2–5%. In most of these cases it presents as a palpable mass.

However, DCIS is now most commonly detected in screening programmes in asymptomatic women by mammographic identification of microcalcification in the breast, and in such series the frequency is approximately 20–25%. Microscopically, a variable number of ducts may be involved, but DCIS in general involves a single duct system within the breast and is not a disease arising as a field change through the breast.

DCIS varies in terms of both the architecture of the process and the cytonuclear grade of the malignant cells. In the past, DCIS was classified according to its architectural growth pattern, including solid, comedo, cribriform, and micropapillary types. In solid DCIS, the ducts are completely filled by a disorderly proliferation of epithelial cells (Fig. 15.12). There is often central comedo-type necrosis in the lumen so that lipid-rich yellow debris may be expressed from the cut surface, similar to toothpaste from a tube. A cribriform architecture is characterized by a geometric 'lacy' network of bridges and trabeculae. The micropapillary pattern consists of a proliferation of epithelial cells, which form small papillary projections into the lumen.

Although the architectural classification system has some value, in many cases a mixture of more than one pattern may be present. There is less variation in the cytonuclear grade of a single DCIS case and the main system of classification of DCIS now, therefore, describes the cytonuclear grade of the tumour nuclei as being high, intermediate, or low grade in appearance. High-grade DCIS is composed of malignant cells with abundant cytoplasm, marked nuclear pleomorphism, and increased mitoses. Low-grade DCIS is formed from small, regular cells, which often form cribriform or micropapillary structures, as described above. Intermediate-grade DCIS shows features less marked than those of high-grade disease and more prominent than those of low-grade DCIS.

Coarse microcalcification in the central necrotic debris, or fine clustered calcification in the luminal secretions, forms useful radiological features for the mammographic detection of DCIS. When DCIS extends along the major ducts as far as the nipple, groups of neoplastic cells may enter the deeper layer of the epidermis and spread within it through the nipple and areola. The affected skin shows reactive inflammatory changes in the dermis. These changes produce a characteristic eczematous appearance named Paget's disease of the nipple (Fig. 15.13) after Sir James Paget who described it in 1874. The carcinoma cells usually form clusters within the epidermis and can be distinguished by their atypia with large nuclei, prominent nucleoli, and abundant cytoplasm. Paget's disease is accompanied by an underlying DCIS which may be small and confined to the nipple ducts or situated deep in the breast; relatively rarely nowadays in the developed world there may also be invasive cancer present.

Usually DCIS is confined to one duct system in the breast, although this may overlap more than one quadrant. Because of the associated microcalcification, DCIS is now frequently identified mammographically when small and there is an increasing trend towards breast-conserving therapy (complete local excision, with tumour-free wide margins, typically with postoperative radiotherapy) for this, as for small invasive cancers. If primary therapy is adequate the long-term prognosis of DCIS is excellent, with a 10-year survival rate of >95%.

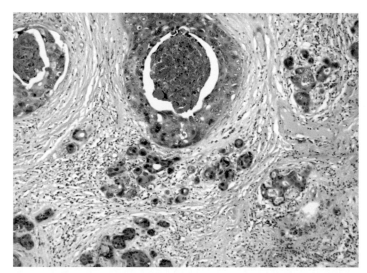

FIG. 15.12 High-grade ductal carcinoma *in situ* (DCIS): duct spaces are completely filled by a solid, neoplastic proliferation of large malignant cells. In this case the DCIS extends into the lobules as 'cancerization' of lobules; this may mimic invasion, but the process in both ducts and lobules has a surrounding myoepithelium (not shown). The DCIS within ducts bears central comedo-type necrosis.

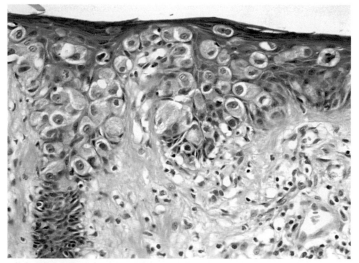

FIG. 15.13 Paget's disease of the nipple: when DCIS extends along major ducts as far as the nipple, groups of neoplastic cells may enter the deeper layer of the epidermis and spread within it through the nipple and areola. In this case, malignant cells with abundant cytoplasm and large nuclei are seen in the basal layers of the nipple.

## Invasive Carcinoma

### Key Points

Histological types of invasive breast carcinoma are as follows:

- Invasive ductal carcinoma, now better called no specific/special type (NST), is the most common (>50%).
- Invasive lobular carcinoma (of which there are several variants) is the second most common type (approximately 15%).
- Tubular carcinoma is much more common in screening than symptomatic practice.
- Medullary-like, mucinous, invasive cribriform, metaplastic and a variety of other types are rare.

A number of different morphological types of invasive breast carcinoma are recognized, with different microscopic features, including tumours with mixed appearances.

### Invasive Carcinoma of No Special Type (NST) (Ductal) (Fig. 15.14)

Over 50% of invasive breast carcinomas fall into this category. Grossly, they form a firm, often hard, moderately defined lump usually measuring 10–40 mm in diameter. They cut like an unripe pear and it is this type that was traditionally referred to as 'scirrhous' carcinoma. Microscopically, the tumour is composed of cords and sheets of large epithelial cells, which infiltrate in a disorganized fashion between dense bands of collagen. The cells vary in size and shape, some tubule formation may be seen, and mitoses are usually present, but there are no special morphological features.

### Invasive Lobular Carcinoma (Fig. 15.15)

This accounts for approximately 10–15% of all invasive carcinomas. Various subtypes of invasive lobular carcinoma are also described. Although overall these tumours may have a scirrhous macroscopic appearance similar to NST carcinomas, more frequently they are softer with an ill-defined outline and may be more difficult both to palpate clinically and to identify macroscopically. Microscopically, they are composed of small to moderately sized, regular epithelial cells with infrequent mitoses. Classically, linear cords of cells infiltrate diffusely as discrete or single cells within fine collagen bands, giving a so-called targetoid or 'single file' pattern. The discohesive growth pattern is a reflection of loss of function of the E-cadherin–catenin cell adhesion system.

### Tubular Carcinomas (Fig. 15.16)

These are uncommon in symptomatic series, accounting for about 2% of invasive carcinomas; this prevalence increases in screened populations to approximately 15% because these are often small impalpable lesions that are detected mammographically as spiculate masses. Grossly these cancers may be less than 10 mm in diameter, firm, and have an irregular star-shaped, stellate outline. Microscopically, there is central elastosis and elongated tubular structures radiate through a cellular fibroblastic stroma. The tubules are lined by a single layer of relatively regular epithelial cells, without an associated myoepithelial layer, and with central luminal spaces present. Mitoses are infrequent. Occasionally a mixture of tubular and invasive cribriform structures is seen and more rarely a 'pure' invasive cribriform carcinoma is diagnosed.

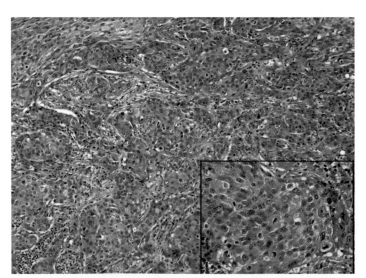

**FIG. 15.14** Invasive breast carcinoma of no special type (ductal): the invasive carcinoma is formed from irregular islands of pleomorphic malignant cells. These have no surrounding myoepithelial cells and diffusely infiltrate into the stroma. The higher-power inset shows the malignant cells in more detail, with numerous mitoses.

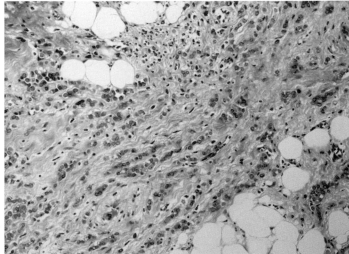

**FIG. 15.15** Invasive lobular carcinoma: this subtype of invasive carcinoma is composed of moderately sized, relatively regular malignant cells. Typically, linear cords of carcinoma cells infiltrate diffusely as 'single files'.

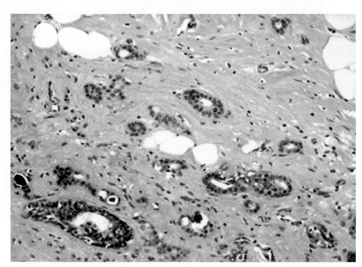

**Fig. 15.16** Tubular carcinoma: this subtype of invasive carcinoma is formed from elongated tubular structures infiltrating through a cellular fibroblastic stroma. The tubules are lined by a single layer of relatively regular cancer cells, without an associated myoepithelial layer, and with central luminal spaces.

### Medullary-like Carcinomas

These are rare. Macroscopically, they are well defined and soft, and usually measure between 10 mm and 40 mm in diameter. Microscopically, they are composed of syncytial masses of large epithelial cells (with indistinct cell boundaries) with a conspicuous lymphoplasmacytoid infiltrate in the stroma and at the periphery, which has a pushing edge. The cells are large and atypical and vary markedly in size and shape with conspicuous mitoses present. This histological subtype of carcinoma is commonly seen in *BRCA1* mutation carriers.

### Mucinous Carcinomas

These are also rare (<1% of invasive carcinomas). Characteristically they have a well-defined gelatinous, jelly-like gross appearance. Histologically, the tumour is composed of clumps of small, relatively regular epithelial cells lying within lakes of mucin.

### Mixed Types of Carcinoma

Combinations of histological patterns occur relatively commonly and these are defined as being of mixed type (and the elements present described) when the lesion is less than 90% 'pure' in type. A lesion may be formed of mixed mucinous and NST carcinoma or mixed lobular and NST carcinoma, and so on. In addition, although pure tubular carcinoma is uncommon in both symptomatic and screening practice, in about 20% of all invasive carcinomas a mixed pattern is seen, where a tubular structure is preserved centrally, but infiltrating NST carcinoma is present at the periphery; some groups classify these forms as tubular mixed carcinomas or tubular variant carcinomas, depending on the presence and proportion of the tubular elements.

Several even rarer patterns of invasive carcinoma may be seen (all <1% of the total) including invasive papillary carcinoma, metaplastic carcinoma (spindled cell, squamous or matrix producing), and very rare salivary gland-type cancers, such as adenoid cystic carcinoma.

## Routes of Spread

> ### Key Points
>
> Breast carcinomas may spread:
> - by direct infiltration of skin, skeletal muscle, and chest wall
> - via the lymphatic system to axillary and internal mammary lymph nodes
> - via the vascular system (haematogenous spread), particularly to lungs, bone, and liver.

Unfortunately, at the time of diagnosis a breast cancer may already be widely disseminated. There are three main ways in which breast cancer may spread from the primary site: by local infiltration, via the lymphatic system, and via the blood. Locally, if a tumour remains undetected and continues to grow it will eventually invade the overlying skin, and the deep fascia and chest wall. This is termed a 'locally advanced primary'. Careful histological studies have shown that lymphatic permeation can be observed at the periphery of many breast carcinomas, and axillary lymph nodes may be involved by metastatic carcinoma in up to 40% of females with apparently 'operable' tumours. Metastatic carcinoma may also be found in internal mammary lymph nodes, especially if the primary tumour is located in an inner quadrant of the breast. Distant metastasis occurs via the bloodstream; many organs may be involved but the most common are lungs, bone and liver.

## Prognosis of Invasive Carcinoma

> ### Key Points
>
> The most important prognostic factors for invasive breast cancer are as follows:
> - Lymph node stage (stage 1: node negative; stage 2: one to three nodes involved; stage 3: four or more positive lymph nodes)
> - Histological grade (1, 2 or 3)
> - Tumour size.

The crude overall mortality rate for symptomatic primary operable breast carcinoma is 40% after 5 years, >60% at 10 years, and approximately 75% at 35 years. Thus, after prolonged follow-up, only a quarter of patients with breast cancer can be considered to be clinically 'cured', whereas three-quarters of an age-matched control population are still alive. However, several pathological factors are known to have an influence on the prognosis of an individual patient.

The size of the tumour at diagnosis is important; not surprisingly the smaller the tumour the better the survival. This is the logical basis for breast cancer screening using mammography to detect tumours at a stage before they are palpable. Although the main route for metastasis to other organs is via the bloodstream, lymphatic invasion occurs simultaneously and gives a good indication of such spread. For all patients with invasive breast carcinoma, axillary lymph nodes should be excised and examined histologically; both the number and, if involved, the level of locoregional lymph nodes bearing metastasis correlate with survival; the more nodes involved and the higher the level in the axilla, the worse the prognosis. Overall, the 10-year survival rate is reduced from 75% in women with histologically uninvolved nodes to 30% in those with metastatic deposits in axillary nodes (Fig. 15.17).

The tumour size and the stage of lymph node involvement are largely time-dependent factors: the longer the tumour has been growing the more advanced it will be. An important biological factor, which probably remains relatively constant, is the degree of tumour differentiation. Both tumour subtype (as described above) and histological grade correlate well with prognosis. The special tumour types such as tubular and mucinous carcinomas carry an excellent long-term survival, infiltrating lobular carcinoma has an intermediate prognosis, and infiltrating NST carcinoma (ductal) has a relatively poor prognosis.

Histological grade is determined by assessing three histological features in combination: the amount of gland (tubule) formation; the size of the tumour cells and degree of nuclear pleomorphism; and the mitotic count. Three grades are defined, ranging from grade 1, typically with much tubule formation, little pleomorphism, and low mitotic counts, through grade 2 to grade 3 cancers. The last typically shows little or no tubule formation, marked pleomorphism, and high mitotic counts. Eighty-five per cent of females with grade 1 tumours are alive 10 years after diagnosis compared with 35% with grade 3 tumours.

The lymph node stage and the histological grade of each tumour are the two most important predictors of survival for patients with invasive breast cancer. Tumour size is the third most valuable feature. These indicators of prognosis may be contradictory, however, e.g. the patient may have a grade 3 but node-negative carcinoma; the former would suggest a poor outcome, whereas the latter a more hopeful prognosis. It is possible to combine these features, in order to incorporate the value of each feature, into a single score to provide the best prediction of tumour behaviour for each female. One such approach is the Nottingham Prognostic Index, but others are used in different centres, e.g. online algorithms, such as Adjuvant! Online (www.adjuvantonline.com) and PREDICT (www.predict.nhs.uk) are widely used in clinical practice; these take into account the histological features described above, and hormone receptor and HER2 status, and apply data from overviews of clinical management to calculate the likelihood of survival and the probable benefit for the patient from a variety of therapies. Using such systems for each individual tumour, the patient can be counselled about the likely behaviour of the tumour and, if systemic therapy is appropriate, the most appropriate treatment selected.

### Predictive Markers in Invasive Breast Carcinoma

Prognostic factors, as described above, are applied to identify how a tumour is likely to behave in terms of tumour recurrence and patient survival, and thus which patients require subsequent systemic therapies. Superimposed on these *prognostic* factors, *predictive* factors are analysed to determine which treatments are most likely to benefit the individual, e.g. in many females with breast cancer the course of the disease may be influenced by alterations in the hormonal background of the patient. This was first demonstrated by Beatson in Glasgow in 1896 when he carried out bilateral oophorectomy in females with advanced breast cancer. The oestrogen receptor (ER) competitor tamoxifen or, more recently, the aromatase inhibitors have been used successfully in the treatment of hormone receptor-positive metastatic disease and high-risk operable disease. Assessment of ER protein in tumour samples provides a good prediction of likely response to endocrine therapy: a favourable response is unlikely if an ER cannot be detected. ER status is routinely examined in tissue sections from all invasive breast cancers using immunochemistry (Fig. 15.18) and about 80% are positive. Thus the likelihood of response to hormone therapy can be predicted and the most appropriate therapy selected.

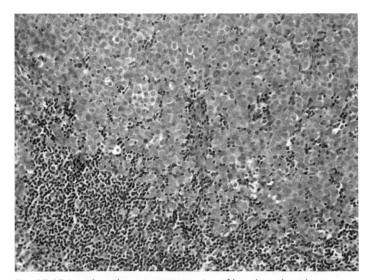

**FIG. 15.17** Lymph node metastasis: section of lymph node with metastatic carcinoma cells seen as large pleomorphic malignant cells (top of image) compared with normal-sized lymphoid cells (bottom of photomicrograph).

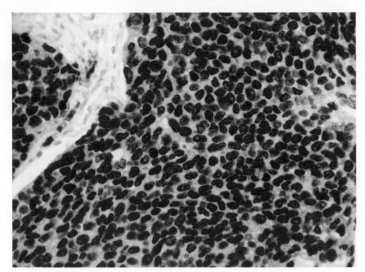

**FIG. 15.18** Oestrogen receptor immunohistochemistry in invasive breast carcinoma. Sheets of invasive breast carcinoma cells stained immunohistochemically with an antibody against the oestrogen receptor. The nuclei of the carcinoma cells all show strong reactivity (as intense brown staining) and this tumour is therefore strongly oestrogen receptor positive, indicating a good chance of response to hormone therapy.

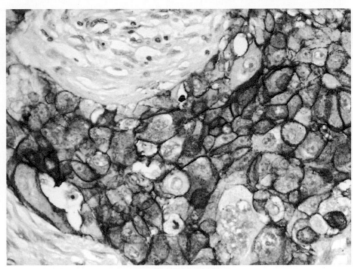

**FIG. 15.19** HER2-positive breast cancer: invasive breast cancer with strong positive staining of HER2 protein on the surface of the cell membranes (3+ staining).

## HER2

HER2 is a member of the human epidermal growth factor receptor family and encodes a transmembrane tyrosine kinase receptor. It is expressed in approximately 15% of primary invasive breast cancers and is associated with a poorer patient outcome in several studies, although it is also more commonly present in tumours with a poor profile in general (e.g. worse histological grade). Targeted drug therapy using humanized monoclonal antibodies against the HER2 protein has been developed and proven invaluable in the treatment of that subgroup of females who have cancers that overexpress the protein on the surface of the tumour cells or amplification of the gene. For example, Herceptin (trastuzumab) has proved efficacious both in females with metastatic cancer and in those with early breast cancer (without metastasis). All invasive breast cancers are now tested for the presence of excess protein on the cell surface by immunohistochemistry (Fig. 15.19) or for amplification of the gene by fluorescent, or chromogenic, *in situ* hybridization (Fig. 15.20).

## Aetiology of Breast Carcinoma

No single causal agent has been found for breast carcinoma, but a number of predisposing factors have been identified (see *Box 15.1*). The incidence of breast cancer, similar to carcinomas in general, increases with age, but the increase occurs earlier than for most cancers, being most rapid between the ages of 30 and 50 years, after which it rises more slowly to a maximum in old age. The strongest aetiological factor is a

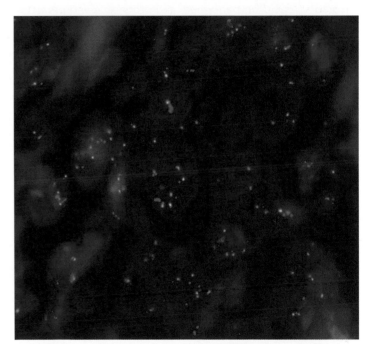

**FIG. 15.20** Fluorescent *in situ* hybridization (FISH) for the *HER2* gene. The number of copies of the *HER2* gene in the tumour cell nucleus is assessed with fluorescence microscopy and the number of signals for the gene (red dots) is counted per cell and compared with the number of signals for chromosome 17 (green dots). A ratio of *HER2* gene to chromosome 17 of more than 2 is considered positive, as seen here.

positive family history; there is a definite increased risk if a female relative, i.e. mother, maternal grandmother, or sister, has had breast cancer. Occasional families exist in which there is a very high incidence of breast cancer, and these

A 61-year-old female attended for routine 3-yearly mammography. A spiculate mass was seen. This was not identified on her previous mammograms. She was recalled for further assessment and the mass was also visible on ultrasound examination but not clinically palpable. The imaging appearances were strongly suspicious of malignancy and the lesion was sampled by needle-core biopsy under ultrasound guidance. Histology showed invasive carcinoma (Fig. 15.21) of provisional (i.e. as assessed on the limited amount of tissue in the core biopsy) grade 1.

The patient elected to have breast-conserving surgery rather than mastectomy. To excise the mass, a marker wire was inserted under ultrasound guidance so that the surgeon could identify the correct area to remove in the operating theatre. After removal, but during surgery, a radiograph was taken of the tissue excised so that it was certain that (1) the tumour had been removed and (2) the margins of excision were sufficiently distant from the edges of the mass. On receipt in the laboratory, the specimen was painted with different coloured inks to mark the different margins (according to sutures positioned by the surgeon during the operation). It was then incised (Fig. 15.22) by the pathologist, in order to obtain good fixation, so that grading could be performed, and prognostic and predictive markers, such as ER and HER2, could be examined in due course on well-fixed tissue.

Histological examination confirmed that the tumour was an invasive breast carcinoma that measured 14 mm in maximum extent. This was of histological grade 1. Low-grade cribriform DCIS was also present. Excision was widely complete by more than 5 mm at all margins. Despite the low histological grade, one of the five axillary nodes removed contained metastatic carcinoma and the tumour was thus of lymph node stage 2 (fewer than four lymph nodes involved). The tumour was also examined by immunohistochemistry to determine whether ER expression and HER2 protein were present; strong, extensive staining for ER was seen (100% of nuclei were positive), indicating that it was probable that the tumour would respond to hormone therapy, such as an aromatase inhibitor. No membrane immunoreactivity for HER2 protein was present and the tumour was therefore regarded as HER2 negative; the tumour would therefore not respond to targeted anti-HER2 therapies such as trastuzumab.

Despite the node metastasis, the patient's Nottingham Prognostic Index Score was 3.28 and her prognosis predicted to be good (Fig. 15.23). More than 83% of patients in this good prognostic group are alive at 10 years' follow-up. Adjuvant! Online (www.adjuvantonline.com/index.jsp) similarly predicts an 82.5% 10-year survival rate without any systemic treatment for such a patient, but also provides the information that 5 years of aromatase inhibitor would confer an additional 2.6% benefit. The addition of a second-generation chemotherapy regimen to the aromatase inhibitor would provide only a further 1.5% benefit (i.e. total 4.1% benefit for the two combined treatments). Based on the histopathological features entered into such algorithms, the breast multidisciplinary team will make recommendations to the patient about her choices for further clinical treatment.

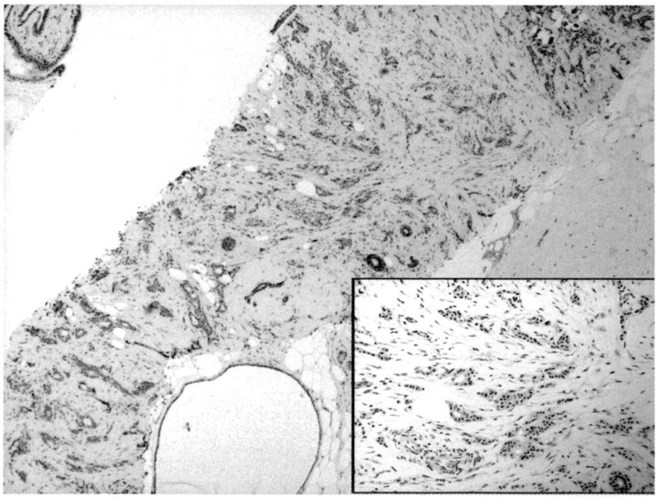

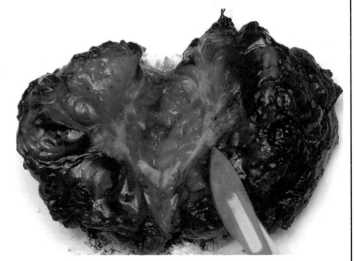

FIG. 15.22 Macroscopic specimen of wide local excision: the wide local excision specimen has been received in the laboratory and the different aspects painted with inks so that the margins can be identified on the histological slide by the various colours. This is undertaken according to orientation sutures placed on the specimen by the surgeon, e.g. the surgeon may mark the medial aspect with a medium-length suture, the lateral with a long suture, and the superior with a short suture according to local protocol. In the incised specimen the invasive tumour can be seen centrally (at the tip of the scalpel blade) as a pale area with an irregular outline within the normal yellow fatty tissue.

FIG. 15.21 Core biopsy of fibrous tissue infiltrated by invasive carcinoma. The tumour is forming tubular structures. An adjacent benign cyst is present (bottom centre). Inset of higher power of the same tumour shows irregular islands of carcinoma with a reactive fibroblastic stroma.

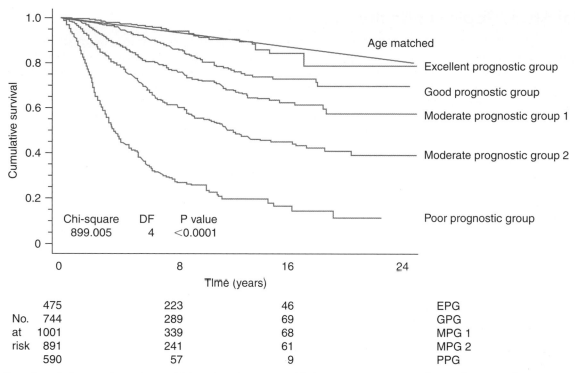

FIG. 15.23 Overall survival curves for patients with invasive primary operable breast carcinoma according to the Nottingham Prognostic Index (NPI) groups from data from the Nottingham Tenovus Primary Operable Breast Cancer Series. Each of the five lines shows survival for females within that range of NPI scores, namely excellent, good, moderate 1, moderate 2, and poor prognostic groups.

patients may have a genetic predisposition (see Special Study Topic 15.2).

Although differences in racial susceptibility have been established (the incidence is lower in China and Japan) this is partly due to environmental factors, because the incidence rises in 'westernized' Japanese females. This does not, however, completely explain the increase in some aggressive 'basal-like' invasive breast carcinomas, which are more common in African–Caribbean and Hispanic females. There is good evidence that exposure to female sex hormones, and oestrogen in particular, is an important factor in the development of breast cancer, but it is not certain

## 15.2 Special Study Topic

### GENETICS OF BREAST CANCER

The development of malignancy is related to abnormalities in structure and/or function of tumour-suppressor genes and oncogenes. A great many genes have been found to show aberrations in invasive breast carcinoma including members of the tyrosine kinase family of growth factors such as epidermal growth factor and *HER2*, as well as *c-myc*, the tumour-suppressor gene *TP53*, and members of the *ras* family. Many of these abnormalities are seen in sporadic cases of breast cancer. Although inherited cases account for only 5–10% of breast cancer, it is clear that some families have a significantly greater risk than the general population

for the development of breast cancer. In particular it is likely that a true hereditary factor is implicated if the disease is diagnosed at a young age, is bilateral, or many family members are affected. In some families with breast cancer, ovarian carcinoma may also be seen and in others both males and females may be affected.

It is clear that there is not a single gene that is mutated in all cases of familial breast cancer. One of the first abnormalities to be identified was a mutation in the tumour-suppressor gene *TP53* (also seen in sporadic breast cancer) on the short arm of chromosome 17. Li–Fraumeni syndrome is a cancer family syndrome with a germline mutation in *TP53* causing breast cancer, but also sarcomas, various childhood malignancies, and gliomas. This autosomal dominant inherited condition is, however, associated with <5% of familial breast cancers.

## Special Study Topic continued . . .

However, breast cancer-associated gene 1 (*BRCA1*) and subsequently gene 2 (*BRCA2*) have been cloned. These are also of autosomal dominant inheritance. *BRCA1* mutation is associated with an overall lifetime risk of 85% of developing breast cancer but the site of the mutation appears to be important with relation to the differing risks of breast and ovarian cancer.

The *BRCA1* mutation appears to be implicated in approximately 45% of cases of familial breast cancer and the *BRCA2* mutation in another 40%. *BRCA2* mutations may also be found in those families in which male breast cancer is also present. Other genetic syndromes account for only approximately another 5% of hereditary breast cancers; it seems likely therefore that combinations of low-penetrance genes are important in the remainder of familial breast cancers.

A female may have several close relatives who have developed breast cancer and, as described above, the likelihood of a genetic aetiology is increased if they did so at a young age. Her statistical risk of developing breast carcinoma can be ascertained by comparison with large epidemiological series. Risks are often quoted in terms of 'relative risk' in comparison to the general population, but for an individual patient this may be difficult to understand and thus unhelpful. For example, a relative risk of 10 times the population does not mean that the patient is at 10 times the risk, of 1 in 12, for the population lifetime risk. In particular, the relative risk differs according to the female's age. Thus a cumulative risk for an individual is more helpful and can give an estimated risk of developing cancer over a lifetime.

The risk of any individual in a breast cancer family of developing carcinoma, however, depends on whether she has inherited the genetic mutation present. If the specific abnormalities can be identified in the affected family member's tissue/blood it can be sought in the individual seeking advice. If a *BRCA1* mutation has indeed been inherited, the risk for the individual approaches 100% over her lifetime. These women may choose to have bilateral preventive/prophylactic mastectomy or to attend high-risk clinics with magnetic resonance imaging (MRI)-based breast screening. If a mutation cannot be identified in the family members or tissue is not available, the absence of an abnormality in the patient does not preclude the presence of an abnormal gene, because present screening techniques will not identify 100% of mutations. In these females risk must be estimated from the epidemiological data.

---

whether there is a systemic effect or an increase in target organ sensitivity. Some other risk factors have been identified; apart from the obvious difference in the incidence in men and women, the risk in women is increased by early menarche and late menopause, whereas early first pregnancy and oophorectomy before the age of 35 years have a protective effect. The balance of epidemiological evidence suggests that long-term users of the contraceptive pill are at an increased risk. Similarly, the higher doses of sex hormones used in older formulations of hormone replacement therapy also increase risk.

### Genomic Assessment of Invasive Carcinoma

In addition to the identification of gene mutations in individuals who potentially have familial cancer, it is evident that sporadic invasive carcinomas can also be subtyped based on the genetic changes seen in the malignant cells (rather than in the germline of the patient). Studies have shown that invasive breast cancers can be defined as having a 'luminal' intrinsic subtype with a better prognosis than those of 'basal' type or those of 'HER2-like' genomic signature. Although the original research describing these intrinsic types was undertaken on nucleic acids extracted from fresh portions of breast cancer, with complex analysis of the profiles of hundreds of genes, subsequent studies have assessed smaller numbers of target genes or applied immunohistochemical examination for specific proteins, to routinely fixed and processed specimens to try to replicate this new system of subtyping, and have proved successful. Luminal-type breast cancers are typically ER positive, with luminal A and luminal B types described, the former having a better prognosis than the latter. Basal-like tumours are typically hormone receptor negative and HER2 negative, and express basal cytokeratins. These tumours are often aggressive and there is an ongoing search for the most appropriate clinical management for these problematic lesions. HER2 lesions typically express HER2 protein and/or show gene amplification, and thus are potentially amenable to HER2-targeted treatments.

## Other Malignant Tumours of the Breast

### Sarcomas

Most types of malignant connective tissue tumour have been described in the breast, but all are rare (<1% of all malignancies). The prognosis of angiosarcoma is now thought to depend on the degree of differentiation of the vascular endothelium. These malignant vascular tumours have an association with radiotherapy and have been described after irradiation following wide local excision for breast cancer in the overlying subcutis. Other sarcomas are exceedingly rare and their clinical behaviour is thus not entirely clear from the published literature; liposarcomas, leiomyosarcomas, and fibrosarcomas appear to behave in an essentially similar fashion to those in other sites in the body.

### Lymphomas

The breast is an unusual primary site of lymphomas, diffuse large B-cell lymphoma being the least rare. Its distinction from carcinoma preoperatively is important in order to avoid unnecessary surgery. Involvement of the breast in disseminated lymphomas and in myeloid leukaemia is more common. For example, young females with Burkitt's lymphoma may develop bilateral breast involvement. Disseminated lymphoma, chronic myeloid leukaemia, and myeloma may rarely present with breast masses before disease elsewhere becomes evident.

## THE MALE BREAST

## Hypertrophy (Gynaecomastia)

### Key Points

- Hypertrophy of the male breast is due to changes in sex hormone levels.
- It is most common in older males (related to chronic liver disease, prostatic cancer treatment, and some other medication) but may occur at puberty.
- Microscopically, an increase in the stroma is seen with duct enlargement and, sometimes, epithelial hyperplasia.

The male and female breasts are essentially similar until the development of secondary sex characteristics at puberty; in some adolescent males one or both breasts may then enlarge. This is known as pubertal hypertrophy and is rarely marked, but may cause pain, discomfort, or embarrassment. It is due mainly to an increase of stroma and enlargement of ducts, but without lobule formation. The hyperplastic duct epithelium may be surrounded by a zone of oedematous, fibrillary stroma. However, it tends to regress and surgical removal is rarely necessary. Similar changes may occur in old age. Both pubertal and senile hypertrophy are due to changes in levels of sex hormones; gynaecomastia occurs in response to high ocstrogen levels, e.g. in chronic liver disease, in prolonged hormonal therapy for prostatic cancer, and reportedly in workers involved in the manufacture of oestrogens. Less commonly, it is induced by digitalis or some other drug. Very rarely hypertrophy results from an underlying endocrine disease such as feminizing tumour of the adrenal cortex. Testicular injury is another extremely rare cause. In chromatin-positive Klinefelter's syndrome (47,XXY), the enlarged breasts show lobules histologically comparable to those of the normal female breast.

## Tumours in the male breast

Tumours in the male breast are rare. Carcinomas are morphologically the same as those in the female organ and similarly the prognosis is poor if spread has occurred to the lymph nodes (and the chest wall). Perhaps surprisingly, they are even more commonly ER positive than female breast cancer. Metastatic tumour, e.g. from a bronchial or prostatic carcinoma, occasionally occurs in the male breast, just as metastases from other malignancies may be seen in the female breast. Thus, as in the female, the male breast may be involved in generalized lymphoid neoplasms and leukaemias.

## SUMMARY

- Benign lesions of the female breast are frequently seen in clinical practice; the most common lesions are fibrocystic change and fibroadenomas.
- The importance of benign lesions lies chiefly in exclusion of malignancy; particular mimics of carcinoma are fat necrosis, radial scars, and sclerosing adenosis.
- Risk factors for breast cancer are female sex, increasing age, northern European or American descent, previous personal or family history of breast cancer, uninterrupted menses, and atypical epithelial proliferative disease.
- Ductal carcinoma in situ is a precursor of invasive tumour (although progression is not invariable) and is often identified mammographically as microcalcifications.
- Invasive breast cancer is of heterogeneous microscopic appearance and variable prognosis.
- The most important features in predicting prognosis of invasive breast carcinoma patients are lymph node stage, histological grade, and tumour size.
- Diseases of the male breast are rare; the most common abnormality is gynaecomastia (hypertrophy) due to changes in sex hormone levels.

## FURTHER READING

Lakhani SR, Ellis IO, Schnitt SJ, Tan PH, van de Vijver MJ, eds. WHO Classification of Tumours of the Breast. 4th edn. Lyon: International Agency for Research on Cancer, 2012.

O'Malley FP, Pinder SE, Mulligan AM, eds. Foundations in Diagnostic Pathology: Breast pathology. 2nd edn. Philadelphia, PA: WB Saunders, 2011.

Royal College of Pathologists/NHS Cancer Screening Programmes. Pathology Reporting of Breast Disease. London NHS Breast Screening Programme (NHS BSP). Publication No. 58, 2005. Available at www.rcpath.org/Resources/RCPath/Migrated%20Resources/Documents/P/PathologyReportingOfBreastDisease-CORRECTED-lowres.pdf and www.cancerscreening.nhs.uk/breastscreen/publications/nhsbsp58-low-resolution.pdf.

# 16

## THE MALE REPRODUCTIVE SYSTEM

Dan Berney and Cathy Corbishley

## OUTLINE OF THE MALE REPRODUCTIVE SYSTEM

The male reproductive system comprises the following structures:

- The testes, in which the seminiferous tubules produce spermatozoa and the interstitial (Leydig) cells produce the male hormone testosterone. Spermatozoa pass from the testis via the rete testis through the epididymis and the vas deferens to the urethra, and thence to the exterior via the penis at ejaculation. Fluid produced from the seminal vesicles, which are posterior to the prostate, are added to the spermatozoa on ejaculation through the penis.

- The prostate gland, which is situated at the base of the bladder and surrounds the prostatic urethra. In the normal male this gland is about the size of a walnut and adds secretions to semen that are necessary for sperm viability. Neither seminal vesicles nor the prostate are a place of storage for sperm.

## THE TESTIS

### Embryology and Congenital Abnormalities

The testis develops embryologically from the genital ridge adjacent to the mesonephros. Germ cells migrate to the genital ridge and are surrounded by proliferating mesothelium to form 'sex cords', which will form the seminiferous tubules with Sertoli cells and germ cells. Sertoli cells are essential 'nurse' cells for spermatogenesis. Surrounding mesodermal stroma forms the Leydig cells. During intrauterine development the testes descend into the scrotum, apparently guided by an anchoring structure composed of undifferentiated mesenchyme, the gubernaculum.

### Cryptorchidism

Cryptorchidism, or maldescent, is the most common congenital abnormality. The testis may reside at any point along its path of descent. Spermatogenesis will proceed satisfactorily only in the lower temperature of the scrotum, and cryptorchidism is therefore a significant cause of male infertility. Maldescent is also an important predisposing factor for testicular germ cell tumours, both within the undescended testis and in the contralateral organ, even if it is normally located in the scrotum. It is therefore important to investigate the position of the testis in male infants and, if possible, to bring any undescended testis down into the scrotum (orchidopexy). Better imaging and laparoscopy now enable the urologist to locate the intra-abdominal testis in a non-invasive manner and to remove it if it cannot be brought down into the scrotum surgically. This will also reveal rare cases of anorchia (congenital absence of the testis) and those of the vanishing testis, where only epididymal remnants are identified at the site of the testis with no remaining testicular tubules present.

### Torsion

Torsion of the testis after infancy is usually ascribed to an unusually long mesorchium, the 'mesentery', which unites the body of the testis with the epididymis. Young males with this condition present with an acute onset of unilateral pain in the scrotum due to rotation of the testis around the mesorchium, with resultant obstruction of the venous return from the testis, which rapidly becomes engorged with blood. Early diagnosis is essential because prompt reversal of the rotation and fixation of the organ results in complete resolution, whereas delay leads to infarction and death of the testis.

## Inflammatory Conditions

Inflammation of the testis (orchitis) may be due to many infective agents. The most common viral cause is mumps in countries with no immunization programme, and orchitis is common in males with this infection. The viraemia in mumps also causes inflammation of other organs besides the salivary glands and testes (e.g. the pancreas and ovary), although clinical symptoms from these organs are uncommon. Mumps orchitis may lead to infertility.

## Infertility

Sperm counts appear to be decreasing in many countries, and this is therefore the main causal factor for many couples with infertility. For some men sperm counts may be improved by simple factors such as avoiding overheating by not wearing tightly fitting underpants. However, males with non-obstructive azoospermia may now undergo testicular sperm extraction (TESE). This involves the removal of a small biopsy of seminiferous tubules under local anaesthesia followed by the extraction of viable spermatozoa for intracytoplasmic sperm injection (ICSI). Biopsy material can be examined later histologically to confirm whether sperm are present or absent.

A number of patients who have had vasectomies for contraceptive purposes are subsequently found to have spermatozoa in their ejaculate, having previously been azoospermic. This may be the result of vasitis nodosa, when spermatozoa released into the tissues at the site of section of the vas deferens elicit a granulomatous inflammatory response, within which epithelial cells from the vas deferens ramify and connect with those of the other portion of transected vas deferens such that continuity is re-established.

For endocrine causes of male infertility see Chapter 17.

## Tumours

Testicular tumours are not common, and yet they represent the most common solid tumour of young males. The vast majority of testicular tumours (>95%) are derived from the germ cells of the testis.

### Aetiology

The association of germ cell tumours and cryptorchidism has been known for many years, although the stated increased risk associated with this abnormality varies considerably in different publications, from a fourfold increase in patients with this condition in some reports, to a fortyfold increase in others. The existence of a proposed testicular dysgenesis syndrome has been proposed, which includes a constellation of pathological conditions – cryptorchidism, low sperm count, and hypospadias –although this syndrome remains hypothetical and is contested by some. There is also a small familial incidence of testicular tumours. The vast majority of testicular tumours show a specific genetic abnormality, namely multiple copies of the long arm of chromosome 12.

The cause or causes of the increasing incidence of testicular tumours in young men in the past 20 years are far from clear. The role of testicular maldescent has been known for many years, but this accounts for only a small percentage of tumours. However, the observations that (1) tumours in males with cryptorchidism may occur in the contralateral testis, (2) there is an established increased risk of tumour in the other testis in patients who have had one tumour, and (3) occasional tumours are familial, all point to a genetic cause in some patients.

The incidence of testicular tumours in western countries has increased considerably over the past few decades, and this has been attributed to an increase in oestrogenic substances in the environment. These may come from a variety of sources, from the administration of oestrogens to mothers at risk of miscarriage to metabolic byproducts of chemicals used extensively in packaging. Support for this proposition is provided by the reported decrease in sperm counts of the typical western male over the past 15 years, which can also be attributed to environmental oestrogenic substances. Similarly, reports of male fish with ambiguous genitalia occurring in water that has been contaminated by chemicals indicate the presence of oestrogenic material in the environment.

## Intratubular Germ Cell Neoplasia

The precursor lesion of testicular germ cell tumours is intratubular germ cell neoplasia, unclassified (IGCNU). It was initially described as carcinoma *in situ* but other rarer forms have also been described, leading to this rather cumbersome name. These cells are recognizable histologically. IGCNU is seen in seminiferous tubules adjacent to most testicular

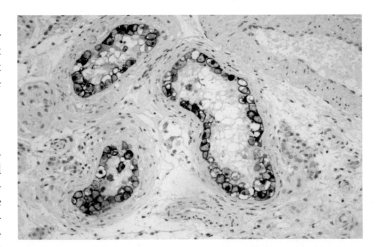

**FIG. 16.1** Seminiferous tubule with intratubular germ cell neoplasia, unclassified (IGCNU): the IGCNU cells stain positively (brown) with an immunohistochemical marker for placental alkaline phosphatase.

germ cell tumours, and it has also been seen in biopsies taken from cryptorchid testes of patients who have subsequently developed a tumour in the same testis (Fig. 16.1).

## Germ Cell Tumours

### Terminology

A number of classifications are in use, particularly in the UK, where an older system, the British Testicular Tumour Panel (BTTP) classification is still used in some centres. We recommend use of the World Health Organization (WHO) classification, which predominates internationally. In both systems the tumours divide neatly into seminomas and non-seminomatous germ cell tumours (NSGCTs).

NSGCTs have the capacity to differentiate into all varieties of mature and malignant-appearing tissues, recapitulating any stage of embryogenesis and thus potentially producing a bewildering spectrum of histological appearances. It is very important clinically to differentiate seminomas from NSGCTs, as they are managed clinically in completely different ways. Both seminomas and NSGCTs are present in approximately 40% of testes containing a germ cell tumour, and these combined tumours are managed clinically as NSGCTs.

Testicular germ cell tumours show unique or unusual features compared with most other solid tumours:

- The peak incidence is younger than most solid tumours: 20–50 years, with NSGCTs presenting at a younger age than seminomas.
- They are uniquely chemo- and radiosensitive, with high cure rates.
- The tumours spread to the para-aortic nodes and NOT the inguinal nodes, following their embryological derivation.
- They may produce serum tumour markers, which can be monitored.
- Their unique chemosensitivity has resulted in many different methods of treatment, including excision of metastases and multiple courses of chemotherapy for resistant cases, with 'cure' even in widely disseminated cases.

### Seminoma

> #### Key Points
>
> - Seminoma has a peak incidence at 40 years.
> - It spreads predominantly via the lymphatic system.
> - It is very radio- and chemosensitive.
> - Most do not produce serum tumour markers.

These tumours occur in middle-aged males with a peak incidence at 40 years and usually present as an enlarged, painless testis. Many patients will not have raised tumour markers. Some have elevated serum lactate dehydrogenase (LDH), but this serum marker may be raised in other conditions. The β subunit of human chorionic gonadotrophin (hCG) may also be mildly raised.

These tumours have a characteristically uniform, slightly lobulated, cut surface (Fig. 16.2), and histologically are composed of large cells with clear cytoplasm and vesicular nuclei with squared edges. They also show many fibrous bands and significantly have an associated lymphocytic infiltrate (Fig. 16.3). Those cases with a raised serum hCG level also contain syncytiotrophoblastic giant cells but, despite this, they have the same prognosis as those tumours not containing giant cells.

They usually spread via the lymphatic system, and enlarged para-aortic abdominal lymph nodes are often the first sign of metastatic spread. Occasionally, lymphadenopathy is the presenting symptom – these patients almost always have an unrecognized primary tumour in the testis. On rare occasions no primary testicular tumour is found,

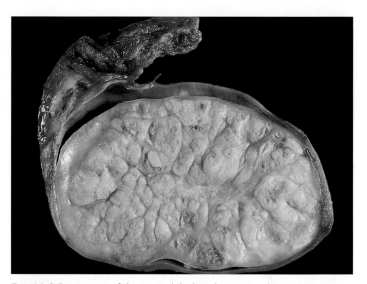

**Fig. 16.2** Seminoma of the testis: lobulated, creamy white tumour replaces most of the body of the testis, but there is no necrosis.

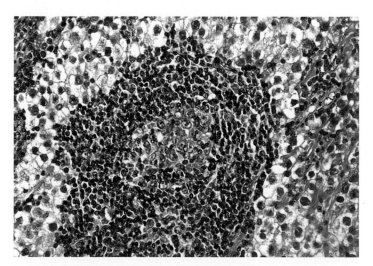

**Fig. 16.3** Seminoma of the testis: tumour cells at the periphery have clear cytoplasm and well-demarcated cell borders. Centrally, there is a lymphoid follicle; this is a common occurrence in these tumours.

and these tumours are thought to have arisen from germ cells in the genital ridge which have not migrated down into the scrotum within the testis and have developed into a tumour in this ectopic site.

Seminomas may be treated in a variety of ways and the options depend on the stage of the disease and also patient choice. Orchidectomy is often curative, and many patients will be followed up expectantly. However, adjuvant treatment will reduce the chances of recurrence. Until recently, this was adjuvant radiotherapy to the para-aortic nodes. The vast majority of centres have now moved to offering patients adjuvant chemotherapy in the form of carboplatin. For metastatic disease, other more intense chemotherapy regimens will be offered. In any case, the overall survival rate in high: well over 95%.

### Non-Seminomatous Germ Cell Tumour

> **Key Points**
>
> - Non-seminomatous germ cell tumour occurs in the 20- to 30-year age group.
> - It spreads via blood vessels.
> - It is not radiosensitive, but responds to appropriate chemotherapy.
> - The majority of tumours secrete α-fetoprotein (AFP) and/or hCG, which can be measured in the serum.

NSGCTs have the potential to differentiate into the whole spectrum of embryonic and extraembryonic tissues. Extraembryonic tissue comprises trophoblast, as seen in the placenta and yolk sac tumour from the organ of that name. These two tissues secrete hCG and AFP, respectively, and patients with tumours containing these histological elements have raised levels of these substances in their serum. In practice, 80% or more of NSGCTs will have raised levels of one of these tumour markers in the serum. Similar to seminomas, the most frequent presentation of NSGCTs is an enlarged, painless testis. These markers help confirm the germ cell nature of any testicular tumour, may aid diagnosis in those patients who present with symptoms arising from a metastasis, and may help in postoperative management to look for evidence of recurrence. Macroscopically, non-seminomatous tumours have a more variable appearance than seminomas. The malignant areas are soft, brownish and often haemorrhagic, whereas the differentiated areas are white and frequently cystic (Fig. 16.4).

The different types of NSGCTs are described below. However, in many cases the tumour is mixed, with any combination of the elements seen.

#### Embryonal carcinoma

This is composed of sheets of anaplastic cells of epithelioid appearance (Fig. 16.5). It recapitulates the most primitive stages of embryonic development and is highly malignant, often associated with areas of vascular invasion.

### Teratomas

Teratomas may contain any adult tissue type, in a bizarre mixture of epithelial and stromal elements such as muscle,

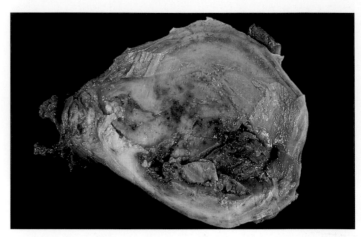

**FIG. 16.4** Malignant teratoma of the testis with extensive haemorrhagic necrosis.

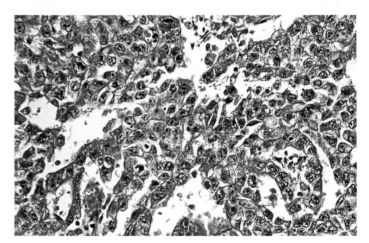

**FIG. 16.5** Embryonal carcinoma – the most common malignant element seen in malignant teratomas. The tumour cells have an epithelial (carcinomatous) appearance.

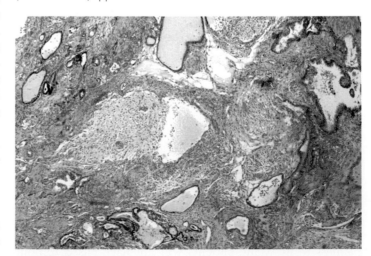

**FIG. 16.6** Teratoma showing a mixture of mature cystic and solid elements including, in this case, many glial elements.

cartilage, or even glial tissue (Fig. 16.6). They may be mature or show immature elements. Even pure teratomas with no malignant-looking elements have the capacity to behave in a malignant fashion and hence require follow-up. However, most cases are mixed with embryonal carcinoma or other elements. They are thus distinct from the teratomas seen in ovarian neoplasms (see Chapter 14, p. 434). Occasionally one of these teratomatous elements becomes malignant in its own right, and obliterates other areas, leading to what is known as 'somatic transformation'. These teratomas tend to behave in an aggressive way and the prognosis is poor.

### Yolk Sac Tumour

This enigmatic line of differentiation is frequently found in NSGCTs, but it is rarely seen in pure form, which tends to occur in prepubescent males. It shows a multitude of patterns, and tends to appear more monomorphic (Fig. 16.7) than embryonal carcinoma, with which it is often associated. It produces AFP as mentioned previously.

### Choriocarcinoma

This differentiation pattern towards placental-type tissue is composed of monomorphic cytotrophoblast cells admixed with syncytiotrophoblastic giant cells (Fig. 16.8). Tumours containing significant quantities of choriocarcinoma are particularly aggressive. Those tumours associated with very high serum levels of hCG often present with grossly haemorrhagic metastases in liver, lungs, or brain, and have a much worse prognosis than other NSGCTs.

### Mixed tumours

It must be emphasized that most NSGCTs are mixtures of the above elements. Some NSGCTs are also combined with seminomatous tumour. In these cases, the treatment is determined by the NSGCT elements.

Treatment after orchidectomy is more likely to include an adjuvant chemotherapy regimen. Follow-up may include further chemotherapy for relapsed disease or excision of retroperitoneal lymph nodes after treatment if persistent masses remain. The choices made after orchidectomy depend on disease stage, serum markers, and tumour factors such as the amount of 'malignant' elements and the presence of vascular invasion. Although the survival rates are lower for NSGCTs than for seminomas, they are still highly favourable, and death from any testicular germ cell tumour is now rare.

## Non-Germ Cell Tumours of the Testis

Approximately 5% of testicular tumours are not of germ cell derivation. They comprise a large and heterogeneous group, which are rarely encountered clinically and are derived from a variety of tissues, including the sex cord and stromal elements described in the embryogenesis of the testis. The

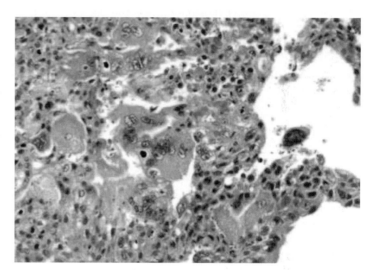

**Fig. 16.8** Choriocarcinoma showing a cytotrophoblast and syncytiotrophoblast.

**Table 16.1** Non-germ cell tumours of the testis

| Tumour derivation | Example |
| --- | --- |
| Sex cord/stromal tumours | Leydig cell tumour<br>Sertoli cell tumour |
| Mesenchymal | Embryonal rhabdomyosarcoma, leiomyosarcoma |
| Mesothelium | Adenomatoid tumour (benign)<br>Malignant mesothelioma of the tunica vaginalis (malignant) |
| Haematopoietic | Malignant lymphoma, leukaemic infiltrates |
| Metastatic | Any source possible: gastrointestinal tract, prostate, kidney |

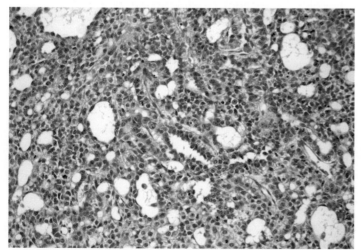

**Fig. 16.7** A yolk sac tumour showing a partially cystic and monomorphic appearance.

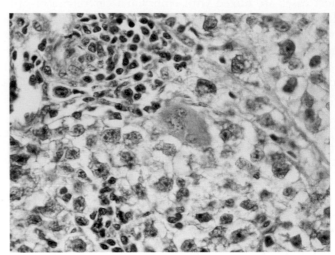
increasing use of ultrasonographic investigations is leading to an increase in the detection of small yet insignificant testicular lesions (*Table 16.1*).

## THE PROSTATE

The prostate gland is positioned at the base of the bladder, and surrounds the proximal urethra. The seminal vesicles, which lie posterosuperiorly, and join the vasa deferentia from the testes, drain into the posterior prostatic urethra adjacent to a small promontory, the verumontanum, which is easily seen at cystoscopy. The seminal vesicles do not store the spermatozoa but, similar to the prostate gland, produce secretions necessary for the nurture of spermatozoa. The prostate is composed of numerous glandular acini, which drain via ducts into the urethra. One of the secretions of these glands is prostate-specific antigen (PSA), which may be detected in blood; elevated levels are found in patients with carcinoma of the prostate, but levels are also raised when the gland is either large or inflamed.

In older men (aged ≥50 years), there is a gradual enlargement of the prostate, a condition known as 'benign nodular hyperplasia'. This may produce severe urinary symptoms such as urgency, frequency, and dysuria and, in extreme cases, acute urinary retention. In this same age group, adenocarcinoma arises in this organ, and is an important cause of death with the ever-increasing longevity of the western male. A detailed description of the lobular anatomy of the prostate would be inappropriate, but it is important to note that benign nodular hyperplasia occurs in the central portions of the gland, the central zone and transitional zone, whereas most carcinomas occur in the peripheral zone. Operations to treat benign nodular hyperplasia (transurethral resection of the prostate [TURP]) remove the central part of the gland only, and do not necessarily remove or even detect coexisting carcinomas. Such surgery is therefore not an effective treatment for this tumour.

Congenital abnormalities of the prostate and seminal vesicle also occur, but are uncommon and rarely of any clinical significance.

### Inflammatory Conditions

Histological examination of prostatic tissue removed for obstructive symptoms will often show a small number of both acute and chronic inflammatory cells associated with prostatic acini, although these are rarely associated with clinical symptoms. Clinically significant, more extensive, acute or chronic inflammation of the prostate is less common.

In some cases of severe chronic inflammation within the prostate there is a significant granulomatous element with multinucleate giant cells and numerous histiocytes. This is a non-specific inflammatory response to prostatic secretions within the stroma after the rupture of ducts. This non-specific granulomatous prostatitis is important clinically because the inflammation produces a firm gland, which may be mistaken for carcinoma at rectal examination, and may also give a raised level of serum PSA, thus adding to diagnostic confusion.

Tuberculosis of the prostate is exceptionally rare but may occur in association with infection of the kidney and bladder in regions with high incidence. The most common infective cause of granulomatous prostatitis is infection with BCG (bacille Calmette–Guérin), which is used as intravesical therapy for superficial bladder cancer.

## Benign Nodular Hyperplasia

### Key Points

- Benign nodular hyperplasia arises through excessive growth of the transitional and central zones of the prostate.
- It produces frequency and dysuria, and occasionally urinary retention.
- It is a significant cause of renal failure in older males, causing obstructive uropathy.
- It may give rise to a significantly raised serum level of PSA.

This common condition in middle-aged and elderly males is almost certainly due to some disturbance in the balance of male hormone production, because it does not occur in castrated males. The condition is caused by an overgrowth of the various stromal and glandular elements of the prostate – glands, smooth muscle, and fibrous tissue – thereby producing glandular and stromal nodules, which may impinge upon the prostatic urethra. The condition affects only the central and transitional zones and, when excessive, may produce a rounded nodule of prostate at the base of the bladder between the ureteric orifices (Fig. 16.10). This acts like a ballcock, obstructing the urethral orifice when bladder pressure rises at micturition. The bladder wall of these patients is thickened and trabeculated. In severe cases, acute or chronic renal failure may occur due to ureteric blockage; this is referred to as obstructive uropathy.

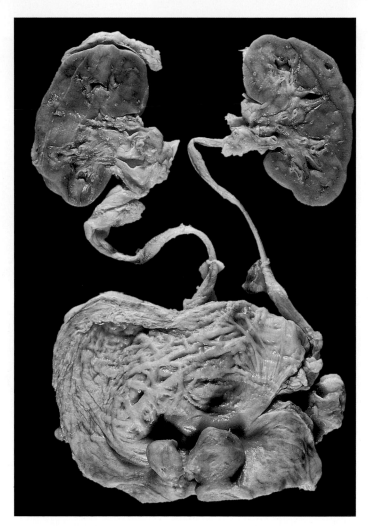

**FIG. 16.10** Benign nodular hyperplasia of the prostate: hyperplasia of the central portion of the gland (middle lobe) projects into the base of the bladder. Obstruction of urinary flow has resulted in thickening of the muscle of the bladder wall, giving a trabeculated appearance, and also leading to a degree of ureteric dilatation and hydronephrosis.

## Carcinoma

### Key Points

- Carcinoma of the prostate usually arises in the peripheral zone, and is not always sampled in TURP specimens.
- It is preceded by prostatic intraepithelial neoplasia (PIN).
- It is a common cause of cancer death but has a variable incidence.
- It has a very variable natural history.
- It is commonly associated with the development of bone metastases.

The vast majority of tumours of the prostate are adenocarcinomas (Fig. 16.11). Other tumours are so much rarer in comparison that they will not be considered here. Prostatic carcinomas vary considerably in their degree of

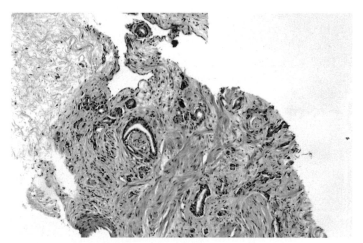

**FIG. 16.11** Carcinoma of prostate gland, seen in a needle biopsy. The tumour can be seen encircling a nerve in the centre. This tumour has a Gleason score of 4 + 3 = 7 (see text).

differentiation, and this in part determines the natural history of the disease. Similar to many other epithelial neoplasms, invasive prostatic carcinoma is preceded by an *in situ* tumour, termed PIN. Carcinoma of the prostate is the second most common malignant cause of death in western males.

## Aetiology and Epidemiology

The pathogenesis of prostate cancer remains largely unelucidated. Genetic abnormalities that increase the probability of development of prostate cancer have been reported, but the increase in risk is slight. The same genes that predispose to breast cancer also predispose to prostate cancer. Breast cancer and prostate cancer show some remarkable similarities in frequency, histology, and treatment of disease.

Prostate cancer shows remarkable geographical and ethnic variability. It is very common in black populations and relatively infrequent in Asian populations, although the adoption of 'western' lifestyles may be changing this. White people show a high incidence but less than black populations. Although the tumour occurs in the same age group as benign nodular hyperplasia, the two conditions are not thought to be causally related.

Studies of the natural history of this tumour are problematic due to its variable biological behaviour. Postmortem studies conducted in the past revealed that many older men who had died of unrelated causes had histological carcinomas in their prostate and that the incidence of these increased with age. Similarly, histological examination of prostatic tissue removed for benign hyperplasia often reveals incidental adenocarcinoma.

As serum PSA levels are often raised in prostate cancer, it has been used, with little evidence, as a screening tool for the detection of cancer. Males with a high serum PSA undergo a transrectal ultrasound-guided biopsy. However, many men with raised serum PSA do not have carcinoma, and also some tumours do not secrete PSA. Imaging has proved problematic for assessment of the prostate, so multiple prostate biopsies have to be taken at the time of transrectal ultrasound scanning (TRUS) to sample the gland. Recently, magnetic resonance (MR)-based imaging has been used in some centres to assist disease localization and staging.

This increased detection in the past 20 years has led to an 'epidemic' of prostate cancer in centres with high uptake of PSA-based screening. However, this has also meant that prostatic carcinomas of little clinical significance are detected, so that most prostate cancers detected by PSA do not spread and the patients die of other causes.

The optimal method of treatment for prostate cancer is also not well understood. Established radical techniques for localized disease include radical prostatectomy in which the entire gland is removed (Fig. 16.12), radical radiotherapy, and brachytherapy (implantation of radioactive seeds into the prostate). However, these techniques are not without sequelae, and they carry a risk of impotence, or even incontinence. In the knowledge that most tumours detected are indolent, there has been an increasing move to treat men

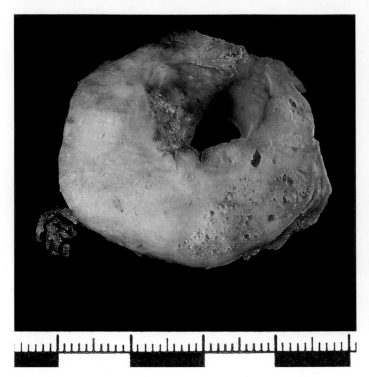

**Fig. 16.12** Carcinoma of the prostate gland in a radical prostatectomy specimen. Prostate cancer may be difficult to identify with the naked eye. However, here the tumour occupies most of the gland on the left of the picture.

by 'active surveillance', which monitors the disease closely and opts for radical treatment only on certain criteria (such as a rising serum PSA).

Growth of prostatic glandular cells – both benign and malignant – requires testosterone and dihydrotestosterone. In the early 1940s it was shown that castration was an effective treatment for some cases of metastatic prostate cancer, and this formed the basis of antiandrogen therapy, which is still employed widely today. However, these methods are almost always only used on males with metastatic tumours, in whom regional therapy will not be curative.

From the above, it will be appreciated that methods to differentiate the indolent from the aggressive cancers are required. Unfortunately, at present, the perfect discriminator does not exist. However, methods employed currently include:

- Serum PSA level
- Stage of tumour on imaging or amount of involved prostate biopsy tissue
- The grade of the tumour: Gleason grading.

Prostate cancer is graded using the Gleason system, originally devised over 40 years ago by Donald Gleason, which grades tumours by the degree of glandular differentiation. In the initial system, tumours were graded from 1 (very well differentiated) to 5 (anaplastic). As many tumours have a variable degree of differentiation, the system attributed primary and secondary grades to those lesions with more than one pattern. Tumours were thus given two Gleason grades.

The first of these was determined by the predominant pattern of differentiation and the second by the next most prevalent pattern: these scores were then added together to give a Gleason score, e.g. Gleason 3 + 4 = 7. If the tumour was uniform, the grade was repeated: Gleason 4 + 4 = 8. This led to a scoring system running from 2(1 + 1) to 10(5 + 5).

However, in the past 20 years it has become apparent that most of Gleason's original scores of 1 and 2 were not tumours, but rather were benign glandular proliferations. The Gleason scoring was therefore modified by the International Society of Urological Pathology in 2005, so that now, especially on needle biopsies, Gleason grades 1 and 2 are not diagnosed; hence, in practice, the scheme runs from 6 to 10. Gleason 3 + 3 = 6 adenocarcinomas have a very favourable prognosis, although sampling errors may occur on needle biopsy, where higher grades are not detected.

It is somewhat surprising, given the above, that Gleason scoring remains the most powerful predictor of how a prostate cancer will behave. Even subtle differences in Gleason score may affect survival, e.g. Gleason 3 + 4 = 7 tumours behave in a more favourable manner than Gleason 4 + 3 = 7 tumours. The Gleason score is therefore essential information in the treatment of the disease and is likely to remain so for the foreseeable future.

Needle biopsies of the prostate gland taken to detect carcinoma are not always easy to diagnose. The malignant cells have the usual criteria of malignancy, but the small tumours detected by screening programmes are often well differentiated. Normal prostatic acini are surrounded by a thin layer of basal cells, which are not present around malignant glands, and their absence can be detected by immunostaining with high-molecular-weight cytokeratins that stain basal cells, but not acinar cells. Prostate cancer cells also have a predilection for infiltrating lymphatics and the spaces around nerves. The presence of perineural infiltration is also an indicator of malignancy.

Examination of radical prostatectomy specimens is performed to confirm the presence of malignancy, and to compare the Gleason score with that seen in previous biopsies. The resection margins are examined carefully to assess whether the tumour has been adequately excised.

## Tumour Spread

Local spread into the base of the bladder is common, and such tumours may be difficult to differentiate from primary bladder cancer. Immunocytochemistry is useful in this situation, because prostatic cancer cells typically express PSA and prostatic acid phosphatase (PSAP). Extension posteriorly into the rectum is uncommon, because there is a dense layer of fascia between the two organs.

Prostate cancer metastasizes primarily via the lymphatics, initially to the pelvic and para-aortic lymph nodes. Some surgeons will sample pelvic lymph nodes by frozen section at the time of radical prostatectomy and cancel the operation if metastasis to local nodes is found. Spread to bones is also common; these metastases are frequently osteosclerotic and radiologically may be mistaken for Paget's disease of bone. Alkaline phosphatase levels will be elevated in both conditions, but PSA only with metastases from prostate cancer. Bone metastases are commonly seen in the lumbar vertebrae and pelvis (Fig. 16.13). This has been attributed to the extensive venous plexus connecting the prostate and this portion of the skeleton, but it is more probable that this is the part of skeleton most commonly seen by urologists in intravenous urography (IVU) and on plain radiographs of

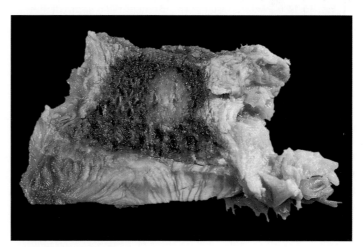

**FIG. 16.13** Osteosclerotic (osteoblastic) metastasis of carcinoma of the prostate gland in a vertebral body.

## PROSTATIC ADENOCARCINOMA: TWO CONTRASTING CASE STUDIES

### Case 1

A 74-year-old male went to his GP complaining of backache. A radiograph of his lumbar spine showed sclerotic areas in his lumbar vertebrae, which were considered most probably to be metastatic prostate carcinoma rather than Paget's disease of bone (Fig. 16.14). This was supported by the findings of a firm, irregular prostate gland on digital rectal examination (DRE) and a raised serum level of PSA. A limited transrectal needle biopsy of the prostate was taken, and this confirmed the

diagnosis of adenocarcinoma of the prostate, Gleason score 5 + 5 = 10 (Fig. 16.15). The patient was treated with hormone therapy and had remission of his symptoms, associated with a rapid fall in his PSA. Hormone therapy controlled his disease for 5 years, until his PSA began to rise again. Alternative combined hormone therapy and chemotherapy controlled the tumour for a further 3 years, before he died from metastatic prostate cancer at age 83.

### Case 2

A 54-year-old male went to see his GP for a health check-up. He gave a family history of his father dying from prostate

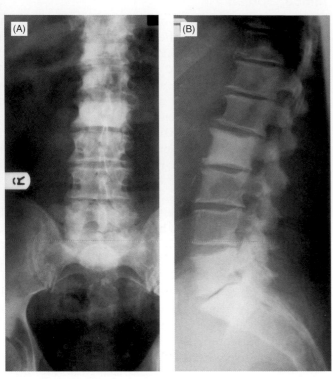

FIG. 16.14 (A) Anteroposterior and (B) lateral radiographs of the lumbar spine. The bodies and posterior elements of L2, L5, and S1 vertebrae are sclerotic. There are also areas of patchy sclerosis in other vertebral bodies and in the right iliac bone. This is the typical appearance of skeletal metastases from prostate cancer.

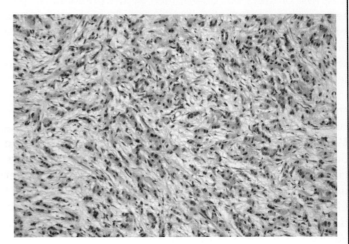

FIG. 16.15 Prostate core showing a Gleason score 5 + 5 = 10 adenocarcinoma with single infiltrating cells and no acinar differentiation.

cancer at age 60. After discussion with his general practitioner he underwent a PSA test, which showed a raised level, and he was referred to a urologist. Examination showed no abnormality and transrectal examination was normal. However, he underwent a transrectal biopsy and three of the twelve cores showed adenocarcinoma, Gleason score 4 + 3 = 7 with perineural invasion (see Fig. 16.11). Imaging suggested that the tumour was limited to the prostate and he underwent a radical prostatectomy, which showed a mutifocal prostate cancer of the same grade as the biopsy. He remains well, 5 years after the operation, and his PSA remains undetectable.

the bladder because whole-body imaging reveals the presence of metastases throughout the skeleton in most of these patients.

# THE PENIS AND SCROTUM

## Congenital Abnormalities

Cryptorchidism has been discussed previously (see p. 463). Important congenital abnormalities of the penis include the following:

- Hypospadias, in which the urethra opens onto the ventral aspect of the penile shaft, after incomplete fusion of the urethral folds during embryological development.
- Epispadias, when the urethra opens onto the dorsal aspect of the shaft; this is frequently associated with bladder exstrophy due to abnormal differentiation of the cloacal membrane.
- Congenital phimosis – foreskin that cannot be retracted.

## Inflammatory Conditions

The penis is involved in many sexually transmitted infections, but discussion of these is to be found in Chapters 18 and 19, and in texts relating to dermatology and microbiology. Viral warts of the penis, condylomata acuminata, are not uncommon and have the same histological appearance and natural history as those seen in the female genitalia (see Chapter 14, pp. 439–441) and around the anus. The foreskin

### Key Points

- Tumours of the penis are uncommon in the UK but are more common in developing countries.
- They are rare in men circumcised in infancy.
- They are associated with human papillomavirus (HPV) infection and lichen sclerosus.
- They spread to inguinal lymph nodes, but these may be enlarged due to peritumoral inflammation rather than metastasis.

may become non-retractable and/or inflamed in adult life. In many cases this is associated with simple balanitis but in some cases there is a specific dermatosis. Lichen sclerosus (see Chapter 14, p. 422) causes thickening of the skin. This condition also goes under the exotic name of balanitis xerotica obliterans.

## Tumours (Carcinoma)

Worldwide, squamous cell carcinoma of the penis is a common tumour, although it is relatively rare in western communities (10 new cases per million population per year in the UK). The tumour usually arises on the internal aspect of the foreskin (prepuce), or on the glans (Fig. 16.16). It may thus not be readily seen and there may be delay in presentation. The tumour is rare in men who are circumcised in infancy. Recent work has shown an association with HPV infection, with similar types to those found in cervical cancer being implicated (see Chapter 14, pp. 439–441). Lichen sclerosus of the penis also increases the risk of development of penile carcinoma. If found early, the disease can be cured by radical circumcision or glansectomy/partial penectomy with reconstruction (penis-preserving surgery).

The tumour may spread by lymphatics to the inguinal lymph nodes. However, lymph node enlargement may be reactive in these cases as a result of inflammation associated with the primary tumour.

Squamous cell carcinoma of the scrotum is very rare, but is of historical interest because it occurred in males who had swept chimneys by crawling through them as children. This finding was originally reported by Percival Pott in the eighteenth century, and was the first description of a tumour being caused by a chemical agent. In the nineteenth century, tumours at the same site were described after exposure to machine oil in factory workers using cotton-spinning machinery; this was known as mule-spinner's carcinoma.

## SUMMARY

- Testicular cancer is a relatively uncommon tumour, which occurs in young males and is increasing in incidence in the UK. Modern chemotherapeutic regimens cure 95% or more of patients, including those with metastatic disease.
- Prostate cancer is a common tumour in older males, and its incidence is also increasing. In theory males can be screened for this tumour by measurement of PSA levels in the blood, but there is considerable debate about the correct way to manage patients with non-metastatic disease. Although some tumours respond to hormone manipulation there is increasing use of radical surgery and radiotherapy, although the effectiveness of these treatments is not satisfactorily established.
- Penile cancer is rare in the western world and is associated with HPV infection in many cases. In those patients who present early, the disease can be cured with penis-preserving surgery.

## FURTHER READING

Eble JN, Santer G, Epstein JI, Sesterhenn IA. *World Health Organization Classification of Tumours. Pathology and Genetics. Tumours of the urinary system and male genital organs.* Lyon: IARC Press, 2004.

Epstein J, Cubilla A, Humphrey P. *Tumors of the Prostate Gland, Seminal Vesicles, Penis and Scrotum.* AFIP Atlas of Tumor Pathology, Series 4, Number 14. Washington DC: American Registry of Pathology, 2011.

Ulbright T, Berney DM. Testicular neoplasms. *In*: Carter D, Greenson JK, Reuter VE, Stoler MH, Mills SE (eds), *Sternberg's Surgical Pathology*, 5th edn. Philadelphia, PA: Lippincott Williams & Wilkins, 2009.

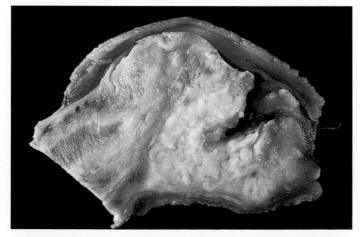

**Fig. 16.16** Carcinoma of the penis, arising beneath the foreskin and destroying much of the glans.

# 17

# ENDOCRINE SYSTEM

Anne Marie McNicol and Alan Foulis

## INTRODUCTION

The endocrine system is very important in maintaining normal homeostasis, and interacting with the central and peripheral nervous systems, and the immune system. It can be considered in two main parts:

1. The classic endocrine system, consisting of the pituitary, thyroid, adrenal, and parathyroid glands, the islets of Langerhans in the pancreas, and the endocrine cells of the testis and ovary. They secrete hormones into the bloodstream and these interact with cells at distant sites.
2. The diffuse endocrine system which comprises cells scattered singly or in small groups within other tissues, such as the gut, lung, and skin. These release chemicals that affect the function of other cells in the local environment – paracrine signalling. The physiological roles of these cells are poorly understood and, consequently, little is known of the diseases that affect them.

Therefore, this chapter deals only with abnormalities of classic endocrine glands.

Endocrine diseases present in two main ways: first, the gland secretes too much or too little hormone, resulting in a specific clinical syndrome; second, there is an increase in size due to hyperplasia or tumour. A mass may be noticed by the patient, or it may cause symptoms due to pressure on local structures. If a malignant tumour develops, symptoms or signs may be related to invasion or metastases. Sometimes there is a combination of hormonal and mass effects.

Some endocrine diseases are familial. These include the autoimmune diseases where the patterns of inheritance have still to be fully defined. There are also a number of syndromes in which specific types of endocrine tumours occur in a familial setting, the most widely recognized being multiple endocrine neoplasia, types 1 and 2 (MEN1, MEN2), which are discussed in more detail on pp. 498–499. The unravelling of their molecular genetic background raises the practical and ethical problems of genetic screening and counselling.

Very few of the diseases discussed in this chapter are common. However, it is important to recognize them, because they may cause significant morbidity if untreated, and, in most instances, they can be treated to good effect.

The final diagnosis in endocrine pathology must in general be based on a combination of clinical, biochemical, and pathological findings. Some recent technical advances have permitted pathology to contribute more specific information.

## Techniques in Endocrine Pathology

These are:

- conventional histopathology
- immunohistochemistry
- electron microscopy
- *in situ* hybridization
- cytogenetics and molecular genetics.

In the past it was difficult to understand the functional aspects of endocrine tissues by histological examination. Immunohistochemistry, *in situ* hybridization, and ultrastructural analysis have made significant advances in our understanding of normal function and the changes that occur in disease. In many instances, these techniques now also contribute to diagnosis.

### Immunohistochemistry

Antibodies to specific hormones or other cellular proteins are applied to tissue sections, and the sites of binding are

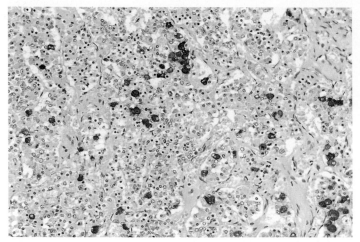

FIG. 17.1 Section of anterior pituitary gland stained by the immunoperoxidase technique with an antibody to adrenocorticotrophic hormone (ACTH). Corticotrophs (ACTH-producing cells) are scattered among immunonegative cells, which produce other hormones.

visualized by histochemical techniques, which generate a coloured signal where the protein is localized (Fig. 17.1). We now know that some tumours produce hormones but do not secrete them, and that others synthesize more than one hormone. We can also show that a tumour is of neuroendocrine origin even when it is not synthesizing known hormones, because it is possible to localize other proteins produced by this type of cell (e.g. PGP9.5, chromogranins, CD56, and NCAM [neural cell adhesion molecule]).

### In Situ **Hybridization**

This technique allows the presence of messenger RNAs (mRNAs) to be demonstrated and can therefore confirm that a tumour is the source of increased circulating hormone even if it does not store sufficient to be detected by immunohistochemistry (Fig. 17.2). The method is based on the natural complementary base pairing of nucleotides. A nucleotide probe (DNA or RNA) complementary to a sequence within the specific RNA binds to it on the tissue section. This probe is labelled so that sites of binding can be detected by immunohistochemistry or autoradiography.

### Electron Microscopy

This has been a powerful tool in endocrine pathology particularly when coupled with immunocytochemistry. Very precise classification of cell types is possible, based on the morphology of neurosecretory granules and the distribution of organelles. It is now possible, however, to gain much of this information by using immunohistochemistry.

## PITUITARY GLAND

The pituitary gland consists of two lobes: the anterior (adenohypophysis) arises from the oral cavity and accounts for about 75% of the weight, and the posterior

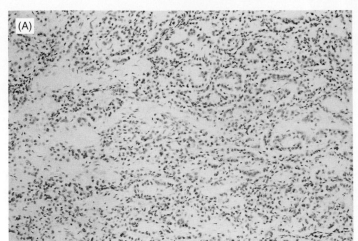

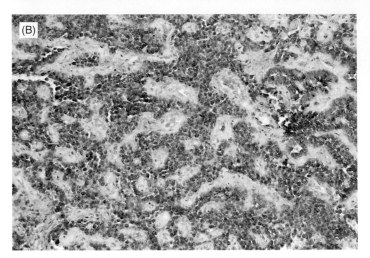

FIG. 17.2 Sections from a pituitary tumour in a patient with hyperprolactinaemia. (A) Immunostaining for prolactin is negative, because the tumour cells are not storing the hormone. (B) In situ hybridization for prolactin mRNA gives a positive signal, confirming that the tumour is producing the hormone.

(neurohypophysis) grows down from the brain and remains connected to the hypothalamus by the pituitary stalk. The gland sits in a bony cavity, the sella turcica, covered by a layer of dura perforated by the pituitary stalk. It lies below the optic chiasma and the cavernous sinuses lie laterally. Any significant enlargement can result in pressure on these structures.

## Anterior Pituitary

The anterior lobe secretes six classic hormones: growth hormone (GH), prolactin (PRL), adrenocorticotrophic hormone (ACTH), thyroid-stimulating hormone (TSH), and the gonadotrophins, follicle-stimulating hormone (FSH) and luteinizing hormone (LH). These are released into the circulation and regulate target organs at distant sites. Other peptides, growth factors and cytokines, that may have paracrine actions, are also produced. The secretion of anterior pituitary hormones is mainly under the control of hypothalamic releasing and inhibiting factors, carried directly in the hypothalamic–pituitary portal system. The primary capillary plexus lies in the median eminence of the hypothalamus where these factors are secreted. Blood passes down venous channels in the pituitary stalk to the secondary capillary plexus in the anterior lobe. There is negative feedback by hormones from the target organs at both pituitary and hypothalamic levels, and also by pituitary hormones on the hypothalamus. Basal levels of many anterior pituitary hormones show a circadian rhythm and may be altered by external stimuli.

## Growth Hormone

The secretion of GH by somatotrophs is regulated by two hypothalamic factors: growth hormone-releasing hormone (GHRH) stimulates whereas somatostatin (SMS) inhibits release. GH has direct effects including stimulation of protein synthesis in liver and muscle, and lipolysis of fat stores. Indirect effects include skeletal growth mediated by insulin-like growth factor 1 (IGF-1) which also exerts negative feedback on GH release from the pituitary.

## Adrenocorticotrophic Hormone

ACTH is produced in corticotrophs from a large precursor molecule, pro-opiomelanocortin (POMC). Its release is stimulated by corticotrophin-releasing factor (CRF) and vasopressin (VP). It regulates the secretion of glucocorticoids by the adrenal cortex; these exert negative feedback on both CRF and ACTH secretion.

## Glycoprotein Hormones

FSH, LH, and TSH are glycoproteins consisting of two subunits. The α subunit is common to all three, but each has a specific β subunit. FSH and LH are produced in the same cells (gonadotrophs). In males, FSH stimulates spermatogenesis and LH regulates Leydig cell function. In females, FSH is involved in regulation of follicle growth, whereas LH is related to ovulation and the development of the corpus luteum. The absolute and relative levels of the two hormones vary with the menstrual cycle. The hypothalamic peptide gonadotrophin-releasing hormone (GnRH) is important in the stimulation of both FSH and LH secretion whereas androgens and oestrogens exert negative feedback.

TSH, secreted by thyrotrophs, stimulates the thyroid follicular cells. Its secretion is stimulated by thyrotrophin-releasing hormone (TRH), with negative feedback from thyroid hormones.

## Prolactin

This stimulates the breast during lactation. Circulating basal levels are similar in males and females, but no specific function has yet been identified in the male. In contrast to the other pituitary hormones, the dominant regulatory influence of the hypothalamus is inhibitory, effected mainly by dopamine.

## *Anterior Pituitary Hyperfunction*

### Key Points

Anterior pituitary hyperfunction is associated with:
- acromegaly
- Cushing's disease
- hyperprolactinaemia
- rarely, hypersecretion of other hormones.

Hyperactivity of the anterior pituitary is usually associated with excess hormone secretion from a pituitary adenoma. Less commonly, excessive release of hypothalamic stimulating factors causes hyperstimulation of the pituitary. Rarely, ectopic release of these peptides from a neuroendocrine tumour at another site (e.g. neuroendocrine tumour of pancreas) results in hypersecretion of pituitary hormones.

### Acromegaly

Acromegaly is caused by excess growth hormone secretion in adult life, usually from a pituitary adenoma. There is overgrowth of soft tissues and bone, with enlargement of the feet and hands, and a characteristic facial appearance with prognathism (a prominent lower jaw) and widening of the nose. Osteoarthritis often results from the irregular bone growth. Nerve entrapment can cause pain and paraesthesia. Internal organs also enlarge, with cardiomegaly and hypertension. There is a twofold increase in mortality if the disease is untreated, mainly from cardiovascular complications. Effects on general metabolism cause abnormal glucose tolerance and sometimes diabetes mellitus (see Case History 17.1). Gigantism occurs when GH excess occurs before the epiphyses have closed.

### Cushing's Disease

Cushing's syndrome (see below) is the result of excessive circulating free glucocorticoids. About 70% of cases are due to hypersecretion of ACTH from the pituitary gland, known as Cushing's disease. Almost all patients have an ACTH-secreting adenoma. Corticotroph hyperplasia is present in a minority possibly caused by excessive secretion of CRF and/or vasopressin by the hypothalamus.

### Hyperprolactinaemia

If prolactin is secreted in excess in a premenopausal woman, the menstrual cycle is abnormal, and the patient presents with amenorrhea, infertility, and occasionally galactorrhoea. In males, hyperprolactinaemia may cause loss of libido or infertility, but is usually asymptomatic, as it is in postmenopausal females. Thus, although prolactin-secreting adenomas are often diagnosed in young females even when small, they do not usually manifest themselves in other patients unless large enough to cause pressure effects.

In contrast to the other hormones, hypersecretion of prolactin has a number of causes other than tumour. Anything that interferes with normal transport of dopamine to the anterior lobe, or with its turnover or metabolism, may result in hyperprolactinaemia (*Box 17.1*). The physiological rise of prolactin in pregnancy and lactation must always be considered in the differential diagnosis.

### Hypersecretion of Other Hormones

TSH-secreting tumours are a rare cause of hyperthyroidism. Gonadotrophin excess is usually asymptomatic.

## *Hypopituitarism*

> **Key Points**
>
> Hypopituitarism is associated with:
> - pressure from a pituitary tumour
> - iatrogenic complications after pituitary surgery or irradiation
> - Sheehan's syndrome.

Deficiency of several hormones is usually caused by destruction of the pituitary gland, stalk, or hypothalamus. In developed countries, the most common cause is now

> **Box 17.1** CAUSES OF HYPERPROLACTINAEMIA
>
> - Prolactin-secreting adenoma of pituitary gland
> - Pituitary stalk pressure, e.g. by another type of tumour
> - Hypothalamic destruction by tumour or inflammation
> - Drug therapy:
>   dopamine receptor antagonists (phenothiazines, metoclopramide)
>   drugs affecting dopamine turnover (methyldopa, reserpine)
> - Primary hypothyroidism
> - Idiopathic
> - Physiological (pregnancy)

## ACROMEGALY

### Clinical History

A 52-year-old male was referred to an oral surgeon because of marked prognathism and distortion of his bite, and was subsequently referred to an endocrinologist. The patient gave a history evolving over 5 years, during which time he had noticed two increases in shoe size. His hands had also increased to the extent where he could no longer wear his ring. He complained of intermittent paraesthesia of his hands in a distribution consistent with carpal tunnel syndrome. He

had been aware, for several years, of excessive sweating and recurrent occipital headaches. He had also been troubled by pain in his hands, knees, and hips, consistent with osteoarthritis. The evolution of the facial changes is shown in Figs 17.3 and 17.4.

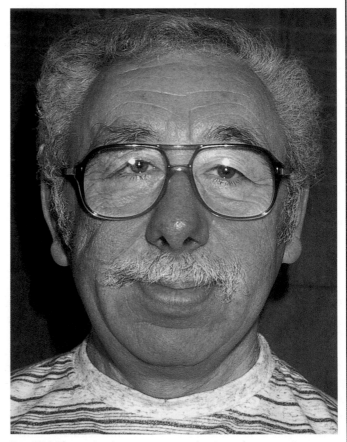

FIG. 17.4 The patient's appearance at the time of presentation in 1996.

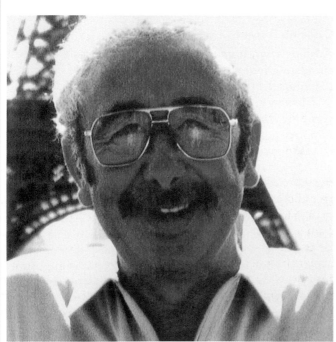

FIG. 17.3 The patient's appearance in 1990.

## Biochemistry

Initial investigations showed raised GH levels of between 12 and 50 mU/L, with an average of 32 mU/L (normal range up to 10 mU/L). IGF-1 levels were also raised. At a GH level of 18.7 mU/L, the IGF-1 level was 701 µg/L (normal 80–360 µg/L). During a glucose tolerance test, the patient exhibited a normal glucose profile, but his GH level failed to suppress. These findings were all consistent with a diagnosis of acromegaly.

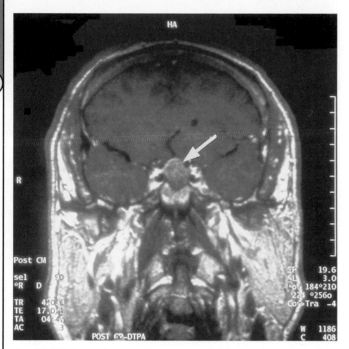

FIG. 17.5 Enhanced magnetic resonance (MR) scan showing the pituitary (arrow).

Magnetic resonance image (MRI) (Fig. 17.5) showed a 2-cm pituitary adenoma with no invasion of the cavernous sinus, but minor displacement of the optic chiasma. The patient's visual fields were normal and, before surgery, he was treated with octreotide subcutaneously, the aim of which was both to reduce GH levels and to shrink the tumour. The pituitary adenoma was removed at trans-sphenoidal surgery, and was confirmed as a GH-producing tumour by immunocytochemistry (Fig. 17.6).

Postoperatively, the GH levels fell to 1.1 mU/L and IGF-1 levels to142µg/L. Over time, the patient felt well although, as is usual, the bony and soft-tissue changes did not fully regress.

(Case history produced with the help of Dr AR McLellan and Professor GM Teasdale.)

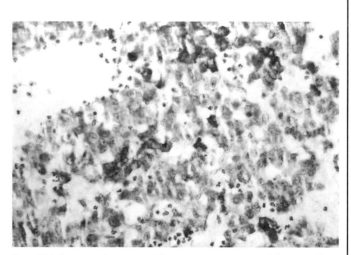

FIG. 17.6 Section of pituitary adenoma immunostained for growth hormone, confirming it as the source of secretion.

---

pressure from an expanding pituitary tumour or damage after pituitary surgery. Sheehan's syndrome (pituitary necrosis secondary to postpartum haemorrhage) is still the leading cause in countries where obstetric services are poorly developed. Irradiation of the pituitary or adjacent structures may also result in hypopituitarism as a late complication. Occasional cases are the result of trauma, inflammation (including autoimmune hypophysitis), or intrasellar tumours other than pituitary adenomas. Histiocytosis X or granulomatous diseases may affect the production of hypothalamic releasing hormones. Suprasellar tumours (e.g. craniopharyngioma) can destroy the hypothalamus or stalk.

The clinical manifestations are variable. Gonadotrophin deficiency usually presents first with amenorrhoea in females, impotence in males, and loss of secondary sex characteristics and libido. Low circulating GH levels are usually asymptomatic. Lack of TSH and ACTH causes hypothyroidism and hypoadrenalism, presenting as nausea, vomiting, hypotension, and occasionally fatal collapse.

Isolated hormone deficiencies are usually the result of genetic abnormalities in the expression of specific hormones.

GH deficiency is a cause of growth retardation and there is occasional lack of ACTH or gonadotrophins.

### Pituitary Adenomas

These are the most common lesions of the anterior pituitary gland, comprising about 10% of intracranial neoplasms in neurosurgical practice. They are found more commonly *post mortem*, indicating that most cause no clinical symptoms because they do not secrete excess hormone. Most are sporadic, but they may occur as part of the MEN1 syndrome (p. 498). They are classified as microadenomas (<10 mm diameter) and macroadenomas (≥10 mm). Small tumours are usually recognized only if they secrete excess hormone. Larger tumours may present even if they are non-functional because of local pressure effects (Fig. 17.7). If they compress the optic chiasma or nerves, visual disturbances may occur (classically bitemporal hemianopia). Headache is not uncommon. Pressure on the para-adenomatous gland may cause atrophy and hypopituitarism.

A minority show aggressive behaviour with spread into the hypothalamus and brain, eventually causing increased

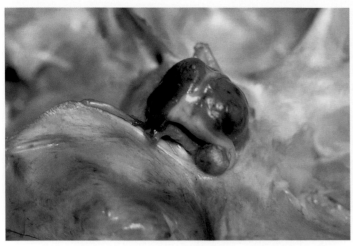

FIG. 17.7 A large non-functional adenoma of the anterior pituitary gland, which has grown up out of the sella turcica and compressed the optic chiasma. The tumour is haemorrhagic and shows cystic change.

Box 17.2 CLASSIFICATION OF PITUITARY ADENOMAS

● Clinical:
    hormone-secreting
    silent/non-functional
● Size:
    <10 mm: microadenoma
    ≥10 mm: macroadenoma
● Behaviour:
    within pituitary fossa
    invasive
● Immunohistochemical:
    evidence of positivity for specific hormones

intracranial pressure, but these are not classified as malignant. Pituitary carcinoma is extremely rare and diagnosed only when metastasis is identified. Lateral spread into the cavernous sinus may make it impossible to remove the tumour fully, leading to continued excessive secretion of hormone. Alternatively, there may be an initial period of remission followed by recurrence when the tumour remnant has grown sufficiently to secrete excessive hormone.

Occasionally haemorrhage into a tumour causes raised intracranial pressure, presenting as a medical emergency (pituitary apoplexy). If the patient survives, there is often regression of the disease because of necrosis of the tumour tissue.

### Classification

Clinicopathological classification of these tumours is the ideal approach. The features to be taken into account are shown in *Box 17.2*. Morphological classification is now based on the immunohistochemical identification of the hormone-producing cell type. If there is clinical or biochemical evidence of raised hormone levels, the tumour is regarded as functional. Some tumours stain positively for a specific hormone, but do not appear to secrete it in excess. These are referred to as non-functional or 'silent' and clinically are usually larger tumours presenting with mass effects (see Fig. 17.7). Assessment of size and behaviour is usually made on the basis of radiological findings. In a minority of tumours subclassification based on further immunohistochemical and ultrastructural analysis is important for diagnosis and prognosis. Such cases should be dealt with by specialist units.

### Aetiology

Pituitary adenomas probably arise as a result of a combination of molecular genetic changes and hormonal stimulation acting as a promoter. Hyperstimulation by hypothalamic releasing factors may play a part in the development of ACTH-producing adenomas in rare cases of Addison's disease and TSH-producing adenomas in hypothyroidism, where reduced negative feedback increases their secretion. Growth hormone-releasing hormone (GHRH) can stimulate somatotroph proliferation in the normal pituitary. A subgroup of GH-secreting tumours has mutations in the gene encoding the α subunit of the stimulatory G protein, Gsα. These inhibit GTPase activity, leading to a permanently activated Gsα, continued elevation of cyclic AMP (cAMP) and therefore uncontrolled stimulus to secretion of GH and somatotroph proliferation. Few of the oncogenes and tumour-suppressor genes important in other tumours have been shown to be involved. The tumour-suppressor genes *TP53* and *MEN-1* do not play a significant role in sporadic tumours. Inactivation of *p16* and retinoblastoma (*RB1*) genes may occur in some tumours, probably by mechanisms other than deletion. The *ras* oncogenes may be involved in the progression to malignancy.

### Other Tumours and Cysts

Small cysts of no clinical importance are common in the remnants of Rathke's cleft at the junction of the anterior and posterior lobes. Occasionally one may enlarge and cause atrophy of the anterior lobe. Craniopharyngiomas – although more commonly suprasellar – may occur in an intrasellar location. Rare tumours may arise from other components of the gland, e.g. fibroma or angioma. Metastatic tumours are uncommon in the anterior lobe.

### Inflammatory Conditions

Inflammatory disease is rare. Acute inflammation is usually a direct extension of infection in neighbouring structures. Granulomatous inflammation, e.g. tuberculosis or sarcoidosis, may involve the gland directly or lead to hypopituitarism if it affects the hypothalamus. Autoimmune hypophysitis is rare compared with autoimmune disease of other endocrine glands. Cytomegalovirus infection may be seen in AIDS (see Chapter 19, p. 544).

### Circulatory Disturbances

Infarction has to affect more than 70% of the gland before clinical evidence of hormone deficiency is seen. In Sheehan's syndrome, the pituitary is particularly vulnerable to hypotension because of the low-pressure portal system and an increase in size in pregnancy. Infarcts may also occur with disseminated intravenous coagulation, long-term ventilation, sickle cell disease, raised intracranial pressure, or diabetes mellitus. Small infarcts are common *post mortem*, but are of no clinical significance.

## Posterior Pituitary

The posterior lobe secretes oxytocin and vasopressin (antidiuretic hormone [ADH]), which are synthesized in the hypothalamus and pass down nerve fibres in the pituitary stalk to be secreted into the peripheral circulation. Oxytocin stimulates uterine contraction in labour and ejection of milk in lactation. There are no known diseases associated with excess or deficiency. Vasopressin regulates fluid balance by stimulating water reabsorption in the kidney. Lack of vasopressin causes diabetes insipidus. Patients have polyuria (often >10 L in 24 hours) and polydipsia. The urine is dilute, even when the patient is deprived of fluid. The disease may be due to mutations in the vasopressin gene, or to destructive lesions of the hypothalamus, including tumours, granulomatous disease, and histiocytosis X. It may also follow head injury or neurosurgical procedures, and, in these cases, may be transient.

# THYROID GLAND

The thyroid gland lies just below the cricoid cartilage, and consists of two lateral lobes linked by the isthmus. It comprises mainly follicles lined by cuboidal epithelium, which store varying amounts of colloid. Colloid contains thyroglobulin, the protein on which the thyroid hormones, thyroxine ($T_4$) and triiodothyronine ($T_3$), are synthesized (Fig. 17.8). This pathway is stimulated by TSH, and there is negative feedback to the pituitary. $T_4$ undergoes deiodination peripherally to produce $T_3$, which is the active hormone with significant regulatory effects on metabolism. It acts via nuclear receptors present in all cells. Diseases that disrupt the synthesis and secretion of these hormones cause widespread metabolic effects.

Scattered among the follicles in the upper two-thirds of each lobe are the C-cells, which secrete calcitonin. These are derived from the ultimobranchial bodies, most probably of neuroectodermal origin. Calcitonin is involved in the regulation of calcium metabolism, but its exact role is unclear.

Patients with thyroid disease may present with general enlargement of the gland (goitre), with a single nodule or evidence of thyroid hormone excess or lack. The latter presentations cause well-recognized syndromes.

## Hyperthyroidism

Often known as thyrotoxicosis, the symptoms and signs are related to a general increase in metabolic activity. It is usually due to autoimmune thyroid disease (Graves' disease) (*Box 17.3*). Patients are hyperkinetic, show emotional lability, and complain of heat intolerance, excessive sweating, and weight loss despite a good appetite. There is tachycardia, increased cardiac output, and palpitations. Older patients may have atrial fibrillation and cardiac failure. Some of these effects are direct whereas others – such as the characteristic eyelid retraction – are due to increased sensitivity

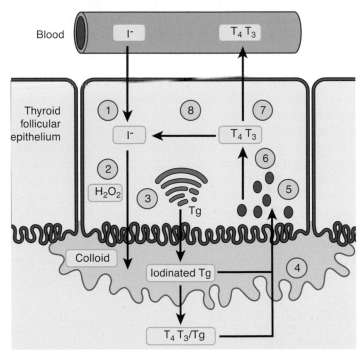

FIG. 17.8 The synthetic pathway and secretion of thyroid hormones. (1) Inorganic iodide is trapped and (2) oxidized within the follicular cells by the action of thyroid peroxidase. (3) It is then secreted into the colloid and undergoes organification close to the cell membrane by the iodination of tyrosyl residues on thyroglobulin (Tg), also secreted by the follicular cells. First, monoiodotyrosine (MIT) and diiodotyrosine (DIT) are produced. Thyroxine ($T_4$) is then formed by the coupling of two molecules of DIT, and triiodothyronine ($T_3$) by coupling of MIT and DIT. When hormone is required, thyroglobulin is (4) reabsorbed and (5) undergoes proteolysis, releasing (6) $T_3$ and $T_4$, which (7) diffuse into the circulation. (8) The excess, along with MIT and DIT, undergoes deiodination.

---

**Box 17.3** CAUSES OF HYPERTHYROIDISM

- Graves' disease – 80%
- Toxic nodular goitre – 10%
- Thyroid adenoma – 5–10%
- Early Hashimoto's thyroiditis
- Thyroid-stimulating hormone (TSH)-secreting pituitary adenoma
- Ingestion of thyroid hormones

to sympathetic stimulation; the levator palpebrae superioris muscle has sympathetic innervation. In some patients with Graves' disease there is proptosis – protuberance of the eyeball due to inflammatory infiltration of the extraocular tissues of the orbit (so-called 'thyroid eye disease').

## Hypothyroidism

In the adult this is called myxoedema and the symptoms depend on the severity of hormone deficiency, which causes a reduction in general metabolic activity. The causes are shown on *Box 17.4*. There is weight gain and general lethargy with cold intolerance. The skin and hair are dry and the accumulation of mucopolysaccharides in the connective tissue results in thickening of the skin, hoarseness, and pain and paraesthesia when nerves are trapped. There is intellectual impairment. Change of mood may progress to psychosis. In severe deficiency, hypothermia and coma can develop. Raised blood cholesterol levels increase the risk of cardiovascular disease.

Cretinism is due to severe hypothyroidism in infancy. Thyroid hormones are critical for normal brain development, and these children show signs of learning disabilities, neuromuscular abnormalities, deaf mutism, and retarded growth. There is a goitre when it is caused by severe iodine deficiency or inherited defects of the enzymes involved in thyroid hormone synthesis. Rarely, thyroid agenesis or hypoplasia occurs, and in these cases goitre is absent. It is extremely important to make an early diagnosis because hormone replacement permits normal development.

## Functional Disorders

### *Non-toxic Nodular Goitre*

#### Key Points
- Non-toxic nodular goitre is the most common thyroid disease.
- It is either endemic or sporadic.
- There is nodular enlargement of the thyroid gland.
- Affected individuals may be either euthyroid or hypothyroid.

Non-toxic nodular goitre is the most common lesion in thyroid pathology. When there is absolute or relative iodine deficiency, reduced levels of thyroid hormones result in increased TSH secretion by the pituitary gland. This induces thyroid hyperplasia in an attempt to increase thyroid hormone output. The demands are usually intermittent and the gland undergoes cycles of growth and involution, resulting in the well-recognized picture of multinodular goitre, with nodules consisting of follicles of varying size, fibrosis, haemorrhage, and focal inflammation. Enlargement is usually asymmetrical, and the gland may weigh up to several hundred grams (Fig. 17.9). Occasionally, simple goitre

> **Box 17.4** CAUSES OF HYPOTHYROIDISM
>
> - Autoimmune thyroid disease:
>     Hashimoto's thyroiditis
>     Primary myxoedema
> - Severe iodine deficiency
> - Dyshormonogenesis
> - Following thyroid surgery or radioiodine therapy
> - Ingestion of goitrogens
> - Hypopituitarism

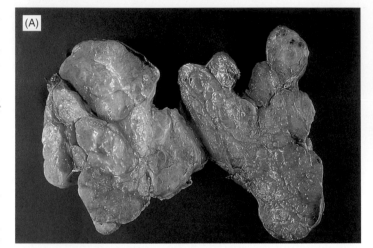

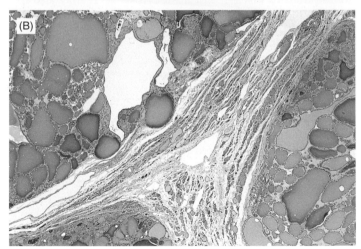

**FIG. 17.9** (A) A cut section through a multinodular goitre showing gross asymmetrical enlargement. (B) Nodularity is obvious on histological assessment.

may produce signs or symptoms suggestive of tumour. When one nodule is larger than the others (dominant nodule) fine-needle aspiration cytology or even thyroid lobectomy may be required to distinguish the two. Occasionally, there may be compression of the trachea, oesophagus, or recurrent laryngeal nerve.

On an epidemiological basis, two forms are defined:

1. Endemic goitre affects more than 10% of the population, occurring in areas with absolute deficiency of

iodine, usually far from the sea, reflecting seafood as the major source of iodine. Endemic areas include the Andes, Himalayas, and Alps. The introduction of iodized salt has reduced the incidence. Goitre usually develops in childhood, and the sexes are equally affected.

2. Sporadic goitre is due to relative lack of iodine in individuals. It reflects inadequate intake, inherited abnormalities in thyroid hormone production, and ingestion of goitrogens, i.e. substances that interfere with hormone synthesis. These include vegetables of the *Brassica* family, excessive fluoride, or drugs such as *p*-aminosalicylic acid and sulphonylureas. Some people also suggest that autoimmune mechanisms may be involved.

## Autoimmune Thyroid Disease

> ### Key Points
>
> - Autoimmune thyroid disease is associated with antibodies to thyroid antigens.
> - The clinical picture varies according to the antibodies produced.
> - Females are more commonly affected than males.

This group of diseases – Graves' disease, Hashimoto's thyroiditis, and primary myxoedema – is characterized by lymphoid infiltration of the gland and the presence of circulating antibodies to various components of thyroid follicular cells (*Table 17.1*), some of which are thought to play an active role in pathogenesis. Thyroid-stimulating immunoglobulins (TSIs) bind to and activate the TSH receptor, causing increased secretion of thyroid hormones, usually in Graves' disease. Other antibodies are thought to stimulate growth, and may be important in goitrogenesis in

TABLE 17.1 Autoantibodies in thyroid autoimmune disease

| Anti-thyroperoxidase | Present in >80% of patients with chronic thyroiditis: also found in 10% of normal adults |
|---|---|
| Anti-TSH receptor | |
| Thyroid-stimulating immunoglobulins | Stimulate activity |
| Thyroid growth immunoglobulin | May stimulate growth |
| Receptor-blocking antibodies | ? Contribute to hypothyroidism |
| Anti-thyroglobulin | Present in approximately 35% of patients with anti-thyroperoxidase antibodies |

TSH = thyroid-stimulating hormone.

Hashimoto's thyroiditis. Receptor-blocking antibodies may contribute to hypothyroidism and to thyroid atrophy in primary myxoedema. These diseases may be familial and are associated with other organ-specific autoimmune diseases (*Box 17.5*).

### Graves' Disease

This is characterized by a diffuse goitre and hyperthyroidism. It mainly affects females aged 20–40 years. The gland is diffusely hyperplastic and hyperaemic, clinically resulting in a bruit on auscultation. In the untreated case, the thyroid epithelium is hyperplastic and there is little colloid storage. Lymphocytic infiltration is usually less marked than in Hashimoto's thyroiditis.

It is unusual now to see the classic histological features of the disease because of effective drug therapy. A minority of patients relapse and come to surgery, but are usually euthyroid at the time of surgery because of treatment with antithyroid drugs, with or without the addition of iodine. Their thyroids show complex histological features, antithyroid drugs inducing more marked follicular hyperplasia, whereas iodine reduces vascularity and increases colloid storage. This emphasizes the importance of a full clinical history in the interpretation of the histological appearances in endocrine disease.

### Hashimoto's Thyroiditis

This is a disease of middle-aged females, in whom it occurs 20 times more commonly than in males. There is a diffuse, firm, painless goitre (Fig. 17.10). Initially, the patient is

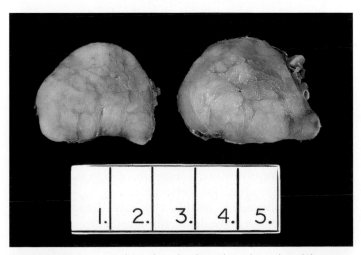

FIG. 17.10 Hashimoto's thyroiditis: the thyroid is enlarged, and the cut surface is pale in contrast to the normal brown appearance.

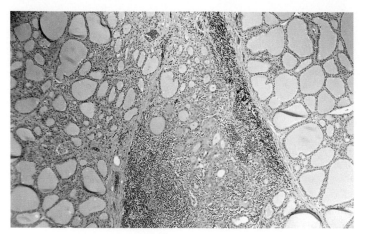

**FIG. 17.11** Hashimoto's thyroiditis showing the diffuse lymphoid infiltrate with destruction of the thyroid epithelium.

usually euthyroid, but 80% become hypothyroid. Occasional patients are hyperthyroid at presentation, presumably due to the presence of TSIs. High-titre antiperoxidase antibody is usually present. The gland is widely infiltrated and replaced by lymphocytes, plasma cells, and macrophages, often with germinal centre formation (Fig. 17.11). The thyroid follicular cells are enlarged with eosinophilic granular cytoplasm due to accumulation of mitochondria (Askanazy or Hürthle cell change). A subgroup of patients show marked fibrosis in the gland. Many of these patients show an abundance of IgG4-positive plasma cells and are thought now to represent a manifestation of IgG4-related disease (see also Chapter 6, p. 122).

### Primary Myxoedema

This disease mainly affects elderly females. The thyroid is atrophic, largely replaced by fibrous tissue with a lymphoid infiltrate. Patients are severely hypothyroid and are the most likely to present with hypothermia and coma.

### Other Forms of Thyroiditis

- *Acute thyroiditis* may occasionally develop in bacteraemia or by local extension of inflammation.
- *Giant cell (de Quervain's) thyroiditis*, also known as *subacute thyroiditis*, presents as a painful goitre. It is probably viral in origin, and there are often preceding general or upper respiratory symptoms and signs. Females are affected three times as often as males. Hyperthyroidism and the presence of thyroid antibodies are usually transient. Although there is an initial acute inflammation, followed by a granulomatous response, the whole process may resolve. Even if some fibrosis persists, there are no long-term functional effects.
- *Riedel's thyroiditis*: in this very rare disease the thyroid is replaced by dense fibrous tissue, which often extends into perithyroidal tissues, mimicking invasive

carcinoma. It may present as goitre or with symptoms related to involvement of the trachea or recurrent laryngeal nerve. Some cases are associated with fibrosclerosis at other sites, and these are now also thought to be part of the IgG4-related disease spectrum (see also Chapter 6, p. 122).

- *Focal chronic thyroiditis* is seen in 15–20% of postmortem examinations of patients with no clinical evidence of thyroid disease. This may represent subclinical autoimmune disease because the incidence is similar to that of thyroid autoantibodies in the general population.
- *Lymphocytic thyroiditis* occurs in children and young adults who present with goitre and sometimes hyperthyroidism. It may be a precursor of Hashimoto's disease.

## Thyroid tumours

### Key Points

Thyroid tumours include:
- follicular adenoma
- follicular carcinoma
- papillary carcinoma
- medullary carcinoma
- anaplastic carcinoma
- lymphoma.

Thyroid tumours usually present as solitary thyroid nodules and most are 'cold' on scan, concentrating radioactive iodine less actively than the surrounding gland. Some 70% of clinically apparent solitary nodules are, however, dominant nodules in a multinodular goitre. The rest are tumours, mostly benign. Thyroid cancer is rare and accounts for less than 1% of all cancers and less than 0.5% of deaths from cancer. Cold nodules in males and younger females should be regarded as more suspicious than those in middle-aged females. Most tumours arise from follicular cells and most are follicular adenomas. There are two types of differentiated carcinomas – follicular and papillary – which develop and behave differently. The C-cells give rise to medullary carcinoma.

### Follicular Adenoma

These are the most common thyroid neoplasms, presenting most frequently in females aged >30 years. They are usually non-functional but may occasionally secrete excess thyroid hormones. They are generally encapsulated and compress the surrounding gland. Haemorrhage, degeneration, and fibrosis may occur. They show a variety of histological appearances but these have no clinical importance. It can sometimes be difficult for a pathologist to distinguish between an adenoma and a hyperplastic (adenomatoid) nodule in a nontoxic goitre, but again this has no clinical significance.

## Follicular Carcinoma

These comprise 15–20% of all thyroid cancers but are more common in areas of iodine deficiency. Their peak incidence is in the fifth decade, a third of cases occurring at age >50 years. They are also more common in females. They metastasize by the vascular route, particularly to bone and lung. The overall survival rate is reported to be about 50%. Two variants are recognized: encapsulated, so-called 'minimally invasive' carcinoma, in which vascular and capsular invasion is seen only on microscopic examination (Fig. 17.12), and 'widely invasive' tumours, in which obvious spread is seen throughout the gland or beyond (Fig. 17.13). The latter have a poorer

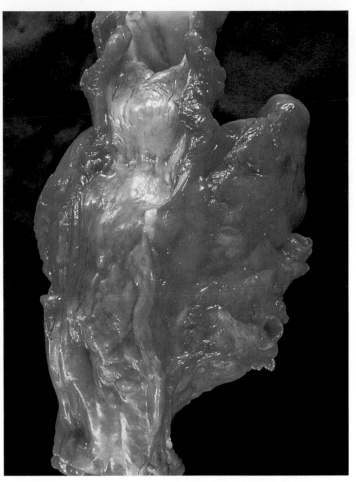

FIG. 17.13 This postmortem specimen shows invasion of the trachea and oesophagus by a follicular carcinoma of thyroid.

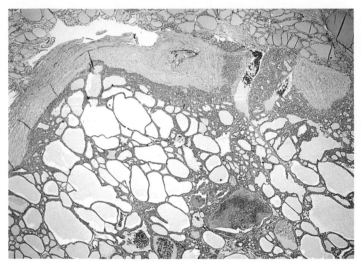

FIG. 17.12 Tongues of tumour are seen breaching the capsule and invading the surrounding gland in this minimally invasive follicular carcinoma of thyroid.

## INVESTIGATION OF A THYROID LUMP

A 32-year-old female presented with a lump in the right side of her neck (Fig. 17.14). She had no other symptoms, but on examination the lump was clearly related to the thyroid gland. A radioiodine scan showed a cold nodule (Fig. 17.14). The thyroid function tests were normal.

Fine-needle aspiration cytology showed the cellular appearances of a follicular lesion (Fig. 17.15). In such cases, surgical removal is necessary to distinguish between follicular adenoma and follicular carcinoma. The pathologist must sample widely the interface of the lesion and normal gland,

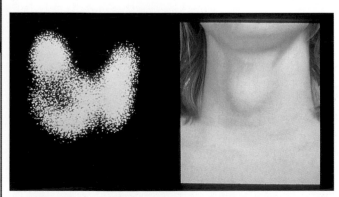

FIG. 17.14 The clinical appearance of the thyroid nodule is shown on the right, with the radioiodine scan on the left.

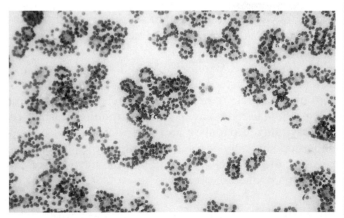

FIG. 17.15 The fine-needle aspiration cytology specimen showed a microfollicular pattern consistent with a follicular neoplasm (Leishman's stain).

and look for penetration of the capsule, or for invasion into vessels within the capsule or in the normal gland. At operation, there was a 3-cm-diameter nodule in the right lobe of the thyroid, and a lobectomy was performed. Histological examination demonstrated both capsular (Fig. 17.16) and

vascular (Fig. 17.17) invasion, the diagnosis being minimally invasive (angioinvasive) follicular carcinoma. The patient went on to have a completion thyroidectomy.

(Case history produced with the help of Drs HW Gray and CJR Stewart.)

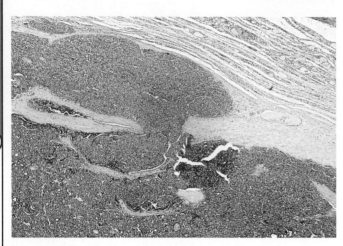

FIG. 17.16 The follicular carcinoma shows capsular invasion.

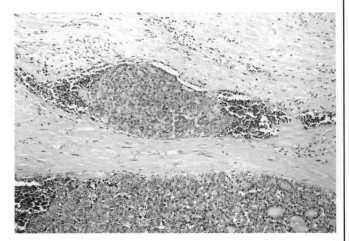

FIG. 17.17 Vascular invasion is also present.

prognosis than the former. In addition, minimally invasive tumours with vascular invasion are more likely to metastasize than those showing only capsular invasion.

### Papillary Carcinoma

All papillary tumours of the thyroid are regarded as malignant. They account for 60–70% of all thyroid cancers, occur in young adults (30–40 years), and are three times more common in females than in males. They have a good prognosis overall with a 5-year survival rate approaching 90%. They are not usually encapsulated and may be multifocal. 40% of patients have metastases in local lymph nodes at presentation, but this does not seem to alter the prognosis. The patient may first present with an enlarged lymph node if the thyroid primary is very small. In the small minority in whom the tumour has spread through the thyroid capsule or there are distant metastases, the prognosis is worse.

The diagnosis of papillary carcinoma is now made on the basis of characteristic cytological features, with clear or grooved nuclei, rather than on architectural features. Many of these lesions show papillary structures (Fig. 17.18); some have mixed papillary and follicular architecture; and a subgroup shows only follicular architecture (the follicular variant of papillary carcinoma). Some have fibrosis and psammoma bodies are present in about half.

### Medullary Carcinoma

These account for 5–10% of thyroid cancer. Up to 20% are familial, forming part of the MEN2 syndrome (see pp. 498–499). Medullary carcinoma is slightly more common in

females. Sporadic tumours are usually unilateral and most present between ages 40 and 60 years. In contrast, familial cases are usually bilateral and multifocal, arising from C-cell hyperplasia, and often present before the age of 25 years. Histologically, they differ from the other thyroid tumours. They consist of cells with an alveolar or trabecular arrangement. They are immunopositive for calcitonin (Fig. 17.19). Amyloid, formed from the calcitonin precursor, is seen in about 50% of cases. They may secrete other hormones such as ACTH or serotonin, which may occasionally result in ectopic hormone syndromes. These tumours show both lymphatic and vascular spread. The overall 10-year survival rate is around 50%.

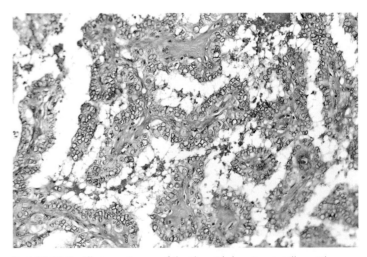

FIG. 17.18 Papillary carcinoma of the thyroid showing papillae with fibrovascular cores and classic optically clear nuclei.

### Other Tumours

Occasionally, in older females, a rapidly growing anaplastic carcinoma occurs. These are highly malignant and usually present as a rapidly growing mass. They probably represent progression of a pre-existing follicular or papillary tumour.

Benign and malignant tumours may rarely arise from the connective tissue or vascular components (e.g. haemangiomas). Occasional metastases are seen, usually from the lung, breast, or gastrointestinal tract.

In 1–2% of patients with Hashimoto's thyroiditis, B-cell lymphoma develops. This may also present as a rapidly expanding mass. Differentiation from anaplastic carcinoma can be made by fine-needle aspiration cytology.

### Aetiology of Thyroid Tumours

The molecular genetic pathways involved differ in follicular and papillary tumours. Mutations in *RAS* oncogenes play a role in some follicular tumours and are said to be associated with metastases. Iodine deficiency seems to favour *RAS* mutation. Other follicular lesions show rearrangement of *PAX8-PPARγ* genes. In contrast, point mutations in the *BRAF* gene are the most common change seen in papillary carcinoma. Chromosomal rearrangements involving the *RET* proto-oncogene on chromosome 10 or *NTRK1* on chromosome 1 also characterize papillary carcinoma, and may in some cases follow irradiation (reviewed in Special Study Topic 17.1). Mutations in the *TP53* tumour-suppressor gene have been identified only in undifferentiated tumours.

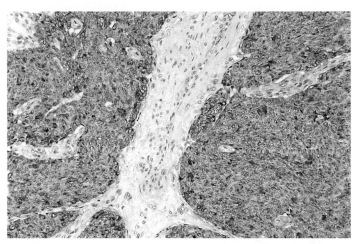

**FIG. 17.19** Medullary carcinoma of thyroid showing immunopositivity for calcitonin (brown).

## 17.1 Special Study Topic

### RADIATION AND THYROID CANCER

The general carcinogenic effects of radiation are well known. Exposure to particulate radiation produces double-stranded breaks in DNA and can therefore result in a number of changes, including deletions and chromosomal inversions or translocations. Increased numbers of thyroid cancers in the survivors of the Hiroshima and Nagasaki atomic bombs, and after therapeutic irradiation of the head and neck, first raised the possibility that radiation might be involved in the pathogenesis of the disease. The thyroid may be exposed to radiation in two ways: first by external irradiation and second by exposure to radioactive iodine. These are discussed separately below.

The thyroid appears to be much more susceptible to radiation-induced tumorigenesis in children than in adults. This may reflect a requirement for hormonal or growth factor stimulation in the pathogenesis, but this aspect remains to be elucidated.

### External Radiation

In the early days of therapeutic irradiation, its long-term effects were not appreciated, and it was used in the treatment of minor conditions in children, including tinea capitis and tonsillar hyperplasia or thymic enlargement. Around 1950, an increased incidence of thyroid cancer in people who had undergone such irradiation in childhood was first reported, and this has been extensively confirmed. Pooling of data from a number of series indicates an average excess relative risk of 7.7 per gray (Gy). In children, it appears that the thyroid has one of the highest risk coefficients observed for any organ, with increased risk at levels as low as 0.1 Gy. The effects of the atomic bombs in Japan were also related to external radiation because the explosions occurred at high altitude and there was little radioiodine fallout.

### Radioiodine exposure

Iodine-131 ($^{131}$I) is given both as a diagnostic tool in thyroid disease and, at higher doses, as a therapeutic agent in hyperthyroidism. There is no evidence to suggest that this results in an increased risk of thyroid cancer. Studies on fallout-induced thyroid cancer after atomic bomb testing support this, and suggest that the increased risk is due to short-lived radioiodines, $^{132}$I and $^{133}$I. However, these studies have been unable to produce a risk coefficient for exposure.

On 26 April 1986, the nuclear reactor at Chernobyl, Ukraine, exploded, releasing 300 MCi of radioactive substances into the atmosphere, including about 40 MCi of $^{131}$I and about 100 MCi of short-lived radioiodines. ($^{133}$I and the precursor of $^{132}$I, tellurium). The southern part of Belarus was most affected. Large doses of radioactive iodine were inhaled and ingested

## Special Study Topic continued . . .

on food, giving high doses to the thyroid. This is an iodine-deficient area, with incomplete iodine supplementation, and this probably raised the thyroid dose. An increase in thyroid cancer in children was noted as early as 1990. The annual incidence rose to more than 40 per million children in Belarus, compared with 1 per million in many countries. In 2005, it was concluded that about 4,000 cases of thyroid cancer were caused by exposure to fallout from the accident. To the contrary, however, there appears to have been little or no increased risk for those exposed as adults. Children may be more susceptible because their thyroid is growing much more rapidly than in adults. Also, they consume more milk than adults, and mammary epithelium concentrates iodine and secretes it in milk. If potassium iodide had been administered at the time as a competitive blocker of radioiodine uptake, it would most probably have reduced the incidence in susceptible groups.

### Tumour Type and Molecular Genetics

Almost all radiation-induced thyroid tumours are papillary carcinomas. Papillary thyroid carcinoma has a number of variants and in the early years after Chernobyl the tumours seen in the children were generally of the solid type and showed an aggressive pattern of behaviour, with lung and lymph node metastases. Nevertheless, death from disease has been rare. After 10 years, fewer of the tumours were of the solid type, and classic and follicular variants were seen more often.

The molecular genetic changes in papillary carcinoma are not fully elucidated. In about 16% of sporadic adult cases, there is oncogenic rearrangement of the *RET* proto-oncogene on chromosome 10q11.2, which encodes a receptor tyrosine kinase. A number of rearrangements have been identified in which the gene loses the ligand binding and transmembrane domains and fuses to another gene at its 5'-end, coming under the regulation of the fused gene. These rearrangements result in ubiquitous expression of the fused proteins, the ability to dimerize and thus become active in the absence of ligand, and translocation to the cytoplasm where they may interact with unusual substances. All of these are probably important in the neoplastic process. In *RET/PTC1*, which accounts for almost all sporadic cases, there is a chromosomal inversion and fusion with the *H4* gene at 10q21. In *RET/PTC 3* there is also an intrachromosomal inversion with the *ELE1* gene, also at 10q11.2. In contrast to sporadic cases, *RET* rearrangements were reported in about 60% of the early post-Chernobyl papillary thyroid carcinomas, and two-thirds of these were *RET/PTC3*. Interestingly, when the distribution of variants changed in the later tumours, the proportion of cases with *RET/PTC1* has increased and with *RET/PTC3* has decreased. This suggests that particular translocations are associated with both tumour phenotype and tumour latency.

The most common molecular genetic change in adult sporadic cases is the V600E mutation in the *BRAF* gene that occurs in about 45% of cases. This mutation has been found only rarely in post-Chernobyl cases. This is evidence that double-stranded DNA breaks are important in radiation-induced thyroid tumours.

### Further Reading

Furmanchuk AW, Averkin JI, Egloff B, *et al*. Pathomorphological findings in thyroid cancers of children from the Republic of Belarus – a study of 86 cases occurring between 1986 (post-Chernobyl) and 1991. *Histopathology* 1992;**21**:401–408.

LiVolsi VA, Abrosimov AA, Bogdanova T, *et al*. The Chernobyl thyroid cancer experience: pathology. *Clinical Oncology* 2011;**23**:261–267.

Williams D. Radiation carcinogenesis: lessons from Chernobyl. *Oncogene* 2008;**27**(suppl 2):S9–18.

Activating mutations in the *RET* gene are involved in medullary carcinoma arising as part of the MEN2 syndrome. This does not play a significant role in sporadic tumours.

## Miscellaneous Disorders

Occasional abnormalities of thyroid descent occur, most commonly lingual thyroid. Thyroglossal duct cysts are situated in the midline and develop from persistence of the lower part of the tubal downgrowth that gives rise to the gland. Amyloid may be seen, either as part of systemic amyloidosis or as an isolated finding.

## ADRENAL GLANDS

The adrenal glands lie above the kidneys and comprise the outer cortex, which is of mesodermal origin, and the inner medulla, derived from neuroectoderm. In the adult, they weigh around 4 g in cases of sudden accidental death. However, stimulation by ACTH causes them to increase in size, and the stress of terminal illness results in an average weight of 6 g at hospital postmortem examination. The cortex and medulla are dealt with separately.

## Adrenal Cortex

The cortex consists of three zones – zona glomerulosa, zona fasciculata, and zona reticularis – which synthesize a range of steroid hormones (Fig. 17.20). The zona glomerulosa, which is dispersed focally below the capsule, secretes the mineralocorticoid aldosterone, and is regulated by the renin–angiotensin system. Aldosterone plays a major role in the regulation of plasma volume and potassium balance, mainly by effects on the kidney. The zona fasciculata produces glucocorticoids, mainly cortisol. These have wide-ranging effects on general metabolism, promoting gluconeogenesis and inhibiting protein synthesis. They have

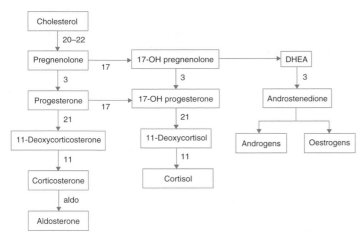

FIG. 17.20 Pathways of adrenal steroidogenesis: the enzymes involved are: 20–22 = 20,22 desmolase (CYP11A); 3 = 3β-hydroxysteroid dehydrogenase; 21 = 21-hydroxylase (CYP21); 11 = 11β-hydroxylase (CYP11B1); aldo = aldosterone synthase (CYB11B2); DHEA = dehydroepiandrosterone.

anti-inflammatory and immunosuppressive effects, particularly affecting T cells. Actions on bone metabolism favour the development of osteoporosis. The gland also secretes sex steroids, probably from the zona reticularis. These are mainly androgens, but may undergo peripheral conversion to oestrogens.

## Adrenocortical Hyperfunction

### Key Points

Disorders associated with adrenocortical hyperfunction are:

- Cushing's syndrome
- primary hyperaldosteronism
  Conn's syndrome
  idiopathic hyperaldosteronism
- adrenogenital syndrome.

There are three main syndromes within this spectrum, relating to the hypersecretion of glucocorticoids, aldosterone, or sex steroids.

### Cushing's Syndrome

This is the result of the excessive secretion of cortisol, although some of the features may be caused by secretion of precursors in the steroidogenic pathway with mineralocorticoid effects. If undiagnosed, or untreated, there is a high morbidity and mortality. It occurs most commonly in females, but may present in males and, rarely, in children. The administration of excessive doses of therapeutic steroids may induce an iatrogenic form of the disease.

The clinical picture is characteristic (Fig. 17.21). Increased protein breakdown leads to loss of muscle bulk, particularly on the limbs; centripetal deposition of fat results in moon face, buffalo hump, and truncal obesity; inhibition of

protein synthesis and abnormal collagen maturation cause abdominal striae. There is hypertension. Osteoporosis may lead to vertebral collapse. Proximal myopathy is common. Diminished glucose tolerance is present, with hyperglycaemia and glycosuria in up to 20% of cases. Wound healing may be delayed. Mental symptoms are common with depression and sometimes psychosis. In some cases, there is

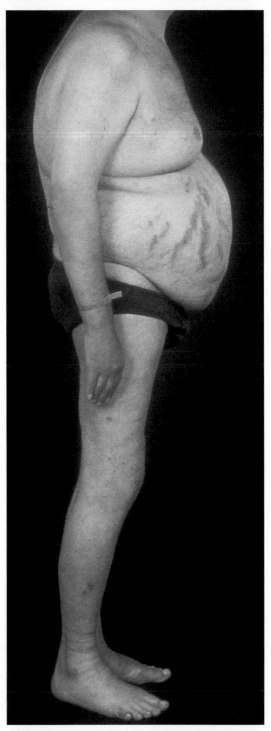

FIG. 17.21 A patient with Cushing's syndrome. Note the characteristic obesity of the neck and trunk and the relative wasting of the limbs. (Courtesy of Professor J.M. Connell, University of Dundee.)

---

**Box 17.6** CAUSES OF CUSHING'S SYNDROME

Pituitary adenoma : 67%
Adrenal tumour: 15%
   Adenoma
   Carcinoma
Ectopic ACTH syndrome: 17%
Ingestion of glucocorticoids

---

also excess secretion of androgens, with hirsutism, amenorrhoea, and virilization.

The main causes are shown in *Box 17.6* and are outlined below.

### Cushing's Disease (Pituitary-dependent Cushing's Syndrome)

This accounts for about 70% of cases. There is excess ACTH secretion from the pituitary, usually from a corticotrophic adenoma (see pp. 479–480). This causes hyperstimulation of the adrenals and bilateral cortical hyperplasia, which may be diffuse or nodular. In diffuse hyperplasia, the gland is increased in weight to between 6 and 12 g and the cortex is broadened. In the less common nodular hyperplasia, obvious nodules visible to the naked eye are present and the glands may be markedly enlarged. Why these nodules develop is unknown but they are more common in longstanding disease. The raised plasma glucocorticoids can be suppressed by high doses of dexamethasone. ACTH levels are usually just above normal, with loss of the circadian rhythm.

### Adrenocortical Tumours with Autonomous Secretion of Cortisol

These cause about 20% of cases in adults, with 80% occurring in women. Approximately half are malignant. In children, adrenocortical tumours cause 50% of cases, and carcinoma is more common. Particularly with malignant tumours, the production of sex steroids also causes virilization (so-called 'mixed' Cushing's syndrome). The excess glucocorticoids suppress ACTH secretion by the pituitary. This results in atrophy of the contralateral adrenal and of the adrenal remnant adjacent to the tumour. If the tumour is removed surgically, the patient must receive glucocorticoids until ACTH secretion is re-established and the remaining adrenal gland regenerates. The raised cortisol levels in these patients cannot be suppressed by dexamethasone. Plasma ACTH levels are low or undetectable.

### Ectopic ACTH Syndrome

In the remaining cases, there is secretion of ACTH by a non-pituitary tumour. These include carcinoid tumours and small cell carcinoma of the lung, thymic carcinoid tumours, and, occasionally, neuroendocrine tumours of the pancreas. Patients with lung cancer may not develop full-blown clinical features because of the other effects of a rapidly progressing tumour. There is bilateral diffuse adrenal hyperplasia and the glands are usually heavier than in Cushing's disease, weighing up to 20 g each. The high glucocorticoid levels are not suppressed by dexamethasone. Levels of ACTH and ACTH precursors are raised, usually to higher levels than in Cushing's disease.

### Hyperaldosteronism

#### Primary Hyperaldosteronism

This is characterized by hypertension, periodic muscle weakness or paralysis, muscle cramps and tetany, nocturia, and polyuria. There is often hypokalaemia, metabolic alkalosis (high serum bicarbonate), high plasma aldosterone, and low renin, indicating autonomous secretion of aldosterone. About a third of patients have an adrenal adenoma (Fig. 17.22), three-quarters in females. This is known as Conn's syndrome. Carcinomas are rare. In the remaining cases, there is bilateral hyperplasia of the zona glomerulosa of unknown cause (idiopathic hyperaldosteronism). Surgical removal of an adenoma can be curative if performed before the vascular changes of hypertension become established.

#### Secondary Hyperaldosteronism

Increased activity of the renin–angiotensin system will stimulate aldosterone secretion. This can occur in kidney disease where there is renal ischaemia (see Chapter 13, p. 393), in oedema, and occasionally with a renin-secreting tumour. Plasma levels of both aldosterone and renin are high.

### Adrenogenital Syndrome

#### Adrenal Tumours

These may secrete sex steroids, more usually androgens. This is more common in carcinomas than in adenomas. In women

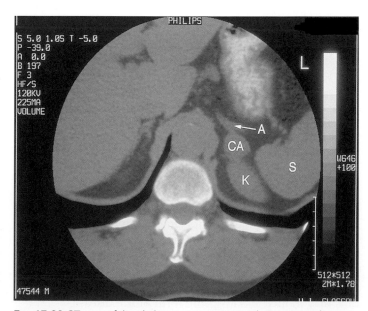

**FIG. 17.22** CT scan of the abdomen in a patient with Conn's syndrome. An adenoma (CA) is seen in the left adrenal, continuous with normal adrenal tissue (A). The kidney (K) and spleen (S) are also shown. (Courtesy of Professor J.M. Connell, University of Dundee.)

it results in virilization (clitoromegaly and hirsutism). Occasionally secretion of oestrogens may cause gynaecomastia and penile and testicular atrophy in males.

### Congenital Adrenal Hyperplasia

This is associated with a group of diseases, which are the result of inherited mutations in the genes encoding the enzymes and other proteins involved in steroidogenesis. Reduction in cortisol secretion causes reduced negative feedback and ACTH secretion is increased in an attempt to produce normal levels of cortisol. This usually also results in an increase in androgen secretion. Intermediate steroids with mineralocorticoid effects may also be secreted in excess. The clinical picture depends on the combination of steroids secreted. The increased stimulation leads to massive adrenocortical hyperplasia. The most common form is 21-hydroxylase deficiency, with a mean incidence of 1 in 14,000. Female infants have clitoromegaly and various degrees of labial fusion. The internal reproductive tract is normal. Males present with precocious puberty. In two-thirds of cases, aldosterone synthesis is also impaired and these infants have features of salt loss with dehydration, vomiting, and hypotensive collapse. Deficiency of 11β-hydroxylase is 20% as common. Deoxycorticosterone accumulates along with androgens, causing hypertension in addition to virilism.

## Adrenocortical Tumours

It has not been clear how common adrenal adenomas are because in the past they were usually diagnosed in life only when they secreted excess hormone. *Post mortem*, nodules can be found in about 5% of adrenals, and clonality studies suggest that the larger lesions are neoplastic. More of these are now being identified in live patients because people have their abdomens scanned in the investigation of other diseases. This raises the problem of what to do with them. At present, if there is no evidence of significant hormone secretion and the lesion is <3 cm in diameter, and does not grow on sequential scanning, most surgeons would not remove it. This approach is based on the low probability of malignant potential and the fact that carcinomas tend to be larger tumours. Functional adenomas may secrete cortisol, aldosterone, or sex steroids. They resemble normal adrenal cortex histologically, tending to have a preponderance of lipid-laden fasciculata-like cells.

### Adrenocortical Carcinoma

This is a rare tumour, with an incidence of only 1–2 per million of the population. Most are obviously malignant at presentation with local spread and/or metastases (Fig. 17.23). The prognosis is poor. The histological distinction between benign and malignant intra-adrenal tumours can be difficult. There is no one feature that distinguishes malignancy and diagnosis is based on multifactorial analysis. Tumours secreting androgens, oestrogens, or intermediate steroids are more likely to be malignant.

Adrenal carcinomas show widespread cytogenetic changes, but the critical molecular genetic events involved in their pathogenesis are still under investigation. The *MEN1* gene does not appear to be involved in sporadic tumours. Abnormalities in *TP53* may play a role in tumour progression. The *RAS* oncogenes are not mutated. Overexpression of IGF-2 has been shown in carcinoma, and IGF-1 and members of the epidermal growth factor and transforming growth factor families may also play a role in regulating growth.

## Adrenocortical Hypofunction

### Key Points

- Acute adrenocortical hypofunction may result from meningococcal septicaemia and other infections.
- Chronic adrenocortical hypofunction may result from autoimmune adrenalitis or tuberculosis.

In both acute and chronic hypofunction, about 90% of the cortex must be destroyed before clinical symptoms are present. Adrenal cortical failure may be the result of primary disease of the adrenal gland, or secondary to lack of ACTH release from the pituitary, most commonly as one aspect of panhypopituitarism.

### Acute Adrenocortical Insufficiency

This is a rare complication of septicaemia, particularly due to meningococcal infection, and is known as Waterhouse–Friderichsen syndrome. It is seen less frequently with other bacteraemic infections, including pneumococci, staphylococci, or *Haemophilus influenzae*. It presents with vomiting,

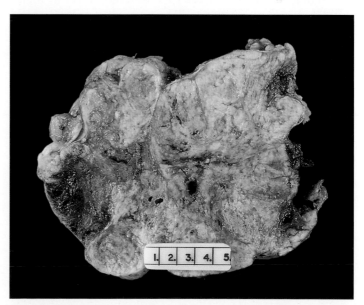

**Fig. 17.23** Adrenocortical carcinoma, showing necrosis and haemorrhage. This tumour was causing Cushing's syndrome.

salt loss with hyponatraemia, hyperkalaemia, hypogly-caemia, and dehydration, causing collapse, hypotension, and sometimes death. Patients often have a high fever and pur-puric rash. There is haemorrhage into the adrenal glands, with extensive cortical necrosis. In the past it was thought that the adrenocortical failure played a major role in the vascular collapse; it is now realized that it is probably a minor component, the major factors being the massive bac-teraemia and endotoxaemia, which result in disseminated intravascular coagulation and shock.

Acute adrenocortical failure superimposed on chronic failure (Addisonian crisis) may occur when increased demands are made on a chronically failing adrenal cortex by, for example, infection or trauma. In addition, lack of cortico-steroid cover in adrenalectomized patients may precipitate adrenal failure, as may the sudden withdrawal of glucocor-ticoids from patients on long-term treatment. It is critically important therefore that patients receiving glucocorticoids should be made fully aware of the risk of discontinuing these drugs. Acute adrenocortical failure may also be part of the acute presentation of congenital adrenal hyperplasia.

### Chronic Adrenocortical Insufficiency (Addison's Disease)

In chronic adrenal insufficiency, there is general lethargy, muscle weakness, hypotension, anorexia, and pigmentation of the skin and mucous membranes. The most common cause of chronic insufficiency in developed countries is now auto-immune adrenalitis, which accounts for 75% of cases. The adrenals are atrophic with an infiltrate of lymphocytes and plasma cells. The medulla is not affected. There is an asso-ciation with other organ-specific autoimmune diseases, such as autoimmune thyroid disease, pernicious anaemia (see Chapter 8, p. 218), vitiligo, and type 1 diabetes mellitus.

The second most common cause is tuberculosis, in which the medulla is also destroyed. This continues to be the major cause in developing countries. The adrenals are enlarged and consist of masses of caseous material often with calcification that may be seen on radiographs. Occasionally amyloidosis, fungal infection, or secondary tumour may result in adrenal failure.

Chronic adrenal insufficiency results in ACTH cell hyperplasia with increased ACTH secretion by the pituitary. Occasionally a pituitary adenoma may form.

## Adrenal Medulla

The main component of the medulla is the phaeochromo-cytes or chromaffin cells, which secrete the catecholamines, adrenaline and noradrenaline. Nerves and ganglion cells are also found. Tumours are the only important pathology.

### Phaeochromocytoma

Phaeochromocytomas (Fig. 17.24) arise from the chromaf-fin cells and produce symptoms related to catecholamine excess, which may at first be intermittent. These include

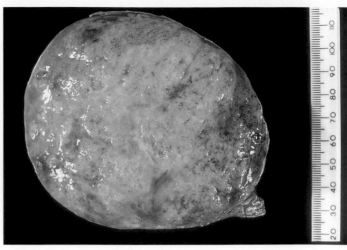

FIG. 17.24 Phaeochromocytoma removed from a patient with hypertension. The normal adrenal can be seen to the bottom right.

hypertension, palpitation, sweating, and sometimes col-lapse. There is hyperglycaemia and glycosuria. They occur in both sexes across a wide age range, but are rare in children. Similar tumours may arise in extra-adrenal paraganglia, most commonly in the organs of Zuckerkandl. Historically, about 10% were thought to be familial, as part of the MEN2 syndrome (see pp. 498–499), von Hippel–Lindau (VHL) syndrome, and neurofibromatosis type 1(NF1). The recent identification of familial cases associated with mutations in the subunits of the succinate dehydrogenase (*SDHx*) genes suggests that up to 30% of cases are familial. In some of these syndromes, phaeochromocytomas are associated with extra-adrenal paragangliomas. Bilateral tumours are present in about half the familial cases. Malignancy is defined by the presence of metastasis and less than 10% of all these tumours are malignant. However, extra-adrenal paragangli-omas, particularly intra-abdominal tumours, are more often malignant than intra-adrenal tumours.

Phaeochromocytomas usually consist of cells arranged in an alveolar or trabecular pattern. It is difficult to pre-dict tumour behaviour on histological grounds. They may occasionally produce ectopic hormone syndromes, secre-ting ACTH or vasoactive intestinal polypeptide (VIP), causing the WDHA (watery diarrhoea, hypokalaemia and achlorhydria) syndrome.

### Other Tumours

Neuroblastoma is a tumour arising in children from the primitive cells of the medulla. Benign tumours may arise from the other components of the medulla, and include neurofibroma and ganglioneuroma, fibroma, and angioma.

Occasionally, pseudocysts may develop, due to haemorrhage into adrenal tumours. Haematopoietic tissue is frequently seen in the adrenal cortex *post mortem*. This may coexist with adipose tissue, the so-called myelolipoma. Metastases are common, particularly from bronchial carcinoma.

# PARATHYROID GLANDS

There are usually four parathyroid glands, lying posterior to the thyroid gland: two at the upper and two at the lower poles. However, one or more may be intrathyroidal, or lie in the lower neck or upper mediastinum close to the thymus. The total weight is 120 mg in adult males and 140 mg in females, the upper limit of normal for an individual gland being 50 mg. They consist of two main cell types: (1) chief cells, which form the main functional group, and are usually eosinophilic, but may also appear clear, depending on the intracellular glycogen content; and (2) oxyphil cells, which are slightly larger, and have a strongly eosinophilic rather granular cytoplasm, due to the presence of large numbers of mitochondria. The number of oxyphil cells increases with age. Stromal fat is seen after puberty, and constitutes up to 30% of the normal adult gland.

The parathyroid glands secrete parathyroid hormone, which regulates serum calcium levels by effects on bone, the kidneys, and the gut. Secretion is controlled by circulating calcium, via the calcium-sensing receptor.

## Hyperparathyroidism

Hyperparathyroidism is classified as:

- primary, when excessive secretion of parathyroid is autonomous
- secondary, when the gland secretes parathyroid hormone in response to increased physiological stimulation, most commonly in renal failure
- tertiary, when autonomous hypersecretion of hormone develops on a background of secondary hyperparathyroidism.

### Primary Hyperparathyroidism

This is a disease of middle age and is slightly more common in females. Patients may present with general tiredness and muscle weakness, and are often now diagnosed at this stage before significant pathology develops. In the past, more people presented with renal calculi and some developed severe bone disease with osteitis fibrosa cystica (see Chapter 12, pp. 353–354). Other complications include duodenal ulceration and acute pancreatitis. Metastatic calcification may cause nephrocalcinosis and renal failure, and may affect the soft tissues, heart, and other organs.

In 80% of patients, there is a single parathyroid adenoma and removal results in cure. In 15–20% of cases, there is enlargement of more than one gland, i.e. primary hyperplasia. Parathyroid carcinoma accounts for only 2–3% of cases. At the time of surgery it is often obvious that a carcinoma is infiltrating the surrounding tissues and the surgeon may have difficulty in removing it. As with other endocrine tumours, it can be difficult for the pathologist to predict malignant behaviour if there is no obvious invasion or metastasis.

However, the recent observation that nuclear staining for the protein parafibromin is reduced or absent in malignant tumours may be helpful in the difficult case.

Primary hyperparathyroidism may occur as part of the MEN1 syndrome. Hyperplasia (Fig. 17.25) may be found in these cases.

### Secondary Hyperparathyroidism

Persistent low serum levels of ionized calcium will result in increased stimulation of parathyroid hormone release and result in hyperplasia. This occurs most commonly in chronic renal failure (see Chapter 13, p. 393), but may also be seen in malabsorption syndromes and with vitamin D deficiency.

Occasionally, a patient with secondary hyperparathyroidism becomes hypercalcaemic. This is referred to as tertiary hyperparathyroidism. It is thought that some cells in a parathyroid gland become autonomous, i.e. insensitive to the controlling effect of $Ca^{2+}$, and an inappropriately high level of hormone results. In some cases an adenomatous nodule may develop.

## Hypoparathyroidism

Deficiency of parathyroid hormone causes hypocalcaemia and hyperphosphataemia. The low calcium causes increased muscular tone and, if severe, tetany. Patients often develop cataracts, and may have psychological changes and convulsions. The most common cause is surgical removal of the glands, sometimes inadvertently during thyroidectomy or head and neck surgery. It forms part of DiGeorge syndrome (see Chapter 2, p. 27), when it is coupled with immunological deficiencies. This is due to hypoplasia or aplasia of both parathyroids and thymus, caused by abnormal development of the third and fourth branchial arches. Very rarely, autoimmune parathyroiditis is the cause, sometimes associated with other autoimmune organ-specific diseases.

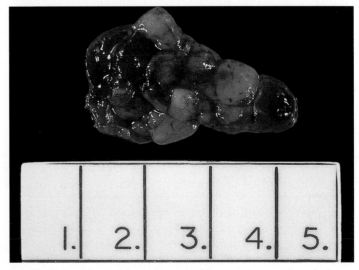

FIG. 17.25 Nodular parathyroid removed from a patient with multiple endocrine neoplasia, type 1 who had hypercalcaemia. The other glands were also nodular, but much smaller.

# DIABETES MELLITUS

## Key Points

- Diabetes mellitus is an extremely common metabolic disorder, which is increasing in prevalence
- It is known as a 'syndrome of inadequate insulin action'
- The type 1 condition is insulin dependent
- The type 2 condition is non-insulin dependent
- Eye, renal, vascular and neurological complications are commonplace.

Diabetes is not a single disease, but rather the pathological and metabolic state caused by inadequate insulin action. A feature common to all types is glucose intolerance. Diabetes is defined clinically as either a fasting plasma glucose level >7.8 mmol/L (140 mg/dL) or a 2-hour post-prandial plasma glucose >11 mmol/L (200 mg/dL).

Insulin is a major anabolic hormone that promotes the uptake of glucose by cells and the formation of intracellular glycogen from glucose. It also stimulates cells to utilize amino acids for protein synthesis rather than for gluconeogenesis, and it promotes the uptake of free fatty acids by adipose tissue. A lack of insulin, therefore, results in a general catabolic state with loss of weight, hyperglycaemia, diminished protein synthesis, increased gluconeogenesis, and hyperlipidaemia due to lipolysis in adipose tissue. Although the renal threshold is usually raised, there is heavy glycosuria, which results in an osmotic diuresis, causing dehydration and thirst. In the liver, excess free fatty acids are converted via acetyl-CoA into ketone bodies, which, in the absence of available glucose, are metabolized for cellular energy. The ketone bodies (acetoacetic acid, β-hydroxybutyric acid, and acetone) dissociate to produce hydrogen ions, with a resultant metabolic acidosis (ketoacidosis). This complex of metabolic disturbances produces hyperosmolarity, hypovolaemia, acidosis, and electrolyte imbalance, which have serious effects on the functions of neurons and result in one form of diabetic coma – ketoacidotic coma. The other major form – hyperosmolar non-ketotic coma – results from massive dehydration and profound hyperglycaemia in the absence of ketoacidosis. Relative or absolute overdosage with insulin causes hypoglycaemic effects, including coma which, unless treated, may be fatal.

## Classification of Diabetes

Over 99% of cases of diabetes are caused by two diseases: type 1 or type 2. Type 2 diabetes is 10 times more common than type 1. The principal differences between the two are detailed in *Table 17.2*. Specific diseases in which diabetes occurs as a secondary event include chronic pancreatitis, haemochromatosis, cystic fibrosis, acromegaly, Cushing's syndrome and glucagon-secreting islet cell tumours.

**TABLE 17.2** The two main diseases that result in diabetes mellitus

| Type 1 diabetes | Type 2 diabetes |
| --- | --- |
| Onset age <40 years | Onset age >40 years |
| Thin patient | Obese patient |
| Affects 1 in 250 of population in the UK | Affects 1 in 25 of population in the UK |
| Liable to ketoacidotic coma | Liable to hyperosmolar non-ketotic coma |
| Always requires insulin for therapy | Does not always require insulin for therapy |
| Concordance rate for monozygotic twins 40% | Concordance rate for monozygotic twins 90% |
| Genetic link with class II MHC antigens | No genetic link with class II MHC antigens |
| Islet cell antibodies present | Islet cell antibodies absent |
| Insulitis present | Insulitis absent |
| B cells destroyed in pancreas | B cells not destroyed in pancreas |
| Islet amyloid absent | Islet amyloid present |

MHC = major histocompatibility complex.

In haemochromatosis, excess iron is taken up by B cells, but not by other islet endocrine cells, resulting in inhibition of insulin synthesis.

## Complications of Diabetes

- Atheroma
- Hypertension
- Diabetic nephropathy
- Diabetic retinopathy
- Bacterial infection
- Peripheral neuropathy.

Coma due to lack of diabetic control is now a relatively rare cause of death, and the mortality and morbidity of diabetes are due to the above complications.

### Cardiovascular Complications

It is customary to speak of diabetic macroangiopathy, most commonly affecting large muscular arteries, and diabetic microangiopathy, affecting arterioles and capillaries. The former is simply atheroma (see Chapter 6, pp. 117–120), which tends to develop early and become severe in people with diabetes of either sex. This – plus the fact that 50% of patients with type 2 diabetes have hypertension – results in 50% of adult diabetic deaths being due to cardiovascular, cerebrovascular, or peripheral vascular diseases. In diabetic patients with peripheral vascular disease, the small muscular arteries of the lower leg and foot are commonly affected. Thus, a toe may be gangrenous in the presence of normal femoral and popliteal pulses due to the fact that relatively small vessels are narrowed by atheroma.

## 17.2 Special Study Topic

### TYPES OF DIABETES MELLITUS

### Type 1 Diabetes

#### Aetiology and Pathogenesis

In this disease, insulin-secreting B cells are selectively destroyed in the pancreatic islets, but A, D, and PP cells are preserved. The process of B-cell destruction appears to take many years, and the patient presents clinically with diabetes when about 80% of the B cells are lost. Islets in which there is active B-cell destruction are inflamed; this is termed 'insulitis' (Fig. 17.26). The infiltrate in the islets consists of lymphocytes (90%) and macrophages (10%). Among the lymphocytes the relative prevalence of subtypes is: CD8-positive cytotoxic T cells > B lymphocytes > CD4-positive helper T lymphocytes.

#### Autoimmunity

Type 1 diabetes is an organ-specific autoimmune disease in which both humoral (islet cell antibodies) immunity and cell-mediated immunity are directed towards the B cells. At clinical presentation at least 80% of patients have circulating cytoplasmic islet cell antibodies. Some 15% of patients develop other organ-specific autoimmune diseases such as thyroiditis, pernicious anaemia, or autoimmune Addison's disease.

#### Genetic Factors

There is a significant link between type 1 diabetes and the class II major histocompatibility complex (MHC) genes – DP, DQ, and DR in humans. People carrying the DR3 allele have a relative fivefold risk of developing type 1 diabetes. The risk for DR4 is sevenfold, and that for DR3/DR4 heterozygotes is fourteenfold. There is an even stronger association with the DQ gene. However, the concordance rate between identical twins is only 40%, indicating the involvement of non-genetic factors in the pathogenesis of the disease.

#### Environmental Factors

If diabetes is an autoimmune disease occurring in a genetically susceptible population, what are the environmental triggers that might precipitate the development of autoimmunity? At least two theories exist.

First, the process may be initiated by an enteroviral infection. Enteroviruses include Coxsackieviruses and echoviruses. Up to 30% of patients presenting with type 1 diabetes have raised antibody titres in serum (usually to Coxsackie B viruses) and approximately 40% of cases have evidence of enteroviral RNA in their peripheral blood at this time. Other viruses that have been implicated are mumps and rubella viruses but there is less evidence for a role for these two.

Second, the type of infant diet may influence the development of the disease.[1] Epidemiological studies have suggested that exposure to cows' milk antigens before 6 months of age may play a part. It is conceivable that an immune response to a bovine antigen in food may precipitate autoimmunity by cross-reacting with an antigen on the pancreatic B cell, but the evidence is not convincing.

#### The Pancreas in Type 1 Diabetes (Fig. 17.27)

At clinical presentation of diabetes, most of the insulin-secreting B cells that remain express interferon-α, a cytokine that is secreted by cells infected by viruses. Second, the endocrine cells in islets that express interferon-α hyperexpress class I MHC molecules. In vitro, interferon-α causes islet

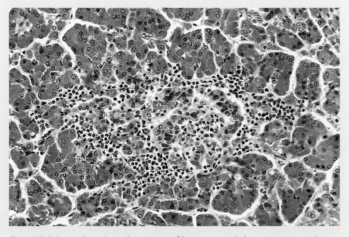

FIG. 17.26 Insulitis: lymphocytes infiltrating and destroying an islet.

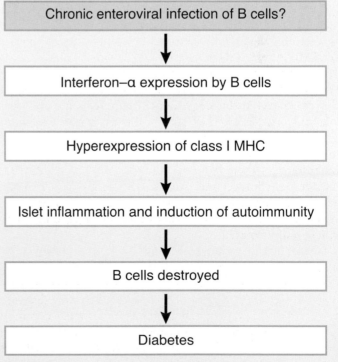

FIG. 17.27 Immune events in the pancreas in type 1 diabetes.

## Special Study Topic continued . . .

endocrine cells to hyperexpress class I MHC; thus it seems likely that secretion of interferon-α by B cells is the initiating abnormality. Enteroviruses consist of an RNA core with a surrounding shell made of capsid proteins. These viruses can cause chronic infection of cells in addition to acute lytic infections. In lytic infections there is much viral capsid protein expressed, but in chronic infection the virus may exist mainly in the form of double-stranded RNA, with little evidence of expressed viral capsid protein. Double-stranded RNA is a potent stimulator of interferon-α secretion.

In most patients with type 1 diabetes occasional B cells express enteroviral capsid protein (Fig. 17.28) and most of the remaining B cells express interferon-α. The B cells expressing the viral protein could represent the 'tip of an iceberg' of a chronic enteroviral infection affecting the majority of insulin-secreting B cells.[2]

In some normal pancreases of people without diabetes, enteroviral capsid protein is seen in B cells but there is no interferon-α expression and no hyperexpression of class I MHC. How the body reacts to chronic enteroviral infection in B cells may determine their fate. Perhaps it requires a particular antiviral response by the innate immune system (interferon-α expression and class I MHC hyperexpression) to provoke an inflammatory cell infiltrate in the islet and the development of autoimmunity. Probably it is the autoimmune response that is ultimately responsible for the destruction of insulin-secreting B cells, leading to type 1 diabetes. If this hypothesis is true, there is the tantalizing possibility that infant immunization against enteroviruses may prevent the disease.

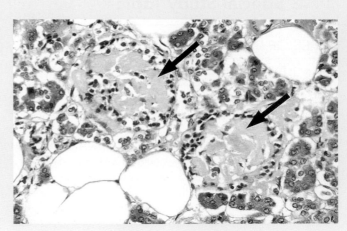

**FIG. 17.29** Amyloid (pink indicated by arrows) largely replacing two islets.

## Type 2 Diabetes

The pancreas at clinical presentation of this disease does not show the same dramatic loss of B cells as that seen in type 1 diabetes. However, in about 70% of cases, amyloid is present within islets (Fig. 17.29). The chemical nature of the amyloid protein has now been determined. It consists of a 37-amino-acid peptide known variously as islet amyloid polypeptide or amylin. This protein is produced by B cells in both normal and diabetic individuals.

Patients with type 2 diabetes, obese people, and 25% of the normal population show resistance to the action of insulin. These people thus have to hypersecrete insulin in order to achieve metabolic homeostasis. Although in many normal people this, possibly genetic, disorder may cause no illness, it is proposed that in a minority there is eventual B-cell exhaustion, with falling insulin secretion and hence the development of type 2 diabetes. Thus, there may be both a qualitative and quantitative insulin insufficiency. The concordance rate for type 2 diabetes among monozygotic twins is 90%, suggesting that the failure of B cells to cope with prolonged insulin resistance may also be genetic. By the time the patient presents with type 2 diabetes, there is a marked reduction in insulin response to a glucose load. The accumulation of amyloid in the islets may reflect longstanding B-cell hyperfunction where the islet amyloid polypeptide has been hypersecreted in parallel with insulin. It is interesting in this regard that amyloid of the same composition is also found in some insulinomas.

## References

1 Ellis TM, Atkinson MA. Early infant diet and insulin-dependent diabetes. *Lancet* 1996;**347**:1464–1465.
2 Richardson SJ, Willcox A, Bone AJ, Foulis AK, Morgan NG. The prevalence of enteroviral capsid protein in pancreatic islets in human type 1 diabetes. *Diabetologia* 2009;**52**;1143–1151.

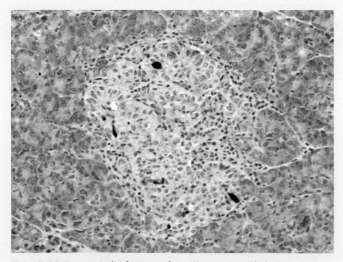

**FIG. 17.28** Enteroviral infection of B cells in type 1 diabetes. The cytoplasm of affected cells stains dark brown on immunohistochemistry, indicating the presence of enteroviral capsid protein.

In diabetic microangiopathy, two types of lesion have been described: first, a thickening of the basement membrane or an accumulation of basement membrane-like material in capillaries; and second, endothelial cell proliferation together with basement membrane thickening. The cause of the microangiopathy is uncertain, but it affects people with diabetes of all types, appears to be related to the duration of the disease, and is aggravated by poor diabetic control. It is responsible for diabetic retinopathy (see Chapter 11, p. 341) and diabetic nephropathy (see Chapter 13, pp. 406–407). Diabetic retinopathy is the most common cause of blindness under age 65 years in developed countries. Renal disease causes 21% of deaths in type 1 diabetes and 11% in type 2 diabetes.

### Infections

There is an increased susceptibility to bacterial and fungal infections in diabetes. Boils, carbuncles, and urinary tract infections – sometimes complicated by pyelonephritis and renal papillary necrosis – are of frequent occurrence, and may precipitate diabetic coma. People with diabetes have an increased risk of tuberculosis, especially of the lungs, and unless treated the disease tends to progress rapidly.

### Other Pathological Effects

Trophic disturbances – such as ulceration of the fingers or toes and neuropathic arthropathy – may develop as complications of diabetic peripheral neuropathy. It is noteworthy that atheroma, diabetic microangiopathy, peripheral neuropathy, and susceptibility to infections all tend to promote gangrene of the extremities in diabetes.

The incidence of diabetic complications in both type 1 diabetes and type 2 diabetes can be reduced by treating hypertension vigorously and ensuring strict control of blood sugar levels.

# THE GONADS

## Testis

The adult testes are paired ovoid organs within the scrotum, weighing 15-20 g each. They comprise mainly the seminiferous tubules, which contain Sertoli cells and germ cells in the various stages of maturation from spermatogonia to spermatozoa. The Sertoli cells secrete growth and inhibitory factors, which play important roles in the maturation of the germ cells and an androgen-binding protein that binds testosterone. Spermatogenesis is mainly under the control of FSH, from the pituitary, and testosterone, secreted by Leydig cells.

### Male Pseudohermaphroditism

Male pseudohermaphroditism is a rare condition in which the karyotype is 46,XY, and the individual has bilateral testes, but has ambiguous or female internal and external genitalia. It is usually due to inherited mutations in one of the genes encoding the enzymes involved in androgen synthesis or in the androgen receptor gene.

### Disorders of Puberty

These comprise two broad groups of precocious puberty and delayed puberty. Precocious puberty may be due to premature activation of the hypothalamic–pituitary–gonadal axis. It may be induced by testosterone secretion from a Leydig cell tumour, or by chorionic gonadotrophin secretion from a tumour. It is also seen in some variants of congenital adrenal hyperplasia (see p. 491) in which the adrenals are secreting large amounts of androgens.

The most common congenital form of delayed puberty is Kallmann's syndrome, which is associated with absent or reduced secretion of GnRH from the hypothalamus, and thus of gonadotrophins from the pituitary. It is usually associated with anosmia or hyposmia. A number of genes have been associated with the syndrome. All play a part in the control of the GnRH-releasing neurons in the hypothalamus and their ability to stimulate FSH and LH production. Hypopituitarism can also result in delayed puberty, but there will probably also be deficiencies in other hormones.

Hypergonadotrophic hypogonadism is usually the result of impaired production of testosterone. It is found in Klinefelter's syndrome (XXY genotype) and the Sertoli cell-only syndrome, in which spermatogenesis does not occur and only Sertoli cells are seen in the tubules.

### Infertility

There are numerous causes of male infertility. Some are related to chromosomal defects, or to primary hypofunction of the hypothalamic–pituitary–gonadal axis. However, secondary changes in the hypothalamic–pituitary–gonadal axis may also be seen in diseases of other endocrine organs, and in chronic diseases of other organs, e.g. kidney and liver. Infertility may also follow on after chemotherapy or exposure to toxic substances.

### Hormonal Aspects of Testicular Tumours

Human chorionic gonadotrophin (hCG) is secreted when choriocarcinoma forms part of a mixed germ cell tumour. Leydig cell tumours can secrete a variety of androgens and other steroids, and in children may result in precocious puberty. Testicular tumours are discussed further in Chapter 16.

## Ovary

The ovaries are paired intra-abdominal organs with complex anatomy, physiology, and biochemistry: their pathology is discussed further in Chapter 14. Their main function is the production and release of the mature oocytes. This requires multiple interactions between the follicles and the stroma, with the production of steroids, peptide hormones, and growth and inhibitory factors.

### Female Pseudohermaphroditism

In the female, this is usually due to the excessive androgen secretion of congenital adrenal hyperplasia (see p. 491); the ovaries are normal (see also Chapter 14, p. 421).

### Infertility

As a result of the complexities of the menstrual cycle, there is a wide range of causes of female infertility, which are discussed in detail in textbooks of gynaecology. Causes include primary ovarian disease and abnormalities of the hypothalamic–pituitary–gonadal axis. In this context, hyperprolactinaemia (see *Box 17.1*) should be considered. As with the male, diseases of other endocrine glands and chronic diseases of other organs may also result in infertility.

### Hormonal Aspects of Ovarian Tumours

It is now recognized that most ovarian tumours have the potential to secrete hormones, although this may not result in the production of clinical symptoms. Sex cord/stromal tumours (see Chapter 14, p. 434) are often associated with hormone production. Excessive oestrogen production from a granulosa cell tumour may result in menstrual disturbances, postmenopausal bleeding, or sexual precocity. Androgen secretion from other variants may result in virilization and hirsutism. In epithelial tumours, hormone production is usually by the stroma, and is most often oestrogens, androgens, and progesterone. Occasional cases of ectopic hormone secretion are found.

### Hormonal Aspects of Non-neoplastic Ovarian Disease

Patients with polycystic ovary syndrome (see Chapter 14, p. 431) present with obesity, oligo- or amenorrhea, hirsutism, and infertility. There is also evidence of excess oestrogen, with endometrial hyperplasia and sometimes even endometrial carcinoma. The ovaries are enlarged and contain multiple cysts. There are multiple abnormalities within the hypothalamic–pituitary–gonadal axis, with raised and fluctuating levels of LH, low levels of FSH, and enhanced sensitivity of gonadotrophs in the pituitary to GnRH.

In older women, stromal hyperplasia may occur and is associated with obesity, hypertension, abnormal glucose tolerance, and virilization.

---

## 17.3 Special Study Topic

### MULTIPLE ENDOCRINE NEOPLASIA SYNDROMES

It has been appreciated for some time that particular combinations of endocrine tumours show familial associations. In these syndromes, tumours occur in more than one endocrine gland in the same individual, and/or in a number of members of the family. These tumours are often preceded by hyperplasia. There are two main types of MEN: types 1 and 2. Both are inherited in an autosomal dominant manner, but the pattern of tumours differs. Familial predisposition to neoplasia is usually associated with the inheritance of a germline mutation in a specific gene. The tumours present at an earlier age than in sporadic cases. Occasionally there is the development of a new mutation in an individual which is then passed on to following generations. Advances in molecular genetic techniques now permit the screening of people at risk once the gene of interest has been identified. This process is easier if a few hotspots for mutation are defined.

### Multiple Endocrine Neoplasia Type 1

This syndrome has a prevalence of between 1 and 10 per 100,000 population. Affected individuals develop hyperplasia or tumours of the parathyroid gland, gastroenteropancreatic (GEP) neuroendocrine tumours, and adenomas of the anterior pituitary gland. In some cases, adrenocortical tumours occur, and tumours of the skin, including lipomas, collagenomas, and angiofibromas. Parathyroid tumours arise in about 95%

of affected individuals, and are usually the first to present clinically, resulting in hypercalcaemia. GEP tumours are seen in about 40%. Benign GEP tumours will often be identified in patients aged <40 years if functional (e.g. insulinoma), whereas malignant tumours in these sites tend to occur later in life. Pituitary tumours usually present at ages >40 years. The age-related penetrance has been calculated as 7% at 10 years of age, 52% at 20, rising to 98% at 40, and 100% at 60.

The gene involved is *MEN1* on chromosome 11q13 encoding a protein comprising 610 amino acids named menin. The gene consists of 10 exons spanning more than 9 kb of genomic DNA. The protein is ubiquitously expressed, and has wide-ranging functions in the regulation of cell proliferation. It is also important in DNA damage-dependent cell cycle arrest or DNA damage repair. More than 450 different mutations have been identified in the coding region in MEN1 families. Most are predicted to give rise to a truncated menin protein, presumably with loss of function. There is no link between particular mutations and the phenotype. In addition, the mutations are scattered throughout the whole of the coding region, with no obvious hotspots. This means that it is difficult to set up a routine genetic screening programme. However, if the particular mutation in a family is known, individuals at risk can be identified by targeting the sequencing to the appropriate part of the gene.

### Multiple Endocrine Neoplasia Type 2

MEN2 has been estimated to have a prevalence of 1 in 35,000 individuals. It is characterized by inherited forms of medullary carcinoma of the thyroid (MTC) and has three subtypes. In

## Special Study Topic continued . . .

type 2a, MTC is accompanied by phaeochromocytoma and parathyroid tumours or hyperplasia, and, in type 2b, by phaeochromocytoma and mucocutaneous neuromas. Some families develop only MTC (familial MTC). The biology of the MTC varies with the subtype. In MEN2b, it develops earlier and pursues a more aggressive course than in MEN2a.

The gene involved is the *RET* (rearranged in transfection) proto-oncogene, localized to chromosome 10q11.2. It consists of 20 exons and encodes a receptor tyrosine kinase. The receptor consists of a large glycosylated extracellular domain containing a number of clustered cysteine residues and calcium-binding motifs, a single hydrophobic transmembrane domain, and a cytoplasmic domain with tyrosine kinase activity. Receptor signalling requires dimerization. The ligands are members of the glial cell-line-derived neurotrophic factor (GDNF) family. In contrast to the *MEN1* gene, a finite number of mutations have been identified and there is a fairly strong genotype/phenotype correlation. This makes familial screening easier. Almost all MEN2a patients have mutations at one of the cysteine residues on the extracellular domain, most at codon 634. This is thought to lead to spontaneous dimerization and activation of the receptor. A cysteine-to-arginine transposition appears to confer a higher risk of developing parathyroid disease. In MEN2b, the mutation is in the intracellular domain, activating tyrosine kinase even in the absence of dimerization. Genetic screening programmes based on analysis of these hotspots are now available. The identification of specific mutations can permit counselling on specific levels of risk for the individual components of the syndrome and a sensible approach to treatment, e.g. prophylactic thyroidectomy is undertaken at an earlier age in individuals with the mutation linked to MEN2b.

### *MENX* and MEN4

Recently, a colony of rats spontaneously developed a syndrome of MENs, comprising those associated with both MEN1 and MEN2. They were found to harbour a germline mutation in the *Cdkn1b* gene, encoding the p27 cell cycle inhibitor. This syndrome has been termed MENX. Screening of patients with clinical features of MEN1, but no evidence of mutations in the *MEN1* gene, has demonstrated mutation in the human homologue, *CDKN1B*, in some cases. Thus, this is a further gene conferring susceptibility to MENs. This is referred to as the MEN4 syndrome.

### Further reading

Pellegata NS, Quintanilla-Martinez L, Siggelkow H, *et al*. Germ-line mutations in p27Kip1 cause a multiple endocrine neoplasia syndrome in rats and humans. *Proceedings of the National Academy of Science of the USA* 2006;**103**:15558–15563.

Raue F, Frank-Raue K. Update multiple endocrine neoplasia type 2. *Familial Cancer* 2010;**9**:449–445.

## SUMMARY

- Most diseases of endocrine glands are uncommon, but they are important to recognize because many can be treated.
- Patients present in one of two ways. They may develop syndromes caused by secretion of too much, or too little, hormone or they may have an increase in size of the gland due to tumour or hyperplasia. This may be noticed by the patient or may cause pressure effects.
- It is very important to integrate the clinical, biochemical, and pathological findings in reaching the final diagnosis.
- Some endocrine tumours occur in a familial setting, including MEN1 and MEN2, in which recognized combinations are found. About 30% of phaeochromocytomas and paragangliomas are familial.
- Autoimmune endocrine disease is most probably caused by interactions between the inherited aspects of an individual's immune system and environmental factors.
- Diabetes mellitus is not a single disease, but is the pathological and metabolic state caused by inadequate insulin action. Type 1 is insulin dependent, whereas type 2 is non-insulin dependent.

## FURTHER READING

Lloyd RV, ed. *Endocrine Pathology: Differential diagnosis and molecular advances*, 2nd edn. New York: Springer-Verlag, 2009.

Melmed S, Polonsky KS, Larsen PR, Kronenberg HM, eds. *Williams Textbook of Endocrinology*. 12th edn. Philadelphia, PA: WB Saunders, 2011.

# 18

# THE SKIN

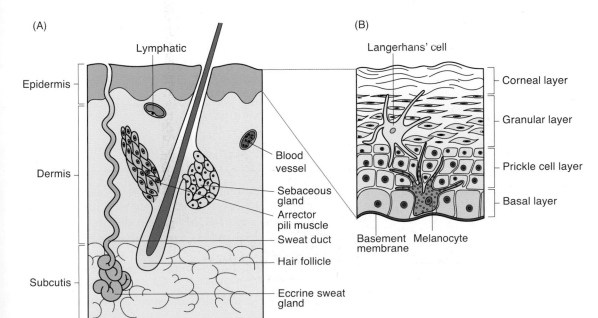

Alan T Evans and Wolter J Mooi

## NORMAL SKIN STRUCTURE AND FUNCTION

The skin is the largest organ of the body, typically weighing 4–5 kg. The epithelial components (epidermis, sweat glands, and pilosebaceous units) originate from the ectodermal layer of the embryo, whereas the mesenchymal tissues of the dermis are derived from mesoderm.

### Normal Functions of Skin

The skin is structurally and functionally complex (*Box 18.1* and *Fig. 18.1*).

---

**Box 18.1** THE FUNCTIONS OF THE SKIN

- Strong mechanical barrier to microorganisms and antigens
- Thermoregulation (dermal vessels and sweat glands) and insulation by fat
- Fluid and electrolyte balance (sweat glands)
- Endocrine function (UV-dependent synthesis of vitamin D)
- Protection from UV radiation (melanin pigment from melanocytes)
- Immune function (epidermal Langerhans' cells)
- Sensory function (touch, temperature, pressure, pain)

---

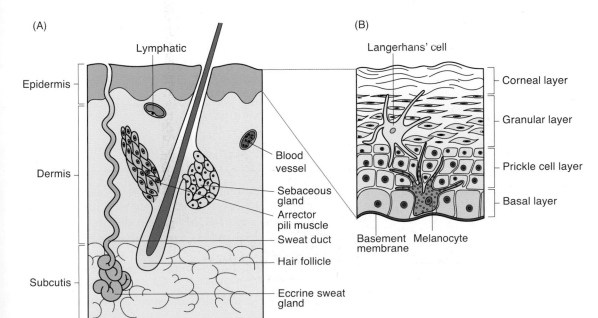

**FIG. 18.1** (A) Diagram depicting the various components of normal skin and (B), in greater detail, the normal epidermis.

## Normal Epidermal Structure

The epidermis is a stratified, keratinizing squamous epithelium with several distinct layers of keratinocytes (Fig. 18.1B). These include, from bottom to top:

- the basal layer of proliferative cells
- the prickle cell layer of polygonal cells with prominent desmosomal attachments
- the granular cell layer of flattened cells rich in keratohyalin granules
- the corneal layer of differentiated keratinocytes shed from the skin surface.

In addition to keratinocytes, the epidermis contains other important cell types:

- Melanocytes are found between the basal layer keratinocytes (Fig. 18.2). They synthesize melanin pigment, which is transferred via branching dendritic processes to adjacent keratinocytes. Melanin is responsible for ultraviolet (UV) protection. Melanocytes are the precursor cells of melanocytic naevi and malignant melanoma.
- Langerhans' cells are dendritic bone marrow-derived cells located in the mid and upper epidermis. They act as sentinels monitoring the epidermal environment for antigens, and are of central importance in initiating a variety of inflammatory dermatoses such as contact dermatitis. They are not identified on routine microscopy, but can be demonstrated immunochemically (Fig. 18.2) and by electron microscopy.
- Merkel cells are neuroendocrine cells responsible for mechanoreception. They are invisible in routinely stained sections, but can be demonstrated immunochemically by staining for cytokeratin 20. They are the precursor cells for an aggressive neuroendocrine carcinoma, which usually arises in sun-damaged skin.

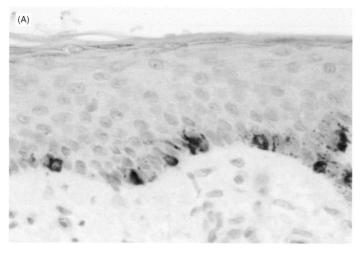

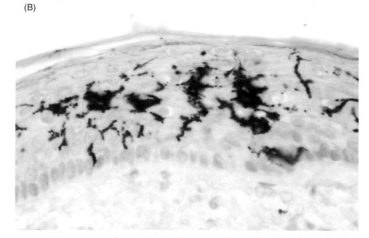

FIG. 18.2 (A) Immunohistochemical staining for S100 protein demonstrates melanocytes distributed among basal epidermal keratinocytes. (B) Highly dendritic Langerhans' cells (shown immunohistochemically by staining for the CD1a antigen) are present throughout the epidermis.

## The Dermis

The connective tissue matrix of the dermis consists largely of type I and III collagen fibres, together with elastic fibres embedded in ground substance composed of hyaluronic acid and chondroitin sulphate. The dermis has two distinct areas. The papillary dermis is a thin, superficial layer of loosely textured fibres rich in small nerves and capillaries orientated at right angles to the skin surface. The underlying reticular dermis is more substantial, with thick bundles of type I collagen lying parallel to the skin surface. The reticular dermis contains the appendage structures (sweat glands and pilosebaceous units). Fibroblasts are the main cell type responsible for synthesizing the various constituents of the dermis and they also produce collagen IV and laminin, which are important components of the basement membrane. More recently it has become apparent that a proportion of dermal spindle cells are, similar to Langerhans' cells, highly dendritic with phagocytic function. These 'dermal dendrocytes' are morphologically similar to epidermal Langerhans' cells and are thought to have a similar role in immune surveillance and antigen presentation.

## DISEASES OF THE SKIN

Skin diseases are common in both general and hospital practice. Over 1,000 skin disorders are described, and new entities continue to be reported. Many skin diseases (especially the inflammatory dermatoses) have confusing names based largely on the macroscopic appearance of the rash; however, recent progress in our understanding of the aetiopathology of the dermatoses will ultimately enable the development of a more rational classification and system of nomenclature.

Many of the rarer inflammatory skin conditions retain confusing nomenclature and it is therefore fortunate that the 10 most common skin diseases account for two-thirds of all dermatology practice!

**TABLE 18.1** A glossary of the terminology used in skin pathology

| Term | Description |
|---|---|
| **Macroscopic term** | |
| Macule | A circumscribed impalpable area of colour change |
| Papule | A small palpable lesion, usually <5 mm diameter |
| Nodule | A larger palpable lesion, usually >5 mm diameter |
| Plaque | A raised flat-topped lesion, usually >5 mm diameter |
| Vesicle | A small fluid-filled blister, usually <5 mm diameter |
| Bulla | A larger fluid-filled blister, usually >5 mm diameter |
| Pustule | A vesicle containing pus |
| Crust | Dried plasma proteins often with inflammatory cells and blood |
| Scale | Dry flaky or powdery surface due to thickened corneal layer |
| Excoriation | Deep (usually self-inflicted) scratch |
| Lichenification | Thickened skin with prominent markings resembling tree bark |
| Purpura | Extravasation of erythrocytes into dermis |
| Alopecia | Loss of hair from normally hirsute area |
| **Microscopic term** | |
| Acanthosis | Epidermal thickening due largely to hyperplasia of the prickle cell layer |
| Hyperkeratosis | Thickened corneal layer |
| Parakeratosis | Retained nuclear staining characteristics in the corneal layer |
| Dyskeratosis | Premature keratinization of epidermal cells |
| Spongiosis | Intraepidermal oedema |
| Acantholysis | Loss of keratinocyte cohesion |
| Lichenoid | Describes inflammation attacking the basal layer |
| Cytoid body | A homogeneous eosinophilic apoptotic keratinocyte |

This chapter concentrates on primary skin disorders, and has three main sections:

- non-infective inflammatory disorders
- infective disorders
- neoplasms.

Conditions may merit discussion because they are commonly encountered, e.g. eczema, psoriasis, and the epidermal tumours. Other rarer conditions, e.g. pemphigus vulgaris and bullous pemphigoid, are included because they illustrate important pathogenic mechanisms.

Some conditions (e.g. lupus erythematosus and necrobiosis lipoidica) may act as useful pointers to underlying systemic disease. A diverse range of skin conditions are induced by drugs.

Dermatopathology employs a number of terms that are specific to the skin, and a glossary of those in common use is provided in *Table 18.1*.

## Non-infective Inflammatory Disorders

For such a large group of diverse diseases it is impossible to provide a comprehensive classification system that is easy to understand and use. Many of the disorders selected for presentation in this section involve the epidermis, which has a limited repertoire of reaction patterns to diverse inflammatory insults. Accordingly, a classification system that utilizes the epidermal reaction pattern provides a straightforward method of categorizing these conditions. Key examples of inflammatory disorders that typify each reaction pattern are provided in *Box 18.2*. These key examples define the essential core content for this area of study.

Some non-infective inflammatory disorders are not centred on the epidermis, but on other skin components including dermal collagen, dermal blood vessels, appendage structures, and subcutaneous fat. These diseases are less important in terms of core knowledge, although a few examples are discussed briefly.

---

**Box 18.2** EPIDERMAL REACTION PATTERNS

- **Spongiotic reaction pattern** (intraepidermal oedema)
  Key example is eczematous dermatitis
- **Psoriasiform reaction pattern** (epidermal hyperplasia with regular rete ridge elongation)
  Key example is psoriasis
- **Lichenoid reaction pattern** (basal layer damage)
  Key examples are lichen planus and lupus erythematosus
- **Vesiculobullous reaction pattern** (intra- or subepidermal blistering)
  Key examples are pemphigus vulgaris and bullous pemphigoid

# The Spongiotic Epidermal Reaction Pattern

## *Eczematous Dermatitis*

### Key Points

Eczematous dermatitis:

- is a reaction pattern and not a specific disease
- may be hereditary (e.g. atopy) or due to environmental causes (e.g. contact dermatitis)
- may have acute and chronic stages
- may be complicated by superimposed bacterial, fungal, or viral infection.

### General

The terms 'eczema' and 'dermatitis' are used interchangeably. Eczema is favoured by dermatologists and dermatitis by pathologists. The generic term 'dermatitis' (i.e. inflammation of the skin) could be applied loosely to any of several hundred inflammatory skin disorders but it should be reserved primarily for describing the pathological changes of eczema.

### Clinical Features

Eczema is not a specific entity, but a common cutaneous reaction pattern occurring in response to diverse insults (Fig. 18.3). The acute stage is characterized by an

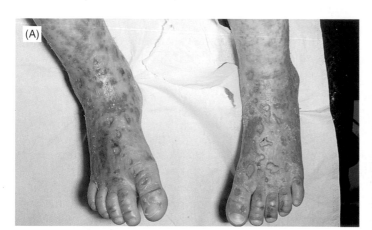

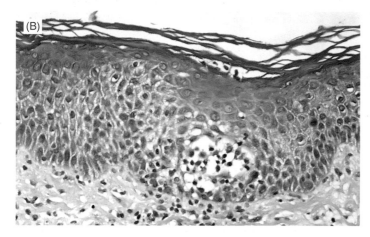

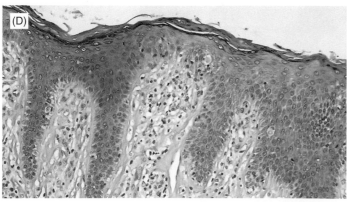

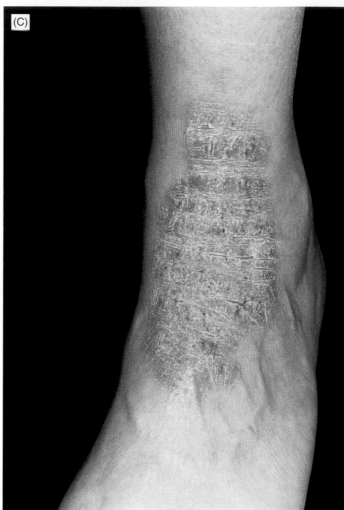

**Fig. 18.3** Acute eczema: (A) note the blisters oozing oedema fluid. (B) The hallmarks of acute eczema are spongiotic intraepidermal oedema (with oedema fluid separating individual keratinocytes) together with intraepidermal aggregates of oedema fluid and lymphocytes known as vesicles. (C) In chronic eczema the skin shows markings resembling tree bark, an appearance termed 'lichenification'. With chronicity the epidermis shows more prominent acanthosis and surface scale. Lymphocytic inflammation is present within the fibrotic dermis; however, by this stage (D) there is less marked epidermal inflammation and spongiosis.

itchy papulovesicular rash with surface oozing and crust. With chronicity, the lesions become thickened with surface scale and accentuated surface markings in the process called lichenification (this is especially likely if there has been repeated rubbing and scratching). The clinical and histological features of eczema can also be complicated by bacterial and viral infection (see Case History 18.1).

### Microscopic Features

Microscopic features of eczematous dermatitis include:

- upper dermal perivascular lymphocytic infiltrate
- spongiosis
- vesiculation
- chronicity leading to acanthosis, surface scale, and dermal fibrosis
- subacute lesions that show a combination of acute and chronic features.

### Clinical Subtypes

Irrespective of the underlying cause, the lesions of eczema show similar pathological features. However, the dermatologist is often able to classify eczema as being either endogenous (due mainly to hereditary factors) or exogenous (due to environmental factors). The most commonly encountered example of endogenous eczema is atopic dermatitis. Filaggrin is a protein that promotes the aggregation of keratin filaments into granules of keratohyalin within the granular cell layer – this process is essential for the skin's barrier function. Mutations in the filaggrin gene are now recognized as the cause of the inherited disorder of keratinization known as ichthyosis vulgaris (a condition characterized by dry scaly skin). More importantly, filaggrin mutations are associated strongly with atopic dermatitis, indicating that defects in barrier function are important in eczema and also in determining susceptibility to other atopic disorders such as asthma. Good examples of exogenous eczema are primary irritant dermatitis and allergic contact dermatitis.

## Atopic Dermatitis

Atopic dermatitis shows the following general characteristics:

- It is a common childhood condition beginning in early infancy.
- There is a strong genetic component reflecting mutations in genes encoding filaggrin.
- There is an excess of IgE formation in response to common allergens.
- There is often a family history of atopy (including hay fever and asthma).
- It usually improves spontaneously in late childhood.
- It may be widespread, but the flexures are often more severely affected.
- Patients are prone to secondary bacterial, fungal, and viral infection.

## Primary Irritant Dermatitis

In primary irritant dermatitis:

- the epidermis is damaged directly
- the condition may be induced by 'physical' stimuli such as direct rubbing or radiation
- the condition may be induced by exposure to chemicals, such as acids, alkalis, detergents, or urine.

## Allergic Contact Dermatitis

Allergic contact dermatitis:

- is a type IV (delayed-type) hypersensitivity reaction (Fig. 18.4)
- requires topical exposure to a sensitizing agent
- common sensitizers are nickel, rubber, plants, and ointments
- antigen is processed (i.e. made more immunogenic) by epidermal Langerhans' cells (Fig. 18.5)
- processed antigen is presented to the T cells
- re-exposure to antigen provokes helper T cells to release inflammatory mediators
- patch testing with common allergens is useful in establishing the diagnosis.

Many other variants of eczema are described. Worthy of note is photoallergic dermatitis, which occurs on sun-exposed sites in response to a topically applied or ingested photosensitizing agent (often a drug). In addition, a diverse range of drugs act as antigens or haptens. Subsequent re-exposure to the drug provokes a dermatitis reaction, which remits only when administration of the drug is discontinued. The presence of eosinophils within an inflammatory dermatosis often reflects a drug-based aetiology.

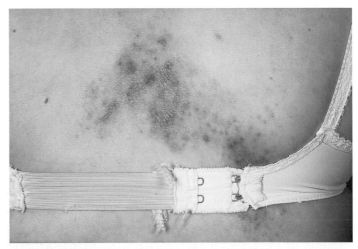

**FIG. 18.4** Contact allergic dermatitis: in this case, the patient is sensitive to nickel in zip fasteners.

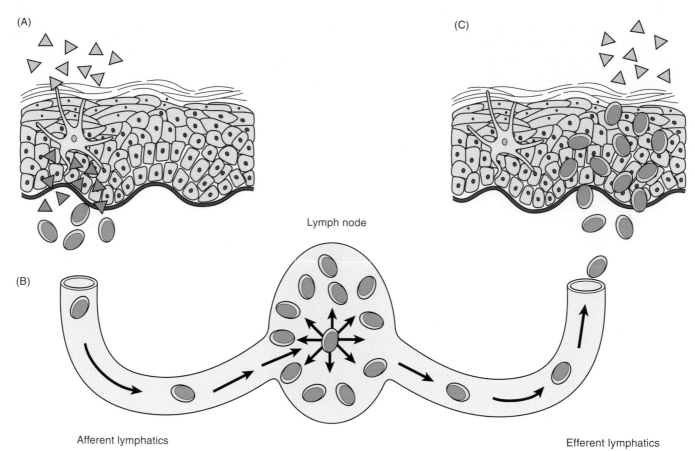

(A)

(C)

Lymph node

(B)

Afferent lymphatics

Efferent lymphatics

FIG. 18.5 Contact allergic dermatitis: the immunopathogenesis of this delayed-type hypersensitivity reaction is presented diagrammatically. Langerhans' cells process antigens (pale blue triangles) applied to the epidermal surface. (A) During processing, proteins are added to the antigen (dark blue triangles) enhancing its immunogenicity before being presented to T lymphocytes (green discs). (B) Sensitized T lymphocytes then migrate to regional lymph nodes, where they undergo clonal expansion. Subsequent exposure to the antigen results in chemical signalling which stimulates the proliferation of specifically sensitized T lymphocytes. (C) Cell adhesion molecules allow these lymphocytes to home into the area of re-exposed epidermis where they elaborate a range of cytokines responsible for eliciting spongiotic dermatitis.

## The Psoriasiform Epidermal Reaction Pattern

### Psoriasis

#### Key Points

Psoriasis:
- is a common dermatosis affecting 1–2% of the population
- has a strong genetic predisposition
- is characterized by increased epidermal turnover
- has a relapsing and remitting course.

#### Clinical Features

Psoriasis is a common inflammatory dermatosis affecting 1–2% of the population. The gender-related incidence is equal. The condition may present as an eruptive guttate eruption in early adulthood, characterized by the appearance of multiple small papules 5–15 mm in diameter, but the condition may develop at any age. The most common type of psoriasis (psoriasis vulgaris) is characterized by well-defined, pinkish-red oval plaques bearing a fine, silver scale. If a few scales are scraped off, then multiple small bleeding points appear on the exposed surface (Auspitz's sign); this reflects the ease of removing the thinned suprapillary epidermal plates to expose ectatic capillaries. Psoriasis follows a chronic relapsing and remitting course. Relapses may be precipitated by a number of factors including common infections, stress, and drugs. Plaque development may also be triggered by local trauma (e.g. in the skin bordering a surgical incision). This effect is known as Koebner's phenomenon, the pathogenic mechanism for which is unclear.

Some patients with chronic psoriasis show nail involvement that varies from minor pitting to extensive destruction (onycholysis) (Fig. 18.6). Approximately 5% of patients develop a seronegative arthropathy (see Chapter 12, pp. 375–376) clinically similar to rheumatoid disease, with involvement of the small joints of the fingers and toes and destruction of the distal interphalangeal joints. In a small proportion of sufferers the arthritis is exceptionally severe, resulting in marked joint deformity and disability.

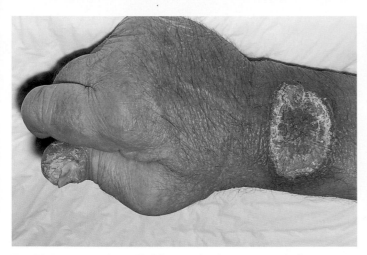

FIG. 18.6 Psoriasis: this well-defined scaly plaque is typical of psoriasis. Note the dystrophic nail changes.

Several other variants of psoriasis have been described, although all show broadly similar histological changes. In generalized pustular psoriasis, fever and systemic upset accompany the appearance of small sterile pustules on an erythematous background. In some cases psoriasis presents with generalized erythroderma which may be difficult to distinguish clinically from cutaneous T-cell lymphoma. These unusual variants of psoriasis may result in metabolic disturbances and leave the patient prone to overwhelming infection.

### Microscopic Features

The microscopic features of psoriasis largely reflect rapid keratinocyte turnover (Fig. 18.7). Typically, the following are seen:

- hyperkeratosis
- parakeratosis
- rete ridge elongation
- suprapapillary plate thinning
- frequent suprabasal mitoses
- dilated dermal capillaries
- Munro's microabscesses (collections of neutrophils) in the stratum corneum.

### Aetiology and Pathogenesis

There is now a considerable amount of detailed information on the aetiology and pathogenesis of psoriasis. A family history of psoriasis is common and linkage analysis studies reveal nine separate loci (*PSORS1–9*) associated with the disease. The susceptibility allele HLA-Cw6 on *PSORS1* has been identified in up to 50% of cases of young patients who present with familial psoriasis with a guttate appearance. Older patients who present with pustular psoriasis typically lack any association with *PSORS1*. These older patients have a higher incidence of HLA-B27 and may have a peripheral arthritis. Factors (such as infections and stress)

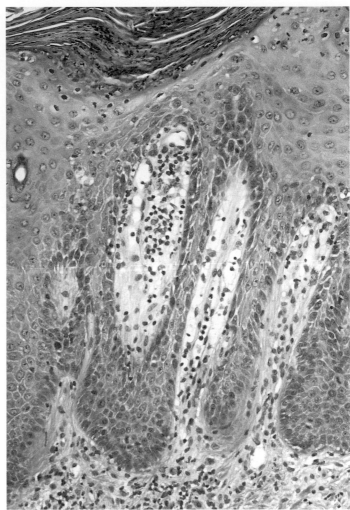

FIG. 18.7 Psoriasis: The epidermis is acanthotic with evidence of clubbing and fusion of rete ridges. Large numbers of neutrophil polymorphs are apparent within parakeratotic surface scale forming Munro's microabscesses.

may trigger psoriasis, supporting a role for environmental factors. In essence, the aetiology of psoriasis appears to be multifactorial.

Established plaques show prominent epidermal hyperplasia due to rapid keratinocyte turnover. In normal skin, the keratinocytes take approximately 50 days to traverse the epidermis before being shed. In psoriatic skin, this journey is completed in only 3–7 days. A unifying theory that explains the complex interplay of enhanced keratinocyte proliferation, changes in the dermal vasculature, and an inflammatory response composed of both lymphocytes and neutrophils is being sought.

There is strong evidence for the role of a T-cell-mediated immune reaction in inducing and maintaining lesions of psoriasis and this is supported by clinical studies that show good responses to anti-lymphocyte therapies, immunomodulators such as ciclosporin, and, more recently, agents that interfere with interleukin 2 (IL-2) receptor binding. In psoriatic lesions skin-specific memory T lymphocytes have been identified and these produce substances such as IL-22 and interferon (IFN)-γ, which are important in regulating epidermal growth and differentiation. The keratinocytes in psoriatic skin are also able to elaborate a range of inflammatory mediators such as IL-1α, IL-1β, and tumour necrosis factor (TNF)-α; these factors play a role in angiogenesis and promote the expression of vascular adhesion molecules, which are important in facilitating the migration of lymphocytes from vessels in the upper dermis into the epidermis. Keratinocytes located within the superficial epidermis also synthesize IL-8, a potent neutrophil chemoattractant, and local elaboration of this cytokine may account for the appearance of corneal microabscesses.

### Other Psoriasiform Dermatoses

Psoriasis is the key example of a dermatosis displaying the psoriasiform epidermal reaction pattern (characterized by regular rete ridge elongation). A number of other skin diseases can show this morphological pattern, e.g. a proportion of patients with Reiter's syndrome develop mucocutaneous lesions, which are difficult to distinguish both clinically and histologically from pustular psoriasis. Psoriasiform epidermal hyperplasia may also be seen in some cases of subacute and chronic eczema (see p. 504), superficial dermatophyte infections (see pp. 522–523), and in association with the cutaneous T-cell lymphoma mycosis fungoides (see p. 533).

## The Lichenoid Epidermal Reaction Pattern

### Lichen Planus

#### Clinical Features

This common skin disease is the prototypic example of an inflammatory dermatosis showing a lichenoid pattern of inflammation centred on the basal epidermis. Lichenoid inflammation is characterized by interface damage with focal basal layer liquefaction and single cell keratinocyte apoptosis, resulting in the formation of cytoid bodies, which at the ultrastructural level comprise an aggregate of keratin filaments. The disease usually presents between the ages of 30 and 60 years, with spontaneous resolution after 1–2 years. The skin lesions are characterized by itchy, scaly, flat-topped violaceous papules (Fig. 18.8), often with fine white surface markings called Wickham's striae. Lesions develop most commonly on the forearms, wrists, hands, and glans penis. The cutaneous lesions often exhibit a symmetrical distribution.

Many patients (up to 70%) have coexisting oral lesions, which may be papular, similar to those on the skin, but may appear as white net-like areas. Some patients with oral lichen planus never develop cutaneous lesions. Oral lesions are often persistent, and chronically ulcerated oral lichen planus is associated with a slightly increased risk of squamous cell carcinoma. Less commonly, there is involvement of other mucous membranes, including the upper respiratory tract, vulval region, and anus. Occasionally,

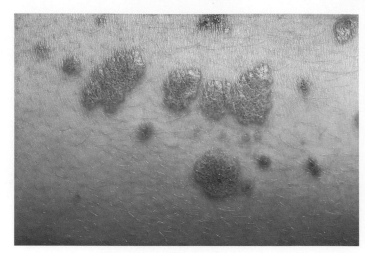

**FIG. 18.8** Lichen planus: itchy, flat-topped, polygonal, and violaceous papules are typical of lichen planus.

lichen planus predominantly involves hair follicle epithelium (lichen planopilaris), leading to destruction of follicular units and alopecia.

#### Microscopic Features

The microscopic features of lichen planus include (Fig. 18.9):

- irregular, 'saw-toothed' acanthosis with hyperkeratosis
- a dense band of lymphocytes and histiocytes at the dermoepidermal junction
- liquefaction degeneration of the basal layer
- the appearance of cytoid bodies in the upper dermis
- melanin pigment incontinence – melanin is released from the damaged basal cells into the dermis.

#### Aetiology and Pathogenesis

The aetiology of lichen planus is unknown; there appears to be a genetic component because affected individuals are

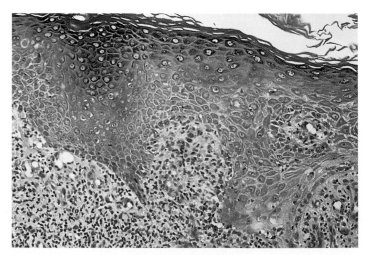

**FIG. 18.9** Lichen planus: the epidermis shows hyperkeratosis, hypergranulosis, and irregular acanthosis. Within the upper dermis there is a dense band-like infiltrate of lymphocytes and histiocytes lying in close association with the basal epidermis.

more likely to be HLA-DR1 and HLA-DQ1 positive. The pathogenesis is almost certainly immune in nature, with most studies suggesting a delayed-type hypersensitivity reaction to an epidermal neoantigen. A well-documented association with viral infections (such as hepatitis B and C, and HIV), and also a range of drugs, suggests that an exogenous antigen may be required to combine with an as yet unidentified self-antigen to initiate the cellular immune response. Increased numbers of epidermal (antigen-presenting) Langerhans' cells, a marked excess of T-helper lymphocytes within the band-like infiltrate, and immunoreactant deposition around the dermoepidermal junction and within cytoid bodies all support an immune mechanism. Activation of CD8+ T lymphocytes with release of cytokines and expression of FasR/FasL within basal keratinocytes suggests that apoptosis is the main mode of cell death in lichen planus.

### Other Lichenoid Dermatoses

Lichen planus is the key example of a dermatosis with a lichenoid pattern of inflammation. Many other conditions show similar features, e.g. some drugs provoke lichenoid eruptions very similar to lichen planus. Other important examples discussed briefly include lupus erythematosus and erythema multiforme. Graft-versus-host disease – a lichenoid dermatosis seen in a well-defined clinical setting – is presented in Special Study Topic 18.1.

### Lupus Erythematosus

> #### Key Points
>
> Lupus erythematosus:
> - is an autoimmune disorder that occurs mainly in young females
> - is associated with antinuclear and anti-DNA antibodies
> - has predominantly cutaneous (discoid lupus erythematosus [DLE]) or multisystem variants (systemic lupus erythematosus [SLE]).

Lupus erythematosus (LE) is an autoimmune disorder of early- to mid-adult life, which occurs mainly in females (gender ratio 2:1). The condition is characterized by the production of autoantibodies directed against 'self'-antigens, most of which are nuclear. Circulating antinuclear antibodies (ANAs) can be detected by immunofluorescence in 90% of patients. In 50% of cases, antibodies to double-stranded DNA are demonstrated (these are associated with renal involvement – see Chapter 13, pp. 404–405 – and their titres reflect disease activity). Some patients elaborate an antibody (anti-Ro/SSA) against a cytoplasmic antigen within epidermal keratinocytes. Anti-Ro/SSA is particularly associated with subacute lupus (see below).

Once the circulating immune complexes localize in the tissues, complement activation is triggered and inflammation results. The mechanism stimulating autoantibody production in LE is unclear. It is proposed that deregulated T-suppressor lymphocytes promote B-lymphocyte over-activity and the overproduction of antibodies against 'self'-antigens. Genetic factors appear important in view of an association with several HLA types, whereas environmental agents (e.g. drugs, viruses, or UV light) may act as the initiating event by provoking cellular DNA damage and antigen exposure. As for many skin diseases, the aetiology is probably multifactorial.

Three major clinical patterns of LE are described, the most common variant being DLE. In most patients the condition is localized and characteristically causes scaly red patches in a 'butterfly distribution' over the nose and cheeks (Fig. 18.10). The condition is often exacerbated by sunlight. Lesions heal slowly with scarring, and scalp involvement results in permanent alopecia. Only 1% of patients with localized DLE progress to SLE but in those patients with generalized DLE (usually with lesions on the trunk and upper limbs) the risk of progression is 5%.

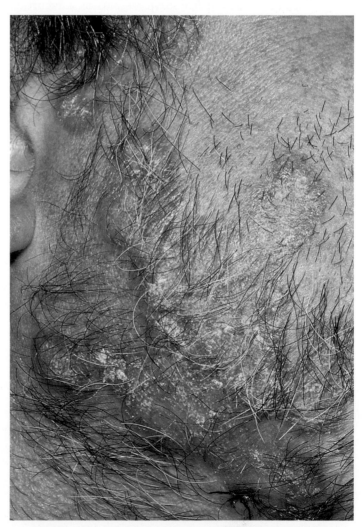

**FIG. 18.10** Chronic discoid lupus erythematosus (CDLE): this is a large plaque of chronic lupus, associated with marked scarring, on the cheek. Sometimes the lesions have a symmetrical 'butterfly' distribution involving the nasal bridge and both cheeks.

### Microscopic Features

The microscopic features of LE include (Fig. 18.11):

- epidermal atrophy and hyperkeratosis
- follicular plugging
- superficial and deep perivascular and periappendiceal lymphocytic infiltrate
- a lichenoid pattern of basal layer liquefaction degeneration
- basement membrane thickening (with chronicity)
- granular basement membrane deposition of IgG, IgM, or C3 on direct immunofluorescence.

SLE is a chronically remitting and relapsing multisystem disorder that may involve the skin, causing DLE-type changes. However, it is the pattern of involvement of other tissues (e.g. kidney, joints, heart, lung, central nervous system, and serosal surfaces) that dominates the clinical picture. With immunosuppressive treatment, the 10-year survival rate now exceeds 90% although renal and/or neurological involvement remains a poor prognostic indicator. Subacute LE (associated with anti-Ro/SSA) presents as a recurring photosensitive rash on the face, trunk, and upper limbs. Visceral involvement is rare.

### Erythema Multiforme

This fairly common self-limiting eruption may present as macules, papules, and blisters. The classic variant begins with erythematous maculopapular lesions, which develop into 'target lesions' with a red margin and a dusky, blistered centre (Fig. 18.12). Most cases resolve within a few weeks. Recurrent episodes are generally associated with underlying herpes simplex infection. Cases with severe oral, conjunctival, and anogenital involvement may prove fatal and this pattern of severe disease is termed Stevens–Johnson syndrome.

A number of factors can precipitate erythema multiforme by provoking a cell-mediated immune response. Triggers include viral infection (e.g. herpes simplex), bacterial infection (particularly *Mycoplasma pneumoniae*), a wide range of drugs, and neoplasms. In 50% of cases a trigger is not identified.

#### Microscopy

Microscopy of erythema multiforme includes (Fig. 18.13):

- a lichenoid pattern of inflammation
- lymphocytes extending into the epidermis
- vacuolar changes at the dermoepidermal junction
- subepidermal blistering
- cytoid bodies above the basal layer
- epidermal necrosis.

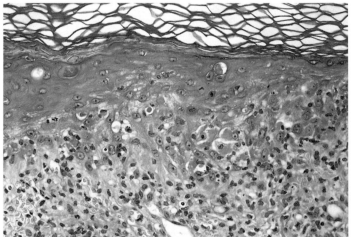

**FIG. 18.12** Erythema multiforme (EM): this is a classic 'target' lesion of EM. Note the central discrete area of blistering.

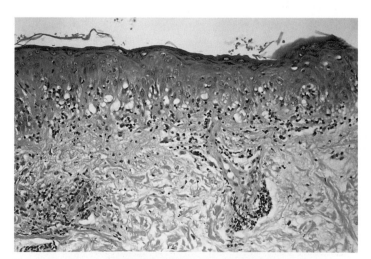

**FIG. 18.11** Chronic discoid lupus erythematosus (CDLE): in this active lesion of lupus the epidermis is atrophic and hyperkeratotic. Numerous lymphocytes are apparent close to the basal epidermis, and this is associated with striking liquefaction degeneration.

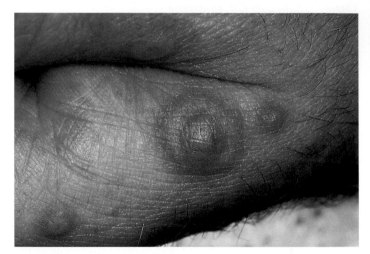

**FIG. 18.13** Erythema multiforme: in EM, the lymphocytic infiltrate tends to obscure the dermoepidermal junction. Lymphocytes infiltrate the epidermis, and scattered eosinophilic cytoid bodies are evident within both the basal and suprabasal layers.

## 18.1 Special Study Topic

### GRAFT-VERSUS-HOST DISEASE

This condition usually develops in an immunocompromised patient given histoincompatible lymphocytes from an immunocompetent donor. Consequently, graft-versus-host disease (GVHD) is usually seen in patients receiving a bone marrow transplant for treatment of marrow aplasia, leukaemia, or one of the primary immunodeficiency states. Acute GVHD ensues in approximately 50% of patients who have received an HLA-matched allogeneic bone marrow transplant. The syndrome is thought to be due to competent donor cytotoxic T lymphocytes attacking recipient epithelial cells that express unmatched minor histocompatibility antigens.

GVHD affects primarily the skin and mucous membranes, gastrointestinal tract, and liver. The cutaneous lesions of acute GVHD are erythematous macules and papules, which may be widespread, but often affect the palms and soles most severely. Microscopy reveals features similar to erythema multiforme, with vacuolar degeneration of the basal epidermis and scattered necrotic eosinophilic keratinocytes involving all the epidermal layers (Fig. 18.14). Typically, one or more lymphocytes can be seen lying in close approximation to a degenerate keratinocyte (this phenomenon is referred to as 'lymphocyte-associated apoptosis' or 'satellite cell necrosis').

Chronic GVHD supervenes in 10% of patients who have received an allogeneic bone marrow transplant. In the chronic phase, cutaneous and oral lesions resembling lichen planus develop. Ultimately, the skin displays marked dermal fibrosis, resembling the sclerodermatous skin changes of progressive systemic sclerosis.

The gastrointestinal tract and liver are commonly involved in GVHD. The oesophagus may become inflamed and, in the chronic phase, fibrosis and stricture formation ensue.

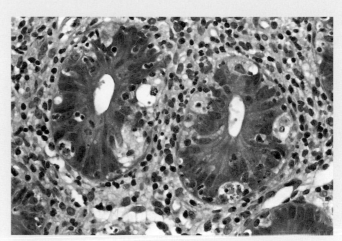

FIG. 18.15 Gastrointestinal tract graft-versus-host disease: in this section from the colon there is nuclear debris around the periphery of the glands. This debris originates from epithelial cells undergoing lymphocyte-associated apoptosis.

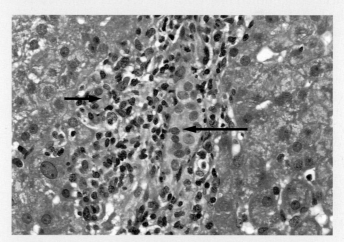

FIG. 18.16 Hepatic graft-versus-host disease: the bile ducts (arrows) in this portal tract are surrounded by lymphocytes. A few lymphocytes infiltrate between the ductal epithelial cells, some of which are undergoing apoptosis.

Colonic involvement manifests primarily as diarrhoea, which reflects lymphocyte-induced apoptosis of the crypt epithelium (Fig. 18.15). The liver exhibits a periportal lymphocytic infiltrate with damage to the epithelial cells lining the bile ducts and to the hepatocytes (Fig. 18.16).

GVHD is associated with a high morbidity and mortality, and patients with this condition are especially prone to overwhelming opportunistic infection.

### Further Reading

Aractingi S, Chosidow O. Cutaneous graft-versus-host disease. *Archives of Dermatology* 1998;**134**:602–612.

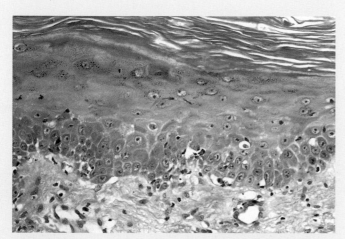

FIG. 18.14 Cutaneous graft-versus-host disease (GVHD): the epidermis shows marked hyperkeratosis, and there is a sparse infiltrate of lymphocytes extending into the epidermis. Note the close relationship between the intrusive lymphocytes and the eosinophilic apoptotic keratinocytes ('satellite cell necrosis').

## The Vesiculobullous Epidermal Reaction Pattern

### General features

> **Key Points**
>
> In bullous disorders:
> - blisters may follow injury due to heat, infections, bites, and drug reactions
> - of the autoimmune type there is immune-mediated attack on cell adhesion molecules
> - the histological features and also the pattern of immunoreactant deposition facilitate diagnosis.

A range of skin conditions are associated with the formation of blisters (more correctly termed 'vesicles' or 'bullae'). Examples include thermal injury, insect bite reactions, drug reactions, and various cutaneous infections by viruses, bacteria, and fungi. Some inflammatory dermatoses (e.g. acute eczema) may cause vesicles and bullae. Similarly, many of the lichenoid disorders (particularly lichen planus and erythema multiforme) may cause blisters reflecting damage to the basal keratinocytes, which anchor the epidermis to the underlying basement membrane and dermis.

The remainder of this section concentrates on primary vesiculobullous disorders, namely pemphigus vulgaris, bullous pemphigoid, and dermatitis herpetiformis. These three acquired conditions share an autoimmune pathogenesis, although the target antigen in each is different. The study of these conditions has furthered our knowledge of the molecules responsible for maintaining the structural integrity of the skin (Fig. 18.17).

Epidermal keratinocytes are held together by adhesion molecules. The intracellular domains of these molecules are linked to the actin and keratin filaments of the cytoskeleton, whereas the extracellular portions are homophilic and bind to other adhesion molecules of the same family or, at the basal layer, to extracellular matrix molecules of the basement membrane.

Of prime importance in maintaining epidermal cell adhesion are the family of calcium-dependent adhesion molecules called the *cadherins*, which are found within desmosomes. One desmosomal cadherin (desmoglein 3) located primarily within the prickle cell layer is the target antigen in pemphigus vulgaris.

The integrin family of cell adhesion molecules also plays a role in keratinocyte–keratinocyte cohesion, but these are mainly of interest because of their location in the hemidesmosomes, which bind basal keratinocytes to basement membrane matrix molecules such as epiligrin, fibronectin, and laminin. Integrins are heterodimers composed of an $\alpha$ and a $\beta$ chain. Although various chains exist, the subtype $\alpha_6/\beta_4$, which is found within the hemidesmosomes of basal cells, is crucial in maintaining epidermal–dermal adhesion because of its affinity for the extracellular matrix ligand laminin. Lying in close association with $\alpha_6/\beta_4$ integrin are the major (230 kDa) and minor (180 kDa) target antigens for bullous pemphigoid. These antigens are distinct from $\alpha_6/\beta_4$ integrin, although it appears to be destroyed by the intensity of the immunologically mediated attack on its neighbours. Disruption of $\alpha_6/\beta_4$ integrin–laminin binding plays a major role in generating the subepidermal bullae seen in pemphigoid.

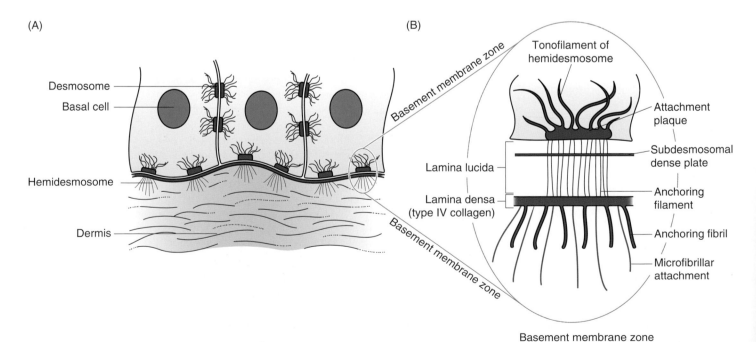

**Fig. 18.17** Diagram illustrating the mechanisms responsible for (A) epidermal–epidermal adhesion and (B) epidermal–dermal adhesion.

## Pemphigus Vulgaris

Four variants of pemphigus are described – all are rare, although pemphigus vulgaris is the most common, accounting for 80% of cases. This disease of middle-aged and elderly people often commences with painful oral blisters and erosions. After weeks or months, fragile bullae develop on the trunk (Fig. 18.18), axillae, groins, scalp, and face. Lesions may also involve the conjunctiva, membranes of the upper aerodigestive tract, lower genitourinary tract, and anus.

The blisters of pemphigus are easily traumatized, leaving shallow erosions that ooze blood and then crust over. New lesions can be induced by gentle friction over apparently normal skin (Nikolsky's sign). Treatment with immunosuppressive agents such as corticosteroids and azathioprine is generally successful. The mortality rate of 5–15% usually reflects overwhelming infection complicating steroid therapy or biochemical derangements seen in very extensive disease.

In pemphigus vulgaris the immune system elaborates IgG autoantibodies against desmoglein 3, which maintains desmosomal attachments in the prickle cell layer. Once antibody–antigen complexes form on the cell surface, the desmosomes are disrupted by components of the complement cascade, and also by proteases liberated from epidermal cells; this results in acantholysis and loss of epithelial integrity. Direct immunofluorescence on fresh biopsy material demonstrates a meshwork of intraepidermal IgG, and most patients have circulating pemphigus antibody, which can be demonstrated by an indirect immunofluorescence technique using monkey oesophagus or human skin as an *in vitro* substrate.

The pathogenic mechanism resulting in the epidermal blistering of pemphigus vulgaris is now established, although the factors that initiate autoantibody production are unclear. Trauma, radiation, burns, chemicals, and drugs may lead to exposure of desmoglein 3 to the immune system. However, an excess of certain HLA types (A10, A26, Bw38, and DR4) suggest that genetic factors are also relevant.

## Microscopy

In pemphigus vulgaris:

- the classic lesion is a suprabasal blister (Fig. 18.19)
- basal keratinocytes remain attached to the basement membrane
- the bulla contains scattered acantholytic keratinocytes (Fig. 18.19)
- inflammation is sparse
- direct immunofluorescence shows deposition of IgG between epidermal keratinocytes (see Fig. 18.21A).

## Bullous Pemphigoid

Bullous pemphigoid is a chronic bullous disorder of elderly people. The condition is more common than pemphigus vulgaris, and has a more benign course. In some patients the disease is localized to the scalp or shins, but in those with more generalized disease blisters develop over the abdomen, groins, and flexor surfaces of the limbs. In contrast to pemphigus, oral involvement occurs in only 10% of cases, and other mucous membranes are affected rarely. The blisters of bullous pemphigoid are larger than those of pemphigus vulgaris and more resistant to trauma (reflecting their subepidermal location), and Nikolsky's sign is negative. Lesions may develop on previously normal skin or on erythematous itchy macules, which precede blistering by weeks or months (so called pre-bullous pemphigoid).

In bullous pemphigoid, IgG autoantibodies are targeted against a major and/or a minor antigen of the hemidesmosomes, which fix basal cells to the basement membrane. These antigens co-localize with $\alpha_6/\beta_4$ integrin–laminin complexes, which suffer collateral damage when immune complexes activate complement, resulting in eosinophil chemotaxis and protease release. The mechanisms triggering the formation of autoantibodies to hemidesmosome antigens are unknown, although the suspected factors are similar to those implicated in causing pemphigus vulgaris (i.e. trauma,

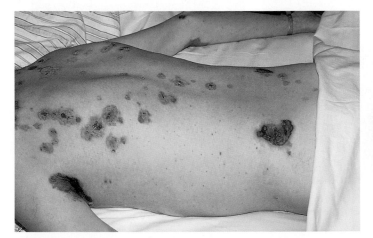

**FIG. 18.18** Pemphigus vulgaris: the fragile blisters of pemphigus vulgaris are often disrupted, leaving shallow erosions.

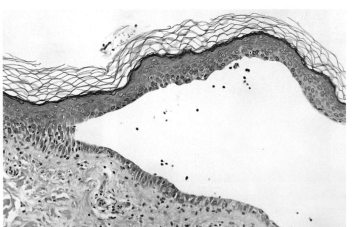

**FIG. 18.19** Pemphigus vulgaris: in this bullous disorder the blister cavity lies above the basal layer, which remains attached to the basement membrane.

burns, radiation, and a range of drugs). The presence of circulating IgG autoantibodies can be demonstrated in 80% of patients, although their titre does not correlate with disease severity or activity.

Microscopy

In bullous pemphigoid:

- the subepidermal bulla contains fibrin and eosinophils
- the blister roof comprises full-thickness epidermis
- there is upper dermal oedema
- there is dermal inflammation with lymphocytes and eosinophils (Fig. 18.20)
- direct immunofluorescence shows linear IgG and/or C3 at the dermoepidermal junction (Fig. 18.21B).

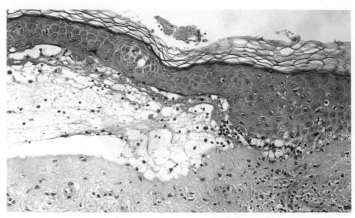

FIG. 18.20 Bullous pemphigoid: in this condition the blister cavity lies beneath the full thickness of the epidermis. Note the large numbers of eosinophil leukocytes within the dermis and bulla.

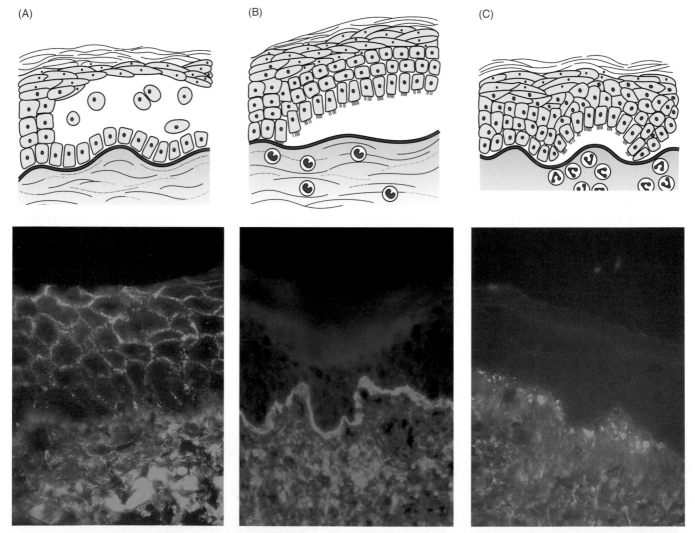

(A)

(B)

(C)

FIG. 18.21 Pemphigus vulgaris: (A) direct immunofluorescence demonstrates a 'chicken-wire' pattern of IgG deposition within the epidermis. The line drawing emphasizes the suprabasal site of bulla formation with preservation of the basal layer. (B) Bullous pemphigoid: direct immunofluorescence demonstrates a linear band of IgG deposition along the basement membrane zone. The line drawing illustrates that the bulla is subepidermal; however, the basement membrane does remain attached to the dermis and forms the floor of the blister – this is not obvious on routine histology. Eosinophils are often the predominant cell type in the inflammatory infiltrate. (C) Dermatitis herpetiformis: direct immunofluorescence shows coarse granules of IgA deposited in the papillary dermis. The line drawing shows a discrete focus of subepidermal blistering associated with an infiltrate of neutrophil polymorphs.

## Dermatitis Herpetiformis

This rare, chronic, blistering disease usually presents in early adulthood. The eruption is characterized by crops of intensely itchy papules and vesicles, which typically develop over the elbows and knees in a symmetrical distribution. Other common sites include the scalp, neck, shoulders, and buttocks. Due to scratching and excoriation, intact vesicles are seen infrequently. Large bullae occur rarely.

Dermatitis herpetiformis is of particular interest because of its strong association with coeliac disease (see Chapter 9, p. 256). Up to 90% of patients with skin lesions have histological evidence of gluten-sensitive enteropathy on small-bowel biopsy, although most are asymptomatic. The pathogenesis of dermatitis herpetiformis is unknown, although direct immunofluorescence studies reveal granular deposits of IgA in the dermal papillae (Fig. 18.21C). It is proposed that IgA antibodies targeted against the gliadin component of gluten also react with connective tissue matrix proteins of the dermal papillae. Once the immune complexes are formed, the complement cascade is activated, generating neutrophil chemotaxins. Neutrophil microabscesses at the tips of the dermal papillae are the microscopic hallmark of dermatitis herpetiformis (see Case History 18.1).

---

### BLISTERING RASH

A 68-year-old male was referred to the dermatology department complaining of intensely pruritic lesions over his elbows (Fig. 18.22). Examination demonstrated excoriated papulovesicles over the extensor aspects of both forearms. Dermatitis herpetiformis (DH) was thought most likely. A fresh (i.e. not formalin-fixed) skin biopsy was submitted for direct immunofluorescence and histopathology investigations.

Blood for antigliadin and antiendomysial antibodies was sent to the immunopathology department. Meanwhile, the patient received a course of dapsone, with rapid relief of pruritis.

Microscopy shows subepidermal blistering with papillary dermal microabscesses typical of DH (Figures 18.23 and 18.24). Granular deposits of IgA within the papillary dermis (similar to those shown in Fig. 18.21C) and positive serology supported this diagnosis.

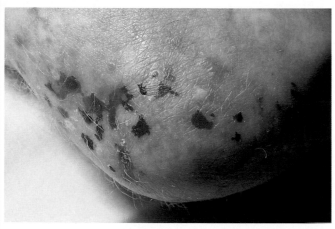

**FIG. 18.22** The typical excoriated papulovesicular rash of dermatitis herpetiformis.

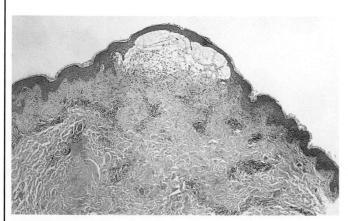

**FIG. 18.23** Scanning magnification demonstrates a discrete focus of subepidermal vesiculation.

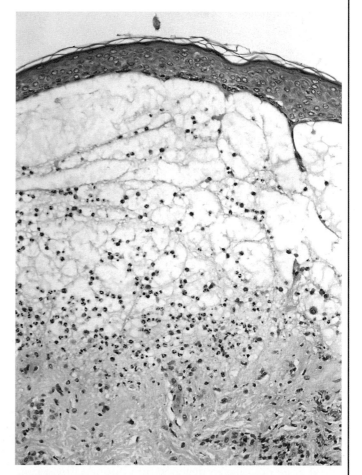

**FIG. 18.24** At higher magnification, large numbers of neutrophil polymorphs are apparent within the blister cavity and within the floor of the blister.

Although the patient was free of gastrointestinal symptoms, an endoscopic biopsy of his distal duodenum revealed subtotal villous atrophy with excessive intraepithelial lymphocytes compatible with gluten-sensitive enteropathy (Fig. 18.25). A gluten-free diet was introduced, and the skin lesions regressed slowly after several months, allowing the dose of dapsone to be reduced.

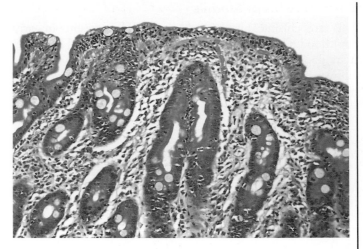

**Fig. 18.25** A biopsy of the distal duodenum demonstrates subtotal villous atrophy together with crypt hyperplasia and a marked increase in intraepithelial lymphocytes. These features are compatible with gluten-sensitive enteropathy.

# INFLAMMATION OF THE DERMIS AND SUBCUTIS

## General

The inflammatory disorders presented so far have centred on the epidermis. However, a range of conditions primarily involve the various components of the dermis or the sub-cutaneous fat. An example of a disease for each component is presented in *Table 18.2*.

**TABLE 18.2** Examples of inflammatory conditions that primarily affect the dermis and subcutis

| Skin component affected | Disorder |
| --- | --- |
| Dermal connective tissue | Granuloma annulare |
| Pilosebaceous units | Acne vulgaris |
| Dermal blood vessels | Leukocytoclastic (allergic) vasculitis |
| Subcutaneous fat | Erythema nodosum |

## Dermal Connective Tissue

### Granuloma Annulare

This common condition of children and young adults generally causes raised annular lesions localized to the dorsal aspects of the fingers and hands. In approximately 15% of patients the lesions are generalized and this pattern is usually seen in older females. Rarely, disseminated granuloma annulare is associated with underlying conditions such as lymphoma or HIV infection. Microscopy demonstrates a central zone of collagen degeneration bounded by a rim of palisading macrophages (Fig. 18.26). A subcutaneous variant (mainly seen on the lower legs of children) may mimic closely a rheumatoid nodule. Necrobiosis lipoidica, although

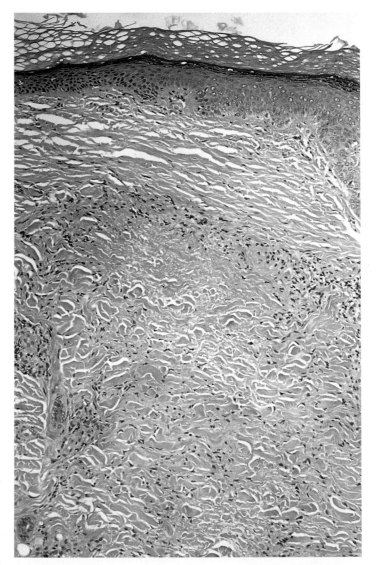

**Fig. 18.26** Granuloma annulare: within the dermis there is a zone of amorphous and eosinophilic collagen degeneration. A rim of histiocytes (tissue macrophages) surrounds the area of collagen degeneration (forming a palisading granuloma).

similar histologically, differs by causing firm reddish-yellow plaques on the lower legs of middle-aged females. Some 60% of patients with necrobiosis lipoidica have, or will develop, diabetes mellitus. The cause of these conditions is unknown although they may reflect an immune complex-mediated vasculitis or delayed-type hypersensitivity reaction.

## Pilosebaceous Units

### Acne Vulgaris

This common inflammatory disorder of the pilosebaceous units of the face and trunk is, to varying degrees, experienced by most adolescents. At puberty, the pilosebaceous units appear particularly sensitive to increased levels of circulating androgens. This stimulatory effect promotes increased keratin production within the pilosebaceous ducts (which become plugged, leading to comedones), whereas enhanced sebum production results in cystic dilatation of the remaining unit. Subsequent colonization of plugged units by *Corynebacterium acnes* may invoke an acute inflammatory response. Rupture of plugged, distended, and infected units releases debris into the dermis, eliciting an intense foreign body granulomatous reaction, which may heal with the formation of scarring.

## Dermal Blood Vessels

### Leukocytoclastic (Allergic) Vasculitis

An acute vasculitis of the small dermal blood vessels is a common cause of purpura. This condition is mediated by immune complex deposition, and common precipitating factors include infections, drugs, and underlying malignancy. Some children with Henoch–Schönlein purpura (a variant of allergic vasculitis) have systemic involvement evidenced by joint pain, gastrointestinal pain and haemorrhage, and glomerulonephritis.

In allergic vasculitis, circulating immune complexes are deposited in the walls of small venules. This leads to complement activation and the production of neutrophil chemotaxins. The neutrophils release lysosomal enzymes, which damage the venules leading to endothelial cell swelling, thrombosis, fibrinoid necrosis, and red cell leakage (purpura) (Fig. 18.27). Many of the neutrophils undergo karyorrhexis. Direct immunofluorescence of early lesions may reveal immunoglobulin and C3 within the walls of damaged vessels.

## Subcutaneous Fat

### Erythema Nodosum

This panniculitis presents as tender red nodules which appear over the lower legs and resolve slowly over a period of several weeks. The condition, which is more common in females, occurs in association with infections (*Streptococcus*

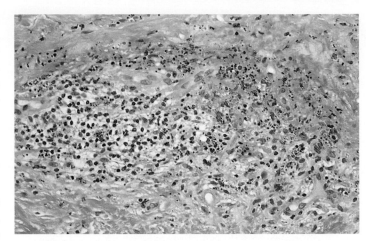

**FIG. 18.27** Leukocytoclastic (allergic) vasculitis: the dermal capillary blood vessels are surrounded by an intense infiltrate of neutrophil polymorphs. Capillary endothelial cells appear swollen and the presence of abundant nuclear debris is in keeping with leukocytoclasis.

and *Yersinia* spp.), chronic inflammatory bowel disease, sarcoidosis, and some drugs. Microscopy reveals chronic inflammation of the subcutaneous tissue, particularly the fibrous septa that divide the fat into lobules. Frequently, there is evidence of venulitis with associated haemorrhage. The aetiology is unclear and, although venulitis may be identified and vascular immunoreactant deposition is occasionally noted, there is no compelling evidence that the condition is primarily the result of an immune complex-mediated vasculitis. A rarer condition is erythema induratum (or nodular vasculitis) which, in some cases, represents an immune response to underlying tuberculosis (a tuberculid reaction). The inflammation in erythema induratum involves both the fat lobules and septal connective tissue; it is often granulomatous and vasculitis is a major feature.

## INFECTIVE DISORDERS

### General Features

A wide spectrum of organisms are capable of infecting the skin. Some cutaneous infecting organisms, such as the superficial dermatophyte that causes athlete's foot, are very common pathogens, whereas others are rare. Precisely what constitutes core knowledge for the reader will largely depend on geographical location. Nevertheless, a combination of inexpensive air travel and holiday packages to remote destinations will continue to ensure that even the most exotic of cutaneous infections will be encountered occasionally. Discussion of infections generally encountered in tropical regions (e.g. protozoa and helminths) is largely beyond the scope of this text, but some of these are discussed in Chapter 19.

Healthy skin is resilient to pathogens unless its integrity is compromised, or the immunocompetence of the host diminished. The types of infection to be discussed include:

- viral infections
- bacterial infections
- fungal infections
- arthropod infestations.

## Viral Infections

### Key Points

- Viral infections may cause a short-lasting rash, which is often vesicular.
- Overwhelming viral infection may occur in immunosuppressed patients, or in those with eczema.
- Some viruses are capable of latent infections, with subsequent reactivation.
- Some viruses cause the formation of tumours, benign or malignant.

### *Herpesvirus Infections*

#### General features

The herpesvirus family comprises several biologically and serologically distinct members. Understanding of this group continues to evolve, with human herpesvirus 8 (HHV8) recently being identified as the causative agent of Kaposi's sarcoma (see Chapter 19, p. 546 ). Three members of this family are associated commonly with skin disease (*Table 18.3*).

#### Herpes Simplex Virus Type 1

Herpes simplex virus type 1 (HSV-1) is associated with a mild or asymptomatic primary oropharyngeal infection

**TABLE 18.3** The spectrum of skin conditions associated with the herpesvirus family

| Herpes virus type | Main clinical association |
| --- | --- |
| Herpes simplex (type 1) | Recurrent herpes labialis (cold sores) |
| Herpes simplex (type 2) | Recurrent genital herpes |
| Varicella-zoster virus | Primary infection is varicella (chickenpox) Reactivation of latent virus causes zoster (shingles) |

in childhood. At the time of primary infection, the virus passes along sensory nerves to infect and lie dormant within the neuronal cells of sensory ganglia. Latent HSV-1 infection is very common, with 80% of the population harbouring the virus within the trigeminal ganglion. Latent virus can be reactivated by several factors such as febrile illnesses, sunburn, menstruation, trauma, and stress. Once reactivated, the virus passes down the sensory nerves, producing tingling and discomfort and followed soon after by a crop of painful vesicles, which resolve in about 1 week without scarring. Typically, the vesicles develop around the lips (herpes labialis) and are known commonly as 'cold sores'. Severe disseminated infection may occur in immunocompromised patients. Widespread primary infection of the skin (eczema herpeticum) is seen occasionally in patients with atopic eczema. This is a severe condition with fever and constitutional upset, which may prove fatal. Eczema herpeticum and the histological features of HSV-1 infection are discussed in more detail in Case History 18.2.

#### Herpes Simplex Virus Type 2

HSV-2 preferentially causes genital lesions, and is transmitted primarily by sexual contact. HSV-2 also lies dormant within sensory ganglia, leaving the host prone to developing intermittent crops of painful vesicles. The factors that trigger reactivation are broadly similar to those for HSV-1. Neonatal HSV-2 infection occurs in 10% of children delivered to women with active herpetic lesions. This severe and potentially fatal infection can be avoided by caesarean section.

#### Varicella-zoster Virus

Varicella-zoster virus (VZV; herpesvirus type 3) causes the very common acute vesicular eruption known as varicella (chickenpox). This highly infectious childhood condition is characterized by crops of vesicles and pustules at varying stages of crusting and healing. When acquired in adulthood, the disease is often more severe, although widespread dissemination with potentially fatal encephalitis or pneumonitis is usually restricted to immunocompromised hosts.

VZV also has the ability to lie dormant within sensory ganglia. Reactivation causes herpes zoster ('shingles'), a fairly common condition seen in adults. Reactivation becomes more likely with increasing age, perhaps reflecting a reduced pool of memory T cells specific for the virus. Patients with immunodeficiency are especially prone to developing herpes zoster, which rarely may disseminate (with potentially fatal results).

## VIRAL SKIN INFECTION

A 19-year-old female, with a long history of flexural atopic eczema requiring topical steroids, was referred urgently to the dermatology department with an extensive eruption over the right foot and ankle (Fig. 18.28), in association with fever and lethargy. Examination confirmed ulcerating papulovesicular lesions and tender groin lymphadenopathy. Eczema herpeticum was suspected, and a diagnostic biopsy was submitted for confirmation. The patient was commenced on the oral antiviral drug, aciclovir.

The biopsy demonstrated vesiculation and an intense lymphocytic infiltrate (Fig. 18.29). Many keratinocytes exhibited classic changes of herpesvirus infection with multinucleation and nuclear pallor (Fig. 18.30). After a few days, a secondary bacterial infection developed, and *Staphylococcus aureus* was cultured from a swab. Treatment with oral flucloxacillin was instituted, and the lesions healed completely after 3 weeks.

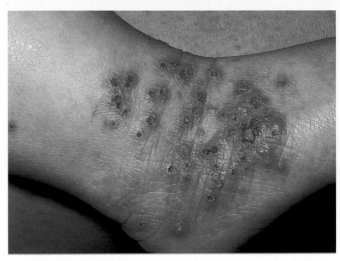

**FIG. 18.28** Numerous ulcerated vesicles are evident over the ankle.

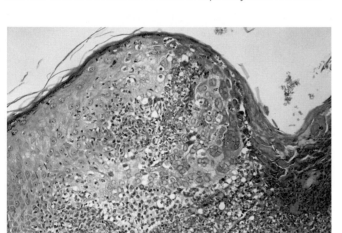

**FIG. 18.29** Scanning magnification shows intense inflammation involving the dermis and epidermis. Loss of nuclear staining and multinucleation can be appreciated even at this power.

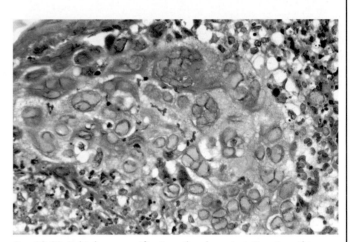

**FIG. 18.30** At higher magnification, the characteristic cytopathic effects of herpesvirus infection are clearly demonstrated. Margination of nuclear chromatin results in the nuclei appearing 'empty', and many of the keratinocytes are multinucleated.

The onset of herpes zoster is heralded by pain and discomfort in the affected dermatome. After a short period the skin becomes erythematous, and crops of vesicles appear. The vesicles often become pustular, crust over, and heal after approximately 14 days. These lesions are mildly infectious, and non-immune individuals (usually children) may contract varicella after exposure to an adult with herpes zoster. Herpes zoster mainly causes lesions on the trunk and abdomen, although cranial involvement is not uncommon. Involvement of the ophthalmic branch of the trigeminal nerve results in ocular complications (including blindness) in 30% of cases. Herpes zoster may be associated with severe persistent pain.

The histopathological changes seen in VZV infection are very similar to those of HSV-1 and HSV-2.

### Human Papillomavirus Infections

#### General Features

The human papillomavirus (HPV) family of DNA-containing viruses incorporates almost 150 types responsible for various warty lesions. Transmission of HPV occurs by direct inoculation of infected desquamated cells onto host skin. HPV replication occurs in the superficial prickle and granular cell layers where infected cells remain shielded from the blood supply (and immune system), allowing lesions to persist for months or years. Eventually, warts tend to regress spontaneously – an event that is associated with lymphocytic infiltration reflecting a cell-mediated immune response. Patients with diminished cellular immunity are especially prone to HPV infection, the resulting lesions being persistent and refractory to treatment.

**TABLE 18.4** The clinical distribution of skin warts typically associated with specific subtypes of the human papillomavirus (HPV) family

| HPV type | Main clinical association |
|---|---|
| HPV-1 | Plantar warts |
| HPV-2 (less often 1, 4, and 7) | Common warts |
| HPV-3 (less often 10) | Plane warts |
| HPV-6 (less often 11) | Anogenital warts |
| HPV-16 (less often 18) | Anogenital warts at risk of neoplastic transformation |

Specific HPV subtypes are associated with different verrucous lesions (*Table 18.4*).

### Common Warts

The common wart (verruca vulgaris) is seen most frequently on the dorsal aspects of the hands and fingers, and on the face. Warts appear as keratotic papules that are 1–10 mm in diameter, and spontaneous involution ensues within months or a few years. Malignant transformation is very rare, except in the verrucae developing in immunosuppressed renal transplant recipients.

*Microscopy*

Microscopy of common warts (Fig. 18.31) typically shows:

- hyperkeratosis and parakeratosis
- irregular epidermal acanthosis and papillomatosis
- superficial vacuolated koilocytes (HPV-infected keratinocytes)
- clumping of keratohyalin granules
- lymphocytic infiltration (if regressing).

### Plantar Warts

This common type of wart occurs on the sole of the foot. Infection is seen in young individuals, and it is probably acquired in communal changing rooms and swimming pools. The lesions resemble common warts, except that they have an endophytic growth pattern and lie largely beneath the markedly hyperkeratotic skin surface.

### Plane Warts

These fleshy, flat-topped warts develop in the same areas as common warts, but show less marked filiform acanthosis. Plane warts have a tendency to occur at sites of trauma (Koebner's phenomenon), and crops of lesions may develop in areas of scratching.

### Anogenital Warts

HPV infection of the anogenital skin is seen primarily in young, sexually active adults. Lesions vary in size from small

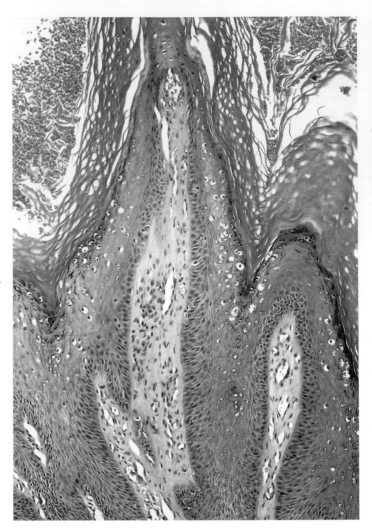

**FIG. 18.31** Viral wart: the epidermis is thrown into folds (papillomatosis), and there is marked hyperkeratosis. Within the superficial layers of the epidermis many of the keratinocytes display nuclear pyknosis and perinuclear haloes. These koilocytes indicate the presence of papillomavirus infection.

inconspicuous papules up to large fleshy condylomata. Malignant transformation is unusual with HPV-6 and -11, whereas HPV-16 and -18 are associated with a significant risk of progression (via dysplasia) to invasive squamous cell carcinoma. Perineal HPV infection is the principal cause of carcinoma of the anal region and vulva. Females with perineal condylomata should have regular smears because they frequently have concurrent HPV infection and dysplasia of the vulva and cervix (see Chapter 14, Special Study Topic 14.1, pp. 439–441).

### Poxvirus Infections

#### General Features

The most famous member of this family is variola (smallpox) which, following its eradication, is of historic interest only. The poxvirus infection seen most commonly is molluscum contagiosum. Much less common is orf, an endemic poxvirus infection of sheep, which occasionally causes large necrotic skin lesions on the hands and forearms of sheep-handlers.

### Molluscum Contagiosum

This common poxvirus infection is associated with dome-shaped, umbilicated papules on the face and limbs of young children. In adulthood, genital lesions occur, reflecting sexual transmission. The lesions typically regress spontaneously within a few months. Extensive crops of persistent lesions may occur in patients with impaired cellular immunity.

#### Microscopy

Microscopy of molluscum contagiosum (Fig. 18.32) includes:

- endophytic hyperplasia of the epidermis
- a central crater
- large eosinophilic viral inclusion bodies
- inclusions (molluscum bodies) that replace the entire cell and are shed onto the surface.

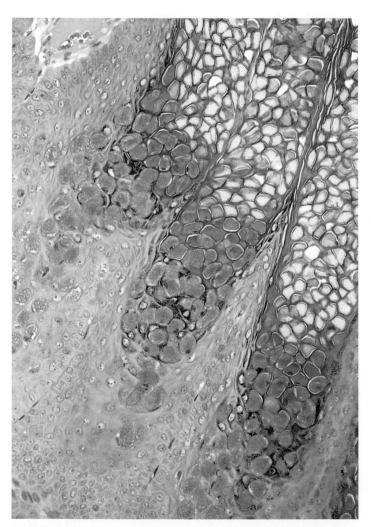

**FIG. 18.32** Molluscum contagiosum: large eosinophilic intracytoplasmic viral inclusions are present within the superficial layers of the epidermis.

## Bacterial Infections

### Key Points

- Bacterial infections are usually due to non-resident flora.
- Pyogenic organisms cause localized abscesses or rapidly spreading cellulitis.
- Mycobacteria cause a wide range of infections, e.g. leprosy.

#### General features

The large numbers of commensal bacteria that colonize the skin surface only occasionally assume pathogenic importance. Of greater importance are bacteria that do not form part of the resident flora and are generally acquired by person-to-person contact. A simple method of classifying the more commonly encountered bacterial infections is presented in *Table 18.5*.

#### Staphylococcal Infections

##### Impetigo

This acute superficial pyogenic infection of the upper epidermal layers, seen most commonly in young children, presents as a pustular eruption on the face or extremities with crusted golden exudate. Impetigo is generally caused by *Staphylococcus aureus*, although group A β-haemolytic streptococci are sometimes isolated.

**TABLE 18.5** Examples of skin conditions associated with various types of bacterial infection

| Bacterium | Main clinical associations |
| --- | --- |
| **Coccobacilli** | |
| *Staphylococcus aureus* | Impetigo |
| | Staphylococcal scalded skin syndrome |
| | Furuncles and carbuncles |
| β-Haemolytic streptococci | Erysipelas |
| | Cellulitis |
| | Necrotizing fasciitis |
| **Mycobacteria** | |
| *Mycobacterium leprae* | Leprosy |
| *Mycobacterium tuberculosis* | Various lesions |
| *Mycobacterium marinum* | Swimming pool granuloma |
| **Spirochaetes** | |
| *Treponema pallidum* | Syphilis |
| *Borrelia burgdorferi* | Erythema chronicum migrans |

### Staphylococcal Scalded Skin Syndrome

This rare condition of infants and young children is caused by a specific *Staphylococcus aureus* (group 2, phage type 71). This organism elaborates an epidermolytic toxin causing widespread erythema and desquamation. After several days, antibodies neutralize the toxin and facilitate healing. In some individuals (particularly adults), potentially fatal staphylococcal septicaemia ensues.

### Furuncles and Carbuncles

These common lesions reflect staphylococcal infection of hair follicles. A furuncle (boil) involves a solitary follicular unit, whereas a carbuncle involves several adjacent follicles. Purulent exudate may discharge through the follicular ostium, although in some cases surgical drainage is required. Furuncles and carbuncles are more common in people with diabetes.

## β-Haemolytic Streptococcal Infections

### Erysipelas and Cellulitis

Erysipelas is a sharply demarcated and rapidly spreading infection of the superficial dermis. The preferential sites are the legs and, less often, the face. Cellulitis is a less well-demarcated and more deeply sited infection of the dermis and subcutaneous fat.

### Necrotizing Fasciitis

This rare and exceptionally severe form of cellulitis is associated with necrosis of the skin, subcutis, fascial connective tissue, and underlying skeletal muscle. The leg and perineum are the usual sites of occurrence and scrotal involvement may occur (Fournier's gangrene). The causal β-haemolytic streptococcus often acts in association with anaerobic bacteria, leading to gas formation in the deep tissues. This rapidly progressive and often fatal infection necessitates early and vigorous surgical treatment.

## Mycobacterial Infections

Mycobacterial infection is associated with chronic granulomatous inflammation within the dermis. Leprosy affects 15 million people in tropical countries. Cutaneous infection with *M. tuberculosis* is now very rare in developed countries. Skin infection with atypical mycobacteria is, in many non-tropical countries, the most common type of mycobacterial infection. A good example is *M. marinum*, which is found in swimming pools and aquaria, and causes persistent warty nodular lesions on the extremities. Infection remains localized to the cooler peripheral skin, reflecting the organism's inability to multiply at body temperature. Mycobacterial infections are discussed further in Chapter 19 (pp. 549–556))

## Spirochaetal Infections

Syphilis is sexually transmitted, with the primary ulcerated chancre developing at the point of inoculation (usually the anogenital region). Erythema chronicum migrans describes a sharply defined spreading lesion caused by infection with the spirochaete, *Borrelia burgdorferi*. This organism is transmitted by a tick bite and, when left untreated, the infection may spread to joints, the nervous system, and the heart (Lyme disease). More recently, it has been proposed that borrelial infection may be associated with some low-grade cutaneous lymphomas in a manner similar to the relationship between infection with *Helicobacter pylori* and primary gastric lymphoma (see Special Study Topic 9.1, pp. 253–254).

# Fungal Infections

## General features

> **Key Points**
>
> - Superficial fungal infections involving epidermis, hair, and nail infections are common.
> - Deep mycoses affect the dermis and subcutaneous fat, and are uncommon in temperate climates.

A wide range of fungi can cause skin infection. The most simple method of classification is into two groups. The first group includes fungi that infect the superficial layers of the skin together with the hair and nails (*Table 18.6*). The second group comprises the deep mycoses that infect the dermis and subcutaneous fat (these are uncommon in temperate climates, and are not discussed further).

The diagnosis of superficial fungal infection may be possible on clinical grounds, although skin scrapings and, in some cases, a biopsy are required. Deeply sited fungal infection is usually diagnosed on biopsy material. Fungi stain magenta pink with periodic acid–Schiff (PAS) (Fig. 18.33), and this facilitates their detection in tissue sections.

**TABLE 18.6** Examples of common superficial fungal skin infections

| Fungus (dermatophytes) | Main clinical associations |
| --- | --- |
| *Epidermophyton* spp. | Tinea pedis and cruris |
| *Microsporum* spp. | Tinea capitis |
| *Trichophyton* spp. | Tinea pedis, cruris, corporis, or capitis; nail infection |

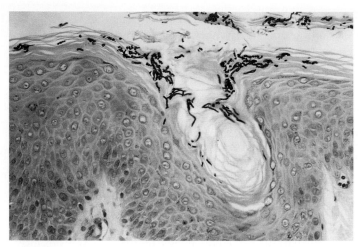

**FIG. 18.33** Superficial dermatophyte infection: large numbers of fungal hyphae are present within the stratum corneum. (Stain: periodic acid–Schiff.)

## Tinea

The various types of dermatophyte infection are classified according to the site involved:

- Tinea capitis is the term given to dermatophyte infection (usually *Trichophyton tonsurans* or *Microsporum canis*) of the scalp, which causes slight scaliness and mild hair loss. A minority of cases develop marked suppurative folliculitis (kerion).
- Tinea corporis reflects infection of non-hirsute skin, tinea cruris affects the groin region, and tinea pedis (or athlete's foot) – the most common dermatophytosis – causes itchy, macerated fissures in the interdigital spaces. These three variants are usually caused by infection with *Trichophyton rubrum*, *Trichophyton mentagrophytes*, or *Epidermophyton floccosum*.
- Fungal infection of the nail (onychomycosis) results in a thickened brittle nail showing yellow–brown discoloration. Onychomycosis is generally due to infection with *T. rubrum* or *T. mentagrophytes*, although *Candida albicans* may infect the fingernails (often after an episode of candidal paronychia).

## Candidiasis

*Candida albicans* – a normal commensal of the oropharynx, gut and vagina – does not usually colonize normal skin. The most common cutaneous infection with *C. albicans* occurs in the intertriginous folds, and is especially likely in obese individuals or in hot humid climates. Chronic mucocutaneous candidiasis, which affects the mucous membranes, skin, and nails, is generally seen in children with defective cell-mediated immunity. In adults, the syndrome is rarer and may point to the presence of an underlying tumour (especially thymoma). Disseminated candidiasis involves multiple organs, with skin lesions being seen in a minority of cases. It is a disease that is associated particularly with immunosuppression, intravenous drug abuse, and broad-spectrum antibiotic treatment.

### Pityriasis Versicolor

This describes a common superficial infection with the unicellular commensal yeast *Malassezia furfur*. Pathogenicity is acquired only when budding occurs in warm humid conditions. Lesions appear as small scaly hypo- or hyperpigmented macules over the torso and upper arms.

## Arthropod Infestations

### General Features

An enormous array of arthropods are capable of causing human disease. Many members are venomous (e.g. spiders, scorpions, wasps, and bees), others act as vectors for microbes (e.g. tick-borne borellial infection), and some (e.g. the scabies mite and various types of lice) infest the skin.

### Scabies

This contagious condition is due to infestation with the mite *Sarcoptes scabiei*, with transmission being facilitated by close physical contact. After mating, gravid female mites tunnel into the corneal layer leaving burrows containing faeces and eggs (Fig. 18.34). Infestation results in an itchy papulovesicular rash involving the interdigital skin, palms, wrists, inframammary folds, and genitals. The itch associated with infestation reflects an allergic reaction to the mite. The complex relationship that exists between the mite and host immune system is emphasized by cases of extensive infestation with crusting and secondary bacterial infection (Norwegian scabies) seen in immunosuppressed and debilitated patients.

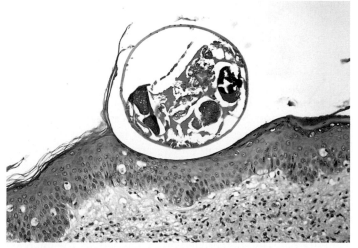

**FIG. 18.34** Scabies: a scabies mite (*Sarcoptes scabiei*) is apparent within the stratum corneum.

### Pediculosis

Lice are blood-sucking insects, the saliva of which elicits an intensely itchy allergic reaction. Three species of louse cause different patterns of infestation:

- *Pediculus humanus capitis* infests the scalp, with outbreaks occurring commonly in schools. The lice and hair shafts bearing attached eggs (nits) are readily identifiable.
- *Phthirus pubis* infests any areas of coarse hair including pubic, axillary, and trunk hair. Transmission is generally by sexual contact.
- *Pediculus humanis corporis* (the body louse) is rarer, except in circumstances of gross overcrowding and poor hygiene (e.g. in times of war). The faeces from this species are an important vector of diseases, such as the rickettsial infection causing typhus. This louse is larger than the other species, and it differs by laying its eggs in the seams of clothing rather than cementing them to hair shafts.

# NEOPLASTIC DISEASES

### Key Points

- Most skin tumours are benign.
- Tumours can arise from epidermal epithelium, adnexae, melanocytes, neuroendocrine cells, and dermal constituents.
- UV light is the main aetiological factor in most skin cancers.
- Awareness and early detection of skin cancers lead to better cure rates.

Of all the tissues of the body, the skin is most directly exposed to the outside world and its plethora of tissue-damaging and mutagenic influences. Not surprisingly, neoplasms of the skin are common and, as a reflection of the complex histology of the skin, constitute an extremely varied group.

Fortunately, the large majority of skin tumours are benign, and the most common malignant ones (basal cell carcinoma and squamous cell carcinoma) are generally cured by simple surgical excision. Some malignant skin cancers, however, are potentially life threatening: the most important of these is melanoma. The much rarer angiosarcoma, Merkel's cell carcinoma, and some primary cutaneous malignant lymphomas are also high-risk malignancies.

As the skin is more easily inspected than practically any other tissue of the body, most cutaneous tumours can be identified when they are small. Indeed, awareness of the benefits of early cancer detection has led to the increasingly early surgical removal of skin cancers, which is reflected in steadily improving cure rates. As small malignant skin tumours may be quite difficult to distinguish from benign ones, it requires considerable clinical experience and

diagnostic acumen to select those lesions that require excision and histological evaluation from the much larger number of lesions that are clinically inconsequential.

## Benign Epidermal Tumours

Benign epidermal tumours constitute a varied group of lesions. Some are entirely benign and banal, but others have a certain premalignant potential; some are easy to recognize for what they are, but others may mimic malignancy. Indeed, as a group, these tumours constitute a major challenge to the student (who needs to become acquainted with the main types), the clinician (who must diagnose them or decide on the need for histological diagnosis and treatment), and the pathologist (who needs to provide the definitive diagnosis). Here, we limit the discussion to the two most important types.

### Seborrhoeic Keratosis

The typical characteristics of seborrhoeic keratosis are that:

- it is a common, benign epidermal tumour
- it protrudes above skin surface
- it is usually pigmented
- it occurs most commonly in middle-aged and elderly individuals
- the sudden emergence of large numbers of lesions may indicate visceral cancer (the Leser–Trélat sign).

This benign tumour of the epidermis occurs most commonly on the trunk of middle-aged or elderly individuals, and usually presents as a pigmented, sharply circumscribed growth with a coarsely granular surface (Fig. 18.35). It often protrudes above the skin surface in its entirety, so that it appears to have been 'stuck on' the skin. The sudden emergence of large numbers of seborrhoeic keratoses may be caused by internal malignant neoplasms, most commonly

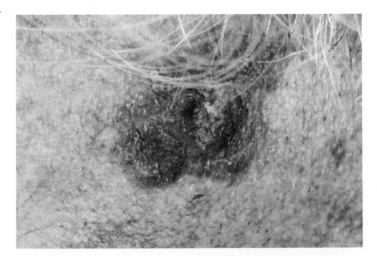

FIG. 18.35 Seborrhoeic keratosis: this slightly raised and brownish benign skin tumour is common in late adult life. This particular example is only slightly raised and brownish; others are dark, broad-based papillomas.

gastrointestinal cancers. This so-called Leser–Trélat sign should incite a search for a possible visceral malignancy. Recent evidence suggests that secretion of growth factors and cytokines by the visceral cancer cells triggers the emergence of these multiple seborrhoeic keratoses.

Histologically, a seborrhoeic keratosis consists of a proliferation of epidermal-type squamous epithelium with some degree of maturation impairment, so that the number of basal-type epidermal keratinocytes is disproportionately increased. Accordingly, the term 'basal cell papilloma' is commonly used as a synonym. In its most common form, the epithelial proliferation assumes an exophytic growth pattern with keratin-filled 'horn cysts' (Fig. 18.36). Clinically, these lesions are usually inconsequential, because malignant transformation is exceptionally rare. If the lesion troubles the patient, it can be removed by simple excision, which is curative.

### Keratoacanthoma

The typical characteristics of keratoacanthoma are that:

- it is a benign epidermal tumour
- it has a central, keratin-filled crater that is bordered by proliferating squamous epithelium
- there is a characteristic rapid initial growth, followed by stabilization and eventual regression
- the lesion has a close histological resemblance to well-differentiated squamous cell carcinoma.

This hyperkeratotic skin nodule most commonly arises in sun-exposed skin and grows rapidly, reaching a size of >1 cm within a few months. The lesions closely resemble squamous cell carcinoma, both clinically and histologically. However, unlike carcinoma, which continues to grow relentlessly when left untreated, the initial quick growth of

keratoacanthoma is followed by a period of stability and, subsequently, regression. The histopathologist, whose task it is to distinguish between keratoacanthoma and squamous cell carcinoma, needs to rely on but a few subtle characteristics of tissue architecture and cellular morphology; in some cases, the distinction may prove impossible. The presence of an exuberant but regular proliferating squamous epithelium surrounding a keratin horn mass on all sides is one of the main histological characteristics of keratoacanthoma.

## Premalignant Epithelial Lesions of the Epidermis

As is the case at many other body sites, the emergence of carcinoma of the skin is preceded by more or less well-defined and recognizable 'precursor' lesions. The two main examples – actinic keratosis and Bowen's disease – are considered here.

### Actinic Keratosis

The typical characteristics of actinic keratosis include:

- an area of epidermal dysplasia with overlying parakeratosis
- the lesions occurring either singly or multiply on sun-damaged skin
- if left untreated, some progressing to carcinoma.

This skin lesion arises in chronically sun-exposed skin (hence its synonym: solar keratosis) in white adults. It presents as a somewhat scaly brownish or erythematous macule, generally <1 cm in size. Multiple lesions are common. Histologically, the key features are those of epidermal dysplasia, evidenced by nuclear atypia associated with impaired epidermal maturation (Fig. 18.37). Although not an integral part of the lesion, the dermis characteristically exhibits marked

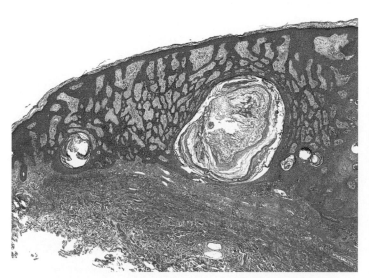

**FIG. 18.36** Seborrhoeic keratosis: an exuberant proliferation of well-circumscribed strands of epithelium resulting in thickening of the involved skin is characteristic. Note the presence of two small cysts filled with horn lamellae.

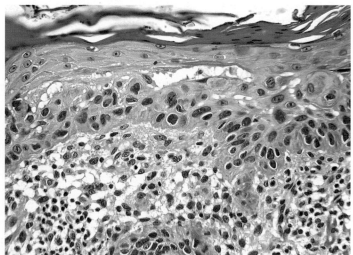

**FIG. 18.37** Actinic keratosis: the epidermis exhibits irregular orientation and increased variation in size and shape of keratinocytes and their nuclei. This is associated with parakeratosis (the presence of blue-staining nuclei in the stratum corneum) and an inflammatory infiltrate within the underlying dermis.

degenerative changes resulting from chronic solar ('actinic') damage. Invasive growth of the atypical epithelium is absent by definition; its development hallmarks the emergence of squamous carcinoma.

When left untreated, some actinic keratoses ultimately evolve into invasive squamous cell carcinomas. To prevent this, excision, cauterization, freezing, or another type of superficial treatment is generally instituted. Such simple treatment is generally curative; however, the keratosis may recur and new ones may emerge, so that regular review is advocated.

### Bowen's Disease

Bowen's disease of the skin:

- equates with epidermal squamous cell carcinoma *in situ*
- occurs in middle-aged and elderly individuals
- typically affects the lower leg, but lesions also occur on the head, trunk, and genitalia
- on microscopy shows high-grade cellular atypia and architectural disorder
- has some lesions that, if left untreated, progress to invasive squamous carcinoma.

Similar to actinic keratosis, Bowen's disease of the skin is an epidermal neoplastic lesion that has not yet acquired the potential to invade the underlying tissues. Presenting clinically as a local reddish discoloration, the lesion is characterized histologically by a pronounced degree of nuclear atypia and disordered maturation, including the presence of abnormal mitotic figures and dyskeratotic cells. The degree of nuclear and architectural atypia markedly exceeds that typically seen in actinic keratosis. Bowen's disease of the epidermis may affect sun-damaged skin – when it is sometimes referred to as bowenoid actinic keratosis – or covered skin lacking clinical and histological evidence of solar damage. The causative factors responsible for the latter examples remain obscure.

## Carcinoma of the Skin

The majority of skin carcinomas arise in the epidermis, the component of the skin that is most directly exposed to the mutagenic influences of the outside world. Carcinomas of skin adnexae are far less common: they are briefly considered on p. 533. However, in the common basal cell carcinoma (see below), the origin from epidermal versus adnexal epithelium is in fact often unclear.

### Basal Cell Carcinoma

Typically, basal cell carcinoma:

- is a slow-growing malignant tumour of keratinocytes
- is common, especially in the sun-exposed skin of white people
- has a risk associated with history of peak exposures to UV radiation (sunburn; tanning equipment)
- causes local tissue destruction by invasive growth, but metastasis is exceptionally rare
- shows a typical 'basaloid' appearance of tumour cells
- shows palisading of nuclei at the periphery of tumour nests.

This non-metastasizing but locally aggressive epithelial neoplasm commonly arises in sun-exposed skin of middle-aged or elderly white individuals. In its most typical form, it appears as a shiny and pearly nodule, at times with central ulceration (so-called 'rodent ulcer') (Fig. 18.38). Other examples form slowly spreading, ill-defined patches of cutaneous thickening or reddish discoloration. Histologically, the tumour cells most commonly form irregular strands and nodules, often with characteristic peripheral tumour cell palisading (Fig. 18.39). Basal cell carcinoma derives its

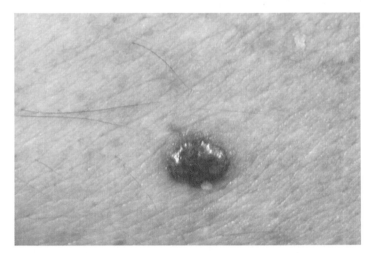

**FIG. 18.38** Basal cell carcinoma: this example manifests itself as a shiny, pigmented skin papule.

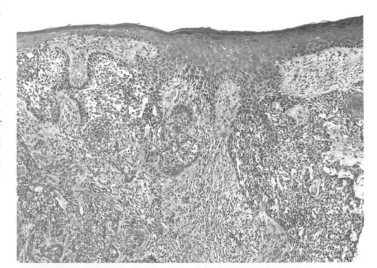

**FIG. 18.39** Basal cell carcinoma: irregular strands of small, darkly stained epithelial cells extend into the dermis. Although there may be a superficial resemblance to seborrhoeic keratosis (see Fig. 18.36), the strands are more irregular and the cellular details (not visible at this magnification) also differ.

name from the histological resemblance of the tumour cells to the basal cells of the epidermis. Variants include a superficial spreading variant, and a poorly circumscribed spindle-cell variant (morphoeic type), which has a bad reputation for extending beyond the clinically apparent borders of the lesion, and an associated tendency to recur locally.

Basal cell carcinoma is generally cured by simple total excision. It is essential to obtain tumour-free surgical margins, because basal cell carcinoma almost never metastasizes but may produce extensive local destruction of tissues if the treatment is inadequate. Especially in anatomically sensitive locations, such as near the eye, nostril, or ear, local recurrence and ingrowth of basal cell carcinoma may ultimately necessitate extensive and mutilating surgery.

## Squamous Cell Carcinoma

Squamous cell carcinoma:

- is a common type of epidermal carcinoma
- arises commonly in the sun-damaged skin of white people
- has a risk related to life-long cumulative UV exposure (rather than history of peak exposures)
- can arise in burn scars, in chronic ulcers, or after exposure to chemical carcinogens
- has the histological features of squamous epithelium, with frequent keratinization, and irregular growth
- is locally aggressive
- may metastasize to regional lymph nodes, and also to distant sites.

Squamous carcinoma arises from the epidermal squamous epithelium, presumably from its basal cell layer. However, it differs from basal cell carcinoma morphologically as well as clinically; the most important difference is the metastatic potential of squamous cell carcinoma.

Again, solar irradiation appears to be a major causative factor, because these tumours arise most commonly in the sun-damaged skin of middle-aged or elderly white individuals (Fig. 18.40), but it is cumulative exposure, rather than a history of peak exposures that correlates most strongly with its incidence. In addition, chronic ulcers, burn scars, immunosuppression, and direct exposure of the skin surface to certain industrial carcinogens are important causative factors in some populations.

Clinically, squamous cell carcinoma most commonly presents as a hyperkeratotic nodule or area of induration. In more advanced stages, ulceration and destruction of underlying tissues may be evident. Histologically, the tumour consists of irregular strands and nodules of atypical squamous epithelium (Fig. 18.41), which penetrate the underlying tissues and induce a desmoplastic stromal response. If there is a predisposing factor such as a chronic ulcer, the diagnosis of carcinoma may be very difficult, because reactive epidermal proliferation and hyperkeratosis at the ulcer margin may closely mimic carcinoma, both clinically and histologically.

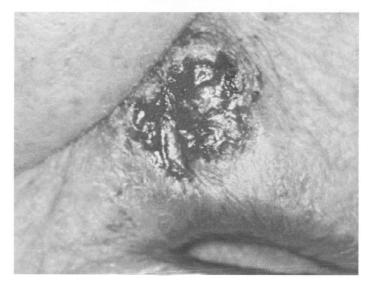

**FIG. 18.40** Squamous cell carcinoma, manifesting itself as an irregular ulcer near the upper lip of an elderly patient.

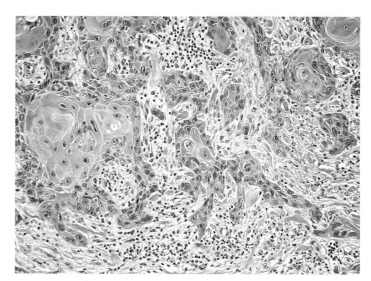

**FIG. 18.41** Squamous cell carcinoma, forming highly irregular strands of atypical epithelial cells, invading the skin and inducing an inflammatory response.

Generally, squamous cell carcinoma of the skin is easily cured by local excision. Metastases are rare, except in the minority of cases that are associated with a chronic ulcer: in these, metastasis occurs in up to a third of cases.

Some squamous cell carcinomas of the plantar or genital skin – designated verrucous carcinomas – consist of very well-differentiated squamous epithelium, and do not form the characteristically irregular cellular strands and nests. Large cell masses, with a 'pushing' rather than an 'infiltrating' pattern of growth, give the erroneous impression that true invasive growth is absent. However, such tumours do grow progressively and destructively, without halting at natural tissue borders, so there is no doubt that these tumours are capable of true invasive growth.

### Merkel Cell Carcinoma

Merkel cell carcinoma is a rare, highly aggressive carcinoma of the skin, thought to arise from the rare epidermal Merkel cells (which play a role in the reception of mechanical stimuli, and have some neuroendocrine properties). Merkel cell carcinoma readily metastasizes to regional lymph nodes and distant sites. It should be distinguished from a variety of tumours, most importantly from skin metastasis of an extracutaneous neuroendocrine carcinoma. This distinction is important, because radical surgery of the skin tumour has the potential of cure if the tumour is primary, but not if it represents a metastasis from an occult visceral primary.

## Melanocytic Naevus

The melanocytic naevus – more generally known as a 'naevus' or 'mole' – is a benign, melanocytic neoplasm, which usually arises in the epidermis and often involves the dermis as well. Many variants of this lesion, which is extremely common in white races, have been recognized, but only the most common and clinically important ones are considered here.

### Common Acquired Naevus

Common acquired naevus is typically:

- very common in white individuals
- a small, symmetrical, well-circumscribed hyperpigmented macule or papule
- a melanocytic proliferation within the epidermis and/or the dermis (Fig. 18.42)
- stable in size, after an initial growth phase, and ultimately disappears spontaneously.

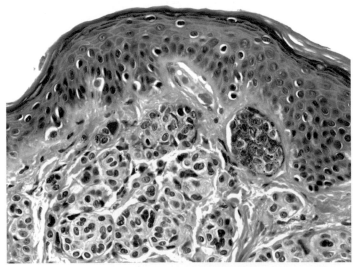

**FIG. 18.42** Common acquired naevus: round to oval nests of melanocytes are present at the dermoepidermal junction, as well as in the upper dermis. The epidermis shows a reactive lengthening of the rete ridges and slight hyperkeratosis.

Melanocytic naevi of the usual type are very common in white people, but less so in black races. At birth, naevi are usually absent (except for the so-called congenital naevi – see below). Most emerge in childhood and adolescence, but some arise in adulthood. After a period of growth, the naevus stabilizes in size and appearance, and after many years gradually loses its pigmentation, diminishes in size, and ultimately disappears so that, in old age, naevi are again absent or scarce. Their main significance derives from their cosmetic effect and the fact that at least half of all cutaneous melanomas (see below) arise in them.

The causative factors responsible for the emergence and disappearance of these very common but enigmatic lesions have remained partly obscure. Sunlight certainly plays a role: marked sun exposure – and especially a history of sunburn in childhood – is associated with increased numbers, and they are uncommon on areas of doubly covered skin, such as the buttock area.

Melanocytic naevi are benign neoplasms: most harbour an activating mutation of the oncogene *BRAF*; others have activating *NRAS*, *HRAS*, or *GNAQ* mutations (all these mutations have a stimulatory effect on the mitogenic MAP kinase pathway). The mechanism by which they at some stage lose their proliferative potential has now been identified as 'oncogene-induced cellular senescence' (OIS), a dominant growth-arrest response that is activated by inappropriate mitogenic signalling – as may originate from abnormal promitogenic proteins encoded by mutated oncogenes – and is thought to play a generic tumour-suppressor role.

The common acquired naevus probably arises most commonly from epidermal melanocytes, which are situated at the junction between the epidermis and dermis. In the first phase of its development, a proliferation of these melanocytes emerges, first in an arrangement of solitary cells arranged side to side, later in the form of cell nests (junctional naevus). The melanocytes of this and subsequent stages of naevus development are often designated 'naevus cells'. Macroscopically, such an early naevus presents as a brown, flat, usually symmetrical, and well-circumscribed macule, reaching a size of up to several millimetres. After some time, the naevus cells extend into the superficial dermis, where they continue to form nests and sheets. This migration into the dermis should not be equated with invasive growth of malignant tumours, because in naevi it is an entirely innocent phenomenon. The lesion is now designated a compound naevus, because it involves both the junction and the dermis.

After a number of years – and for reasons unknown – the junctional component disappears, so that all naevus cells are now intradermal (intradermal naevus). At the base of the naevus, the melanocytes usually become smaller and/or elongated and lose their pigmentation (so-called 'maturation'). After further passage of time, the intradermal naevus cells also gradually diminish in number and disappear altogether, so that, ultimately, the skin returns to normal.

## Spitz Naevus

This naevus type, which is most common in childhood and adolescence, but which may also occur later in life, most often presents as a symmetrical reddish or skin-coloured nodule, with a predilection for the face and extremities. Its importance lies in its close histological resemblance to melanoma, which may lead to overdiagnosis and overtreatment of this essentially innocent lesion. Several variants of Spitz naevus have been recognized: these include the pigmented spindle cell naevus (also known as Reed naevus) which, in its most characteristic form, presents as a small, symmetrical, pitch-black nodule, raising clinical suspicion of nodular melanoma (see below) – a suspicion that may be compounded by the somewhat alarming histology of this exuberant and densely cellular naevus. However, similar to the classic Spitz naevus, the Reed naevus is harmless.

## Congenital Naevus

About 1% of newborn white babies are born with a clinically detectable melanocytic naevus. In contrast to acquired naevi – which are usually smaller than 1 cm across – such congenital naevi are much more variable in size and shape, and occasionally cover large parts of the body (so-called giant congenital naevi) (Fig. 18.43).

Clearly, extensive congenital naevi cause significant cosmetic problems and, in addition, there is a small risk of malignant transformation. Various surgical procedures are currently used in order to eradicate as much as possible of the giant congenital naevus, preferably within the first few weeks or months of life.

## Blue Naevus

In contrast to the naevus types discussed so far, this enigmatic melanocytic tumour appears to arise within the dermis rather than the epidermis. The naevus is often slightly bluish when viewed from the skin surface, because the pigmentation is deeply located in the skin and covered by the opaque normal overlying skin tissue (the resultant colour shift toward blue is known as the Tyndall effect). In contrast to most intradermal naevus cells, some melanocytes of blue naevi possess slender dendrites and actively produce melanin.

## Melanoma

Characteristically:

- melanoma is a malignant tumour of melanocytes
- at least half of all melanomas arise in a melanocytic naevus
- the treatment is primarily surgical, but novel targeted therapies carry promise in a palliative setting and as adjuvant therapy
- the chance of cure is closely related to tumour thickness
- metastases occur in nearby skin and subcutis (satellites/in-transit metastases), regional lymph nodes, and distant sites
- there are four main subtypes: superficial spreading melanoma; nodular melanoma; lentigo maligna melanoma; and acral lentiginous melanoma.

Malignant melanoma, or simply melanoma – the adjective 'malignant' being omitted because there is no such thing as a benign melanoma – is a malignant tumour of melanocytes. Clinically, melanomas are flat or raised lesions, and are often irregular in shape and colour. They occasionally bleed, and may produce an itching or burning sensation. These signs or a history of recent change in a previously stable mole calls for excision and histological evaluation.

Melanomas vary widely in macroscopic and histological appearance. Four main subtypes are recognized (Table 18.7). Superficial spreading melanoma in its most characteristic form presents as an irregularly shaped and coloured, slowly

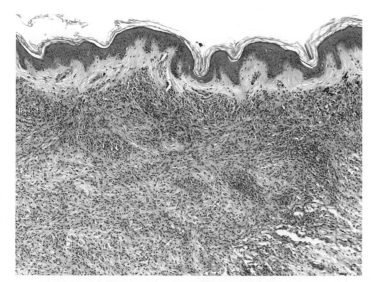

**FIG. 18.43** Congenital naevus: large numbers of naevus cells occupy almost the entire thickness of the dermis. Such deep penetration of tissues is common in congenital naevi, but rare in acquired naevi.

**TABLE 18.7** The clinical and aetiological characteristics of melanoma

| Melanoma type | Site | Remarks |
|---|---|---|
| Superficial spreading melanoma | Anywhere | Most common type of melanoma in white people |
| Nodular melanoma | Anywhere | Usually rapidly growing |
| Lentigo maligna melanoma | Sun-damaged skin of elderly white people | Precursor lesion: lentigo maligna (Hutchinson's freckle) |
| Acral melanoma | Volar skin or nail bed | Most common type of melanoma in black people |

growing lesion with a flat periphery (Fig. 18.44). Part of the lesion may become raised, and in the course of time may show accelerated growth and ulceration. Typical histology is shown in Fig. 18.45. Nodular melanoma usually grows rapidly from the start, forming a nodule that is commonly – but not always – pigmented. If the tumour is totally devoid of pigment (amelanotic melanoma), the initial clinical impression is often that of a trivial, benign lesion. Lentigo maligna melanoma arises in the sun-exposed skin of middle-aged or elderly white people, and is most common on the face and the dorsa of the hands. The melanoma derives its name from the precursor lesion, lentigo maligna (also known as 'Hutchinson's freckle'), a proliferation of atypical melanocytes within the atrophic epidermis of sun-damaged skin, which produces a slowly enlarging, irregularly shaped pigmentation. Acral melanoma arises in the skin of the palms of hands, soles of feet, or subungually. In contrast to the previous three main melanoma types, which are rare in non-white individuals, the incidence of acral melanoma is roughly equal amongst the various races.

The treatment of melanoma is primarily surgical, and the prognosis primarily depends on tumour stage (the presence or absence of regional or distant metastases). In the absence of any signs of metastatic disease, its thickness (measured in millimetres – Breslow's thickness) and the presence of ulceration and intradermal mitotic activity predict prognosis. Ulcerated, thicker, and mitotically active tumours do worse.

Melanoma has a propensity to produce small tumour deposits in the direct vicinity of the primary tumour. To avoid the outgrowth of these so-called 'satellites' – which may be undetectable at the time of resection of the primary tumour – melanoma is excised with a wide margin of surrounding skin and subcutis. Usually, a skin margin of 1 cm is used for all invasive melanomas with a thickness up to 2 mm; for thicker melanomas, even wider margins are used.

Metastases occur primarily in regional lymph nodes and pass via the bloodstream to a wide variety of organs. Superficial metastases that occur between the primary tumour and the regional nodes, and which are presumably caused by outgrowth of tumour emboli within lymph vessels, are known as 'in-transit metastases'.

Melanoma with regional lymph node metastases is still potentially curable by radical surgery. To assess melanoma prognosis optimally, and select patients who might benefit from regional lymph node dissection, it is possible to identify the lymph node in the regional lymph node basin that is the first to receive the lymph from the site of the primary tumour – and, potentially, tumour cell emboli travelling in it. This is done by injecting a small amount of radioactive or blue-coloured fluid at the site of the primary tumour, and subsequently identifying the first regional lymph node to become radioactive and blue. This so-called 'sentinel lymph node' is investigated thoroughly for the presence of metastatic melanoma by the pathologist. If no metastasis is found in the sentinel node, it is unlikely that more distant nodes of that lymph node basin contain metastases, so that a lymph node dissection need not take place.

When distant metastases (i.e. metastasis beyond the body region of the primary melanoma) manifest themselves, there are no longer any curative options. However, targeted therapies such as those blocking the activity of the abnormal protein encoded by a mutated *BRAF* gene (the same mutation is commonly present in benign naevi, see above) or novel immunotherapeutic approaches that enhance T-cell responses, have in recent years led to – sometimes substantial and prolonged – remissions in selected melanoma patients with inoperable metastatic disease.

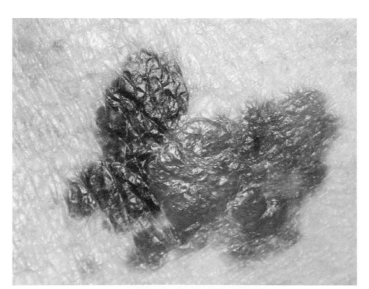

FIG. 18.44 Superficial spreading melanoma: this lesion shows several of the key features of melanoma: irregular shape, marked variation in colour, and irregular surface with loss of skin lines in some places.

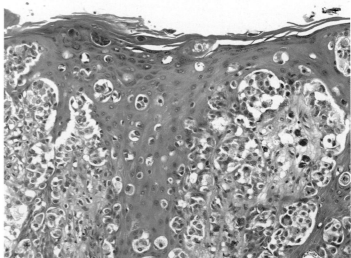

FIG. 18.45 Superficial spreading melanoma: atypical melanocytes are seen throughout the thickness of the epidermis, which contrasts with the more regular nests of melanocytes at the dermoepidermal junction, seen in most naevi (compare with Fig. 18.42).

## CASE HISTORY 18.3

### A SUSPICIOUS MOLE

A 35-year-old female visited her GP because she had recently noticed a dark mole on her upper thigh; the mole was enlarging and gave a slightly burning sensation (Fig. 18.46). The patient's father had a history of melanoma on the back, which had been removed 2 years previously.

On inspection, a pitch-black, symmetrical, oval, non-ulcerating papule of 0.8 cm diameter was seen. The number and features of the patient's other naevi were considered to be within normal limits. The lesion was considered to be suspicious of nodular melanoma and was excised

with a margin of 2 mm, in order to obtain a histological diagnosis.

Histological examination revealed the characteristic features of a pigmented spindle cell naevus (PSCN, Reed naevus) (Fig. 18.47). This naevus subtype can present as a pitch-black papule that is clinically indistinguishable from a small, nodular, pigmented melanoma. The burning sensation was probably derived from the mild inflammatory response caused by the shedding of melanin pigment from the lesion. The GP reassured the patient that the lesion was entirely benign, and that there was no relation to her father's history of melanoma.

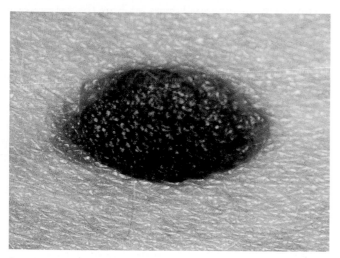

FIG. 18.46 The skin lesion of this patient manifested itself as a raised, darkly pigmented, symmetrical nodule. Because of the pitch-black colour, there was some concern that the lesion could be a heavily pigmented nodular melanoma.

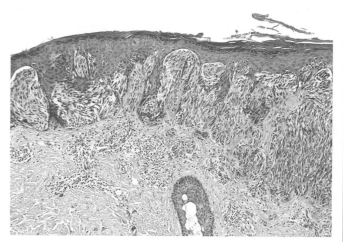

FIG. 18.47 Histology of the lesion shows many confluent nests and sheets of melanocytes at the dermoepidermal junction, associated with epidermal hyperplasia and hyperkeratosis. The histology is characteristic of pigmented spindle cell naevus (PSCN), a benign lesion.

### Familial Dysplastic Naevus Syndrome

A high incidence of melanoma is found in some families; the melanoma patients – or those who later develop melanoma – often have an abnormally large number of naevi, which vary markedly in size, shape, and colour, and occur at sites where naevi are normally rare. Histologically, these so-called dysplastic naevi show a number of distinctive features, the most important of which are cytological and architectural atypia, and some associated inflammation and fibrosis. Family members with such large numbers of clinically and histologically abnormal naevi have a markedly increased lifetime risk of melanoma, so that close follow-up is essential. Any change in a previously stable naevus is suspicious of malignant change, necessitating removal. In this way, many 'early melanomas' can be removed, which results in a markedly improved life expectancy for these patients.

It is important to note that very similar dysplastic naevi also occur as solitary lesions in individuals with a negative family history for melanoma and that, in this

context, melanoma risk hardly exceeds that of the general population.

The dysplastic naevus syndrome phenotype may result from different genotypes. Particularly intriguing is the finding of involvement of the *INK4A* gene in some families, because the protein p16, encoded by this gene, is a potent proliferation inhibitor (acting by blocking CDK4's proliferation-promoting kinase activity) that is abundantly present in the large majority of common naevi, but is absent from many melanomas. Further evidence incriminating p16 in melanomagenesis derives from recent studies of p16 knockout mice which, under certain conditions, exhibit an increased incidence of melanoma.

## Various other Skin Tumours

### Dermatofibroma

This common and innocent intradermal proliferation of mesenchymal cells with characteristics of histiocytes as well as fibroblasts (hence its alternative designation cutaneous fibrous histiocytoma) presents as a firm, skin-coloured, or slightly hyperpigmented nodule, usually <1 cm in size, and most commonly located on the extremities. It has been hypothesized that the lesion represents a response to tissue damage rather than a neoplasm, but the identification of karyotypic aberrations in a substantial number of these lesions indicates that the lesion is neoplastic. It is important not to confuse dermatofibroma with the rare dermatofibrosarcoma protuberans, which shares some of its histological features, but diffusely invades surrounding tissues and has a notorious propensity for local recurrence and relentless local invasive growth.

## Vascular Tumours

### Haemangioma

Haemangiomas of the skin are benign tumours of endothelium, which are especially common in childhood. Capillary haemangiomas produce large numbers of small vessels (Fig. 18.48); cavernous haemangiomas consist of large, gaping vascular spaces. Large and flat congenital haemangiomas are commonly referred to as port wine stains. In contrast, the so-called 'strawberry haemangioma' of the neonate is a raised lesion, which sometimes grows rapidly to produce a disfiguring exophytic lesion, but it generally regresses spontaneously after a number of years so that a conservative approach is warranted. Pyogenic granuloma, which is a haemangioma rather than a granuloma, produces a reddish nodule with a wet surface, caused by erosion of the overlying epidermis. Some of these lesions arise after trauma, and it is still a matter of debate whether these represent true neoplasms or exuberant reactive endothelial proliferations.

### Kaposi's Sarcoma

Kaposi's sarcoma is a locally aggressive endothelial tumour (Fig. 18.49) that occurs in several clinical settings, the best known of these being the association with AIDS (see Chapter 19, p. 546). However, the tumour may also affect HIV-negative individuals, especially elderly males, transplant recipients, and children in certain regions of Africa. The tumour is closely associated with the presence of human herpesvirus type 8, which plays an important causal role in its pathogenesis.

Clinically, the lesion often presents initially as one or several small macules, but may later progress to mass lesions (nodular phase) with ulceration of the overlying epidermis. Involvement of internal organs, such as the respiratory and digestive tracts, is common.

### Angiosarcoma

Angiosarcoma of the skin is a rare, malignant tumour of vascular endothelium, which most commonly arises on chronically sun-exposed skin in elderly people. The tumour usually presents as an ill-defined area of cutaneous thickening, induration, and discoloration, but later develops protuberant and locally aggressive masses. The tumour often extends far beyond the clinically apparent borders, responds poorly to therapy, and, because of these properties, carries a dismal prognosis. Other cutaneous angiosarcomas arise on the basis of chronic lymphoedema, such as may develop in the arm after axillary lymph node dissection and radiotherapy for breast carcinoma (Stewart–Treves syndrome). Again, the prognosis is poor.

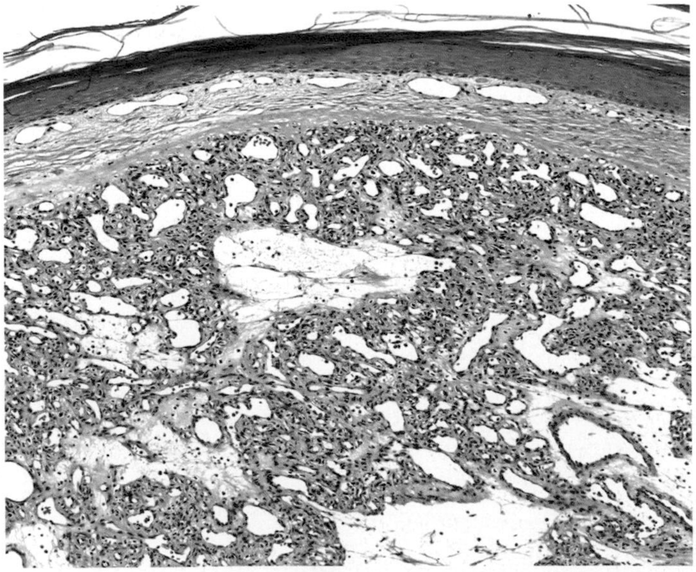

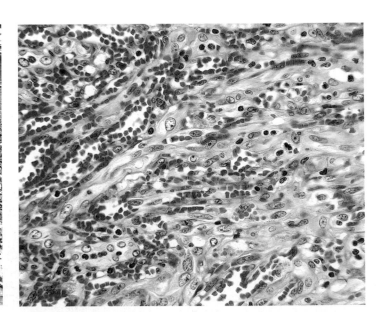

**FIG. 18.48** Cutaneous haemangioma: a benign tumour characterized by an accumulation of regular vessels, which may be small or large, and lined by (usually) flat endothelial cells.

**FIG. 18.49** Kaposi's sarcoma, showing an irregular mass of elongated atypical endothelial cells alternating with slit-like spaces filled with blood.

## Cutaneous Lymphoma

Cutaneous lymphoma may be of either T-cell or B-cell origin. The main type of primary cutaneous T-cell lymphoma is mycosis fungoides (MF). The initial stage of MF – which may last for many years – is characterized by the formation of patches, which are vexingly difficult to distinguish clinically and histologically from a number of inflammatory skin diseases. Permeation of the epidermis by monoclonal atypical T cells constitutes the essential diagnostic feature. The early, patch stage of MF is followed by the emergence of indurated plaques and, later, nodules and larger tumours. A variant of cutaneous T-cell lymphoma, characterized by generalized skin reddening (erythroderma) and involvement of lymph nodes and blood, is known as Sézary's syndrome. A variety of other lymphoma types including B-cell lymphomas may arise, or become manifest clinically, in the skin: these rare tumours fall outside the scope of this chapter.

## Metastasis to the Skin

It should be borne in mind that carcinomas of internal organs may grow into, or metastasize to, the skin. Breast cancer may involve the skin by direct local extension or lymphatic spread. Skin metastasis of renal carcinoma is of special significance: for unknown reasons, renal carcinoma more commonly metastasizes to the skin than carcinomas of many other organs. As the primary tumour of renal carcinoma may stay asymptomatic for a long period of time, metastases rather than the primary tumour may produce the first symptoms.

## Tumours of Skin Appendages

Characteristically:

- the tumours of skin appendages comprise a highly heterogeneous group
- the large majority are benign
- some are associated with specific syndromes.

The hair follicles and sweat glands give rise to an extraordinary variety of neoplasms. The large majority are benign, and precise subtyping of these is generally of little consequence – which explains why general designations such as 'benign eccrine sweat gland tumour' are commonly used. The significance of some variants derives mainly from the possible confusion with malignant tumours, or from the association with some specific syndromes. Some adnexal tumours (the carcinomas in the list below) are malignant.

The basis of the histological classification of these neoplasms is by way of their phenotypic resemblance to adnexal structures, from which they have presumably arisen (*Table 18.8*). Thus, there are eccrine and apocrine sweat gland tumours, and tumours of the pilosebaceous unit.

**TABLE 18.8** Histological classification of neoplasms

| Adnexal structure | Tumour presumably arising from it |
|---|---|
| Eccrine sweat gland | Syringoma |
| | Nodular hidradenoma |
| | Microcystic adnexal carcinoma |
| Apocrine sweat gland | Cylindroma |
| | Apocrine carcinoma |
| Pilosebaceous unit | Infundibular cyst ('epidermal cyst') |
| | Trichofollicular cyst |
| | Pilomatrixoma ('Malherbe's tumour') |
| | Pilar tumour ('proliferating trichilemmal cyst') |

### Eccrine Sweat Gland Tumours

Syringomas usually present as multiple small papules on the upper cheek. Histologically, they are found to consist of a proliferation of small epithelial cells arranged in small islands and strands, resulting in a superficial resemblance to basal cell carcinoma. Nodular hidradenoma – which probably arises from the distal portion of the sweat duct – produces a solitary nodule consisting of large masses of epithelium. Malignant eccrine sweat gland tumours are rare and comprise a varied group of lesions, including microcystic adnexal carcinoma, most of which occur on the face and have a bad reputation for local recurrence and destructive growth, so that early complete surgical removal is essential.

### Apocrine Sweat Gland Tumours

Situated mainly in areas where apocrine glands are numerous (axillae, groins, midline of back), these rare neoplasms exhibit a baffling variability of appearances. Cylindromas occur multiply on the skin of the face (usually forehead) and scalp but, in contrast to syringomas of the face, which remain small, these tumours can grow to form disfiguring masses ('turban tumour'). Histologically, closely adjacent islands of small epithelial cells, with little adjacent stroma, result in a jigsaw-like appearance. Apocrine carcinomas are exceedingly rare.

### Tumours of the Pilosebaceous Unit

Simple epithelial cysts within the dermis or subcutis, lined by an attenuated layer of stratified squamous epithelium, are often designated 'epidermal cysts'; however, these lesions do not originate from the epidermis but from the hair follicle infundibulum, and are therefore properly termed 'infundibular cysts'. The cyst wall may rupture, inducing a granulomatous inflammatory response. The resultant swelling and pain may draw attention to the lesion. A histologically

## 18.2 Special Study Topic

### XERODERMA PIGMENTOSUM AND DNA REPAIR

The basic defect in the rare inherited disorder xeroderma pigmentosum (XP) is a failure to repair DNA damage by nucleotide excision. This defect uncovers the devastating effects of the genetic damage that the skin incurs naturally, but which in healthy individuals is repaired quickly and effectively, so that it does not lead to significant cell and tissue damage. The fact that most of this damage is sun induced is evident from the extreme photosensitivity of the skin in XP patients and the approximately 2,000-fold increase in the incidence of skin cancers, including squamous cell carcinomas, basal cell carcinomas, and melanomas. Some of these malignant tumours appear at an early age, even in childhood. The distribution of lesions reflects the aetiological role of sunlight exposure – the face, dorsa of hands, but also arms and legs being most severely affected. In these patients, the extensive skin damage and multiple tumours often necessitate major surgical procedures. Avoidance of sun exposure is obviously an essential part of the clinical management.

The basic molecular mechanisms underlying this rare disease have been the subject of intense research interest. It has become clear that, at the genetic level, a variety of defects may cause very similar phenotypic effects: at least seven genetically distinct subgroups of XP have thus far been identified. This is a reflection of the fact that nucleotide excision repair is not a single enzyme activity, but is brought about by a multiprotein complex, each component of which needs to function adequately in order to achieve effective nucleotide excision repair.

The link between genotype (defective nucleotide excision repair resulting in accumulation of UV-induced mutations) and phenotype (emergence of large numbers of sunlight-induced cancers) is easily understood, but it should be added that not all defects in nucleotide excision repair are equally complete and severe, e.g. Cockayne's syndrome, another very rare form of defective nucleotide excision repair, is not associated with an elevated skin cancer risk. In this syndrome, the defect in nucleotide excision repair affects only the small minority of genes that are actively transcribed, but bulk genomic DNA repair remains intact, which no doubt explains why there is no cancer predisposition in that syndrome.

Pilomatrixoma, or Malherbe's tumour, is a benign hair follicle tumour that may be recognized clinically because, as a result of extensive calcification, it is as hard as stone. Finally, the rare so-called pilar tumour, or 'proliferating trichilemmal cyst', is of interest, because it may produce an alarmingly large tumour of the scalp, usually in elderly females, and histologically may be misdiagnosed as carcinoma if a small biopsy is taken from the centre. However, the tumour is entirely benign, as becomes evident when the expansile growth pattern of the edge of the tumour is appreciated.

Hypertrophy and hyperplasia of sebaceous glands of the skin of the nose, of a poorly understood but probably non-neoplastic nature, result in a disfiguring nasal swelling known as rhinophyma. The benign sebaceous adenoma and malignant sebaceous carcinoma are both very rare. In addition to the obvious importance of early recognition and removal of sebaceous carcinoma, there is an added level of clinical significance in that some sebaceous tumours are associated with increased incidence of visceral carcinomas, due to germline mutations in DNA mismatch-repair genes (Muir–Torre syndrome).

---

similar cyst, which most commonly involves the scalp but is characterized by trichilemmal rather than epidermal type keratinization, is known as a trichilemmal cyst.

## SUMMARY

Dermatopathology can appear to be a daunting subject with a myriad of seemingly obscure diagnoses compounded by complex terminology and pathogenic mechanisms that often remain poorly understood. At a basic level it is reassuring to know that a relatively small group of well-defined disorders account for the bulk of dermatology practice.

As is the case in all areas of pathology, the subject becomes infinitely more manageable when diseases with similar morphological characteristics are grouped together in a classification, e.g. there are many hundreds of non-infective inflammatory disorders but the majority can be placed into one of only a few broad groups according to the morphological reaction pattern displayed by the epidermis

(see *Box 18.2*). The logical classification for cutaneous neoplastic disease, as for other organ systems, reflects the cell of origin and examples of tumours derived from the epidermal cells (principally the keratinocytes and melanocytes), dermal constituents, adnexal structures, and lymphoid elements have been presented.

Currently, the classification of most cutaneous disease relies largely on histological and clinical characteristics but this is likely to change in the future as the detailed molecular genetic abnormalities underpinning disorders are unravelled, linking conditions formerly believed to be unrelated, e.g. mutations in the filaggrin gene recently found to be responsible for a common inherited type of dry scaly skin (ichthyosis vulgaris) are now implicated strongly in the pathogenesis of the clinically distinct conditions atopic dermatitis and asthma.

It is crucial to remember that accurate diagnosis of cutaneous disease demands close correlation of the pathological findings with the clinical picture and also with the results of other investigations such as microbiology, immunofluorescence studies, and molecular genetics. Diseases with diverse but distinctive clinical patterns can share very similar histological features and it is therefore fortunate that there is no other area of medicine where the organ of interest is so accessible to inspection. At the very least the pathologist needs to be made aware of several pieces of information including the site of the biopsy, any relevant history (such as a recent infection or exposure to drugs), together with the duration, distribution, and description of the abnormality. Specialist multidisciplinary meetings of dermatologists and dermatopathologists, when diagnoses can be reviewed – and if necessary revised, in the light of more detailed information – are now central to effective patient management.

## FURTHER READING

Calonje JE, McKee PH, Brenn T, Lazar AJ, McKee PH. *McKee's Pathology of the Skin*, 4th edn. Philadelphia, PA: Saunders, 2011.

Weedon D. *Weedon's Skin Pathology*, 3rd edn. Edinburgh: Churchill Livingstone, 2009.

# 19

# INFECTIONS

Runjan Chetty and Sebastian B Lucas

## INTRODUCTION

Infectious diseases are caused by living organisms that invade and damage organ function – they are commonly termed 'pathogens'. The means by which pathogens produce disease are almost infinitely variable. The previous chapters have detailed the standard common organ infections such as bacterial pneumonias, viral hepatitis, helicobacter gastritis, and bacterial dysentery. Here, some multisystem infections and parasitic diseases that are encountered both globally and in Europe are described.

In the scale of human disease, infections are the most common causes of illness and death. In industrialized countries with well-resourced health systems, cardiovascular disease causes approximately half of all deaths, and cancer another quarter. Specific infections make up much of the remainder. However, many deaths are ultimately from an infection coming at the end of a clinical course (e.g. bronchopneumonia after a stroke, Gram-negative sepsis after leukaemia). In resource-poor countries, where most of the world's population lives, infections are the dominant diseases from birth.

The list of infectious agents of humans is both long and expanding. With improved clinical observations and epidemiology, more refined methods of microbiological isolation and, in the 1990s, the advent of molecular technology to identify RNA and DNA, new infectious diseases are continually being described (Table 19.1). These infections are not entities that had not existed before – they simply had not been identified previously. The rate at which infectious diseases spread is highly conditional on environmental and social circumstances. The extreme example of this is HIV/AIDS, which emerged from being a limited infection in central Africa during the 1970s to the main cause of death in many poor countries by the year 2000.

As well as 'new diseases', several ancient diseases have begun to re-emerge as major public health problems, long after the medical establishment had considered them to be declining. Tuberculosis and falciparum malaria are good examples of this re-emergence.

TABLE 19.1 Some examples of important infections of humans that have been newly identified since 1975

| Year identified | Agent | Disease |
| --- | --- | --- |
| 1975 | *Cryptosporidium* spp. | Diarrhoea |
| 1977 | *Legionella* spp. | Pneumonia |
| 1977 | Ebolavirus | Haemorrhagic fever |
| 1982 | *Borrelia burgdorferi* | Lyme disease |
| 1983 | *Helicobacter pylori* | Gastritis |
| 1983 | HIV | AIDS |
| 1985 | Microsporidia | Diarrhoea |
| 1989 | Hepatitis C virus | Chronic liver disease |
| 1994 | HHV-8 | Kaposi's sarcoma |
| 2003 | Coronavirus | Viral pneumonia (SARS) |
| 2012 | Coronavirus | Viral pneumonia (MERS) |

SARS = severe acute respiratory syndrome; HHV = human herpes virus; MERS = Middle East respiratory syndrome.

# PATHOGENESIS OF INFECTIOUS DISEASES

The general pathogenic mechanisms are listed in Box 19.1. Many pathogens cause disease directly, for example by toxin production. However, a large number of intracellular pathogens activate the immune system, which then damages host tissues as a by-product of attempting to eliminate the pathogen; this is termed 'immunopathology'. The body's repair mechanisms – which include scarring – may then cause further and chronic organ damage.

Infections may be further subdivided into those that attack at the first or repeated presentations, and those that enter and lie latent within host cells and re-emerge at a later period (latent infections).

## Classification of Infectious Agents

Classically, all infectious agents have been regarded as containing either RNA or DNA. However, this definition may be upset by the phenomenon of the transmissible spongiform encephalopathies (e.g. Creutzfeldt–Jakob disease), which can 'infect' animals and humans, but this does not involve the transmission of nucleic acids (see Chapter 11, p. 323). The major categories of infections are viruses, bacteria, chlamydiae, rickettsiae, mycoplasmas, fungi, protozoa, helminths, and arthropods. The last three categories are collectively termed 'parasitic infections' (*Tables 19.2–19.6*).

## Overview of Immunosuppression and Infections

The normal host defence systems against infection begin with the external skin cover, and the external and internal mucosal surfaces (such as conjunctiva, airways, and gut). Behind these physical barriers are complex systems of interacting cells and their secretions such as antibodies and cytokines, and the complement system. It is not an exaggeration to state that most of these internal defence systems have evolved in response to infectious challenges from the environment. Thus, when these defences malfunction, as a result of either inherited or acquired defects, infection is the consequence and the major focus of clinical management.

---

**Box 19.1** SUMMARY OF HOW PATHOGENS CAN CAUSE DISEASE

- Pathogen–cell contact and damage to the cell
- Invasion of the cell and damage to the cell
- Release of toxins that damage nearby cells
- Induction of systemic inflammatory responses
- Obstruction of, or damage to, blood vessels
- Induction of local acute inflammation
- Induction of immune-mediated antibody responses
- Induction of cell-mediated immune responses
- Space-occupying lesion in an organ
- Induction or promotion of malignant tumours

---

**TABLE 19.2** Virus infections and their tissue tropisms

| Region/tissue | Infection |
|---|---|
| Respiratory tract | Influenza virus |
| | Measles virus |
| | RSV (respiratory syncytial virus) |
| | Adenovirus |
| | Coronavirus |
| Skin | HPV (human papillomaviruses) |
| | Herpes simplex and herpes zoster |
| Mucosae | Herpes simplex |
| | HPV |
| | EBV (Epstein–Barr virus) |
| Salivary gland | Mumps virus |
| Liver | Hepatitis viruses A, B, and C |
| Gut | Rotavirus |
| Central nervous system | Poliovirus |
| | JC virus |
| | Arboviral encephalitis |
| | Herpes simplex |
| T cells | HIV (human immunodeficiency viruses) |
| | HTLV-I (human T-cell lymphotrophic virus type I) |
| B cells | EBV |
| Any organ | CMV (cytomegalovirus) |

**TABLE 19.3** Bacterial infections and subtypes

| Subtype | Infecting organism/infection |
|---|---|
| Pyogenic | *Staphylococcus aureus* (pneumonia, sepsis) |
| | *Streptococcus pneumoniae* (pneumonia) |
| | *Pseudomonas* spp. (sepsis) |
| | *Klebsiella* spp. (sepsis) |
| | *Neisseria meningitis* (meningitis) |
| | *Neisseria gonorrhoea* (gonorrhoea) |
| Intestinal infections | *Escherichia coli* (enteritis) |
| | *Shigella* spp. (dysentery) |
| | *Salmonella* spp. (typhoid) |
| | *Helicobacter pylori* |
| Mycobacteria | *M. tuberculosis* (tuberculosis) |
| | *M. avium-intracellulare* (atypical infection) |
| | *M. leprae* (leprosy) |
| Clostridia | *Clostridium perfringens* (gas gangrene) |
| | *Clostridium tetani* (tetanus) |
| Chlamydia | *Chlamydia trachomatis* (pelvic inflammatory disease, trachoma) |
| Mycoplasma | *Mycoplasma pneumoniae* (atypical pneumonia) |
| Spirochaetes | *Treponema pallidum* (syphilis) |
| Actinomycetes | *Actinomyces* spp. (actinomycosis) |

**TABLE 19.4** Fungal infections and their locations

| Location | Infection |
|---|---|
| Skin surface | Dermatophytes (tinea) |
| Mucosae | *Candida albicans* |
| | *Aspergillus* spp. |
| Subcutaneous | Mycetoma-causing species |
| Systemic | *Cryptococcus neoformans* |
| | *Histoplasma capsulatum* |

**TABLE 19.5** Protozoal infections and their habitat

| Habitat | Infection |
|---|---|
| Lymph node and systemic | *Toxoplasma gondii* |
| | *Leishmania* spp. |
| Skin and systemic | *Leishmania* spp. |
| Intraerythrocytic, central nervous system | *Plasmodium falciparum* |
| Intestine | *Entamoeba histolytica* |
| | *Cryptosporidium parvum* |
| | *Giardia lamblia* |
| Liver | *Entamoeba histolytica* |

**TABLE 19.6** Helminth infections and the habitat of helminths

| Habitat | Infection |
|---|---|
| Bladder, liver and gut | *Schistosoma* spp. |
| Intestine | *Necator* and *Ankylostoma* spp. (hookworms) |
| | *Ascaris lumbricoides* (gut roundworms) |
| | *Trichuris trichiura* (whipworm) |
| | *Strongyloides stercoralis* |
| | *Enterobius vermicularis* (pinworm) |
| Any organ | *Echinococcus granulosus* (hydatid cyst) |

Immunosuppression may be classified as primary (inherited) or acquired, the latter category being by far the most important. The primary conditions also include genetically determined malfunctions of the complement system and leukocytes (*Box 19.2* and *Table 19.7*).

## Overview of Viral Infections

Viruses are intracellular pathogens that use the host cell metabolism for their replication. There are hundreds of species of viruses, which contain either RNA or DNA in their core. The viruses vary in size from 20 nm to 30 nm, and they tend to infect certain cells, i.e. they exhibit tissue tropism. Once inside host cells, the infection may be abortive (viral replication is incomplete), latent (the infection persists but without continuous replication), or persistent (replication produces new virions). Viruses cause disease in many ways, and these are summarized in *Box 19.3*.

---

**Box 19.2** CAUSES OF IMMUNOSUPPRESSION THAT PREDISPOSE TO INFECTIONS

**Primary inherited conditions**
- Agammaglobulinaemia
- Common variable immunodeficiency
- Isolated IgA deficiency
- DiGeorge syndrome (thymic deficiency)
- Severe combined immunodeficiency disease (SCID)
- Wiskott–Aldrich syndrome
- Inherited complement deficiencies
- Inherited leukocyte function defects

**Acquired conditions**
- HIV/AIDS
- Malnutrition
- Extremes of age
- Cirrhosis
- Cancer (solid, lymphoma, and leukaemia)
- Steroid therapy, anticancer chemotherapy, and transplant immunosuppressive therapy
- Autoimmune diseases
- Diabetes mellitus

---

**Box 19.3** PATHOGENESIS OF VIRAL DISEASES

- Entry into a cell via a receptor
- Replication using host cell enzymes or by incorporation into the cell nuclear DNA (e.g. human papillomavirus [HPV])
- Interference with host cell metabolism (e.g. polio)
- Damage to the host cell membrane (e.g. measles, HIV, herpes simplex virus [HSV])
- Direct cytolytic effect of the virus, killing the cell (e.g. cytomegalovirus [CMV], HIV, HSV)
- Damage to mucosal cells, permitting secondary infection (e.g. influenza, measles)
- Damage to host immune cells, permitting opportunistic infections (e.g. HIV)
- Presentation of viral antigen on the host cell surface, inducing attack by host lymphocytes (e.g. hepatitis B)
- Induction of cell proliferation and transformation, producing cancer (e.g. HPV, EBV)

**TABLE 19.7** Immunodeficiency conditions and consequent infections – some representative examples

| Defect | Infections (more common and severe) |
|---|---|
| Reduced number of polymorphonuclear neutrophils | Pyogenic bacteria (*Staphylococcus, Pseudomonas* spp.); fungi (*Candida, Aspergillus* spp.) |
| Defective oxidative burst in leukocytes (chronic granulomatous disease) | Pyogenic bacteria; mycobacteria: many species |
| Interferon-γ receptor deficiency | Mycobacteria: many species |
| Complement defect | Neisseria infections (gonococcus, meningitis) |
| B-cell defect (defective IgG production) | Pyogenic bacteria (*Haemophilus* spp., staphylococci, streptococci) |
| Isolated IgA deficiency | Intestinal giardiasis |
| CD4+ T-helper cell | Virus: CMV, herpes |
| | Bacteria: pyogenic bacteria |
| | Mycobacteria: many species |
| | Fungi: *Candida* spp., cryptococci, *Pneumocystis jirovecii* |
| | Protozoa: *Leishmania donovani* |
| Iatrogenic immunosuppression (e.g. transplantation, steroids) | Mycobacteria: many species |
| | Pyogenic bacteria |
| | Fungi: *Aspergillus* spp. |
| | Protozoa: *Entamoeba histolytica* |
| | Worms: *Strongyloides stercoralis* |

# HIV/AIDS

## Key Points

- HIV/AIDS is caused by a retrovirus, the human immunodeficiency virus (HIV).
- It is a global pandemic.
- HIV destroys the cell-mediated immune system.
- It permits opportunistic infections, in addition to Kaposi's sarcoma and lymphomas.
- AIDS is ultimately fatal, although HIV can temporarily be controlled using chemotherapy.

## History and Epidemiology of the HIV/AIDS Pandemic

AIDS is a disease characterized by profound immunosuppression which leads to opportunistic infections, secondary neoplasms, and neurological disorders. In 1981, clinicians in the USA noted unusual frequencies of hitherto rare conditions – *Pneumocystis jirovecii* pneumonia and Kaposi's sarcoma – in previously well males. These males were homosexual, and had these fatal diseases as a consequence of depleted T-helper cells (CD4+ phenotype): the disease complex was termed the 'acquired immune deficiency syndrome', or AIDS. By 1984, the aetiology of this immunosuppression had been determined as a retrovirus, the modes of

viral transmission described (*Box 19.4*), and the geographical spread of the infection was being investigated.

The viruses that cause AIDS are the HIVs, of which type 1 (HIV-1) is globally distributed, and the second much less frequent type (HIV-2) is mainly restricted to West African countries or people therefrom.

This fatal disease is pandemic. In the year 2011, about 34 million people were living with HIV/AIDS and 1.7 million people died from illnesses related to their infection. Over 90% of infected people live in sub-Saharan Africa, south and east Asia, and South America. In many parts of Africa,

> **Box 19.4** MODES OF TRANSMISSION OF HIV INFECTION
>
> - Heterosexual intercourse
> - Anal sexual intercourse
> - Mother-to-child transplacental and perinatal transmission
> - Intravenous drug users who share contaminated needles
> - Blood transfusion and infected blood products (e.g. factor VIII concentrates)
> - Accidental percutaneous injury with infected blood (e.g. to healthcare workers)
> - To infant via breastfeeding

a quarter of the adult population is infected with HIV, and parts of Asia are similarly affected. In such hyperendemic areas, life expectancy is decreasing, as a consequence of increasing numbers of young adults and infected babies dying of AIDS. In the UK over 6,000 new infections are registered annually, and up to 73,000 of the population have a diagnosed infection.

Over time, the HIV in a person mutates from an M-trophic to a T-trophic strain. This is significant because T-trophic strains are more virulent and T-cell cytolytic.

## 19.1 Special Study Topic

### PATHOGENESIS OF HIV/AIDS

Most adult infections are from the transmucosal passage of HIV virions in body fluids, across the cervical, penile, and rectal mucosae. HIV has a surface glycoprotein molecule, gp120, which binds to the CD4 receptor on host cells. More recently, two co-receptors for gp120 have been described, the binding of one of which is also necessary for HIV infection to occur. CCR5 which is present on macrophages, Langerhans' cells, and CD4+ T cells; and CXCR4 which is restricted to T cells. There are polymorphisms in the CCR5 receptor which may account for the very small number of people who have been significantly exposed to HIV infection yet do not appear to be susceptible. M-trophic HIV strains use CCR5, whereas T-trophic strains use the CXCR4 receptor.

An M-trophic virus enters a susceptible mucosal Langerhans' dendritic (antigen-presenting) cell via the surface CD4 and CCR5 receptors; a CD4+ T cell fuses with the dendritic cell and becomes infected; the infected T cell passes to the local lymph nodes where it activates and infects more CD4+ T lymphocytes, and within days the infection is widely disseminated to lymphoid tissue throughout the body. The other main cell infected by HIV is the macrophage, also via its CD4 surface receptor. This is how infection can spread to the brain, through the microglia (brain macrophages) (Fig. 19.1).

Vertical transmission occurs in up to 25% of pregnancies in HIV-infected mothers in the absence of anti-HIV treatment; this may be via the placenta or the fetal mucosae. In infections by blood, HIV virions directly infect CD4+ T cells.

Once inside a susceptible cell, the HIV RNA genome is transcribed into a matching DNA via a reverse transcriptase enzyme. This can remain in the cytoplasm but, when the cell divides, the HIV DNA enters the nucleus and becomes integrated into the host cell DNA as a provirus. Transcription, productive infection, and then host cell death occur when the cell is activated by cytokines or antigen. Infected T cells die by cytolysis, although the precise mechanisms are unclear.

Immune resistance to HIV infection involves B-cell activation (with lymph node hyperplasia) and natural killer (NK) cells killing infected T cells by apoptosis, but these do not eliminate the infection, which progressively destroys the cell-mediated immune system by destruction of T-helper cells faster than they can be replaced. The huge turnover of HIV and T cells is indicated in *Box 19.5*. This implies that anti-HIV chemotherapy can reduce productive infection and retard the disease, but cannot eliminate the infection completely.

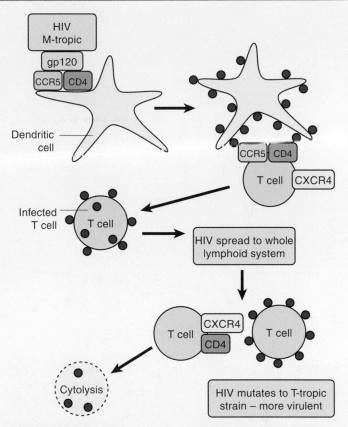

**FIG. 19.1** Human immunodeficiency virus (HIV) infection. HIV enters the Langerhans' dendritic cell, via gp120 binding to the receptors CD4 and CCR5; HIV then spreads to the T cells via the same receptors, and throughout the lymphoid system. Over time, the virus mutates and enters T cells via CD4 and CXCR4 receptors.

---

**Box 19.5** KINETICS OF HIV IN THE LATENT PHASE OF INFECTION

- $10^{10}$ HIV viral particles produced per day in the body
- $10^9$ CD4+ T cells produced and destroyed per day
- A large pool of infected CD4+ T cells with half-life of 1 day (viral DNA integrated)
- A small pool of CD4+ cells latently infected with half-life of <7 days (DNA not integrated)
- A small pool of very long-lived latently infected CD4+ T cells (half life >4 months) with integrated DNA
- Long-lived HIV-infection in brain microglia (DNA integrated)

## Special Study Topic continued . . .

Although the HIV destroys the T-cell system, patients are asymptomatic but can infect others. The peripheral blood CD4+ T-cell count is used as a surrogate marker of bodily cell-mediated immunocompetence. The normal values are 500–2,000/mm$^3$; the count drops transiently during acute infection, and then progressively during the latent phase. Conversely, blood viral loads peak during acute infection then drop, and rise again in the latent phase (Fig. 19.2).

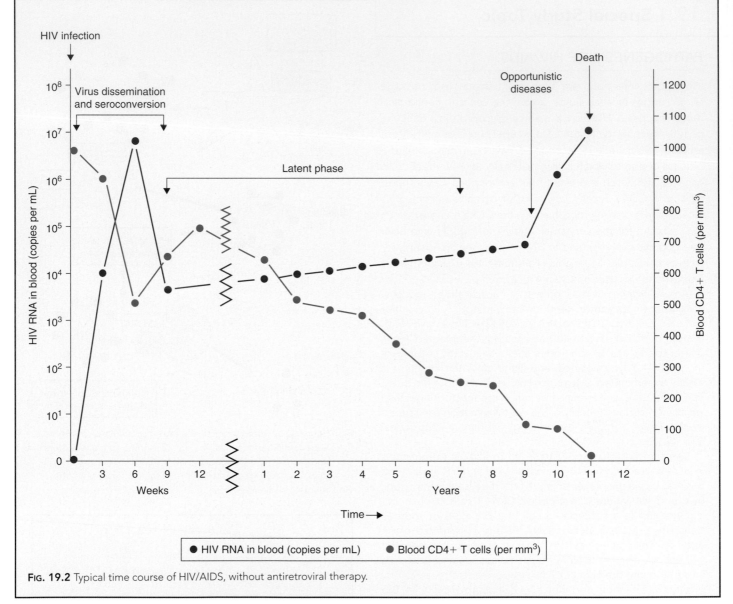

FIG. 19.2 Typical time course of HIV/AIDS, without antiretroviral therapy.

## Natural History and Clinical Features of HIV/AIDS

The natural history of HIV/AIDS is summarized in Fig. 19.3. About half of those individuals infected have a seroconversion illness that mimics acute infectious mononucleosis. During the latent phase, a proportion develop persistent generalized lymphadenopathy (PGL), which is a reactive hyperplasia affecting all lymph nodes. Histologically, there is follicular germinal cell hyperplasia of the B-cell follicles, reacting to virus in the follicle dendritic cells. The lymph nodes later atrophy.

General constitutional symptoms develop years after infection, with weight loss, lassitude, fever, and diarrhoea. These may result from the HIV viral damage to various organs (e.g. gut mucosal HIV infection), but are also attributable to one or more secondary infections; once there is an identified opportunistic disease, the patient is said to

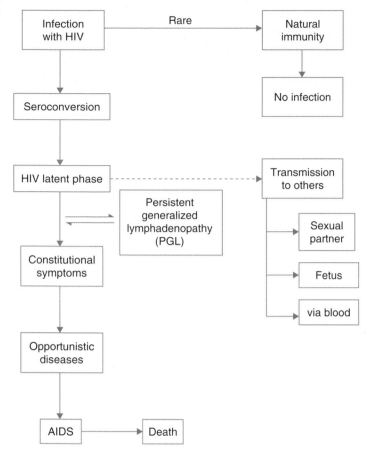

**FIG. 19.3** Overview of HIV infection and clinical outcome.

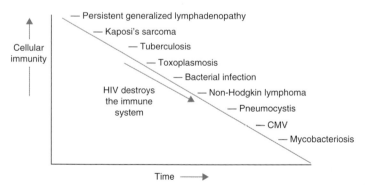

**FIG. 19.4** The progression of HIV disease. As the immune system is destroyed, the more virulent opportunist infections (e.g. tuberculosis) develop earlier, and the less virulent (e.g. *M. avium-intracellulare*) later.

have AIDS, indicating a state of severe cellular immuno-suppression. Without treatment, survival is no more than months. Opportunistic diseases are of varying virulence, and Fig. 19.4 outlines how the more virulent (e.g. tuberculosis) present earlier, when patients have a less-damaged immune system.

Patients may present at several time points during the HIV/AIDS sequence (*Box 19.6*).

The list of opportunistic infections and tumours that are important in HIV-infected adults and children is long, and every organ may be involved. Multiple pathologies are common in the terminal phase of the disease (*Box 19.7*).

---

**Box 19.6** HOW PEOPLE PRESENT WITH HIV DISEASE

- Primary infection, seroconversion illness
- Asymptomatic through incidental HIV screening
- With persistent generalized lymphadenopathy
- With non-specific constitutional illness
- With a specific opportunistic infection, neoplasm, or HIV dementia
- As they are dying of opportunistic disease and wasting
- If infants: failure to thrive and opportunistic infections

---

**Box 19.7** IMPORTANT OPPORTUNISTIC DISEASES IN HIV/AIDS

Viral infections:
- Cytomegalovirus
- Herpes simplex
- JC virus
- Molluscum contagiosum

Bacterial infections:
- *Mycobacterium tuberculosis*
- *Mycobacterium avium-intracellulare*
- *Streptococcus pneumoniae*
- Non-typhoid salmonella infections
- *Treponema pallidum* (syphilis)

Fungal infections:
- *Pneumocystis jirovecii (carinii)*
- *Candida albicans*
- *Cryptococcus neoformans*

Protozoal infections:
- *Cryptosporidium parvum*
- *Leishmania* spp.
- *Toxoplasma gondii*
- Microsporidia

HIV-associated tumours:
- Kaposi's sarcoma
- B-cell non-Hodgkin's lymphoma: cerebral and extracerebral
- Mucosal squamous cell carcinomas: cervix, anus, conjunctiva

Other HIV-associated diseases:
- Central nervous system: HIV encephalitis and dementia
- Gut: mucosal HIV infection and malfunction
- Kidney: HIV-associated nephropathy (HIVAN)

# The Pathological Features of HIV/AIDS

## Viral Infections

### Cytomegalovirus

> **Key Points**
>
> - Cytomegalovirus is a latent infection, which is reactivated in HIV/AIDS.
> - It infects endothelial and epithelial cells.
> - It causes damage to the gut, lung, retina, and brain.

Cytomegalovirus (CMV) is a DNA herpes virus, and latently infects most people. It is acquired transplacentally, during infancy, by respiratory droplet infection, and via sexual intercourse. It reactivates in states of immunosuppression – particularly HIV/AIDS – and also in transplant recipients. By infecting the endothelial and epithelial cells it causes cytolytic cell damage and focal necrosis. Common presentations in HIV/AIDS are a pneumonitis, intestinal lesions with diarrhoea, confusional states from encephalitis, and, importantly, visual defects. Retinal CMV infection is a significant cause of blindness in HIV disease, and is the reason why many patients are given prophylactic anti-herpesvirus therapy. Morphologically, the nucleated layers of the retinal epithelium show the characteristic CMV nuclear and cytoplasmic inclusions, with necrosis.

CMV infection is diagnosed by finding the viral inclusions in biopsies (Fig. 19.5) and virological identification in samples of blood and cerebrospinal fluid (CSF).

### Herpes Simplex

This is representative of the large group of human herpes DNA viruses, which includes herpes simplex virus (HSV) types 1 and 2, herpes zoster, CMV, Epstein–Barr virus (EBV), and human herpes virus 8 (HHV8 – the cause of Kaposi's sarcoma).

HSV is transmitted by direct contact with infected lesions, mainly through sexual intercourse. It primarily affects the genital skin and mucosae, but it is also neurotropic, and can disseminate to internal organs. Whether or not there is clinical primary infection, latent infection is thereafter lifelong, and HSV reactivates in immunosuppression.

The skin and mucosal lesions are painful and erosive. Typically, they are on the penis and vulva, and around the mouth ('cold sore'). Pathologically, the epithelial cells contain characteristic nuclear inclusions of virus (Fig. 19.6), associated with cytolytic necrosis and inflammation. Similar pathology is seen in the skin lesions of chickenpox, caused by herpes zoster.

In HIV/AIDS, severe HSV skin and mucosal ulceration can occur, involving the genitalia, mouth, and oesophagus. It can also cause necrotizing encephalitis and ulcerating conjunctival keratitis; both these lesions also occur in people without evident immunosuppression.

### JC Virus

This is a papovavirus that everyone acquires as a latent infection in childhood. In late HIV disease it can reactivate, and cause a characteristic cytolytic infection of brain oligodendrocytes. This results in white matter necrosis and is termed 'progressive multifocal leukoencephalopathy' (PML) (see Chapter 11, p. 314).

### Molluscum Contagiosum

This is a poxvirus infection that produces multiple small white nodules on the skin. It is normally common in childhood, and is more florid in people with HIV.

## Bacterial Infections

The mycobacterial infections (*M. tuberculosis* and *M. avium-intracellulare*) are described in later sections of this chapter. Streptococcal infection causes both pneumonia

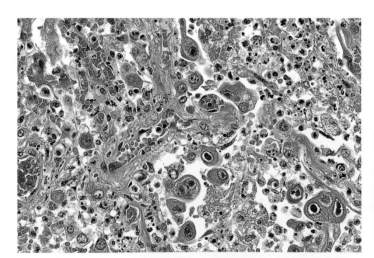

**FIG. 19.5** Cytomegalovirus (CMV) pneumonitis: there are large intranuclear viral inclusions in alveolar epithelial cells.

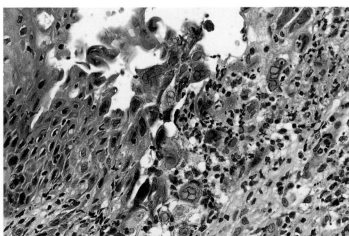

**FIG. 19.6** Herpes simplex virus (HSV) of the penis: the squamous mucosa is eroded and there are multinucleated cells, the nuclei of which contain blocks of HSV virions.

and septicaemia; non-typhoid salmonella infections cause enteritis and septic shock.

## Fungal Infections

### Pneumocystis jirovecii

This is a ubiquitous fungus in the environment (although it was once classified as a protozoan parasite) to which everyone is exposed. Similar to many infections of very low virulent potential, it causes disease only in those significantly immunosuppressed (*Box 19.8*; see also Fig. 19.4). Although it is now seen mainly in those with HIV infection (adults and children) and transplant recipients (especially renal transplants), there have been epidemics in infancy that relate to malnutrition.

The infection can present rapidly with shortness of breath and prostration. A chest radiograph shows fluffy fine shadows in the perihilar zones or throughout the lung fields.

On pathological examination, the lung in pneumocystis pneumonia is solid, pale brown, and dry (Fig. 19.7). Microscopically, the alveoli are filled with masses of cysts, thus preventing gas exchange. The cysts are 3–4 μm in

| Box 19.8 CONDITIONS PREDISPOSING TO *PNEUMOCYSTIS JIROVECII* PNEUMONIA |
| --- |
| • HIV infection |
| • Malnutrition in infancy |
| • Steroid and anticancer chemotherapy |
| • Immunosuppression for preventing organ transplant rejection |

diameter, and contain small nuclei (Fig. 19.8). There is often a mild interstitial lymphoplasmacytic infiltrate (interstitial pneumonitis). Aided by chemotherapy, macrophages phagocytose the fungi to clear the alveoli. However, if the infection persists or returns, there is progressive intra-alveolar organization and interstitial fibrosis. The diagnosis of pneumocystis pneumonia is made by identifying the organisms in sputum or bronchial lavage specimens, or by lung biopsy. Standard treatment is with co-trimoxazole, which enables the lung to return to normal. However, in those with continuing immunosuppression, prophylactic therapy needs to be maintained. If and when pneumocystis pneumonia returns, it tends to cause progressive lung damage, with fibrosis and even cavitation.

### Cryptococcus neoformans

| Key Points |
| --- |
| • *Cryptococcus* sp. is a ubiquitous fungus in the environment. |
| • It infects humans via the respiratory tract. |
| • It disseminates in people with cell-mediated immune defects. |
| • It spreads from the lungs to the brain, lymphoreticular system, and skin. |
| • It is a common cause of cerebral confusional states in HIV/AIDS. |
| • It is usually fatal if not treated. |

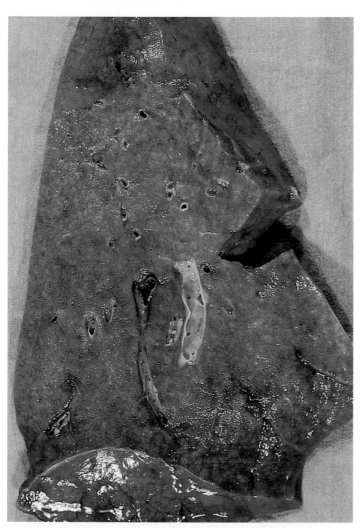

FIG. 19.7 *Pneumocystis jirovecii* pneumonia: there is complete consolidation of the lung.

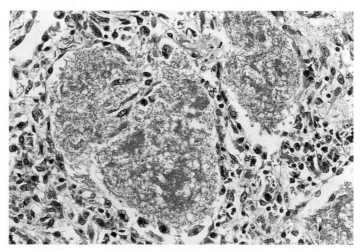

FIG. 19.8 *Pneumocystis jirovecii* pneumonia: the alveoli are filled with numerous tiny cysts with nuclear dots. Interstitial inflammation is present.

This fungus is present globally in bird droppings and the soil. Infection is acquired by inhalation, but clinical disease is uncommon in people who are not immunocompromised. The primary lesion is a pneumonia: it may be localized (a 'cryptococcoma' that can present as a mass on chest radiograph) or, more commonly, as a diffuse process causing breathlessness. HIV-infected patients are prone to developing cryptococcal meningoencephalitis, presenting with confusion or focal neurological signs.

Pathologically, in HIV disease, the fungus elicits a minimal cellular reaction, so within the consolidated lung one sees alveoli filled with yeast. The brain shows milky, thick meninges and mucoid holes in the grey and white matter (resembling Swiss cheese – Fig. 19.9). Histologically, the fungal yeasts have a mucoid capsule; they lie in unactivated macrophages or free in parenchyma and spaces around vessels.

Diagnosis is based on seeing the yeasts in tissue samples (e.g. CSF or biopsies), supported by antibody detection of antigen in blood or CSF (the CrAg test). Modern antifungal

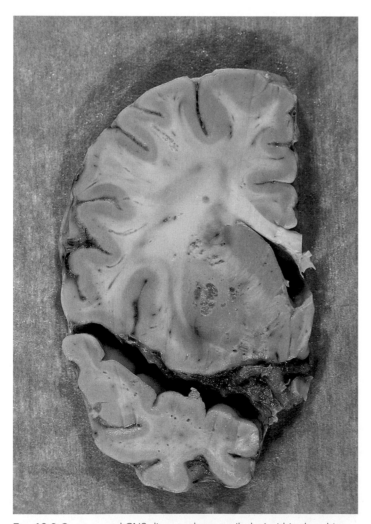

**FIG. 19.9** Cryptococcal CNS disease: there are 'holes' within the white and grey matter – these are large accumulations of *Cryptococcus neoformans*.

therapy can clear the disease, but it always recurs if prophylactic therapy is not continued.

### Protozoal Infections

*Leishmania*- and *Toxoplasma*-mediated infections are described elsewhere in this chapter (see pp. 563–564 and 566–567).

### *Cryptosporidium* sp.

*Cryptosporidium parvum* is a gut parasite of cattle that can be transmitted to humans via contaminated water. In non-immunocompromised people it causes self-limiting diarrhoea. However, in immunocompromised patients, chronic cholera-like diarrhoea results, with malabsorption. *C. parvum* infects the small and large bowel mucosae, the parasites residing in large numbers just within the enterocyte surface membrane; small intestinal villi are blunted and there is an enteritis.

Several species of microsporidia (e.g. *Enterocytozoon bieneusi*) have been newly described in people with severe HIV-associated immunosuppression, and globally are a common cause of diarrhoea. The parasites reside within the enterocyte cytoplasm. As with *Cryptosporidium* sp., the exact pathogenesis of the diarrhoeal disease is unclear.

Diagnosis of both infections is by finding the parasites in faeces, or by gut biopsy (see Fig. 19.12). No specific therapy is available, but anti-HIV chemotherapy often eradicates the infections.

### HIV-associated Tumours

#### Kaposi's Sarcoma

Kaposi's sarcoma (KS) – which was first described in 1872 – is a peculiar proliferation of endothelial cells affecting the skin, mucosal surfaces, lymph nodes, and many internal organs. Although HIV infection greatly increases the frequency of KS, it is not a necessary factor in the lesion's development. In 1994 a virus, human herpesvirus type 8 (HHV8), was found to be the significant factor; this is globally distributed and is transmitted by sexual intercourse, and vertically to children.

In all organs, KS (see Chapter 18, p. 532) develops as a red flat lesion (macule on the skin), and then thickens to plaques and infiltrative red nodules (Fig. 19.10). It behaves as a space-occupying lesion and causes significant local oedema (e.g. in the subcutis and lung). Histologically, the mature lesion is a spindle-cell tumour with red blood cells between the endothelial tumour cells.

#### Lymphoma

HIV-associated lymphomas comprise B-cell, high-grade tumours (see Chapter 8, p. 200), located in extranodal sites. They are 100-fold more common in HIV-infected people than in the normal population, and many are associated with EBV infection. Cerebral lymphoma (see Chapter 11, p. 334) presents with focal neurological signs

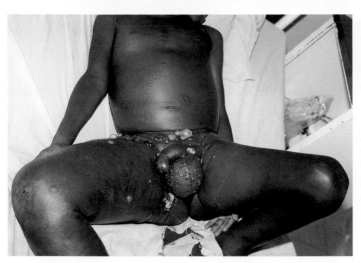

FIG. 19.10 Kaposi's sarcoma: there are widespread nodular lesions around the pelvis, with leg oedema, in an HIV-Infected young man.

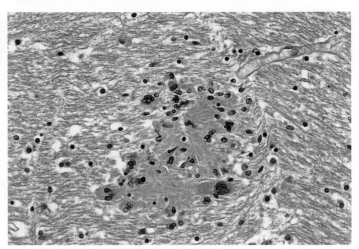

FIG. 19.11 HIV encephalitis: microglia and giant cells are present in the cerebral white matter

and confusion; pathologically, there are one or more tumour masses within the brain, the malignant cells spreading out from the blood vessel walls. Elsewhere, tumours present as oral and intestinal ulcerating lesions, and with pulmonary and retroperitoneal masses. A common histological pattern is high-grade B-cell lymphoma similar to that of Burkitt's lymphoma.

### Mucosal Squamous Cell Neoplasms

Intraepithelial and invasive squamous cell neoplasms of the cervix and anus are aetiologically associated with human papillomavirus (HPV) infections (see Chapter 14, pp. 439–441). People who are co-infected with HIV have a significant risk of developing intraepithelial neoplasia at these sites, which are often detected by screening. However, invasive malignant lesions are less frequent than expected. In central Africa, conjunctival carcinoma (associated with UV light exposure) is also more common in those with HIV infection.

### Neurological Disease in HIV/AIDS

In addition to common central nervous system (CNS) diseases such as toxoplasmosis, cryptococcosis, progressive multifocal leukoencephalopathy (PML), and lymphoma, HIV-associated dementia is a late phenomenon (see Chapter 11, pp. 319–325 for a full discussion of dementia). It appears to be caused by cortical neuronal loss and abnormalities of the dendritic connections. Morphologically, there is cerebral atrophy, and the characteristic HIV encephalitis comprises multiple nodules of infected microglia and microglial giant cells in the white matter (Fig. 19.11). By secreting toxic cytokines, these lesions also affect neural function.

### Skin Disease in HIV/AIDS

The skin lesions in HIV/AIDS include herpetic ulceration, molluscum contagiosum nodules, cryptococcal nodules, mycobacterial infections, lymphoma, Kaposi's sarcoma, and a pruritic maculopapular rash (particularly in Africans).

### Renal Disease in HIV/AIDS

Many opportunistic diseases can affect the kidney (e.g. cryptococcosis, CMV infection of the tubules, pyaemic bacterial infection, tuberculosis, lymphoma), but one specific entity is important – HIV-associated nephropathy (HIVAN). Clinically, this condition presents with renal failure and nephrotic syndrome. Pathologically, it is characterized by focal segmental glomerulosclerosis (FSGS) with a typical 'collapsing' appearance (collapsing glomerulopathy, see Chapter 13, p. 398) and interstitial inflammation with tubular atrophy and dilatation. It appears to be caused directly by HIV, and is significant because it is an ethnically restricted opportunistic disease in HIV/AIDS: it occurs only in people of African descent.

### Paediatric HIV Disease

This is common in many poor parts of the world because, without antiretroviral chemotherapy during pregnancy and delivery, about 25% of fetuses are infected if the mother is HIV infected. The clinical and pathological features are

---

**Box 19.9** FEATURES OF PAEDIATRIC HIV DISEASE

- Failure to thrive
- Lymphadenopathy (PGL)
- Diarrhoea and wasting, with opportunistic parasitic infections
- *Pneumocystis jirovecii* pneumonia
- Bacterial infections, particularly pneumonia
- Lymphoid interstitial pneumonia (LIP) and measles pneumonitis
- Thymic atrophy
- HIV encephalitis and neurodevelopmental delay

listed in *Box 19.9*. Without specific treatment, the mortality rate in children is 50% by the age of 3 years, and few survive 5 years. Malaria is not aggravated by HIV infection.

## Treatment of HIV/AIDS

This hugely complex area comprises specific antiretroviral therapy (ART), e.g. by inhibiting the reverse transcriptase enzyme, in addition to specific therapy for opportunistic infections and tumours, and prophylaxis against opportun-

---

**Box 19.10** HIV THERAPY

- Antiretroviral therapy (ART) slows down HIV virion production and prolongs life
- ART permits partial restoration of CD4+ T-cell counts and immune status
- ART prevents or enables the patient to eliminate many opportunistic diseases
- Specific prophylaxis (e.g. co-trimoxazole against *Pneumocystis jirovecii*) prolongs life
- All of these therapies have potentially severe toxic side effects (e.g. marrow suppression, liver damage, atherogenesis, redistribution of body fat stores)

---

istic infections. The major clinicopathological points of HIV therapy are listed in *Box 19.10*.

### Immune Reconstitution Inflammatory Syndrome

Immune reconstitution inflammatory syndrome (IRIS) or immune recovery or immune restoration syndrome is an inflammatory reaction in HIV-infected patients which occurs paradoxically with ART or highly active antiretroviral therapy (HAART). The syndrome may be evoked with the start or re-commencement of treatment or a change in the treatment regimen to more active ART drugs. With the restoration of immunity following treatment, there is an over-zealous inflammatory or immune-related response to specific infectious or non-infectious antigens.

The most frequently encountered infections are *Mycobacterium tuberculosis* (TB), cryptococcal meningitis, varicella-zoster, herpesviruses, CMV, *Pneumocytis jirovecii* pneumonia (PCP), and hepatitis B and C. Other conditions such as *Mycobacterium avium* complex (MAC) and latent cryptococcal infection have also been reported. The non-infectious sequelae include rheumatoid arthritis and other autoimmune diseases. Indeed, in a third group of patients their innate immune make-up (specific HLA alleles such as HLA class II, interleukin-1 (IL-1), IL-6, tumour necrosis

---

**CASE HISTORY 19.1**

### HIV/AIDS IN AFRICA

A 35-year-old African male presented to his local hospital in West Africa with a 6-month history of weight loss and intermittent diarrhoea with watery stools (not bloody). Direct examination of the faeces showed oocysts of *Cryptosporidium* spp. (Fig. 19.12), and serology confirmed the clinical suspicion of infection with HIV-1. His blood CD4+ T-cell count was 55/mm³. He thus had AIDS.

Being relatively wealthy, the patient could afford to be treated with antiretroviral drugs; his diarrhoea ceased and he put on weight. His CD4 count rose to 200/mm³, but

he became intolerant of the anti-HIV drugs and stopped them. He also stopped taking regular co-trimoxazole prophylaxis therapy. After 2 months his weight had fallen again, and he was readmitted with fever and a cough. a chest radiograph showed pneumonia, and blood culture indicated a *Streptococcus pneumoniae* bacteraemia. Antibiotics suppressed this infection.

Six months later, he was admitted for the last time, fitting and in coma. Despite empirical anti-toxoplasmosis therapy, the patient died. *Post mortem*, the swollen brain showed a large haemorrhagic mass in the basal ganglia; histology confirmed *Toxoplasma gondii* as the cause (Fig. 19.13).

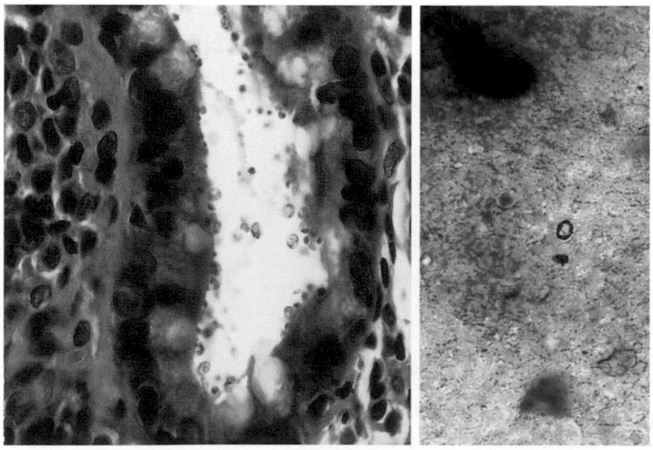

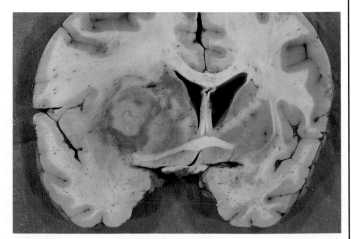

**FIG. 19.12** Cryptosporidiosis. Right: oocysts of *Cryptosporidium* sp. in the faeces (Ziehl–Neelsen staining). Left: rectal crypt lined by numerous parasites.

**FIG. 19.13** Cerebral toxoplasmosis. There is a haemorrhagic necrotic lesion compressing the surrounding brain.

## Clinicopathological Points

1. Treating HIV infection and reducing the viral infection load permits partial recovery of the cell-mediated immune system, and thereby indirectly treats several of the opportunistic infections, including cryptosporidiosis, for which there is no specific therapy.

2. Simple prophylactic antibiotics – if taken consistently – can prevent several bacterial infections, pneumocystis pneumonia, and reactivation of toxoplasmosis.
3. During the course of HIV disease, patients have multiple pathologies.

factor [TNF]-$\alpha$) predisposes to the development of IRIS to specific antigens.

An increase in the CD4 cell count and/or a rapid drop in viral load usually accompany IRIS. Although most cases occur in patients who have low CD4 counts and high viral load levels when ART is started, IRIS can occur at any CD4 level. The clinical manifestations usually occur within the 4–8 weeks after commencement of therapy.

# BACTERIAL INFECTIONS

## Mycobacterial Infections

Mycobacteria are aerobic Gram-positive bacilli with a thick waxy cell wall. They are often referred to as acid-fast bacilli (AFBs) because once a stain colour has bound to the wall, it is resistant to decolorization by acid. The standard stain is red carbol fuchsin, the basis of the classic Ziehl–Neelsen (ZN) stain for mycobacteria (see Fig. 19.21). Most mycobacteria are environmental saprophytes (including *M. avium-intracellulare*) and reside in water and soil. However, two species are essentially human adapted, transmitted directly from human to human, and the cause of much human disease: these are *M. tuberculosis* and *M. leprae*, the aetiological agents of tuberculosis and leprosy respectively.

### Tuberculosis

#### Epidemiology

Tuberculosis (TB) is a typical epidemic infection, which affects large numbers in a susceptible population with high mortality and then becomes less virulent over decades and centuries as humans adapt to it. Thus, it accounted for a quarter of adult deaths in the mid-nineteenth century in British cities. Although the incidence subsequently reduced greatly (*Box 19.11*), the frequency of UK cases has risen again since the early 1990s due to overseas immigrants being infected with TB, in addition to HIV co-infection and poverty. In tropical countries, TB has, for more than a century, been a major cause of mortality, but this has now been made even worse by the HIV/AIDS pandemic.

#### Sequence and Pathogenesis of TB Infection

Acquisition of TB is usually by inhalation of bacilli from a patient with cavitating pulmonary TB, and this gives rise to primary TB (Fig. 19.14). The lung lesion is in any lobe, and is usually subpleural. The initial polymorphonuclear leukocyte inflammatory response cannot contain the bacilli, at which point monocyte-derived macrophages phagocytose them. Within hours, bacilli are carried in cells to the draining hilar lymph nodes and the characteristic inflammatory reaction develops in both lung and nodes (the primary complex – Fig. 19.14). There is necrosis of the lesions, which macroscopically are yellowish and are thus termed 'caseous (cheesy) necrosis' (Fig. 19.15). The factors responsible for this necrosis are unclear, but they involve delayed-type (type IV) hypersensitivity phenomena (*Box 19.12*) and coincide with skin test positivity for tuberculous infection. Around the necrosis there are formed granulomas, a product of cell-mediated immunity (CMI) where, after antigenic stimulation and co-presentation with MHC class II molecules, T-helper cells secrete cytokines to active macrophages. Activated macrophages – which morphologically are known as epithelioid cells – have more potent products that are able to kill or neutralize virulent agents such as *M. tuberculosis* (oxide radicals and proteases – Figs 19.16 and 19.17).

#### Primary TB

Tuberculous disease that occurs within 5 years of infection is classified as 'primary TB'. The primary lung/node complex is usually subclinical, and heals spontaneously with fibrous scarring and even dystrophic calcification.

As part of the primary infection there is a bacillaemia with dissemination of infection to many organs (see Fig. 19.14).

---

**Box 19.11** EPIDEMIOLOGY OF TUBERCULOSIS

- 2 billion people infected (a third of the global population)
- 8 million new cases each year globally
- 3 million deaths each year in England and Wales, 8,000 new cases per year (and rising)

These also usually heal, but they may progress or reactivate later to cause 'end-organ TB'. Bone, adrenal gland, kidney, and brain are typical sites, with caseous granulomatous destructive lesions: if they form a tumour-like mass of necrosis, they are called 'tuberculomas'.

The lung apex zone is frequently a site of such dissemination, and bacilli here may remain latent in macrophages for years and even decades. Subsequently, they may reactivate to cause post-primary pulmonary TB. Pleuritis and progressive bronchopneumonic disease can occur in a small proportion of those with primary TB, but this occurs more frequently if they are co-infected with HIV.

If there is a heavy bacillaemia in primary infection and CMI is poor, miliary TB may result (it is called 'miliary' because the lesions resemble seeds – see Fig. 19.19). This represents multiorgan haematogenous dissemination of infection, forming 1- to 3-mm necrotic foci with a poor granulomatous CMI response. The lungs are typically involved. If there is meningeal spread, then death always occurs in the absence of treatment.

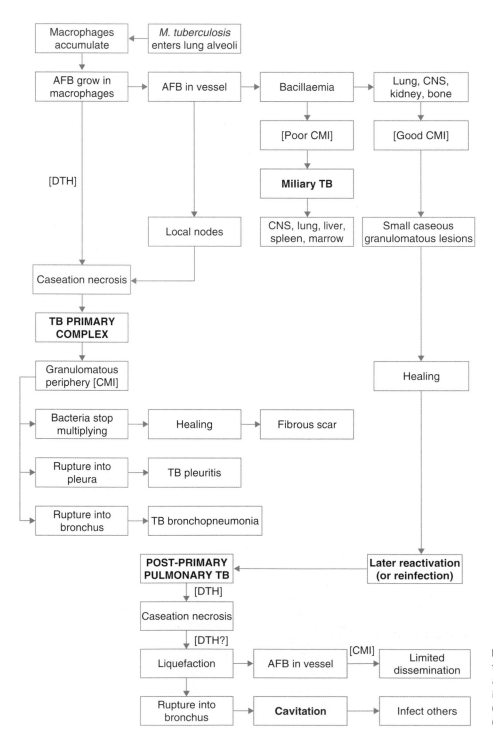

FIG. 19.14 The typical development of tuberculosis (TB): primary complex, miliary TB, and subsequent post-primary pulmonary TB. The immunopathological inputs are indicated: CMI (cell-mediated immunity) and DTH (delayed-type (type IV) hypersensitivity). AFB = acid-fast bacilli.

## Post-primary Pulmonary TB

This is the characteristic form of adult pulmonary TB, and such patients are the source of *M. tuberculosis* infection – they have 'open TB'. The pathogenesis is either reactivation of a previous lesion, or reinfection with a new bacillus, or *M. tuberculosis* infection for the first time. These proportions depend on environmental circumstances. Some 5–10% of those with healed pulmonary primary lesions reactivate later in life, often precipitated by a change in immunological status (*Box 19.13*). Patients present with cough, often haemoptysis,

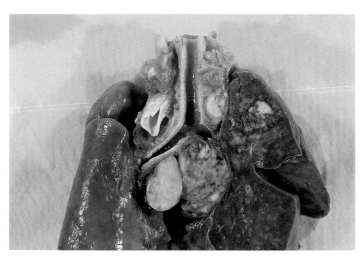

FIG. 19.15 Primary tuberculosis in a child. There is a small lung lesion near the left apex, and large caseating hilar lymph node masses are present.

---

**Box 19.13** CONDITIONS PREDISPOSING TO REACTIVATION OF TUBERCULOSIS LESIONS

- HIV infection
- Alcoholism and liver cirrhosis
- Malnutrition
- Diabetes
- Steroid and immunosuppressive therapy
- Old age

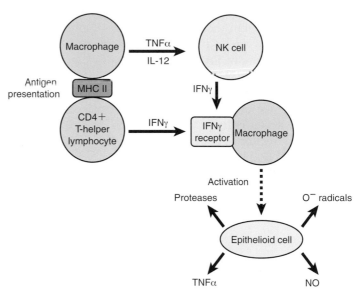

FIG. 19.16 Schematic outline of cell-mediated immunity: macrophages present antigens to a CD4+ T cell via MHC class II molecules, whereas cytokines activate macrophages, which become epithelioid cells. The alternative activation route via natural killer (NK) cells is indicated. IFN = interferon; IL = interleukin; TNF = tumour necrosis factor.

---

**Box 19.12** IMMUNOPATHOLOGICAL RESPONSES TO *M. TUBERCULOSIS* INFECTION

Cell-mediated immunity (CMI):
- involves activation of macrophages to epithelioid cells, forming granulomas
- requires T cells
- is effective in controlling mycobacteria, or killing them
- prevents dissemination of bacilli

Delayed-type (type IV) hypersensitivity (DTH)
- appears at the time of caseation in primary infection
- also manifests as a positive skin test to tuberculoprotein (e.g. Mantoux test)
- causes mass necrosis of *M. tuberculosis* infected tissue
- rapidly controls spread of infection, but at the cost of mass tissue necrosis
- is responsible for liquefaction necrosis of lung lesions
- pathogenesis is not well understood, but involves different T-cell subsets from those involved in CMI

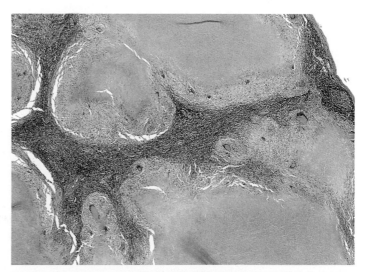

FIG. 19.17 Caseation (pink areas) of a lymph node in primary tuberculosis, with surrounding giant cell granulomas.

and feeling generally ill. The chest radiograph usually has upper zone shadows, and sometimes also cavitation.

The pathological features are as follows. Typically, the lesions are in the apex of the lung, the site of previous seeding of infection. There is an aggressive necrotizing granulomatous pneumonia, and crucially the necrotic material becomes liquefied. If the material communicates with an airway, the necrotic debris is coughed up, along with large numbers of AFBs. This leaves a cavity in the lung, lined by granulomatous inflammation (Fig. 19.18). Peripheral to this is a fibrotic lining, and the whole lesion is termed 'fibrocaseous TB'. There is some passage of bacilli from the lung to local nodes and other internal organs, but this is much less prominent than occurs in primary infection.

Robert Koch – who discovered the tubercle bacillus – described a feature of TB infection in guinea-pigs that helps to explain the difference between primary and post-primary lung lesions. When *M. tuberculosis* is injected into the hind limb of a guinea-pig, a local nodule develops and the draining lymph nodes enlarge with caseation. If a second subcutaneous infection is injected into the other hind limb 4–6 weeks later, a nodule develops rapidly, ulcerates, and sloughs off; the local node is unaffected. Thus, the tissue reaction is more aggressive the second time round, indicating greater delayed-type (type IV) hypersensitivity (DTH). A similar

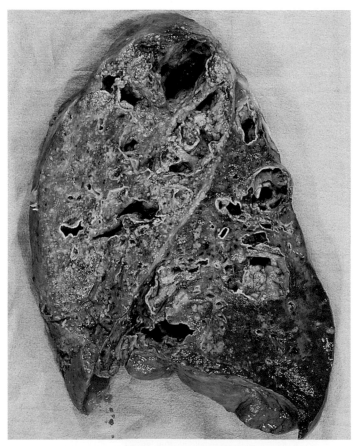

**Fig. 19.18** Post-primary pulmonary tuberculosis: cavitating lesions are present at the apex and elsewhere in the lung.

phenomenon occurs if the second injection is not live bacilli but is sterile tuberculoprotein.

Adults acquiring tuberculosis for the first time also tend to develop a post-primary rather than a primary type response, unless they are HIV-infected.

With proper anti-tuberculous treatment, the mortality rate of adult pulmonary TB is <10%. Although the granulomatous inflammation subsides, the cavities and scarring remain. Full anti-TB therapy takes several months to complete. Failure to complete the course may permit renewal of infection and, worse, the development of drug-resistant strains of *M. tuberculosis*.

It is important to identify and treat the disease rapidly, because the lung cavity lining is a rich source of bacilli that can infect others. One complication is massive haemoptysis because the inflammation may erode into a bronchial artery. Chronically, colonization of the cavity by an aspergilloma (see later) may occur.

### Diagnosis of TB

The main diagnostic methods are direct examination of sputum, tissue, CSF, and so on for AFBs and culture of suspected material (culture has higher sensitivity and enables identification of which particular *Mycobacterium* sp.). Tissue is obtained by knife biopsy, fine-needle aspiration of peripheral nodes, and CT-guided biopsy of, e.g. deep lymph nodes. It is essential that such material be submitted for culture as well histology. Increasingly, polymerase chain reaction (PCR) technology is used for rapid sensitive diagnosis on fresh tissue material and, furthermore, for the rapid identification of sensitivity to rifampicin, the main antituberculosis drug.

### Tuberculosis in HIV/AIDS

HIV is now the major risk factor for reactivation of previous TB infection: indeed, instead of a lifetime risk of 5–10% reactivation, there is a 10% per annum risk of disease. Similarly, primary infections in HIV-infected people are much more aggressive than in non-infected people.

Patients present with fever, severe malaise, weight loss, and diarrhoea, and the tuberculous disease is usually disseminated. Any organ can be affected, including the lung with miliary nodular disease, lymph nodes, intestine, and meninges. If presentation is relatively early during the course of HIV disease, the pathology is granulomatous and AFBs are relatively sparse. However, in the state of terminal immunosuppression, the lesions are non-reactive ('anergic TB'): there are no epithelioid cells, giant cells, or granulomas, just necrotic macrophages and huge numbers of bacilli (Figs 19.19 and 19.20). Patients die in a state of toxic shock, probably related to the release of the cytokine tumour necrosis factor α (TNFα).

This pathology is not unique to those with HIV infection. It also occurs in people severely immunosuppressed by other means (see *Box 19.2* and *Table 19.7*).

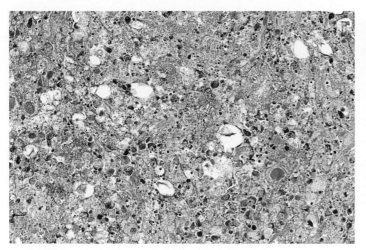

FIG. 19.19 Pulmonary lesions: necrotic macrophages and no granulomas.

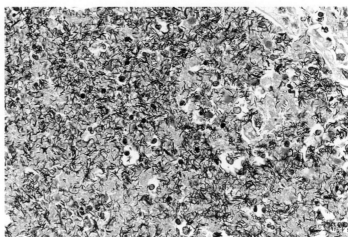

FIG. 19.20 Acid-fast staining to show vast numbers of tubercle bacilli (Ziehl–Neelsen stain).

## TUBERCULOSIS IN A HOMELESS INTRAVENOUS DRUG USER

A 35-year-old unemployed white male lived in a central London doorway and was known to be injecting heroin regularly. He had not been seen for several days until he was found by the police, slumped on a park bench. He was incoherent, and was taken to the police station where initially he was thought to be on a heroin 'high'. However, when next morning his conscious level was worse and his breathing was obviously fast and shallow, he was brought to the hospital accident and emergency department.

He was very thin. A chest radiograph showed widespread fine nodularity: the differential diagnosis was bacterial or tuberculous lung disease. His blood pressure was 80/55 mmHg. A sample of sputum contained numerous AFBs on Ziehl–Neelsen staining. Blood toxicology showed traces of heroin metabolites, but this was insufficient to account for the male's mental status. As a result of his lifestyle and presumed TB infection, the blood was also tested for HIV and hepatitis B and C virus infections: he was HIV negative, but HBV and HCV positive.

He was commenced on intravenous anti-TB therapy and oxygen by mask. He appeared to improve, with rising blood $PO_2$ and blood pressure, but on the fifth day of treatment he went into cardiorespiratory failure, and then asystole. Despite resuscitation measures – which were undertaken despite his being a TB risk to healthcare workers – the male died.

*Post mortem*, he had miliary TB of the lung (Fig. 19.21) and hilar lymph nodes. Histology showed poor granuloma formation and abundant AFBs in the lesions (see Figs 19.19 and 19.20); the lung was very oedematous. There were no old calcified lung lesions. The liver appeared macroscopically normal, but on histology there was stage 3 fibrosis and chronic portal inflammation, consistent with HCV infection at the pre-cirrhotic phase. The results of sputum culture were returned 2 weeks later and showed the presence of *M. tuberculosis*, with normal drug sensitivity.

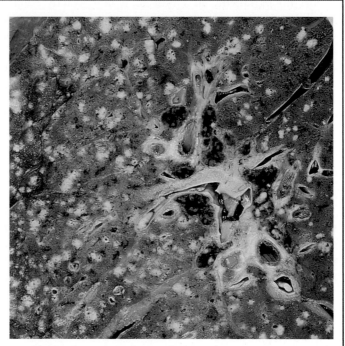

FIG. 19.21 Miliary tuberculosis in the lung: there are numerous small white necrotic lesions in the parenchyma and the hilar lymph nodes.

## Clinicopathological Points

1. Malnourished intravenous drug users are at high risk of acquiring TB.
2. This patient's infection had the morphology of severe primary TB, rather than a reactivation lesion.
3. Despite appropriate chemotherapy, patients with advanced TB may die in shock – perhaps due to an excessive immunological reaction initiated by the anti-TB drugs rapidly killing the large bacillary load.
4. Incoherence in drug users may be due to medical illness, and not to toxic substances.

## Mycobacterium avium-intracellulare

The patterns of *Mycobacterium avium-intracellulare* (MAI) clinical pathology are listed in Box 19.14.

---

**Box 19.14** PATTERNS OF *MYCOBACTERIUM AVIUM-INTRACELLULARE* CLINICAL PATHOLOGY

- Immunocompetent patients: neck lymph node infection
- Immunocompetent patients with damaged lungs: necrotizing bronchopneumonia
- Immunosuppressed patients (e.g. HIV): widespread infection of macrophages

---

Humans are constantly infected with MAI through food and water supplies but, until the HIV pandemic, clinical disease was uncommon. Pre-AIDS, the major disease was a granulomatous necrotizing lymphadenitis affecting the cervical nodes, mainly in children, which exactly resembled TB pathologically. Infection is acquired by mouth. Treatment – after culture identification of the pathogen – is surgical drainage, but chemotherapy is not required.

Chronic bronchopulmonary infection occurs in already damaged lungs (e.g. by TB or bronchiectasis). The MAI colonize poorly drained or aerated lung zones, causing granulomatous necrotizing inflammation similar to TB itself, with progressive lung destruction. The preferred treatment is surgery plus chemotherapy.

The most frequent MAI disease is now part of HIV/AIDS. Towards the terminal phase of disease (see Fig. 19.4), such patients present with fever, diarrhoea, and lymphadenopathy. The standard work-up includes bone marrow biopsy and blood culture to look for MAI infection, because there is bacillaemia and AFBs are present within macrophages throughout the lymphoreticular system: bone marrow, lymph nodes, gut mucosa, spleen, and liver. Nodules and sheets of highly parasitized cells without granuloma formation are seen. As MAI is of low virulence, there is usually no necrosis (Fig. 19.22). Antibiotic treatment is both difficult and expensive.

## Leprosy

---

### Key Points

- Leprosy is caused by *Mycobacterium leprae*.
- It is the most common global cause of peripheral neuropathy.
- It is characterized by infection of the peripheral nerves and skin.
- It has an immunopathological spectrum of disease.
- It is treatable and curable if diagnosed early.

---

Today, leprosy is uncommon in the UK (up to 30 new patients present each year), but globally there are still

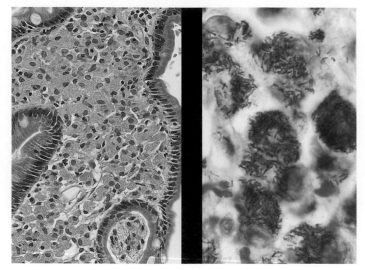

**FIG. 19.22** *Mycobacterium avium-intracellulare* infection. Left: duodenal biopsy with macrophages filling the lamina propria (haematoxylin and eosin stain). Right: the cells contain many acid-fast bacilli (Ziehl–Neelsen stain).

up to one million sufferers in the tropics and subtropics, with 600,000 new cases a year, particularly in India. This is markedly fewer than two decades ago, due to determined global case finding and treatment, and mass bacille Calmette–Guérin (BCG) immunization (BCG may not prevent TB in the tropics, but it is effective in preventing leprosy). Leprosy is important because it is the most common cause of peripheral nerve disease and, if diagnosed early, is curable and the feared deformities are preventable.

Leprosy is the result of infection by *Mycobacterium leprae*, which, apart from a few monkeys and armadillos in the wild, affects only humans. This bacillus has never been cultivated in the laboratory, although the mouse footpad supports growth and may be used for drug resistance testing. The habitat and mode of infection of the bacterium are still unclear, but it is probable that bacilli are inhaled from secretions from the respiratory tract of patients with the lepromatous form of the disease (see below).

The leprosy bacillus targets Schwann cells of the peripheral nerves, and is also phagocytosed by macrophages. Control of bacillary replication is via classic CMI, and many of those infected never develop clinical disease (Fig. 19.23). Those who develop the clinical disease (with an incubation period of several years) generally have either:

- lepromatous leprosy: there are large numbers of organisms and little CMI, indicating a specific immune defect to leprosy
- tuberculoid leprosy: there is granuloma formation (i.e. good CMI) and few or no evident infectious organisms.

### Clinical Features

In lepromatous leprosy there are multiple symmetrical reddish patches and nodules on the skin, which may be tender,

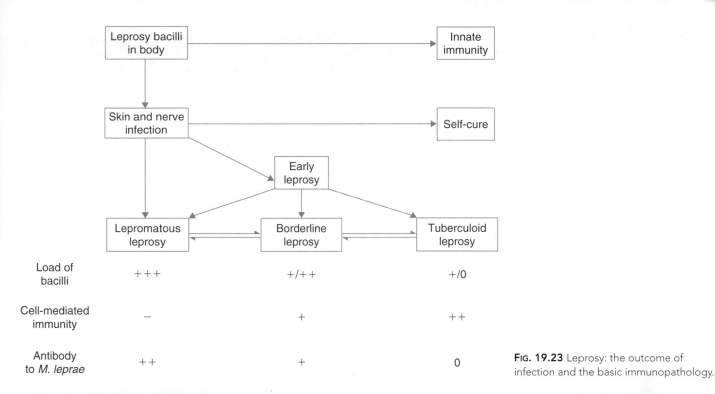

| | Lepromatous leprosy | Borderline leprosy | Tuberculoid leprosy |
|---|---|---|---|
| Load of bacilli | +++ | +/++ | +/0 |
| Cell-mediated immunity | − | + | ++ |
| Antibody to *M. leprae* | ++ | + | 0 |

FIG. 19.23 Leprosy: the outcome of infection and the basic immunopathology.

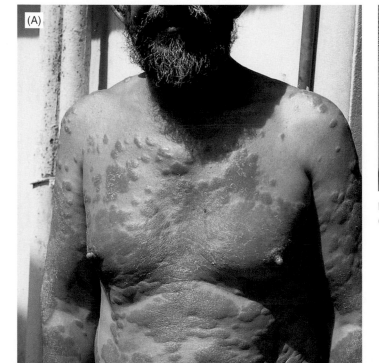

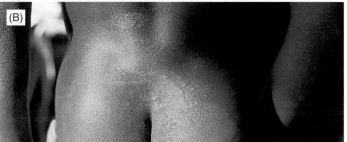

FIG. 19.24 Clinical leprosy: (A) widespread nodular lepromatous lesions; (B) tuberculoid leprosy with few, hypopigmented, flat lesions.

but not itchy. The peripheral nerves are progressively thickened and damaged, producing glove-and-stocking anaesthesia of the hands and feet (Fig. 19.24A).

In contrast, in tuberculoid leprosy the skin lesions are few and asymmetrical, with a raised margin and hypopigmented centre; they are often anaesthetic (Fig. 19.24B). The peripheral nerves are thickened; damage may be acute with relatively sudden anaesthesia or motor damage.

In advanced leprosy, the surface lesions may be destructive (e.g. of the nose) and disfiguring, but the effects of nerve damage are more important. Sensory anaesthesia permits trauma to feet and hands, secondary ulceration, and osteomyelitis; motor nerve damage causes paralyses such as ulnar nerve palsy and claw hand.

## Pathology

In lepromatous leprosy, there are abundant mycobacteria in masses of macrophages in the skin, and also often in dermal and peripheral nerve Schwann cells (Figs 19.25 and 19.26). The bacilli are non-toxic, and can be detected by incising a skin lesion, smearing some of the dermal 'juice' on to a slide, and staining for AFBs (this is called 'taking a slit skin smear'). Nerves in this form of the disease may undergo progressive fibrosis, resulting in glove-and-stocking anaesthesia. Other organs may also be infected by leprosy bacilli, such as the testes (with chronic atrophy causing gynaecomastia), iris (causing iritis), and larynx.

Tuberculoid leprosy – so called because it shares some histopathological features with TB – is characterized by granulomas in and around nerves in the skin (Fig. 19.27), and bacilli are detected only with difficulty. Destructive granulomas affect the endoneurium of peripheral nerves, causing anaesthesia and motor damage, whereas in some patients a major peripheral nerve may undergo caseous-type necrosis causing irreparable damage.

## Management

The disease may be diagnosed from the typical skin and neurological features, supported by slit skin smears. For patients in industrialized countries, a skin or nerve biopsy

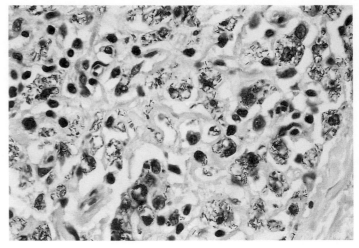

**Fig. 19.26** Lepromatous leprosy: the macrophages contain many acid-fast leprosy bacilli (Wade–Fite stain).

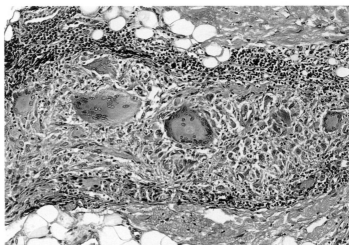

**Fig. 19.27** Tuberculoid leprosy: skin biopsy showing a deep nerve disrupted by a giant cell granulomatous infiltrate.

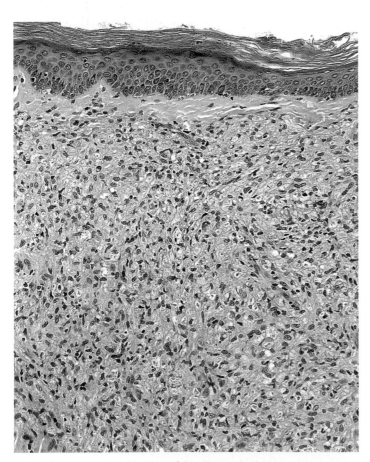

**Fig. 19.25** Lepromatous leprosy of the skin: packed macrophages are present under the epidermis.

is always performed for proper confirmation and accurate subtyping of the disease.

Proper treatment of leprosy involves multidrug therapy with rifampicin and other mycobactericidal or static drugs. Most of the bacteria are rapidly killed, but it may take years for all the leprosy bacillus antigen in lepromatous patients to be cleared. In those patients with chronic disabilities due to neuropathy, plastic surgery may be beneficial (e.g. tendon transfer), and good care of anaesthetic feet can prevent ulceration.

## Syphilis

Syphilis is a systemic infection caused by *Treponema pallidum*. It is transmitted mainly by sexual intercourse (sexually transmitted syphilis), and less commonly via the placenta (congenital syphilis).

The organism is a spirochaete, of length 4–14 μm and diameter 0.2 μm, which cannot be grown in culture (Fig. 19.28). It invades the penile and vulvovaginal

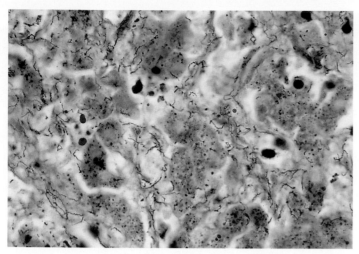

**FIG. 19.28** Spirochaetes of *Treponema pallidum* in congenital syphilis (Warthin–Starry stain).

mucosae directly and, at that site, the primary lesion – a chancre – develops. Within hours of infection, spirochaetes disseminate via lymphatics and the bloodstream, and reactive lymphadenopathy develops. Thereafter, the disease sequence is unpredictable, but a proportion of patients go on to develop secondary and tertiary syphilis, which have distinct clinical pathologies (Fig. 19.29).

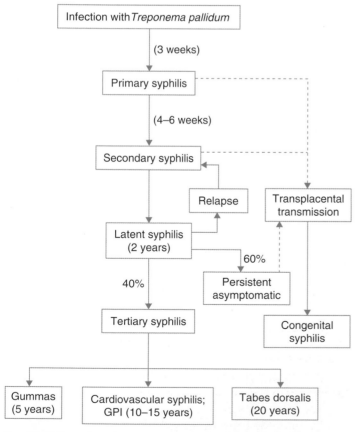

**FIG. 19.29** Sequelae of events in untreated syphilis, with time scales and approximate proportions. GPI = general paralysis of the insane.

## Clinical and Pathological Features

The primary lesion or chancre is a punched-out ulcer, which heals within weeks with minimal scarring. Histologically, there is associated epithelial hyperplasia, a plasmacytic perivascular inflammatory infiltrate, oedema, and abundant spirochaetes. A characteristic feature of primary and secondary syphilis lesions is a reactive swelling of vascular endothelial cells: this is termed 'endarteritis obliterans' (and is also found in other infections such as TB).

In secondary syphilis, the mucosal surfaces develop erythematous rashes (condylomata lata), with generalized lymphadenopathy, representing a reaction to the initial haematogenous spread of infection. Histologically, they resemble primary lesions.

There are three basic forms of tertiary lesion: the gumma, cardiovascular lesions, and neurosyphilis. Gummata are necrotic lesions of varying size (up to centimetres) that appear in the skin, testis, liver, and bones (e.g. the nose, with collapse). Histological examination shows the presence of necrotic granulomas, similar to those of TB, and spirochaetes are rarely identified.

The *cardiovascular lesions* are arteritis affecting the media of large vessels; there is chronic inflammation and destruction of the elastic elements critical for maintenance of the artery diameter. Thus, the classic lesion is proximal thoracic aortitis, which can manifest as an aneurysm (the rupture of which is usually fatal), dilatation of the aortic valve ring with aortic regurgitation, or coronary artery stenosis with myocardial ischaemia.

*Neurosyphilis* (see Chapter 11, p. 312) comprises meningitis, tabes dorsalis, and general paralysis of the insane (GPI). The meningovascular inflammation is an example of endarteritis obliterans, and can cause ischaemic cerebral lesions. There may also be small meningeal gummata. Tabes dorsalis is a degeneration of the posterior spinal columns and dorsal nerve roots; it results from chronic inflammation of the nerve roots. GPI is a cerebral atrophy characterized by loss of neurons, a microglial cell reaction, and visible spirochaetes in the tissues.

*Congenital syphilis* is rare, but is a cause of abortion, fetal hydrops, or newborns with hepatosplenomegaly and pneumonia. Abundant spirochaetes are present in the lesions. Later, central nervous system, bone, and mucocutaneous lesions may develop.

## Diagnosis

Although the primary and secondary lesions have distinct histopathology and usually evident spirochaetes, the mainstay of diagnosis is serological. The screening tests are the rapid plasma reagin (RPR) and Venereal Disease Research Laboratory (VDRL) tests – these detect autoantibodies and are not specific. Specific tests are the treponemal haemagglutination assay (TPHA) and treponemal immobilization test (TPI).

# FUNGAL INFECTIONS

Most fungi are saprophytes living in the soil, and humans are constantly exposed to infection, particularly through the respiratory tract. A few potential pathogens, such as *Candida* sp., are also part of the normal human flora. In nature they usually grow in a mycelium composed of elongated branching cells 5–10 μm across, called hyphae; in humans, they may change their growth morphology and form rounded cell yeasts.

## *Candida* sp.

*Candida albicans* is part of the normal flora of the mouth and gut, and some 10% of females have the infection in the vagina. Clinical disease is common and precipitated by a wide range of immunological defects (*Box 19.15*). The more common superficial infections involve the mouth, vagina, and oesophagus. The fungus proliferates in, and invades, the squamous epithelium, causing local irritation and even ulceration. Grossly, the mucosal surfaces are thickened and pale (Fig. 19.30). Histologically, *Candida* sp. is characterized by having both hyphae and yeast forms in tissue (Fig. 19.31).

In severe infections, there is haematogenous dissemination of *Candida* sp.; this is particularly common in leukaemic patients and is a cause of septic shock. The main organs involved are the kidney, liver, lung, brain, and meninges. There are multiple small abscesses within which are clumps of yeasts.

## *Aspergillus* spp.

There are many *Aspergillus* species in the environment, of which *A. flavus* is the most common pathogen. Infection is by inhalation. Clinical disease occurs only if the patient has abnormal defences against infection, or has a structurally abnormal lung. The three main clinicopathological patterns of aspergillosis are indicated in *Box 19.16*.

Aspergilloma is a mass of fungal hyphae growing in a lung cavity that communicates with the airways; it does not invade the lung. The aetiology of the cavity is most commonly previous TB. The condition presents with cough and haemoptysis, and the only curative treatment is to resect the cavity.

---

**Box 19.15** CONDITIONS ASSOCIATED WITH CANDIDIASIS

- Diabetes
- Oral contraceptive pill
- Pregnancy
- Insufficient neutrophil polymorphs
- Phagocyte defects
- Anticancer and transplantation therapy
- Leukaemia
- HIV disease

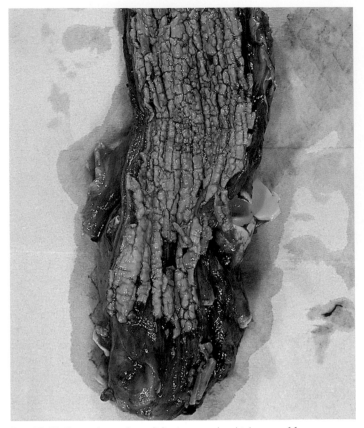

**FIG. 19.30** Oesophageal candidiasis: note the thick coat of fungus on the mucosa.

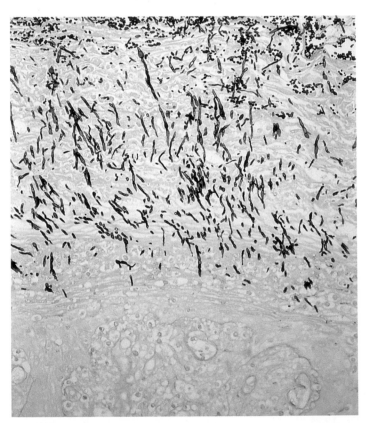

**FIG. 19.31** Oesophageal candidiasis: fungal hyphae (black) are invading the mucosa (Grocott's silver stain).

Bronchopulmonary aspergillosis is a type III hypersensitivity (antigen–antibody) reaction (see Chapter 2, pp. 24–25) that takes place across the bronchial epithelium, reacting to fungal antigens in the airways. Clinically, patients suffer from asthma and eventually bronchiectasis (see Chapter 7, p. 186). The airways are plugged with mucus and eosinophils, and the mucosa is oedematous and inflamed.

Invasive aspergillosis occurs in patients with depleted neutrophil leukocytes, e.g. patients with leukaemia and those receiving cancer chemotherapy. The condition presents with poor lung function, infiltrates on the chest radiograph, and septic shock. The infection is highly necrotizing, with large clusters of aspergillus hyphae invading the bronchial mucosa (Fig. 19.32) and pulmonary arteries, which thrombose, leading to lung infarction. Haematogenous spread may affect other organs, producing areas of necrosis.

## Mycetoma

Mycetoma is a subcutaneous fungal disease that is caused by certain environmental fungi, and is contracted by injury through the skin, mainly in tropical countries. It is a chronic soft-tissue infection that gradually spreads with swelling and dysfunction of the affected limb. There are deep abscesses and fibrosis, sinuses that discharge through the skin, and osteomyelitis if the underlying bone is involved (Fig. 19.33). Visible grains of fungi discharge through the skin sinuses, which may be taken and viewed directly under the microscope to make the diagnosis.

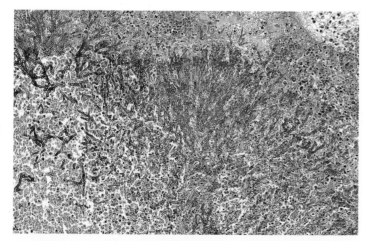

**FIG. 19.32** Invasive aspergillosis: fungal hyphae are infiltrating the bronchial wall.

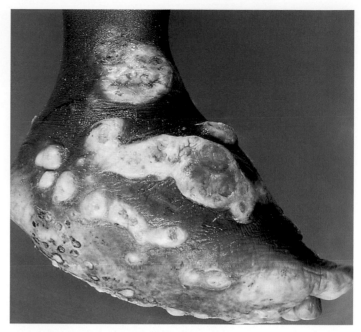

**FIG. 19.33** Mycetoma of the foot: the foot is swollen and there are discharging sinuses.

# PARASITIC INFECTIONS

Parasitic diseases result from infection by protozoa (single cell organisms), helminths (worms), and some arthropods. They range from the rapidly fatal through the chronically morbid, to the incidental and asymptomatic. About 20 genera of protozoa afflict humans, and about 100 species of worms. Some infections are restricted to humans, and others are zoonoses (infections of animals), where humans are infected incidentally but not at a critical stage in the parasite's lifecycle. One protozoal infection alone, *Plasmodium falciparum*, is a major public health problem for a third of the world's population, and in Africa it kills an estimated one million children each year.

Parasitic diseases are not synonymous with tropical diseases, which incorporate the natural results of poverty, overcrowding, malnutrition, and lack of clean water and adequate disposal of excreta. In industrialized countries many parasites are endemic at low levels (e.g. amoebae and hydatid cysts), and several at high levels (e.g. *Toxoplasma gondii* and threadworms). Each year, a fifth of the global population flies to distant countries: visitors to endemic zones can bring back their newly acquired parasites before the incubation period is over, and present clinically at home.

## Parasite Pathophysiology

The intensity of infection often determines whether an infection is symptomatic. In the absence of effective host resistance, protozoa can replicate within the host and build up fatal intensities, e.g. in cerebral malaria. Conversely, most worms do not multiply in the human host, but increase in numbers by repeated infections (the life cycles are not detailed here, but details may be found in standard texts on parasitology).

Resistance to parasitic infection is a vast and complex subject. Many intracellular protozoal infections are subject to control by host cell-mediated immunity; extracellular infections tend to elicit antibody responses that modulate the degree of infection. In worm infections, both cell-mediated and antibody-mediated immune mechanisms are important – examples are strongyloidiasis and schistosomiasis.

The pathogenic mechanisms by which parasites cause disease vary greatly, e.g. in schistosomiasis the damage is immunopathological, with secondary scarring. The lesions of amoebiasis are entirely due to direct cytotoxic tissue damage.

A few parasites are associated with the development of malignant tumours: examples are *Schistosoma haematobium* with squamous cell carcinoma of the bladder, and *Plasmodium falciparum* malaria with Burkitt's lymphoma (high-grade B-cell lymphoma). The parasites do not directly produce any carcinogenic agent; rather they appear to act as tumour promoters, or cause immunosuppression.

## Protozoal Infections

### *Malaria*

> **Key Points**
>
> - Malaria is a mosquito-transmitted infection.
> - It is endemic in tropical regions, but travellers can present anywhere.
> - *Plasmodium falciparum* infects only the red blood cells.
> - It causes anaemia by red cell rupture.
> - It causes cerebral malaria (coma) with significant mortality.

The main and most pathogenic of human malarias is that caused by *Plasmodium falciparum*. This disease was once endemic in Europe, but the UK now has about 2,000 imported cases of falciparum malaria each year, with a fatality rate of about 1%. In the tropics – and particularly in Africa and south-east Asia – more than two billion people live in zones at risk for malaria. About 90% of deaths from malaria occur in sub-Saharan Africa.

In malarial zones, at birth there is maternal antibody-mediated immunity from infection. Thereafter, in areas of regular transmission, children are the main sufferers (malaria is a major cause of childhood mortality in the tropics), and survivors acquire immunity, the nature of which is not well understood. By adulthood, clinical episodes of infection are uncommon, unless the person loses his or her immunity by moving away from an endemic zone. In contrast, visitors (e.g. European tourists) to malarial areas have no

immunity, and unless they take antimalarial prophylaxis they are liable to become infected. The clinical features of malaria are detailed in *Box 19.17* (and also Fig. 19.34).

### The Lifecycle of *Plasmodium falciparum*

The anopheline mosquito is the vector for malaria. The multiplication of parasites occurs in the liver (without clinical

> **Box 19.17** CLINICAL FEATURES OF MALARIA (SEE ALSO FIG. 19.34)
>
> - Fever: classically, a peak occurs every 2 days
> - Normocytic anaemia
> - Hepatosplenomegaly
> - Prostration
> - Renal failure and shock
> - Pulmonary oedema
> - Hypoglycaemia and acidosis
> - Cerebral malaria, coma leading to death
> - In pregnancy: increased abortion, stillbirth, maternal death, and small fetuses
> - Effects of chronic infection: Burkitt's lymphoma, massive splenomegaly

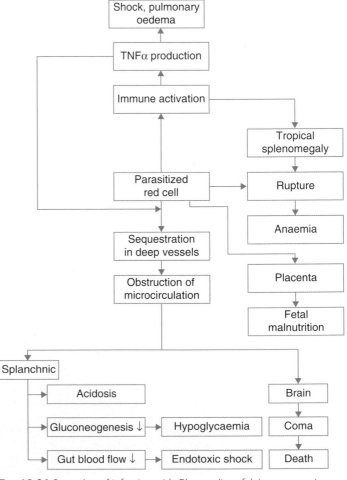

**FIG. 19.34** Sequelae of infection with *Plasmodium falciparum* causing malaria. TNF = tumour necrosis factor.

effects), and then by repeated intraerythrocytic cycles of division (schizogony) and red cell rupture. The incubation period is about 2 weeks, but this may be prolonged.

## Pathology and Pathogenesis of Malaria

Malaria is an intraerythrocytic infection. As a result of red cell rupture at schizogony, there is haemolytic anaemia, the haemoglobin level often falling to <5 g/dL. Parasitaemia rates may be up to 50% of circulating red cells, the trophozoites being visible as small rings, accompanied by some dark-brown haemozoin pigment (Fig. 19.35; see also Fig. 19.39). This pigment is the product of the parasite's metabolism of haemoglobin.

The liver and spleen are moderately enlarged, and dark in colour. The colour derives from the accumulation of haemozoin pigment in the macrophages, phagocytosed from ruptured red cells (Fig. 19.35). Macrophage hyperplasia accounts for some of the organomegaly, along with congestion of the small vessels and sinusoids. The hypoglycaemia, which is particularly prominent in children with malaria, is associated with reduced glycogen stores in the liver.

The kidney and lung may fail in severe falciparum malaria. The kidneys may show the effects of shock (acute tubular necrosis; see 'Septic shock', pp. 573–575), and some very severely affected patients also develop 'blackwater fever', with haemoglobinuria that colours the urine dark red, and casts of haemoglobin that are visible in the tubules.

The pulmonary alveoli may become oedematous, and in some severely affected patients there is shock lung (hyaline membrane disease). There is no specific alveolitis or pneumonia in malaria, and the manifestations are part of the systemic cytokine-mediated effects of shock.

The parasite has a particular affinity for the maternal sinuses of the placenta, and high parasite counts are noted there. This adversely affects fetal nutrition, with resulting high fetal mortality and low birthweight.

Cerebral malaria is the key pathogenic puzzle in falciparum malaria, and is a major cause of death in infected children and adults. Clinically, there is a rapidly deteriorating conscious level and coma, sometimes with focal neurological

signs. With effective treatment and support, recovery may be equally rapid, with no evidence of residual neurological damage in most patients.

In those who die from cerebral malaria, the brain is mildly swollen and very congested, and on slicing it often shows multiple petechial haemorrhages in the white matter (Fig. 19.36). Histologically, the small vessels are packed with parasitized red blood cells, and some vessels have ruptured to cause the haemorrhages. This vascular packing phenomenon is termed 'sequestration'. The probable pathogenesis is indicated in Fig. 19.37. The parasitized cells

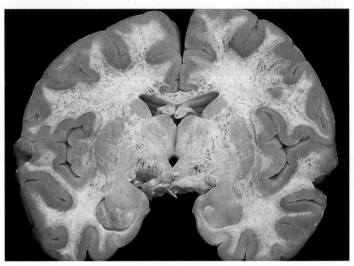

FIG. 19.36 Cerebral malaria in a child: mild swelling, grey cortex (from the haemozoin pigment), and petechial haemorrhages in the white matter.

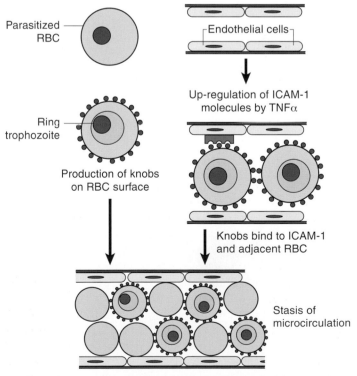

FIG. 19.37 Pathogenesis of sequestration in falciparum malaria. ICAM = intercellular cell adhesion molecule; RBC = red blood cell; TNF = tumour necrosis factor.

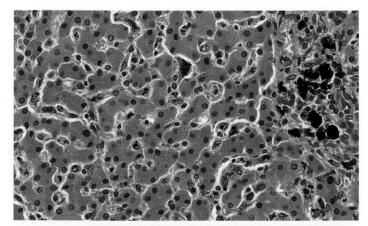

FIG. 19.35 Malarial liver: note the extensive brown haemozoin pigment in Kupffer cells and portal macrophages.

develop 'knobs' on the surface membrane, comprising cell and parasite proteins (Fig. 19.38). These bind to adhesion molecules on the endothelial cells; the most studied of these is intercellular adhesion molecule-1 (ICAM-1). This is up-regulated in malaria, perhaps as a result of increased systemic TNF-α production. The result is stagnation of blood flow and secondary ischaemia of the brain, producing coma. If the stagnation is severe enough, the capillary ruptures and a petechial haemorrhage results.

### Chronic Effects of Falciparum Malaria

Children in Africa who are chronically infected by falciparum malaria are liable to develop a high-grade B-cell lymphoma (Burkitt's lymphoma) if they are also infected early in life with EBV. EBV causes B-cell proliferation and transformation if it is not controlled, and malaria contributes to reduced cell-mediated control of EBV.

Some adults in endemic zones may develop massive splenomegaly with secondary hypersplenism (anaemia and

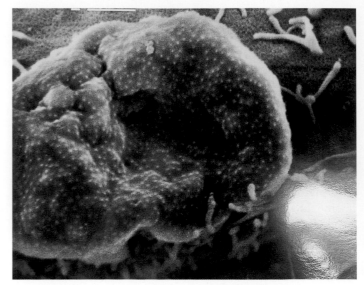

FIG. 19.38 Red cell with falciparum malaria: this scanning electron micrograph shows the tiny knobs on the red cell surface.

## IMPORTED MALARIA

A 60-year-old English female visited the East African coast for a 2-week holiday, and took chloroquine as antimalarial prophylaxis only for the duration of the trip. Two weeks after returning to the UK, she felt unwell and feverish. Although her general practitioner considered influenza, not knowing about her visit to Africa, she was admitted to hospital in a coma that developed over one morning. A blood sample taken in accident and emergency showed *Plasmodium falciparum* trophozoites in her red blood cells (a 30% parasitaemia) (Fig. 19.39).

Immediate intravenous quinine was started, followed by an exchange blood transfusion; this reduced the malaria parasitaemia to 1% within 2 days. However, the woman died from cardiorespiratory failure on the third day, without having regained consciousness. *Post mortem*, the liver and spleen were found to be enlarged and dark brown in colour, the heart flabby (but not infarcted), and the lungs oedematous.

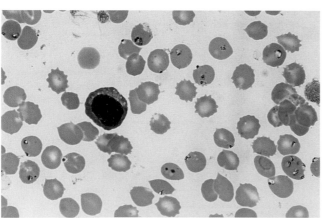

FIG. 19.39 *Plasmodium falciparum* infection of red cells: the blood smear shows many ring forms in red cells (Giemsa stain).

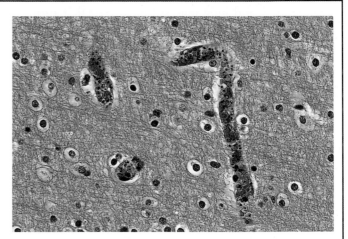

FIG. 19.40 Cerebral malaria: the capillaries are packed with sequestered parasitized red cells.

The brain was swollen, with flattening of gyri, and was plum coloured. On coronal slicing, the brain showed ventricular compression and numerous petechial haemorrhages in the white matter. Microscopy confirmed cerebral malaria, with parasitized red cells packed in the capillaries and venules (Fig. 19.40).

### Clinicopathological Points

1. Falciparum malaria in East Africa (and elsewhere) is often chloroquine resistant; thus prophylaxis was inadequate.
2. Effective antimalarial chemotherapy and exchange transfusion reduce the parasite load in the circulation, but do not immediately flush out the sequestered parasitized red cells in the brain vessels.
3. Fatality can be rapid as in this case, through microvascular ischaemia and impaired nutrition of the brain.

cytopenias) (see Chapter 8, pp. 213–215). Splenomegaly is essentially a lymphoreticular reactive hyperplasia to chronic infection that is idiosyncratic (there is an inherited tendency). There are high immunoglobulin levels in the blood, but parasite numbers are very few. This condition is also referred to as 'tropical splenomegaly syndrome'.

### Diagnosis and Treatment

Diagnosis of acute malaria is by microscopic examination of the blood film. Treatment requires one or more antimalarial drugs to which the parasite is not resistant (resistance to the cheaper drugs such as chloroquine is spreading). In the UK, patients with high blood parasite counts are often also given an exchange blood transfusion.

### Leishmaniasis

Leishmaniasis is a group of diseases caused by protozoa of the genus *Leishmania*. With few exceptions, these are zoonoses (i.e. diseases acquired from animals, the main hosts being canines and small mammals), and transmission is from the bite of sandflies, the vector of infection. The distribution is tropical and subtropical, but includes the Mediterranean littoral; this is why many cases are imported by travellers to the UK.

Three broad groups of diseases are apparent (*Table 19.8*). Morphologically, the parasites are identical, but the species does in part determine the pattern of disease. All are intracellular parasites, and the control of infection is by CMI, similar to what happens with *M. tuberculosis* infection (see Fig. 19.16). Hence, HIV/AIDS alters the clinical pathology of leishmaniasis.

The parasites – which are known as amastigotes in the human part of the lifecycle – are 2–3 μm in size, and divide by binary fission in macrophages.

Cutaneous leishmaniasis is a localized, self-healing condition. An ulcer develops at the site of the infected sandfly bite. The parasites multiply and the inflammatory response is necrotizing. CMI then develops with a granulomatous response, the parasites are controlled and eliminated, and

the ulcer heals with scarring some weeks or months after infection. The diagnosis is confirmed by finding parasites in smears and biopsies from the lesion, with *in vitro* cultivation and PCR-based testing, which can confirm the species. Chemotherapy is still with agents containing antimony (antimonials), and is effective in reducing skin scarring by accelerating healing.

Mucocutaneous leishmaniasis is a variant of cutaneous leishmaniasis, caused specifically by *L. brasiliensis*. In some patients, there is spread of the skin infection to a squamomucosal junction, characteristically on the lips and nose. The resulting inflammation can be very destructive and cause gross disfigurement by bone, soft-tissue, and skin necrosis.

Visceral leishmaniasis – also known as kala-azar – affects only a small proportion of the many people infected with *L. donovani*: these are people who have not generated a sufficient specific cell-mediated immune response to suppress the infection initially. Thus, visceral leishmaniasis represents a relatively anergic state and the parasites disseminate throughout the macrophages of the lymphoreticular system. In this it has a parallel with disseminated *Mycobacterium avium-intracellulare* infection in immunosuppressed patients. Clinically, there is hepatosplenomegaly, lymphadenopathy, fever, and cachexia, with anaemia and pancytopenia (*Box 19.18*). In infected patients, the spleen can weigh up to 3 kg; indeed, visceral leishmaniasis is one of the few causes of massive splenomegaly (*Box 19.19* and see Chapter 8, pp. 213–215). As a consequence of both splenomegaly and marrow involvement, there is anaemia and cytopenia (hypersplenism).

The incubation period for leishmaniasis is several months and, if untreated, the patient usually dies from secondary

---

**Box 19.18 PATHOLOGY OF VISCERAL LEISHMANIASIS**

- Macrophages filled with parasites
- Organs involved: liver (Kupffer cells), spleen, lymph nodes, bone marrow, and gut mucosa
- Anaemia and pancytopenia
- Hypergammaglobulinaemia (B-cell stimulation) of IgG and IgM
- Secondary bacterial infections: pneumonia and septic shock

---

**Box 19.19 DIFFERENTIAL DIAGNOSIS OF MASSIVE SPLENOMEGALY**

- Visceral leishmaniasis
- Chronic myeloid leukaemia and myelofibrosis
- Lymphoma
- Storage diseases, e.g. Gaucher's disease
- Chronic falciparum malaria
- Hydatid cyst

---

**TABLE 19.8** Leishmaniasis: the diseases, parasite species and geographical distribution

| Disease | Parasite | Distribution |
| --- | --- | --- |
| Cutaneous leishmaniasis | *Leishmania infantum* | Mediterranean |
| | *L. major* | Middle East, Asia |
| | *L. mexicana* | South and Central America |
| Mucocutaneous leishmaniasis | *L. brasiliensis* | South and Central America |
| Visceral leishmaniasis (kala-azar) | *L. donovani* | Africa, Asia, Mediterranean |

bacterial infection. As a result of the high parasite loads, the macrophage defence system is effectively paralysed, permitting sepsis.

The diagnosis of visceral leishmaniasis is made by identifying parasites in spleen (e.g. splenic aspirate), liver, or bone marrow biopsy (Fig. 19.41). Serological identification of specific antibody is usually positive. Chemotherapy is effective.

Not surprisingly, individuals co-infected with HIV and *Leishmania* sp. suffer severe acute visceral leishmaniasis, which is virtually impossible to cure in the face of absent CMI. However, immunosuppression from HIV and other causes (e.g. chronic lymphocytic leukaemia, steroid therapy) can also result in latent leishmania infections becoming clinically overt. This can occur years or decades after infection, the parasites having presumably remained within macrophages in small, subclinical numbers. Both cutaneous and visceral disease can result from this re-emergence of infection.

### Giardiasis

> **Key Points**
>
> - Giardiasis is caused by *Giardia lamblia*.
> - It appears as a luminal infection of the upper small bowel.
> - It does not invade tissues.
> - It causes diarrhoea and malabsorption.
> - It may mimic coeliac disease.
> - It is readily diagnosable and treatable.

Infection with *Giardia lamblia* is common, and cosmopolitan. It is important as a treatable cause of acute and chronic diarrhoea and weight loss. The transmission route is faecal–oral, i.e. people ingest oocysts from the faeces of infected individuals via contaminated food and water (including water supplies), and sexual practices. The life-cycle is vegetative, with binary fission of the parasites in the upper small bowel lumen. The organism does not invade tissues. The trophozoites measure $20 \times 15\ \mu m$, and the cysts in faeces are smaller.

Only a minority of those patients with *Giardia* sp. are symptomatic. They have abdominal pain and diarrhoea of varying severity; a proportion may also suffer from malabsorption. Children and those with IgA deficiency are particularly susceptible.

The parasites attach to the small bowel enterocyte brush border, and can be present in large numbers (Fig. 19.42). The gut villi may be normal or blunted, but only rarely are as flat and inflamed as in coeliac disease. The pathogenesis of giardiasis is unclear; the damage to the mucosa may be mechanical, there may be toxic damage, or an immune injury may play a role.

In diagnosis, the cysts may be found in the faeces, but this is unreliable. A duodenal biopsy, performed in the work-up of patients with upper gastrointestinal tract and malabsorption symptoms, is a common means of obtaining the diagnosis.

### Amoebiasis (Entamoeba histolytica)

> **Key Points**
>
> - Amoebiasis is caused by distinct invasive and non-invasive (benign) species of *Entamoeba* sp.
> - It causes proctocolitis with bloody diarrhoea.
> - It can spread to the liver to cause a liver abscess.
> - The gut and liver symptoms can mimic those of many other diseases.
> - It is treatable and curable.

Amoebiasis is a potentially severe disease caused by *Entamoeba histolytica*, an infection of the large bowel that is transmitted via the faecal–oral route. About 10% of the global population is infected, with higher prevalence in the tropics and subtropics, but the disease is endemic at all latitudes.

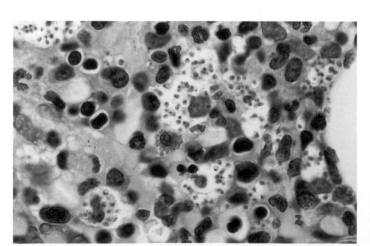

**FIG. 19.41** Visceral leishmaniasis: bone marrow biopsy with many parasites in the macrophages.

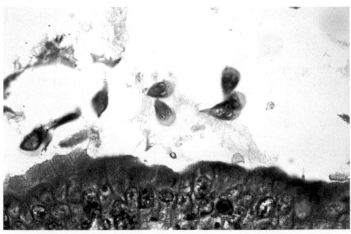

**FIG. 19.42** Giardiasis: six pear-shaped parasites are present near the enterocyte surface.

However, only a small proportion of those infected have significant disease. The explanation has recently become evident. Although the parasites are morphologically identical, there are two genetically distinct species of *Entamoeba*: one species never invades tissues, is now known as *E. dispar*, and is the more common infection; the other species can invade the gut epithelium and is called *E. histolytica*. The lifecycles are vegetative, with binary fission and release of infective cysts into the faeces. The trophozoites in the gut lumen and liver are 20–30 μm in size, and the cysts are smaller.

## Clinical Features

*Entamoeba dispar* may be asymptomatic, or a cause of mild lower gut diarrhoea. It is commonly identified in homosexual men. Conversely, *E. histolytica* is potentially fatal, causing painful diarrhoea with blood in the stool; this mimics idiopathic inflammatory bowel diseases such as ulcerative colitis and Crohn's disease, and bacterial colitis. This may resolve spontaneously, or persist and progress to more severe mucosal ulceration. If untreated, up to 5% of patients – and especially those who are pregnant or receiving steroids – suffer colon perforation and peritonitis, which has a high mortality.

If the parasites spread to the liver via the portal veins (Fig. 19.43), one or more liver abscesses will develop. There is tender hepatomegaly, fever, leukocytosis, and cholestatic jaundice. Clinically, the symptoms and signs are very similar to those of a bacterial liver abscess or hepatocarcinoma. If untreated, a liver abscess is fatal, because it perforates through the liver capsule into the peritoneum, or less commonly across the diaphragm into the pleural cavity. It is important to note that the absence of current colonic disease does not exclude liver amoebiasis; some gut infections are subclinical.

## Pathological Features

The colorectal lesions are focal erosions or deeper ulcers that undermine the mucosa (Fig. 19.44). Ulcers may become very large with just residual islands of oedematous mucosa, and they may perforate through the muscularis into the serosa and the peritoneal cavity. The amoebae are seen on the surface epithelium, damaging enterocytes, and at the advancing edge (Fig. 19.45). They do not induce an acute inflammatory response. Characteristically they phagocytose erythrocytes. An important difference at colonoscopy between amoebic ulcers and those of ulcerative colitis and bacterial dysentery is that they are focal, rather than being a diffuse mucosal disease; conversely, they can mimic Crohn's disease.

In the liver, the abscess does not contain true pus (i.e. no polymorphonuclear leukocyte accumulation), but

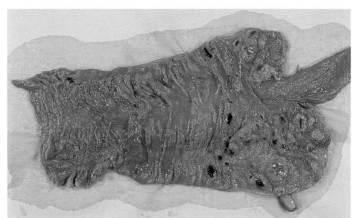

FIG. 19.44 Amoebiasis: this image shows the terminal ileum (right), caecum, and ascending colon (left). Many ulcers are present, predominantly in the caecum.

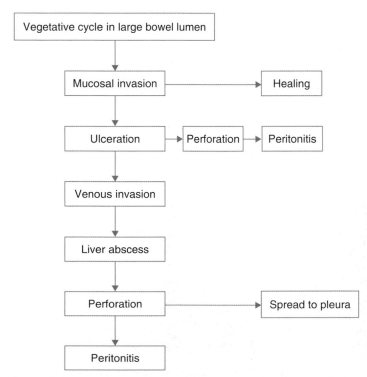

FIG. 19.43 Sequelae of infection with *Entamoeba histolytica*.

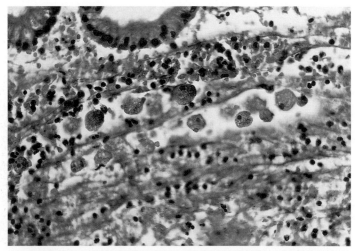

FIG. 19.45 Amoebiasis: trophozoites (many with phagocytosed red cells) can be seen invading under the colonic mucosa.

rather comprises dead liver tissue, fluid and fibrin exudate, and blood; it is said to resemble anchovy sauce in texture. Abscesses are 4–12 cm in diameter, with a necrotic, irregular periphery (Fig. 19.46). The amoebic trophozoites destroy and phagocytose hepatocytes.

### Pathogenesis of Amoebiasis

Pathogenic amoebae cause direct tissue damage by secreting an ionophore called 'amoebapore' (a 28-kDa protein). This is released after direct contact with host cells' receptors, and causes a 2-nm membrane lesion through which cell contents and ions are able to leak (Fig. 19.47). The cell dies and may be phagocytosed by the parasite. In addition, the parasites secrete tissue proteases, which also enable invasion and entry into small veins. There appears to be no immunopathological component to amoebic disease. However, there are some unresolved puzzles; although those patients receiving steroids have severe disease, amoebiasis is neither more common nor more severe in people with HIV/AIDS.

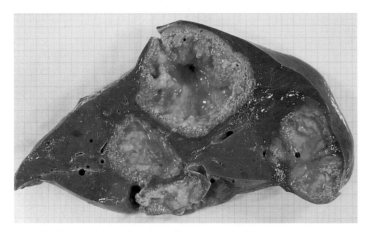

**FIG. 19.46** Amoebiasis: four liver abscesses are present.

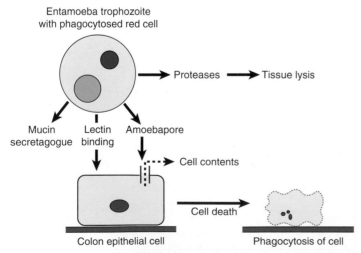

**FIG. 19.47** The pathogenesis of intestinal amoebiasis: the parasites secrete a potent ionophore ('amoebapore') which results in lysis of the cell.

### Diagnosis and Treatment

Although antibodies to *E. histolytica* are present in the serum of most patients with invasive gut and liver disease, the main diagnostic tools are examination of faeces for parasite trophozoites or cysts, a colorectal biopsy, or direct microscopic examination of a surface scrape of a rectal ulcer. For suspected liver abscess, a fine-needle aspirate or biopsy identifies the parasites (or provides an alternative diagnosis). Metronidazole is used effectively to treat the invasive condition. A liver abscess may also need to be aspirated if it is considered to be near to the point of rupture.

### Toxoplasmosis

**Key Points**

- Toxoplasmosis due to *Toxoplasma gondii* is acquired from undercooked meat, or from cat faeces.
- It is a common infection globally.
- The primary infection is usually asymptomatic or a cervical lymphadenitis.
- A latent infection may reactivate because of immunosuppression (e.g. HIV).
- Reactivated toxoplasmosis causes cerebral lesions and myocarditis.

Infection with *Toxoplasma gondii* is one of the frequent opportunistic infections in patients with HIV/AIDS. It is a common latent infection around the world, with evidence of infection in between 10% and 90% of the adult population (about 40% prevalence in the UK).

The lifecycle is complex. The sexual phase of the cycle takes place in the mucosal lining of the intestine of felines, with the excretion of oocysts in faeces. A wide range of intermediate hosts ingests the oocysts, which form latent cysts in many tissues including muscle (cells contain hundreds of 2-μm parasites). Humans are infected by eating cysts in undercooked infected meat, or by oocysts direct from cats and possibly from contaminated water supplies.

### Clinical Pathology

The pathological forms of toxoplasmosis are outlined in Fig. 19.48.

The most common consequence is a subclinical latent infection, where tissue cysts reside in brain and muscle where they cause no significant pathology, but they may reactivate if the person becomes immunosuppressed. Acute acquired toxoplasmosis presents as fever, malaise, lymphadenopathy, and splenomegaly. As suspicion of lymphoma is common, lymph node biopsy is frequently performed in tandem with serology. Characteristically, the node shows reactive follicular hyperplasia and numerous small non-necrotic granulomas, but rarely – if ever – any detectable parasites. Congenital toxoplasmosis follows transplacental transmission in about 30% of women who acquire toxoplasma

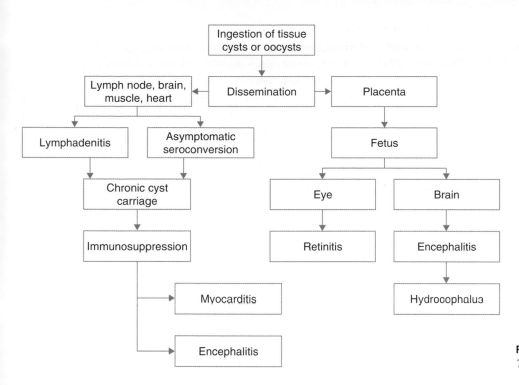

FIG. **19.48** Sequelae of infection with *Toxoplasma gondii.*

infection in pregnancy. During the first trimester this results in abortion, and as pregnancy progresses the risk of severe fetal disability declines. The classic tetrad is hydrocephalus or microcephaly, chorioretinitis, and cerebral calcification. Histologically, there is an encephalitic reaction against the parasites. Milder sequelae include learning disability and epilepsy.

Ocular toxoplasmosis occurs after congenital toxoplasmosis, or as a reactivation in immunocompromised hosts. The retina and choroid are mainly involved, causing blurred vision and pain. There is acute retinal necrosis.

Toxoplasmosis in the immunocompromised host reflects the reactivation of latent infection in tissue cysts when CMI declines. Currently, the most common cause is HIV/AIDS, and CNS disease is the major focus. The prevalence of cerebral toxoplasmosis depends on the infection level in the population co-infected with HIV. Patients present with focal cerebral lesions or confusion. Imaging can suggest the diagnosis supported by serology, but often treatment is given empirically. The main differential diagnosis is cerebral lymphoma. Grossly, the acute lesions are haemorrhagic, necrotic and space occupying which, with oedema, cause cerebral compression (see Fig. 19.13). Histologically, there are cysts, free parasites, necrosis, and vasculitis (Fig. 19.49). With treatment, the lesions regress. Toxoplasmosis can also present in HIV/AIDS as a myocarditis with heart failure.

The diagnosis of toxoplasmosis is made by a combination of clinical, imaging, morphological, and serological investigations. Parasites may be visible in tissues – and confirmed by immunocytochemical labelling. Serology detects both IgM (evidence of active infection) and IgG (chronic/past

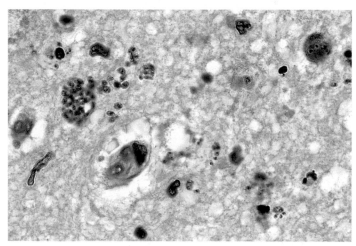

FIG. **19.49** Cerebral toxoplasmosis: a cyst is breaking up (left), with many tiny parasites spreading through the brain.

infection) antibodies, but has yet to provide high sensitivity and specificity.

## HELMINTH INFECTIONS

There are more than 100 parasitic worm infections of humans; these may be subclassified into roundworms (nematodes), trematodes (flatworms, flukes), and cestodes (tapeworms). Globally, the most common are the parasites of the intestinal lumen: hookworms, ascarids and whipworms in the tropics, and pinworms in temperate zones (see *Table 19.6*). The clinicopathological effects of intestinal nematode worms are summarized in *Table 19.9*. The infections that are discussed in more detail are those with more systemic clinical pathology – namely, schistosomiasis, hydatid disease, and strongyloidiasis.

## Schistosomiasis

### Key Points

- Schistosomiasis is caused by the blood flukes *Schistosoma haematobium*, *S. mansoni*, and *S. japonicum*.
- The disease is caused by the effects of eggs deposited in the tissues.
- It results in cystitis, enteritis, and chronic liver disease.
- It is the common cause of portal hypertension in the tropics.
- It is the common cause of bladder cancer in endemic zones.

The three major schistosome worms affect 10% of the world's population in the tropics and Middle East, and are significant causes of chronic gut, bladder, and liver disease. The lifecycle is complex because snails are required as an intermediate host. Humans are infected through the skin from small cercariae (larvae) in fresh water, which pass to the lungs and mature; worms then migrate via the bloodstream to their main location in deep veins. The lifecycle is completed when eggs are excreted in faeces or urine into water, taking about 40 days from infection. The adult worms are 10–15 mm long, and feed on red cell haemoglobin. Males fertilize female worms, and hundreds of eggs are excreted by each female per day. The eggs are 90–160 μm long, depending on the species.

### Clinical and Pathological Features

After infection, there may be a local dermatitis where the cercariae penetrated the skin. Once the worms start laying eggs, some people infected for the first time develop an acute systemic disease (Katayama's syndrome) (*Box 19.20*).

TABLE 19.9 Pathology of the major intestinal nematode worm infections

| Parasite | Location | Effect |
|---|---|---|
| Hookworms | Small bowel | Mucosal erosion and bleeding, normocytic anaemia |
| *Ascaris* spp. | Small and large bowel | Intestinal obstruction |
| Whipworms | Colorectum | Dysentery, anaemia |
| Pinworms | Appendix, colorectum | Perianal pruritis |
| *Strongyloides* spp. | Small bowel | Diarrhoea |

This is a serum sickness-type illness that is associated with a humoral antibody response to new egg antigens.

Schistosomiasis is mainly a chronic disease, and the clinical pathology depends on the species involved (Fig. 19.50).

### Box 19.20 ACUTE SCHISTOSOMIASIS (KATAYAMA'S SYNDROME)

- Fever and blood eosinophilia
- Abdominal pain
- Diarrhoea
- Cough and infiltrates on chest radiograph
- Urticaria
- Lymph node, liver, and spleen enlargement

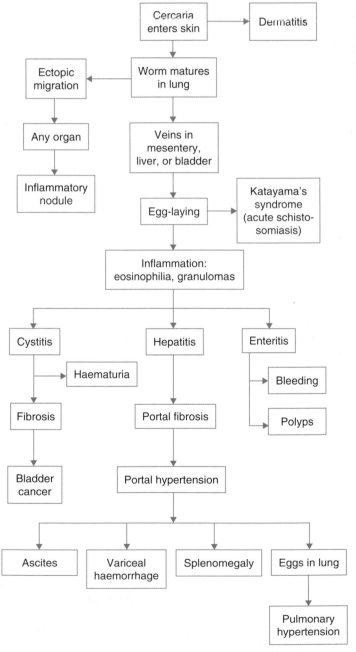

FIG. 19.50 Sequence of clinicopathological events in schistosomiasis.

## Schistosoma haematobium Infection

This species is found in the Middle East and Africa. It classically causes painful cystitis with haematuria. New lesions are the foci of inflammation around eggs as they traverse the urothelial mucosa. Histologically, there are many eosinophils around the eggs (Fig. 19.51). As the lesions become more chronic, cystoscopy reveals nodules and 'sandy patches'; these represent granuloma formation, secondary fibrosis, and calcification of eggs that have not been excreted. In chronic severe infections, the bladder wall becomes so fibrosed that it does not empty properly, and bacterial bladder infections persist.

Ureteric obstruction may arise from inflammation around eggs laid in the lower ureter, and cause hydronephrosis. Intestinal disease is similar to that caused by *S. mansoni*.

The most important complication of chronic infection is squamous cell carcinoma of the bladder, not the standard transitional cell carcinoma of industrialized countries (*Box 19.21*). This condition is a major disease in those parts of the world endemic for *S. haematobium* (Egypt, Middle East, and tropical Africa). It usually presents late, filling the bladder space, with invasion through the muscle wall. Its pathogenesis is probably through bacterial cystitis, squamous metaplasia of urothelium, and catabolism of dietary nitrates/nitrites into carcinogenic nitrosamines.

## S. mansoni and S. japonicum

Patients present with gut and/or liver disease (*Box 19.22*). These infections cause bloody diarrhoea: the eggs cross the mucosa, and erosions result. Focally, infection intensities can build up with formation of inflammatory polyps containing large numbers of eggs.

The most important condition is the liver disease, hepatosplenic schistosomiasis. Eggs that are carried to the liver induce granulomas in the small portal veins, with hepatomegaly. There is haemozoin pigment (similar to that formed in malaria) in the macrophages and Kupffer's cells. The granulomas cause fibrosis of the portal tracts in a characteristic pattern still known as Symmers' clay pipestem fibrosis (Figs 19.52 and 19.53). However, this is not true cirrhosis because the architecture of the liver lobules is intact.

---

**Box 19.22** CLINICAL PATHOLOGY OF *SCHISTOSOMA MANSONI* AND *S. JAPONICUM*

- Small and large bowel inflammatory erosions
- Portal hepatitis
- Chronic liver fibrosis (but not cirrhosis)
- Portal hypertension
- Splenomegaly
- Variceal haemorrhage

---

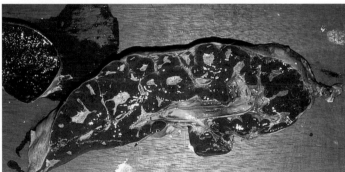

FIG. 19.52 *Schistosoma mansoni*: chronic liver infection has caused marked fibrosis around the main portal tracts.

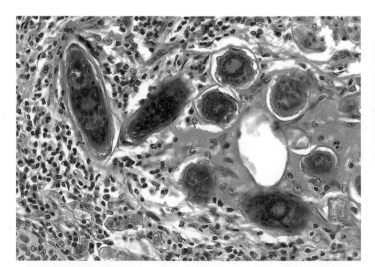

FIG. 19.51 *Schistosoma haematobium*: live eggs in mucosa.

---

**Box 19.21** CLINICAL PATHOLOGY OF *SCHISTOSOMA HAEMATOBIUM*

- Cystitis with haematuria
- Proctitis and distal colitis
- Progressive bladder fibrosis
- Ureteric obstruction by granulomatous inflammation
- Bladder squamous cell carcinoma in chronically infected people

---

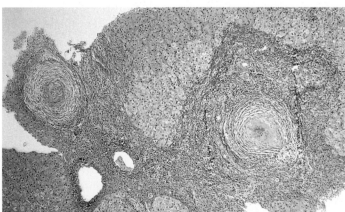

FIG. 19.53 *Schistosoma mansoni*: chronic liver infection with two granulomas surrounded by concentric fibrous rings, and increased portal fibrosis tissue linking them (van Gieson's stain)

The clinical effects in chronic infection are those of portal hypertension, and variceal haemorrhage is common. However, unlike in cirrhosis in which the vascular architecture is damaged, in this disease liver metabolism is better preserved, so hepatic coma does not result from the breakdown of blood in the gut. Schistosomiasis is not associated with the development of liver or intestinal cancer.

As a product of portal hypertension and portosystemic venous anastomoses, eggs laid in mesenteric veins can pass to the lungs. There, they lodge in the pulmonary arterioles, induce granuloma formation and fibrosis, and can thereby cause pulmonary hypertension.

More importantly, adult worms do not always migrate to veins in the 'classic' body locations around the bladder, intestine, and upstream from liver. Rather, they can locate in 'ectopic' sites such as the brain and spinal cord, skin, retroperitoneum, lymph nodes, and genitalia. As a consequence, schistosomal granulomatous nodules may be found in various places, often mimicking a neoplasm. The most serious of these ectopic schistosomiases are space-occupying lesions in the brain, and inflammatory lesions in and around the spinal cord. The latter are not uncommon and are a cause of spinal paralysis.

### Pathogenesis

The pathology in schistosomiasis comes essentially from the host reaction to parasite eggs. The adult worms elicit no reaction because they coat themselves in host red cell antigens. The eggs live for only 3 weeks, and around half are excreted and half retained in the body. In the process of excretion or retention they cause the disease spectrum. The main determinants of disease severity are the intensity and chronicity of infection. Travellers who acquire schistosomiasis do not develop chronic severe disease, in contrast to those who build up infection levels from years of exposure (*Box 19.23*).

### Diagnosis and Treatment

The diagnosis is made by identifying the eggs in samples of faeces, urine, or tissue biopsies. Schistosome serology is specific and useful, but remains positive after effective therapy. Treatment with praziquantel is standard for all species; this kills the adult worms but does not affect the host reaction to eggs in tissues.

---

**Box 19.23** PATHOGENESIS OF SCHISTOSOMIASIS

- Host reaction to eggs in tissues
- Acute inflammatory response with eosinophils
- Erosion of mucosal surfaces as eggs are excreted
- T-cell-mediated response with granuloma formation around eggs
- Subsequent fibrosis related to healing of granulomas
- Organ dysfunction secondary to fibrosis

---

## Hydatid Disease

**Key Points**

- Hydatid disease is caused by larvae of the tapeworm *Echinococcus granulosus*.
- It results in cysts in the liver, peritoneum, and lung.
- The cysts act as space-occupying lesions.
- The diagnosis is confirmed by radiology and fine-needle aspiration.
- It is treated by surgery and chemotherapy.

*Echinococcus granulosus* is a tapeworm that is widely prevalent, irrespective of latitude. It is endemic at low levels in the UK and at high levels in Africa and the Middle East.

This is a zoonosis by which humans are accidentally infected and develop the intermediate cystic stage of the lifecycle of the tapeworm. The definitive hosts are canines, with worms in the intestine and eggs excreted in the faeces. The usual intermediate hosts are bovines, sheep, and camels; when their offal, containing cysts, is eaten by dogs, the lifecycle continues.

Ingested tapeworm eggs hatch in the duodenum and pass to the liver via the portal veins. Growing at a rate of up to 2 cm a year, a hydatid cyst develops which may reach over 20 cm in final size (Fig. 19.54). The eggs can also reach other organs and result in cysts there (*Box 19.24*).

### Pathology

The form of hydatid cyst is similar in all organs. The parasite generates a soft white laminated acellular membrane, which is 1–2 mm thick. Outside this, the host reacts with a fibrous wall that helps to contain the cyst and stop it from rupturing. Within the membrane is a thin germinal membrane from which bud myriads of scolices (singular scolex), which are the heads of future adult tapeworms (Fig. 19.55). The scolices have characteristic suckers and a ring of curved

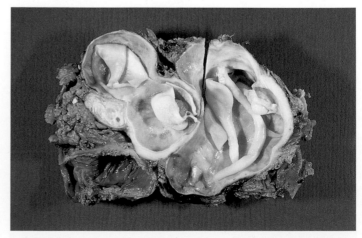

**FIG. 19.54** Hydatid cysts in the mesentery, causing intestinal obstruction.

**Box 19.24** ORGANS AFFECTED BY HYDATID DISEASE, AND THE EFFECTS

- Liver (>70% of patients): enlargement, discomfort, bile duct obstruction
- Peritoneal cavity: abdominal swelling, adhesions and intestinal obstruction
- Lung: shortness of breath, abnormal chest radiograph
- Brain: cerebral compression, epilepsy
- Kidney: compression, hydronephrosis
- Spleen: moderate-to-massive splenomegaly
- Bone: fracture, collapse
- Any organ (in endemic zones, this is in the differential diagnosis of all tumours)

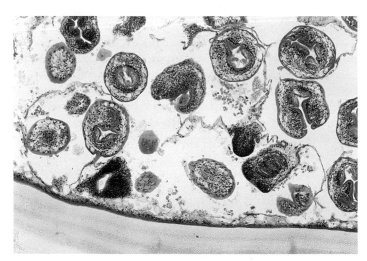

FIG. 19.55 Hydatid cyst: this histology image shows the pale-staining laminated membrane (bottom), germinal membrane (red line), and numerous scolices within the cyst.

hooklets. Often, a cyst membrane generates internal daughter cysts, and the whole structure contains much colourless watery fluid.

The cyst acts like an expanding benign tumour. Over many years or decades, if untreated, cysts die and collapse. Spontaneous, traumatic, or iatrogenic rupture may occur, with secondary spread of infection to adjacent organs or body cavities. There is a risk of a type 1 anaphylactic shock reaction, which is potentially fatal, if hydatid cyst antigen enters the bloodstream to react with specific antibodies. This risk modifies the approach to treatment, but it is not a bar to performing fine-needle aspiration (FNA) of suspected cysts for diagnosis: large studies have demonstrated the safety of the procedure.

### Diagnosis and Treatment

Clinical suspicion and radiology are the main indicators of a hydatid cyst. Serology is reasonably sensitive and specific. FNA is often used to confirm the diagnosis, and often makes it when unsuspected. The scolices and hooklets are readily identified on cytological preparations.

The ideal management is to remove the cyst if possible; single liver cysts form a major presentation. Care must be taken when opening the cyst not to spill its contents, before sucking the parasitic material out. If cysts are multiple, or in the peritoneal cavity, bone, or lung, then chemotherapy (albendazole) is available but is slow in effect, and it is uncertain whether it ultimately sterilizes a hydatid cyst.

## Strongyloidiasis

**Key Points**

- Strongyloidiasis is caused by *Strongyloides stercoralis*.
- *Strongyloides stercoralis* infects the intestinal mucosa.
- It is almost unique among worms by proliferating in humans, with life long infection.
- It causes diarrhoea.
- During immunosuppression, it can disseminate in the body and precipitate septic shock.

Strongyloidiasis is caused by the nematode *Strongyloides stercoralis*. This worm is endemic in the tropics and subtropics and, because of its lifecycle, it can be a lifelong infection and is potentially fatal. Importantly, people infected previously (e.g. soldiers in the Far East during the Second World War) can present decades later with acute illness for the first time. Humans are infected by larvae in the soil, deposited from human faeces. The larvae penetrate the skin and migrate to the small intestine and lodge in mucosal crypts. The female lays eggs, which immediately hatch into larvae in the bowel lumen. These are able to re-invade the bowel or perianal skin, so keeping an autoinfection cycle going. Should the patient become immunosuppressed (*Box 19.25*), this autoinfection cycle can rapidly generate massive infection (hyperinfection) with millions of parasites throughout the whole intestine, and haematogenous dissemination of larvae to all organs including the liver, lungs, and meninges.

**Box 19.25** CONDITIONS THAT PREDISPOSE TO HYPERINFECTION WITH *STRONGYLOIDES STERCORALIS*

- Steroid therapy
- Organ transplantation and therapeutic immunosuppression
- Old age (a common cause for decline in immunity)
- HTLV-1 co-infection
- Cancer, particularly HTLV-1-associated T-cell lymphoma
- Malnutrition

## Clinical Features

The infection may be asymptomatic, or the cause of periodic skin itch. If the gut infection intensity builds up, it causes diarrhoea and weight loss. If there is massive infection (hyperinfection), it precipitates multiple organ failure with fulminant diarrhoea, septic shock, pneumonia, and meningitis, accompanied by a high blood eosinophil count.

The sequelae of infection with *Strongyloides* sp. are indicated in Fig. 19.56.

## Pathology

With mild infection there are focal erosions of small bowel mucosa, with adult worms in the mucosal crypts accompanied by chronic inflammation and local eosinophilia. Adult worms are typically 2.5 mm long. The disease may be segmental in the bowel, reminiscent of Crohn's disease.

In hyperinfection, the intestine is extensively ulcerated and there are abundant worms (Fig. 19.57). Acute pneumonia and shock lung, inflammation, and enlargement of the liver and meningitis follow. Some of this is in reaction to the larvae (250 μm long), which are disseminated in blood vessels; the intestinal lesions also permit the entry of Gram-negative bacteria, producing bacteraemia and septic shock.

One notable and intriguing co-infection is that of HTLV-I (human T-lymphotrophic virus type I) and *Strongyloides* sp.

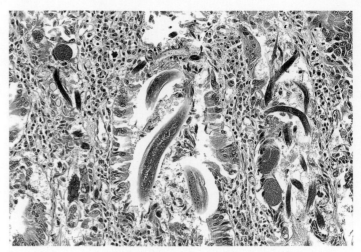

FIG. 19.57 *Strongyloides* hyperinfection: there is a heavy infection of the small bowel, with adult and larval worms in the mucosa.

This is important in West Africa and the Caribbean, and in people who have originated from those areas. HTLV-1 is the cause of a high-grade T-cell lymphoma in a proportion of those infected; it appears that strongyloides co-infection can accelerate the malignant transformation. Conversely, the immunological damage of HLTV-1 infection can precipitate hyperinfection in those with subclinical strongyloides infection.

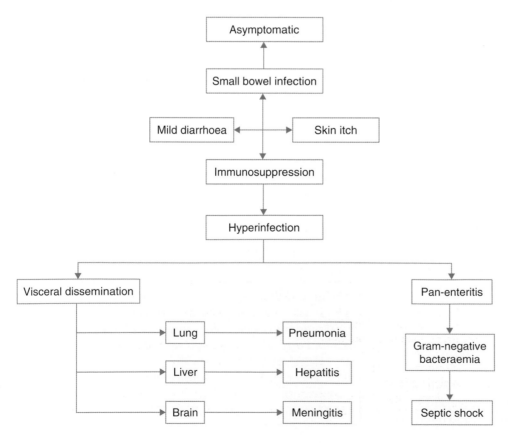

FIG. 19.56 Sequelae of infection with *Strongyloides stercoralis*.

# SEPTIC SHOCK

Shock is the end-result of many clinical processes, and is defined as the hypoperfusion of critical organs such that their function and integrity is compromised. This may be either reversible or irreversible (and then generally fatal). Because modern hospital medicine sustains severely ill patients who might previously have died without interventions; older and frailer patients undergo major operations; more patients undergo organ transplantation with subsequent immunosuppression; and intensive care facilities are expanding in size and complexity, an increasing number of patients are encountered in various states of shock. This section deals with the pathogenesis of one such type – septic shock (Box 19.26). Further details on shock in general may be found in Chapter 6, pp. 106–109.

## Aetiology

The aetiology of septic shock is most commonly infection by Gram-negative bacilli that produce endotoxins (hence the term 'endotoxic shock'). These include *Escherichia coli*, and *Pseudomonas*, *Klebsiella*, and *Enterobacter* spp. Initially, the infection is localized to an organ or cavity, such as appendicitis, pneumonia, or peritonitis after bowel surgery. If the host defences and medical interventions such as antimicrobial drugs and surgical resection are unable to contain the infection, the systemic inflammatory and cytokine effects then involve other organs, and there is often dissemination of infection with bacteraemia and then septicaemia ('bacteraemia' indicates bacterial infection in the blood without major clinical disease, whereas 'septicaemia' also involves shock). Gram-positive bacteria, some systemic fungal infections, and severe falciparum malaria infection also initiate similar pathophysiological processes to Gram-negative septic shock.

## Pathogenesis

Shock caused by endotoxin-producing Gram-negative bacteria has been the most comprehensively studied. Endotoxin is a lipopolysaccharide (LPS) structural component of the outer cell wall of these bacilli. In contrast to bacterial exotoxins (e.g. that produced by *Clostridium perfringens*, a cause of tissue gangrene), which are secreted by intact bacteria, LPS is released as the bacilli disintegrate. LPS comprises a long-chain toxic fatty acid (lipid A), which is common to all Gram-negative bacteria, and a variable polysaccharide carbohydrate chain that includes the O antigens, unique to each species. Similar LPS-like complex molecules are present in the walls of other bacteria and fungi.

LPS binds to circulating monocytes, tissue macrophages, and endothelial cells, and activates them. This is obviously a useful evolutionary adaptation in the cellular defence against infection. The key event that turns a local infection into septic shock is the progressive production of TNF-α by LPS-activated macrophages. TNF-α causes macrophages and many other cells in the body (e.g. liver) to secrete interleukin 1 (IL-1) which, depending on the concentration, damages tissues directly. Thereafter, a series of cytokine cascades generates further interleukins (IL-6 and IL-8), with production of the acute phase responses and nitric oxide (NO), and can activate the clotting system to initiate disseminated intravascular coagulation (DIC). The cardiac output falls due to pump failure, peripheral vascular resistance falls, tissues are underperfused, capillaries leak resulting in tissue oedema, and critical capillary/epithelium interface in the lung alveoli is damaged (Fig. 19.58).

The features of septic shock can be reproduced by the injection of endotoxin lipopolysaccharide alone.

### Clinical Features

As can be predicted from the pathophysiology, the clinical aspects of septic shock comprise fever, systemic hypotension, increasing oxygen requirement to maintain blood $PO_2$, infiltrates on a chest radiograph, generalized oedema, oliguric renal failure, and jaundice. Chronologically there is a division into three stages. In the initial phase, the body's normal compensatory mechanisms maintain critical organ perfusion. This is succeeded by a progressive phase in which tissue hypoperfusion results in organ failure, particularly cardiorespiratory failure, exacerbated by toxic endothelial damage and fluid leakage; metabolic acidosis and renal shutdown occur. Patients can recover from this phase. The final, irreversible, phase follows when critical organ cellular injury is too severe for regeneration or compensation, even if the organs were to be reperfused adequately.

### Pathological Features

The critical organs damaged in shock are the lungs, heart, kidneys, intestine, liver, and brain. The morphologies are not unique to septic shock, and may be seen in shock from other aetiologies. In the case of the lung, shock lung has a broadly similar morphology whether it follows from sepsis, drug toxicity, or external trauma such as high-pressure ventilation and oxygen toxicity. With regard to the heart, the clinical syndrome of 'electromechanical dissociation (EMD)' is a common pre-death observation. The ECG records electrical

---

**Box 19.26** CLASSIFICATION OF SHOCK: THE FIVE MAJOR TYPES

- Cardiogenic: from ventricular failure (e.g. infarction, tamponade)
- Hypovolaemic: from haemorrhage or plasma loss (e.g. burns)
- Septic: from infection, usually bacterial
- Anaphylactic: from type I immunological hypersensitivity reactions
- Neurogenic: from spinal cord injury

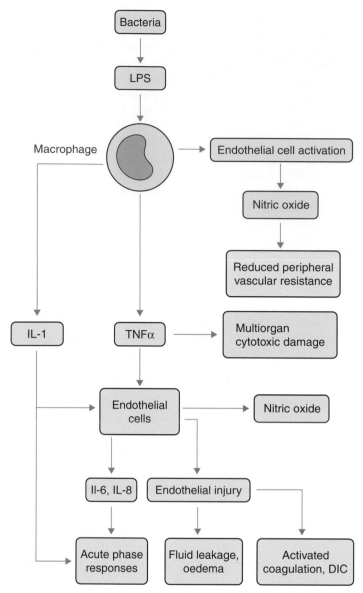

FIG. 19.58 The course of events in septic shock. DIC = disseminated intravascular coagulation; IL = interleukin; LPS = lipopolysaccharide; TNF = tumour necrosis factor.

impulses, but the cardiac output measured both clinically and by echocardiography is slight. This results from overt ischaemic damage to myocytes and probably from direct toxic functional damage by TNF and other cytokines. Finally, as the result of the overactivation of the cytokine and cellular defence systems in the progressive and final stages of septic shock, there is an increased susceptibility to more bacterial infections (e.g. bronchopneumonia).

Whether the patient can recover from septic shock will depend on control of the initiating and subsequent infection events, the degree of damage suffered by the critical organs, and their capacity to recover with cellular regeneration. Kidney tubular damage (acute tubular necrosis), pulmonary alveolar damage, and liver necrosis are, in principle, recoverable lesions provided that appropriate intensive care support is available. If the integrity of the intestinal mucosa is damaged, the consequent invasion by Gram-negative bacteria from the luminal faeces perpetuates and worsens the septic shock. The loss of cardiac myocytes from ischaemic and toxic damage, and loss of cerebral cortex neurons, are, of course, irreversible.

### Outcome of Septic Shock

The mortality rate of septic shock ranges from 25% to 75% according to age (the older the patient, the poorer the outcome), the underlying cause, and patient management. In clinical practice, the outcome is often determined by the degree of acute cardiac muscle damage (on top of any pre-existing heart disease) and the capacity of the lung alveolar lining cells to regenerate while the fibrosing response is inhibited. It must be remembered that modern intensive care itself, with positive-pressure ventilation, high inhaled oxygen concentrations, and powerful toxic drugs including inotropes, can incur and may reinforce the pathology of shock: the balance between undertreatment and overtreatment is often difficult to negotiate.

## SEPTIC SHOCK

A 67-year-old female had mitral stenosis with reduction of cardiac output. About 20 years ago, she had a mitral valvotomy to relieve the stenosis, but a definitive artificial valve replacement was now required. The operation was technically successful, but she was slow in waking up from anaesthesia.

In intensive care, 2 days after surgery, her respiratory function deteriorated, requiring increasing concentrations of oxygen and ventilation pressures to maintain the $PO_2$ in blood. Her chest radiograph showed diffuse infiltration. Her blood pressure fell, and increasing doses of inotropic drugs were needed to keep the systolic blood pressure at 100 mmHg. Daily blood cultures were taken, and on the fourth postoperative day a Gram-negative pseudomonas bacillus was isolated. The patient developed oliguric renal failure and, despite antibiotic therapy, she died from cardiorespiratory failure 7 days after surgery.

*Post mortem*, the mechanical mitral valve was properly *in situ*, without any superimposed endocarditis. The kidneys had pale and oedematous cortices, characteristic of acute tubular necrosis. The lungs were heavy, consolidated, and mucoid in appearance, with multiple 1- to 2-mm grey foci. The liver had micronodular cirrhosis. Histologically, the lungs were bronchopneumonic; numerous small pulmonary arteries were thickened due to dense intramural infiltration of Gram-negative bacilli; there was secondary luminal thrombosis and surrounding infarction of the lung (Fig. 19.59). The kidneys showed features of DIC (Fig. 19.60). The undiagnosed cirrhosis (a recognized infection risk factor) predisposed her to septic shock.

## Clinicopathological Points

1. The undiagnosed liver cirrhosis (probably alcoholic in aetiology) was the reason why the patient did not clear the anaesthetic drugs rapidly, so delaying recovery.

2. The pseudomonas bacteraemia was probably acquired from nosocomial infection of the intravascular lines necessary for intensive care support.

3. *Pseudomonas* sp. characteristically causes a vasculitis, resulting in occlusive thrombosis and infarction.

4. The septic shock precipitated DIC, which contributed to renal failure.

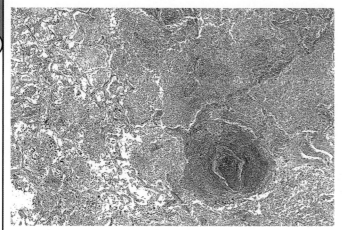

FIG. 19.59 Lung: a small pulmonary artery (lower half) is thickened by infiltrating pseudomonas bacilli, and is thrombosed. The surrounding lung is infarcted.

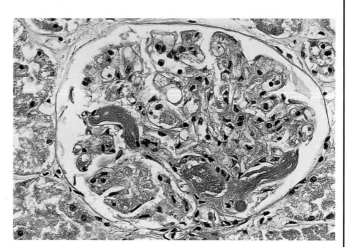

FIG. 19.60 Kidney: thrombi are present in the glomerular capillaries, indicating disseminated intravascular coagulation.

## SUMMARY

This chapter outlines the basic clinicopathological features and epidemiological aspects of a range of infectious diseases that are encountered in Europe. Virus infections (particularly HIV and its complications), bacteria, fungi and parasitic protozoa, and worms are included. As a result of increasing travel and migration, it is important that diseases acquired only outside Europe are understood, as well as global infections. The emphasis throughout is on pathogenesis, i.e. understanding why the infections affect some people but not others, and how they cause disease and sometimes death.

## FURTHER READING

Cohen J, Powderly WG, Opal SM. *Infectious Diseases*, 3rd edn. Edinburgh: Mosby, 2010.

Mandell GL, Bennett JE, Dolin R. *Mandell, Douglas and Bennett's Principles and Practice of Infectious Diseases*, 7th edn. Edinburgh: Churchill Livingstone, 2009.

Ward KN, McCartney AC, Thakker B. *Notes on Medical Microbiology*. Edinburgh: Churchill Livingstone, 2008.

# INDEX

Figures in **bold** denote figures and tables separate from the corresponding text.